Occupational Therapy and Physical Dysfunction

For Elsevier

Commissioning Editor: *Rita Demetriou-Swanwick*
Development Editor: *Catherine Jackson*
Project Manager: *Elouise Ball*
Designer/Design Direction: *Kirsteen Wright*
Illustration Manager: *Bruce Hogarth*

Occupational Therapy and Physical Dysfunction

Enabling occupation

SIXTH EDITION

Edited by

Michael Curtin BOccThy MPhil EdD
Course Co-ordinator, Occupational Therapy, School of Community Health, Charles Sturt University, Albury, NSW, Australia

Matthew Molineux BOccThy MSc PhD
Associate Professor, School of Occupational Therapy & Social Work and Centre for Research into Disability and Society within Curtin Health Innovation Research Institute, Curtin University of Technology, Peth, WA, Australia

Jo-anne Supyk-Mellson MSc DipCOT
Senior Lecturer, Directorate of Occupational Therapy, School of Health, Sport and Rehabilitation Sciences, University of Salford, Manchester, UK

Foreword by
Anne Turner
Marg Foster
Sybil E. Johnson

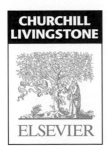

CHURCHILL LIVINGSTONE
ELSEVIER

Edinburgh   London   New York   Oxford   Philadelphia   St Louis   Sydney   Toronto   2010

CHURCHILL LIVINGSTONE
ELSEVIER

First Edition © Longman Group Limited 1981
Second Edition © Longman Group Limited 1987
Third Edition © Longman Group Limited 1992
Fourth Edition © Pearson Professional Limited 1996
Fifth Edition © Elsevier Limited 1999

Sixth edition © 2010, Elsevier Limited. All rights reserved.

ISBN 978 0 08 045084 1

British Library Cataloguing in Publication Data
A catalogue record for this book is available from the British Library

Library of Congress Cataloging in Publication Data
A catalog record for this book is available from the Library of Congress

Notice
Neither the Publisher nor the Editors assume any responsibility for any loss or injury and/or damage to persons or property arising out of or related to any use of the material contained in this book. It is the responsibility of the treating practitioner, relying on independent expertise and knowledge of the person, to determine the best treatment and method of application for the person.

The Publisher

ELSEVIER your source for books, journals and multimedia in the health sciences
www.elsevierhealth.com

Working together to grow libraries in developing countries

www.elsevier.com | www.bookaid.org | www.sabre.org

ELSEVIER   BOOK AID International   Sabre Foundation

The publisher's policy is to use **paper manufactured from sustainable forests**

Printed in Italy by Printer Trento S.r.l.

Contents

Contributors ix

Foreword xiii

Preface xv

Section 1 Occupation and occupational therapy in context 1

   1 **Defining occupational therapy** 3
     Clare Wilding

   2 **The nature of occupation** 17
     Matthew Molineux

   3 **Occupational therapy: a disability perspective** 27
     John Swain and Sally French

   4 **Contesting assumptions in occupational therapy** 39
     Karen Whalley Hammell

Section 2 An overview of occupational therapy practice 55

   5 **Occupational reasoning** 57
     Joan C. Rogers

   6 **Understanding models of practice** 67
     Jo-anne Supyk-Mellson and Jacqueline McKenna

   7 **Process of assessment and evaluation** 81
     Clare Hocking

   8 **Writing occupation-focused goals** 95
     Julia Bowman and Lise L. Mogensen

   9 **Enabling skills and strategies** 111
     Michael Curtin

Section 3 Essential foundations for occupational therapy 125

   10 **The art of person-centred practice** 127
     Thelma Sumsion

   11 **Occupation in context** 135
     Gail Elizabeth Whiteford

   12 **Enabling communication in a person-centred, occupation-focused context** 151
     Sue Baptiste

13 Analysis of occupational performance 161
Gill Chard

14 Psychosocial support 189
Jacqueline McKenna

15 Advocating and lobbying. 211
Valmae Rose, Kevin Cocks and Lesley Chenoweth

16 Educational strategies 221
Tammy Hoffmann

17 Health promotion and occupational therapy 239
Rachael Dixey

18 Working with groups 253
Claire Craig and Linda Finlay

Section 4 Working with and within communities 265

19 Community development. 267
Nick Pollard, Dikaios Sakellariou and Frank Kronenberg

20 Developing partnerships to privilege participation 281
Roshan Galvaan, Peliwe Mdlokolo and Robin Joubert

21 Working towards inclusive communities 297
Hanneke van Bruggen

22 Community-based rehabilitation: opportunities for occupational
therapists in an evolving strategy 313
Kirsty M. Thompson, Christina L. Parasyn and Beth Fuller

23 Entrepreneurial opportunities in the global community. 327
Marilyn Pattison

Section 5 Working with the individual 339

24 Enabling engagement in self-care occupations. 341
Helen van Huet, Tracey Parnell, Virginia Mitsch and
Annette McLeod-Boyle

25 Leisure 357
Ben Sellar and Mandy Stanley

26 Play 371
Karen Stagnitti

27 Work rehabilitation 391
Catherine Cook and Sue Lukersmith

28 Home modification: occupation as the basis for an
effective practice 409
Catherine Bridge

29 Toward universal design 431
    Leslie C. Young, Andrew Phillip Payne and Sharon Joines

30 Assistive devices for enabling occupations 453
    Helen Pain and Sue Pengelly

31 Wheelchairs: posture and mobility 469
    Rachel L. McDonald

32 Driver assessment and rehabilitation within the context of
    community mobility 489
    Marilyn Di Stefano and Wendy Macdonald

33 Orthotics for occupational outcomes 507
    Natasha Lannin and Iona Novak

34 Biomechanical strategies 527
    Janet Golledge

35 Skills for addressing sensory impairments 543
    Farieda Adams and Michelle Morcom

36 Moving and handling strategies 553
    Maggie Bracher and April Brooks

37 Optimising motor performance following brain impairment 579
    Annie McCluskey, Natasha Lannin and Karl Schurr

38 Cognitive and perceptual strategies 607
    Carolyn A. Unsworth

39 Strategies for sensory processing disorders 637
    Deborah Windley

    Index 653

Contributors

Farieda Adams BSc PGDipHT
Head Occupational Therapist, Leeds Teaching Hospitals Trust, Leeds, UK

Sue Baptiste MHSc OTReg(Ont)
Professor, School of Rehabilitation Science, McMaster University, Hamilton, Ontario, Canada

Julia Bowman BAppSc(OT)Dist MAppSc(OT)Res
Lecturer, School of Biomedical and Health Sciences, University of Western Sydney, Sydney, NSW, Australia

Maggie Bracher DipCOT MScErg
Lecturer/Back Care Advisor, School of Health Sciences, University of Southampton, Southampton, UK

Catherine Bridge PhD MCogSc BAppSc
Associate Professor, Centre for Health Assets Australasia (CHAA), University of New South Wales, Sydney, NSW, Australia

April Brooks MSCP
Clinical Physiotherapy Specialist in Patient Handling, Portsmouth City (Teaching) NHS Trust and Hampshire Primary Health Care NHS Trust, Portsmouth, UK

Gill Chard PhD BSc(Hons) DipCOT
Professor and Head of Department, Department of Occupational Science and Occupational Therapy, Brookfield Health Sciences, University College Cork, Cork, Ireland

Lesley Chenoweth BSW MSW PhD
Professor of Social Work, School of Human Sciences and Social Work, Griffith University, Meadowbrook, QLD, Australia

Kevin Cocks
Director, Queensland Advocacy Inc., Brisbane Transit Centre, Brisbane, QLD, Australia

Catherine Cook PhD MAppSc BAppSc
Senior Lecturer, School of Biomedical and Health Sciences, University of Western Sydney, Penrith South, NSW, Australia

Claire Craig MA(Oxon) BSc(Hons) PGCE FHEA
Senior Lecturer, Occupational Therapy, Sheffield Hallam University, Sheffield, UK

Michael Curtin BOccThy MPhil EdD
Course Co-ordinator Occupational Therapy, School of Community Health, Charles Sturt University, Albury, NSW, Australia

Marilyn Di Stefano BAppSc(OccTher) GradDipErgnomics PhD Cert Erg
Senior Lecturer, School of Occupational Therapy, La Trobe University, Melbourne, VIC, Australia

Rachael Dixey PhD BA(Hons)
Professor and Group Head, Health Promotion, Leeds Metropolitan University, Leeds, UK

Linda Finlay PhD BA(Hons) DipCOT
Academic Consultant, Open University, Milton Keynes, UK

Sally French DipGradPhys DipTP BSc(Hons) MSc PhD
Associate Lecturer, Open University, UK

Beth Fuller MPH BOT
Disability Program Coordinator, Nossal Institute for Global Health, The University of Melbourne, Carlton, VIC, Australia

Roshan Galvaan BSc(OT) MSc(OT) UCT
Senior Lecturer, Faculty of Health Sciences, University of Cape Town, South Africa

Janet Golledge MA DipCOT
Senior Lecturer, Faculty of Health and Life Sciences, York St John University, York, UK

Karen Whalley Hammell PhD MSc OT(C) DipCOT
Honorary Research Associate, Department of Occupational Science and Occupational Therapy, University of British Columbia, Vancouver, British Columbia, Canada

Clare Hocking PhD MHSc AdvDipOT DipOT
Associate Professor, School of Occupational Science and Occupational Therapy, Auckland University of Technology, Auckland, New Zealand

Tammy Hoffmann PhD BOccThy(Hons)
Lecturer, Division of Occupational Therapy, School of Health and Rehabilitation Sciences, University of Queensland, Brisbane, QLD, Australia

Sharon M.B Joines PhD
Ergonomist, Assistant Industrial Design Professor, College of Design at NC State University, Raleigh, NC, USA

Robin Joubert NatDipOT BA DEd
Associate Professor and Head of School of Audiology, Occupational Therapy and Speech-Language Pathology, University of KwaZulu Natal, Durban, South Africa

Frank Kronenberg BScOT BAEd
International Guest Lecturer and Consultant in Occupational Therapy Without Borders, and Director, Shades of Black Works, uBuntourism, Cape Town, South Africa

Natasha Lannin PhD BSc(OT) GradDip
Senior Research Fellow, Rehabilitation Studies Unit, Sydney Medical School, The University of Sydney, Sydney, NSW, Australia

Sue Lukersmith BAppSc
Director, Lukersmith and Associates, Woodford, NSW, Australia

Annie McCluskey PhD MA DipCOT
Senior Lecturer, Occupational Therapy, The University of Sydney, Sydney, NSW, Australia

Wendy Macdonald BSc(Hons)Psychology GradDipPsych PhD
Associate Professor, Centre for Ergonomics and Human Factors, La Trobe University, Melbourne, VIC, Australia

Rachael L. McDonald PhD BAppSc PGDip
Senior Lecturer, Department of Occupational Therapy, School of Primary Health Care, Monash University, Melbourne, VIC, Australia

Jacqueline McKenna MSc PGCEPR BSc(Hons) DipCOT
Senior Lecturer, Directorate of Occupational Therapy, University of Salford, Salford, Manchester, UK

Annette McLeod-Boyle BOccThy ThC(Hons) GCertEd MOccThy
Lecturer, Occupational Therapy, School of Community Health, Charles Sturt University, Albury, NSW, Australia, and Occupational Therapist, Sub Acute Service, Northeast Health Wangaratta, Wangaratta, VIC, Australia

Peliwe Mdlokolo BSc(OT)
Occupational Therapy, School of Audiology, Occupational Therapy and Speech-Language Pathology, University of Kwa-Zulu Natal (Westville Campus), Durban, South Africa

Virginia Mitsch BAppSc MOT
Occupational Therapist, South West Brain Injury Rehabilitation Service, Albury, NSW, Australia

Lise L. Mogensen BAppSC(Hons)OT
Social Justice and Social Change Research Centre, University of Western Sydney, Sydney, NSW, Australia

Matthew Molineux BOccThy MSc PhD
Associate Professor, School of Occupational Therapy & Social Work and Centre for Research into Disability and Society within Curtin Health Innovation Research Institute, Curtin University of Technology, Perth, WA, Australia

Michelle Morcom BScOT
Occupational Therapy Department, Mater Health Services, Brisbane, QLD, Australia

Iona Novak PhD MSc(Hons) BAppSc
Head of Research, Cerebral Palsy Institute, University of Notre Dame, Sydney, NSW, Australia

Helen Pain MSc DipCOT
School of Social Sciences, University of Southampton, Southampton, UK

Christina L. Parasyn BAppSC(OT) MSS
Policy Officer, Disability Inclusive Development, AusAID (Australian Agency for International Development), Australia

Tracey Parnell BAppSc MOT
Lecturer, Occupational Therapy, School of Community Health, Charles Sturt University, Albury, NSW, Australia

Marilyn Pattison DipCOT(UK) BAppSc(OT) MBA
Managing Partner, MPOT Occupational Therapy, Risk Management and Rehabilitation Services, Adelaide, SA, Australia, and Executive Director of World Federation of Occupational Therapists

Andrew Phillip Payne MAarch PhD
Professor of Architecture, Savannah College of Art and
Design, Savannah, Georgia, USA

Sue Pengelly DipCOT BA(Hons) MBA PGCE ILTM
Lecturer in Occupational Therapy, Cardiff University,
Cardiff, UK

Nick Pollard BA DipCOT PGCE MA MSc
Senior Lecturer in Occupational Therapy, Sheffield
Hallam University, Sheffield, UK

Joan C. Rogers PhD OTR/L FAOTA
Professor, Occupational Therapy, University of
Pittsburgh, Pittsburgh, Pennsylvania, USA

Valmae Rose BOccThy(Hons)
Educative Officer, ACROD Limited (Queensland Division),
Lutwyche, QLD, Australia

Dikaios Sakellariou BSc MSc
Lecturer, Department of Occupational Therapy, School of
Healthcare Studies, Cardiff University, Cardiff, UK

Karl Schurr MAppSc BAppSc
Senior Physiotherapist in Neurology, Bankstown-
Lidcombe Hospital Stroke Unit, Sydney, NSW, Australia

Ben Sellar BAppSc(Hons)
PhD Candidate, Centre for Research into Social
Inclusion, Macquarie University, Sydney, Australia
and Casual Lecturer, Occupational Therapy Program,
University of South Australia, Adelaide, SA, Australia

Karen Stagnitti BOccThy PhD
Associate Professor, Occupational Science and Therapy,
Deakin University, Geelong, VIC, Australia

Mandy Stanley BAppSc MHlthSc(OT) PhD
Senior Lecturer, Occupational Therapy Program, School
of Health Sciences, University of South Australia,
Adelaide, SA, Australia

Thelma Sumsion PhD OTReg(Ont)
Associate Professor, School of Occupational Therapy,
The University of Western Ontario, London, Ontario,
Canada

Jo-anne Supyk-Mellson
Senior Lecturer, Directorate of Occupational Therapy,
School of Health, Sport and Rehabilitation Sciences,
University of Salford, Manchester, UK

John Swain PhD
Professor of Disability and Inclusion, Northumbria
University, Newcastle upon Tyne, UK

Kirsty M. Thompson BAppSc PhD
Director, Inclusive Development, cbm, Melbourne, VIC,
Australia

Carolyn A. Unsworth BAppSc PhD AccOT OTR
Associate Professor, School of Occupational Therapy, La
Trobe University, Bundoora, VIC, Australia

Hanneke van Bruggen BSc HonDscie FfWOT
Executive Director of ENOTHE (European Network of
Occupational Therapy in Higher Education)

Helen van Huet BAppSc
Lecturer, School of Community Health, Faculty of
Science, Charles Sturt University, Albury, NSW, Australia

Gail Elizabeth Whiteford BAppSc MHSc PhD
Pro Vice Chancellor (Social Inclusion), Macquarie
University, Sydney, NSW, Australia

Clare Wilding BAppSC MAppSc PhD AccOT
Courses Manager, School of Community Health, Faculty
of Science, Charles Sturt University, Albury, NSW,
Australia

Deborah Windley DipCOT MRes
Senior Lecturer, Occupational Science and Occupational
Therapy Group, Leeds Metropolitan University, Leeds,
UK

Leslie C. Young MS
Director of Design, The R.L. Mace Universal Design
Institute, Chapel Hill, NC, USA

'To everything there is a season and a time to every purpose under heaven …
A time to get and a time to lose, a time to keep and a time to cast away …'

Ecclesiastes 3:1

And so it is for the original team of editors of this text. As *Occupational Therapy and Physical Dysfunction* grows into its sixth edition the time has come for us to pass it on to a new editorial team.

When we first developed and edited the book (entitled *The Practice of Occupational Therapy*) in 1981 it was a reflection of the thinking of the time. The subsequent editions, culminating in edition five, published in 2002, delivered a series of texts for pre-registration students during the last 20 years of the 20th century and the first few years of the 21st century. The early editions reflected the position of the occupational therapy profession in the UK during those years, when the vast majority of occupational therapists worked within statutory services and most were embedded within organisations beholden to the medical model and medical thinking. The publication of these early editions probably coincided with the period when the identity of the profession was at its poorest, with many occupational therapists lacking the ability to define the uniqueness of their profession and unable to identify its bespoke theory base. In all fairness it may well have been that these did not actually exist.

Annie's explorations of the profession against the theories of human development show it to have been, at that time, in a period of 'late childhood'. In the latter half of the 20th century occupational therapy was endeavouring to hold on to its heritage of 'doing' while applying it formulaically through mechanical and psychological processes that adhered to the paternalistic medical environment. Occupational therapists embraced the development and use of technical machinery and theories from other professions in order to prove themselves to be scientific in their approach in the absence of their own theory base. Edition one reflects this thinking with detailed descriptions of how to use rehabilitation equipment including wire twisters and electronic cycles, how to play remedial games and how to measure for and use walking aids. The book was, in effect, a 'workshop manual' for occupational therapists working in statutory care. Our theory, such as it was, was purely medical. We articulated no value base, had no outcome measures and the word occupation was sadly lacking from the proposals for intervention. Occupational therapy in physical dysfunction was clearly focused on fixing performance components, with some brief exploration of the use of activities of daily living to help people live with long-term limitations.

Edition two (1987) was fairly similar. Thinking had not moved far and although there was now talk of community (rather than domiciliary) practice and a hint at the need to consider the psychological aspects of a physical disability, by today's standards thinking remained old-fashioned. Chapters were based around diagnoses and the focus was on treating a disability rather than focusing on the individual's needs for meaningful engagement. The concept of working with groups or communities was not considered.

Edition three (1992) showed some green shoots in terms of modern thinking within the profession. This edition contained Annie's first attempt at a philosophy and the tracing of the history of the profession. On a personal basis this edition was the catalyst that began her professional interest in the development of the profession and the basis for its function. For the first time there was recognition of the profession's challenge to its relationship with medical model thinking but the mention of occupation remained elusive.

In edition four (1996) Averil Stewart's foreword felt the text contained 'evidence of critical and logical thinking' that showed a 'progression in thinking'. While by today's standards these progressions seemed small, the introduction of discussion of professional models showed the grass roots understanding of the developing theories of occupation. Averil commended us for 'leading the way', a flattery that seems to emphasise how very much the profession has further advanced in the last 15 years.

Finally, in 2002 edition five reflected the growth of occupational science and debated its relationship to occupational therapy. The chapter on philosophy was reflective, as were those presenting theoretical frameworks. There was a distinct move away from the micro concerns on performance components and a reflection by all contributors of the occupational focus of practice, although at that time this was indeed a struggle for some contributors for whom this was a new way of thinking.

What a delight then to see where the new editorial team has taken edition six. Concepts of human occupation and the theories and evidence that support these are at the heart of this text – no questions, no debate; the profession knows what it is! Occupation-based practice is accepted as the benchmark for occupational therapy. The language of occupation is embedded and gone is the diagnosis-based layout. In reflecting the globalisation of practice the book draws from contributors around the globe. Not only are the group of contributors international many come with world-wide professional reputations that will only enhance the credibility of this truly exciting new text. It is a particular delight to see contributions from people well known within disability rights movements, a true reflection of a person-centred perspective. The text also reflects the hugely fast-moving changes that have taken place in the profession in the last seven years. Work with communities, as well as individuals, is presented.

When Annie originally met with the new team to discuss the handing over of the text there was an awareness of their need for continuity and we were extremely grateful for that. However we are also delighted that they have felt in no way hide bound by the structures of what has gone before. Rather we feel we have been able to cast the new team off on a journey that has made the text fit for the 21st century, and for that we are forever grateful. The text remains true to its aim, which is to provide a foundation text for pre-registration students that explains and debates the concepts, theories and practises of our profession.

To Michael, Matthew and Jo we extend a huge thank you and our warmest congratulations. Taking on an existing text is no mean feat. Letting go of a project that has been part of our lives for over a quarter of a century is like watching a child leave home – exciting, scary and potentially fraught with concerns. Having read the text we are delighted that, like a child that successfully flees the nest and makes much of her life beyond home, we have passed this project on to a team of able, astute and professionally grounded editors who have made this book their own. We hope they will enjoy and learn from their future journey as much as we enjoyed and learnt from our journey.

Annie Turner DipCOT MA FCOT
Professor of Occupational Therapy,
University of Northampton

Marg Foster TDipCOT MMedSci FCOT
Retired Occupational Therapy Subject Manager,
University of Derby

Sybil Johnson DipCOT DMS
Retired

Preface

Occupational Therapy and Physical Dysfunction has played a key part in pre-registration occupational therapy education in the United Kingdom for almost 30 years and was edited throughout that time by Annie Turner, Marg Foster and Sybil Johnson. The book was developed to provide a British perspective on working with people whose occupational performance and engagement was affected by physical dysfunction. It began as a collection of lecture notes on key topics and has been continually developed since the first edition was published in 1981.

Occupational therapy knowledge and practice have developed significantly over the last three decades, and continue to evolve at a rapid rate. Leaders within occupational therapy and occupational science have encouraged a return to occupation as the core of occupational therapy practice. This has been complemented by developments such as the International Classification of Functioning Disability and Health (ICF) and the Ottawa Charter for Health Promotion. As a result, the relationship between occupation and health and well-being has received unprecedented attention.

As new editors of this book we have attempted to respond to the internal and external influences on the profession. To that end we have developed a book that demonstrates how an occupational perspective can be implemented in occupational therapy practice. This has resulted in numerous changes from previous editions, which include:

- A new title for the book *Occupational Therapy and Physical Dysfunction: Enabling Occupation*. Although the focus of the book remains on working with people with physical impairments, the new title of the book reflects the primacy of occupation in occupational therapy practice.

- Consideration of individuals, groups and communities – occupational therapists have a history of working with individuals but growing attention needs to be given to impacting on systems for the benefit of whole groups, communities and societies.

- A focus on strategies – rather than focusing on discrete diagnostic categories the book presents a range of strategies that, with the use of professional reasoning, can be transferred across practice settings.

- An international perspective – wherever occupational therapists work, global issues can and do influence professional knowledge and practice and so it is important to capture occupational therapy practice in a variety of social, political and geographical contexts.

- Inclusion of practice scenarios – the practice scenarios provide authentic examples to illustrate the application of theory to practice.

- New chapter features – the introduction of chapter summaries and key points provide readers with a quick overview of each chapter.

- To convey values and attitudes that are truly person-centred or inclusive, as far as possible we have tried to include appropriate language in chapters[1]. For example:
  o The term 'disabled person' is used in preference to 'person with a disability' to recognise that disability is caused by attitudinal and environmental barriers rather than a person's impairment. This is in line with the Social Model of Disability and the Affirmation Model of Disability, which has been promoted by the disability movement[2].

---

[1] When using direct quotes the original terminology will be retained rather than the preferred terminology for this book.

[2] French, S., & Swain, J. (2004). Whose tragedy? Towards a personal non-tragedy view of disability. In J. Swain, S. French, C. Barnes & C. Thomas (Eds.), *Disabling barriers – enabling environments* (2nd ed., pp. 34–40). London: Sage Publications.

Oliver, M. (1990). *The politics of disablement*. London: MacMillan.

Shakespeare, T., & Watson, N. (1997). Defending the social model. *Disability and Society*, 12(2), 293–300.

Thomas, C., & Corker, M. (2002). A journey around the social model. In M. Corker & T. Shakespeare (Eds.), *Disability/postmodernity: embodying disability theory* (pp. 18–31). London: Continuum.

It is acknowledged that other countries do use the term 'person with a disability' to emphasise the person rather than the disability, and indeed, this is the term favoured in the recent United Nations 2006 *Convention of the Rights of Persons with a Disability*. Our choice of 'disabled person' is not to cause offence to those who choose to use the alternative phrase. However, we prefer the phrase 'person with an impairment' and to focus on the *abilities* of a person. In our choice of terminology we are reminded of one of the slogans put forward by a disability organisation in the United Kingdom, 'don't *dis* my ability'; that is what we have tried to respect in the language we have used in this book.

○ Where possible we have used the term 'person' to refer to the individual engaged in a collaborative relationship with, and requiring the services of, an occupational therapist. At times, however, the term 'client' is used to ensure clarity.

○ The term 'practice setting' is used in place of 'clinic' to recognise that occupational therapists work in a variety of work places. This type of terminology is also preferred to emphasise that a lot of the work occupational therapists do does not have a medical focus.

○ The term 'occupation' is used rather than activity or function (unless in reference to the World Health Organisation's ICF).

○ 'Professional reasoning', which encompasses 'occupational reasoning', is used rather than 'clinical reasoning', as the term 'clinical' has medical connotations and we believe that the reasoning of occupational therapists is broader than just the medical.

The chapters in this book are set out in five sections. Each section of the book has a specific focus:

Section 1: Occupation and Occupational Therapy in Context

Occupational therapy is a profession that has developed over a relatively long period of time, during which it has been subject to many forces. While some of these are easily identifiable others are not. It is vital, therefore, that occupational therapists take a critical and reflective stance regarding their work and the influences on that work. The individuals, groups and communities occupational therapists work with are subject to a range of contextual influences and so it is important to not only recognise those but to acknowledge how they shape professional concepts and processes. For example, the constructions of 'disability' and 'a helping profession' bring with them particular ways of seeing the world, and these need to be explicated before they can be considered. Similarly, occupational therapists often find themselves working in settings which may not share person-centred or occupation-focused perspectives and these work settings can cause tensions. Theories and research about human occupation and the relationship between occupation and health are developing and how these inform practice must be considered.

Section 2: An Overview of Occupational Therapy Practice

Occupational therapy practice continues to evolve and develop as we move into the 21st century. Advanced and novice practitioners are continually adapting and evolving assessment and enabling skills and strategies, along with the developing evidence base, to facilitate occupational performance and engagement of people with whom we work. This section presents the professional reasoning skills and the professional knowledge base required for practice. The section then moves on to cover the process of doing assessments and evaluations, developing occupation-focused goals, and finally the implementation of relevant and appropriate enabling strategies. This section sets the scene for Sections 3, 4 and 5.

Section 3: Essential Foundations for Occupational Therapy

Whether working with individuals, groups or communities there are many strategies that traverse occupational therapy practice. This section covers key strategies that we feel all occupational therapists must consider when working with people. These strategies are essential to considering people, and the occupational nature of the work occupational therapists do, in a holistic manner. They are also essential to promoting the rights of the people we work with to live in inclusive and occupationally just societies. The strategies covered in this section are not exhaustive of all essential strategies used by occupational therapists; but these challenge occupational therapists to think outside the box when working with people who require their services.

Section 4: Working with and within Communities

Over recent years there has been a concerted push for occupational therapists to move toward working with communities, in an effort to create occupationally just societies, enabling health and well-being of all community members. This has meant moving out of our comfort zone of working with individuals on a one-to-one basis, to unknown role emerging practice areas. A lot of this work has been done in majority world countries and emerging economies, where the issues that face large populations of disabled and unwell people are too enormous to be dealt with in an individual manner. However, there is no reason why these approaches cannot be used in minority world countries. This section provides a rationale for occupational therapists engaging in this type of work and various examples of practice, such as working with displaced people, connecting with rural people, establishing collaborative partnerships with relevant organisations, and enhancing a community's capacity to deal with occupational issues. Occupational therapists are challenged to consider different ways of working and of promoting the core message that 'occupation is essential for health and well-being'.

Section 5: Working with the Individual

When working with individuals a number of approaches need to be considered, and all have a place within person-centred occupation-focused occupational therapy. The ultimate goal of occupational therapy is to enable people to participate in occupations and so it is essential to consider the occupations that are important to each individual. When choosing strategies an occupational therapist may, in collaboration with the person, choose to focus on modifying the environment or the equipment used to facilitate occupational engagement. When there is potential to improve the person's capacities and abilities, specialised strategies that address these may be appropriate. Alternatively a combination of methods may be employed to address occupational issues.

We are grateful to the contributors from around the world who have enthusiastically given their time to share their expertise in writing the chapters for this book. Each contributor was given a loose structure and a broad outline for their chapter. They were given the freedom to present their chapter in a way that suited their style and their material. This is why there is some variance of style between the chapters. We wanted to celebrate the individuality of each contributor. A number of additional occupational therapists have contributed practice scenarios to illustrate how the theory in the chapters can be applied in practice.

Working with people who have difficulties with occupational performance and engagement is complex. Our aim for this book is to provide a reference for occupational therapists to support their practice, to stimulate reflection on the knowledge, skills and attitudes which inform practice, and to encourage development of occupation-focused practice.

It is an honour to be editors of this sixth edition. We trust the book will be useful to readers as they engage with the challenges facing occupational therapists and people who have difficulties with occupational performance and engagement.

Michael Curtin
Matthew Molineux
Jo-anne Supyk-Mellson

Section **One**

Occupation and occupational therapy in context

Section One

Occupation and occupational
Defining occupational therapy in context

Clare Wilding

Chapter One

Defining occupational therapy

Clare Wilding

CHAPTER CONTENTS

The importance of a clear and recognisable
definition. 4

Threats inherent in being inarticulate 4

Benefits of a clear definition. 5

Problems of articulation 5

Occupation: core philosophy but
peripheral reality?. 5

Challenges to clearly articulating
occupational therapy 7

Over-inclusive definitions 8

Problems of 'fit': epistemological
difference 9

Ways of describing and defining
occupational therapy 10

Giving up 'function': becoming 'experts
in occupation' 10

Promoting the 'health through
occupation' message 11

Towards a clearer articulation of
occupational therapy 12

SUMMARY

Consistent with the concept that occupation is
the foundation stone of occupational therapy,
this chapter makes a case for the importance of
acknowledging the central position of occupation
in all definitions of occupational therapy. Having
a clear and easily recognisable definition of
occupational therapy is imperative if the
profession is to survive the current challenges,
such as competition for limited resources, other
professions widening the scope of their practice,
and pressure for generic rather than specialist
workers. However, even though a chorus of
occupational therapy leaders has urged the
profession to state clearly and explicitly what
occupational therapy stands for, occupational
therapists have struggled to achieve this aim. The
chapter explores a number of reasons why
occupational therapists have experienced
difficulty describing occupational therapy and
concludes that, even though there are challenges
to defining occupational therapy, this profession
can be better articulated by consistently using
the word 'occupation' and by explaining the
occupational therapy meaning of this term.

KEY POINTS

- It is vital to professional survival that occupational therapists represent and promote occupational therapy accurately and effectively.
- Enabling occupation is a core and foundational philosophical value of occupational therapy.
- Occupational therapists may have experienced difficulty defining occupational therapy due to their making errors, albeit inadvertently, in their articulation of the profession.
- Using 'occupation' as a key descriptor of occupational therapy should assist occupational therapists to overcome articulation difficulties and experience a stronger sense of professional identity.
- Occupational therapists need to promote the idea that health, well-being, survival, and life satisfaction can be achieved through engaging in occupation and that occupational therapists have unique and expert skills in enabling occupational engagement and occupational performance.

The importance of a clear and recognisable definition

Since the beginnings of occupational therapy, there has been uncertainty about what might be the best way to describe, and thus define to ourselves and to others, the nature of occupational therapy. Anecdotally, many occupational therapists and occupational therapy students fear being asked to explain what occupational therapy is, precisely because they find it challenging to do so; they are unsure about how best to explicate this complex profession to others. However, even though it has been challenging for occupational therapists to define occupational therapy, it is a very important task, since a clear and memorable definition may mean that the profession can thrive, develop, and move forward into the future. By contrast, in a worst-case scenario, if occupational therapists fail to promote and represent their profession adequately, it may mean that occupational needs, issues, and concerns are not addressed adequately and appropriately. Such a situation could result in a consequent loss of health, well-being, and quality of life for individuals, families, communities, organizations, and societies. Thinking about the importance of having a good definition is a necessary place to start, since being aware of what is at stake can provide the motivation needed to push through the challenges and reach a solution.

Threats inherent in being inarticulate

In the current economic rationalist and evidence-based climate there are many reasons why occupational therapists should be able to state clearly what it is they do and why occupational therapy is of value. Competition for scarce health dollars is fierce and, therefore, occupational therapy must be able to demonstrate that it is effective and that it provides a necessary and unique service (Fisher 1998, Pierce 2001). In competitive health environments, it may be essential that occupational therapists are able to articulate their distinctive contribution to health care, lest they be replaced by cheaper (yet inferior) workers. Lack of clarity about occupational therapy's role in health care may mean that occupational therapists never realise the powerful contribution they have to make to individuals, groups, and societies (Reilly 1962).

Many authors (Ambrosi & Schwartz 1995, Asmundsdottir & Kaplan 2001, Hughes 2001, Pollard & Walsh 2000, Wallace 1986) have argued that occupational therapists need to improve their ability to promote the profession so that its profile is strengthened and it is better recognised and understood. Indeed, for over four decades, alarm has been expressed that occupational therapists' apparent inability in professional representation could easily sound the death knoll for the profession (Kornblau 2004, Reilly 1966/1984, Wallace 1986, Woodside 1971). Occupational therapy leaders have been challenging occupational therapists for years to better explain what occupational therapy is, and to describe how it can be of service to society, in order for the profession to thrive, or even just to survive (Barker 1984, Creek & Ormston 1996, Fisher 1998, Nelson 1996, Reilly 1962, Wallace 1986).

Speaking of the health care system, Atwal and Caldwell (2003) asserted that clients may suffer and their care might be compromised if professionals are unable to clearly articulate the contribution their profession makes to health care. In order for multidisciplinary teams to provide a safe and ethical treatment plan for their clients, relevant information from all team members must be received, and so occupational therapists should make their role more widely understood and strengthen their professional image (Atwal & Caldwell 2003). In some instances, occupational therapists are reliant upon other people to refer or to direct individuals to occupational-therapy services. If the worth of occupational therapy is not recognized, then people who need occupational therapy services may remain unaware that a service exists that can fulfil their needs.

Occupational therapists themselves are also believed to suffer through experiencing difficulty in being able to define occupational therapy. Moore et al (2006) found that a major cause of job dissatisfaction amongst Australian occupational therapists was that other health professionals and occupational therapy clients did not understand the occupational therapy role. Dissatisfaction with the professional image of occupational therapy may result in therapists leaving the profession (Moore et al 2006). An earlier survey of occupational therapists (Bailey 1990) found that 'lack of respect for occupational therapy by other professionals ... lack of understanding of occupational therapy by other professionals' (p. 25), 'role conflict with physical therapy' (p. 26), and 'being disillusioned with occupational therapy' (p. 27) were amongst the reasons given for therapists leaving occupational therapy. A literature review of factors that contributed to work stress amongst occupational therapists revealed that a lack of professional identity, low status of occupational therapy, and feelings of being undervalued by colleagues were significant work-related stressors (Lloyd & King 2001). Poor definition and articulation of occupational therapy can lead to role incompatibility, role conflict, and role ambiguity, which all contribute to the experience of 'role stress' (Hughes 2001). Therefore, role stress and potentially burnout, and loss of occupational therapists from the profession, might occur as a result of being inarticulate about the profession.

Benefits of a clear definition

In contrast to the threat posed if members of a profession are inarticulate about their profession's skills and purpose, there can be benefits when professionals are more eloquent about their profession's contribution. Being able to articulate what and why professionals do what they do, allows distribution of knowledge and understanding, and, in addition, the knowledge base of the professions can be contributed to and grow (Butler et al 2001). Furthermore, being able to explain practice to others can assist in organisational growth, since innovative individuals can pass on their knowledge to others, thus moving the whole organisation to a higher and more effective level of understanding and performance (Butler et al 2001).

Being able to define one's profession and its purpose may also enable better teamwork. For example, Jones' (2005) ethnographic research found that many multidisciplinary teams do not work effectively together, but rather that individuals work 'in parallel'. This situation can result in service provision that is less effective than it could be and some client issues are not addressed. Jones (2005) advocated that for interprofessional teams to be effective they each need to be aware of their own and other disciplines' boundaries and strengths, and that professionals should be articulate about their professional philosophy, theory, and knowledge, so that they can be aware of what they can and cannot do. Another study found that if professional roles were better defined, there could be a better working environment and more interprofessional collaboration, ultimately resulting in more benefit to service recipients (Crozier 2003).

Problems of articulation

While there is clearly a need for occupational therapists to be assertive advocates of their unique role and purpose, it has been reported that therapists appear to have tremendous difficulty in communicating what occupational therapy is (Kronenberg et al 2005, Thornton & Rennie 1988) and that this problem is very widespread (Fisher 1998). One major issue has been occupational therapists' inability to define themselves as different from other professions. This situation is threatening since, when there is considerable overlap between two professions and fiscal resources are scarce, then only one group may be supported (Bing 1981, Woodside 1971). Additionally, inability to clearly define the boundaries of occupational therapy has left the profession defenceless against other professions making 'incursions' into the professional domain of occupational therapy (Kornblau 2004, Wallace 1986, p. 93). In order to compete effectively, it appears that occupational therapists need to become better and more direct communicators of the unique services that occupational therapy can provide.

Occupation: core philosophy but peripheral reality?

The discussion turns now to exploring the unique features of occupational therapy. What are the constituents of occupational therapy that make it distinctive from other professions? Why is one type of therapy labelled 'occupational', and another type is called 'physical therapy' or 'speech therapy' or 'psychological therapy'? Many occupational therapist authors (Crepeau et al 2003, Molineux 2004, Reilly 1962, Rogers 2005, Schwammle 1996, Townsend & Polatakjo 2007, Wilcock 2000) state that the exclusive contribution that occupational therapy brings to multidisciplinary health care, must be a profound understanding of enabling occupation.

Occupational therapists' utilisation of occupation within their therapy is complex. Knowledge of occupation is employed as a *means* to facilitate the development of health in people (Pollock & McColl 2003) and in this sense occupation may be conceptualised as being used therapeutically. Occupational therapists also aspire to the goal of facilitating occupational engagement and performance as the *end*, or outcome of therapy. Schwammle (1996) encouraged occupational therapists to concern themselves with enabling their clients to achieve a state of 'occupational competence', which in turn provides them with a sense of control and achievement that can increase a person's sense of well-being. Occupational therapy practice which focuses on occupation as means and/or end of practice is purported by leaders of occupational therapy to be the kind of occupational therapy toward which therapists ought to be striving (Fisher 2003, Reilly 1962). Occupational therapy that aims to use occupation as means and end may be described as *occupation-focused*. This kind of therapy is built upon the theoretical assertion that 'there is a 3-way link between occupation, health, and survival, in that occupation provides the mechanism for people to fulfil basic human needs essential for survival and health; to adapt to environmental changes; and to develop and exercise genetic capacities in order to maintain health and to experience physical, mental, and social well-being' (Wilcock 2006, p. 51).

There is overwhelming support for the concept of occupation as the core domain of concern for occupational therapy; however, there has also been conflict about this assertion, as it appears that not all authors agree with this perspective. In the most direct attack against occupation, Mocellin (1996, p. 16) stated that 'the notion of 'health through occupation' is no longer useful nor is it likely to provide the necessary foundation for the further advancement of the profession'. Other occupational therapists have been less directly confrontational but have nevertheless tended to push an occupational focus to the background of practice, in favour of foregrounding concepts that are more consistent with a medical model (Wilcock 2006). Having a medical focus rather than an occupational one may have resulted in therapists focusing on remedying performance components rather than addressing occupation itself, which Molineux (2004) warned is highly problematic, as it can lead to issues of role blurring, role overlap, and role ambiguity. Other examples of occupational therapy becoming narrowed and 'medicalised,' rather than occupation-focused include highlighting 'functional independence' (Crabtree 2000) or activities of daily living (Thornton & Rennie 1998) as the ultimate goals of occupational therapy. Such weightings detract from having a more encompassing and complex conceptualisation of occupation as a whole phenomenon. Similarly, Persson et al (2001, p.16) concluded that occupational therapy will become a meaningless and

ineffective practice if therapists 'focus exclusively on the micro perspective' to the exclusion of bigger picture occupational issues.

Chevalier (1997) concurred that occupational therapists experience difficulty agreeing about what occupational therapy is, but he did not think that this was necessarily a detrimental position to be in. Chevalier proposed that occupational therapists should celebrate their diversity as signifying that occupational therapy is an energetic profession and he contended that occupational therapy philosophy is broad enough to allow a variety of different perspectives. Whilst such a view may be attractive, since it silences disagreement, and it is certainly inclusive of all perspectives, nevertheless, it also propagates the idea that occupational therapy has no clear unifying goal and, thus, that occupational therapy is undefined and indefinable. Such a situation renders it impossible to clearly articulate occupational therapy purposes and practice.

Even though there have been some voices that de-emphasise the centrality of occupation to occupational therapy, many more occupational therapy leaders and academics (Baum & Baptiste 2002, Crabtree 1998, Fisher 1998, Law et al 2002, Nelson 1996, Reilly 1966/1984, Wilcock 2000) have advocated that occupational therapy must have as its basis a fundamental focus on occupation and, in particular, on the concept of enabling occupation. Nelson (1996) recommended that a focus on occupation would unite occupational therapy and ensure its continued survival. Other authors attest that occupation-focused practice is occupational therapy's unique contribution to health care (Asmundsottir & Kaplan 2001, Reilly 1962) and that being the best at providing this exclusive perspective will certify the professional survival of occupational therapy in a fiercely competitive health environment (Pierce 2001).

When occupational therapy practice is centred on occupation, it is most consistently aligned with occupational therapy's philosophical base (Fisher 1998, Katz 1985, Molineux 2004, Wilcock 2000); indeed, occupation-focused practice enables occupational therapy to achieve its full potential (Crabtree 2000). Occupation-focused practice may result in more satisfying practice for individual occupational therapists (Molineux 2004, Wilding 2008) and considering occupation may assist therapists' interventions to be more meaningful when dealing with complex issues (Persson et al 2001). Perhaps most importantly, Yerxa (2000) claimed that occupation-focused practice enables occupational therapy to be a true, self-defining profession.

Challenges to clearly articulating occupational therapy

Many occupational therapists have expressed that it is difficult to describe occupational therapy (Fisher 1998, Kronenberg et al 2005, Schwartz 2003). One reason for the difficulty explaining occupational therapy arises from the language that is used to describe occupational therapy practice. The issue of what language to use to describe occupational therapy is confounded by different therapists advocating the use of different and sometimes conflicting nomenclature, throughout the history of occupational therapy. For example, in 1971, Diasio asserted that occupational therapists ought to change the name of the profession to acknowledge that they are 'generalists in activities' (p. 241). Part of the difficulty in deciding what language to use to describe occupational therapy is that the profession is very complex and multifaceted, and it is, therefore, extremely difficult to define (Creek et al 2005).

Occupational therapists may also experience difficulty explaining their profession because of issues that arise due to being a predominantly female profession (Pollard & Walsh 2000). For example, the 'feminine' profession of occupational therapy has experienced difficulty in accommodating the 'male demands for scientific rigour' espoused by the 'masculine' profession of medicine, and 'thus medicine has still to recognise the value of [occupational therapists'] work' (Pollard & Walsh 2000, p. 426). Diasio (1971, p. 240) considered that occupational therapy lacked status due to being perceived to be a 'women's profession'. In addition, female values of care may result in occupational therapists sacrificing their own independence in favour of promoting the independence of others and, as a consequence, occupational therapists fail to speak up on their own behalf to advocate for the profession of occupational therapy (Pollard & Walsh 2000). Being female may also account for a tendency towards passiveness, and quiet acceptance of, and compliance with, prevailing discourses that tend to disregard occupational therapy values and concerns (Wilding 2008).

An explanation, which is somewhat paradoxical, is that the more experienced therapists become, the less articulate they are about their decision-making (Butler et al 2001). When investigating what it meant to be an articulate practitioner, these authors found five levels of articulation: novice, advanced beginner, competent, proficient, and expert. Butler et al found that as tacit knowledge accumulated, the less articulate professionals became about their practice. In a different study of a novice therapist's and an experienced therapist's professional reasoning processes, Gibson et al (2000, p. 24) found, in accordance with Butler et al's findings, that the experienced therapist had more difficulty articulating her reasoning process. Despite the reasons that may underpin this situation, it is likely to be problematic for the profession of occupational therapy that its highest-level practitioners are unable to clearly express what their practice is about and why they do what they do.

In a study I conducted with a group of 15 occupational therapists working in an acute, hospital setting in Melbourne, which explored the therapists' articulation of their profession, a range of reasons emerged explaining why the therapists experienced difficulty in describing occupational therapy (Wilding 2008). One articulation problem was that the participating therapists tended to focus on diversity within occupational therapy rather than commonality, which meant that their definitions were too lengthy and the central focus of occupational therapy was not clear. Another significant difficulty was that medical model concepts of health and ways of practicing tend to dominate health systems, and this can make it difficult for occupational therapists to be understood and to practice in occupation-focused ways. 'Nellie's story' is an amalgam of the participating therapists' explanations of how they described occupational therapy and the challenges they faced in doing so (Practice Scenario 1.1). This story has been previously presented and discussed in Wilding and Whiteford (2007).

Practice Scenario 1.1
Nellie's story

When Nellie is asked to explain occupational therapy she sighs deeply, rolls her eyes and laughs nervously. She thinks to herself, 'oh no, do I have to explain this again? I find it difficult. I wish that people just knew'. A nurse asked me just the other day on the ward when I came up. She'd sent the referral and she goes, 'Now what does OT do?'

Well, what is occupational therapy? That's the million-dollar question isn't it? I normally say that I'm here to find out how you were managing prior to coming to hospital and get an idea on how you're managing at the moment, just to see if there's anything you might need in the way of equipment or services to make it easier for you when it's time to go home and I will throw in there like your showering or cooking and cleaning.

My main job is to see how you function with your everyday activities prior to coming into hospital. To see how you're going now and what your current function is like and then to make recommendations to see whether you need to go home, whether you need equipment for home or whether you might need some rehabilitation and I also have quite a large role in education, on how to get back to your activities. Educate you on restrictions and the functional sort of implications that they might have. Yeah, I'd talk to them a bit about home set up and how that's part of my role in terms of making sure they are safe to be able to do their everyday activities.

I tend to use the word 'activities' rather than 'occupations' because I think it's more a lay term. I think a lot of people think occupation means work. I probably don't use the jargon as much. I probably say the difficulties you're having in performing some of the everyday tasks and then give like brushing your hair or feeding as an example.

I also tend to use the word 'function'. To me, 'function' means how they're doing things as well. So it is similar to occupation. So how they're doing things, but how they're functioning. Function as in can you do this, can you do your showering? How are you actually functioning? Function means your ability to perform a task. Functional independence I will describe as being able to go about and perform the task you need to do as you were doing pre-morbidly. However, I also think 'function' to patients isn't something they understand, as it's a bit like 'occupation'. I think where we use an example makes more sense to patients. It's also funny that I hear the physiotherapists talking a lot about 'function' these days. And the physio's will also say that they help patients with their functioning. Sometimes people still look at me a bit blankly and I'll just say something like, even though I tend to try and avoid it, but I'll say a physiotherapist works in muscular physical movement, what we do is work with function rather than specifically targeting physical movement.

Then I'll usually explain that in mental health I look at things like their safety in the community, their ability to achieve daily activities. Then I might say paediatrics might look at children's ability to look at improving their handwriting through postural activities, and I just give a couple of different examples. Because I think if you just give one example it gives that person a very narrow image of what OT is when there is a lot more out there but it's usually a mouthful! I think people sometimes wonder why they asked in the first place.

I also include specific aspects of my role that are determined by the setting that I work in. For example, in the acute hospital I say that I look at how to improve their safety or independence and that my job is to ensure a safe and effective discharge. I might also say, 'I run the groups,' since this is in my job description. Sometimes my job is all about preventing deconditioning. I do education about managing. I do equipment. I'm involved with referring to post acute care for support from services. I also assist people to die comfortably at home through working with the patient and the families to provide equipment or strategies so that they're comfortable and able to manage. But often I'm still referred to just give the relaxation tapes out.

Over-inclusive definitions

As Nellie's story illustrates, a mistake that occupational therapists might sometimes make, is including too much detail about the particular tasks and duties that they do: for example, that occupational therapists consider safety and independence; they focus on performing activities of daily living; they aim to prevent deconditioning; they provide equipment, education, and referral; they facilitate discharge; and, they perform specific therapeutic treatments. Sometimes therapists can include unnecessary information about occupational therapy processes or philosophical beliefs, such as: occupational therapists aspire to be holistic; diversity is celebrated; occupational therapists desire to empower and motivate their clients; and, therapists seek to build their clients' confidence. While these lists of tasks, processes, and values are not untrue in relation to what occupational therapy is, having a very lengthy description of occupational therapy can mean that the core message of being occupation-focused therapists can become diluted and, thus, the listener can become confused and have difficulty remembering exactly what occupational therapy is.

When the diversity of occupational therapy is emphasised, the profession's common focus upon occupation can become obscured. A decade ago,

Townsend (1998) advocated that language can be used effectively by occupational therapists to unite the profession because it can demonstrate that the common ground of the profession is about being person-centred and about occupation. Thus, it seems important that occupational therapists should reach agreement about how to describe practice so that they do not confuse others and work at cross purposes to their aim of promoting occupational therapy, by having too many varied descriptors of occupational therapy.

Occupational therapists may have adopted lengthy and detailed descriptions of occupational therapy because a straightforward definition of occupational therapy might appear to be far too simple. Occupational therapists may have tended to describe the diversity of occupational therapy in order to help to illustrate the complexity and worth of the profession. Even though the complexity, difficulty, and challenge of elegant occupational therapy practice is hidden from view, since it occurs in the minds of therapists (Yerxa 2000), the value of occupational therapy may still be easily seen in the difference that it makes to the survival, health, well-being, and life satisfaction of people. There is an increasing body of evidence that highlights that addressing the occupational needs of clients can be truly transformative, health-restorative, and health-enhancing (Clark 1993, Clark et al 2004, De Vries et al 2004, Golledge 2004, Hayley & McKay 2004, Jackson et al 1998, Jackson & Schkade 2001).

Problems of 'fit': epistemological difference

Occupational therapists have also faced difficulty trying to describe occupational therapy because the philosophy and orientation of occupational therapy is radically different from that of medicine, and yet the medical model is the dominant system of thought and practice in Western societies, so much so that it has achieved status as the 'folk model' of disease (Engel, 1977, p. 130). Therefore, it is almost as if occupational therapists are speaking a completely different language to everyone else. Indeed, occupational therapy professional jargon is quite different to other health professions' idiom. Others may speak of medical conditions, medications, and physiological and anatomical mechanisms by which disease, injury, and curing of disease and injury

occurs within the body, while occupational therapists speak of how occupational performance is functional or dysfunctional according to each individual's experience. Philosophically, theoretically, and practically, occupational therapy does not fit at all well with medicine's philosophy, theory, and practice; the focus of the medical model is about curing illness and injury, primarily through the methods of medication and surgery. In contrast, the focus of occupational therapy is about enabling people to engage in their chosen occupations and meeting people's occupational needs (Christiansen & Baum 1997, Crepeau et al 2003, Kielhofner 2004, Townsend 1997). Non-occupational therapists have no framework for understanding occupational concepts, in part because they do not have the same understanding of the word 'occupation,' and also because they have a different concept of what 'health' is than do occupational therapists.

Historically, occupational therapy benefited from an alliance with medicine since this partnership brought with it increased status and support for the development and growth of the fledgling profession of occupational therapy (Schwartz 2003b). However, as well as the benefits, the association with medicine has created some problems for contemporary occupational therapy practitioners. Most notably, the difficulty caused by a close allegiance to medicine is that when occupational therapists try to 'fit' into the medical model, their practice can become distorted into something that is quite different from that described by the philosophy of occupational therapy. For example, within the medical model, health problems are theorised to be located in either the mind or the body, and the precise sites of disorder are sought. When occupational therapists attempted to match this type of thinking, practice moved away from a holistic consideration of occupational performance and engagement, to become specialised according to medical classifications (Bryden & McColl 2003) and occupational therapists 'split' into those therapists working in the area of physical disabilities and those working in psychosocial dysfunction (Schwartz 2003).

When occupational therapists try to fit with medical model practices they focus on impairments, and this narrows and limits occupational therapy (Baum et al 2002). Other ways in which occupational therapy can be limited by medical model thinking is to focus on 'function' and 'independence' (Crabtree 1998). Occupation-focused practice can become very constrained in medically dominated health services (Bryden & McColl 2003, Jongbloed & Wendland 2002, Pollard & Walsh 2000). Changing occupational therapy practice into a 'medicalised hybrid' can have significant negative consequences for being able to clearly describe and define occupational therapy; since this type of practice falls between the definitions of both medicine and of occupational therapy and there is no easy way to name it. Additionally, because such practices do not match with occupational therapy philosophy and theory, and evidence illustrating the efficacy of these practices may be missing, they can also be impossible to defend.

Ways of describing and defining occupational therapy

As has been discussed, the common core of occupational therapy practice is about enabling people to engage in a range of occupations and building people's capacity and ability to perform occupations. These are fundamental occupational therapy concepts and actions that are explained and elaborated by many authors (Christiansen & Baum 1997, Crepeau et al 2003, Fisher 1998, Kielhofner 2004, Law et al 2002, Townsend 1997, Townsend & Polatajko 2007). Thus, in defining occupational therapy it would seem highly appropriate to emphasise that occupational therapists enable occupational engagement and occupational performance. And, additionally, there are also pitfalls about describing occupational therapy that would be best to avoid, such as including too much description of the diversity of occupational therapy (since this detracts from the core definition).

Giving up 'function': becoming 'experts in occupation'

Returning to the study of occupational therapists' articulation of their practice in an acute setting (Wilding 2008), in their practice prior to the study, the therapists used to actively avoid describing their practice using the word 'occupation,' as they felt that they would be misunderstood by others. Instead they used 'function' as an alternative for 'occupation'. The use of function as synonymous with occupation is somewhat ubiquitous in occupational therapy; for example, several authors use these terms interchangeably (Baum & Baptiste 2002, Burke & Kern 1996, Pierce 2001). Indeed, the use of 'function' in

occupational therapy has been so pervasive that it has been posited that the terms 'occupation', 'purposeful activity', and 'function' may be substituted for each other without causing problems (AOTA 1997). However, as the therapists in my study reflected more critically upon their descriptions of occupational therapy, they realised that 'function' was not in fact synonymous with 'occupation' and that describing their practice as being 'about function' was far less powerful than describing it as being about 'enabling occupation'. Additionally use of the word 'function' within a range of professions seems to have constrained occupational therapy from being able to highlight its unique role and contribution in health-service provision. If the distinctive contribution of occupational therapy remains unrecognised by significant groups (especially funding bodies) then the profession will continue to experience difficulty presenting its profile and perceived relevancy. Subsequently, the therapists experimented with using the words 'occupation' and 'doing' (as a lay-person's version of occupation), and began to think of themselves as 'experts in occupation'. Describing themselves and occupational therapy in this way had a profound and transformative effect upon the therapists' senses of professional confidence, professional esteem, and professional identity, as illustrated by 'Katrina's story' (Practice Scenario 1.2). Parts of this story have been previously presented and discussed in Wilding and Whiteford (2008).

Practice Scenario 1.2 Katrina's story

Sometimes I have to explain 'function'. Not all of my patients grasp 'function' and so I usually end up explaining function with a sentence. Perhaps it's not so useful for us to use the word function, because function is movement function or body function or emotional function or social function. It just means the ability to function, it means that the machine works well, that the body works well so we want to kind of differentiate between general kind of function, like my body is healthy in terms of I don't have sickness, it's functioning, I'm able to digest my food, I'm able to breathe, oxygen gets pumped around my body so the system's functioning, but we want to talk about, we want to differentiate that I'm able to do the activities that are meaningful to me, which is our occupation.

The other day I was writing my notes and I kept thinking, the sticker proclaims we are the 'occupational therapist'. And yet we never see 'occupation' in our notes! I think that if we started using 'occupation' as a heading that it would actually make more sense. I think people would understand what we're talking about more, because it would then fit with why we're called occupational therapists. It makes sense that occupational therapists would talk about 'previous occupational performance' and 'current occupational performance'. And after these headings, you wouldn't just talk about work; you'd talk about the patient's activities of daily living and everything, so then other people would understand that occupation means everything that meaningfully occupies people.

I have been substituting 'function' with 'occupation' in the notes and saying 'doing' with the patient. And I have been able to do it quite successfully. I've heard the term before that occupational therapists are '**experts in doing**'. And all of a sudden that made sense to me, that's our role! We're experts in the doing side of things. And actually, yeah, we are, that's what we were trained to do. And that's actually quite empowering to know you're an expert in that area. Whereas before then, I thought we knew a lot about a lot of things, but not necessarily felt that we were experts in one area. I thought the doctors are experts in medication and physios are experts in exercise. We sort of do a bit of this and a bit of that, but it makes sense that occupation is our focus; that's what our expertise is in. It's not the physio, its not the medical, it's the doing, the next bit, and I think in my role that's made a lot of sense and so I know where to target my intervention.

I have been trying out different words to describe occupational therapy that perhaps I haven't used previously – I've used 'occupation' with patients' families. I say, 'OT is making sure that patients can get back into their occupations and when OT's talk about occupations we're not just talking about work, we're talking about all the things people do like showering and dressing and things like that'. I've used the word occupation where I hadn't been previously and that's where the title comes from and I'm thinking to myself 'yeah, that's where the title comes from'. And my clients say, 'Oh that's why it's occupational therapy!' So I think using occupation has helped me and others understand why we're called occupational therapists. Previously we were giving some explanations about function and I just think that sometimes why we are called occupational therapists didn't gel with people. I think that has changed and that's improved their understanding because they're able to think: 'Occupational therapy? Oh they're the ones that do that work about occupations'.

It is important to note that the therapists used the word occupation, but that they also explained occupational therapists' understanding of occupation; for example, as **all** the activities that occupy a person's time and life, as opposed to the common, but narrow, understanding of occupation as employment. The therapists also used headings in their report writing that highlighted that occupation is the focus of their concern. For example they used the headings: occupational performance, occupational history, and occupational engagement. Similarly, Hughes (2001) suggested using strategies of increasing opportunities and support to use occupational-therapy language and theory, receiving additional supervision, and working more closely with other occupational therapists as a means to combat role stress experienced by occupational therapists in many health-care settings.

When 'occupation' is used as a descriptor for occupational therapy and occupation-related terms are used as primary labels for work, one's own sense of professional identity can be changed dramatically. By deciding to declare one's self as an *occupation*-al therapist, that is, a therapist whose core concern is about enabling occupation and engaging people in health-restoring occupations, a therapist may experience a transformed professional identity and a corresponding increase in satisfaction and clarity of purpose. Therapists may also develop increased confidence and an improved sense of internal power as they move from being 'professionals who enable clients' functioning in order to facilitate discharge' to becoming 'experts in occupation'.

Language shapes practice, and for this reason it is essential to choose the language that best suits the direction in which one wishes one's practice to proceed. The use of 'function' sets occupational therapists along a course that is aligned more closely with medicalised practices, since a focus on 'function' emphasises the working (or non-working) of performance components. Whereas, use of the word 'occupation' stresses that occupational therapy practice is not limited merely to occupational function, but rather it encompasses all of the array of features of occupation, which is a very broad and complex phenomenon.

Promoting the 'health through occupation' message

The use of occupational terminology would seem to meet goals of making the profession readily communicable to others and also acting as a boost to professional identity. In contrast to the narrow perspective of occupational therapy practice that is conveyed by words such as 'function' and 'independence,' the use of occupation-focused language also helps to transmit a more complex perception of occupational therapy, since it encapsulates concepts of 'wholeness, fulfillment, and personal authenticity' (Crabtree 1998, p. 207). 'Occupation' can be used as a clear 'brand' for the profession of occupational therapy and its specific use within the profession can be explained so that others may appreciate that occupation can have a broad meaning. Indeed, I believe that occupational therapists *must* continue to explain again and again and again what occupation means in the context of occupational therapy. It is not enough to describe it once and expect that everyone will immediately remember.

Occupational therapists use the word 'occupation' in a specialised way and the concept of enabling health, well-being, and life satisfaction through engaging in occupation is not the most common understanding of how health is created. It appears that in order for occupational therapy to be taken seriously and to become better known, a whole world of people need to realise that ill-health and illness can be caused not only by micro-organisms and body system failures, but also by what they do everyday; that people can influence their health, not only by taking a pill or receiving surgery, but also through engaging in 'ordinary' occupation. Thus, occupational therapists need to continually explain occupation and its benefits. Repeatedly using the word occupation and explaining it may begin to slowly help others understand what occupational therapy really is. Another benefit of using occupation in communications is that by doing so, occupational therapists are continually linking what they do with the name of the profession and this type of consistency appears to have benefit to helping both others and ourselves better understand *and remember* what occupational therapy is.

When it is remembered that an occupation-focused perspective is the unique contribution that occupational therapy makes to society and to health-care service delivery, the importance of highlighting occupation and the 'health through occupation' message becomes clearly apparent. If individuals, families, organisations, societies, and occupational therapy are to thrive in the future, occupational therapists must promote the message that what people do every day can impact their health,

well-being, survival, and life satisfaction, and, in addition, occupational therapists are the professionals who should be consulted to achieve a healthy life through everyday doing. If this relationship does not become common knowledge there may not be a place for occupational therapy, and this would be a tremendous loss to people and to society. For occupational therapists to demonstrate their valuable and unique contribution to society, they need to be giving a clear and loud message that occupation can affect health and that occupational therapists are the people who are best equipped to help others achieve health and well-being through occupation.

Towards a clearer articulation of occupational therapy

This exploration of occupational therapists' articulation of occupational therapy has shown that it is vital that occupational therapists become better communicators about what occupational therapy is and why this profession is essential to society. It is also clear that occupational therapists have experienced considerable difficulty in explaining occupational therapy well. In part, this problem of articulation has occurred because therapists have used the wrong language to describe their practice and they have mistakenly tried to demonstrate the value of occupation through highlighting the complexity and diversity of occupational therapy in over-inclusive definitions, rather than allowing acts of health-enhancing transformation through occupation to 'speak for themselves'. The purpose of pointing out these errors of action is not to apportion blame or to invoke guilt, but rather to demonstrate that there may be ways of changing our descriptions of occupational therapy so that others more readily understand and remember what occupational therapy is and how it serves society.

The study in which I have been recently involved (Wilding 2008) illustrated that when occupational therapists working in an acute setting focused more overtly on occupation, they were able to overcome the identity discord they had previously experienced. By choosing to practice in an occupation-focused way and describing themselves as 'experts in occupation' the participating occupational therapists were able to align their practice with occupational therapy philosophy and their identity became clear; they are *occupation*-al therapists whose role is to enable people's meaningful and health-restorative engagement in, and performance of, occupation. In addition, using occupation-focused idiom appears to assist occupational therapists to keep their eyes firmly on the vision of occupational therapy as about enabling health through the medium of engaging in occupation. If other words are used to describe occupational therapy then alternative meanings of these words seem to distract and confuse occupational therapists as to their purpose and role.

Language is clearly an important vehicle through which to present and promote occupational therapy's philosophical principles and core concepts. The most significant of these is occupation, and its essential relationship to health and well-being. It is hoped that this chapter will not only be thought provoking, but also that it might serve as a catalyst for action. Active engagement in consolidating our collective identity, enhancing our profile and ensuring public representations of occupational therapy that are consistent with what we actually value, may be seen as a responsibility for all members of the profession.

References

Ambrosi, E., & Schwartz, K. B. (1995). The profession's image, 1917–1925, Part I: Occupational therapy as represented in the media. *American Journal of Occupational Therapy*, 49, 715–719.

American Occupational Therapy Association. (AOTA). (1997). Statement – Fundamental concepts of occupational therapy: Occupation, purposeful activity, and function. *American Journal of Occupational Therapy*, 51, 864–866.

Asmundsdottir, E. E., & Kaplan, S. (2001). Icelandic occupational therapists' attitudes towards educational issues. *Occupational Therapy International*, 8(1), 63–78.

Atwal, A., & Caldwell, K. (2003). Ethics, occupational therapy and discharge planning: Four broken principles. *Australian Occupational Therapy Journal*, 50, 244–251.

Bailey, D. M. (1990). Reasons for attrition from occupational therapy. *American Journal of Occupational Therapy*, 44, 23–29.

Barker, J. (1984). Into the 21st century – Are we ready? (Sylvia Docker Lecture). *Australian Occupational Therapy Journal*, 31, 98–105.

Baum, C., & Baptiste S. (2002). Reframing occupational therapy practice. In: M. Law, C. M. Baum, & S. Baptiste (Eds.), *Occupation-based practice: Fostering performance and participation* (pp. 3–15). Thorofare, New Jersey: Slack.

Baum, C., Berg, C., Seaton, M. K., & White, L. (2002). Fostering occupational performance and participation. In: M. Law, C. M. Baum, & S. Baptiste (Eds.). *Occupation–based practice: Fostering performance and participation* (pp. 27–36). Thorofare, New Jersey: Slack.

Bing, R. K. (1981). Occupational therapy: revisited: A paraphrastic journey. *American Journal of Occupational Therapy*, 35, 499–518.

Bryden, P., & McColl, M. A. (2003). The concept of occupation: 1900 to 1974. In: M. McColl, M. Law, D. Stewart, L. Doubt, N. Pollock, & T. Krupa. *Theoretical basis of occupational therapy* (pp. 27–38). Thorofare, New Jersey: Slack.

Burke, J. P., & Kern, S. B. (1996). Is the use of life history and narrative in clinical practice reimbursable? Is it occupational therapy? *American Journal of Occupational Therapy*, 50, 389–392.

Butler, J., Kay, R., & Titchen, A. (2001). Articulating practice. In: J. Higgs, & A. Titchen (Eds.), *Professional practice in health, education and the creative arts* (pp. 199–211). Oxford: Blackwell Science.

Chevalier, M. (1997). Occupational therapy and the search for meaning. *British Journal of Occupational Therapy*, 60, 539–540.

Christiansen, C., & Baum, C. (1997). *Occupational therapy: Enabling function and well-being* (2nd ed.). Thorofare, New Jersey: Slack.

Clark, F. (1993). Occupation embedded in a real life: Interweaving occupational science and occupational therapy. *American Journal of Occupational Therapy*, 47, 1067–1077.

Clark, F. A., Jackson, J., & Carlson, M. (2004). Occupational science, occupational therapy and evidence-based practice: What the Well Elderly Study has taught us. In: M. Molineux (Ed.), *Occupation for occupational therapists* (pp. 200–218). Oxford, UK: Blackwell Publishing.

Crabtree, J. (1998). The end of occupational therapy. *American Journal of Occupational Therapy*, 52, 205–214.

Crabtree, J. (2000). What is a worthy goal of occupational therapy? *Occupational Therapy in Health Care*, 12(2/3), 111–126.

Creek, J., & Ormston, C. (1996). The essential elements of professional motivation. *British Journal of Occupational Therapy*, 59, 7–10.

Creek, J., Ilott, I., Cook, S., & Munday, C. (2005). Valuing occupational therapy as a complex intervention. *British Journal of Occupational Therapy*, 68, 281–284.

Crepeau, E. B., Cohn, E. S., & Schell, B.A.B. (2003). Occupational therapy practice. In: E. B. Crepeau, E. S. Cohn, & B. A. B. Schell (Eds.). *Willard & Spackman's occupational therapy* (10th ed.) (pp. 27–30). Philadelphia, Pennsylvania: Lippincott Williams & Wilkins.

Crozier, K. (2003). Interprofessional education in maternity care: shared learning for women-centred care. *International Journal of Sociology and Social Policy*, 23(4/5), 123–138.

De Vries, G., Kikkert, M., Schene, A., & Swinkels, J. (2004). Dutch study indicates: Extra occupational therapy is cheaper and has a positive effect with patients with depression. *WFOT Bulletin*, 49, 20,19.

Diasio, K. (1971). The modern era – 1960 to 1970. *American Journal of Occupational Therapy*, XXV, 237–242.

Engel, G. (1977). The need for a new medical model: A challenge or biomedicine. *Science*, 196(4286), 129–136.

Fisher, A. (1998). Uniting practice and theory in an occupational framework. *American Journal of Occupational Therapy*, 52, 509–521.

Fisher, A. G. (2003). Why is it so hard to practice as an occupational therapist? (Guest editorial). *Australian Occupational Therapy Journal*, 50, 193–194.

Gibson, D., Velde, B., Hoff, T., Kvashay, D., Manross, P. L., & Moreau, V. (2000). Clinical reasoning of a novice versus an experienced occupational therapist: A qualitative study. *Occupational Therapy in Health Care*, 12(4), 15–31.

Golledge, J. (2004). Therapeutic occupation following stroke: A case study. In: M. Molineux (Ed.), *Occupation for occupational therapists* (pp. 155–168). Oxford: Blackwell Publishing.

Hayley, L., & McKay, E. (2004). 'Baking gives you confidence': Users' views of engaging in the occupation of baking. *British Journal of Occupational Therapy*, 67, 125–128.

Hughes, J. (2001) Occupational therapy in community mental health teams: a continuing dilemma? Role theory offers an explanation. *British Journal of Occupational Therapy*, 64, 34–40.

Jackson, J. P., & Schkade, J. K. (2001). Occupational adaptation model versus biomechanical–rehabilitation model in the treatment of patients with hip fractures. *American Journal of Occupational Therapy*, 55, 531–537.

Jackson, J., Carlson, M., Mandel, D., Zemke, R., & Clark, F. (1998). Occupation in lifestyle redesign: The well elderly study occupational therapy program. *American Journal*

of Occupational Therapy, 52, 326–336.

Jones, M. (2005). Cultural power in organisations: The dynamics of interprofessional teams. In: G. Whiteford, & V. Wright–StClair (Eds.), *Occupation and practice in context* (pp. 179–194). Marrickville, NSW: Elsevier Churchill Livingstone.

Jongbloed, L., & Wendland, T. (2002). The impact of reimbursement systems on occupational therapy practice in Canada and the United States of America. *Canadian Journal of Occupational Therapy*, 69, 143–152.

Katz, N. (1985). Occupational therapy's domain of concern reconsidered. *American Journal of Occupational Therapy*, 39, 518–524.

Kielhofner, G. (2004). *Conceptual foundations of occupational therapy*, (3rd ed.) Philadelphia: FA Davis.

Kornblau, B. (2004). A vision for our future (Presidential address). *American Journal of Occupational Therapy*, 58, 9–14.

Kronenberg, F., Algado, S. S., & Pollard, N. (2005). Preface. In: F. Kronenberg, S. Algado, & N. Pollard (Eds.). *Occupational therapy without borders: Learning from the spirit of survivors* (p. xv–xvii). Edinburgh: Elsevier Churchill Livingstone.

Law, M., Baum, C., & Baptiste, S. (Eds.). (2002). *Occupation-based practice: Fostering performance and participation*. Thorofare, New Jersey: Slack.

Lloyd, C., & King, R. (2001). Work-related stress and occupational therapy. *Occupational Therapy International*, 8(4), 227–243.

Mocellin, G. (1996). Occupational therapy: A critical overview, part 2. *British Journal of Occupational Therapy*, 59, 11–16.

Molineux, M. (2004). Occupation in occupational therapy: A labour in vain? In: M. Molineux (Ed.). *Occupation for occupational therapists* (pp. 1–14). Oxford: Blackwell Publishing.

Moore, K., Cruickshank, M., & Haas, M. (2006). Job satisfaction in occupational therapy: A qualitative investigation in urban Australia.

Australian Occupational Therapy Journal, 53, 18–26.

Nelson, D. L. (1996). Why the profession of occupational therapy will flourish in the 21st century. *The American Journal of Occupational Therapy*, 51, 11–24.

Persson, D., Erlandsson, L.-K., Eklund, M., & Iwarsson, S. (2001). Value dimensions, meaning and complexity in human occupation – A tentative structure for analysis. *Scandinavian Journal of Occupational Therapy*, 8, 7–18.

Pierce, D. (2001). Occupation by design: Dimension, therapeutic power, and creative process. *American Journal of Occupational Therapy*, 55, 249–259.

Pollard, N., & Walsh, S. (2000). Occupational therapy, gender and mental health: An inclusive perspective? *British Journal of Occupational Therapy*, 63, 425–431.

Pollock, N., & McColl, M. A. (2003). How occupation changes. In: M. McColl, M. Law, D. Stewart, L. Doubt, N. Pollock, & T. Krupa (Eds.). *Theoretical basis of occupational therapy* (pp. 63–80). Thorofare, New Jersey: Slack.

Reilly, M. (1962). Occupational therapy can be one of the great ideas of 20th century medicine. *American Journal of Occupational Therapy*, XVI, 1–9.

Reilly, M. (1966/1984). The challenge of the future to an occupational therapist. *American Journal of Occupational Therapy*, XX(5), 221–225, reprinted in *Occupational Therapy in Health Care*, 1(1), 89–98.

Rogers, S. L. (2005). Portrait of occupational therapy. *Journal of Interprofessional Care*, 19(1), 70–79.

Schwammle, D. (1996). Occupational competence explored. *Canadian Journal of Occupational Therapy*, 63, 323–330.

Schwartz, K. B. (2003). The history of occupational therapy. In: E. B. Crepeau, E. S. Cohn, & B. A. B. Schell (Eds.). *Willard and Spackman's occupational therapy* (10th ed., pp. 5–13). Philadelphia: Lippincott Williams & Wilkins.

Thornton, G., & Rennie, H. (1998). Activities of daily living: An area of occupational therapy expertise.

Australian Occupational Therapy Journal, 35, 49–58.

Townsend, E (ed) (1997). *Enabling occupation: An occupational therapy perspective*, Ottawa, Ontario: Author.

Townsend, E. (1998). Occupational therapy language: Matters of respect, accountability and leadership. *Canadian Journal of Occupational Therapy*, 65, pp. 45–50.

Townsend, E. A., & Polatajko, H. J. (2007). *Enabling occupation II: Advancing an occupational therapy vision for health, well-being, and justice through occupation*. Ottawa, Ontario: Canadian Association of Occupational Therapists.

Wallace, C. (1986). Whither occupational therapy? (1986 Sylvia Docker Lecture). *Australian Occupational Therapy Journal*, 33, 93–100.

Wilcock, A. A. (2000). Development of a personal, professional and educational occupational philosophy: An Australian perspective. *Occupational Therapy International*, 7(2), 79–86.

Wilcock, A. A. (2006). *An occupational perspective of health* (2nd ed.). Thorofare, New Jersey: Slack.

Wilding, C. (2008). Identifying, articulating, and transforming occupational therapy practice in an acute setting: a collaborative action research study. Unpublished PhD thesis. Charles Sturt University, Albury, NSW.

Wilding, C., & Whiteford, G. (2007) Occupation and occupational therapy: Knowledge paradigms and everyday practice. *Australian Occupational Therapy Journal* 54:185–193.

Wilding, C., & Whiteford, G. (2008). Language, identity and representation: Occupation and occupational therapy in acute settings. *Australian Occupational Therapy Journal*, 55, 180–187.

Woodside, H. H. (1971). The development of occupational therapy 1910–1929. *American Journal of Occupational Therapy*, XXV, 226–230.

Yerxa, E. J. (2000). Occupational science: A renaissance of service to humankind through knowledge. *Occupational Therapy International*, 7, 87–98.

Chapter Two

2

The nature of occupation

Matthew Molineux

CHAPTER CONTENTS

Introduction 17

Defining occupation. 18

The nature of occupation. 19

   Occupation as active engagement 19

   Occupation as purposeful. 20

   Occupation as meaningful. 20

   Occupation as contextualised. 21

   Occupation as human 22

Occupation and health: just a good idea?. . .22

Conclusion. 24

SUMMARY

Occupation is a concept that remains controversial within occupational therapy. Some occupational therapists feel it is vague, poorly defined, and widely misunderstood. Others, however, feel that the ambiguity of 'occupation' is useful given the diversity of human experiences it seeks to label. As a result many theorists and researchers have attempted to explore occupation in order to define it. While there is no suggestion that research into occupation is not needed and important, the desire for a single universally accepted definition may be misguided. Occupation is complex and so will be hard to define succinctly, but to force a snappy definition on the construct is likely to be too simplistic. This chapter acknowledges that many definitions have been articulated, but proposes 'the nature of occupation' as a more useful way of understanding occupation.

Furthermore, this chapter draws attention to the growing evidence that supports an occupational view of humans and health.

KEY POINTS

- Occupation is a complex and multifaceted phenomenon that can not be succinctly defined.
- Occupations are those experiences that are active, purposeful, meaningful, contextualised and human.
- Occupational therapists must ensure they consider the nature of occupation in all their work with individuals, groups and communities.
- There is a wealth of theoretical and research literature which supports the idea of occupation and the link between occupation and health.
- Occupational therapists must be aware of relevant literature and use it regularly to support and describe their practice.

Introduction

Since the founding of the modern profession, occupation has held a central place within occupational therapy. While its prominence has waxed and waned over the decades, it has, nonetheless, been the concept that has (or should have) provided unity in, and distinctiveness to, the profession. Despite this, occupational therapists have continued to struggle to adequately define occupation in a way that is true to its complexity, yet understandable by many. The result has been that there are almost as many definitions of occupation as there are occupational therapists. It is proposed here that rather than continuing to seek a succinct sentence to explain occupation it is more useful to recognise the key characteristics of occupation. These can be used to explain occupation, although it will take more than a few sentences, and to remind occupational therapists of the factors to consider when working with individuals, groups or communities. This chapter will begin with a discussion of the nature of occupation, and end with a reminder of the literature which supports the idea of occupation, and the link between occupation and health.

Defining occupation

To understand the relationship between engagement in occupation and health in order to use occupation in a therapeutic way, it is necessary to define terms. However, there is a dilemma in relation to occupation, one that could be construed as a significant weakness of the occupational therapy profession. It is that, despite the central place of occupation within both the profession of occupational therapy and the discipline of occupational science, there is no single, widely accepted definition of occupation. Within occupational therapy, the main difficulty with definition has centred on the fact that 'occupation' is understood by almost all those outside of the profession as meaning 'paid employment', when it actually means much more than that within professional discourse. It is possible, however, to view the ambiguity of the term in a positive light, as it highlights the all-encompassing use of the word within the profession. Breines (1995), for example, suggested that this very ambiguity was one of the key reasons why it was chosen by the founders of the profession. Furthermore, occupation is complex and multifaceted (Yerxa et al 1989) and, hence, seeking a shared and easily understood definition is likely to be fraught with difficulties. Such a definition may not capture the intricacy of occupation and so may even impede the development of theory and practice (Yerxa 1988).

The debates which have occurred, and those which continue around this definition, are indicative of 'healthy, evolving scholarship that pushes understanding forward' (Pierce 2001, p. 138). Rather than inhibiting our ability to explore and study occupation (American Occupational Therapy Association 1995), it is argued that this situation frees us from the normal constraints of positivistic science and enables a true *exploration* of the concept. A generative or inductive approach to understanding occupation is less limiting and more likely to ensure its multidimensional nature remains intact.

In the spirit of healthy scholarship and debate, and in an attempt to begin to illuminate the complexity of occupation, Table 2.1 presents a sample of definitions of occupation from the professional literature. Although there are many other definitions in the literature, these provide a useful starting point, and highlight some interesting issues. For example, one of the complaints of occupational therapy practitioners is that too often colleagues refer to occupational therapy merely because the person needs 'something to do'. Implicit in this is the idea that as humans all that is necessary to ensure health and happiness is for a person to be kept busy, and for time to be filled. However, the choice of words of the American Occupational Therapy Association (1997) question this assumption, as their definition suggests that time needs to be *fulfilled*, not merely filled. This suggests that it is not just a case of being occupied and busy, but being engaged in something that contributes to happiness or satisfaction.

Table 2.1 Sample definitions of occupation
'behaviours whereby humans, collectively and individually, make their place in the physical, temporal and social world' (Kielhofner 1992, p. 50)
'the ordinary and familiar things that people do everyday' (American Occupational Therapy Association 1995, p. 1015)
'the activities people engage in throughout their daily lives to fulfil their time and give their life meaning' (American Occupational Therapy Association 1997, p. 864)
'comprises all the ways in which we occupy ourselves individually and as societies' (Townsend 1997, p. 19)
'our occupations are all the active process of looking after ourselves and others, enjoying life, and being socially and economically productive over the lifespan and in various contexts' (Townsend 1997, p. 19)
'specific "chunks" of activity within the ongoing stream of human behaviours which are named in the lexicon of the culture' (Yerxa et al 1989, p. 5)
'an occupation is a specific individual's personally constructed, nonrepeatable experience' (Pierce 2001, p. 139)

The definitions presented in Table 2.1 also highlight that occupations have both solitary and collective dimensions, in that individuals engage in occupations alone, with others around them, or as part of a group (Kielhofner 1992, Townsend 1997). Occupational therapists are well attuned to the importance of what some might see as the everyday and the mundane occupations that are part of life, such as washing and dressing, cooking, and cleaning the house. However, it is important to recognise, that understanding occupation in that way is a two-edge sword. As the definition from the American Occupational Therapy Association (1995, p. 1015) suggests, occupations can be 'ordinary and familiar' and it is vital to recognise that occupational therapy can make very significant contributions for people whose ability to engage in the ordinary and familiar has been disrupted. For example, for a person who has had a stroke, being able to wash and dress independently may no longer be an everyday, perhaps taken-for-granted, undertaking. It may be something to work towards and savoured once achieved, as it signifies a step forward, closer to discharge from hospital. Conversely, an occupation may not be ordinary and familiar as some occupations occur rarely, but are nonetheless an important part of life. Imagine a couple trying to plan for their only daughter's wedding while detained in a refugee detention centre with its inherent restrictions and limitations. The wedding is likely to be a once in a lifetime event and yet is an occupation that is fundamental to their parental role.

Readers are likely to be able to identify other issues from the limited definitions of occupation that are presented in Table 2.1, such as the role of culture in legitimising occupations (Yerxa et al 1989); it is worth reflecting on the explicit and implicit meanings in any explanations of occupation.

The nature of occupation

It is proposed here that rather than attempting to choose a single definition to guide our understanding of occupation, it is more fruitful to consider the *nature* of occupation. In doing so, it is possible to identify that occupation has five key characteristics or factors: active engagement, purpose, meaning, contextual, and human. Each of these will now be discussed drawing on existing occupational science and occupational therapy literature.

Occupation as active engagement

Occupation is a process that is manifested in some form of doing (Cynkin 1979, Meyer 1922/1977, Schkade & Schultz 1992, Simon 1993, Townsend 1997). It is an active process in that it not only occupies time and space, but it requires investment of energy, interest and attention (American Occupational Therapy Association 1972, Breines 1995). It is easy to understand how types of doing which are manifested in physical activity can be viewed as occupation. It is also the case that occupation can include instances of mental doing (American Occupational Therapy Association 1995, Breines 1995). For example it is clear how the physical (and mental) activity of building a fence can be construed as occupation. It requires physical engagement to cut the wood, dig the holes for fence posts, and nail the fence panels in place. Necessarily, it also requires mental engagement – planning, problem solving, judgement, concentration, and so on. In contrast, consider a person lying on the grass in the park gazing at the clouds on a summer day. By conventional wisdom this would not be considered a physical activity. It might also be the case that some would not consider this activity to involve any mental doing. Think, however, about what might be taking place while the person is lying there gazing at the clouds and the blue sky. The individual might be making a mental list of the shopping needed for the coming week, he or she might be trying to distinguish patterns within the clouds, it might be an opportunity for a songwriter to compose lyrics; the possibilities are endless. While the individual may not be engaged in any physical doing, in all likelihood there is some mental activity taking place, no matter how seemingly trivial; so lying gazing at the clouds is an occupation. Some might suggest that there are situations when a person is truly 'doing' nothing, where no physical or mental activity is taking place; meditation for example. It is true that while meditating the individual is not likely to be making a mental shopping list for the week ahead, but meditation does require mental activity. In order to meditate it is necessary to not only achieve the meditative state, but also to maintain it; both are examples of mental doing.

Mental and physical doing can exist concurrently or in isolation (Breines 1995). That is to say, an occupation can include one or both facets and still be considered an occupation. In fact where they both exist within the same occupation the two may not be related. It is possible to separate mental doing from the physical doing that is taking place simultaneously. I was very aware of this when working as a cleaner in a sheet metal factory. While I was physically involved in sweeping and cleaning, I was mentally reminiscing about the night before, or planning the week ahead.

Implicit in the idea of occupation as active engagement is the belief that occupation necessitates the use of our inherent capacities and abilities. As such, engagement may involve drawing on our sensorimotor, cognitive, and psychosocial abilities and characteristics (American Occupational Therapy Association 1994, 2002, Canadian Association of Occupational Therapists 1991, 1993, Schkade & Schultz 1992). The extent and combination of the use of these attributes will not only vary from person to person, but also from occupation to occupation, as well as between different instances of the same occupation.

Occupation as purposeful

All human endeavours have some reason or purpose. This is evident in the many attempts to classify occupations, which have generally reflected the purpose of the occupation for the individual. At an abstract level, there is general agreement that what people do can be broadly classified into self-care, productivity, and leisure occupations. The purpose of self-care or self-maintenance occupations is to look after oneself, productivity occupations enable one to be socially and/or economically productive, and leisure occupations are the means by which people enjoy life (American Occupational Therapy Association 1994, 2002, Townsend 1997, Wilcock 1998, Yerxa et al 1989). These abstract descriptions of occupations can be operationalised as concrete occupations such as showering and dressing in the morning before work (self-care or self-maintenance), volunteering at the local hospice one day each week (productivity), or reading a book (leisure), and so on.

Furthermore, Wilcock (1993, 1995, 1998) has suggested that occupations serve three main purposes for humans that go beyond the easily recognisable reasons for engagement. These purposes share some similarities with Maslow's (1970) hierarchy of human needs, although Wilcock takes an occupational perspective. First, occupation provides the means by which humans can meet survival needs such as obtaining food and shelter. Second, occupation not only induces and enables development of skills necessary for successful living, but also provides the means by which these skills are maintained. Finally, Wilcock (1993) has argued that occupation prompts and rewards the use of individual capacities so that the organism can flourish, and reach potential. As such, occupation plays a central role in the healthy survival of individuals.

In addition, occupation serves two particular purposes for the collective human species. First, because occupation provides the means by which humans are able to express their innate social nature, it enables the collective development of shared configurations of occupations, which in turn enable groups of humans to establish themselves as recognisable communities (Cynkin 1979, Wilcock 1998). Second, occupation is the means by which the species as a whole ensures its survival. Humans, both individually and collectively, can make two types of responses to environmental challenges, those that are adaptive and those that are not. The simple yet persuasive theory of survival of the fittest indicates clearly that those responses that are adaptive will confer survival benefits on individuals and these will then be passed down the generations, thereby ensuring continuation of the species. Maladaptive responses, i.e. those that are inflexible and adversely impact upon health (Wood 1993), will not enable individuals to respond in a way that ensures survival. For this reason, some authors have gone so far as to suggest that one defining characteristic of occupation is the extent to which it is adaptive (Clark et al 1991, Schkade & Schultz 1992, Wood 1993, Yerxa 1992).

Occupation as meaningful

Just as occupation has purpose, it always has meaning to the individual engaged in it, and it is often rich with such meaning (American Occupational Therapy Association 1997, 2002, Clark et al 1991, Hammell 2004). As a result, while we might be tempted to classify, define and understand occupation according to its outward appearance, this may overlook its essence (Clark et al 1991, Yerxa 1988). The centrality of meaning in occupation is highlighted by the idea that occupations have meanings that are both unique and dynamic. They are unique because each person makes sense of his or her existence in a very individual manner. Given that existence in the world is experienced as engagement in occupation, it stands to reason that the meaning ascribed to seemingly similar instances of doing will be unique to each individual. Furthermore, given that the job of living requires us to be in constant interaction with our human and non-human surroundings, we as individuals are constantly changing. The meaning of occupation is dynamic, therefore, because just as we as humans are in a constant state of flux, so too is the meaning we ascribe to occupations within our repertoire. To fully appreciate engagement in any given occupation, it is crucial to tap into the subjective experience of that engagement (Clark et al 1991, Hammell 2004, Persson et al 2001, Wood 1995, Yerxa 1988, Yerxa et al 1989). Pierce (2001, p. 139) drew particular attention to subjectivity as a key characteristic of occupation when she proposed that 'an occupation is the experience of a person, who is the sole author of the occupation's meaning'.

Meaning is what motivates occupational performance (Fisher 1998), and it is important to appreciate that *actual* meaning may not be congruent with *apparent* meaning. Given that the meaning attached to an occupation can be derived from a myriad of sources (Carlson 1996, Yerxa et al 1989), it is possible that the easily recognisable source of meaning bears no resemblance to the actual meaning for the individual. Jackson (1995) provided a clear example in her story of a young man, diagnosed as HIV positive, baking cookies with his occupational therapist. To the onlooker it might seem that the meaning of the occupation rests in the young man's interest in cooking or his need to cook in order to live independently. In her paper, however, Jackson revealed that the occupation was one that the young man had performed with his grandmother who had recently died. The significance of this for the young man lay in the fact that his grandmother was one of the few people who knew, and accepted, him as gay. Given the narrow-minded views of most of the people in the young man's small rural community, this acceptance was especially powerful. Hence, engagement in the occupation of baking held special symbolism and meaning for him.

Occupation as contextualised

Many authors within occupational therapy and occupational science suggest that humans exist within a multitude of contexts – physical, social, cultural, chronological, developmental, life cycle, disability status, institutional, legal, political, economic, temporal, historical – and that these impact on occupation, and occupations can in turn shape the same contexts (American Occupational Therapy Association 1994, 2002, Canadian Association of Occupational Therapists 1991, 1993, Clark et al 1991, Farnworth 2003, Larson 2004, Pierce 2001, Yerxa 1988). Some authors go so far as to suggest that for an occupation to be considered as such, it must be sanctioned by the sociocultural world (Cynkin 1979, Fidler & Fidler 1978, Yerxa et al 1989). It follows that to understand occupation it is necessary to understand the contexts within which occupations occur. The reasons for this are twofold as the relationship between humans, occupations and contexts is complex and non-linear. First, occupation is the way in which humans respond, ideally in an adaptive way, to the challenges presented by the environments. To this end, it is necessary to understand the situation that gives rise to a particular occupation if we are to fully comprehend the occupation itself (Clark et al 1991, Law et al 1998). Second, contexts go beyond merely eliciting occupations; they can either facilitate or inhibit the resultant occupations (American Occupational Therapy Association 1994, Canadian Association of Occupational Therapists 1991, 1993). For example, social norms dictate that one response to a noisy fellow patron in the cinema is more acceptable than another: asking the person to be quiet rather than becoming physically aggressive. Alternatively, the presence of a ramp at the cinema might facilitate the participation of a person who must use a wheelchair in order to mobilise independently.

There is one more context that must be taken into account when understanding occupation; the occupational history of the individual (Clark et al 1991). It has been suggested that it is through occupations, and the organisation of these occupations, that individuals distinguish themselves from others (Cynkin 1979), with each person having a unique occupational history. Furthermore, this history of past occupational engagement influences the form and pattern of future occupational engagement (Black 1976, Carlson 1996, Russel 2001, Wilcock 1995). The relationship between past and future occupations may be quite simple – having ridden a bike as a child, I am able to ride a bike as an adult. Previous experience of the occupation has provided me with the necessary skills, abilities, and confidence, to undertake the occupation again with little effort. However, the relationship may be more complex, as in the example given earlier of the young man baking cookies. Here, he not only had the skills, but due to his personal occupational history, baking cookies had special significance for him, as it allowed him to re-connect with his past.

Occupation as human

It has been implied indirectly in the preceding sections that occupation is a uniquely human characteristic. While it is acknowledged that all species engage in different forms of doing, it is generally suggested that engagement in occupations is a key characteristic that distinguishes humans from other species (Clark et al 1991, Cynkin 1979, Wilcock 1998, Yerxa 1988, Yerxa et al 1989). Yerxa (2000a, 2000b) exemplified this view by coining the phrase 'homo occupacio' to describe the human species. While this may be nothing more than a case of evolutionary arrogance, the belief that humans alone are occupational is widely held within the literature. Various authors have argued this from different perspectives. Wood (1993) used evidence from primatology to suggest that there is a biological basis for the occupational nature of humans, and that it is through the process of evolution that we have emerged as occupational beings. Fortune (1996) has used evidence from anthropology to demonstrate the change in the symbolic nature of the proto-occupations of Neanderthals to the occupations of modern humans. Taking a wider view, Wilcock (1998) argued that engagement in occupation is innate and inborn and is part of our species' common characteristics, and so is a constituent aspect of our humanity.

Of particular interest in this debate is the extent to which humans and other species engage in occupation. It is clear that non-human species engage in activities that are aimed at ensuring survival of both the individual and the species, but humans seem to go beyond basic survival needs in terms of their engagement in occupation (Wilcock 1998). It is true that humans engage in a wide range of occupations that are unrelated to basic needs such as shelter and sustenance. An occupational view of humans requires a broader view of what constitutes survival needs. The fact that these wide-ranging occupations enable individuals to develop their skills and abilities, and flourish, is vital to human survival (Wilcock 1998).

To summarise, given the myriad of definitions of occupation in the literature it is proposed that it is more useful to consider those characteristics that constitute the nature of occupation. Occupation is viewed as those experiences which humans engage in that necessitate active engagement, have purpose, individual meaning, and are contextualised. Given that occupational therapy was founded on a belief in the health benefits of occupation, it is noteworthy that this does not feature explicitly in most of the published definitions, although it does feature in research and theoretical literature.

Occupation and health: just a good idea?

At the time the modern occupational therapy profession was founded, the idea of occupation and its impact on health was just that, an idea. Founders of the profession had personal experience of the positive impact of engaging in occupation and worked to promote those ideas (Peloquin 1991a, 1991b). A reliance on 'good ideas' is no longer acceptable and in fact the history of occupational therapy includes calls to strengthen the evidence base of the profession (Reilly 1962, Rogers 1984). The need and importance of developing the evidence to support occupational therapy practice is readily understood in the current climate of evidence-based practice, although that framework can lead to a narrow focus on just one particular type of evidence. In the spirit of evidence-based medicine, it is right that practitioners and funders of health and social care are concerned with the evidence to support (or not) a particular intervention (Sackett et al 1996). This, however, is only one sort of evidence with which occupational therapists must be concerned. Several decades ago Rogers (1984) identified the three components of the knowledge base which should underpin occupational therapy practice:

1. Knowledge of normal occupational functions
2. Knowledge of ineffective performance in occupational functions
3. Knowledge of the therapeutic properties of occupation.

Although many occupational therapy researchers and practitioners are primarily concerned with the third of these types of knowledge, the profession is in need of all three. After all how can an occupational therapist devise an appropriate intervention programme if the way in which that occupation is typically performed is not understood, or if the mechanisms of poor occupational performance are not delineated?

Occupational therapy students, practitioners, educators and researchers might believe there to be very little 'evidence' to support the occupation and health philosophy, but that is not the case. It does not require a particularly complex search of information sources to identify a large number of theoretical and research-based papers which are useful in supporting the philosophy and practice of occupational therapy. While it is not possible, nor desirable given the rate at which the literature grows, to provide a comprehensive review of all the relevant literature, this section will provide a taste of the papers which occupational therapists could use to support or critique their practice.

Wood (1993) has presented convincing arguments as to why it is not only appropriate, but valuable, to consider occupation from an evolutionary perspective. Drawing on time use data for humans and non-human primates, she has argued that there is evidence of a phylogenetic history of human occupation. Furthermore, it has been demonstrated that non-human primates, if given the opportunity and choice, will engage in what have been called proto-occupations, i.e. 'the activities of nonhuman primates that are similar in form to the occupations of humans but lack their complexity' (Wood 1993, p. 516). For example, in research into feeding-enrichment programmes, captive non-human primates have been found to engage in less maladaptive behaviour when provided with the opportunity to participate in species-typical feeding proto-occupations (Bloomsmith et al 1988, Chamove 1996). It has also been found that when challenges arise from the environment, non-human primates adapt through proto-occupation. Observation of a troop of monkeys living in a natural habitat in Japan revealed that the monkeys invented new proto-occupations, in this case 'sweet potato washing' and 'wheat washing', to enable them to make best use of the food resources available (Kawai 1965). More recently, the study of captive non-human primates has suggested a synergistic relationship between the physical and social environments, with the latter mediating the impact of the former on occupational engagement (Wood 2002).

In terms of the human research that has been completed, it is clear that there are different experiences of engagement in activity. One study compared the performance of elderly female nursing home residents in two situations; when performing an occupation or a rote exercise (Yoder et al 1989). Another study compared the performance of elderly nursing home residents in three conditions; kicking a balloon to keep it off the floor (materials-based occupation), kicking their leg in the air while imagining that they were keeping a balloon off the ground (imagery-based occupation), or flexing and extending their knee as many times as possible (rote exercise) (DeKuiper et al 1993). In these research projects it has been shown that when humans engage in experiences which are, or which more closely resemble, occupations they perform a greater number of repetitions, report greater enjoyment, have an increased pain tolerance, and show a better quality of performance. Slightly different research has shown that memory for the steps involved in a task is improved when children actually perform the occupation, rather than just observe it (Hartman et al 2000). In addition, it is interesting to note that when given the choice, people chose to engage in a task which more closely resembles an occupation than a rote exercise (Zimmerer-Branum & Nelson 1995).

The first assumption underpinning the occupational therapy profession is that humans are occupational beings. Having reviewed some of the literature relating to this, it is time to turn to the next key assumption – the relationship between occupation and health.

Law et al (1998) undertook a critical review of the literature to examine the extent of support for the suggestion that health is determined by engagement in occupation. Given the complexity of the relationship between the person, the environments in which they exist and the occupations in which they engage, Law and her colleagues limited the review to the effect of occupation on health and well-being. A literature search was undertaken and the reference lists from the articles identified were also searched for research papers published between 1980 and 1996 which addressed the effect of occupation on health and well-being. Using protocols for which inter-reviewer reliability was established, the team reviewed a total of 23 articles, most of which were not from the occupational therapy literature. The results of this review are encouraging as the authors found that there was some '… compelling support for the influence of occupation on health and well-being' (Law et al, p. 84). The research reviewed highlighted that humans experience greater stress, and demonstrate physiological changes and decreased health when occupation is removed.

It was also found that capacity and participation in occupations were significantly related to quality of life. While this critical review is useful and provides a helpful summary of the literature published between 1980 and 1996, research has continued and there have been a number of interesting publications since 1996 that have shed further light on the benefits of engagement in occupation for humans.

At the risk of taking a reductionist approach, it could be argued that the research discussed earlier in relation to improved performance when people engage in an occupation compared to a rote exercise suggests that occupational engagement has physical benefits. Following principles of training and practice, it seems reasonable to extrapolate that if the number of repetitions is greater in the occupation condition then there will be greater improvement in performance components such as muscle strength, range of movement, and eye–hand co-ordination. While Fisher (1998) suggests that there is growing evidence which negates the generalisability of skills improved through exercise or remedial activities, it would seem that there is at least some benefit in engagement in occupation over non-occupations. However, there are other rewards which occupation bestows. The literature points clearly to the way in which occupation has significant social benefits. Occupations enable people to establish and maintain relationships with other individuals, or to be accepted as a member of a group or society (Laliberte-Rudman et al 1997, Rebeiro et al 2001, Taylor & McGruder 1996, Unruh et al 1999). Making choices about engaging in occupations is a means by which individuals can carefully control their interactions with others when disability presents barriers to positive social encounters (Clark 1993, Laliberte-Rudman 2002, Magnus 2001).

Conclusion

While acknowledging that no single definition of occupation is widely accepted, this chapter has proposed one way of understanding this important construct. Through an examination of the published literature it is possible to delineate several characteristics that capture the complexity of occupation: it is active, purposeful, meaningful, contextualised, and human. Despite the belief that, and the growing evidence for, a link between occupation and health, a clear link between occupation and health is not generally found within definitions of occupation. Although much energy is expended in trying to find a universal definition of occupation, it is probably more fruitful to have a shared understanding of the *nature* of occupation. This will ensure occupational therapists have a basis on which to discuss their work with individuals, groups and communities. Furthermore, it should ensure that when working with people the complexity of occupation will not be forgotten.

This chapter has also challenged the idea that there is little research to support the idea of occupation and the link between occupation and health. Although it was not the intention to provide a comprehensive overview of the existing research, this chapter did demonstrate that there is literature that occupational therapists can, and should, use to describe and support their practice. In this age of evidence-based practice it is imperative that occupational therapists use relevant literature to underpin their practice. If, as it should be, practice is focused on occupation, then the supporting literature base must include material that supports the idea of occupation and the occupation–health link, as well as that which is focused on particular intervention strategies or approaches.

References

American Occupational Therapy Association. (1972). Occupational therapy: Its definition and functions. *American Journal of Occupational Therapy*, 26(4), 204.

American Occupational Therapy Association. (1994). Uniform terminology for occupational therapy (3rd ed.). *American Journal of Occupational Therapy*, 48(11), 1047–1054.

American Occupational Therapy Association. (1995). Position paper:

Occupation. *American Journal of Occupational Therapy*, 49(10), 1015–1017.

American Occupational Therapy Association. (1997). Fundamental concepts of occupational therapy: Occupation, purposeful activity, and function. *American Journal of Occupational Therapy*, 51(10), 864–866.

American Occupational Therapy Association. (2002). Occupational therapy practice framework:

Domain and process. *American Journal of Occupational Therapy*, 56(6), 609–639.

Black, M. (1976). The occupational career. *American Journal of Occupational Therapy*, 30, 225–228.

Bloomsmith, M., Alford, P., & Maple, T. (1988). Successful feeding enrichment for captive chimpanzees. *American Journal of Primatology*, 16(2), 155–164.

Breines, E. (1995). Understanding 'occupation' as the founders did. *British Journal of Occupational Therapy*, 58(11), 458–460.

Canadian Association of Occupational Therapists. (1991). *Occupational therapy guidelines for client-centered practice*. Toronto: CAOT Publications.

Canadian Association of Occupational Therapists. (1993). *Occupational therapy guidelines for client-centered mental health practice*. Toronto: CAOT Publications.

Carlson, M. (1996). The self-perpetuation of occupations. In: R. Zemke & F. Clark (Eds.), *Occupational science: the evolving discipline* (pp. 143–157). Philadelphia: F.A. Davis.

Chamove, A. (1996). Enrichment in primates: Relevance to occupational science. In: R. Zemke & F. Clark (Eds.), *Occupational science: the evolving discipline* (pp. 177–180). Philadelphia: F.A. Davis.

Clark, F. (1993). Occupation embedded in a real life: Interweaving occupational science and occupational therapy. *American Journal of Occupational Therapy*, 47(12), 1067–1078.

Clark, F., Parham, D., Carlson, M., Frank, G., Jackson, J., Pierce, D., Wolfe, R., & Zemke, R. (1991). Occupational science: Academic innovation in the service of occupational therapy's future. *American Journal of Occupational Therapy*, 45(4), 300–310.

Cynkin, S. (1979). *Occupational therapy: toward health through activities*. Boston: Little, Brown & Co.

DeKuiper, W., Nelson, D., & White, B. (1993). Materials-based occupation versus imagery-based occupation versus rote exercise: A replication and extension. *Occupational Therapy Journal of Research*, 13(3), 183–197.

Farnworth, L. (2003). Time use, tempo and temporality: Occupational therapy's core business or someone else's business. *Australian Occupational Therapy Journal*, 50(3), 116–126.

Fidler, G., & Fidler, J. (1978). Doing and becoming: Purposeful action and self-actualization. *American Journal of Occupational Therapy*, 32(5), 305–310.

Fisher, A. (1998). Uniting practice and theory in an occupational framework. *American Journal of Occupational Therapy*, 52(7), 509–521.

Fortune, T. (1996). The proto-occupation/occupation interface: An exploration of human occupation and its symbolic origins. *Journal of Occupational Science: Australia*, 3(3), 86–92.

Hammell, K. (2004). Dimensions of meaning in the occupations of daily life. *Canadian Journal of Occupational Therapy*, 71(5), 296–305.

Hartman, B., Kopp Miller, B., & Nelson, D. (2000). The effects of hands-on occupation versus demonstration on children's recall memory. *American Journal of Occupational Therapy*, 54(5), 477–483.

Jackson, J. (1995). Sexual orientation: Its relevance to occupational science and the practice of occupational therapy. *American Journal of Occupational Therapy*, 49(7), 669–679.

Kawai, M. (1965). Newly-acquired pre-cultural behaviour of the natural troop of Japanese monkeys on Koshima Islet. *Primates*, 6(1), 1–30.

Kielhofner, G. (1992). *Conceptual foundations of occupational therapy*. Philadelphia: F.A. Davis.

Laliberte-Rudman, D. (2002). Linking occupation and identity: Lessons learned through qualitative exploration. *Journal of Occupational Science*, 9(1), 12–19.

Laliberte-Rudman, D., Cook, J., & Polatajko, H. (1997). Understanding the potential of occupation: A qualitative exploration of seniors' perspectives on activity. *American Journal of Occupational Therapy*, 51(8), 640–650.

Larson, E. (2004). The time of our lives: The experience of temporality in occupation. *Canadian Journal of Occupational Therapy*, 71(1), 24–35.

Law, M., Steinwender, S., & Leclair, L. (1998). Occupation, health and well-being. *Canadian Journal of Occupational Therapy*, 65(2), 81–91.

Magnus, E. (2001). Everyday occupations and the process of redefinition: A study of how meaning in occupation influences redefinition of identity in women with a disability. *Scandinavian Journal of Occupational Therapy*, 8(3), 115–124.

Maslow, A. (1970). *Motivation and personality* (second ed.). New York: Harper & Row.

Meyer, A. (1922/1977). The philosophy of occupation therapy. *American Journal of Occupational Therapy*, 31(10), 639–642.

Peloquin, S. (1991a). Occupational therapy service: Individual and collective understandings of the founders, Part 1. *American Journal of Occupational Therapy*, 45(4), 352–360.

Peloquin, S. (1991b). Occupational therapy service: Individual and collective understandings of the founders, Part 2. *American Journal of Occupational Therapy*, 45(8), 733–744.

Persson, D., Erlandsson, L.-K., Eklund, M., & Iwarsson, S. (2001). Value dimensions, meaning, and complexity in human occupation – A tentative structure for analysis. *Scandinavian Journal of Occupational Therapy*, 8(1), 7–18.

Pierce, D. (2001). Untangling occupation and activity. *American Journal of Occupational Therapy*, 55(2), 138–146.

Rebeiro, K., Day, D., Semeniuk, B., O'Brien, M., & Wilson, B. (2001). Northern Initiative for Social Action: An occupation-based mental health program. *American Journal of Occupational Therapy*, 55(5), 493–500.

Reilly, M. (1962). Occupational therapy can be one of the great ideas of 20th century medicine. *American Journal of Occupational Therapy*, 16(1), 1–9.

Rogers, J. (1984). Why study human occupation? *American Journal of Occupational Therapy*, 38(1), 47–49.

Russel, E. (2001). The occupational career revisited. *Journal of Occupational Science*, 8(2), 5–15.

Sackett, D., Rosenberg, W., Gray, J. A. M., Haynes, R., & Richardson, W. (1996). Evidence based medicine: what it is and what it isn't. *British Medical Journal*, 312(7023), 71–72.

Schkade, J., & Schultz, S. (1992). Occupational adaptation: Toward a holistic approach for contemporary practice, Part 1. *American Journal of Occupational Therapy*, 46(9), 829–837.

Simon, C. (1993). Use of activity and activity analysis. In: H. Hopkins & H. Smith (Eds.), *Willard and Spackman's occupational therapy* (8th ed.) (pp. 281–292). Philadelphia: J. B. Lippincott.

Taylor, L., & McGruder, J. (1996). The meaning of sea kayaking for persons with spinal cord injuries. *American Journal of Occupational Therapy*, 50(1), 39–46.

Townsend, E. (1997). Occupation: Potential for personal and social transformation. *Journal of Occupational Science: Australia*, 4(1), 18–26.

Unruh, A., Smith, N., & Scammell, C. (1999). The occupation of gardening in life-threatening illness: A qualitative pilot project. *Canadian Journal of Occupational Therapy*, 67(1), 70–77.

Wilcock, A. (1993). A theory of the human need for occupation. *Journal of Occupational Science: Australia*, 1(1), 17–24.

Wilcock, A. (1995). The occupational brain: A theory of human nature. *Journal of Occupational Science: Australia*, 2(2), 68–73.

Wilcock, A. (1998). *An occupational perspective of health*. Thorofare: Slack.

Wood, W. (1993). Occupation and the relevance of primatology to occupational therapy. *American Journal of Occupational Therapy*, 47(6), 515–522.

Wood, W. (1995). Weaving the warp and weft of occupational therapy: An art and science for all times. *American Journal of Occupational Therapy*, 49(1), 44–52.

Wood, W. (2002). Ecological synergies in two groups of zoo chimpanzees: Divergent patterns of time use. *American Journal of Occupational Therapy*, 56(2), 160–170.

Yerxa, E. (1988). Oversimplification: The hobgoblin of theory and practice in occupational therapy. *Canadian Journal of Occupational Therapy*, 55(1), 5–6.

Yerxa, E. (1992). Some implications of occupational therapy's history for its epistemology, values, and relation to medicine. *American Journal of Occupational Therapy*, 46(1), 79–83.

Yerxa, E. (2000a). Confessions of an occupational therapist who became a detective. *British Journal of Occupational Therapy*, 63(5), 192–199.

Yerxa, E. (2000b). Occupational science: A renaissance of service to humankind through knowledge. *Occupational Therapy International*, 7(2), 87–98.

Yerxa, E., Clark, F., Jackson, J., Parham, D., Pierce, D., Stein, C., & Zemke, R. (1989). An introduction to occupational science, a foundation for occupational therapy in the 21st century. *Occupational Therapy in Health Care*, 6(4), 1–17.

Yoder, R., Nelson, D., & Smith, D. (1989). Added-purpose versus rote exercise in female nursing home residents. *American Journal of Occupational Therapy*, 43(9), 581–586.

Zimmerer-Branum, S., & Nelson, D. (1995). Occupationally embedded exercise versus rote exercise: A choice between occupational forms by elderly nursing home residents. *American Journal of Occupational Therapy*, 49(5), 397–402.

Chapter Three

3

Occupational therapy: a disability perspective

John Swain and Sally French

CHAPTER CONTENTS

Introduction 28

From the standpoint of disabled people. . . .28

    Contrasting perspectives: the social
    model of disability 30

    Contrasting perspectives: the affirmative
    model of disability 31

Changing therapy: client-centred. 32

Changing therapy: citizen-centred 34

Conclusion. 35

SUMMARY

This chapter analyses occupational therapy from the viewpoints and experiences of disabled people. We begin with a section entitled *From the standpoint of disabled people*, setting the scene in terms of disabled people's critical stance towards professional intervention and the unequal power relations between service users and service providers. We turn, then, to ideas and beliefs about the meaning of 'disability' and contested understandings of 'the problem'. In particular we focus on the individual medical and tragedy models that dominate professional intervention, and challenge these with the social and affirmative models that have been generated by disabled people. This provides the basis for critical reflection on the provision and practice of occupational therapy, 'the solutions'. The shift towards 'client-centred therapy' is examined in terms of the inherent power relations. We conclude by suggesting a move away from a client-centred approach towards a citizen-centred approach in which service users are involved in the formulation and running of the services themselves, at all stages, including the production of knowledge about what disability is and what services, if any, are required.

KEY POINTS

- Disability can be viewed in a variety of ways and this has given rise to conflict between occupational therapists and disabled people.
- Occupational therapists need to embrace the principles of the Social Model of Disability and the Affirmative Model of Disability if they are to move away from an individualistic, tragic and charitable way of working and thinking.
- Social Model of Disability highlights the social and political nature of disability.
- Acceptance of the Affirmative Model of Disability leads to the rehabilitation goals of striving for physical independence and normality being far less tenable.
- Although disabled people value the skills and expertise of occupational therapists, they want their own expertise to be recognised and to work in a spirit of collaboration.
- Occupational therapists are encouraged to move away from a client-based model of service to a citizen-based model, in which users are involved in the formation and running of services at all stages.
- When there is choice and control on the part of the disabled person, and a true working partnership with an occupational therapist, creative and satisfactory ideas emerge leading to very positive experiences.

Introduction

It is clear from the title 'occupational therapist' that the role involves the use of occupation in rehabilitation. On the National Health Service, United Kingdom, web site, occupational therapy is defined as follows (www.nhscareers.nhs.uk, 2008):

> Occupational therapy is the assessment and treatment of physical and psychiatric conditions using specific purposeful activity to prevent disability and promote independent function in all aspects of daily life…..They work with people of all ages to help them overcome the effects of disability caused by physical or psychological illness, ageing or accident.

A rather broader definition is provided by the World Federation of Occupational Therapists (www.wfot.org.au, 2008):

> Occupational therapy is a profession concerned with promoting health and well being through occupation. The primary goal of occupational therapy is to enable people to participate in the activities of everyday life. Occupational therapists achieve this outcome by enabling people to do things that will enhance their ability to participate or by modifying the environment to better support participation […] Occupational therapists believe that participation can be supported or restricted by physical, social, attitudinal, and legislative environments. Therefore, occupational therapy practice may be directed to changing aspects of the environment to enhance participation.

Until the Second World War occupational therapists mainly worked with people who were labelled as mentally ill, where occupation of one kind or another was prescribed to lift depression and improve morale and self-esteem. Following the Second World War the interests of occupational therapists expanded to include people with physical diseases and impairments. Here the rationale behind the prescribed occupation was to strengthen muscles, restore co-ordination and mobilise joints in order to improve or maintain physical function and, if possible, to return or approximate the person to 'normal' (French 2008). I (Sally) have clear memories of working as a physiotherapist in the early 1970s where the patient with, for instance, a fractured femur, a stroke or an arthritic hip, would first attend physiotherapy for a session in the hydrotherapy pool or on the weight and pulley system, and then go to the occupational therapy department to use a range of machines including looms and carpentry equipment. Occupational therapists also aim to improve independence in basic living skills by assessing people for assistive devices and home modifications, such as stair lifts and wheelchairs, and helping them to use them.

On the surface there does not seem anything wrong with the role of the occupational therapist as described above. We all know that occupation, particularly if it is of our own choosing, can lift our mood and improve self-esteem, and activities such as digging, using a sewing machine and sawing wood can, if carefully chosen, have specific physical effects. It can also be important to have the correct tools and house adaptations in order to cook, wash, climb the stairs, and go out. Why then have disabled people become critical of occupational therapists and what, if anything, do they want from them instead?

In this chapter we will attempt to answer these questions by using the direct voice of disabled people who have experienced therapy and who have analysed the meaning of disability. We shall begin, then, with a section headed *From the standpoint of disabled people*. We then examine different, contrasting understandings of disability with particular emphasis on the perspectives of disabled people themselves. Finally we turn to the implications for the practice of occupational therapy. Here we review recent developments, particularly under the impetus of client-centred practice, and the possibilities that are generated specifically from the viewpoint of disabled people themselves.

From the standpoint of disabled people

As the title of this chapter suggests, disability can be viewed in a variety of ways. This has given rise to conflict between occupational therapists and disabled people, as their perceptions of disability are frequently at odds. As you read the following two quotations from disabled people who have received occupational therapy, think about the differing ways in which occupational therapists and disabled people may view disability:

What concerns me most of all is this focus on trying to make me 'normal'. I get that from all the therapists. I get a lot of referrals of 'this may help' and 'that may help'. They had a massive case conference before the adaptations – it was a case of 'how normal can we make her first? Are the adaptations necessary?' They deliberately didn't widen the bathroom door upstairs to try and make me walk to the toilet. I very deliberately leave the feet off my wheelchair to keep my legs moving – it's definitely helped to maintain the muscle tone – but they don't like this. I can't feel them so I have to be very careful as I've been known to run over my own feet. They don't like it for safety reasons, but you make choices – I go sailing and that could be dangerous [...] Nobody thinks about the real world, it's all very purist. I want therapists to be flexible and realistic. I want them to say, 'What sorts of things would help you to lead a full life in the context of your impairment?' It's either, 'You're disabled so what can we do to make you better?' or, 'You're OK'. Nobody says, 'What would make a better life?' That's what I would like. (Kate)

(French 2004a, p. 103)

I've often thought about OTs in rehab, if only they could think about the context from which their patients came. I was received as head of department of a girls' comprehensive school, head of physical education, and this OT said to me, 'Now you've really got to learn to type because that's what you'll be doing'. She negated the whole context of my professional life – I was just a patient. Just because someone has had an accident or an illness doesn't mean that they've changed one iota. I went in as a gymnast and a sports person, that hadn't changed; it was just that I couldn't do it anymore. There was no acknowledgement of what my life was about or how to shape my new future. They had a routine, it was almost like, 'She's got fingers; she can type'. I couldn't identify with it, there was no link with anything to do with me. (Sandy)

(French 2004a, p. 99)

In the first quotation Kate is critical of a central aspect of the role of occupational therapists and the thinking that underpins it – that of trying to approximate disabled people to what is regarded as 'normal', however much time, effort and stress is involved. The power of the occupational therapist over Kate comes across in this quotation, as she had more say over the adaptations, even though it is Kate's home. It is clear that Kate wants to be treated as a unique individual, not a patient or client. She wants to be able to take risks like any other adult and for her life to be seen in its wider social context. Most of all she wants somebody to consult her rather than tell her what she needs. There are similar themes in the quotation from Sandy. She feels stripped of her identity as a physical education teacher and angry that she has no choice over her treatment. She cannot identify with the activity of typing and feels she is being treated as one patient among many, rather than as an individual with a unique history who is trying to rebuild a meaningful future.

In an interview for French and Swain (2006), Arlene provided a number of examples from her experiences with occupational therapists that clearly reflected those of Kate and Sandy. These were sometimes laced with humour:

It has taken thirteen years to get anything. OTs come and go and invariably they treat you in the same way which is that they know best. You can tell them you can't use equipment and they take no notice. One OT came out and gave me a bed raiser thing. It was a big blow up thing. And it went under your pillow and you pressed the button and it sat you in the up position which is where I've got to be to sleep, but unfortunately in a single bed it also shoves you straight onto the floor. So as you press the button to go in the up position it pushes you off the bed. She said 'I'll leave this here' and I said 'I'm sure it doesn't work' and I pressed it while she was here [...] and shot straight onto the dog's bed. I wasn't hurt but if she had listened in the first place I wouldn't have ended up sharing a bed with a dog. (Unpublished interview data)

Arlene thus provides an example of resistance in the power relationship between therapist and client, in this case determining the provision of equipment. Her resistance takes the form of demonstrating the inappropriateness of the equipment. All professional relationships contain elements of power and the question of power is inescapable in a therapeutic

29

relationship (Falardeau & Durand 2002). Palmadottir (2003), in a study exploring clients' perspectives on the outcome of occupational therapy practice, found that clients had little power in their relationships with therapists, lacked information and were unclear about the objectives of the intervention, let alone feeling they have a say in defining the goals.

Contrasting perspectives: the social model of disability

Underlying the policy and practice of all the health and caring professions, including occupational therapy, are ideas and beliefs about the meaning of disability. Two interacting models of, or ways of viewing, disability have prevailed within these professions for as long as they have existed. The first is the individual model which views disability in terms of disease and impairment – the problem is seen as being within the individual. According to this perception of disability disabled people have something wrong with them that needs to be fixed or corrected so that they can be as much like other people as possible. The main way in which they are identified is by their impairment or disease. Indeed, as Ballantyne and Muir (2008) argue, access to occupational therapy services is dependent upon having a defined problem or deficit. The second is the tragedy model where disabled people are viewed as unhappy, inferior, and a burden to their families and society. As Parens and Asch (2000, p. 20) state:

> There are many widely accepted beliefs about what life with disability is like for children and their families......They include assumptions that people with disabilities lead lives of relentless agony and frustration and that most marriages break up under the strain of having a child with a disability.

These models of disability are not peculiar to occupational therapy, but have dominated society throughout history and the world. Knowledge is shaped by social and political forces, and professionals, government, and the media have had the power to define disability in terms of individual pathology. This view of disability has, however, recently been challenged by the collective voice of disabled people with some resulting changes in policy. Charity advertising, for instance, has been compelled to become more positive in recent years

and professions such as occupational therapy are beginning to reflect on the growing criticisms of their practice from disabled people (Ballantyne & Muir 2008).

The individual model of disability has been challenged by the social model. Rather than viewing disability as being caused by impairment, the social model views disability as resulting from a disabling society in terms of the built environment, the social structures which underpin society, and the behaviour and attitudes that disabled people encounter in their interactions with others. The social model thus highlights the social and political nature of disability. In this model disability is viewed as lying outside rather than within the individual. The social model of disability has gathered strength over the past 30 years with the growth of the disabled people's movement which resulted, in the United Kingdom, in the passing of the Disability Discrimination Act in 1995 and subsequent changes to the built environment such as ramps and bleeper crossings. There is also now an academic discipline, Disability Studies, which analyses disability in much the same way as Women's Studies analyses the social and political situation of women. Occupational therapists, however, are only minimally exposed to Disability Studies. In the time I (Sally) spent teaching occupational therapy students (1994–1999) only one three-hour slot in the entire three-year course was devoted specifically to the subject.

Although the individual model has been criticised by disabled people this does not, of course, mean that disabled people do not want and expect an excellent health care service. The problem lies with the way the individual model can dominate disabled people's lives. This tends to be most intense during childhood as the following quotations illustrate:

> Looking back from the age of nine to sixteen the primary aim of that school was to 'therup' me. It had nothing to do with education really.
>
> (Davies 1992, p. 37)

> For young people the disadvantages of medical treatment need to be weighed against the possible advantages. Children are not usually asked if they want speech therapy, physiotherapy, orthopaedic surgery, hospitalisation, drugs, or cumbersome and ugly 'aids and appliances'. We are not asked whether we want to be put on daily regimes or programmes which use hours of precious play-time. All these things are

just imposed on us with the assumption that we share our parents' or therapists' desire for us to be more 'normal' at all costs. We are not even consulted as adults as to whether we think those things had been necessary or useful.

(Mason & Rieser 1992, p. 82)

Kate, in the quotation earlier, was not saying that she did not want to be helped by occupational therapists, but that she wanted them to take her unique lifestyle into account when making decisions about her home adaptations and to work in partnership with her as an equal. Sandy too wanted therapy to be geared to her individual aspirations so that it would be meaningful to her. Again, this would involve her working in an equal partnership with the occupational therapist.

Contrasting perspectives: the affirmative model of disability

The tragedy model of disability has been described in our formulation of the affirmative model (Swain & French 2000). We are both disabled, Sally from birth and John since middle age, yet neither of us identify with the notion that our lives are tragic or 'lesser' because of our impairments. We have noticed too that challenging the tragedy view is a common theme in the writings of disabled people. This is evident in the following quotations. As you read them you may like to make a note of the underlying themes which are being expressed:

I do not wish for a cure for Asperger's Syndrome. What I wish for is a cure for the common ill that pervades too many lives, the ill that makes people compare themselves to a normal that is measured in terms of perfect and absolute standards, most of which are impossible for anyone to reach.

(Halliday Wiley 1999, p. 96)

I cannot wish that I had never contracted ME [myalgic encephalopathy], because it has made me a different person, a person I am glad to be, would not want to miss being and could not relinquish even if I were cured.

(Wendell 1996, p. 83)

I am never going to be able to conform to society's requirements and I am thrilled

because I am blissfully released from all that crap. That's the liberation of disfigurement.

(Shakespeare et al 1996, p. 81)

I can't imagine being hearing, I'd need a psychiatrist, I'd need a speech therapist, I'd need some new friends, I'd lose all my old friends, I'd lose my job.....It really hits hearing people that a deaf person doesn't want to become hearing. I am what I am.

(Shakespeare et al 1996, p. 184)

There's nothing about my old life I miss at all, apart from being able to play my guitar. I've discovered that I have an extremely strong marriage and I get far more satisfaction from my work as a counsellor than from any other job I've had. I'm as confident now as I've ever been and my life is so much richer. I've always been a positive person and having a stroke didn't change that.

(Boazman 2002, p. 94)

These are just a few quotations from many similar ones we could have chosen. A major theme in the quotations is that being disabled is not necessarily viewed as a problem and that life may become better or be just as good following disablement by the opening of different opportunities, discoveries and insights. None of this is to imply that disability is *never* viewed as a tragedy by disabled people but to challenge the idea that it inevitably is. Neither does the affirmative model deny that living in a disabling environment can be difficult and frustrating. Although the social model of disability – involving changes to the environment and people's behaviour – is relatively easy to grasp, the idea that disability is something to be embraced and celebrated is, we have found, more difficult for non-disabled people to accept. As Oliver (1993, p.50) states:

... ideologies are so deeply embedded in social consciousness generally that they become 'facts'; they are naturalised. Thus everyone knows that disability is a personal tragedy for individuals so 'affected'; hence ideology becomes common sense.

Once an affirmative model of disability is accepted, however, the rehabilitation goals of striving for physical independence and 'normality' become far less tenable. If disability is viewed as 'out there' in the environment and if disabled people are comfortable with themselves, where does that leave the occupational therapist? Clearly if the social model and the affirmative model of disability are accepted, the work of the occupational therapist, as it presently stands, is seriously challenged. This can make it difficult for occupational therapists to examine and accept these models because it impinges directly on a role which may be valued and hard won. In the NHS definition of occupational therapy given at the start of this chapter, for instance, disability is said to be caused by 'physical or psychological illness, ageing or accident', rather than any social or political process, and that occupational therapists help disabled people overcome what are deemed to be their problems.

Changing therapy: client-centred

In addressing the challenges raised in the social model and affirmative model perspectives, we need to look first at recent developments in occupational therapy. Occupational therapy is, of course, not a static entity but a changing arena of service provision within a shifting social and historical context. The mandates for change are generated by research, legislation, organisational policy, and stakeholder agendas. They find expression under such umbrella concepts as psychosocial occupational therapy (Cara & MacRae 2005), evidence-based practice (Addy 2006) and, crucially, client-centred practice (Sumsion 2006).

At the simplest level this is an expansion of forms of intervention, professional contexts in which occupational therapists work with the client population. This is expressed in an introductory text, as follows (Sabonis-Chafee & Hussey 1998, p. 7):

> Recently, OT has expanded to include even more diverse services such as assistive technology, aquatics, animal-assisted therapy, ergonomics, and community integration. The OT practitioner works with clients who have a physical, cognitive, or psychological or psychosocial impairment. ... The recipients of OT services are as diverse as the world itself.

The medical approach, however, is clearly adhered to and propagated.

Client-centred approaches represent a far more fundamental shift in occupational therapy, as is clearly shown in the following definition proposed by Sumsion (2000, p. 208):

> Client-centred occupational therapy is a partnership between client and the therapist that empowers the client to engage in functional performance and fulfil his or her occupational roles in a variety of environments. The client participates actively in negotiating goals, which are given priority and are at the centre of assessment, intervention and evaluation. Throughout the process the therapist listens to and respects the client's needs and enables the client to make informed decisions.

This definition is similar to the principles laid out by Stewart et al (2003, pp. 5–6). They state:

> Patient-centred care presupposes several changes in the mindset of the clinician. First, the hierarchical notion of the professional being in charge and the patient being passive does not hold here. To be patient-centred the clinician must be able to empower patients, share the power in the relationship, and this means renouncing control which traditionally has been in the hands of the professional. This is the moral imperative in patient-centred practice.

This notion of an equal partnership from the standpoint of occupational therapists seems to reflect, at least to an extent, good practice from the viewpoint of disabled service users. In interviews for French and Swain (2006), disabled people were asked for examples of positive experiences of occupational therapy. David had generally had good experiences. He told us:

> Best thing about the OTs is that they actually come and talk to you, about what your requirements are. My general experience is good with OTs, so though they have a bit of background knowledge about a range of impairments, they do actually, in my experience, listen to what your requirements are. ... So actually it has always been good. They come and see you in your own environment and they'll chat to you about what

your needs are and they'll put that down into a report. (Unpublished interview data)

Arlene, whose experiences we have already referred to above, had few examples of what she thought to be good practice:

I've only met one OT that's any good and that's the one that's given me ... everything I need. At first she was a bit wary of me and I was definitely wary of her but she's just left her post she's gone to work in Devon. Before she left we got on really well because she actually listened to me and that made the difference. ... She knew what she was talking about and did listen to the disabled person, which makes the difference – just the listening. (Unpublished interview data)

Dawn, the mother of a disabled child provided us with a further example:

She makes recommendations that are clearly based on what she believes to be right and she listens and she's prepared to alter according to family circumstances. An example of that would be when she originally looked at our old house for rails around the house she made the recommendation, came back for comments and took on board what I had to say, and made some alterations. She's also got off the fence and written to local authorities, complained and pleaded with them to alter curbs, pavements, roads around the house. It is not part of her brief really but she is prepared to do that.

(French & Swain 2006, pp. 78–79)

It is clear from these quotations that, although disabled people value the skill and expertise of occupational therapists, they want their own expertise to be recognised and to work with therapists in a spirit of collaboration. Though the actual term 'client-centred' is not used the principles of good practice are clearly similar. The promotion of client-centred practice is founded on the recognition that, as eloquently expressed by Kate, Sandy and Arlene, clients experience little power in the relationship with their therapists.

Sumsion (2006) recognises the question of power in therapist–client relationships as central to changing therapy practice. She states that, 'It is the transfer of power to the client that moves the inter-action from the static medical perspective to one focused on the client's needs' (2006, p. 41). This argument focuses on the inherent power imbalance within the professional–disabled service user relationship: professional power to control disabled people's bodies, the access of professionals to a whole range of social opportunities (work, housing, social security) and the power of professionals to engage in processes whereby disabled clients can be labelled as being different, needy and helpless (Marks 1999).

So how might client-centred practice relate to the social and affirmative model perspective of disability? First, it is necessary to point out that these models of disability and impairment are not models of professional intervention. They are, in essence, models of 'the problem' (i.e. the disabling society and the dominant presumptions about disabled people and their lives as being tragic). There are associated general implications and principles for the practice of occupational therapy but the models are not blueprints. There are few, but nevertheless a growing, number of references to the social model within occupational therapy literature. Writing in 1996 about the responses of the occupational therapy profession to the perspectives of the disabled people's movement, Craddock (1996, p. 75) stated:

... a review of the British Journal of Occupational Therapy *revealed that only in 1994 did the profession in this country start to assess the impact of the disability movement and the debate regarding the implications of its perspective for occupational therapy practice has hardly begun.*

In more recent occupational therapy literature, a connection is typically made between client-centred practice and the social model. Pengelly (2006, p. 43), for instance, writes about 'how the social model and client-centred approach can be integrated into therapists' clinical reasoning throughout the problem-solving process and during the implementation of recommendations'. She argues that once the social model is taken to inform practice, the focus for intervention becomes the removal of barriers, which include the built environment, attitudes and organisations. Whilst emphasising the importance of the social model in informing practice, she does add a caveat that 'this should be used within the holistic and client-centred framework embodied in OT models of practice' (Pengelly 2006, p. 62).

The idea that the social model is easily compatible with the holistic and client-centred frameworks is, however, questionable. The holistic framework is provided by consideration of the impact of environmental and personal factors as they are thought to relate to the client's functioning. As long ago as 1996 Craddock rightly questioned the holistic tradition as an adequate response to the social model of disability in occupational therapy practice. She wrote, 'The holistic approach of treating the whole person in the context of his or her environment has not required us to challenge the official definitions of all our interventions as treatment' (Craddock 1996, p. 76). Indeed, at its simplest, it can be argued that a holistic approach to clinical practice takes the individual model into the whole of disabled people's lives (French 2004b).

As we have suggested above, client-centred practice, in principle, supports increasing the client's power within occupational therapy. Nevertheless, it does not resolve the inherent tensions between the social and individual models of disability. As Kielhofner (2005, p. 493), the guest editor of a special edition of *The American Journal of Occupational Therapy* addressing the implications of the social model, states:

> ... from a disability studies perspective, such an approach still focuses on the individual rather than on society's collective response to the individual. Importantly, choosing what to do within occupational therapy is not the same as the disability community deciding whether it wants occupational therapy services or what role it would like occupational therapy to play in addressing the needs of the members of their community.

As Kielhofner recognises, from the social model perspective disability is essentially political and questions of control lie at the heart of its implications, not just within occupational therapy, but in determining lifestyle and quality of life – independent living from the perspective of disabled people. Hammell (2006) recognises that occupational therapists have discussed client-centred practice for over two decades, justified by the claim that the approach emanates from and empowers disabled clients' perspectives. However, she goes on to state:

> It is therefore particularly ironic that although occupational therapists have debated and

> refined their own definitions of client-centred practice ..., little effort has been expended in exploring the meaning of client-centred practice with clients.

> (Hammell 2006, p. 155)

Rather than the social model being adopted by the occupational therapy profession as a supposed foundation for clinical practice, it can be seen as providing fundamental challenges to generate critical reflection. This stance is taken by Clark (2006, p. 243) who states, 'There is a need to understand the nature of the argument posed by the disability movement, even if one does not fully accept them, so as to reflect critically on our clinical practice'. Notwithstanding the more recent developments within occupational therapy that are compatible with the social model, caution is required towards any claims from professionals that they adhere to a social model of disability. The challenges reach into all aspects of the provision of occupational therapy, including the participation of disabled people in the provision of occupational therapy, the management of the profession, policy-making and, as recognised in the following quotation, professional training:

> Only through such reflection can members of the nondisabled community, including professionals who offer services to disabled persons, generate insight into their own deeply embedded attitudes about disability. Importantly ... this reflective process should begin in the context of our professional educational programs.

> (Kielhofner 2005, p. 491)

Again, however, the question of control arises. Who teaches the disability elements of the professional educational programmes? The provision of Disability Equality Training has been one of the main strategies of the disabled people's movement in propagating the social model of disability (Mason 2000) and, perhaps not surprisingly, such training is planned and delivered by disabled people.

Changing therapy: citizen-centred

Taking on this notion of critical reflection, Ballantyne and Muir (2008) set out their responses, as occupational therapy educators, to the social and affirmative model of disability and impairment. They argue that if the occupational therapy profession is to change in response to the social model and the affirmative model of disability, then a change of policy is required from the top of the profession. They do not believe that it is possible for individual professionals to make changes of any magnitude because they are limited by the culture in which they work and the overall policy directives. If a person cannot access the service without demonstrating a defined 'problem', for example, it is unlikely that the individual occupational therapist, whatever his or her attitudes and beliefs, will be able to escape the dictates of the individual model. Ballantyne and Muir (2008) state that:

> ... occupational therapists will find a tension between the dynamic driving service provision, which is essentially individualised and problem based, and a view of impairment and disability as integral positive elements of a person's personal and collective identity.

They advocate working with disabled people in an equal partnership in order to bring about social and political change and, in so doing, move away from a client-based model of service towards a citizen-based model. In a citizen-based model service users are involved in the formulation and running of the services themselves at all stages, including the production of knowledge about what disability is and what services, if any, are required. Some of the traditional skills of the occupational therapist are likely to remain useful, but all goals of intervention need to be fully negotiated with the disabled person. Neither Kate, Sandy, nor Arlene, for instance, were against being helped by occupational therapists, but they were frustrated and dissatisfied at having so little say regarding the way attempts were made to help them; attempts which ultimately proved counterproductive. Despite the usefulness of the skills occupational therapists already possess, it is the case that in order to join disabled people in their ongoing quest for full citizenship, they need to look outwards to the disabling society and to accept that, as individuals, disabled people may be very happy with who they are and have no wish to aspire to 'normality' or to strive for a narrowly defined concept of independence. Although a focus on occupation in the home in order to undertake basic skills of daily living may, for some, be important, this type of intervention has a limited effect if society at large remains inaccessible and disabling to large number of citizens. Molineux (2004, p. 1) believes that occupational therapists find it difficult to attend to the needs of their clients because of '... the dominance of the medical model, coupled with the significant political, institutional and financial pressures, which characterise modern health and social care'.

Conclusion

The topic for this chapter is 'perspectives on disability'. We have attempted to demonstrate that this is not an academic exercise. It is a political concept with people having contrasting personal, collective and institutional interests. Based on his investigation of occupational therapy practitioners, Abberley (1995, p. 222), a disabled academic, concludes that, 'occupational therapy, despite what may be the best intentions on the part of its practitioners, serves to perpetuate the process of disablement of impaired people'. In so doing he clearly lays down the gauntlet for occupational therapists on behalf of disabled people. Along the same lines, Davis (2004) observes that professionals providing services for disabled people are preoccupied not with a struggle for social change or equalising opportunities in any fundamental way, but with enhancing their own career opportunities and power.

We have attempted to demonstrate the demands and mandate for not just client-centred but for client-controlled intervention, and a citizen-based model of services, including occupational therapy. In this light we conclude with some advice based on experience from disabled people, who we quoted earlier in this chapter. They suggest that when there is choice and control on the part of the disabled service user and a true working partnership with the occupational therapist, creative and satisfactory ideas emerge which can lead to very positive experiences. For David this was when occupational therapists recognised his agenda and took his side (French & Swain 2006, p. 79):

> When I was being offered accommodation by the local authority and the housing association it was very useful to have the OT there who could say 'Well no, that's not actually suitable

for this person'. That I found useful because I felt very pressured to just take somewhere to live whenever I was offered somewhere.

A final quote from Arlene provides a succinct statement of the implications of perspectives of disability as generated by disabled people (French & Swain 2006, p.79):

Remember that the person you are going in to, it's their home environment and it's never an extension of the hospital ward. You are not in control. You have got to respect the person that you are going in to. Treat them with dignity and listen to what they say because the disabled person is living the disability and they are the experts.

References

Abberley, P. (1995). Disabling ideology in health and welfare: The case of occupational therapy, *Disability and Society*, 10, 221–232.

Addy, L. (Ed.) (2006). *Occupational Therapy Evidence in Practice for Physical Rehabilitation*. Oxford, Blackwell.

Ballantyne, E., & Muir, A. (in press) In Practice: from the viewpoint of occupational therapy. In: S. French, & J. Swain (Eds.). *Disability on equal terms: understanding and valuing difference in health and social care* (pp. 142–149). London, Sage.

Boazman, S. (2002). I had no way of communicating that I was still a bright, intelligent whole human being. *Good Housekeeping*, November, 93–94.

Cara, E., & MacRae, A. (2005). *Psychosocial occupational therapy: a clinical practice* (2nd ed.). Thomson Delmar Learning, New York.

Clark, A. (2006). A reflective challenge. In: L. Addy, (Ed.). *Occupational therapy evidence in practice for physical rehabilitation* (pp. 1–23). Oxford, Blackwell.

Craddock, J. (1996). Responses of the occupational therapy profession to the perspective of the disability movement, Part 2. *British Journal of Occupational Therapy*, 59(2), 73–77.

Davies, C. (1992). *Life times: a mutual biography of disabled people*. Farnham, Understanding Disability Educational Trust.

Davis, K. (2004). The crafting of good clients. In: J. Swain, S. French, C. Barnes, & C. Thomas, (Eds.). *Disabling barriers – enabling environments*, (2nd ed.) (pp. 203–205). London, Sage.

Falardeau, M., & Durand, M. J. (2002). Negotiation-centred versus client-centred: which approach should be used? *Canadian Journal of Occupational Therapy*, 68, 135–142.

French, S. (2004a). Enabling relationships in therapy practice. In: J. Swain, J. Clark, K. Parry, S. French, & F. Reynolds. *Enabling relationships in health and social care: a guide for therapists* (pp. 132–149). Oxford, Butterworth-Heinemann.

French, S. (2004b). Defining disability: implications for physiotherapy practice. In: S. French, & J. Sim (Eds.). *Physiotherapy: a psychosocial approach* (2nd ed.) (pp. 253–273). Oxford, Elsevier.

French, S. (2008). How did we get here? In: S. French, & J. Swain *Reflecting on disability: a guide for therapists* (pp. 41–65). Oxford, Elsevier.

French, S., & Swain, J. (2006). Housing: the user's perspective. In: Clutton, J. Grisbrooke, & S. Pengelly. (Eds.) *Occupational therapy in housing: building on firm foundations* (pp. 64–82). London, Whurr Publishers.

Halliday Wiley, L. (1999). *Pretending to be Normal: Living with Asperger's Syndrome*. London, Jessica Kingsley.

Hammell, K. W. (2006). *Perspectives on disability and rehabilitation: contesting assumptions; challenging practice*. Edinburgh, Churchill Livingstone Elsevier.

Kielhofner, G. (2005). Rethinking disability and what to do about it: disability studies and its implications for occupational therapy. *The American Journal of Occupational Therapy* 59(5), 487–496.

Marks, D. (1999). *Disability: controversial debates and psychosocial perspectives*. London, Routledge.

Mason, M. (2000). *Incurably human*. London, Working Press.

Mason, M., & Rieser, R. (1992). The limits of medicine. In: R. Rieser, & M. Mason (Eds.). *Disability equality in the classroom: a human rights issue* (pp. 82–83). London, Disability Equality in Education.

Molineux, M. (2004). Occupation in occupational therapy: a labour in vain. In: M. Molineux (Ed.). *Occupation for occupational therapists* (pp. 49–60). Oxford, Blackwell Publishing.

Oliver, M. (1993). Disability and dependency: a creation of industrial societies? In: J. Swain, V. Finkelstein, S. French, M. Oliver (Eds.). *Disabling barriers – enabling environments*. London, Sage Publications.

Palmadottir, G. (2003). Client perspectives on occupational therapy in rehabilitation services. *Scandinavian Journal of Occupational Therapy*, 10, 158–166.

Parens, E., & Asch, A. (2000). *Prenatal testing and disability rights*. Washington, Georgetown University Press.

Pengelly, S. (2006). The social model and clinical reasoning. In: S. Clutton, J. Grisbrooke, & S. Pengelly (Eds.). *Occupational therapy in housing: building on firm foundations* (pp. 43–63). London, Whurr Publishers.

Sabonis-Chafee, B., & Hussey, S. (1998). *Introduction to occupational therapy*, (2nd ed). St. Louis, Mosby.

Shakespeare, T., Gillespie-Sells, K., & Davies D. (1996). *The sexual politics of disability: untold desires*. London, Cassell.

Stewart, M., Brown, J. B., Weston, W. W., et al. (2003). *Patient-centred medicine: transforming the clinical method*. Abingdon, Radcliffe Medical Press.

Sumsion, T. (2000). A revised occupational therapy definition of client-centred practice. *British Journal of Occupational Therapy*, 63(7), 304–309.

Sumsion, T. (Ed.) (2006). *Client-centred practice in occupational therapy: a guide to implementation*, Edinburgh, Churchill Livingstone.

Swain, J., & French, S. (2000). Towards an affirmation model of disability. *Disability and Society*, 15(4), 569–582.

Wendell, S. (1996). *The rejected body: feminist philosophical reflections on disability*. London, Routledge.

Chapter Four

4

Contesting assumptions in occupational therapy

Karen Whalley Hammell

CHAPTER CONTENTS

Introduction .40

Challenging 'thinking as usual' 40

Taking a global perspective 41

Contesting assumptions 41

The nature of the occupational therapy
profession .41
Outcome assessment: who assesses
our client-centredness? 42
Services: client-centred and needs-led or
therapist-centred and bureaucracy-led? 42
Services: client-centred and needs-led or
economic-led? 42
Services: needs-led or discriminatory? 42
Services: client-centred and needs-led?
Taking a sceptical approach 43

The nature of occupational therapy's
goals 43
Striving for normality 43
Striving for physical independence 44
Enhancing quality of life 45
Normality, independence and quality
of life: taking a sceptical approach 45

The nature of occupation 45
We can influence our health by hands and
willpower .45
Work is supportive of health 45
Humans participate in occupations as
autonomous agents 46
Occupations are goal-directed and
socially sanctioned 46
Productive occupations contribute to life's
meaning .46

Occupations enable economic
self-sufficiency 47
Occupations are divisible into categories 47
A balance of occupations is beneficial
to health and well-being 47
Individuals interact with the environment
through occupation 48
Humans need to master the
environment 48

Assumptions informing occupational
therapy: taking a sceptical approach 49

Occupational rights: occupation, health
and well-being 49

Human rights, occupational rights
and well-being 49

Values, knowledge and skills in
occupational-therapy practice 50

SUMMARY

Occupational therapy is underpinned by shared assumptions concerning the nature of occupation, our profession and our goals. Because assumptions, by definition, are those ideas that we assume to be 'right' or 'common-sense', or that we take for granted, they are rarely subjected to critical scrutiny. This chapter aims to promote a culture of healthy scepticism among occupational therapists by unmasking and contesting the specific values reflected in our shared assumptions and by demonstrating that these assumptions, although appearing benign and benevolent, may serve economic and political interests rather than those of disabled people. Returning to occupational therapy's core assumption – that engagement in occupation can positively influence well-being – the chapter supports calls for a renewed vision for occupational therapy: one committed to 'occupational rights' – the right of all people to engage in meaningful occupations that contribute positively to their own well-being and the well-being of their communities.

KEY POINTS

- Occupational therapy theory and practice are informed by shared assumptions that are rarely challenged or contested.
- Much of what occupational therapists regard as 'knowledge' comprises quotes from distinguished occupational therapists rather than research evidence.
- The values underpinning occupational therapy's dominant assumptions are specific to middle-class, minority world theorists.
- Although occupational therapy declares itself to be person-centred and needs-led, little evidence supports this assertion.
- Occupational therapy's claims to be person-centred and needs-led are contested by our role of resource gatekeeper, private practices and our support of societal injustices.
- Occupational therapy's goals of enhancing normality and increasing independence may meet the needs of social conformity and political ideals of individualism rather than the needs of people.
- Occupational therapy's assumptions about occupation are culturally specific and not universal.
- Occupational therapy's assumptions about occupation may serve to protect and reinforce the political and social status quo.
- Occupational therapy could contribute to the well-being of all individuals and communities – not solely those impacted by illness or impairment – by a closer focus on occupational rights.

An enormous difference to the way we live our lives can be created by a shift in perceptions about things we have always taken for granted or never questioned.

(Coleridge 1999, p. 165).

Introduction

This chapter is about *assumptions*: those ideas that we assume to be 'right' or 'common-sense', or that

we take for granted. Occupational therapy is based on shared assumptions concerning the nature of our profession (client-centred and needs-led), the nature of our goals (for example, increasing physical independence to enhance quality of life) and the nature of occupation (for example, that engagement in occupation positively influences health).

More particularly, this chapter is concerned with *contesting assumptions*: with interrogating the validity of occupational therapy's shared assumptions and with challenging occupational therapists' steadfast refusal to accept received ideas. Fundamentally, this chapter aims to encourage an occupational therapy culture of healthy scepticism in conjunction with an innovative rethinking of our role in society.

Challenging 'thinking as usual'

A recent and influential occupational therapy text claims that occupational therapists, like all professionals, 'have some basic assumptions that, by definition, are not questioned, but rather are held to be true. They are challenged only when there is a large accumulation of prevailing evidence to suggest that the assumptions are no longer tenable' (Townsend & Polatajko 2007, p. 20). But is such lack of intellectual rigour acceptable? If we do not search for contesting evidence, how shall we find it? Clearly, if we neither question nor challenge our professional assumptions, they will survive indefinitely, even if they are demonstrably erroneous or inadequate. Moreover, critics observe that the more powerful our beliefs and assumptions become and the greater their longevity, the greater their ability to survive contact with contesting evidence (Childs & Williams 1997, Taylor 1999).

Occupational therapy claims to be a scientific discipline that draws its knowledge base from the insights of occupational science. A truly scientific discipline is one that assures 'a culture of healthy scepticism: a readiness to doubt claims and assumptions about the 'rightness' of any particular theory or intervention' (Brechin & Sidell 2000, p. 12). Regrettably, it is claimed that professional knowledge perpetuated within occupational therapy consists 'primarily of a collage of "quotes" derived from distinguished and respected occupational therapists 'as if these are somehow correct or "true"' (Mocellin 1995, p. 503). It is certainly evident that much of the 'knowledge' that occupational therapists take for granted comprises claims made by a small number of our élite forerunners: beliefs about occupation that may appear to constitute 'common-sense' but that may have little supporting evidence (Hammell 2004a, Law et al 1998, Suto 2004). Because of this habit of substituting authority for evidence (Mocellin 1995), assumptions about occupational therapy's core knowledge are rarely critically appraised or contested. While they remain uncontested, these beliefs and assumptions are said to resemble the dogma of a fundamentalist faith (Mocellin 1995).

Duncan et al (2007, p. 200) note that 'robust academic argument is new to occupational therapy: to date, there has been a notable lack of scholarly articles presenting counter-arguments to theoretical ideas'. Intellectual integrity, however, depends upon sustaining a critical stance: an unwillingness to accept ready-made clichés, or what the powerful or conventional have to say (Said 1996). In particular, professionals are exhorted to guard against the received ideas handed down in their own profession and against being too confident in ideological straightjackets (Said 1979). Intellectual integrity requires us to challenge the beliefs and assumptions inherent in our field, to raise questions, confront dogma, unmask conventional and accepted ideas, take nothing for granted and be unwilling 'to let half-truths or received ideas steer one along' (Said 1996, p. 23). Thus, Kronenberg et al (2005) contend that if occupational therapists are to live up to their self-defined mandate of enabling participation in meaningful occupations, 'they must think critically [and] become aware of the value patterns embedded in our theories' (p. xvi). We must take nothing for granted.

Taking a global perspective

It is relevant to the subject matter of this chapter to recognize that the area of the world self-described as 'first', 'Western' or 'developed' constitutes only about 17% of the global population and is more appropriately termed the *minority* world. For the same reason, what is often labelled the 'developing' or 'third' world constitutes approximately 83% of the global population and is, in reality, the *majority* world (Penn 1999). Thus, Western occupational therapists and theorists are members of a minority population, with values and assumptions that are specific to a minority of people. *Ethnocentrism*, the belief that one's own culture is superior to others

and is the standard by which all other people should be judged (Leavitt 1999), is manifested in the assumption that one's own assumptions and values are universal, rather than specific.

The most influential theories and models within occupational therapy have arisen in the United States (e.g. Reilly, Yerxa and Kielhofner), Canada (e.g. Law, Townsend, Polatajko and colleagues), the United Kingdom (e.g. Hagedorn and Creek) and Australia (e.g. Chapparo, Ranka, Whiteford and Wilcock). Clearly, all these influential thinkers have something in common: they all reside in the minority world. Hence, their theories and models tend to reflect minority viewpoints, values and assumptions that are shaped by their cultural background (the specific socio-political and socio-cultural milieu in which they live) and a complex interaction of personal variables such as education, professional and employment status, economic circumstances, 'race', ethnicity, and social class/caste. While occupational therapy's oft-cited theorists reflect considerable homogeneity on many of these variables, their viewpoints, values, and assumptions are unlikely to be shared by the majority of the world's people.

Thus, the Eastern-influenced Kawa model of occupation (Iwama 2006) is perceived to be not solely innovative, but 'a direct challenge to the implicit, assumed universality and dominance of the occupational models developed in the Western world' (Townsend & Polatajko 2007, p. 279).

Contesting assumptions

It is not possible, within the limited space of a single chapter, to introduce and interrogate all the evidence that contests occupational therapy's core assumptions; and, indeed, this is not the role of this chapter. Rather, I intend to encourage a culture of healthy scepticism by raising questions about the validity and universality of occupational therapy's assumptions. These assumptions will be divided into three sections: the nature of the profession, the nature of the profession's goals, and the nature of occupation.

The nature of the occupational therapy profession

The occupational therapy profession has long proclaimed itself to be client-centred and needs-led (American Occupational Therapy Association 2002,

Canadian Association of Occupational Therapists & Health Service Directorate 1983, College of Occupational Therapists 2000, 2001, 2005). Indeed, the assumption that occupational therapists practice in a client-centred manner is central to our professional self-image.

If we aspire to healthy scepticism and are committed to confronting conventional dogma we must now ask: Is there any evidence to support the premise that occupational therapists practice consistently in a person-centred, needs-led manner? And if so, whose evidence is this: service providers' or service users'?

Outcome assessment: who assesses our client-centredness?

Reports from disability researchers suggest that disabled people frequently perceive their therapists to be superior, coercive, controlling, domineering, and manipulative (Abberley 1995, 2004, Kemp 2002, Swain et al 2003). Even occupational therapists' own research reveals evidence of therapists using such strategies of professional domination as persuasion, intimidation, and coercion (Moats 2007). Intriguingly, occupational therapists' claims to practice in a client-centred manner have rarely been tested by assessing clients' satisfaction with the client-centredness of their services (McKinnon 2000). Like most professionals, occupational therapists like to evaluate the outcomes of their own services (McKnight 1981), despite obvious conflicts of interest (Abberley 1995, Hammell 2006).

Services: client-centred and needs-led or therapist-centred and bureaucracy-led?

Although proclaiming publicly that occupational therapy services 'shall be client-centred and needs-led' (College of Occupational Therapists 2005, 3.2.3), individuals perceive occupational therapists to be accountable, not to their clients, but to their employers (Hammell 2006).

Anxious not to 'rock the boat' of the institutional environments in which they work (and thus to protect their own employment status, career prospects and financial self-interests), occupational therapists habitually collude in the denial of equipment, services and resources that clients need (Barbara & Curtin 2008, Hammell 2007). Although acknowledging that 'resources will never be infinite' (e.g.

College of Occupational Therapists 2001, 3.2.2), occupational therapists frequently act, not as advocates for the resources clients need, but as willing gatekeepers to those resources (Davis 1993, Swain et al 2003). For example, when bureaucrats determine that certain categories of disabled people are ineligible to receive certain categories of wheelchairs, occupational therapists habitually enforce these edicts rather than taking action through the media, and political and legal systems to ensure that disabled people's opportunities to participate in occupations are not limited by inappropriate equipment (Hammell 2007). It should, therefore, not be surprising that rehabilitation therapists are perceived by disabled people to be preoccupied with pursuing their own professional self-interests and with preserving the political and social status quo as agents of the State (Barnes & Mercer 2003, French & Swain 2001, Schriner 2001).

Services: client-centred and needs-led or economic-led?

Occupational therapy's Codes of Ethics proclaim values such as justice and equality, for example, 'occupational therapists are committed to providing services to all individuals in need of those services' (American Occupational Therapy Association 2000). Yet, the assumption that occupational therapy is a client-centred, needs-led profession is challenged by private practices that offer restricted services to specific people, based, not on need, but on economics (Hammell 2006). The reality that in South Africa, 80% of physiotherapists work in the private sector, serving 20% of the population – the privileged élite (Cornielje & Ferrinho 1999) – demonstrates that this is not a needs-led profession. But what are we to conclude from the preponderance of private occupational therapy practices and of the incongruity between private practices and our ethical principles of beneficence (the duty to assist those in need), justice (the duty to ensure fair and equitable distribution of service provision) (College of Occupational Therapists 2000, French 2004, Jonsen et al 1998) and our espoused commitment to 'client-centred and needs-led' practice (College of Occupational Therapists 2005, 3.2.3)?

Services: needs-led or discriminatory?

The assumption that occupational therapy is a client-centred, needs-led profession also has been contested by recent historical evidence. In apartheid South Africa, people were classified according to their skin colour and this determined the 'rights' to which they were entitled (Bozalek 2000). Rather than asserting the equal rights of all disabled people, South African therapists accepted, and thus reinforced, the social and political status quo (Cornielje & Ferrinho 1999, Swartz 2004). It was only at the Truth and Reconciliation hearings that privileged white health professionals were forced to acknowledge their own complicity in the oppression of the black majority (Bozalek 2000). Occupational therapists are not impartial bystanders to political, legal, economic, social, and cultural injustices, but active participants in enforcing specific policies, practices, rules, and regulations that directly impact those whose well-being we claim to have at heart (Hammell 2006).

Services: client-centred and needs-led? Taking a sceptical approach

Occupational therapy's claim that it is client-centred, is both politically expedient and beneficial for the profession's public image. However, when it is stated that occupational therapy is a client-centred profession, we ought to consider: Who is making this claim? What evidence supports this claim? Whose evidence is this? Whose evidence is not presented?

As a profession, we cannot indulge in smugness or complacency. If our practice does not place human need above the imperatives of politics, policies, employers or our own self-interests, then ours is not a client-centred profession, despite protestations to the contrary (Hammell 2006, Townsend 1998).

The nature of occupational therapy's goals

Among the assumptions that inform occupational therapy practice is a sense of the 'rightness' and the beneficence of certain goals. These goals include enhancing normality and increasing physical independence: goals that are assumed to positively influence quality of life. The assumption that these goals are legitimate and beneficial appears to be self-evident; and, indeed, it is precisely the 'common-sense' nature of occupational therapy's assumptions that assures their uncritical acceptance and reproduction. However, because this chapter is committed to scepticism, let us examine whether these goals are, indeed, benevolent and beneficial for disabled people.

Striving for normality

It is often believed that the primary aim of rehabilitation is to restore a disabled person to 'normality' (whatever normality is understood to mean within a given social and cultural environment); and failing this, to restore the person to a state that is as close to 'normality' as possible (Oliver 1996, Stalker & Jones 1998). Kielhofner (2004, p. 241) noted that rehabilitation enforces 'a version of normalcy that pressures disabled persons to fit in by appearing and functioning as much like non-disabled persons as possible'. Occupational therapists have largely failed to contest the assumption that 'normality' is an appropriate goal for people who have impairments and, indeed, have created their own 'norms' (goals) such as 'normal' posture, 'normal' gait and 'normal' handwriting that constitute favoured forms of physical function.

The ideology of 'normality' is also central to the International Classification of Functioning, Disability and Health (ICF) (World Health Organization 2001) which provides a framework for classifying human function in terms of deviations from 'normal' expectations (Barnes 2003, Pfeiffer 2000). Because of its inclusion of *action* and *participation* the ICF has been uncritically embraced by many occupational therapists as if it is somehow 'correct' (Hammell 2004b). It is rarely acknowledged that the purpose of the ICF is *not* to enable the assessment of human needs, but to *classify* deviations from assumed norms in every area of human life: hence its title (Hammell 2004b, 2006).

Norms are neither neutral nor objective (Baylies 2002, Douard 1995, Thomson 1997). 'In any society, what constitutes 'normality' is fluid and flexible, according to how the dominant value systems change and develop' (Corbett 1997, p. 94). To be 'normal' is to conform to what is usual or standard within the dominant population. Indeed, *to be 'normal' is to conform*. Thus, critics claim that normalising goals reflect an effort to induce social conformity rather than enhance capabilities (Sandahl 2003, Stiker 1999). Through their pursuit of 'normality' it is claimed that the rehabilitation professions act as agents of the State, protecting the political and social status quo by individualising problems that are the consequence of environmental factors, demonising difference, justifying the unequal distribution of life opportunities, and inducing individuals to strive to attain those 'norms' of physical function valued by the dominant population (French 1994, French & Swain 2001, Hammell 2006). Moreover, disability theorists claim that the goal of 'norming' the non-standard is often pursued at the expense of function, comfort and expediency (French 1994, Meekosha 1998, Miller et al 2004) that sometimes constitutes abuse (Middleton 1999, Priestley 2003, Swain et al 2003).

Striving for physical independence

There is a traditional assumption that rehabilitation constitutes teaching skills to enable the highest level of physical independence (Swain et al 2003), as if this is a goal to which all people aspire, or 'ought' to aspire, irrespective of culture, role demands or personal values (Hammell 2006).

Physical independence, self-sufficiency and individualism are prized in the minority world and are often unchallenged by therapists who assume that their own belief in the importance of independence is universally shared (Penn 1999). Cross-cultural research shows that this is not a universal aspiration (e.g. Katbamna et al 2000, Wirz & Hartley 1999). Minority world values of independence and self-reliance are alien to those cultures who value social relationships, interdependence, reciprocity and belonging (Iwama 2005a, Lim 2004). Indeed, in societies that value reciprocal obligations and harmonious relationships, 'contentment derived from the well-being of others constitutes an especially salient aspect of quality of life' (Ruff & Singer 1998, p. 8). Further, a wealth of studies among people with illnesses and impairments from Bangladesh to the USA has noted the importance of being able to contribute to others within relationships that foster perceptions of value, connecting and belonging (e.g. Bloom 2001, Lyons et al 2002, Rebeiro et al 2001, Waldie 2002).

Although Western societies value and promote independence, they also promote globalisation: a process that demonstrates the interdependence of all the world's peoples (Steger 2003). For example, that self-declared bastion of self-reliance, individualism and independence – the United States – depends for its materialistic lifestyle upon resources withdrawn from the rest of the world (Elliott 2006).

Minority world occupational therapists place a high value on physical independence in self-care

activities, irrespective of the costs of time and effort for disabled people (Marks 1999), and irrespective of research demonstrating that disabled people often choose to live interdependently, preferring to reserve their time and energies for activities that have personal value and significance (Holcomb 2000, Yerxa & Locker 1990). Importantly, an obsession with physical independence often limits occupational therapy to a process of re-learning the juvenile skills of self-care and mobility, leaving adults ill-equipped to re-engage with their complex lives (Hammell 2006). Abberley (2004) contends that occupational therapists share a disempowering ideology of self-reliance and independence that is out of step with disabled people's needs. Indeed, physical independence in everyday tasks is a preoccupation 'with which occupational therapists have become fixated' (Whiteford & Wilcock 2000, p. 332). This preoccupation manifests itself, for example, in those forms of assessment wherein the capacity to perform a task without physical assistance is accorded a higher score than when assistance is either required or chosen (Johnston & Miklos 2002, Law 1993).

Importantly, because occupational therapists tend to view dependence on others as 'a state of being requiring amelioration' (Iwama 2005b, p. 131), they reinforce cultural stereotypes that those who are 'dependent' are parasitic and burdensome, thus effectively demeaning and devaluing those who depend on us. However, research evidence demonstrates that the ability to contribute to others is associated with lower levels of depression, higher self-esteem and fewer health problems (e.g. Anson et al 1993, Schwartz & Sendor 1999, Stewart & Bhagwanjee 1999). Thus, it may be said that engagement in occupations that support interdependence may positively influence well-being. Moreover, Bunting (2004, p. 322) claims that paying attention to others' needs, or caring, 'is the most deeply engaged experience of our lives'.

Contrary to Western, egocentric ideology, research demonstrates that interdependence is 'an indispensable feature of the human condition' (Reindal 1999, p. 354), that we are all connected closely to others and engaged in interdependent relationships of reciprocal care (Ruff & Singer 1998, Walmsley 1993). Communities are built, not on individualism and independence, but on a sense of belonging and interdependence. Thus, rather than extolling individualism, Bunting (2004, p. 322) contends that we should acknowledge and assert 'that we are all interdependent, and it is in that web of dependence that we find our deepest contentment'. Recognising the importance of interdependent living, many disabled people re-define 'independence,' not as the ability to live without assistance, but as the quality of control they have over their lives and their ability to make decisions and enact choices (Clare 1999, Richardson 1997).

Enhancing quality of life

Occupational therapists often assume that by improving disabled people's physical independence they will somehow enhance their quality of life. This is an admirable goal, but not one that enjoys a supportive evidence base (Hammell 2004c). Countering 'common-sense' assumptions, a large volume of research demonstrates that perceptions of quality in living do not correlate with the degree of physical independence (Hammell 2004d). Moreover, neither the severity of a physical impairment nor the degree of physical independence is predictive of psychological distress (e.g. Hartkopp et al 1998, Krause et al 2000, Post et al 1998).

Normality, independence and quality of life: taking a sceptical approach

In taking a sceptical approach to the assumption that normality and physical independence are legitimate preoccupations for the occupational therapist, one might query: Whose values do these goals reflect? Should occupational therapists be encouraging disabled people to conform to the norms of the dominant population or assisting disabled people to attain the rights and opportunities reserved for those deemed normal? Should occupational therapists strive to enhance people's physical independence, or their ability to make decisions and enact choices?

The nature of occupation

Occupational therapists hold many assumptions about occupation. Indeed, these are core assumptions that constitute our profession's raison d'être. Further, 'occupational therapy's staunchest proponents have imbued occupation with a universal quality that makes it and its profound beneficial meanings seem appropriate and applicable to all people, irrespective of culture' (Iwama 2004, p. 3). Because we are committed in this chapter to challenging the beliefs and assumptions inherent in our field, to raising

questions, confronting dogma, unmasking conventional and accepted ideas, taking nothing for granted and being unwilling to let received ideas steer us along (Said 1996), let us take a sceptical approach to some of these core assumptions.

We can influence our health by hands and willpower

One of occupational therapy's most frequently cited gems of received wisdom is Reilly's (1962, p. 2) claim that 'man, through the use of his [sic] hands as energized by mind and will, can influence the state of his own health'. The word *ableism* springs to mind here, being a term that refers both to the assumption that everyone's abilities match certain ideological norms, and the consequent social practices that presume and privilege able-bodiedness. The assumption that everyone can use their hands if they have the mind and will neatly encapsulates ableism: the conjecture that everyone has hands and the ability to use them if they so desire.

Even if we speculate that Reilly used 'hands' as a metaphor for 'abilities,' there remains a problem with the assumption that all people have the opportunity to engage in life-enhancing occupations, and, indeed, that occupations are inherently life-enhancing. Most of the world's population has little or no choice, control or opportunity to exercise will, and their daily occupations are associated with unremitting drudgery, high risks of injury, illness and premature death (Mocellin 1995).

Work is supportive of health

The assumption that engagement in occupation positively influences health is easily subsumed under a political ideology that values *work* above every other form of human endeavour. Indeed, paid work has long been viewed as a measure of rehabilitation success. Yerxa (1998, pp. 416–417) asserted that 'work is supportive of health even under poor conditions': a naïve belief that betrays its roots in middle-class, minority world culture and that overlooks the political and economic factors shaping the lives of the majority of people. Moreover, even in the affluent West, the assumption that paid employment contributes positively to health is declared to be fraudulent, camouflaging the stress, depression and despair experienced by many caught up in a work culture they equate to 'enslavement' (Bunting 2004). Further, engagement in work such as prostitution does not contribute to either health or well-being. The reality that almost 20% of British workers claim their work is very or extremely stressful is leading to a 'crisis in human sustainability' (Bunting 2004, p. 178) wherein workers are unable to invest time and energy in human relationships, community, or political activities.

The associated assumption – that 'unemployment' is inherently problematic (e.g. Yerxa 1998) – is contested by Mocellin (1996, p. 14) who reiterates the observation that 'the problem of the unemployed is not that they are "idle" but that they are poor'. Although eagerly promoting political ideologies that glorify paid labour, the occupational therapy profession has paid little attention to the occupational needs of those mired in poverty; many of whom are also in (poorly) paid employment.

When the occupational therapy profession promotes work as the consummate form of occupation we collude with specific political ideologies and with a consumer culture that encourages us to earn more money so we can acquire more stuff. While the opportunity to work should be a right afforded to everyone, it should not be imposed by occupational therapists as an objective for everyone (Ville & Ravaud 1996). It seems plausible that our health is impacted by those occupations in which we engage, but a sceptical approach demands caution against accepting conventional ideas that mask specific political ideologies and that reflect minority world, middle-class values.

Humans participate in occupations as autonomous agents

Yerxa (1992, p. 79) claimed that each individual is 'active, capable, free, self-directed, integrated, purposeful, and an agent who is the author of health-influencing activity'. The claim that 'humans participate in occupations as autonomous agents' is reiterated by Townsend and Wilcock (2003, pp. 253, 255) and may, indeed, be a reality for those humans whose occupations are not constrained on the basis of gender, class, caste, race, religion, education, ethnicity, culture, geographic location, or other axes of difference or power. However, the claim has no basis in reality for women incarcerated in brothels; for disabled and elderly people confined in institutions; for those whose caste dictates engagement in specific, degrading occupations; for refugees, or those enduring conditions of slavery, for example. Moreover, the implicit value placed on autonomy

tacitly advances an individualist ideology that is considered normal, indeed admirable, in Western culture but that is not universally shared (Iwama 2006).

Occupations are goal-directed and socially sanctioned

Received wisdom informs us that occupation constitutes those pursuits that are 'goal-directed (purposeful), and socially-sanctioned' (Yerxa et al 1989, p. 5). This implies that productivity is somehow more valuable and important than activities pertaining to leisure or self-care (Suto 1998). Disability theorists claim that by prioritising productive activities, those that contribute to the social and economic fabric of communities (Canadian Association of Occupational Therapists 2002, Townsend & Polatajko 2007), occupational therapists again act as agents of the State, actively perpetuating ideologies that celebrate status and materialism, denigrating those deemed 'dependent' or 'unproductive,' and reinforcing the economic and social status quo (French & Swain 2001).

The definition of occupation embraced by occupational scientists invokes a manner of being occupied that is socially valued. Darnell (2002) contends that this is problematic and ethnocentric, reflecting specific cultural values derived from a particular Western European social, political and economic system. Further, the assumption that occupations ought to be socially sanctioned is contested by disability theorists who have unmasked rehabilitation's political role in reinforcing the demands of social conformity and a consumer economy (Imrie 1997, Stiker 1999). Moreover, occupational therapists' preoccupation with *doing* socially sanctioned activities is rendered problematic by researchers who have found that an important component of living well with a serious illness or impairment lies, not in doing goal-directed, purposeful activities that require social sanction, but in taking time to be contemplative, appreciate nature and enjoy being with special people (e.g. Berterö & Ek 1993, Bloom 2001, Hammell 2004a).

Productive occupations contribute to life's meaning

Part of the conventional dogma perpetuated within occupational therapy states that productive occupations – those that contribute to the social and economic fabric of communities (Canadian Association of Occupational Therapists 2002, Townsend & Polatajko 2007) – contribute to life's meaning. And work may, indeed, be an indispensable component of life's meaning for those whose jobs are safe, rewarding and well-paid. Bauman (1998, p. 34) observed that work that is rich in gratifying experiences such as self-fulfilment, meaning, pride and self-esteem is 'the privilege of the few, a distinctive mark of the elite'. Indeed, the assumption that occupation 'enables the expression and management of self-identity' (Canadian Association of Occupational Therapists 2002, p. 35) reflects the values of a global minority. Moreover, when paid work is promoted as the route to self-respect and social acceptance, this implicitly undermines the value of unpaid work, such as volunteerism and the care of others (Bunting 2004).

The doctrine, promoted by occupational therapists, that work is an essential source of status, social hierarchy, satisfaction, value and identity, emerged only recently in Western culture and is already collapsing (Ville & Winance 2006). Eastern modes of thought (Kupperman 2001) and research findings (Kelly & Kelly 1994) demonstrate that work is not universally perceived to be central to life's meaning, or to contribute to life satisfaction (Clayton & Chubon 1994, Ville & Ravaud 1996).

Occupations enable economic self-sufficiency

It is claimed that engagement in occupation 'enables humans to be economically self-sufficient' (Yerxa et al 1989, p. 5). This assumption neatly side-steps the global reality that economic self-sufficiency is not guaranteed to all those who work. Indeed, the majority of the global population toil from childhood to death in conditions of unrelenting poverty.

Occupations are divisible into categories

A common assumption is that occupations can be divided into categories such as self-care, productivity and leisure (Canadian Association of Occupational Therapists 2002, Townsend & Polatajko 2007) or self-maintenance, work, leisure, and play (American Occupational Therapy Association 1995). Indeed, the Canadian Association of Occupational Therapists (2002) claims that self-care, productivity, and leisure are the 'purposes' of

occupation. The typical ordering of these categories is neither random nor alphabetical (Suto 2004), but a reflection of the values and priorities of physically independent, employed theorists (Hammell 2004a). Moreover, the assumption that leisure and work are divisible is culturally specific (Darnell 2002, Primeau 1996) and alien to members of simple societies (Horna 1994, Storman 1989) and farming communities. Indeed, many members of the global population lack a word to describe the concept of 'leisure' (Kelly & Kelly 1994).

The decision to list and prioritise particular categories of occupation reflects a specific, minority-world 'doctrine of individualism' (Young 2003) that specifically excludes those activities motivated by love and concern for the well-being of others. It is obvious, for example, that care of others cannot be made to fit any of the three privileged categories because these are not *self*-maintenance activities, nor are they socially or economically productive, or experienced as leisure. Rather, they are an expression through occupation (time, energy, interest) of a sense of connectedness to others (Hammell 2004e): the precise sort of inter-dependence that correlates highly with quality of life, but that is denigrated by rehabilitation's fixation with independence.

Occupation is, perhaps, most usefully defined as being anything that people do in their daily lives (McColl et al 1992): a definition that does not privilege 'occupations' over 'activities' (as advocates of taxonomic codes propose) (e.g. Townsend & Polatajko 2007) nor preclude those activities such as meditation, grooming a horse, feeding an ill parent or rocking a baby that are not concerned with care of the self, are not productive (contributing to the social and economic fabric of communities) (Canadian Association of Occupational Therapists 2002, Townsend & Polatajko 2007) or consistently experienced as leisure.

A balance of occupations is beneficial to health and well-being

'One of the most widely cited philosophical beliefs in occupational therapy is that a balance of occupations is beneficial to health and well-being' (Christiansen 1996, p. 432). Although this assumption may be valid, it is unsubstantiated by research (Christiansen & Baum 1997), 'fails to define work, leisure, or what constitutes a balance; does not specify the aspects of health that are promoted; and is not seriously subjected to the possibility of disconfirmation' (Clark et al 1991, p. 306).

The idea that occupational therapists can classify an individual's daily patterns of activity and judge whether an occupational balance exists is inherently problematic. Due to age, culture, socioeconomic status, or lifestyle, the same occupation may be experienced by some people as leisure and by others as productive (or work). Moreover, people define their occupations differently at different times, dependent upon such factors as their mood and goals, the context and the presence of other people (Canadian Association of Occupational Therapists 2002, Primeau 1996, Shaw 1984), making it impossible to classify someone else's occupations. In addition, the assumption that occupational therapists are able to determine occupational imbalance among people whose time use reflects values that differ from their own is clearly contentious (Hammell 2004e). Finally, because there is little agreement on what constitutes 'leisure' (Primeau 1996) and evidence that the concept of leisure is an ableist (Aitchison 2003) and class-bound concept (Suto 2004) that is alien to many members of the global population (Kelly & Kelly 1994), how might a balance of leisure time be judged?

Individuals interact with the environment through occupation

The Model of Human Occupation (Kielhofner & Forsyth 1997), the Canadian Model of Occupational Performance and Engagement (Canadian Association of Occupational Therapists 2002, Townsend & Polatajko 2007) and the Person-Environment-Occupation Model (Law et al 1996) share an assumption that individuals interact and engage with, but are divisible from, their environments. This assumption reflects specific, minority-world perspectives. Eastern ways of thinking understand the individual to be inseparable from the environment, perceiving the indivisibility, interconnectedness and 'oneness' of all life (Chuang 1964, Kupperman 2001). Thus, humans do not engage with the environment through occupation because they are already inseparable from the environment (Iwama 2005b).

Humans need to master the environment

An associated assumption is that 'humans have a drive for efficacy: a biologically driven need to act on the environment' (Yerxa et al 1989, p. 7). Indeed, humans are believed to have an innate urge to achieve *mastery* over the environment (Kielhofner & Burke 1980). Expanding this theme even further, Wilcock (1993, p. 20) claimed that one of the major functions of occupation is to 'develop skills, social structures and technology aimed at superiority over[…]the environment'. The assumption that humans are entitled to dominion over the world – to rule over the Earth, dominate and subdue it – and, thus, have an innate need for mastery over their environment is specific to Judeo-Christian belief systems, derived from Genesis (Iwama 2005b, Steger 2003) and is alien to those societies who value living in balance and harmony within the environment (Iwama 2006). Among all the assumptions highlighted in this chapter, this is the one most in need of critical interrogation.

Because occupational therapists assert that the environment has social, cultural, political, legal, and economic, as well as physical, dimensions (Canadian Association of Occupational Therapy 2002), what are the implications of extolling superiority and mastery over the environment? Domestic abuse, for example, reflects, in part, a perceived entitlement to exert mastery and superiority over one's domestic social environment. Indeed, 'mastery' is a transparently patriarchal term, derived from 'master': a man who has control of people or things. The urge to exert superiority is manifest in humans' willingness to exploit inequities of wealth and power to enslave, prostitute and exploit other humans (i.e. members of their global social environment) (Mocellin 1995).

And what of the physical environment? Currently, 20% of the global population exploit (master and control) 86% of the world's resources. Indeed, the United States, with just 6% of the world's population consumes between 30 and 40% of the planet's natural resources (Steger 2003). This is not only detrimental to the well-being and sustainability of the world's poorest people but is environmentally unsustainable. Human mastery over the environment has caused cataclysmic environmental degradation, including global warming, polluted waterways, massive deforestation, depleted oceans, and a loss of biodiversity (Steger 2003).

In taking a sceptical stance towards the assumption that an entitlement to superiority, mastery, and control over the environment is not only innate, but worthy of facilitation by occupational therapists, we should recognise that this assumption reflects unchallenged cultural values of materialist capitalism and globalisation that are not only exploitative, but unsustainable.

Assumptions informing occupational therapy: taking a sceptical approach

Earlier, I cited the claim that a truly 'scientific' discipline is one that assures 'a culture of healthy scepticism: a readiness to doubt claims and assumptions about the 'rightness' of any particular theory or intervention' (Brechin & Sidell 2000, p. 12). I hope that the critiques sketched in this chapter will have underscored the importance to occupational therapy of a culture of healthy scepticism and will have raised doubts about the 'rightness' of the assumptions that occupational therapists tend to take for granted. Importantly, these assumptions have neither been negated nor 'disproved'. Indeed, much of what we believe about our theories and practices may be justifiable. However, fostering a culture of healthy scepticism within our profession will enable us to challenge the veracity of our assumptions, contest the universality of their application and insist on a supportive evidence base derived from a broad range of perspectives. It will help us to make our practice less ethnocentric, more evidence-based and more relevant, not just for disabled people, but for all those who are denied their right to engage in meaningful occupations.

Occupational rights: occupation, health and well-being

Let us pause and ponder: what lies at the core of occupational therapy? Clearly, it is the belief 'that there is a relationship between occupation, health and well-being, [although] there is little evidence in the occupational therapy literature to support this belief' (Law et al 1998). Moreover, we are currently unable to say with any certainty which dimensions of health are influenced, by which forms of occupation, in which circumstances, by which people and in which phases of their lives. Rather than focusing solely on ill and impaired health (and remaining stranded in the health-care system), Watson (2004) proposes that occupational therapists should be promoting *well-being*. Indeed, it is claimed that 'the

ultimate goal of occupational therapy services is wellbeing, not health' (Christiansen 1999, p. 547). This requires that we also ponder: if engagement in occupation influences human well-being, why are occupational therapists so preoccupied with 'physical dysfunction?' Why is it that we are not concerned about the well-being of all people? Clearly, an exclusive focus on specific individuals is inadequate and 'occupational therapists could and should be working towards the improvement of quality of life for populations of people who would benefit from improved participation in meaningful occupations' (Watson 2004, p. 62).

Hasselkus (2004, p. xv) claimed that 'the focus of occupational therapy needs to be on the *right* of all people to occupational engagement and enrichment'. The principle of *occupational rights* (Hammell 2008) – the right of all people to engage in meaningful occupations that contribute positively to their own well-being and the well-being of their communities – might provide a useful cornerstone for the future practice of occupational therapy.

Human rights, occupational rights and well-being

It is claimed that occupational therapists need to acknowledge the relationship between human rights and health (Watson & Fourie 2004). *Human rights* are 'a set of principles based on social justice; a standard by which the conditions and opportunities of human life can be evaluated' (Armstrong & Barton 1999, p. 211). The concept of human rights centres on two essential elements: freedom and well-being. *Freedom* – 'the right of every human being to participate in the shaping of decisions affecting their own life and that of their society' (Kallen 2004, p. 15) – is directly linked to our ethical principle of autonomy (Jonsen et al 1998) and of person-centred practice. *Well-being* refers to a state of overall contentment with one's physical/mental health, self-esteem, sense of belonging, personal and economic security, and opportunities for self-determination and meaningful occupation (Hay et al 1993, Wilcock et al 1998). Definitions of well-being abound, but Hay et al (1993, p. 5) suggest a definition that parallels the themes identified within this chapter: 'Well-being is the pursuit of personal aspirations and the development and exercise of human capabilities, within a context of mutual recognition, equality, and interdependence'. The idea of interdependence is important because 'the universality of human rights requires that each person act with due regard for other persons' freedom and well-being as well as her [sic] own (Honderich 1995, p. 776). Well-being is not an individualistic, egocentric issue, but one of collective care and mutual responsibility.

Because well-being is unattainable in conditions of oppression and poverty, well-being is clearly a political notion and a matter of social and distributive justice (Hay et al 1993, Honderich 1995). It is because human health and well-being are impacted by the occupations in which we are able, or compelled, to engage that occupational rights are associated with human rights.

Clearly, the idea of *occupational rights* is closely associated with that of *occupational justice*: 'equitable opportunity and resources to enable people's engagement in meaningful occupations' (Wilcock & Townsend 2000, p. 85). This requires our profession's political engagement with those issues that impact people's equitable opportunity to participate in occupations that influence individual and community well-being, such as literacy, education, poverty, exploitation and marginalisation.

If we agree with the premise that 'the focus of occupational therapy needs to be on the *right* of all people to occupational engagement and enrichment' (Hasselkus 2004, p. iii), many of the assumptions outlined in this chapter are not just unsubstantiated, but irrelevant.

Values, knowledge and skills in occupational-therapy practice

The sceptical approach to dogma articulated in this chapter suggests that occupational therapy's assumptions reflect, not universal 'truths', but the specific value-system of an élite group of people in the minority world, and of the political, social and economic environment in which they are encultured. These assumptions pervade what we consider to be the 'knowledge' of our profession and inform our approach to practice. If occupational therapy aspires to be an accountable, competent, evidence-based profession we have to challenge our beliefs and assumptions, raise questions, confront dogma, unmask conventional and accepted ideas, take nothing for granted and be unwilling to let received ideas steer us along (Said 1996). We cannot be smug or complacent. And we need to assert that occupational therapists have a far larger role to play in supporting human well-being than our traditional niche as 'extras' in the health-care system.

References

Abberley, P. (1995). Disabling ideology in health and welfare: the case of occupational therapy. *Disability and Society*, 10(2), 221–232.

Abberley, P. (2004). A critique of professional support and intervention. In: J. Swain, S. French, C. Barnes, & C. Thomas (Eds.). *Disabling barriers – enabling environments* (2nd edn). London, Sage, pp. 239–244.

Aitchison, C. (2003). From leisure and disability to disability leisure: developing data, definitions and discourses. *Disability and Society*, 18, 955–969.

American Occupational Therapy Association (1995). Position paper: occupation. *American Journal of Occupational Therapy*, 49, 1015–1018.

American Occupational Therapy Association (2000). Code of ethics. *www.aota.org/*.

American Occupational Therapy Association (2002). Occupational therapy practice framework: domain and process. *American Journal of Occupational Therapy*, 56(6), 609–639.

Anson, C. A., Stanwyck, D. J. & Krause, J. S. (1993). Social support and health status in spinal cord injury. *Paraplegia*, 31, 632–638.

Armstrong. F. & Barton, L. (1999). 'Is there anyone there concerned with human rights?' Cross-cultural connections, disability and the struggle for change in England. In: F. Armstrong, & L. Barton (Eds). *Disability, human rights and education. Cross-cultural perspectives*. Buckingham, Open University Press, pp. 210–229.

Barbara, A. & Curtin, M. (2008). Gatekeepers or advocates? Occupational therapists and equipment funding schemes. *Australian Occupational Therapy Journal*, 55, 1, 57–60.

Barnes, C. (2003). Review of: T. B. Ustun et al. (Eds). Disability and culture: universalism and diversity. Hogrefe & Huber, Seattle on behalf of the WHO. *Disability and Society*, 18(6), 827–833.

Barnes, C. & Mercer, G. (2003). *Disability*. Cambridge, Polity.

Bauman, Z. (1998). *Work, consumerism, and the new poor*. Buckingham, Open University Press, pp. 34.

Baylies, C. (2002). Disability and the notion of human development: questions of rights and capabilities. *Disability and Society*, 17(7), 725–739.

Berterö, C. & Ek, A–C. (1993). Quality of life of adults with acute leukaemia. *Journal of Advanced Nursing*, 18, 1346–1353.

Bloom, F. R. (2001). 'New beginnings': A case study in gay men's changing perceptions of quality of life during the course of HIV infection. *Medical Anthropology Quarterly*, 15, 38–57.

Bozalek, V. (2000). Feminist postmodernism in the South African context. In: B. Fawcett, B. Featherstone, J. Fook, & A. Rossiter (Eds). *Practice and research in social work. Postmodern feminist perspectives*. London, Routledge, pp. 176–191.

Brechin, A. & Sidell, M. (2000). Ways of knowing. In: R. Gomm, C. Davies (Eds). *Using evidence in health and social care*. London, Sage, pp. 3–25.

Bunting, M. (2004). *Willing slaves. How the overwork culture is ruling our lives*. London, Harper-Collins.

Canadian Association of Occupational Therapists (CAOT) & the Health Services Directorate (1983). *Guidelines for the client-centred practice of occupational therapy*. Ottawa, Health Services Directorate.

Canadian Association of Occupational Therapists: CAOT (2002). *Enabling occupation. An occupational therapy perspective*. (2nd edn). Ottawa, Canadian Association of Occupational Therapists.

Childs, P. & Williams, P. (1997). *An introduction to post-colonial theory*. London, Prentice-Hall.

Christiansen, C. (1996). Three perspectives on balance in occupation. In: R. Zemke, & F. Clark (Eds.). *Occupational Science: the evolving discipline*. Philadelphia, FA Davis, pp. 431–451.

Christiansen, C. (1999). Defining lives: Occupation as identity: An essay on competence, coherence, and the creation of meaning. *American Journal of Occupational Therapy*, 53, 547–558.

Christiansen, C. & Baum, C. (1997). *Occupational therapy: Enabling function and wellbeing*. Thorofare, NJ, Slack.

Chuang, Tzu. (1964). *Basic writings*. (Trans. B. Watson). New York, Columbia University Press.

Clare, E. (1999). *Exile and pride. Disability, queerness and liberation*. Cambridge, Mass, South End Press.

Clark, F., Parham, D. & Carlson, M. et al. (1991). Occupational science: academic innovation in the service of occupational therapy's future. *American Journal of Occupational Therapy*, 45, 300–310.

Clayton, K. S. & Chubon, R. A. (1994). Factors associated with the quality of life of long-term spinal cord injured persons. *Archives of Physical Medicine and Rehabilitation*, 75, 633–638.

Coleridge, P. (1999). Development, cultural values and disability: the example of Afghanistan. In: E. Stone (Ed.). *Disability and development*. Leeds, Disability Press, pp. 149–167.

College of Occupational Therapists (COT) (2000). *Code of ethics and professional conduct for occupational therapists*. London, Author.

College of Occupational Therapists (COT) (2001). Code of ethics and professional conduct for occupational therapists. *British Journal of Occupational Therapy*, 64(12), 612–617.

College of Occupational Therapists (COT) (2005). Code of ethics and professional conduct for occupational therapists. *British Journal of Occupational Therapy*, 68(11), 527–532.

Corbett, J. (1997). Independent, proud and special: calibrating our differences. In: L. Barton, & M. Oliver (Eds). *Disability studies: Past, present and future*. Leeds, The Disability Press, pp. 90–98.

Cornielje, H. & Ferrinho, P. (1999). The sociopolitical context of CBR developments in South Africa. In: R. L. Leavitt (Ed.). *Cross-cultural rehabilitation. An international perspective*. London, WB Saunders, pp. 217–226.

Darnell, R. (2002). Occupation is not a cross-cultural universal: Some reflections from an ethnographer. *Journal of Occupational Science*, 9(1), 5–11.

Davis, K. (1993). The crafting of good clients. In: J. Swain, V. Finkelstein, S. French, & M. Oliver (Eds). *Disabling barriers – enabling environments*. London, Sage, pp. 197–200.

Douard, J. W. (1995). Disability and the persistence of the 'normal,' In: S. K. Toombs, D. Barnard, & R. A.

Carson (Eds). *Chronic illness. From experience to policy*. Bloomington, Ind, Indiana University Press, pp. 154–175.

Duncan, E. A. S., Paley, J. & Eva, G. (2007). Complex interventions and complex systems in occupational therapy: an alternative perspective. *British Journal of Occupational Therapy*, 70(5), 199–206.

Elliott, L. (2006). Sinking into 'ecological debt'. *Guardian Weekly*, April 21–27, p. 27.

French, S. (1994). The disabled role. In: S. French (Ed.). *On equal terms. Working with disabled people*. Oxford, Butterworth Heinemann, pp. 47–60.

French, S. (2004). Reflecting on ethical decision-making in therapy practice. In: J. Swain, J. Clark, K. Parry, S. French, & F. Reynolds. *Enabling relationships in health and social care*. Oxford, Butterworth-Heinemann, pp. 29–43.

French, S. & Swain, J. (2001). The relationship between disabled people and health and welfare professionals. In: G. L. Albrecht, K. D. Seelman, & M. Bury (Eds). *Handbook of disability studies*. London, Sage, pp. 734–753.

Hammell, K. W. (2004a). Using qualitative evidence to inform theories of occupation. In: K. W. Hammell, & C. Carpenter (Eds). *Qualitative research in evidence-based rehabilitation*. Edinburgh, Churchill Livingstone, pp. 14–26.

Hammell, K. W. (2004b). Deviating from the norm: A sceptical interrogation of the ICF. *British Journal of Occupational Therapy*, 67(9), 408–411.

Hammell, K. W. (2004c). The rehabilitation process. In: M. Stokes (Ed.). *Physical management in neurological rehabilitation*, (2nd ed). Edinburgh, Elsevier, pp. 379–392.

Hammell, K. W. (2004d). Exploring quality of life following high spinal cord injury: a review and critique. *Spinal Cord*, 42(9), 491–502.

Hammell, K. W. (2004e). Dimensions of meaning in the occupations of daily life. *Canadian Journal of Occupational Therapy*, 71(5), 296–305.

Hammell, K. W. (2006). *Perspectives on disability and rehabilitation*.

Edinburgh, Churchill Livingstone Elsevier.

Hammell, K. W. (2007). Client-centred practice: Ethical obligation or professional obfuscation? *British Journal of Occupational Therapy*, 70(6), 264–266.

Hammell, K. W. (2008). Reflections on ... well-being and occupational rights. *Canadian Journal of Occupational Therapy*, 75(1), 61–64.

Hartkopp, A., Brønnum-Hansen, H., Seidenschnur, A.-M. & Biering-Sørensen, F. (1998). Suicide in a spinal cord injured population: its relation to functional status. *Archives of Physical Medicine and Rehabilitation*, 79(11), 1356–1361.

Hasselkus, B. R. (2004). Foreword. In: R. Watson, & L. Swartz (Eds). *Transformation through occupation*. London, Whurr, pp. xiii–xv.

Hay, D., Clague, M., Goldberg, M. et al. (1993). *Well-being: a conceptual framework and three literature reviews*. Vancouver, BC, SPARC of BC.

Holcomb, L. O. (2000). Community reintegration and chronic spinal cord injury. *SCI Nursing*, 17(2), 52–58.

Honderich, T. (Ed.). (1995). *The Oxford Companion to Philosophy*. Oxford, Oxford University Press.

Horna, J. (1994). *The study of leisure*. Toronto, Oxford University Press.

Imrie, R. (1997). Rethinking the relationships between disability, rehabilitation and society. *Disability and Rehabilitation*, 19(7), 263–271.

Iwama, M. K. (2004). Revisiting culture in occupational therapy: A meaningful endeavour. *OTJR: Occupation, Participation and Health* 24(1), 2–3.

Iwama, M. K. (2005a). Occupation as a cross-cultural construct. In: G. Whiteford, & V. Wright–St. Clair (Eds). *Occupation and practice in context*. Marrickville, NSW, Elsevier, pp. 242–253.

Iwama, M. K. (2005b). Situated meaning. An issue of culture, inclusion and occupational therapy. In: F. Kronenberg, S. S. Algado, & N. Pollard (Eds). *Occupational therapy without borders*. Edinburgh, Churchill Livingstone Elsevier, pp. 127–139.

Iwama, M. K. (2006). The *Kawa* (River) Model: Client centred rehabilitation in cultural context. In: S. Davis (Ed.). *Rehabilitation: The use of theories and models in practice*. Edinburgh, Churchill Livingstone, Elsevier, pp. 147–168.

Johnston, M. & Miklos, C. (2002). Activity-related quality of life in rehabilitation and traumatic brain injury. *Archives of Physical Medicine and Rehabilitation*, 83(Supp 2), S26–S38.

Jonsen, A. R., Siegler, M. & Winslade, W. (1998). *Clinical ethics*. (4th ed.) New York, McGraw Hill.

Kallen, E. (2004). *Social inequality and social justice. A human rights perspective*. Basingstoke, Palgrave.

Katbamna, S., Bhakta, P. & Parker, G. (2000). Perceptions of disability and care-giving relationships in South Asian communities. In: W. I. V. Ahmad (Ed.). *Ethnicity, disability and chronic illness*. Buckingham, Open University Press, pp. 12–27.

Kelly, J. R. & Kelly, J. R. (1994). Multiple dimensions of meaning in the domains of work, family and leisure. *Journal of Leisure Research*, 26, 250–274.

Kemp, L. (2002). Why are some people's needs unmet? *Disability and Society*, 17(2), 205–218.

Kielhofner, G. (2004). *Conceptual foundations of occupational therapy*, (3rd ed). Philadelphia, FA Davis.

Kielhofner, G. & Burke, J. P. (1980). A Model of Human Occupation, Part I. Conceptual framework and content. *American Journal of Occupational Therapy*, 34(9), 572–581.

Kielhofner, G. & Forsyth, K. (1997). The Model of Human Occupation: an overview of current concepts. *British Journal of Occupational Therapy*, 60, 103–110.

Krause, J. S., Coker, J., Charlifue, S. & Whiteneck, G. (2000). Health outcomes among American Indians with spinal cord injury. *Archives of Physical Medicine and Rehabilitation*, 81(7), 924–931.

Kronenberg, F., Algado, S. S. & Pollard, N. (2005). Preface. In: F. Kronenberg, S. S. Algado, & N. Pollard (Eds.). *Occupational therapy without borders*. Edinburgh,

Churchill Livingstone, Elsevier, pp. xv–xvii.

Kupperman, J. J. (2001). *Classic Asian philosophy*. Oxford, Oxford University Press.

Law, M. (1993). Evaluating activities of daily living: directions for the future. *American Journal of Occupational Therapy*, 47(3), 233–237.

Law, M., Cooper, B., Strong, S., Stewart, D., Rigby, P. & Letts, L. (1996). The Person-Environment-Occupation Model: A transactive approach to occupational performance. *Canadian Journal of Occupational Therapy*, 63, 9–23.

Law, M., Steinwender, S. & Leclair, L. (1998). Occupation, health and well-being. *Canadian Journal of Occupational Therapy*, 65(2), 81–91.

Leavitt, R. L. (1999). Moving rehabilitation professionals toward cultural competence: strategies for change. In: R. L. Leavitt (Ed.). *Cross-cultural rehabilitation. An international perspective*. London, WB Saunders, pp. 375–385.

Lim, K. H. (2004). Occupational therapy in multicultural contexts. Letter to the editor. *British Journal of Occupational Therapy*, 67, 49–50.

Lyons, M., Orozovic, N., Davis, J. & Newman, J. (2002). Doing-being-becoming: Occupational experiences of persons with life-threatening illnesses. *American Journal of Occupational Therapy*, 56, 285–295.

McColl, M. A., Law, M. & Stewart, D. (1992). *Theoretical basis of occupational therapy*. Thorofare, NJ, Slack Inc.

McKinnon, A. L. (2000). Client values and satisfaction with occupational therapy. *Scandinavian Journal of Occupational Therapy*, 7, 99–106.

McKnight, J. (1981). Professionalised service and disabling help. In: A. Brechin, P. Liddiard, & J. Swain (Eds). *Handicap in a social world*. Sevenoaks, Hodder & Stoughton, pp. 24–33.

Marks, D. (1999). *Disability. Controversial debates and psychosocial perspectives*. London, Routledge.

Meekosha, H. (1998). Body battles: bodies, gender and disability. In: T.

Shakespeare (Ed.). *The disability reader: Social science perspectives*. London, Cassell, pp. 163–180.

Middleton, L. (1999). *Disabled children: challenging social exclusion*. Oxford, Blackwell.

Miller, P., Parker, S. & Gillinson, S. (2004). *Disabilism. How to tackle the last prejudice*. London, Demos.

Moats, G. (2007). Discharge decision-making, enabling occupations, and client-centred practice. *Canadian Journal of Occupational Therapy*, 74(2), 91–101.

Mocellin, G. (1995). Occupational therapy: A critical overview, Part 1. *British Journal of Occupational Therapy*, 58, 502–506.

Mocellin, G. (1996). Occupational therapy: A critical overview, Part 2. *British Journal of Occupational Therapy*, 59, 11–16.

Oliver, M. (1996). *Understanding Disability. From theory to practice*. Basingstoke, Macmillan.

Penn, H. (1999). Children in the majority world: is outer Mongolia really so far away? In: S. Hood, B. Mayall & S. Oliver (Eds). *Critical issues in social research. Power and prejudice*. Buckingham, Open University Press, pp. 25–39.

Pfeiffer, D. (2000). The devils are in the details: the ICIDH2 and the disability movement. *Disability and Society*, 15(7), 1079–1082.

Post, M., de Witte, L., van Asbek, F., van Dijk, A. & Schrijvers, A. (1998). Predictors of health status and life satisfaction in spinal cord injury. *Archives of Physical Medicine and Rehabilitation*, 78(4), 395–402.

Priestley, M. (2003). *Disability. A life course approach*. Cambridge, Polity.

Primeau, L. (1996). Work and leisure: transcending the dichotomy. *American Journal of Occupational Therapy*, 50, 569–577.

Rebeiro, K. L., Day, D., Semeniuk, B., O'Brien, M. & Wilson, B. (2001). Northern Initiative for Social Action: An occupation-based mental health program. *American Journal of Occupational Therapy*, 55, 493–500.

Reilly, M. (1962). Occupational therapy can be one of the great ideas of 20th century medicine. *American Journal of Occupational Therapy*, 26, 1–9.

Reindal, S. M. (1999). Independence, dependence, interdependence: some reflections on the subject and personal autonomy. *Disability and Society*, 14(3), 353–367.

Richardson, M. (1997). Addressing barriers: disabled rights and the implications for nursing of the social construct of disability. *Journal of Advanced Nursing*, 25, 1269–1275.

Ruff, C. D. & Singer, B. (1998). The contours of positive human health. *Psychological Inquiry*, 9(1), 1–28.

Said, E. W. (1979). *Orientalism*. London, Routledge.

Said, E. W. (1996). *Representations of the intellectual*. New York, Random House.

Sandahl, C. (2003). Queering the crip or cripping the queer? In: R. McRuer, & A. L. Wilkerson (Eds). *Desiring disability: Queer theory meets disability studies*. Durham, NC, Duke University Press, pp. 25–56.

Schriner, K. (2001). A disability studies perspective on employment issues and policies for disabled people. In: G. L. Albrecht, K. D. Seelman, M. Bury (Eds). *Handbook of disability studies*. London, Sage, pp. 642–662.

Schwartz, C. E. & Sendor, M. (1999). Helping others helps oneself: response shift effects in peer support. *Social Science and Medicine*, 48, 1563–1575.

Shaw, S. M. (1984). The measurement of leisure: a quality of life issue. *Society and Leisure*, 7, 91–107.

Stalker, K. & Jones, C. (1998). Normalization and critical disability theory. In: D. Jones, S. Blair, T. Hartery, & R. Jones (Eds). *Sociology and occupational therapy: an integrated approach*. Edinburgh, Churchill Livingstone, pp. 171–183.

Steger, M. B. (2003). *Globalization*. Oxford, Oxford University Press.

Stewart, R. & Bhagwanjee, A. (1999). Promoting group empowerment and self-reliance through participatory research: a case study of people with physical disability. *Disability and Rehabilitation*, 21(7), 338–345.

Stiker, H.-J. (1999). *A history of disability*. (Trans. W. Sayers). Ann Arbor, University of Michigan Press.

Storman, W. (1989). Work: true leisure's home? *Leisure Studies*, 8, 25–33.

Suto, M. (1998). Leisure in occupational therapy. *Canadian Journal of Occupational Therapy*, 65, 271–278.

Suto, M. (2004). Exploring leisure meanings that inform client-centred practice. In: K. W. Hammell, & C. Carpenter (Eds). *Qualitative research in evidence-based rehabilitation*. Edinburgh, Churchill Livingstone, pp. 27–39.

Swartz, L. (2004). Rethinking professional ethics. In: R. Watson, & L. Swartz (Eds). *Transformation through occupation*. London, Whurr, pp. 289–300.

Swain, J., French, S. & Cameron, C. (2003). *Controversial issues in a disabling society*. Buckingham, Open University Press.

Taylor, G. (1999). Empowerment, identity and participatory research: using social action research to challenge isolation for deaf and hard of hearing people from minority ethnic communities. *Disability and Society*, 14(3), 369–384.

Thomson, R. G. (1997). *Extraordinary bodies: Figuring physical disability in American culture and literature*. New York, Columbia University Press.

Townsend, E. (1998). *Good intentions overruled. A critique of empowerment in the routine organization of mental health services*. Toronto, University of Toronto Press.

Townsend, E. A. & Polatajko, H. (2007). *Enabling occupation II: advancing an occupational therapy vision for health, well-being & justice through occupation*. Ottawa, ONT, CAOT Publications ACE.

Townsend, E. & Wilcock, A. (2003). Occupational justice. In: C. Christiansen & E. Townsend (Eds.). *Introduction to occupation: The art and science of living*. Thorofare, NJ, Prentice Hall, pp. 243–273.

Ville, I. & Ravaud, J.-F. (1996). Work, non-work and consequent satisfaction after spinal cord injury. *International Journal of Rehabilitation Research*, 19, 241–252.

Ville, I. & Winance, M. (2006). To work or not to work? The

occupational trajectories of wheelchair users. *Disability and Rehabilitation*, 28(7), 423–436.

Waldie, E. (2002). *Triumph of the challenged. Conversations with especially able people*. Ilminster, Somerset, Purple Field Press.

Walmsley, J. (1993). Contradictions in caring: reciprocity and interdependence. *Disability, Handicap and Society*, 8(2), 129–142.

Watson, R. (2004). A population approach to transformation. In: R. Watson, & L. Swartz (Eds). *Transformation through occupation*. London, Whurr, pp. 51–65.

Watson, R. & Fourie, M. (2004). International and African influences on occupational therapy. In: R. Watson & L. Swartz (Eds). *Transformation through occupation*. London, Whurr, pp. 33–50.

Whiteford, G. E. & Wilcock, A. A. (2000). Cultural relativism: occupation and independence reconsidered. *Canadian Journal of Occupational Therapy*, 67(5), 324–336.

Wilcock, A. A. (1993). A theory of the human need for occupation. *Occupational Science*, 1, 17–24.

Wilcock, A. A. & Townsend, E. (2000). Occupational justice. Occupational therapy interactive dialogue. *American Journal of Occupational Therapy*, 7(2), 84–86.

Wilcock, A. A., van der Arend, H. Darling K, et al. (1998). An exploratory study of people's perceptions and experiences of wellbeing. *British Journal of Occupational Therapy*, 61(2), 75–82.

Wirz, S. L. & Hartley, S. D. (1999). Challenges for Universities of the North interested in community based rehabilitation. In: E. Stone (Ed.). *Disability and development. Learning from action and research on disability in the majority world*. Leeds, Disability Press, pp. 89–106.

World Health Organisation (2001). *International Classification of Functioning, Disability and Health*. Geneva, World Health Organisation.

Yerxa, E. J. (1992). Some implications of occupational therapy's history for its epistemology, values and relation to medicine. *American Journal of Occupational Therapy*, 46(1), 79–83.

Yerxa, E. J. (1998). Health and the human spirit for occupation. *American Journal of Occupational Therapy*, 5, 412–418.

Yerxa, E. J. & Locker, S. (1990). Quality of time use by adults with spinal cord injuries. *American Journal of Occupational Therapy*, 44(4), 318–326.

Yerxa, E. J., Clark, F., Frank, G., Jackson, J., Parham, D., Pierce, D., Stein, C. & Zemke, R. (1989) An introduction to occupational science: A foundation for occupational therapy in the 21st century. *Occupational Therapy in Health Care*, 6, 1–17.

Young, R. J. C. (2003). *Postcolonialism*. Oxford, Oxford University Press.

Section **Two**

An overview of occupational therapy practice

5

Occupational reasoning

Joan C. Rogers

CHAPTER CONTENTS

The case method 58

Conceptual frameworks for occupational
performance and engagement 58

Phases of the occupational therapy
process 59

    Assessment 59

    Diagnosis 60

    Intervention 61

    Re-assessment 61

Occupational reasoning strategies 61

    Comparative analysis 62

    Hypothesising 63

    Conditional reasoning 63

    Inferential reasoning 63

    Argumentative reasoning 64

    Reframing 64

    Evidence-based reasoning 64

    Application of strategies 64

Sharpening occupational reasoning 64

Conclusion 65

SUMMARY

As humans, it is our nature to think. Our thinking
may be based on information or beliefs; it may
be reality-based or distorted; it may be culturally
appropriate or prejudicial. As occupational
therapy students, we learn a systematic method
of thinking to ensure quality thinking in regard to
assessment and intervention. We call this
thinking *occupational reasoning*. As therapists,
we refine our occupational reasoning so that
quality decisions are made expeditiously. This
chapter explores occupational reasoning. The
case method is introduced to establish the need
for a systematic method of thinking. Then, the
role of a conceptual framework in transforming
the case method to the occupational therapy
process is presented. Thinking strategies that are
used throughout the occupational therapy
process are described: comparative analysis,
hypothesising, conditional reasoning, inferential
reasoning, argumentative reasoning, reframing,
and evidence-based reasoning. The chapter
concludes with suggestions for students and
therapists to improve their occupational
reasoning.

KEY POINTS

- Occupational reasoning is a systematic method
  of thinking about the occupational performance
  and engagement of humans that supports the
  occupational therapy process.
- From an historical perspective, the addition of
  occupational reasoning into the thinking patterns
  of occupational therapists enhanced
  occupational therapy's professionalism and
  autonomy.
- Each phase of the occupational therapy process
  involves multiple reasoning strategies to make
  decisions about assessment, diagnosis,
  intervention, and re-assessment.
- Common reasoning strategies used by
  therapists are: comparing clients to textbook or
  real people, explaining facts through
  hypothesising, linking antecedents (ifs) with

consequences (thens), projecting beyond the facts, debating all facets, re-interpreting and applying research findings to individual clients.

- To improve their occupational reasoning, students and therapists may 'think aloud' about what they are doing and why and share this thinking with more experienced therapists.

The case method

In 1969, Line challenged occupational therapists to discard their old ways of clinical thinking and embrace the case method, a scientific form of reasoning. The 'old ways of thinking' Line alluded to were: (1) physician prescription of occupational therapy, in which physicians make decisions about occupational therapy goals and interventions; (2) standard operating procedures, which specify that all clients having a particular diagnosis receive a standard, predetermined treatment; and, (3) customary thinking, whereby clients are treated in a certain way because 'we have always done it this way'. These strategies limit the need for occupational therapists to think by allocating problem solving to prescriptions written by physicians or encoded in formal or informal traditions. By replacing prescribed thinking with the case method, occupational therapists assume responsibility for the thinking that guides their practice.

The case method provides a generic structure for professional thinking, and as such it supports the reasoning of many professions, including medicine and physical therapy. Each profession makes the process its own by the *concepts* it selects to think about in relation to clients and the *actions* it takes to benefit clients (Holm 1986). Physicians, for example, think about clients' medical status and prescribe medications, surgery, or psychotherapy. Physical therapists focus on clients' physical status and use exercise as their professional tool. Occupational therapists concentrate on occupational performance and engagement, and use daily occupations when working with clients. It is the interaction of occupational performance and engagement with the case method that results in the occupational therapy process and, in turn, it is occupational reasoning that underlies the occupational therapy process.

The case method provides a structure for problem-setting and problem-solving by organising information about individual clients and relating it to occupational therapy knowledge. It facilitates the process whereby therapists learn what they need to

know about clients to make informed decisions about the strategies that may assist the clients. This learning is accomplished collaboratively with clients in *four overlapping and interdependent phases*. First, therapists gather information about clients so that they can understand their clients' occupational challenges and what they might be able to do to assist them. Second, therapists organise and interpret the information gathered and diagnose problems. Third, therapists plan outcomes and actions to assist clients to achieve the outcomes. Fourth, therapists evaluate the actions taken to see if they accomplished the outcomes. These four phases are labelled assessment, diagnosis, intervention, and re-assessment, respectively, and comprise the occupational therapy process.

Conceptual frameworks for occupational performance and engagement

Each phase of the occupational therapy process is guided by the conceptual framework of occupational performance and engagement selected by the therapist. Application of an occupational therapy framework to the case method transforms into the occupational therapy process. Occupational therapy, like many professions, uses many conceptual frameworks. In this context, conceptual framework is intended to be all inclusive of related terms such as theory, model, frame of reference, or paradigm. Holm (1986) grouped occupational therapy frameworks into five fundamental classifications: acquisitional, biomechanical, developmental, occupational behaviour, and rehabilitation. Each framework guides therapists to evaluate different aspects of occupational performance and engagement, diagnose different occupational challenges, intervene using different approaches and procedures, and evaluate improvement in occupational performance and engagement differently.

Some frameworks (e.g. biomechanical) focus only on the enablers of occupation, that is, on factors within clients. From the perspective of the International Classification of Functioning, Disability and Health (ICF) (World Health Organization 2001), they address body structures and functions and their impairments. Other frameworks (e.g. rehabilitation) highlight clients performing their valued daily living activities. In the language of the ICF, they address activities and their limitations. Still other frameworks use a panoramic lens to capture clients performing occupations where they are typically performed, whether the location is the home, school or workplace. Thus, they emphasise participation and its restrictions as defined in the ICF.

Occupational therapy needs different conceptual frameworks of occupational performance and engagement to serve the differential needs of clients. During the acute stage of a burn injury, the biomechanical framework may be the most appropriate to guide intervention aimed at preserving range of motion and strength and preventing scar tissue formation. However, upon discharge from acute care the acquisitional or developmental framework may be more applicable for managing return to work or school despite disfigurement and pain. Strategies implemented under the biomechanical framework, such as active range of motion exercises and wearing pressure garments may still be employed. Hence, the various frameworks of occupational performance and engagement are not necessarily mutually exclusive and it is often appropriate to operate from different, but compatible, frameworks, simultaneously or sequentially. Commonly, intervention for people who have had a stroke includes constraint induced movement therapy for the paralysed extremity and assistive technology devices (e.g. one-handed knife) for use by the non-paralysed extremity. Constraint induced movement therapy emanates from an acquisitional framework and assistive technology from a rehabilitation framework. As depicted in Figure 5.1, the conceptual framework selected by the therapist influences each step of the occupational therapy process.

Phases of the occupational therapy process

Although each phase of the occupational therapy process is discussed separately, there are no clear distinctions between assessment, diagnosis, intervention, and re-assessment. The process is divided into phases to highlight key decisions that are required to support occupational reasoning. The occupational framework selected by the therapist permeates each phase.

Assessment

The purpose of assessment is for therapists to learn about the client's occupational performance and engagement so that they can formulate a diagnosis to direct intervention and re-assessment. Data are gathered about occupational performance and engagement through questioning, testing, and observing. Data may also be collected from the client's medical or school records or from case conferences; however, these data have their origins in questioning, testing, or observing. Questioning may be done orally through interviews or in writing through questionnaires. Interview tools like the Canadian Occupational Performance Measure (Law et al 2005) and questionnaires, like the Health Assessment Questionnaire (Fries et al 1982) are formal, standardised measures that yield information about clients' perceptions of their performance. If clients are unwilling to provide data (e.g. clients who are paranoid), unable to provide data (e.g. infants or clients who are comatose), or unable to provide reliable data (e.g. clients with severe dementia), proxies become the best source of information. Proxies who live with clients, spend considerable time with them, or are their caregivers are preferred.

Testing involves examining clients' performance under standardised conditions. This is accomplished by having clients demonstrate how they perform activities (e.g. cooking, typing) or how they perform components of those activities, such as the physical or cognitive actions that enable or restrict activities. Tests like the FIM™ Instrument (Uniform Data System for Medical Rehabilitation 1997) and the Performance Assessment of Self-Care Skills (Rogers & Holm 1989a) are activity measures and require therapists to observe and describe the client's performance in terms of independence–dependence. Tests such as the Keitel Function Test (Eberl et al

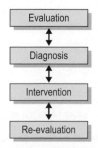

FRAME OF REFERENCE

Evaluation

Diagnosis

Intervention

Re-evaluation

Figure 5.1 • The occupational therapy process

1976), Mini-Mental State Examination (Folstein et al 1975), and Geriatric Depression Scale (Yesavage 1988) are impairment measures used to indicate the extent to which physical, cognitive, and affective factors, respectively, may be negatively influencing performance. For most observational measures, clients are requested to perform the desired activities during a scheduled assessment. Hence, clients may demonstrate bathing in the middle of the afternoon, even though they may usually bathe at bedtime. This procedure allows therapists to use their time efficiently. However, observation may also be carried out informally during daily activities. Settings like assisted living facilities, nursing homes, and schools are particularly suited for informal observation.

Commonly, an occupational therapy assessment incorporates more than one data-gathering method. Therapists may use interviewing to assess perceived performance problems and observation to assess actual performance problems. The conceptual framework selected by the therapist identifies the concepts to be assessed and suggests how data should be organised to facilitate interpretation. However, it does not indicate the method to be used to assess each concept, the extent to which each concept warrants assessment, the tool to be used to measure each concept, the order in which the concepts should be measured, or the means to validate data and resolve inconsistencies.

Diagnosis

As assessment data are 'fitted' to the conceptual framework, the therapist develops a working image of *this* client's occupational performance and engagement. The endpoint of assessment is an occupational diagnosis that defines the client's occupational problem(s) (Rogers 2004). Clients come to

occupational therapy because they have a problem or need. They may report that they are unable to bathe themselves or prepare their meals adequately. Although professional judgement may not be required to recognise a bathing or cooking impairment, to diagnose a bathing or cooking impairment does require occupational therapy knowledge, judgement, and skill.

The occupational diagnosis marks the transition between assessment and planning outcomes and strategies. Hence, the diagnosis must contain sufficient information to provide sound direction. To do this, the occupational diagnostic statement should give an indication of: the nature of the impairment, the presumed cause of the impairment, the evaluative cue supporting the impairment, and, if applicable the health condition(s) associated with the impairment (Rogers 2004). Unlike medicine, which has the ICD-10 (World Health Organization 2005), psychiatry, which has the DSM-IV-TR™ (American Psychiatric Association 2000), and nursing, which has NANDA International (2007), occupational therapy lacks a diagnostic taxonomy. Occupational therapy does not have a label, for example, to distinguish a limitation in dressing associated with cognitive impairment from a limitation in dressing associated with physical impairment. Because of this deficiency, the occupational therapy diagnosis is formulated as a descriptive statement.

As portrayed in Table 5.1, the occupational diagnostic statement has four components – descriptive, cue, explanatory, and health condition (Rogers 2004, Rogers & Holm 1991). The descriptive component identifies the occupational challenge to be targeted for intervention and against which the success of the intervention will be measured. In Table 5.1, the diagnostic statement specifies an inability to write. The cue component identifies the observable sign or signs of the problem. It indicates

Table 5.1 Occupational therapy diagnostic statement

Component	Phrase	ICF
Descriptive	Unable to write telephone messages without pain	d170.3 Writing. Severe difficulty
Cue	As evidenced by increase in number of Tylenol® taken per day	
Explanatory	Inflammation of the metacarpal phalangeal joint of the right thumb	b280 14.2 Pain in upper limb, moderate
Health condition	Rheumatoid arthritis	ICD M05.3

the significant slice of evaluative data that led the therapist to know that a writing limitation was present. The explanatory component gives the reason the therapist hypothesises as the cause of the writing limitation. In the example, insufficient hand strength to hold a writing utensil is thought to be the cause of the writing limitation. The health condition component addresses factors arising from pathology that need to be taken into account in the intervention plan. For a writing limitation secondary to rheumatoid arthritis, therapists would want information about pain, joint deformity, and the use of disease-modifying medications. ICF and ICD-10 codes have been added to Table 5.1 to illustrate their potential usefulness for developing an occupational diagnostic taxonomy.

Occupational diagnostic decisions centre on: formulating plausible hypotheses; determining the support for each occupational diagnosis, including the validity of the explanatory component, which often determines the intervention; and, prioritising occupational diagnoses.

Intervention

The intervention phase responds to the question: How will occupational therapy intervention help alleviate this client's problem or achieve the targeted outcomes? In the intervention phase, data from the occupational diagnosis and assessment phase are used to formulate intervention outcomes and plans to achieve them. Outcome statements are devised that describe occupational performance and engagement after occupational therapy intervention has had its effect. For Mrs. Trippit, a receptionist who exhibited a writing limitation, an occupational goal might be to enable message taking without difficulty. At the beginning of therapy, Mrs. Trippit could not hold a pen long enough to write telephone messages because of hand weakness and pain. An outcome statement might read: within one week (estimated time required for change), Mrs. Trippit will write (desired action) three telephone messages within five minutes, completely and legibly, and report no difficulty holding the pen or pain interference (performance criteria). Occupational outcomes specify how therapists will know if the strategies they plan are achieving the intended results; hence, they must be observable and measurable.

Having determined the endpoint of therapy, the therapist moves to deciding the techniques, and modalities that can be brought to bear on the problem. Of the feasible strategies, which are most appropriate for *this* client with *this* health condition? If insufficient hand strength is the cause of Mrs. Trippitt's writing limitation, then weak hand strength must be improved or circumvented to alleviate the problem in writing. For some clients with rheumatoid arthritis, a restorative approach to improve hand strength may be appropriate, while for other clients a compensatory approach incorporating assistive technology (e.g. enlarged pen for better grasp) may be preferable. For pain interference, a biomechanical approach may be beneficial, namely a rigid or soft thumb post splint to protect the inflamed metacarpal–phalangeal joint of her right thumb. Selecting the most judicious intervention to use with a client, from available options, is the pivotal decision for the intervention phase. Decision-making includes deciding on the therapy: dose (how intense?), frequency (how often?), and duration (how long?).

Re-assessment

The purpose of re-assessment is to ascertain if targeted outcomes have been achieved. To do this, therapists compare clients' current occupational performance and engagement to that predicted at the outset of therapy. Improvement, stability, or deterioration is based on the same measures that were used during assessment to determine that there was a problem. When data indicate that the outcomes were achieved, more advanced outcomes may be proposed or the client may be discharged. When data indicate that the outcomes were not achieved, the time for achieving the outcomes may be extended, outcomes may be revised to reflect more achievable ones, a different intervention may be initiated, or the client may be discharged from services because maximum benefit has been achieved.

Occupational reasoning strategies

Although the occupational therapy process outlines the phases that therapists progress through when working with clients, it does not indicate how therapists select, analyse, synthesise, and evaluate data to make decisions. The sequential and iterative cognitive processes therapists use to assess, diagnose, intervene, and re-assess occupational performance

Table 5.2 Decisions central to occupational reasoning

Phase	Decisions
Assessment	• What concepts should be assessed? • How extensively should each concept be assessed? • What method(s) should be used? • What assessment tools should be used? • In what order should the assessment tools be used? • How should data be validated and inconsistencies resolved?
Diagnosis	• What are the client's occupational diagnoses? • Which occupational diagnosis is best supported by assessment data? • How should occupational diagnoses be prioritised?
Intervention	• What occupational therapy interventions could be used? • What occupational therapy interventions should be used for this client? • How intense should each intervention session be? • How many times per week should intervention be? • How long should each intervention be?
Re-assessment	• Was each stated goal achieved? • Should intervention be terminated? • Should intervention be continued or changed? • Are new outcomes appropriate?

and engagement are collectively called occupational reasoning. Although it is easy to delineate the phases in the occupational therapy process, describing the dynamics of moving forward and backward from one phase to another, while continuing to advance toward diagnostic and therapeutic decisions, is extremely complex. As is apparent from Table 5.2, in which key decisions involved in the occupational therapy process are outlined, efficient and effective management of these decisions requires considerable professional expertise. Although we do not know exactly how occupational reasoning occurs, research on health care professionals, including occupational therapists, has furnished some indications of its dynamics. We will discuss common thinking strategies that therapists use in occupational reasoning:

comparative analysis, hypothesising, conditional reasoning, inferential reasoning, argumentative reasoning, reframing, and evidence-based reasoning (Pesut & Herman 1999).

Comparative analysis

Comparative analysis involves examining similarities and differences between new clients and textbook scenarios or former clients to gain insight about diagnoses and strategies to apply to new clients (Holm & Rogers 1989). During didactic education, students use textbook scenarios to develop images of impairment in 'typical' clients with a particular diagnosis. They learn to expect clients with severe strokes to have hemiplegia and have difficulty with bilateral activities; clients with obsessive compulsive disorder to manifest disordered thinking and make unusual repetitive movements; children with autism to exhibit rocking and other self-stimulating behaviours and to be unaware of their environment, and so on. They also learn an array of occupational therapy strategies appropriate for the occupational challenges associated with these health conditions and the results that can be expected from their application.

These textbook descriptions of typical clients, strategies, and outcomes serve as prototypes for client comparisons. When students engage in fieldwork, they compare the characteristics of their clients to the defining features of these prototypes. Students' reasoning goes something like this: 'My client had a left hemisphere stroke with resultant hemiplegia, and, therefore, if I work with my client using the same strategies used for people following a stroke, I learned about in the classroom, I will get the same outcomes in the same time limits.'

As students observe and work with 'real' people, prototypes are modified based on the occupational performance and engagement, and recovery patterns observed in 'real' clients. Students develop a cognitive or client library based on their caseload. In future encounters with clients with stroke, these stored clients replace the prototypes for comparisons. As professional experience accumulates, students not only add more clients to their cognitive library, they organise their library for easy retrieval. For example, within the stroke library, clients may be classified according to: those with and without sensory impairment, with and without lower-extremity involvement, and with and without a flaccid upper extremity. The functionality of these classifications for comparative reasoning becomes evident when Mrs. Swanson, who has no lower-extremity impairment, is able to grasp large objects in the affected extremity, but has no sensation in the affected hand, comes to occupational therapy. Using comparative reasoning, therapists search for the client in their cognitive library that provides the best, although not perfect, match for Mrs. Swanson. The reference client(s) would be called to mind and would provide therapists with guidance about the most enabling strategies.

Therapists use multiple classification principles to organise their cognitive client libraries, not just diagnosis. For instance, they may classify based on culture or religious beliefs. When a Muslim person who has had a stroke, is assigned to them, they might call to mind past clients who were Muslim, not just those with stroke. These reference clients would remind them to be sensitive to gender (preference for males working with males), fasting schedules (during Ramadan fasting sun up to sun down), and dress (female preference for head scarf) among other factors.

Comparative analysis may be used within, as well as between, client comparisons. During re-assessment, a client's present occupational performance and engagement may be compared to the predicted outcome status. Similarly, actual engagement may be compared two or more times: preadmission, admission, interim, and discharge. These comparisons allow therapists to know if occupational therapy intervention is having the anticipated effect on occupational performance and engagement.

Hypothesising

To hypothesise is to give an explanation for a set of facts that can be tested through the use of experimentation. Early in the assessment phase, therapists may put forth several diagnostic hypotheses (Elstein & Schwarz 2002). An occupational diagnosis is an educated guess, which is based on foundational knowledge. It explains a set of data about a client's occupational performance and engagement and can be tested. Data collection is guided by hypotheses and data are organised to support or dispute each hypothesis (Rogers & Holm 1989). By interviewing Mrs. Ming, the therapist may ascertain that she is dependent in dressing. Observation of Mrs. Ming performing dressing activities, leads the therapist to

think that the reason Mrs. Ming has difficulty dressing is due to hand weakness and lack of range of motion at the shoulder. The therapist then evaluates Mrs. Ming's hand strength and upper extremity joint range of motion to ascertain if the hypothesis about the cause of the dressing limitation is viable. Hand strength might be evaluated by testing grip strength on a dynamometer and pinch strength on a pinch meter. Range of motion might be evaluated with the Keitel Function Test. The results of these impairment tests would be compared to normal values for strength and movement to ascertain if they are deficient. If both values are deficient, the therapist's hypothesis about the cause of dressing dependency remains highly probable. However, it still needs to be tested through such means as progressive active and passive range of motion exercises.

Conditional reasoning

Conditional reasoning reflects an 'if–then' thinking strategy in which antecedents are linked to their consequences. When therapists link diagnoses or impairments to activity limitations or participation restrictions, conditional reasoning may be used. For example: if Mrs. Jones is hearing voices, then she may have difficulty concentrating on typing and will make errors; and if Mr. Book is visually impaired, then he is at risk for falls.

Inferential reasoning

Inferential reasoning involves drawing conclusions from facts. Facts have been or can be verified through observation or examination. Inferences are derived from facts. Therapists commonly make inferences about activity limitations based on facts about impairments. For example, a therapist may reason that because goniometry indicated that Mr. Goodman's external rotation at the hip was severely restricted, he would be dependent in donning socks. 'Dependence in donning socks' is a conclusion that was logically derived from the fact of restricted hip external rotation (movement restricted to: 0 to 20 degrees). This conclusion could be examined through performance testing, and if it were shown to be valid, 'dependence in sock donning' would become a fact rather than an inference. Because the therapist's inference fails to take into account adaptive techniques that circumvent decreased hip motion, such as a sock aid, it may be invalid.

Argumentative reasoning

Argumentative reasoning examines the reasons that support and fail to support a position or action. For example, a therapist may weigh the advantages and disadvantages associated with a home programme plus bi-weekly or monthly hospital-based sessions, for a client who lives in a rural area and has a severe upper-extremity crush injury. Advantages of bi-weekly sessions are that the therapy is supervised, occupation can be graded more effectively, and there is frequent opportunity to monitor infection and progress. The disadvantages are that bi-weekly sessions are expensive, the client lacks insurance, and the client may cancel sessions, especially in wintry weather. The advantages for bi-weekly sessions become disadvantages for monthly sessions and vice-versa for its disadvantages. Explicating the strengths and weaknesses of each stance heightens awareness of all factors that need to be taken into account, facilitates collaboration between therapists and clients, and fosters making quality decisions (Rogers 1983). This strategy is also beneficial for considering risks and benefits associated with client preferences.

Reframing

Reframing involves reinterpretation. It provokes a new view or perspective. For instance, a therapist may reason that Mr. Brown's failure to follow instructions consistently is due to dementia, and, hence, focus on caregiver training. However, after additional sessions, the therapist realises that Mr. Brown has a hearing impairment. Replacing oral instructions with written ones addresses the inconsistency. This solution was made possible by framing the problem as an auditory versus cognitive impairment. Importantly, reframing shapes what we do as well as how we think. Reframing is employed every time a therapist switches a conceptual framework when working with a client.

Evidence-based reasoning

Evidence-based reasoning is similar to comparative analysis, except that clients are compared with study samples versus prototype or actual clients. Assuming that the study meets criteria for internal validity, therapists question its external validity: Can the findings be generalised to this client in my practice? To answer this question, key characteristics, related to

clients (e.g. age, diagnosis), therapists (e.g. competence in specific strategies) and settings (e.g. hospital, school) are matched to those of study subjects. Suppose that following a home-safety programme for community-dwelling older people, a participant asks you about the benefits of hip protectors for preventing hip fractures. Because the daily activities of community-dwelling older adults are more extensive than those living in nursing homes, place of residence would be a key variable on which to match. By reading research, especially systematic reviews and meta-analyses, therapists stock their evidence-based library.

Application of strategies

A therapists' use of these reasoning strategies is highly dependent on their foundational and evidence-based knowledge, professional experience, and reasoning skill. Experienced therapists (experts) formulate more salient hypotheses, and formulate them earlier in the occupational therapy process, than novices (e.g. students and new practitioners). Novices need more data before they can recognise patterns, potentially because they have more difficulty sorting relevant and irrelevant data. Drawing on their professional experience, the thinking of experts is more automatic and less effortful. Experts reserve the more laborious 'if–then' thinking and hypothesis testing for unfamiliar situations or when the 'usual intervention' approach fails. Novices, lacking this depth of experience, rely on more deliberate problem solving. Each repetition of the occupational therapy process incorporates multiple occupational reasoning strategies.

Sharpening occupational reasoning

Professional self-talk provides an approach to improving one's occupational reasoning. It refers to the stream of thoughts that therapists communicate to themselves about a client, before, during, and after they interact with clients (Newell & Simon 1972, Rogers 1982). While it encompasses the occupational reasoning strategies discussed above, the emphasis is on thinking about your thinking while you are thinking. It encourages therapists to identify the thinking strategies that they usually use in practice and to reflect on their adequacy. By sharing self-talk, students can learn best-practice reasoning skills from their supervisors, and therapists can learn them from expert therapists.

Conclusion

Occupational reasoning underlies each professional decision. Although this chapter emphasised thinking skills commonly associated with the scientific method, other perspectives may also be usefully applied to elucidate the decision-making process. Quantitative and qualitative studies of occupational reasoning will advance the science, art, and practice of the occupational therapy process.

References

American Psychiatric Association (2000). *Diagnostic and statistical manual of mental disorders*, (4th ed.), Text revision. Washington, DC, American Psychiatric Association.

Eberl, D. R., Fasching, V., Rahlfs, V. et al (1976). Repeatability and objectivity of various measurements in rheumatoid arthritis: a comparative study. *Arthritis & Rheumatism* 19, 1278–1286.

Elstein, A. S. & Schwarz A. (2002). Clinical problem solving and diagnostic decision making: Selective review of the cognitive literature. *British Journal of Medicine*, 324, 729–732.

Folstein. M. F., Folstein, S. E. & McHugh, P. R. (1975). 'Mini-Mental State': A practical method for grading the cognitive state of patients for the clinician. *Journal of Psychiatric Research*, 12, 189–198.

Fries, J. F., Spitz, P. W. & Young, D. Y. (1982). The dimensions of health outcomes: the health assessment questionnaire, disability and pain scale. *Journal of Rheumatology*, 9(5), 789–793.

Holm, M. B. (1986). Frames of reference: guides for action – occupational therapist. In: H. Schmid (Ed.). *Project for independent living in occupational therapy (PILOT)*. Rockville, MD, American Occupational Therapy Association, pp. 69–78.

Holm, M. B. & Rogers, J. C. (1989). The therapist's thinking behind functional assessment II. In: C. B. Royeen (Ed.). *AOTA self study series: assessing function*. Rockville, MD, American Occupational Therapy Association.

Law, M., Baptiste, S. & Carswell A. et al (2005). *The Canadian Occupational Performance Measure*, (4th ed.). Toronto, CAOT Publications ACE.

Line, J. (1969). Case method as a scientific form of clinical thinking. *American Journal of Occupational Therapy* 23, 308–313.

NANDA International (2007). *Nursing diagnoses: definitions & classification 2007–2008*, (7th ed.). Philadelphia: NANDA International.

Newell A. & Simon, H. A. (1972). *Human problem solving*. Englewood Cliffs, NJ, Prentice-Hall.

Pesut, D. J. & Herman, J. (1999). *Clinical reasoning: The art & science of critical & creative thinking*. Albany, Delmar.

Rogers, J. C. (1982). Teaching clinical reasoning for practice in geriatrics. *Physical & Occupational Therapy in Geriatrics*, 1(4), 29–37.

Rogers, J. C. (1983). Clinical reasoning: the ethics, science, and art. *American Journal of Occupational Therapy*, 37, 601–616.

Rogers, J. C. (2004) Occupational diagnosis. In: M. Molineux (Ed.). *Occupation for occupational therapists* (pp. 17–31). Oxford, UK, Blackwell.

Rogers, J. C. & Holm, M. B. (1989a). *Performance assessment of self-care skills*. Pittsburgh, PA, University of Pittsburgh, Department of Occupational Therapy.

Rogers, J. C. & Holm, M. B. (1989b). The therapist's thinking behind functional assessment. I. In: C. B. Royeen (Ed.). *AOTA self study series: assessing function*. Rockville, MD, American Occupational Therapy Association.

Rogers, J. C. & Holm, M. B. (1991). Occupational therapy diagnostic reasoning: a component of clinical reasoning. *American Journal of Occupational Therapy* 45(11), 1045–1053.

Uniform Data System for Medical Rehabilitation (1997). *The Guide for the Uniform Data Set for Medical Rehabilitation (Including the FIM Instrument)*, Version 5.1. Buffalo: UDSMR.

World Health Organization (2001). *International Classification of Functioning, Disability and Health*. Geneva, World Health Organization.

World Health Organization (2005). *International Statistical Classification of Disease and Related Health Problems*, 10th Revision, (2nd ed). Geneva, World Health Organization.

Yesavage, J. A. (1988). Geriatric depression scale. *Psychopharmacology Bulletin*, 24, 709.

6

Understanding models of practice

Jo-anne Supyk-Mellson and Jacqueline McKenna

CHAPTER CONTENTS

Introduction .67

The mysteries of models 68

The established wisdom 68

Understanding terminology. 69

Pondering the puzzle 70

Sheltering from the semantic storm 71

   The Umbrella Framework for
   Understanding Models 71

Conclusion. .77

SUMMARY

This chapter will focus on the importance of the acquisition and understanding of key concepts within professional knowledge for occupational therapists, specifically discussing models and their application in practice. Although there is agreement around the definition of some terms, such as concept, philosophy and theory, there continues to be a lack of clarity around terms such as paradigm, approach, orientation, frame of reference, and model. These terms are often used interchangeably and meanings continue to reflect the conceptual orientation of the author. Standard definitions do not exist and, to date, the profession has not reached a consensus. Whilst supporting Duncans' (2006) assertion that shared terms and definitions are unlikely to work, this chapter suggests that unless basic terminology and semantics relating to models of practice are consistent, simple, and understandable, information is potentially inaccessible and the acquisition of conceptual knowledge and its application is ultimately impeded. The Umbrella Framework for Understanding Models (UFUM) provides a simple conceptualisation of the models of practice utilised by occupational therapists, aiming to enhance clarity and enable the acquisition of professional knowledge.

KEY POINTS

- There is confusion within our professional terminology around models of practice, resulting in much debate and a continuing lack of clarity.
- The Umbrella Framework for Understanding Models provides a simplified conceptualisation of models of practice used by the occupational therapist, splitting them simply into generic and intervention models.
- A sound understanding of models of practice underpins the development of the essential skills required for their practical application.
- A better understanding will reduce the theory–practice gap – real or perceived.

Introduction

Definitions of occupational therapy include enabling individuals to learn (College of Occupational Therapists 2006) and the facilitation of skill acquisition which relies heavily upon engaging service users in teaching–learning activities (Greber et al 2007). Indeed, according to the College of Occupational Therapists (2005, p. 3), one of the ten key roles of the occupational therapist is that of:

Training, developing, mentoring, teaching, informing and educating health care professionals, students, patients and carers.

As we embrace lifelong learning, the occupational therapist will function as both a learner and a teacher throughout training and practice. Our own learning experience may enable understanding of the process of learning and could assist in the development of the knowledge and skills required when we teach others. According to Hagedorn (1997a) teaching skills are an essential component of the generic core skills of the occupational therapist, necessitating a knowledge of the learning styles and techniques which can be utilised in order to facilitate learning for the promotion of occupational engagement. In our roles as occupational therapy lecturers, we have been involved in designing and developing elements of education which have focused on models of practice and their application in the practice setting by the occupational therapist. The study of relevant theories, including models of practice, supports evidence-based intervention and the challenge lies in facilitating the application of theoretical knowledge to the practice environment.

A quest for clarity, logic, usefulness, and essentials, has informed the development of education approaches around models and their application in practice. Learner feedback has consistently suggested that learning about models of practice is a confusing experience, indeed, in our experience, when past and present learners are asked which elements of their training programme presented the most memorable challenges; inevitably models of practice are cited. Difficult learning experiences in this area often have repercussions with therapists suggesting that avoidance of the subject matter following graduation is common. This ill ease with models may impact on the individual and their practice for many years. In the current environment of evidence-based practice and continuing professional development, a sound understanding of theoretical models and the ability to apply models of practice in health and social care is an essential component of competent 21st century practice.

The mysteries of models

Over a number of years we have asked learners to define or describe the concept of 'a model of practice'. Responses have included that models are; recipes, guides, theories, frameworks, structures, outlines, systems and maps. None of these are essentially incorrect but neither are they explanatory enough to be truly helpful in establishing learner understanding. Perhaps it is useful to look back to 1985 when Krefting summarised the purpose of models as structures which outline what to do, how to do it, and why to do it. Models endeavour to simplify the big picture, making the complex more explicit and more readily understood. The value of a model which structures knowledge and informs intervention is not disputed; however, terminology continues to confuse and learners waste valuable time and energy wrestling with terms which appear to vary from author to author, causing significant frustration and confusion.

The use of the term eclecticism to describe the application of several models of practice can reflect a well-informed, evidence-based, synthesised, individualised, and multi-faceted approach to occupational therapy intervention. That said, it is not uncommon to find the overuse of the term eclecticism as a convenient and misguided coverall for the loosely informed reasoning which arises from either a poorly articulated or inadequate knowledge base and a lack of confidence in the use of our professional vocabulary.

Learner groups have identified several common barriers to learning about models. These include: limited confidence in their grasp of key concepts; frustration with the apparent complexity of the concepts and terms involved; confusion with terminology, language, and semantics; and an overriding sense that they have 'not quite cracked the puzzle' or 'solved the mystery'.

Middleton (2000) has highlighted similar difficulties and has described ambiguous language as being the enemy of understanding. This chapter aims to simplify semantics, probing the professional language issues which appear to maintain the mysteries of models. This will enable the development of essential professional knowledge and skills whilst reducing anxiety and topic avoidance.

The established wisdom

This chapter in no way intends to undermine the received wisdom regarding theoretical and professional terminology. However, the absolute necessity for a structured and robust research-driven evidence base, which informs, supports and structures practice cannot be underestimated. There are some difficulties within our profession in distinguishing between the wisdom which is drawn from opinion, that which is drawn from shared assumptions and tacit knowledge, and that which is drawn from empirical evidence. We suggest that our profession's reliance on the former contributes, in part at least, to the perceived confusion around models of practice, as different writers and experts express different opinions and utilise varying terminology. Absolute homogeneity is neither desirable nor achievable (Duncan 2006, Hagedorn 1997a), but for the trainee or novice therapist some consistency would be helpful.

It is suggested that the willingness of occupational therapists to act on their shared philosophy and beliefs has led to the development of knowledge and techniques which are almost inherited or passed on through professional generations, becoming part of the 'mythology' of occupational therapy (Kelly & Mcfarlane 2007). This is where the cognitive wrestling begins as the protagonists attempt to make enough sense of theory to enable its translation into practice. The perceived theory–practice gap between university education and the realities of the practice environment appears widest at this point. This might be explained by considering the key players in the scenario: the academic, the student and the practitioner. The academic: who rejects myth, relying upon evidence and science to explore, order and structure theory and its application – albeit in the splendid isolation of an educational establishment. The student on placement: who lacks confidence in his/her own knowledge and claims, in an attempt to avoid difficult questions, that they haven't been taught a particular theory, whilst in reality he/she is wrestling with its application in the real world. The busy practitioner: who struggles to express in explicit and formal language his/her 'theory in use' relying on what Kelly and Mcfarlane (2007) termed the 'mystical' aspects of their practice, whilst trying to deal with the difficulties of explaining to a student exactly how to be a competent and successful practitioner.

Grappling with complex concepts is demanding for academics, students and practitioners, but it is no excuse for avoidance. Finlayson (2007) recalls her own resistance to theoretical aspects of her occupational therapy education, and her struggle to see value and purpose in what appeared at the time to be abstract. She noted some years later the recognition of the absolute importance of theory for definition, focus and interpretation of practice and its research. Achieving an appreciation of the purpose and value of theoretical material will enhance the learning experience, assist in application of theory and support achievement of learner occupational goals. Our experience in teaching this complex subject area has allowed us to develop ways to enhance this learning experience which will support engagement of students, facilitating deeper learning, the achievement of occupational goals and the development of a well-structured knowledge base (Biggs 2003).

Understanding terminology

Duncan (2006) summarises the issues around the defining and understanding of terminology, and cites that the complexity of issues presented by varied use of similar terms can be frustrating for students and practitioners trying to make sense of the theoretical influences of the profession. The interchangeable use of terms like applied frame of reference, model of practice, and approach over the past thirty years has served to muddy the waters. Kielhofner (2002) asserts that models of practice occur naturally in the field, reflecting the practical needs and considerations of our profession, as therapists attempt to organise their practice knowledge. He describes conceptual practice models as a way to organise unique occupational therapy theory; whereas Mosey (1970) states that a frame of reference organises existing theory for use in practice leading to confusion and misinterpretation. New terminology will continue to develop as interventions and newer models emerge leading to continuing variations in meanings, influenced in addition by the context of their use (Feaver & Creek 1993), and the conceptual bias and presage of the theorist. Indeed, Kelly and Mcfarlane (2007) suggest that even the published theories of our profession might amount to unverified assumption and personal experience, adding to the confusion for a novice who needs to establish some facts at a basic level. Pierce (2001) describes the apparently irresistible urge of scholars to puzzle over the definitions of the primary concepts of occupation and activity within the profession. Just as the lack of differentiation between these terms impeded the profession's development, debates around the disentangling of terminologies should be concerned with identifying acceptable, flexible and clear ways in which to explain conceptual models as they are designed to be – frameworks to guide thinking, support therapists, and encourage confidence in clinical decision-making and professional reasoning.

As a profession which takes pride in the application of person-centred practice, Brooke et al (2007) criticise the use of categorisation systems. Whilst acknowledging that these are helpful to therapists, the language employed may result in conceptual barriers between therapists and the individuals with whom they work. Again, semantics may lead to miscommunication and misinterpretation by the people we are working with, interfering with the therapeutic relationship and compromising the therapeutic process (Iwama 2005).

According to Rogers (1951) and Burnard (2005) in simple terms, an understanding of what is being expressed requires clarification of its meaning. So when the therapist or learner is presented with a model, to assume understanding of the concept of a model may be unwise and it might be pertinent to take a literal Rogerian approach to learning and ask:

What do you mean when you say it's a model?

How can you help me understand what you mean?

There are a number of possible descriptions of a model, after all meanings are individual and relative. In particular, when introducing a new concept, understanding should not be assumed. The model introduced could be interpreted as a built miniature of a large structure, as in 'a model village' or as an example of perfect behaviour, as in 'a model student' or even as the model Kate Moss on the cover of Cosmopolitan, rather than a theoretical construct which explains the practice of occupational therapy, as in 'The Model of Human Occupation' (Kielhofner 1995). This may seem overly literal but highlights how semantics can cause confusion and hinder learning. It also might assist in determining meaning within the current context and may help occupational therapists to achieve some consensus in their understanding. Therapists want to use the correct terminology; they want to be 'right', but have difficulty early in their education and career accepting the evolving nature of knowledge and the fact that there is often not one 'right answer' (Hagedorn 1997a). Given that differences do and will continue to exist, it is understandably difficult to establish what constitutes correctness in this context, and learners can become distracted and frustrated by a terminological debate as they struggle with the challenge of confusion. The acquisition of this professional knowledge underpins the integration of theory and practice, supporting professional (occupational)

reasoning and the development of the essential skills required for competent practice. Therefore, improving learner understanding of this is of vital importance.

Pondering the puzzle

Occupational therapy paradigms and core values are constantly shifting, being evaluated and adapted to meet the continual changes in health and social care. This reflects the flexibility and management of change required by therapists on a daily basis. As far back as 1984, in her Eleanor Clarke Slagle lectureship, Gilfoyle discussed the transformation of the profession following decades of identity crisis and a questioning of our value system. This has been echoed over the years (Hagedorn 1997a, Wilcock 2001), and attempts have been made to clarify our values, core beliefs, and philosophical bases scientifically to provide a concrete evidence base for occupation-focused practice. The resulting models of practice aim to clarify and unify the profession's belief system, translating the complexity of occupational analysis and performance into a variety of remarkably similar frameworks to help guide practice and steer the (novice) therapist through the occupational therapy process. Models developed to date are still open to change and more will continue to be developed. Gilfoyle and Christiansen (1987) painted a realistic picture when they claimed that within the science of occupation, concepts will continue to develop, with emerging ideas becoming part of a broader understanding. Understanding this evolution within the profession, utilising a sound evidence base, and promoting the ability to learn, re-learn, and adapt through enquiry is at the forefront of occupational therapy education. The evolution of new models is essential for the profession to remain dynamic (Finlay 1997). Universal agreement may not support progressive development which is important in the ever-changing world of health and social care. To remain dynamic therapists need to embrace the opportunity to change along with evolving models (Finlay 1997). Educators need to encourage objectivity, critical analysis and a flexible problem-solving approach in students to prepare them for future adaptability and flexibility when choosing or rejecting models to meet the demands of the health care system and the emerging roles for occupational therapists, as we move rapidly into the 21st century.

Academic and philosophical debate continues regarding the shifts and evolutions in paradigm and values (Duncan 2006, Hagedorn 1997a, Wilcock 2001) yet rather than allowing these complex definitions to interfere with learning, it is important to be equipped with the tools to solve the puzzle of professional terminology to reduce the anxiety surrounding the apparent complexity of models to see them for what they really are – tools to bring meaning to complex theoretical debates and to provide a structure for occupational therapy intervention.

Kortman (1995) considered the terminology used to label theoretical frameworks in occupational therapy and concluded that most terms were interchangeable. The interchangeable nature of existing terminology continues to confuse and hinder our learning.

Occupational therapy focuses on complex dynamic relationships between people, occupations and environments (Law et al 1998). Models of practice should function as tools to be used in therapeutic alliances, enabling engagement in meaningful occupations in chosen environments (Strong et al 1999). The evolution of models of practice over the last 25 years has created much development within the profession. That said, our key principles and concepts, whilst being repackaged, renamed, remarketed, and re-jargonised, ultimately remain true to the essentials of occupational therapy philosophy – holistic person-centred practice – and our models remain occupation-focused tools for intervention. This is what matters; this is what learners need to understand. Ignoring tautological issues, semantics, and the current trend for buzz words for the sake of enhanced clarity and simplicity which aids learning, is reasonable and necessary. This debate is, of course, more complex than is suggested here but must be reserved for another day. That said, Brooke et al (2007) support the view that conceptual models should be examined, critiqued and debated to ensure clarity of purpose. Categorisation systems and frameworks designed for use through the occupational lenses of therapists, may not match with the service users' view of their occupations; therefore, causing the perceptual barriers and disconnections sometimes experienced in the therapeutic relationship. In order to work competently the occupational therapist must be able to conceptualise, plan, implement, communicate, and evaluate occupational performance interventions.

Sheltering from the semantic storm

The practical solution proposed here is to conceptualise models of practice using the structure of an umbrella, building on the single model conceptual structure postulated by Greber et al (2007). Our new conceptualisation aims to offer a broad overview by including a range of models used by occupational therapists. A basic framework of existing occupational therapy models is utilised and semantics are simplified, assisting students and therapists to conceptualise the interplay between occupational therapy philosophy and 'generic' and 'intervention' models. This conceptualisation assists with the clarification of links between core principles and therapeutic tools, integration of theory and practice, and supports professional reasoning.

Within the umbrella framework, the term *generic model* is used to describe occupational therapy models which are the models commonly used to provide structure to the practice of occupational therapy, providing frameworks which operationalise the core values of occupation-focused, person-centred, and holistic practice. *Intervention models* meanwhile describe the principles and tools of 'hands on' practice, what the occupational therapist actually does once a general picture or baseline has been established in order to achieve occupational goals. These intervention models also include tools and techniques, facilitating application of specific therapeutic strategies.

The Umbrella Framework for Understanding Models

Using the Umbrella Framework for Understanding Models (UFUM), the top point of the umbrella is the starting point for this conceptualisation represented in Figure 6.1. Clarification of philosophical principles provides a foundation for the structure and analysis of new and existing concepts and methods (Ikiugu & Schultz 2006). The professional philosophy broadly encompasses existentialism, pragmatism, phenomenology, and the principles of humanistic psychology, linking clearly to the principles of holistic, person-centred practice and the enablement of meaningful activity, which overarch occupational therapy practice. Occupation is central to the values and principles of occupational therapy,

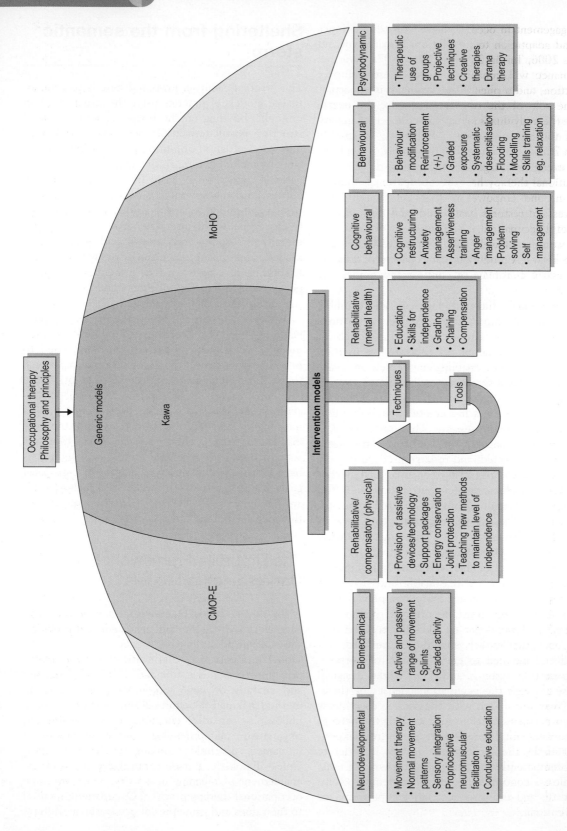

Figure 6.1 • Overview of generic and intervention models

and engagement in occupation requires interaction with and adaptation to the environment (Ikiugu & Schultz 2006, Turpin 2006). Enabling occupational performance will enhance health, well-being and satisfaction, and a phenomenological view suggests that the role of the occupational therapist is to manage the individual's interaction with and perception of the environment in order to achieve this (Turpin 2006).

According to Hagedorn (1997b, pp. 32–33) 'occupational therapy has three purposes; enabling, enhancing and empowering [...] Our philosophy promotes and restores health and well being using purposeful occupation'.

The concept of well-being and its reliance on a balance between productivity, self care and leisure is well established (McColl et al 2003). However, therapists are not primarily concerned with any impairment, but with the ability of the individual to engage in meaningful and purposeful occupations within their specific context and within the environment of the individual. The transactional relationship between the person, the occupation and the environment essentially describes the basis for occupational therapy theory. The dynamic interdependence of personal (physical, psychological, socio-cultural, cognitive-neurological) and environmental (physical, social, economic, political) components (McColl et al 2003), and their impact upon successful engagement in meaningful occupations is at the very core of occupational therapy practice.

The generic models form the main body or cover of the umbrella, literally covering all, and are applied broadly. The intervention models sit underneath the generic models, as the spokes or ribs of the umbrella, providing focused interpretation of the problem and its management, and they can be applied equally within any generic model. The intervention models, in turn, offer shelter to the next level, described as 'tools' by Kramer and Hinojosa (1999) and described in this conceptualisation as tools and techniques. The tools can be seen as the umbrella handle, literally allowing the therapist to get 'hands on' and actualise the related theory into specific interventions. These include specific applications which sit within each intervention model and facilitate the skill acquisition necessary for the achievement of occupational goals.

In order to prevent the therapist becoming exposed to the elements, it is essential for the occupational therapist to shelter under the cover of the umbrella, ensuring the overarching philosophy and core occupational principles remain aligned to all levels of theory and central to all practice. This is supported by Greber et al (2007) who suggest that achieving occupational goals relies upon the therapist operating from within the boundaries of the overarching structure.

Generic models provide a framework for professional reasoning, validating and guiding practice (Hagedorn 1997a). They focus on the central constructs of occupational therapy, occupational form, function, and performance (Duncan 2006), ensuring that practice remains occupation-centred. The framework shown in Figure 6.2 is intended to highlight that generic models can be used across all domains of occupational therapy practice; they provide holistic guidance for people with any condition that has an impact on occupational performance and engagement (or are applicable to anyone with occupational interruption). Occupational therapists can choose from these generic models and apply them in practice across all therapeutic environments from acute physical care to community mental health. Themes are unsurprisingly familiar as all have been developed from a shared evidence base, with shared underpinning philosophies and core beliefs. Some are more person-centred and holistic than others, yet all are different enough to offer choice and flexibility for the therapist. Generic models are simply structures which use an evidence base to guide the occupational therapy process. They might also offer standardised tools to assist in this process, providing effective assessment and outcome measures to support and enhance objectivity. They are not rigid laws and should not narrow the view we have of an individual's situation or dysfunction, but merely provide a viewing lens. The overall generic picture will remain in focus whilst the intervention model guides and shapes the strategies employed, providing processes and procedures which will meet the individual's needs and provide a rationale for practice.

Reed and Sanderson (1983) refer to models which can be applied across a range of practice areas as generic. As discussed these are numerous and ever-developing. However, occupational therapists should not limit themselves to those models included here, as new and developing theories and models will enhance professional knowledge and encourage debate. However, for those attempting to grasp the basic concepts, the three more commonly used and established generic models are used within the UFUM to demonstrate how the generic models link

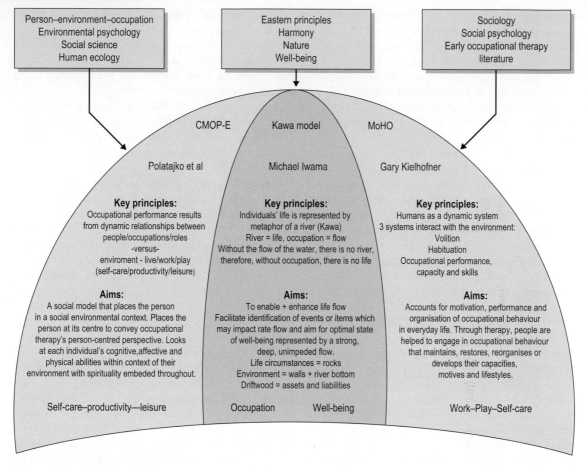

Figure 6.2 • Generic models

with the intervention models. These include: The Canadian Model of Occupational Performance and Engagement (Polatajko et al 2007), Model of Human Occupation (Kielhofner 1995), and The Kawa Model (Iwama 2006). Figure 6.2 illustrates the key features and principles of each of these models in a simple way which may help as an aide memoire when conceptualising how generic models and intervention models compliment each other as suggested within The Umbrella Framework. In addition to this summary of the generic models, the key features of the intervention models are described in Table 6.1. This table identifies key theorists, simplifies key concepts/principles and identifies some specific techniques which can be used within each of the intervention models. This table provides minimal detail of each intervention model and is intended to clarify the conceptualisation of The Umbrella Framework rather than provide detailed information

on each of the models. Readers are directed to the indicative authors referred to for further explanation of key theories underpinning each intervention model as a sound evidence base.

The intervention models including tools and techniques act as structures and principles for therapeutic intervention, rather than as theoretical guides to the occupational therapy process. These models may be more specific to set boundaries and guidelines regarding expected intervention to meet the intervention goals identified by the generic model. They can be likened to the use of a repair handbook for a specific model of car rather than a general manual for diagnosing mechanical problems – a car mechanic may use a general guide to mechanical engines to assist in identifying particular problems with a faulty car. However, he may then need more specific details regarding a particular model when attempting to solve the problems identified. He may

Table 6.1 Intervention models

	Neuro-developmental	Biomechanical	Rehabilitative/ compensatory (physical/psychological)	Psychodynamic	Cognitive behavioural	Behavioural
Key theorists	Bobath Rood Ayres Peto Knott & Voss Brunnstrom	Baldwin Taylor Lient	Dutton Trombly Hagedorn Maslow Tuke & Pinel Allen Hulme & Pullen	Freud Jung Alder Erikson Bowlby Tuckman Yalom	Skinner Beck Ellis Kelly Bandura	Pavlov Thorndyke Skinner Watson
Key concepts/ principles	Derived from neurological learning theory and normal human development Principles based on motor control, neuro-muscular facilitation and sensory integration	Views body as a functioning machine. Purely physical, functional focus Reductionist medical model explaining function physiologically and anatomically. Focus on strength, range of movement, endurance and with reduction of secondary disability	Restores independence through use of compensation strategies and techniques Promotes personal independence Used when return to premorbid functional level is not possible Involves the teaching and learning process To compensate for residual disability by means of aids, appliances or environmental adaptations Maintain dignity and quality of life Personal perspective on recovery	Based on psychoanalytic theories of the mind, personality, psychosexual development and group dynamics. Focusing on emotions and motivations and capacity for self-exploration, knowledge and change Emotions/interpersonal relationships are a source of anxiety and conflict. Unresolved conflicts can manifest as emotional or mental health problems Therapeutic relationship is of utmost importance Defence mechanisms impact function	Thinking, emotion and behaviour are linked. Faulty cognitive appraisal affects feelings and behaviour Behaviour will only change if negative patterns of thinking are changed Analysis of: antecedents beliefs consequences self-perception self-efficacy	All behaviour is learnt. Behaviour can be unlearned or modified Learning can be conditioned – as it occurs in response to stimulus and reinforcement Behaviour can be viewed as a sequence of responses Behavioural analysis: antecedents behaviour consequences

Table 6.1 Intervention models—cont'd

	Neuro-developmental	Biomechanical	Rehabilitative/compensatory (physical/psychological)	Psychodynamic	Cognitive behavioural	Behavioural
Aims of the model	To reduce abnormal movement patterns and increase normal movement through facilitation To improve psychosocial adjustment	To improve performance generally, focus on muscle strength, range of movement, endurance, exercise tolerance and physical mobility	Maximise and maintain the potential of retained, undamaged abilities Restore functional ability to previous level, or as close to this as possible. The combined and co-ordinated use of medical, social, educational and vocational measures for training and retraining the individual to the highest possible level of functional ability (World Health Organisation 1974)	Interventions are generally supportive of ego strength. Supportive interventions maintain ego defences and their functioning Exploration of defences and conflicts and expression of feelings will support insight development and strengthen the ego Use of therapeutic groups	To help individual to recognise negative emotions and their connection to negative thoughts and behaviours Challenge and replace negative thoughts Use techniques to develop coping skills and strategies, improve communication with others and problem solve	Learning programme designed to meet individual needs Addresses behavioural excesses and/or deficits by setting precise behavioural objectives and using reinforcement Desirable behaviours are increased Undesirable/maladaptive behaviours decreased/extinguished Skill acquisition increases the behavioural repertoire
Tools/techniques	Movement therapy Normal movement patterns – inhibition of abnormal patterns Sensory integration Proprioceptive neuro-muscular facilitation (PNF) Conductive education	Active and passive range of movement Provision of splints – static and dynamic Graded activities	Provision of assistive devices/technology Support packages Energy conservation Joint protection Teaching adaptive techniques to maintain independence Education Skill development Grading Compensation	Therapeutic use of groups Projective techniques Creative therapies Drama/music therapy	Cognitive restructuring Anxiety management Assertiveness training Anger management Problem solving Scripting	Behavioural modification Reinforcement (+/−) Contracts Graded exposure Systematic desensitisation Flooding Modelling Skills training, e.g. relaxation, social skills Sequencing, chaining Education

To avoid being overly prescriptive, the application of each intervention model is guided by its own theoretical base. However, intervention models are not mutually exclusive and can be used in combination depending on the needs of the individual and informed by occupational reasoning.

then need to look in a more specific handbook pertaining to the particular make and model of vehicle, this is the difference between the general guide (generic model) and the specific handbook (intervention model) which will suggest possible techniques to solve the problem. Each intervention model provides a perspective from which the therapist views the individual, establishing the assumptions that are used to measure performance and identify dysfunction. The intervention model relies upon these theoretical assumptions to inform the selection and application of specific interventions. Intervention tools and techniques are unlikely to be exclusive to occupational therapy but are congruent with occupational therapy theory (Greber et al 2007), and aligned to both the generic and intervention models selected.

Intervention models described within the UFUM include the biomechanical, neurodevelopmental, rehabilitative/compensatory, psychodynamic, cognitive, and behavioural models. Examples might include: an addiction service which favours a behavioural intervention model and utilises contracts, reinforcement, and skills training in order to address behavioural deficits or excesses that impact occupational performance. Trombly (1995) describes a neurodevelopmental intervention model with individuals with central nervous system damage. She then goes on to describe specific techniques such as Proprioceptive Neuromuscular Facilitation (PNF) or sensory integration (tools/techniques), which are available to meet the person's needs within the guidelines of the intervention model and will support occupational goals.

Overlap may occur and a number of intervention models may be applied within an individualised package of care, attention must be paid to principles, limits and to any contraindications across models in order to ensure the most efficacious treatment is provided.

When the occupational therapist is planning intervention to support a person with a new diagnosis of rheumatoid arthritis, he/she may decide to offer advice on joint protection and energy-conservation techniques, using the rehabilitative intervention model. This process will be supported with the provision of night-resting splints from the biomechanical model. Further intervention may include teaching relaxation techniques to support pain control using strategies from the behavioural intervention model, and the use of the cognitive behavioural model, wherein techniques will challenge

negative thoughts and support motivation. This effective overlap of intervention models works well to meet the individual's needs, supporting a person-centred and holistic philosophy, and evidences the application of an eclectic approach.

Conclusion

According to Steward (1995, p. 359) using models too rigidly as 'route maps rather than speculative illustrations', can impede the development of professional knowledge and understanding. We do not advocate such rigidity, but recognise that therapists have choice which must be informed and requires the application of professional reasoning skills. This can be daunting for a novice or inexperienced therapist who lacks confidence in her own knowledge and is unable to rely upon professional reasoning for decision-making. Hodgetts et al (2007) found that the value of theoretical knowledge and its application to practice becomes clear following graduation, as practitioners begin to rationalise and validate their interventions. This idea is supported by Kortman (1995) who stated that practitioners build their own conceptual frameworks from exposure and access to theories and models, and that this is essential in order to link theory to practice. Ousey (2001) emphasises the importance of partnerships between academia and practice to reinforce this link and bridge the gap, whilst facilitating effective exposure to theoretical models in the practice environment. There is an expectation that students and novice practitioners will have the ability to effectively transfer knowledge they have gained in the classroom directly into practice without difficulty (Camsooksai 2002). A failure to transfer and integrate this knowledge is referred to as the theory–practice gap (Rolfe 1998). Whether this gap is real or perceived matters little, the acquisition and transfer of skills and knowledge from the academic to the practice environments is essential for the support of safe and effective practice.

Whilst acknowledging that simplification of models can distort the real picture (Steward 1995), we have found that simplification of semantics and use of this conceptualisation of how generic models and intervention models fit together improves understanding at a basic level for all parties. This facilitates deeper learning, and clearer and more confident expression, transmission, and sharing of this knowledge for all learners and therapists, ultimately enhancing practice. According to Steward (1995, p. 360) who was discussing the purpose of simplified, rational and somewhat reductionist models, 'novice practitioners may need this approach in the early stages of practice to enable them to participate safely in the therapeutic process'. It is essential to understand how therapeutic tools relate to the concepts of the profession (Greber et al 2007) and sound reasoning relies on the synthesis of theory and therapy.

The challenge of explaining what occupational therapy is remains just that, a challenge, and an inability to articulate our unique contribution to others continues to have serious implications for the profession (Wilding & Whiteford 2007). It is essen-tial to be able to represent and promote occupa-tional therapy, and to be able to articulate the purpose and focus of our profession in order to faci-litate a better understanding of it. In order to justify our own occupational reasoning not only to people we work with – carers and other professionals – but also to the profession and its evidence base, a clear understanding of underpinning theories and their application is vital. Any conceptualisation may be criticised for adding to the semantic confusion. However, any strategy which facilitates or promotes 'joined up thinking', and aids clarity, can only serve to support learning and confidence, ultimately enhancing reasoning and benefiting the profession.

References

Biggs, J. (2003). *Teaching for quality learning at university*, (2nd ed). Oxford, Open University Press.

Brooke, K. E., Desmarais, C. D. & Forwell, S. J. (2007). Types and categories of personal projects: a revelatory means of understanding human occupation. *Occupational Therapy International*, 14(4), 281–296.

Burnard, P. (2005). *Counselling skills for health professionals*, (4th ed). United Kingdom: Nelson Thomas Ltd.

Camsooksai, J. (2002). The role of the lecturer practitioner in interprofessional education. *Nurse Education Today*, 6, 466–475.

College of Occupational Therapists (2005). *10 key roles*. London, COT.

College of Occupational Therapists (2006). *Recovering ordinary lives*. London, COT.

Duncan, E. (Ed.). (2006). *Foundations for practice in occupational therapy*, (4th ed). London, Elsevier.

Feaver, S. & Creek, J. (1993). Models for practice in occupational therapy: Part 2 What use are they. *British Journal of Occupational Therapy*, 56(2), 59–69.

Finlay, L. (1997). *The practice of psychosocial occupational therapy*, (2nd ed). Cheltenham, Stanley Thornes.

Finlayson, M. (2007). Why theory matters – editorial. *Canadian Journal of Occupational Therapy*, 74(4), 291.

Gilfoyle, E. M. & Christiansen, C. H. (1987). The quest for truth and the key to excellence. *American Journal of Occupational Therapy*, 41(1), 7–8.

Greber, C., Ziviana, J. & Rodger, S. (2007). The four quadrant model of facilitated learning (part 1) – using teaching and learning approaches in occupational therapy. *Australian Occupational Therapy Journal*, 54, S31–S39.

Hagedorn, R. (1997a). *Foundations for practice in occupational therapy*, (2nd ed). Edinburgh, Churchill Livingstone.

Hagedorn, R. (1997b). *Occupational therapy perspectives and processes*. London, Churchill Livingstone.

Hodgetts, S., Hollins, V., Triska, O., Dennis, S., Madill, H. & Taylor, E. (2007). Occupational therapy students' and graduates' satisfaction with professional education and preparedness for practice. *Revue Canadienne d'Ergotherapie*, 74(3), 148–160.

Ikiugu, M. N. & Schultz, S. (2006). An argument for pragmatism as a foundational philosophy of occupational therapy. *Canadian Journal of Occupational Therapy*, 73(2), 86–97.

Iwama, M. (2005). Situated meaning: an issue of culture, inclusion and occupational therapy. In: F. Kronenberg, S. A. Algado, N. Pollard (Eds) *Occupational therapy without borders – learning from the spirit of survivors* (pp. 127–139).

Edinburgh, Churchill Livingstone, Elsevier.

Iwama, M. K. (2006). *The Kawa model – culturally relevant occupational therapy*. London, Churchill Livingstone.

Kelly, G. & Mcfarlane, H. (2007). Culture or cult? The mythologocal nature of occupational therapy. *Occupational Therapy International*, 14(4), 188–202.

Kielhofner, G. (1995). *A model of human occupation – theory and application*. Maryland, USA, Williams and Wilkins.

Kielhofner, G. (2002). *A model of human occupation – theory and application*. Maryland, USA, Williams and Wilkins.

Kortman, B. (1995). The eye of the beholder: models in occupational therapy. *British Journal of Occupational Therapy*, 58(12),115–122.

Kramer, P. & Hinojosa, J. (1999). *Frames of reference for paediatric occupational therapy*. Baltimore, Lippincott, William and Wilkins.

Krefting, L. H. (1985). The use of conceptual models in clinical practice. *Canadian Journal of Occupational Therapy*, 52(4), 173–178.

Law, M., Baptiste, S., Carswell, A., McColl, M. A., Polatajko, H. & Pollock, N. (1998). *Canadian occupational performance measure*. (3rd ed). Canada, CAOT publications ACE.

McColl, M.A., Law, M., Stewart, D., Doubt, L., Pollock, N. & Krupa, T. (2003). *Theoretical basis of occupational therapy*, (2ⁿᵈ ed). New Jersey, Slack.

Middleton, M. J. (2000). *Can classrooms be both motivating and demanding? The Role of the Academic Press*. Michigan, University of Michigan.

Mosey, A. C. (1970). *Three frames of reference for mental health*. Thorofare, NJ, Slack.

Ousey, K. (2001). Promoting evidence based education in tissue viability. *Nursing Standard*, 15(30), 62–66.

Pierce, D. (2001). Untangling occupation and activity. *American Journal of Occupational Therapy*, 55, 138–146.

Polatajko, H., Townsend, E. & Craik, J. (2007). Canadian model of occupational performance and engagement (CMOP–E). In: E. A. Townsend, & H. J. Polatajko. *Enabling occupation II: Advancing an occupational therapy vision of health, well-being and justice through occupation*, (p. 23). Ottawa, ON: CAOT Publications ACE.

Reed, K. & Sanderson, S. (1983). *Concepts of occupational therapy*. Baltimore, Williams and Wilkins.

Rogers, C. R. (1951). *Client-centred therapy*. Great Britain, Constable & Company Ltd.

Rolfe, G. (1998). The theory practice gap in nursing: from research-based practice to practitioner-based research. *Journal of Advanced Nursing* 28(3), pp. 672–679.

Steward, B. (1995). Models of practice: maps and models. *British Journal of Therapy and Rehabilitation*, 2(7), 359–362.

Strong, S., Rigby, P., Stewart, D., Law, M., Letts, L. & Cooper, B. (1999). Application of the person environment occupation model: a practical tool. *Canadian Journal of Occupational Therapy*, 66(3), 122–133.

Trombly, K. (1995). *Occupational therapy for physical dysfunction*, (4th ed). Baltimore, Williams and Wilkins.

Turpin, M. (2006). Recovery of our phenomenological knowledge in occupational therapy. *American Journal of Occupational Therapy*, 61(4), 469–473.

Wilcock, A. A. (2001). Occupational science: the key to broadening horizons. *British Journal of Occupational Therapy*, 64(8), 412–417.

Wilding, C. & Whiteford, G. (2007). Occupation and occupational therapy: knowledge paradigms and everyday practice. *Australian Journal of Occupational Therapy*, 54, 185–193.

Chapter Seven

Process of assessment and evaluation

Clare Hocking

7

CHAPTER CONTENTS

Introduction 82

Getting the right information:
complexities and contexts 82

An occupational focus 83

Occupation-based assessment. 84

When to assess 85

Steps in the process: screening,
assessment and evaluation. 85

    Screening 85

    Assessment 87

    Evaluation 87

How to elicit information 88

    Selecting and using standardised
    assessments. 88

    Professional responsibility and
    standardised assessments 89

    Non-standardised assessments. 90

Conclusion. 91

SUMMARY

Assessment means gathering information about people, the occupations that concern them, and the environments in which the occupations occur. While assessment processes are influenced by the context of practice, occupational therapists focus on occupation rather than impairment and take into account people's experience of participating in the occupation. Assessment entails synthesising information gained through observation, interview, examination, and self-ratings. The findings inform therapists about how to work with the person, family, group or community; what aspect of occupation is problematic and the reasons for this; what the person or group aspires to do; and what might make a difference. Assessment encompasses screening the need and priority for intervention, initial assessment, which informs negotiation of goals and planning of strategies, monitoring progress and evaluation of outcomes. Professional and ethical considerations include consent processes, documentation and reporting, using evidence to evaluate assessment tools, and ongoing review of assessment strategies.

KEY POINTS

- Assessment means gathering information about people, the occupations of concern, and the environments in which the occupations occur.
- The information about people that is of interest to occupational therapists includes their occupational history; occupations that shape and express their identity; their capacities, skills and knowledge in relation to the occupation of concern; and their aspirations for participation in occupation.
- To select an effective enabling strategy, therapists sometimes need to investigate what is causing the occupational concern. This may require assessment of the nature or severity of impairments.
- As well as assessing individuals, occupational therapists assess family groups, work groups and their managers, children and their teachers,

communities that have an occupational need, and occupational structures in society, etc.

- Assessment strategies include observation, dialogue, self-rating and examination, and may be standardised or non-standardised.
- Assessment encompasses screening, assessment, monitoring progress and evaluation of outcomes, and continues throughout the occupational therapy process.
- The outcomes of assessment are having a sense of how to work with the people concerned, an agreed plan of action to enhance participation in targeted occupations, and identified ways of determining whether sufficient progress has been made.
- Occupational therapists are responsible for ensuring assessment processes are conducted professionally and ethically.

Introduction

When Albie Sachs, a South African political activist, opened a parcel delivered to his home he tripped the mechanism to a bomb and blew his hands off. He was not the first, nor the last, to receive a parcel-bomb designed to silence those working to end apartheid and counted himself lucky not to lose his eyes. He knew all too well that his injuries were mild compared with the atrocities experienced by many black activists. In the course of the rehabilitation that followed, Albie spent countless hours with an occupational therapist, learning to fit and use prosthetic arms and tie his shoe laces. He was issued a cardholder to enable him to resume weekly card games with his friends.

On discharge, he dispensed with the arms, bought slip-on shoes, and discovered that lodging his cards between the pages of a book was more effective. Whilst careful not to disparage the occupational therapy he had received, Albie, now a judge in South Africa's Constitutional Court, made it clear that resuming his campaign of exposing organised police violence was a far higher priority than independence in personal care (Sachs 2004).

To my mind, Judge Sachs' story is a failure of assessment. That is, the information collected was weighted towards his medical treatment (the prostheses) and the rehabilitation team's understanding of what was needed (independence in ADL). As they should, the assessment findings drove the rehabilitation goals and strategy. However, the information gathered and goals set bore no relationship to Judge Sachs' essence, his political conscience, or his

robust attitude of getting on with the job despite ongoing threats to his safety and the inconvenience of being deprived of his hands.

Getting the right information: complexities and contexts

Assessment is about getting the right information to understand what is going on, what outcomes are significant to the person or people concerned, and acceptable ways of achieving those outcomes. As Judge Sachs' story suggests, assessment is complex because there can be multiple perspectives on what is going on, and what is important and acceptable. Getting it right means working in partnership with people and making judgements about which information is most important, how to get it, and when there is sufficient information to determine a course of action.

There are multiple influences on the assessment process. Of primary importance is the understanding that occupational performance is the product of the person, the occupation(s) and the environment(s) in which it occurs (Kielhofner 2007). That means gathering data about all three components. By making an effort to get to know the person or group they are assessing, therapists ensure they address occupations that are valued and meaningful, such as Judge Sachs' political activities. Moreover when therapists address what is important, people will feel more inclined to share information, concerns, performance limitations and personal aspirations. That preparedness encompasses more than the problem at hand; to work effectively therapists rely on individuals divulging relevant but very personal information, such as feeling that carers sometimes help too much or that the person available to assist is a same-sex partner. The sensitivity that therapists employ in gathering information about people will, in turn, influence their preparedness to coach the therapist through cultural practices. This may include how they perform occupations, make decisions, and convey agreement or disagreement, and how the therapist ought to behave as a visitor, convey respect for high-status individuals, negotiate gender boundaries, and so on. Along with knowledge of the person, knowledge of the occupation and environment underpins the therapist's understanding of the presenting problem, and can help identify barriers and enablers to performance and possible solutions.

Equally influential on the process and outcome of any assessment is the profession's commitment to person-centredness, evidence-based practice, and ethical practice. Being person-centred means the tailoring of an assessment to the person, group, organisation or community with the occupational performance concern. It also means recognising that individuals may have extensive or life-long experience of the issue and its context, or at the other extreme, very limited knowledge of it, such as a person with a newly acquired impairment or a group facing a situation they have not previously encountered. Therapists must vary their approach accordingly, acknowledging some individuals as experts and guiding others to become co-investigators of issues those individuals may be only vaguely aware of.

Another influence is the link many have made between rigorous assessment processes and evidence-based practice (Harris et al 2005, Schofield 2006, Welch & Lowes 2005, Wilby 2005), along with the accumulating evidence of therapists' assessment practices (Blenkiron 2005, Chard 2006, Diamantis 2006). Thoughtfully determining what to assess and ensuring that 'every client [has] a clearly recorded assessment of need' (College of Occupational Therapists 2005, p. 529) provides evidence of person-centredness, professional reasoning and ethical conduct. Additionally, practicing ethically compels therapists to take into account 'the needs, wishes, feelings and choices of clients' (College of Occupational Therapists 2005, p. 529) and ensure they have consented to being assessed. Recognising the need for consent implies people have a legitimate choice about engaging in an assessment, having been given sufficient information about its purpose, what it will involve and how the information generated is likely to be used. Skill in conducting assessments, synthesising data from multiple sources, and professional reasoning is also vital (Wilby 2005), affecting the accuracy of information gained and the sense therapists and clients make of it.

A fourth potent influence on any assessment is the health, disability, educational, vocational, corrections or community context in which it occurs, because that determines the nature of the outcome sought, whether that be independence, risk reduction, alleviation of carer burden, inclusion, employability or productivity, self responsibility, empowerment, community development or something else. The service context also shapes therapists' priorities, practices, attitudes, resources and workloads, all of which have a bearing on the assessment process.

An occupational focus

Having considered the contextual influences, let us turn to the question of what it is that should be assessed and why. Since the early 1990s, occupational therapists have been urged to conduct 'top-down' assessments, meaning that they should focus directly on the things people want and need to do rather than leaping ahead to identify and measure components that may be interrupting performance. To illustrate what is meant by top-down, a therapist might ask a girl who wants to learn to ride a bicycle as well as her friends to demonstrate what happens when she tries to ride. This is a radically different approach to 'bottom-up' assessment, where the therapist would have synthesised knowledge of the performance requirements of bicycle riding and the likely impact of the child's health condition, to decide which aspects of body structure or function to evaluate. The assessment might then have focused on the girl's balance reactions, the degree of spasticity in her lower limbs, or some other impairment thought to be contributing to the performance problem. A top-down approach has been mandated in the American Occupational Therapy Association's (2002) practice framework, which specifies that data gathering begin with building up a profile of the person and in analysing occupational performance.

Several advantages of occupationally focused assessment have been proposed. Firstly, by assessing what the person does do, wants to do, and what happens when he or she attempts to do it, therapists make very evident the relevance of the assessment (Batavia 1992) and the intended outcome of occupational therapy strategy (Trombly 1993). There is clarity in starting 'where you mean to finish' (Molineux 2004, p. 9). Secondly, it has been noted that if they begin by measuring performance components, therapists may overlook critical issues, such as not knowing how to perform the occupation (Polatajko et al 1999), not wanting to (Fisher 1992), or being prevented from performing the occupation by environmental barriers (Roulstone 1998). Occupation-based assessments are less prone to such omissions, because observing performance encompasses opportunities to notice problems stemming from a lack of know-how, motivation, or resources, or from environmental barriers. Moreover, observing actual performance will likely make evident any 'deficits in performance components and their impact on function' (Payne & Howell 2005, p. 279).

Starting from and focusing on occupation aligns with the World Health Organisation's (WHO) emphasis on participation, as outlined in the International Classification of Functioning, Disability and Health (ICF) (World Health Organisation 2001). It also acknowledges that the relationship between impairment of body structure and function and activity limitations is complex, so that change in a performance component may not reduce limitations or enhance people's participation in occupation (Hocking 2003).

Supporting this shift in practice, established and newly developed standardised assessments are being recognised as or developed to directly measure some aspect of occupation. For instance, the Assessment of Motor and Process Skills has been identified as top-down (Payne & Howell 2005) and both the Activity Card Sort – Hong Kong version (Chan et al 2006) and Preschool Activity Card Sort (Berg & LaVesser 2006) measure participation in everyday occupations. There is also intensive work amongst occupational therapy researchers internationally to develop assessments that focus on occupation. Recent examples include the Play Assessment for Group Settings (PAGS) (Lautamo et al. 2005) which measures the play performance of 2- to 8-year-olds, an interest checklist to evaluate the leisure occupations of older Scandinavian people (Nilsson & Fisher 2006) and an Assessment of Computer-Related Skills, which assesses adults' computer abilities (Fischl & Fisher 2006). Other researchers are generating new knowledge of occupation and the settings in which people carry out the majority of their occupations. In one such study 10 people, aged 99 years, were interviewed about their experience of daily occupations (Häggblom-Kronlöf et al 2007) while in another study 80–90-year-old people were asked about the meaning their home holds for them (Dahlin-Ivanoff et al 2007). The results from studies such as these will assist therapists to identify what to ask people and understand what their responses mean. Dahlin-Ivanoff and colleagues, for example, suggest that knowing what people's homes mean to them is essential to assessing whether strategies intended to support occupational performance and well-being will have the desired effect.

As therapists increasingly conduct occupation-based assessments, goals that address impairments, such as improving motor or intrapersonal ability, or strategies focusing at that level (Dekker 1995) may disappear from practice. Another flow-on effect might be a shift in terminology, from talking about 'functional' assessments to more accurately referring to measurement of occupational performance (Wikeby et al 2006). Similarly, guided by the ICF's emphasis on participation, occupational therapists might more confidently speak of assessing people's level of participation in preferred and necessary occupations, the quality or ease of their performance, or the barriers encountered and their effect. Additionally, rather than advocating borrowed concepts such as 'quality of life components' (Schofield 2006, p. 482), therapists might measure people's status on occupations that matter to them.

Nonetheless, therapists will at times assess impairments, perhaps to assist with differential diagnosis of a health condition, such as whether a clumsy child has developmental coordination disorder or cerebral palsy (Missiuna et al 2006a). Another reason might be to identify the perceptual dysfunction disrupting a person's occupational performance, to clarify whether to employ remedial or compensatory strategies. A further reason might be to determine whether an individual has the potential to develop particular skills, such as those required to make sense of, physically manage, and emotionally cope with assistive technologies, and thereby achieve educational goals (Copley & Ziviani 2005).

Occupation-based assessment

Top-down occupationally focused assessment processes might well proceed from the meaning of occupation to its place in people's lives and its observable features (Hocking 2001). Occupational meanings encompass the relationship between the things people do and their identity, which includes understandings about the kind of person they are, who they might become in the future, the things they do, the way they do them, and contexts they do them in. Occupational identity also encompasses beliefs about what is important to do, understanding about occupational roles and skills, and knowledge and aptitudes for occupation. In this sense, occupation is the vehicle for developing one's identity, expressing spirituality, experiencing meaning in living and achieving one's life purpose. Because occupation exists in a social context, the extent to which these meanings align with others' views is also important.

The nature of occupation refers to what is achieved by participating in it. Does it provide relaxation, generate an income, express love for one's children or respect of one's elders, maintain the environment, or get food on the table? In this regard, occupational therapists are concerned with identifying performance that is disrupted by occupational challenges, whether the environment supports or impedes a successful outcome, and the ways in which others help or hinder important abilities.

The observable features of an occupation relate to how the person, environment, and occupation combine. Depending on the issue of concern, occupational therapists assess the context and requirements of performance: the steps involved and actions required, what standard of performance is expected, whether necessary resources are available and accessible and where, when and how often the occupation occurs. This is the basis for understanding whether the occupation or its context can be modified to support performance. Assessing the person encompasses assessing what actually happens: how skillfully the occupation is performed, the time and effort required, satisfaction with the outcome, and so on. Therapists also look for indications of capacity to improve the quality of performance. As was previously mentioned, if the cause of the problem remains unclear, the assessment of the underlying performance components may also be indicated.

When to assess

The discussion to this point has shown that assessment is complex, and spans what people do, why they do it, where it happens, and what is achieved. When occupational therapists conduct an assessment is perhaps more straightforward, because the answer is, 'At every step in the occupational therapy process'. The purpose of gathering information, however, progresses from whether to accept a referral (screening), to what the problem is (assessment), to what was achieved (evaluation of outcomes) and whether the outcome is satisfactory (re-negotiation of goals or discharge) (see Table 7.1). To illustrate the different purposes of assessment at each step, key questions are identified.

A couple of the questions in Table 7.1 warrant further comment, because they do more than inform the therapeutic process. The purpose of screening is to establish whether there are needs that are relevant to occupational therapy. Therapists may also be called on to determine how beneficial their involvement is likely to be (Mozley et al 2007) and to screen out people with a poor prognosis. That is, service priorities or contractual obligations rather than assessment results may determine service delivery. Similarly, one purpose of both initial assessment and outcome measures may be to 'record the severity of the person's disability and function' (Corr & Siddons 2005, p. 202). Creating this record may relate more to determining eligibility for services or monitoring the progression of a long-term health condition than informing the occupational therapy process.

Recognising that assessment continues throughout the occupational therapy process also suggests that it is a dynamic process. That is, rather than following a predetermined plan of information gathering, most therapists will explore aspects of participation in occupation 'as they become relevant and meaningful during the course of the assessment' (Wilby 2005, p. 41), and continue to gather information as intervention progresses.

Steps in the process: screening, assessment and evaluation

Whilst assessment never stops, it is concentrated in the initial phases of the occupational therapy process and once intervention is complete. These different stages of assessment are now considered in more detail.

Screening

Screening refers to identification of 'clients who need more detailed assessment and therapy intervention' (Cooke et al 2005, p. 69). The purpose of screening is to avoid wasting the time and resources of both the people referred and services receiving referrals, and to prioritise referrals. As such, therapists have an ethical responsibility to 'obtain relevant information to enable them to determine the appropriateness of the referral' (College of Occupational Therapists 2005, p. 529). The screening process is the beginning of getting to know the people referred, ensuring they have a sense of what occupational therapy can realistically offer, and establishing a therapeutic alliance. As for all phases

Table 7.1 Questions addressed by assessment findings at each step of the occupational therapy process

Step in the occupational therapy process	Questions assessment findings address
Screening	• Does occupational therapy have anything to offer? • Is what occupational therapy has to offer welcomed? • Is intervention likely to be beneficial? (Mozley et al 2007)
Assessment	• What is the occupational performance issue? • What are its causes? • What might help? • What abilities, skills and resources are available? • How severe is the disability? (Corr & Siddons 2005)
Identification of needs	• What are the person(s)' needs? • Does the extent of those needs warrant intervention? • Is this the best place to service those needs? • Is referral to another service warranted?
Negotiation of goals	• What does the person(s) want? (College of Occupational Therapists 2005) • What do others want? • Can the goals be legally and ethically supported? • What has priority?
Intervention planning and implementation	• Are things progressing as expected? • Are observations consistent with previous understandings? • If not, why not?
Evaluation of outcomes	• What was achieved? • Was that enough?
Re-negotiation of goals or discharge	• Are further needs apparent? • If so, can occupational therapy address them?

of the assessment process, screening should address meaningful occupations deemed important by the individual, family, school, workplace, or community, whether that be 'making nan or roti bread, eating with chop sticks, playing with dolls, using a wok or earth for cooking, tying a turban or using running water to bathe' (Fisher 2005, p. 224).

To obtain the information they need to determine whether a referral is appropriate, occupational therapists have four data-gathering strategies available to them: observation, evaluation, dialogue – more formally referred to as an interview – and self-rating (Corr & Siddons 2005). In determining how to proceed, occupational therapists consider a range of factors including people's health status, their cognitive and communication abilities, the practicalities of observing them participating in the occupation of concern, and the availability of suitable standardised screening tools. There is a range of tools available. One example is the FirstSTEp

Screening Test for Evaluating Preschoolers, which identifies children who are at risk of developmental delays that are predictive of school-related problems (Miller 1993). Another example is the Occupational Therapy Adult Perceptual Screening Test (OT-APST), which is used to screen adults who have experienced a stroke or acquired a brain injury for agnosia, apraxia, acalculia, and impairments in constructional and visuospatial skills that may disrupt a whole range of activities of daily living (Cooke et al 2005). Note, however, that these and perhaps the majority of standardised screening tools that occupational therapists use assess performance components indicative of difficulty with occupation, rather than occupation itself. This reality points to a sorely needed area of knowledge development for the profession.

Whatever the means by which data are gathered, when screening results in acceptance of a referral, it also initiates the process of negotiating the broad goals of assessment and intervention (Copley & Ziviani 2005). In the case of specialist services, such as those providing wheelchair and seating systems or assistive technologies, goals will be relatively circumscribed compared with general rehabilitative or lifestyle redesign services, or community development initiatives. From an evidence-based practice perspective, this initial assessment is also the point at which therapists begin to look for indicators that strategies will prove beneficial (Mozley et al 2007).

Assessment

Having determined that referral to occupational therapy is indicated, a more extensive process of data gathering begins. The picture the therapist gains of the person, the context and occupation of concern sets the stage for relevant goals addressing valued occupational outcomes. In turn, occupation-focused goals support the development of strategies that are perceived to address the issue, and to be achievable and tolerable. Moreover occupation-focused strategies are likely to elicit ongoing effort because, as changes in performance become evident, they provide markers of development, learning, enhanced skill or know-how, increased ease or satisfaction, or whatever the intended outcome.

Two important ethical considerations are only gathering information that will be used and not overstating the significance or trustworthiness of findings, given that they potentially inform life-changing decisions such as discharge destination or withdrawal of a driving license. Other considerations include where to conduct the assessment, with some evidence indicating that people with cognitive deficits perform better in their own home (Bottari et al 2006), and whether the same assessment can be used as a reassessment once intervention is completed. A final point to consider is the nature of the assessment itself (Hocking 2001). That is, is 'being assessed' a scientific exercise where one person objectively observes another or a supportive experience of cooperative problem solving? Does it involve attempting simulated activities and unfamiliar tasks or self-chosen, familiar occupations? Are the assessment activities and the way they are administered consistent with the person's cultural practices and worldviews, or foreign and irrelevant to their cultural context?

Having gathered relevant information, occupational therapists are expected to report their assessment methods and findings in full (College of Occupational Therapists 2005, Gibson et al 2004). That includes representing the views of the person (Gibson et al 2004) and providing an interpretation of results, so that others can understand what they mean (Corr & Siddons 2005). Careful consideration must also be given to who has a right to know the assessment results and the recommendations arising from them, what the people who have been assessed and their carers are told, and how best to convey that information (Welch & Lowes 2005).

Assessment results determine what happens next. If things do not progress as expected, initial assumptions and findings come into question and further assessment following new lines of inquiry may be necessary. That might involve, for example, reviewing the therapeutic approach, revisiting assumptions about how and why the occupation is performed, checking whether the targeted occupations and outcomes are valued and supported by significant others, or assessing whether previously unnoticed impairments, lifestyle factors or environmental barriers are impeding progress.

Evaluation

To evaluate something means to appraise it, and often, to find out how much of it there is. In the context of occupational therapy 'it' refers to the occupational goals and the extent to which they were achieved. Individuals, families, groups and organisations that receive occupational therapy value this information because it provides feedback on what has been accomplished, helping people to realise how far they have progressed and feel satisfied with their efforts. This motivational boost can help people sustain the occupational performance strategies they have learned or lifestyle changes they have made. Evaluation results also assist therapists and their clients to determine whether intervention is complete, and if not, whether new goals or different ways of intervening need to be explored.

There are a number of additional reasons for knowing what was accomplished. The recording of evaluation results completes the clinical record, showing the progression from presenting issues to therapy to outcomes. Occupational therapists also report evaluation results to others: the referral source or health insurer who will decide whether to refer people to occupational therapy in the future, a therapist the person is being referred to who will decide whether to act on that referral, a community that will decide whether occupational therapy input helps move things forward and so on. Whatever the audience, therapists must carefully consider how to present evaluation findings. In some cases, specific observations of improved performance skills and more favourable outcomes, or reporting the removal of risk factors and barriers will suffice. Equally, therapists may seek people's subjective account of whether performance or outcomes of occupation are enhanced, confidence or satisfaction with performance increased, or discomfort associated with performance diminished. In other cases, objective measures of change will be sought.

In both setting goals and in evaluating and reporting outcomes, therapists make an implicit judgement about how much change might be possible, often using experience with previous clients as a benchmark. Supplementing those practice-based insights, the professional literature offers two kinds of information. Firstly, therapists who design a strategy sometimes report its effectiveness. An example is Logan et al's (2006) strategy to improve outdoor mobility amongst people who had experienced a stroke. They reported a 77% success rate, measured by achievement of goals, with maintenance of results after 10 months. Key indicators of lack of success were also identified. While the authors caution that therapists who have not been trained in their methods may not achieve equivalent results, the findings nonetheless give an indication of what might be realistic with similar populations.

Secondly, therapists might draw on findings from randomised controlled trials. One such is Graff and colleagues' (2006) study of the efficacy of an occupational therapy strategy for people over 64 years of age, diagnosed with dementia and living in the community. Designed to improve independence in meaningful occupations and reduce caregiver burden, the results show clinically relevant improvement that was sustained over 12 weeks, despite limitations in learning ability due to dementia. Studies such as this are useful in indicating the magnitude of change that might be achieved with a similar level of input and the timeframe over which change can be expected to be sustained, as well as identifying potentially suitable evaluation tools. Using this information as a benchmark, therapists and clients can judge whether the outcome of therapy is disappointing, reasonable or commendable.

How to elicit information

In addition to being clear about the purpose of conducting an assessment and where it fits into the occupational therapy process, therapists must decide how best to elicit the information they need. That includes choosing between standardised and non-standardised assessments. This section of the discussion addresses the relative strengths and weaknesses of each.

Selecting and using standardised assessments

Standardised assessments generally require the person or group being assessed to respond to set questions, be interviewed about set topics, rate their experiences on a set scale, or engage in a set task, sometimes within a set timeframe. Assessors are required to administer the assessment and record and score the findings in a prescribed way. The objects used and how they are arranged may be specified. There may or may not be normative data, which enable an individual's results to be compared with the 'normal' population.

There are many reasons to opt for standardised assessments. An obvious advantage is that the developer has done a great deal of work on the therapist's behalf, determining what task or tasks to ask people to do and which aspects of performance to direct attention towards. Many also have a conceptual framework that guides interpretation of findings and some identify cut-off scores, that is, scores that indicate a possible problem or a severe problem warranting intervention. The developers of standardised assessments attend to their validity, meaning that the assessment does assess what it was intended to assess, and face validity, which means that the assessment tasks or items are perceived as relevant to whatever is being assessed. Test developers also attend to reliability, ensuring that the result would be much the same if the assessment was administered at another time (test–retest reliability) or by another person (inter-rater reliability) – unless an actual change has occurred in the person being assessed.

Safety concerns, for both the therapist and the person being assessed, may be another reason to opt for a standardised assessment, such as choosing a standardised virtual driving assessment over an on-road test (Lee 2006). It seems that local practice is also influential. Recent surveys in the US and Canada (Korner-Bitensky et al 2006) and Sweden (Larsson et al 2006), for example, reveal wide variations between countries in the assessment tools therapists prefer.

The decision to use a particular standardised assessment tool is determined, firstly, by whether it addresses the aspect of occupation of concern. An equally important consideration is whether the assessment was developed or adapted for use with people of the same age, demographic profile, cultural background, and language as the person or group to be assessed. In some cases there are published reports of the assessment's use with a relevant client group, such as Payne and Howell's (2005) evaluation of using the Assessment of Motor and Process Skills (AMPS) with children. In other cases, therapists must make a judgement based on the developer's claims and the information given about participants in the studies undertaken to develop the assessment or generate validity, reliability or normative data. For example, the 62 participants in a study to examine the psychometric properties of the Child Occupational Self Assessment (COSA) are described as between 8 and 17 years old, having 'adequate ability to communicate self-perceptions' and including boys and girls, half of whom were receiving occupational therapy (Keller et al 2005, p. 121). A therapist considering using the COSA with a child who had recently immigrated from a non-Western country such as Japan or Thailand, or one with very different experiences such as being schooled at home, or a member of a minority racial group would need to make judgements about language capability, the possible impact of cultural difference, and the relevance of assessment items that assume normative life experiences. An additional pragmatic consideration is whether therapeutic application of an assessment has been reported (see for example Edwards et al 2006, Fisher 2005), or whether its use is confined to research.

Equally important to establishing whether an assessment is applicable to a particular client, is the strength of its psychometric properties. There is a wealth of information published each year about both new and existing assessment tools (see for example Berg & LaVesser 2006, Chan et al 2006, Lautamo et al 2005, Nilsson & Fisher 2006). Therapists looking for assistance in identifying or choosing between standardised assessments might also usefully consider published reviews. For instance, Missiuna et al (2006b) investigated the alignment between standardised assessments commonly used with children with developmental coordination disorder and the ICF. Similarly, Harris and colleagues (2005) reviewed a range of outcome measures designed to evaluate how the lives of people with a disability are impacted by mobility-related assistive devices, concluding that none adequately addressed participation outcomes. Guided by this review, therapists might justifiably decide to use a more broadly focused assessment of participation, or conduct a non-standardised interview about what clients did day-to-day and how introduction of a mobility aid changed that. Where relevant reviews are not available, evidence-based approaches to critically evaluating assessment tools are available to guide therapists through a rigorous process of evaluation (see for example Jerosch-Herold 2005).

Professional responsibility and standardised assessments

The strength of evidence on an assessment's occupational focus and psychometric properties, however, does not absolve therapists of their professional responsibilities in the assessment process. Rather, therapists are responsible for recognising and responding to issues, the first of which is to use standardised assessments ethically. That means that therapists must recognise the limitations of their knowledge and expertise (College of Occupational Therapists 2005), including their proficiency in administering an assessment, which affects its reliability, and whether they administer it in the same way as other therapists, which is the basis of interrater reliability.

As well as ensuring their actions do not nullify psychometric properties, therapists are charged with bringing their professional skills and judgement to all assessment processes, including standardised assessments. For example, the Canadian Occupational Performance Measure (COPM) has been endorsed as encompassing cultural occupations, but that possibility depends entirely on therapists' skills (Fisher 2005). Similarly, any variation in the way an assessment is administered rests entirely on the therapist's expertise. For example, the COPM is designed to be administered with the person with the occupational concern or a family member or carer. Administering it with whanau (extended family) might be more culturally fitting in some contexts in New Zealand, in acknowledging others' knowledge of the person and cultural constraints on individuals claiming strengths for themselves, but make the therapist more than ordinarily responsible for documenting the process and appraising the reliability of the results. A related concern is that therapists retain responsibility for recognising when items in standardised assessments are embedded in culturally specific occupational opportunities, putting individuals with different life experiences at a disadvantage. The Touch Inventory for Elementary School-Aged Children (TIE), for example, assumes children being screened for tactile defensiveness have experience of 'fingerpainting, walking barefoot or standing in line' (Brown & Brown 2006, p. 242).

Having adopted a standardised assessment into practice, therapists must remain open to reviewing that decision as occupational therapy theory and broader assessment practices change over time. The renewed focus on occupation rather than performance components, for example, seems to be bringing about a gradual shift towards more occupationally focused standardised assessments (Diamantis 2006). It has also been suggested that standardised assessments that have the capacity to encompass 'occupations related to all aspects of daily life' (Lexell et al 2006, p. 241), such as the COPM, are more suited to practice that acknowledges the complexities of occupation than assessments that evaluate a predetermined selection of occupations. Critical reflection on practice may also support a shift in practice. Diamantis (2006), for example, strongly questioned occupational therapists' continued use of several common visual perceptual assessments, citing insufficient evidence of their utility as outcome measures.

Looking outside the profession, standardised assessments published from the 1990s seem to indicate a fundamental shift in thinking from relying on direct observation or measurement by the health practitioner to valuing and trusting the observations and experience of people who have seen or experienced the nature of the impairment and its impact on participation in a range of environments. An example might be the Pediatric Evaluation of Disability Inventory (PEDI), which parents complete, versus the Denver II, where the health practitioner attempts to elicit certain behavioural responses from the child, generally in a clinic or office environment. Observing this shift in practice suggests that newer assessments might better align with occupational therapy's commitment to person-centredness, which acknowledges people as experts in their own life. In addition, involving adults and even children in bringing their experience to standardised assessment processes has been claimed to foster self-determination (Keller & Kielhofner 2005, Keller et al 2005).

Non-standardised assessments

While any assessment process demands a high level of professional judgement, non-standardised assessments are particularly demanding because therapists are responsible for both the means of assessment and the trustworthiness of the findings. Non-standardised assessments include printed checklists and report formats as well as standard interview questions and tasks, such as getting dressed or making a cup of tea. Therapists report using these assessments because they have been developed locally to suit a particular client group, and because they are available, familiar and comfortable and therapists know what they are looking for. These features make them quick and easy to administer. Therapists are also drawn to the flexibility of non-standardised assessments, whereby 'only parts which are relevant' are used (Blenkiron 2005, p. 154). This 'pick and mix approach' is specifically excluded by most standardised assessments (Corr & Siddons 2005, p. 204). Flexibility also means that assessment and enabling strategies can be intermingled; with possible solutions being trialled as performance issues are identified. This blending of assessment and on-the-spot problem solving is a prominent feature of dynamic performance analysis (Polatajko et al 1999) and typical of established practices such as pre-discharge home-assessment visits, which aim to both assess safety and independence in personal and domestic tasks and generate strategies to enable people to cope (Welch & Lowes 2005). Using non-standardised methods to gather information, however, means that the quality of the data is entirely dependent on the expertise of the therapist (Wilby 2005), while the repeatability of the assessment depends on detailed documentation of the assessment process.

Reasons cited for using non-standardised assessments include the cost of acquiring standardised assessments, lack of knowledge about how to administer them, lack of time to evaluate which would be most suitable (Blenkiron 2005) and managers who do not actively support changes in practice (Chard 2006). Opting for non-standardised assessments also seems to be driven by therapists' discomfort with administration protocols that require them to suspend efforts to engage with and encourage people, to wait and watch while they struggle with tasks and fail, and to resist intuitions about ways to modify tasks, instructions or questions to elicit a more adaptive response (Managh & Cook 1993). From an occupational perspective, non-standardised assessments might be more likely to use actual occupational performance as a point of comparison; typically, what the person concerned could previously do. In contrast, the normative data provided for standardised assessments tend to be impairment-focused, for example the degree of unilateral neglect (Cooke et al 2006), or to address performance components such as grip strength.

Non-standardised assessments have limitations. Those suggested by Welch and Lowes (2005) are the frequent lack of rationale for what is included and what is left out, and the reliance on local therapists to update assessment practices to keep pace with emerging professional concerns, such as person-centred or occupationally focused practice, and new evidence, including the things clients and carers are concerned about. Furthermore, compared with standardised assessments, locally developed assessment processes do not generate strong evidence of therapy outcomes and the overall efficacy of services provided, and it is difficult to relate the results of efficacy studies to local practice because the similarities and differences are unknown (Bowman

2006). To be fair, however, standardised assessments do not always provide a clear rationale for their content, and may not be revised in a timely fashion to reflect shifts in the profession's philosophy or available evidence.

Conclusion

Occupational therapists conduct assessments to understand what occupations mean to people, the roles those occupations serve in their lives, and what is happening when participation is disrupted or dysfunctional. Assessment processes are complex. They span the most intimate to the most public occupations, the mundane requirements of everyday living to spiritual expression, and every occupational setting people might create or enter. Running through this diversity is a consistent demand for high levels of ethical and professional behaviour, which requires constant updating of therapists' knowledge and skills in evaluating and administering standardised assessment tools, and in devising trustworthy non-standardised assessment processes. The imperative for the best possible assessment practices lies in the consequences for individuals, groups and society with an occupational concern; and that therapists ensure they implement effective strategies that achieve important occupational outcomes.

References

American Occupational Therapy Association (2002). Occupational therapy practice framework: domain and process. *American Journal of Occupational Therapy,* 56, 609–639.

Batavia, A. I. (1992). Assessing the function of functional assessment: a consumer perspective. *Disability and Rehabilitation,* 14(3), 156–160.

Berg, C. & LaVesser, P. (2006). The preschool activity card sort. *OTJR: Occupation, Participation and Health,* 26(4), 143–151.

Blenkiron, E. L. (2005). Uptake for standardised hand assessments in rheumatology: why is it so low? *British Journal of Occupational Therapy* 68(4), 148–157.

Bottari, C., Dutil, É., Dassa, C. et al. (2006). Choosing the most

appropriate environment to evaluate independence in everyday activities: home or clinic? *Australian Occupational Therapy Journal,* 53, 98–106.

Bowman, J. (2006). Challenges to measuring outcomes in occupational therapy: a qualitative focus group study. *British Journal of Occupational Therapy,* 69(10), 464–472.

Brown, G. T. & Brown, A. (2006). A review and critique of the Touch Inventory for Elementary School-Aged Children (TIE). *British Journal of Occupational Therapy,* 69(5), 234–243.

Chan, V. W. K., Chung, J. C. C., & Packer, T. (2006). Validity and reliability of the Activity Card Sort – Hong Kong Version. *OTJR: Occupation, Participation and Health,* 26(4), 152–158.

Chard, G. (2006). Adopting the assessment of motor and process skills into practice: therapists' voices. *British Journal of Occupational Therapy,* 69(2), 50–57.

College of Occupational Therapists (2005). College of Occupational Therapists: code of ethics and professional conduct. *British Journal of Occupational Therapy,* 68(11), 527–532.

Cooke, D. M., McKenna, K. & Fleming, J. (2005). Development of a standardized occupational therapy screening tool for visual perception in adults. *Scandinavian Journal of Occupational Therapy,* 12, 59–71.

Cooke, D. M., McKenna, K., Fleming, J. et al (2006). Australian normative data for the

Occupational Therapy Adult Perceptual Screening Test. *Australian Occupational Therapy Journal*, 53, 325–336.

Copley, J. & Ziviani, J. (2005). Assistive technology assessment and planning for children with multiple disabilities in educational settings. *British Journal of Occupational Therapy*, 68(12), 559–566.

Corr, S. & Siddons, L. (2005). An introduction to the selection of outcome measures. *British Journal of Occupational Therapy*, 68(5), 202–206.

Dahlin-Ivanoff, S., Haak, M., Fänge, A. et al. (2007). The multiple meaning of home as experienced by very old Swedish people. *Scandinavian Journal of Occupational Therapy*, 14(1), 25–32.

Dekker, J. (1995). Application of the ICIDH in survey research on rehabilitation: the emergence of the functional diagnosis. *Disability and Rehabilitation*, 17(3/4),195–201.

Diamantis, A. D. (2006). Use of standardised tests in paediatrics: the practice of private occupational therapists working in the United Kingdom. *British Journal of Occupational Therapy*, 69(6), 281–287.

Edwards, D. F., Hahn, M. G., Baum, C, et al. (2006). Screening patients with stroke for rehabilitation needs: validation of the post-stroke rehabilitation guidelines. *Neurorehabilitation and Neural Repair*, 20(1), 42–48.

Fischl, C. & Fisher, A. G. (2006). Development and Rasch analysis of the assessment of computer-related skills. *Scandinavian Journal of Occupational Therapy*, 13, 1–10.

Fisher, A. (1992). Functional measures, part 2: selecting the right test, minimizing the limitations. *American Journal of Occupational Therapy*, 46, 278–281.

Fisher, S. (2005). The Canadian Occupational Performance Measure: does it address the cultural occupations of ethnic minorities? *British Journal of Occupational Therapy*, 68(5), 224–234.

Gibson, F., Sykes, M. & Young, S. (2004). Record keeping in occupational therapy: are we meeting the standards set by the College of Occupational Therapists?

British Journal of Occupational Therapy, 67(12), 547–550.

Graff, M. J. L., Vernooij-Dassen, M. J. M., Thijssen, M. et al. (2006). Community based occupational therapy for patients with dementia and their caregivers: randomised controlled trial. *British Medical Journal*, 333(1196), DOI:10.1136/bmj.39001.688843.BE

Häggblom-Kronlöf, G., Hultberg, J., Eriksson, B. G. et al (2007). Experiences of daily occupations at 99 years of age. *Scandinavian Journal of Occupational Therapy*, 14(3), 192–200.

Harris, A., Pinnington, L. L. & Ward, C. D. (2005). Evaluating the impact of mobility-related assistive technology on the lives of disabled people: a review of outcome measures. *British Journal of Occupational Therapy*, 68(12), 553–558.

Hocking, C. (2001). The issue is: implementing occupation based assessment. *American Journal of Occupational Therapy*, 55(4), 463–469.

Hocking, C. (2003). Creating occupational practice: a multidisciplinary health focus. In: G. Brown, S. Esdaile, S. Ryan (Eds.). *Becoming an advanced healthcare practitioner* (pp. 189–215). London, Butterworth-Heinemann.

Jerosch-Herold, C. (2005). An evidence-based approach to choosing outcome measures: a checklist for the critical appraisal of validity, reliability and responsiveness studies. *British Journal of Occupational Therapy*, 68(8), 347–353.

Keller, J. & Kielhofner, G. (2005). Psychometric characteristics of the Child Occupational Self Assessment (COSA), part two: refining the psychometric properties. *Scandinavian Journal of Occupational Therapy*, 12, 147–158.

Keller, J., Kafkes, A. & Kielhofner, G. (2005). Psychometric characteristics of the Child Occupational Self Assessment (COSA), part one: an initial examination of psychometric properties. *Scandinavian Journal of Occupational Therapy*, 12, 118–127.

Kielhofner, G. (2007). *Model of human occupation: theory and application.* (4th ed). Baltimore, Lippincott Williams & Wilkins.

Korner-Bitensky, N., Bitensky, J., Sofer, S. et al. (2006). Driving evaluation practices of clinicians working in the United States and Canada. *American Journal of Occupational Therapy*, 60(4), 428–434.

Larsson, H., Lundberg, C., Falkmer, T. et al. (2006). A Swedish survey of occupational therapists' involvement and performance in driving assessments. *Scandinavian Journal of Occupational Therapy*, 14(4), 215–220.

Lautamo, T., Kottorp, A., Salminen, A.-L. (2005). Play assessment for group settings: a pilot study to construct an assessment tool. *Scandinavian Journal of Occupational Therapy*, 12, 136–144.

Lee, H. C. (2006). Virtual driving tests for older adult drivers? *British Journal of Occupational Therapy*, 69(3), 138–141.

Lexell, E. M., Iwarsson, S. & Lexell, J. (2006). The complexity of daily occupations in multiple sclerosis. *Scandinavian Journal of Occupational Therapy*, 13, 241–248.

Logan, P. A., Walker, M. F. & Gladman, J. R. F. (2006). Description of an occupational therapy intervention aimed at improving outdoor mobility. *British Journal of Occupational Therapy*, 69(1), 2–6.

Managh, M. F. & Cook, J. V. (1993). The use of standardized assessment in occupational therapy: the BAFPE-R. *American Journal of Occupational Therapy*, 47, 877–884.

Miller, L. (1993). *FirstSTEp Screening Test for Evaluating Preschoolers.* London, Harcourt Assessment.

Missiuna, C., Gaines, R. & Soucie, H. (2006a). Why every office needs a tennis ball: a new approach to assessing the clumsy child. *Canadian Medical Association Journal*, 175(5), 471–473.

Missiuna, C., Rivard, L. & Bartlett, D. (2006b). Exploring assessment tools and the target of intervention for children with developmental coordination disorder. *Physical and Occupational Therapy in Pediatrics*, 26(1/2), 71–89.

Molineux, M. (2004). Occupation in occupational therapy: A labour in vain? In: M. Molineux, (Ed.). *Occupation for occupational therapists* (pp. 1–14). Oxford, UK, Blackwell Publishing.

Mozley, C. G., Schneider, J., Cordingley, L. et al. (2007). The care home activity project: does introducing an occupational therapy programme reduce depression in care homes? *Aging & Mental Health*, 11(1), 99–107.

Nilsson, I. & Fisher, A. G. (2006). Evaluating leisure activities in the oldest old. *Scandinavian Journal of Occupational Therapy*, 13, 31–37.

Payne, S. & Howell, C. (2005). An evaluation of the clinical use of the Assessment of Motor and Process Skills with children. *British Journal of Occupational Therapy*, 68(6), 277–280.

Polatajko, H., Mandich, A. & Martini, R. (1999). Dynamic performance analysis: a framework for understanding occupational performance. *American Journal of Occupational Therapy*, 54, 65–72.

Roulstone, A. (1998). *Enabling technology: disabled people, work and new technology*. Buckingham, UK, Open University Press.

Sachs, A. (2004). *April Award presentation*. Cape Town, South Africa, Occupational Therapy Association South Africa Congress.

Schofield, P. (2006). Measuring outcome in psychiatric rehabilitation. *British Journal of Occupational Therapy*, 69(10), 481–483.

Trombly, C. (1993). Anticipating the future: assessment of occupational function. *American Journal of Occupational Therapy*, 47(3), 253–257.

Welch, A. & Lowes, S. (2005). Home assessment visits within the acute setting: a discussion and literature review. *British Journal of Occupational Therapy*, 68(4), 158–164.

Wikeby, M., Pierre, B. L. & Archenholtz, B. (2006). Occupational therapists' reflections on practice within psychiatric care: a Delphi study. *Scandinavian Journal of Occupational Therapy*, 13, 151–159.

Wilby, H. J. (2005). A description of a functional screening assessment developed for the acute physical setting. *British Journal of Occupational Therapy*, 68(1), 39–44.

World Health Organisation (2001). *International classification of functioning, disability and health*. Geneva, WHO.

8

Writing occupation-focused goals

Julia Bowman and Lise L. Mogensen

CHAPTER CONTENTS

Background 95

Occupation-focused plans: an overview. . . .97

Referral to occupational therapy 97

Assessing the person–environment–
occupation fit 98

Writing occupation-focused aims 100

Setting occupation-focused goals 100

Writing SMART goals. 101

Selecting occupation-focused
strategies 105

Evaluating the person–environment–
occupation fit 106

Conclusion. 107

SUMMARY

Planning the implementation of enabling
strategies is an essential process in the practice
of occupational therapy. It is much more than a
sequence of steps therapists employ to provide a
service to their clients. It is an organisational
structure that facilitates the professional
reasoning process for conducting assessments,
identifying goals, selecting strategies and
evaluating outcomes. This chapter provides a
linear structure for developing occupation-
focused enabling strategies. This approach has
been specifically developed to assist therapists
to identify and write occupation-focused aims
and goals, and to link strategies and evaluation
methods directly to the outcome. If occupational
therapy strategies are not carefully planned, they
may lack focus on occupation, fail to directly
address goals, and be ineffective in achieving
desired occupational engagement outcomes.
Therefore, planning is a skill all therapists must
be competent in to ensure appropriate and
effective service provision to the people who use
their services.

KEY POINTS

When writing occupation-focused goals
occupational therapists need to:

- Collaborate with each person and consider the
  person–environment–occupation fit.
- Focus on occupation and tailor the goals to a
  person's unique occupational needs.
- Apply the principles of the International
  Classification of Functioning Disability and
  Health (ICF).
- Use assessment and goal setting to identify the
  desired outcome of strategies.
- Use SMART goals to direct occupation-focused
  strategies.
- Incorporate appropriate outcome measures to
  quantify change over time in a person's body
  structure and functions, activity or
  participation.
- Include clear documentation of each step of the
  process.

Background

Occupational therapists have claimed for nearly
80 years that occupation as a therapeutic medium
is core to their practice (Emerson 1998, Rebeiro
& Cook 1999). Today, the World Federation of

Occupational Therapists describes occupational therapy as a profession 'concerned with promoting health and well being through occupation' (World Federation of Occupational Therapists 2007). As such, it is important that occupational therapy strategies clearly reflect occupation as their central focus.

Occupational therapists believe the person, the environment and the occupations the person engages in are closely interrelated. Consequently, therapists need to be aware of factors that may influence this finely balanced relationship. The Person–Environment–Occupation (PEO) Model (Law et al 1996) acknowledges the complexity of people performing occupations within broad environments. As such it provides a sound theoretical framework to assist therapists to account for these inter-related constructs when planning strategies. The PEO assumes that the person, the environment and the occupations the person does, interact continuously across time and space. Therefore, the greater the congruence between these elements, the closer the individual is to their desired level of occupational engagement. The PEO model directs therapists to think about strategies that target the person, occupation and environment in different ways. Therapists are also challenged to identify multiple options to elicit change in occupational engagement. As the relationship between the person, environment and occupation is dynamic and constantly changing, the PEO model advocates the ongoing monitoring of strategies to ensure progress toward goal attainment is being made.

Another model designed to assist the intervention planning process is the International Classification of Functioning Disability and Health (ICF) developed by the World Health Organisation (WHO) (World Health Organisation 2002). The ICF framework was designed to facilitate the conceptualisation, classification and measurement of disability. Within this framework, disability is recognised as a multidimensional experience with participation viewed as a component of health rather than a consequence of disease. Use of the ICF by therapists promotes an integrated approach to the gathering and sharing of information, professional decision-making, and evaluating the efficacy and effectiveness of interventions (Australian Institute of Health and Welfare 2003). As such, the ICF has specific application to the intervention planning process in occupational therapy. According to the ICF framework, a person's level of participation is conceived as a dynamic interaction between health conditions, and personal and environmental factors (see Figure 8.1).

Once therapists have a clear understanding of the ICF framework they can use it to guide intervention planning. Through the assessment and goal-setting process therapists identify the desired outcome of intervention. Consideration is then given to the aspect of health (body structure and function, activity or participation) that will be targeted by the strategy. Appropriate strategies are selected to facilitate goal achievement, and finally outcome measures are used that evaluate performance at the target level of health (Australian Institute of Health and Welfare 2003).

To construct enabling strategies that are tailored to meet a person's unique occupational needs therapists require sound professional reasoning skills. Professional reasoning is essentially the way therapists think about what to do and about their ability to develop and modify their actions and plans during all phases of intervention planning and delivery (Early 2001). Therapists use a combination of deductive and inductive reasoning to aid the strategy planning process. Deductive reasoning (for example, scientific, procedural, hypothetical or diagnostic reasoning) is used to apply general knowledge, theories and scientific evidence to specific practice

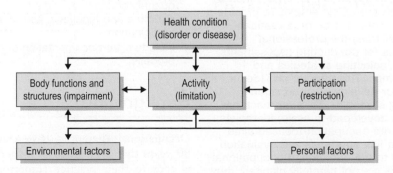

Figure 8.1 • Interactions between the components of the ICF

situations. Inductive reasoning (for example, inter-active, conditional, or narrative reasoning) is used by therapists to assist them in understanding each person and help each therapist to learn from specific practice situations (American Occupational Therapy Organisation 1998). It has been well established that therapists integrate information from a variety of sources when planning strategies for individuals (for example, Early 2001, Fawcett 2002, Hagedorn 1997, 2001, Neistadt 1995, 1998, Radomski 2002). Therefore, therapists must effectively synthesize the information gathered in order to:

- formulate sound aims and set goals that are person-centred

- propose strategies to achieve desired occupation-focused goals

- make decisions about each person's progress, and

- evaluate the overall effectiveness of their strategies.

Detailed documentation of each step of the process is essential to maintain a record of process, change, and development. Documentation may occur in different formats such as file notes, assess-ment forms, progress reports, outcome measure score sheets, and evaluation forms. Not only is docu-mentation and record keeping a legal requirement, it is an effective means of communicating progress and status to the individual and to members of the interprofessional team. Record keeping promotes continuity and supports effective evaluation of occu-pational therapy services. Without adequate docu-mentation from the occupational therapist, other members of the interprofessional team may assume that assessments, strategies and evaluations have not taken place, and there may be uncertainty about the person's current circumstances.

Occupation-focused plans: an overview

In occupational therapy literature, the occupational therapy process has been described both in a linear fashion (for example Early 2001, Radomski 2002) and in a cyclical fashion (for example Hagedorn 1997, Schultz-Krohn & Pendleton 2006). In reality, the process does not take place in a linear or cyclical fashion, but is influenced by many changing and intervening factors. However, a linear approach is the most suitable method to facilitate knowledge

and skill acquisition in student and novice therapists. Therefore, this chapter will describe each step of the process in a tangible and linear way.

Developing enabling strategies is pertinent in all occupational therapy settings. The process is col-laborative and involves the person, their family and other team members (American Occupational Therapy Association 1998). However, enabling strategies are also multifaceted with several steps that require careful consideration. As such, the occupational therapist is typically the initiator and facilitator of each step in the process. These steps include accept-ing and prioritising referrals, conducting assess-ments, identifying the occupational aims and goals, followed by the selection of occupation-focused strategies and the evaluation of the effectiveness of the plan as a whole (Early 2001, Radomski 2002). Clear links between these steps should be evident in the plan. An overview of the process is illustrated in Figure 8.2. Each step of the occupational therapy process will now be described in more detail. Two practice scenarios have also been included to illus-trate the occupational therapy process in practice.

Referral to occupational therapy

Referrals are verbal or written requests for service. Therapists use a variety of methods to screen refer-rals. Therapists have a responsibility to effectively

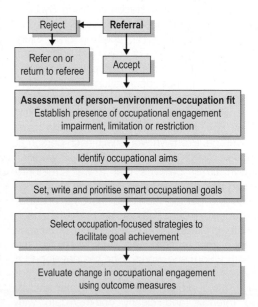

Figure 8.2 • Steps in the intervention planning process

manage their case loads. They should establish and use a method of prioritising people referred to them. Once a referral has been accepted the therapist will proceed with relevant assessments to establish the balance between the person, environment, occupation, and impairment, limitation or restriction in occupational engagement. This is illustrated in Practice Scenario 8.1.

Practice Scenario 8.1 Bronwyn

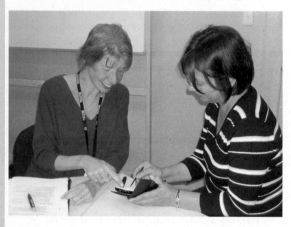

Figure 8.3 • Bronwyn McFarlane (left), occupational therapist at Brain Injury Unit, Royal Rehabilitation Centre, Sydney, assists her client to schedule her next therapy appointment using her Personal Digital Assistant (PDA)

Bronwyn is employed as a senior occupational therapist in a community rehabilitation centre in Sydney, and works with people aged 15–65 years who have a traumatic brain injury (TBI), acquired brain injury (ABI) and/or dual diagnoses of brain injury and mental health problems. The focus of occupational therapy services is to enhance occupational engagement through prescription of equipment and assistive devices, environmental modification and community-based self-care, productivity and leisure skills training. On average, Bronwyn works with each person at least once per week for a period of 8 to 12 weeks.

Bronwyn firmly believes that a well-structured intervention plan that has been developed in collaboration with the person facilitates the best occupational engagement outcomes. As such, she has been instrumental in establishing management processes to enhance the rehabilitation experience for the people with whom she works. She has developed a triage system to assist her in the management of her caseload. This approach allows her to systematically prioritise referrals and clearly communicate with people about access to community occupational therapy services. The success of this system has seen its adoption and implementation by other allied health disciplines.

Bronwyn's planning and implementation of enabling strategies is guided by the Person–Environment–Occupation model. To ensure a thorough approach to assessment, she has devised an initial assessment form and related interview questions to capture the concepts of the person–environment–occupation interaction. Occupation-focused rehabilitation goals are set collaboratively between Bronwyn and the people with whom she works, forming the key component of the intervention plan. Part of this process includes the formal documentation of goals in a contract which is signed by each individual. Bronwyn believes that formal recognition of agreed goals helps to maintain a person's focus and motivation.

Occupation-focused enabling strategies are carefully selected by Bronwyn to specifically address each person's goals. She describes the importance of spending time with each person to discuss how the strategy relates to goal achievement (e.g. Goal example #2, page 101, highlights the strategies Bronwyn may use to assist a young person to understand the steps required to successfully integrate back into his high school community after sustaining TBI). She asserts this step is integral to the person's satisfaction and perceived benefit of occupational therapy services.

Bronwyn monitors progress in occupational engagement toward goal achievement on a weekly basis with each person. This assists Bronwyn to plan sessions, and modify goals or strategies if required. The main outcome measure used by Bronwyn is the Goal Attainment Scale (GAS) (Kiresuk & Sherman 1968). She selected the GAS because of its focus on individual goals.

The practices of innovative therapists like Bronwyn clearly illustrate how employment of simple yet effective strategies helps to ensure that intervention plans are occupation-focused, collaborative, and systematic, and, as such, have intrinsic meaning to each individual.

Note: Goal examples 1 and 2, page 101, are the types of goals that Bronwyn may develop when working with her clients.

Assessing the person–environment–occupation fit

Thorough occupational therapy assessment facilitates the development of effective occupation-focused enabling strategies that will result in improved engagement in daily occupations and enhance quality of life (Fawcett 2002). The purpose of assessment in occupational therapy is to establish a clear picture of an individual's person–environment–occupation fit and identify the presence of any impairment, restriction or limitations in occupational engagement (Practice Scenario 8.2). Therapists analyse the specific skills and abilities the person requires to meet intrinsic needs and achieve their goals. Additionally, therapists identify enabling or constraining environmental factors within the occupational engagement context. Occupational therapists are encouraged to use more standardised instruments to ensure their assessments are as valid and reliable as possible and to enable the evaluation of outcomes (Fawcett 2002). However, it is important to remember that the assessment process should be viewed as the starting point for identifying aims and setting goals, and not as an end in itself (Hagedorn 1997). Box 8.1 summarises the key steps in the assessment of an individual's person–environment–occupation fit.

Practice Scenario 8.2 Alicia

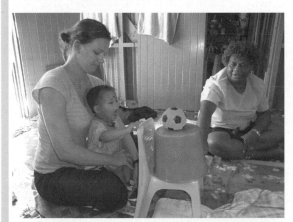

Figure 8.4 • Alicia Frost (left), occupational therapist from The Spastic Centre of New South Wales, Australia working in Fiji with a Community Rehabilitation Assistant (right) encouraging a child with mild cerebral palsy to engage in play occupations

Alicia practices in the area of paediatrics, working with clients aged 0–18 years who have been diagnosed with cerebral palsy, spina bifida, autism, and complex physical disabilities. Alicia travelled to Fiji to participate in a rehabilitation project sponsored by

Australian Volunteers International and the Fiji Crippled Children's Society. Alicia's role in Fiji was to teach the local Community Rehabilitation Assistants how to plan and use occupation-focused interventions with the children and families with whom they work. The aim was primarily to educate families and the local community in physical impairment and to enhance the children and their families' participation in daily occupations and community activities.

Alicia found working in Fiji to be an experience that really tested her ability to adapt her conventional planning framework to suit this culturally different environment. This often meant taking a very pragmatic approach regarding enabling strategies. She regularly had to make do with the limited resources, and had to travel significant distances through difficult terrain to see children in their home, school or community environment. Many of the children she worked with had mild physical impairments. Children with more severe impairments were often restricted to their homes due to mobility and access issues, as well as local cultural beliefs. This restriction meant that family members were typically involved in implementing play-based strategies with the child.

Alicia conducted occupational assessments in the child's own environment, where possible. However, standardised assessments were rarely used in Fiji, mainly because they were often not available, nor in many instances were they applicable. As a result, Alicia relied heavily on her professional reasoning skills to establish each child's story, occupation history and impairment, and limitation or restriction in occupational engagement. After identifying occupational-engagement issues, realistic and achievable goals were set collaboratively with the child, their family, and the community rehabilitation assistant.

The setting of goals with the Fijian children and their families was quite different to what Alicia had previously experienced. Many families had never had any dealings with rehabilitation providers and thus had few expectations. Consequently, Alicia found initially she had to be quite directive in the goal-setting process, recommending strategies that focused on the child's basic occupational needs, such as feeding, drinking, positioning, and other self-care activities. In this environment it was essential that goals that could be easily monitored and subjectively evaluated by the family were set, as the child would not be reviewed by an occupational therapist or community rehabilitation assistant for at least 6 months. Thus, designing sustainable home programmes for the children was an important part of the occupational therapy role in Fiji to ensure ongoing intervention. Additionally, Alicia often had to draw on her creativity when devising strategies appropriate for the children she worked with. Alicia tells a story of modifying an adult-sized wheelchair for a small child using gaffer tape, a very large screw driver and some scraps of foam for seating.

Alicia's experience in Fiji highlights that irrespective of work setting or resource availability, therapists' understanding of the person–environment–occupation interaction is fundamental to the development of a successful intervention plan.

Note: Goal examples 3 and 4, page 102, are the types of goals that Alicia may develop when working with children, either as part of her role at the Spastic Centre or her role in Fiji.

Writing occupation-focused aims

Identifying occupation-focused aims is a shared effort between the occupational therapist, the individual and, often, their family. Aims are established as a result of the synthesis of information collected from both objective and subjective assessments. The purpose of aims is to provide a broad and overarching statement about the person's desired occupational engagement outcome. Therefore, articulation of clear aims sets the course, or provides direction for the implementation of strategies. As aims are broad, overarching statements, they contain few specific details, and, as such, they are difficult to address with one particular strategy. For example, an individual's aim may be to return home and live independently after having a stroke. Clearly this aim must be structured to provide detail regarding how the desired outcome will be achieved. Writing detailed occupational goals fulfils this task. Box 8.2 summarises the key steps that should be followed when establishing occupational aims.

Setting occupation-focused goals

Goal-setting is the cornerstone of the occupational therapy process as goals are a prerequisite to selecting appropriate enabling strategies and evaluating outcomes (Hagedorn 2001). Occupational therapy goals must directly address the identified aims (Neistadt 1998). Therefore, the purpose of goal setting is to operationally define the specific desired outcomes and describe the factors involved in achieving the outcomes. Clearly articulated goals can provide an effective snapshot of the overall intervention plan.

Goals can be either long term or short term. Long-term goals have been described as the destination of therapy, while short-term goals are the pathways to get there (Foto 1996). Short-term goals, where practical, should employ strategies that facilitate the person's engagement in occupation at an activity or participation level. However, short-term goals may address issues at the level of body function and structure. If this is the case, it is important that therapists clearly articulate how short-term goals contribute to the achievement of long-term occupation-focused goals.

Occupational therapists should work collaboratively with individuals to set goals. Research has shown that increased motivation in individuals is related to active participation in identifying goals

Box 8.1

Assessment of the person–environment–occupation fit

Key steps

- Gather information prior to meeting the person
- Gather information from the person, family and caregivers
- Establish occupational engagement history
- Establish person–environment–occupation fit
- Identify occupational impairment, restrictions, limitations, or deprivation
- Use occupational analysis to identify component skills required to perform desired daily self-care, productivity or leisure occupations
- Evaluate enabling or constraining effects of the environment
- Measure baseline occupational engagement prior to commencement of intervention

Box 8.2

Establishing occupation-focused aims

Key steps

- Synthesise information collected through subjective and objective assessments
- Determine what the individual would like to achieve as a result of the implementation of enabling strategies
- Construct a statement that broadly describes the person's desired occupational engagement outcomes and provides direction for the intervention

(Latham 2004, Locke & Latham 2002). Individuals are also more committed if they have been involved in goal setting and, as a result, make significant gains in self-care and living skills occupations (Neistadt 1995). Therefore, issues identified during the assessment phase should be considered carefully when setting goals.

To assist individuals to prioritise their goals, the occupational therapist should explore issues related to the general health, safety, independence, social support networks, and cultural and social values. The therapist should also seek to understand individuals' views of their current situation and their expectations for the future. Synthesis of this information into appropriate occupation-focused goals can be a complex process. Thus, it is important that occupational therapists follow a systematic method to assist them to write goals that are clear and measurable, and reflect the wishes of the people for whom the goals are directed. Selection of a valid and reliable method will also help them to avoid setting goals that are vague and ambiguous.

Tools such as the Canadian Occupational Performance Measure (COPM) (Law et al 1990) and the Goal Attainment Scale (GAS) (Kiresuk & Sherman 1968) were developed to assist therapists to collaboratively set and prioritise goals with the people with whom they are working. Due to its abstract nature, collaborative goal setting may appear to be challenging when working with children less than 10 years of age. Occupational therapists working with young children have traditionally prescribed goals or identified goals in collaboration with parents or teachers. However, in recent years the use of tools like the Perceived Efficacy and Goal Setting System (PEGS) have been effective in assisting children aged 5–9 years to select and prioritise their own goals (Missiuna & Pollock 2000, Missiuna et al 2006).

Writing SMART goals

Goals should be documented in the intervention plan. Currently there is no universally agreed method to guide therapists in writing goals (Levack et al 2006, Siegert et al 2004). Several studies have shown that there is a need for occupational therapists to become skilled at writing clear, occupation-focused goals (Bowman 2006, Bowman & Llewellyn 2002, Neistadt 1995, Northern et al 1995). To assist occupational therapists to write appropriate occupation-focused goals, a structured method was recently developed based on the SMART goal concept com-

monly described in psychology, education, and rehabilitation literature (Mogensen 2005). Although some therapists hold the belief that goals should be short, single-sentence statements, Mogensen argues that for goals to be useful, they must be comprehensive, and address several criteria. The SMART goal method addresses five domains (**S**pecific, **M**easurable, **A**ctivity-based, **R**eview and **T**imeframe) and clearly illustrates the steps required for writing useful goals. The requirements of each domain will be described in detail below. Each criterion will be demonstrated within an example of a short-term goal. Goals 1 & 2 are the types of goals that Bronwyn may develop (Practice Scenario 8.1) and Goals 3 & 4 are the types of goals that Alicia may develop (Practice Scenario 8.2).

Specific (S)

Writing specific goals reduces the chance of ambiguity and of discrepancies, and avoids individual interpretation of achievement expectations. To be *specific*, a goal must address three criteria. The goal must:

1. include a verb that describes the person's desired occupational engagement outcome in terms of *observable behaviour*, for example, the person will *walk* (desired performance behaviour)

2. include the *conditions* that are required for performing or maintaining the goal behaviour (for example, with use of equipment, assistance, independently, with verbal cues, or requires supervision)

3. state the performance *context*, meaning the environment within which the desired behaviour should be performed (for example, the hospital ward or rehabilitation gym, the person's home, work place, or local shops).

Example goal 1 Ms Jones will be able to independently (**criterion S2**) schedule rehabilitation appointments (**criterion S1**) using a Personal Digital Assistant (PDA) (**criterion S2**) at the end of each treatment session at the Outpatient Rehabilitation Centre (**criterion S3**).

Example goal 2 Mark will return to full-time attendance (**S1**), with support from a teacher's aide and selected peers during school hours (**S2**), at his pre-injury High School (**S3**) with a rest break after each teaching session (**S2**).

Example goal 3 *Matthew will be able to request food or drink at meal times **(S1)** in his home environment **(S3)**. Assisted by one of his parents **(S2)**; Matthew will be using the Picture Exchange Communication System (PECS) (Bondy & Frost 1994) instead of screaming **(S2)**.*

Example goal 4 *Luana will be able to play ball **(S1)** with her older brother and sister **(S2)** in her home environment **(S3)**.*

Measurable (M)

A goal must be measurable to objectively determine whether the strategy has had an effect. The goal should indicate how achievement will be measured. Outcome measures can be standardised instruments or self-determined scales. It is particularly important that the method selected to measure the person's behaviour targets the appropriate level (body function and structure versus activity versus participation) of that behaviour. For example, if the person wants to be able to walk from their house to the local shops and back, the measure should determine an increase in distance walked within an acceptable timeframe. To be *measurable*, a goal must address two criteria. The goal must:

1. state *how* performance will be *measured* (for example, using a standardised outcome measurement instrument or by measuring distance, time, and frequency, or the reduction in the level of pain experienced or the number of cues or level of assistance needed)

2. specify the *criteria for an acceptable standard of the behaviour performed*. The goal should specify how much, how fast, how long, how often or how accurate the behaviour needs to be (for example, within 10 seconds, in 30 minutes, no more than two prompts, within 10 seconds after verbal prompt, for at least 20 minutes, to complete within 10 minutes on five consecutive occasions, eight out of ten correct responses or with 80% accuracy, on each occasion, on five consecutive occasions, daily).

Example goal 1 *Ms Jones will be able to independently schedule rehabilitation appointments using a PDA at the end of each treatment session at the Outpatient Rehabilitation Centre. *Ms Jones's progress will be monitored by her occupational therapist by comparing the number of weekly appointments programmed into the PDA without prompting versus*

the number of appointments attended on time **(M1)**. *Ms Jones expects to able attend 100% of planned appointments on time whilst using the PDA* **(M2)**.

Example goal 2 Mark will return to full-time attendance, with support from a teacher's aide and selected peers during school hours, at his pre-injury High School with a rest break after each teaching session. *Mark will gradually increase duration **(M1)** of daily attendance from 2 hours to 7 hours **(M2)** and decrease duration **(M1)** of rest breaks per session from 15 minutes to 5 minutes **(M2)**, without increasing levels of fatigue **(M2)** on the visual analogue scale (VAS) and the Fatigue Severity Scale (FSS) (Krupp et al 1989) **(M1)**.*

Example goal 3 Matthew will be able to request food or drink at meal times in his home environment. Assisted by one of his parents, Matthew will be using the PECS instead of screaming *50% of the time **(M2)** within 4 weeks and 100% of the time **(M2)** within 8 weeks.* Matthew's mother will record daily the *number of times Matthew correctly uses the PECS to request food or drink* **(M1)**.

Example goal 4 Luana will be able to play ball with her older brother and sister *for 15 minutes daily **(M2)** in her home environment.* Luana's progress will be monitored by family members according to *the amount of time she is able to sustain play with the ball* **(M1)**.

Activity-based strategies (A)

Activity-based strategies are those that will effect behaviour change and lead to goal achievement. A strategy must be selected to address the specific occupational impairment, limitation or restriction at the appropriate level of body function and structure, activity or participation. To be *activity-based* the goal must address one criterion. The goal must:

1. state *how* the person will achieve the goal by describing a strategy (for example, by wearing a compression bandage, participate in weekly relaxation groups, use self-calming techniques, practice or part practice of an activity/task such as sit to stand).

Example goal 1 Ms Jones will be able to independently schedule rehabilitation appointments using a PDA at the end of each treatment session at the Outpatient Rehabilitation Centre. *Ms Jones will receive training in using the PDA and time-*

management strategies (A). Ms Jones's progress will be monitored by her occupational therapist by comparing the number of weekly appointments programmed into the PDA without prompting versus the number of appointments attended on time. Ms Jones expects to be able to attend 100% of planned appointments on time whilst using the PDA.

Example goal 2 Mark will return to full-time attendance, with support from a teacher's aide and selected peers during school hours, at his pre-injury High School with a rest break after each teaching session. Mark will gradually increase daily attendance from 2 hours to 7 hours and decrease rest breaks per session from 15 minutes duration to 5 minutes. *His daily attendance will increase from 2 hours to 3 hours after 2 weeks, 4 hours after 4 weeks, 5 hours after 6 weeks, 6 hours after 8 weeks and 7 hours after 10 weeks (A). Duration of rest breaks will decrease to 10 minutes after 4 weeks and 5 minutes after 10 weeks, w*ithout increasing levels of fatigue on the visual analogue scale (VAS) and the Fatigue Severity Scale (FSS).

Example goal 3 Matthew will be able to request food or drink at meal times in his home environment. Assisted by one of his parents, Matthew will be using the PECS instead of screaming 50% of the time within 4 weeks and 100% of the time within 8 weeks. *Matthew's parents will be trained to teach Matthew how to use the PECS to identify and select desired items of food or drink (A).* Matthew's mother will record the number of times Matthew correctly uses the PECS to request food or drink.

Example goal 4 Luana will be able to play ball with her older brother and sister for 15 minutes daily in her home environment. *Luana's siblings will be taught how to provide physical assistance to facilitate Luana in playing with a large, light ball (A).* Luana's progress will be monitored by family members according to the amount of time Luana is able to sustain play with the ball. After 2 months *a second daily play session will be added using the same strategy (A).*

Review (R)

The review domain focuses on the regular monitoring of the person's progress towards achievement of the desired goal outcome. When planning the intervention program a schedule for review and administration of outcome measures should be specified. It

is essential that baseline measures are taken prior to commencement of strategies to enable review of occupational performance progress. Scheduled reviews also assist the therapist to determine whether the goal is realistic and if the strategies are suitable or whether modification is required (for example, increase the timeframe for goal achievement) (see Practice Scenario 8.2). To ensure review of progress occurs, the goal must address one criterion:

1. The goal includes planned *progress review(s)* (for example, within one week, weekly, after four sessions or 3 months).

Example goal 1 Ms Jones will be able to independently schedule rehabilitation appointments using a PDA at the end of each treatment session at the Outpatient Rehabilitation Centre. Ms Jones will receive training in using the PDA and time management strategies. Ms Jones's progress will be monitored *once a week (R)* by her occupational therapist by comparing the number of weekly appointments programmed into the PDA without prompting versus the number of appointments attended on time. Ms Jones expects to be able to attend 100% of planned appointments on time whilst using the PDA.

Example goal 2 Mark will return to full-time attendance, with support from a teacher's aide and selected peers during school hours, at his pre-injury High School with a rest break after each teaching session. Mark will gradually increase duration of daily attendance from 2 hours to 7 hours and decrease duration of rest breaks per session from 15 minutes duration to 5 minutes. His daily attendance will increase from 2 hours to 3 hours after 2 weeks, 4 hours after 4 weeks, 5 hours after 6 weeks, 6 hours after 8 weeks and 7 hours after 10 weeks. Duration of rest breaks will decrease to 10 minutes after 4 weeks and 5 minutes after 10 weeks, without increasing levels of fatigue on the VAS and the FSS. *Mark's re-integration programme and fatigue/energy levels will be reviewed weekly (R) by the community rehabilitation occupational therapist using the FSS. Ongoing progress will be monitored collaboratively by his teacher and the school counsellor on a daily basis (R) using a VAS for fatigue.*

Example goal 3 Matthew will be able to request food or drink at meal times in his home environment. Assisted by one of his parents, Matthew will be using the PECS instead of screaming 50% of the time *within 4 weeks* **(R)** and 100% of the time *within 8 weeks* **(R)**. Matthew's parents will be trained to teach Matthew how to use the PECS to identify and select desired items of food or drink. *Matthew's mother will record daily* **(R)** the number of times Matthew correctly uses the PECS to request food or drink. *His progress and achievement will be reviewed during fortnightly visits by his occupational therapist* **(R)**.

Example goal 4 Luana will be able to play ball with her older brother and sister for 15 minutes daily in her home environment. Luana's siblings will be taught how to provide physical assistance to facilitate Luana in playing with a large, light ball. Play time with the ball will increase from 2 minutes to 4–5 minutes *after 3 weeks* **(R)**, then to 8–10 minutes *after 5 weeks* **(R)**, and 15 minutes *after 6 weeks* **(R)**. Luana's progress will be monitored by family members according to the amount of time Luana is able to sustain play with the ball. After 2 months a second daily play session will be added using the same strategy. Once Luana is able to play for *15 minutes twice daily* **(R)**, the family will work on gradually extending the time to 30 minutes play per session over another 2 months.

Timeframe (T)

Timeframe refers to the overall expected time limit for goal achievement. If no timeframe is set for achieving the desired goal outcome there is no direction for intervention intensity. This may cause costs to inflate unnecessarily. Additionally, a person's motivation may decline if there is no view to goal completion. The *Timeframe* domain includes one criterion:

1. The goal includes the *timeframe* within which the *desired outcome should be achieved* (for example, by a specified date, in one week, or by the last week of term 3).

Example goal 1 By December 15 **(T1)**, Ms Jones will be able to independently schedule rehabilitation appointments using a PDA at the end of each treatment session at the Outpatient Rehabilitation Centre. Ms Jones will receive training in using the PDA and time management strategies. Ms Jones's progress will be monitored once a week by her occupational therapist by comparing the number of weekly appointments programmed into the PDA without prompting versus the number of appointments attended on time. Ms Jones expects to be

able to attend 100% of planned appointments on time whilst using the PDA.

Example goal 2 By the end of second semester **(T1)**, Mark will return to full-time attendance, with support from a teacher's aide and selected peers, during school hours at his pre-injury High School with a rest break after each teaching session. Mark will gradually increase daily attendance from 2 hours to 7 hours and decrease rest breaks per session from 15 minutes duration to 5 minutes. His daily attendance will increase from 2 hours to 3 hours after 2 weeks, 4 hours after 4 weeks, 5 hours after 6 weeks, 6 hours after 8 weeks and 7 hours after 10 weeks. Duration of rest breaks will decrease to 10 minutes after 4 weeks and 5 minutes after 10 weeks, without increasing levels of fatigue on VAS and the FSS. Mark's re-integration program and fatigue/energy levels will be reviewed weekly by the community rehabilitation occupational therapist using the FSS. Ongoing progress will be monitored collaboratively by his teacher and the school counsellor on a daily basis using a VAS for fatigue.

Example goal 3 In 2 months **(T)**, Matthew will be able to request food or drink at meal times in his home environment. Assisted by one of his parents, Matthew will be using the PECS instead of screaming 50% of the time within 4 weeks and 100% of the time within 8 weeks. Matthew's parents will be trained to teach Matthew how to use the PECS to identify and select desired items of food or drink. Matthew's mother will record daily the number of times Matthew correctly uses the PECS to request food or drink. His progress and achievement will be reviewed during fortnightly visits by his occupational therapist.

Example goal 4 Within 2 months **(T)**, Luana will be able to play ball with her older brother and sister for 15 minutes daily in her home environment. Luana's siblings will be taught how to provide physical assistance to facilitate Luana in playing with a large, light ball. Play time with the ball will increase from 2 minutes to 4–5 minutes after 3 weeks, 8–10 minutes after 5 weeks and 15 minutes after 6 weeks. Luana's progress will be monitored by family members according to the amount of time Luana is able to sustain play with the ball. After 2 months a second daily play session will be added using the same strategy. Once Luana is able to play for 15 minutes twice daily, the family will work on

Box 8.3

Writing SMART goals

Key steps

Specific

- Describe the person's desired occupational performance outcome in terms of *observable behaviour using a verb*
- State the *conditions* that are required for performing or maintaining the goal behaviour
- State the engagement *context*, that is, the environment within which the desired behaviour will be performed

Measurable

- State *how* engagement will be *measured*
- Specify the *criteria for an acceptable standard of the behaviour performed*

Activity-based

- State *how* the person will achieve the goal by describing an intervention activity that addresses the desired engagement outcome

Review

- State when progress reviews are planned

Timeframe

- State timeframe within which the desired outcome should be achieved

---

gradually extending the time to 30 minutes play per session over another 2 months.

Following a structured method like the SMART goal concept clearly assists in planning of strategies and evaluation. Without specific goals, the occupational therapy process is likely to become directionless and may continue indefinitely (Ward & McIntosh 1997). Box 8.3 summarises the key steps required for writing SMART goals.

Selecting occupation-focused strategies

Strategies in occupational therapy focus on the acquisition, remediation, improvement or maintenance of occupational performance, so that participation in life tasks, activities and occupational roles may be achieved (Early 2001). The process of selecting appropriate occupation-focused strategies is informed by the therapist's professional reasoning skills, knowledge of occupation and conceptual models of practice (Hagedorn 2001, Turner 2002). When guided by the concepts of the PEO model and the ICF, occupational therapists should take into consideration the transactional dynamics of the interdependent person–environment–occupation fit, and the concepts of activity, participation, and occupational roles when selecting strategies.

Occupational engagement means different things to different people. Each person has a unique set of attributes such as life experiences, cultural traditions, values and beliefs that influence their life roles and occupations. Other issues to consider when selecting strategies include age, gender, interests, skills, and abilities (Foster 2003, Law et al 1996). Strategies should be appropriate to these attributes to ensure that activities are meaningful to the individual. Meaningful activities have face validity and are more likely to be intrinsically motivating. Ultimately, strategies should be selected specifically to address the aims and goals of therapy. Further to this, the therapist needs to carefully match the strategy so that it targets the appropriate level of body function and structure, activities or participation. The format of strategies must also be carefully considered in order to facilitate the best outcome (for example, one-on-one therapy versus a group approach).

Occupational engagement takes place within the context of an environment. Considerations should be given not only to an individual's physical and social environment, but also their socio-economic, institutional, and cultural environments (see Practice Scenario 8.2) (Law et al 1996). Time and environment have a strong influence on strategies. The management, availability, and allocation of time present a constant challenge for occupational therapists. When planning a programme for an individual, the time of sessions must be carefully considered. For example:

1. What time of the day is the most suitable for the individual and his particular condition?

2. How much time can the person realistically spend on strategies?

3. Is it important to establish a routine for the individual?

4. Does timing of the session influence availability of the most suitable location for therapy, such as the school or workplace?

Environments can have enabling or restricting effects on a person. For example, a person may be able to transfer from their wheelchair into a hospital bed where adjustable equipment and ample space are available, but have difficulty with the same task in their own home. At times, the environment may be more adaptable to change than the person. For example, an individual with a chronic or progressive illness or disability may not expect improvement at the body function level. In this case, it would be appropriate to consider environmental modifications to achieve an occupational engagement outcome at the activity or participation level. When selecting environmental stategies, it is important to consider the individual's current personal situation and the likelihood of any changes both in the short and long term.

Therapists need to prioritise strategies that are occupation-focused and facilitate change in occupational engagement. However, there are times where body function and structure must be addressed first to enable or improve occupational engagement at an activity or participation level. For example, increasing a person's muscle strength and joint range of motion may be necessary before he can dress himself. Also, improving sitting balance may be required before the person could sit at a table to eat a meal with his family. Where body function and structure is targeted by strategies, the link to activity and participation level goals should be explicit.

An important component of planning is to ensure occupation-focused strategies are, where possible, evidence based. For therapists this means keeping up to date with the research being conducted within their practice area and implementing strategies that are supported by scientific evidence. The key steps in selecting occupation-focused strategies are summarised in Box 8.4.

Box 8.4

Selecting occupation-focused strategies
Key steps
The enabling strategies should:

- Be based on formal assessment findings, and target occupational aims and goals
- Appropriately target either: body function and structure, activity, or participation
- Address individual attributes related to person–environment–occupation fit
- Consider time available, approach and location

Evaluating the person–environment–occupation fit

There is increasing pressure for occupational therapists to demonstrate that the strategies they have selected achieve desired changes in occupational engagement and are cost-efficient (Bowman 2006, Bowman & Llewellyn 2002, Gutman & Mortera 1997, Kay et al 2001, Landry & Mathews 1998). Previously, the allocation of occupational therapy services was largely based on therapists' personal and professional judgements and values. Now, it is important to be responsive to all stakeholders in the health care system – that is, the individuals and their families, those who pay for the service, and those who employ the therapists to provide the service (Foto 1996). As such, evaluation of the outcome of strategies is a contemporary practice issue for all therapists. It is important then that therapists are competent in the skill of outcome measurement. An outcome can be defined as 'a characteristic or construct that is expected to change owing to a strategy, intervention or program' (Finch et al 2002, p. 271). For example, range of motion may increase at a person's wrist joint as a result of wearing a splint, or a person may be able to independently catch the bus as a result of community travel training. Outcome measurement is the process of quantifying change in a characteristic or construct, using valid and reliable instruments (Austin & Clark 1993, De Clive-Lowe 1996). For example, an increase in range of motion can be measured using a goniometer, and a person's ability to independently catch the bus could be measured using the Goal Attainment Scale (Kiresuk & Sherman 1968). Knowledge of the key steps in the evaluation process is essential if therapists are to choose and effectively use appropriate outcome measures with the people who use their services. A number of authors have described in detail the outcome measurement process and issues to consider when selecting outcome measures appropriate to specific people (for example Dittmar & Gresham 1997, Finch et al 2002, Law 2001, Law et al 2005). The key steps described in the literature are summarised in Box 8.5.

It is important to ensure when evaluating a person's progress toward goal achievement that the outcome measure selected specifically quantifies change brought about by the strategies used with that person. Where possible, outcome measures

Box 8.5

Evaluating person–environment–occupation fit
Key steps
Choosing an appropriate outcome measure

Therapists should ensure the following characteristics of the outcome measure are suitable for each person with whom they are working:

- Population of people with whom the therapist is working – age, sex, diagnosis
- Person–environment–occupation attributes and characteristics
- ICF level – body function and structure, activity, or participation
- Type – descriptive, discriminative, predictive, or evaluative
- Focus – generic versus specific
- Administration – therapist observation (objective) versus person self-report (subjective)
- Psychometric properties – validity, reliability, sensitivity, responsiveness, and interpretability
- Feasibility – cost, training requirements, administration time, and burden

Using the outcome measure

Before using the selected outcome measure therapists should establish:

- Who the outcome measure can be used with
- How frequently the outcome measure will be used
- Whether they know how to use the measure
- Whether they understand administration instructions
- Whether they know how to score the measure
- Whether they are able to interpret the scores
- Whether they are able to explain what the scores mean to others
- How and where they will report the findings of the outcome measure

should be used that reflect a person's participation in daily occupations. Therapists should also develop the habit of reporting outcomes to others in occupational terms. This will reinforce the central role that occupation plays in occupational therapy practice.

Conclusion

This chapter has demonstrated how collaborative, occupation-focused planning is the foundation of occupational therapy practice. A strong emphasis has been placed on the need to consider the person, their occupational roles and their physical and social environment when planning an intervention programme. Collaboration was highlighted as essential to ensure therapy has intrinsic meaning to each individual to enhance their motivation to achieve their goals. Intervention planning was described in this chapter as a linear process to enhance the clarity of the requirements at each step of the process. The importance of linking each step of the process has also been stressed. Conducting subjective and objective assessments was illustrated to form the basis for identifying the broad overarching aims of intervention. SMART goals were clearly articulated and prioritised, leading to the selection of occupation-focused strategies to address impairment, limitation or restriction in occupational engagement. The importance of selecting appropriate outcome measures to measure change in occupational engagement was also described. Two practice scenarios have been used to demonstrate application of planning principles in two areas practice. In summary, occupational therapists need to be skilled in all areas of planning to ensure services provided are effective, person-centred, and occupation-focused.

References

American Occupational Therapy Association (1998). Standards for practice for occupational therapy. Online. Available: http://www.aota.org/general/otsp.asp 31 Jan 2007.

Austin, C. & Clark, C. R. (1993). Measures of outcome: For whom? *British Journal of Occupational Therapy*, 56(1), 21–24.

Australian Institute of Health and Welfare (AIHW) (2003). *ICF Australian user guide. Version 1.0. Disability Series*. AIHW Cat. No. DIS 33. Canberra, AIHW.

Bondy, A. & Frost, L. (1994). *PECS: The Picture Exchange Communication System training manual*. Cherry Hill NJ, Pyramid Educational Consultants.

Bowman, J. (2006). Challenges to measuring outcomes in occupational therapy: A qualitative focus group study. *British Journal of Occupational Therapy*, 69(10), 464–472.

Bowman, J. & Llewellyn, G. (2002). Clinical outcomes research from the occupational therapist's perspective. *Occupational Therapy International*, 9(2), 145–166.

De Clive-Lowe, S. (1996). Outcome measurement, cost-effectiveness and clinical audit: The importance of standardised assessment to occupational therapists in meeting these new demands. *British Journal of Occupational Therapy*, 59(8), 357–362.

Dittmar, S. S. & Gresham, G. E. (1997). *Functional assessment and outcome measures for the rehabilitation professional*. Aspen, Gaithersburg.

Early, M. B. (2001). The occupational therapy process: An overview. In: L. W. Pedretti, M. B. Early (Eds). *Occupational therapy: Practice skills for physical dysfunction*, (5th ed). (pp. 21–28). St Louis, Mosby.

Emerson, H. (1998). Flow and occupation: A review of the literature. *Canadian Journal of Occupational Therapy*, 65, 37–44.

Fawcett, A. L. (2002). Assessment. In: A. Turner, M. Foster, & S. E. Johnson (Eds). *Occupational therapy and physical dysfunction: Principles, skills and practice*, (5th ed). (pp. 107–144). Edinburgh, Churchill Livingstone.

Finch, E., Brooks, D., Stratford, P. W. et al. (2002). *Physical rehabilitation outcome measures: A guide to enhanced clinical decision making*, (2nd ed). Hamilton, B C Decker.

Foster, M., (2003). Skills for practice. In: A. Turner, J. Foster, & S. Johnson (Eds) *Occupational therapy and physical dysfunction: Principles, skills and practice*, (5th ed). Edinburgh, Churchill Livingstone.

Foto, M. (1996). Outcome studies: The what, why, how, and when. *American Journal of Occupational Therapy* 50(2), 87–88.

Gutman, S. A. & Mortera, M. (1997). Applied scientific inquiry: An answer to managed care's challenge? *American Journal of Occupational Therapy*, 51(8), 704–709.

Hagedorn, R. (1997). *Foundations for practice in occupational therapy* (2nd ed). New York, Churchill Livingstone.

Hagedorn, R. (2001). *Foundations for practice in occupational therapy*, (3rd ed). Edinburgh, Churchill Livingstone.

Kay, T. M., Myers, A. M. & Huijbregts, M. P. J. (2001). How far have we come since 1992? A comparative survey of physiotherapists' use of outcome measures. *Physiotherapy Canada* 53, 268–275, 281.

Kiresuk, T. J. & Sherman, R. E. (1968). Goal attainment scaling: A general method for evaluating comprehensive community mental health programs. *Community Mental Health Journal*, 4(6), 443–453.

Krupp, L., LaRocca, N., Muir-Nash, J. & Steinberg, A. D. (1989). The Fatigue Severity Scale: Application to patients with multiple sclerosis and system lupus erythematosis. *Archives of Neurology*, 46, 1121–1123.

Landry, D. W. & Mathews, M. (1998). Economic evaluation of occupational therapy: Where are we at? *Canadian Journal of Occupational Therapy*, 65(3), 160–167.

Latham, G. P. (2004).The motivational benefits of goal-setting. *Academy of Management Executive*, 18(4), 126–129,

Law, M. (2001). *All about outcomes: An educational program to help you understand, evaluate, and choose adult outcome measures (CD–ROM)*. Thorofare, NJ, Slack.

Law, M., Baptiste, S., McColl, M. A. et al. (1990). The Canadian Occupational Performance Measure: An outcome measure for occupational therapy. *Canadian Journal of Occupational Therapy*, 57, 82–87.

Law, M., Cooper, B., Strong, S. et al. (1996). The Person-Environment-Occupation model: A transactive approach to occupational performance. *Canadian Journal of Occupational Therapy*, 63(1), 9–23.

Law, M. C., Baum, C. M. & Dunn, W. (2005). *Measuring occupational performance: Supporting best practice in occupational therapy*. (2nd ed.). Thorofare, NJ, Slack.

Levack, W., Taylor, K., Siegert, R. J. et al. (2006). Is goal planning in rehabilitation effective? A systematic review. *Clinical Rehabilitation*, 20, 739–755.

Locke, E. A. & Latham, G. P. (2002). Building a practically useful theory of goal-setting and task motivation. *American Psychologist*, 57(9), 705–717.

Missiuna, C. & Pollock, N. (2000). Perceived efficacy and goal setting in young children. *Canadian Journal of Occupational Therapy*, 67(2), 101–109.

Missiuna, C., Pollock, N., Law, M. et al. (2006). Examination of the Perceived Efficacy and Goal Setting System (PEGS) with children with disabilities, their parents and teachers. *American Journal of Occupational Therapy*, 60(2), 204–214.

Mogensen, L. (2005). *The development, content validity and inter-rater reliability of the S.M.A.R.T. Goal Evaluation Method (SMART–GEM): A new rating scale for evaluating clinical treatment goals*. Campbelltown, Unpublished Thesis, University of Western Sydney.

Neistadt, M. E. (1995). Methods of assessing client's priorities: A survey of adult physical dysfunction settings. *American Journal of Occupational Therapy*, 49(5), 428–436.

Neistadt, M. E. (1998). Introduction to evaluating and interviewing. In: M. E. Neistadt, E. B. Crepeau (Eds). *Willard and Spackman's occupational therapy*, (9th ed.) (pp. 151–168). Philadelphia, Lippincott.

Northern, J., Rust, D., Nelson, C. et al. (1995). Involvement of adult rehabilitation patients in setting occupational therapy goals. *American Journal of Occupational Therapy*, 49(3), 214–220.

Radomski, M. V. (2002). Planning, guiding and documenting therapy. In: M. V. Radomski, C. A. Trombly (Eds). *Occupational therapy for physical dysfunction*, (5th ed.). (pp. xvii, 1155). Philadelphia, Lippincott Williams & Wilkins.

Rebeiro, K. L. & Cook, J. V. (1999). Opportunity not prescription: An exploratory study of the experience of occupational engagement. *Canadian Journal of Occupational Therapy*, 66, 176–187.

Schultz-Krohn, W. & Pendleton, H. M. (2006). Application of the occupational therapy practice framework to physical dysfunction. In: L. W. Pedretti, H. M. Pendleton, & W. SchultzKrohn (Eds). *Occupational therapy: Practice skills for physical dysfunction*, (6th ed.) (pp. 28–52). St Louis: Mosby.

Siegert, R. J., McPherson, K. M. & Taylor, W. J. (2004). Toward a cognitive-affective model of goal-setting in rehabilitation: is self-regulation theory a key step? *Disability and Rehabilitation*, 26(20), 1175–1183.

Turner, A. (2002). Occupation for therapy. In: A. Turner, M. Foster, & S. E. Johnson (Eds). *Occupational therapy for physical dysfunction*. Edinburgh, Churchill Livingstone.

Ward, C. D. & McIntosh, S. (1997). The rehabilitation process: A neurological perspective. In: R. Greenwood, M. P. Barnes, T. M. McMillan et al. (Eds). *Neurological rehabilitation*. Hove, Psychology Press.

World Federation of Occupational Therapists (2007). What is occupational therapy? Online. Available: http://www.wfot.org.au/information.asp 21 Feb 2007.

World Health Organisation (2002). *Beginners guide towards a common language for functioning, disability and health: ICF.* Online. Available: http://www3.who.int/icf/beginners/bg.pdf 15 Feb 2007.

Chapter Nine

9

Enabling skills and strategies

Michael Curtin

CHAPTER CONTENTS

Introduction 111

Focus on occupation 112

Complexity of occupational therapy
practice 113

The concept of enabling 115

Enabling skills 116

Enabling strategies 116

Conclusion 120

SUMMARY

The concept of enablement is core to the practice of occupational therapy, and underpins the overall goal of enabling people to achieve their occupational potential and be engaged in occupations that promote health and well-being. To achieve this goal, occupational therapists work in a complex and unique way with each individual, embracing scientific, ethical, and artistic thinking to plan, implement and evaluate relevant and appropriate strategies. The manner in which therapists work with people involves the use of at least ten enabling skills: adapt, advocate, coach, collaborate, consult, coordinate, design/build, educate, engage, and specialise. The skills are used in a multitude of different ways when implementing six different strategies commonly employed by occupational therapists: remediation, compensation, education, community development, transformation, and redistributive justice. These strategies embrace the traditional therapy focus of the profession, when working with individuals or small groups, as well as the more recent political focus, in which occupationally just societies are created for all community members.

KEY POINTS

- Occupation and its relationship with health and well-being, underpin the practice and focus of occupational therapy.
- The overall goal of occupational therapy is to enable people to engage in occupations that promote health and well-being.
- Occupational therapists have to become *wise* practitioners, embracing scientific, ethical, and artistic thinking in the planning, implementation, and evaluation of strategies.
- The enabling skills and strategies used by occupational therapists are complex.
- The concept of enablement is the core foundation of occupational therapy.
- Occupational therapists draw on at least ten skills, as proposed by Townsend et al (2007), and six different strategies to enable people.

Introduction

[Occupational therapists] can stand on the rock that is our ethos and from there proclaim our view: time, place and circumstance open paths to occupation. Occupation fosters dignity, competence and health. Occupational therapy

is a personal engagement. Caring and helping are vital to the work. Effective practice is artistry and science. Our profession takes this stand for the sake of persons and their occupational natures. We engage – we involve and occupy ourselves and commit to mutual promise – so that others may also engage. [...] We enable occupations that heal. We co-create daily lives. We reach for hearts as well as hands. We are artists and scientists at once. [...] This is our character; this is our genius; this is our spirit.

(Peloquin 2005, p. 623)

Peloquin's statement eloquently embraces the focus and impact of occupational therapy interventions. She captures the importance of the occupational nature of our work and, in so doing, emphasises the fundamental belief underpinning all occupational therapy interventions, that occupation fosters dignity, competence, and health.

This chapter will illustrate what it means to have an occupational focus to the skills and strategies that occupational therapists use when working with people. Initially, a justification will be given as to why occupational therapists need to focus on occupation when working with people, followed by a discussion of the complexity of occupational therapy practice and the multitude of factors that must be considered when developing occupation focused enabling strategies. This section will include a discussion of the concept of 'wise practice'. The concept of enablement is then presented as this is considered the essence that underpins all the skills and strategies of occupational therapists. Finally, the essential skills of occupational therapists and suggested strategies are briefly covered, providing an introduction to the more detailed illustration of these throughout the remaining chapters of this book.

Focus on occupation

Baum (2003) and Wilcock (2005) state that the occupational therapy profession is underpinned by the principles of occupation and participation, and that both of these principles are central to the definition of health. This belief in occupation is shared by many leaders within the profession, who promote the move away from biomedical practice to an occupation-focused practice; a move that

encourages occupational therapists to take an active role in building healthy communities by promoting engagement in meaningful and purposeful occupations for all citizens (Finlayson & Edwards 1997, Moyers 2005, Schwartz 2003, Wilcock 2003).

Wilcock (1998b, 2003, 2005) proposes that occupational therapists need to focus on occupational ill-health or dysfunction. She identifies three occupational problems that impact on health: occupational imbalance, occupational deprivation, and occupational alienation (Table 9.1). Other authors focus on different occupational problems, such as occupational injustice (Townsend et al 2007, Wilcock & Townsend 2000) and occupational apartheid (Kronenberg & Pollard 2005) (Table 9.1). The one thing that all these problems have in common is the focus on occupation; the everyday tasks and activities that people do. Christiansen (1999) suggests that competence in performing and engaging in occupations contributes to a person's identity, and that the development of a satisfactory identity is essential to a person's feelings of coherence and well-being. This is because occupations that people engage in are fundamentally driven by each individual's aspirations, needs, and environments, and relate to each individual's purposeful and meaningful use of time (Turner 2001). Hence, when using an occupational lens, people are considered to be healthy when they have the choice and ability to actively participate in all aspects of daily living (Christiansen 2006, Crepeau et al 2003, Moyers 2005).

Engagement in occupations is dependent on the dynamic and complex interaction between the type of occupation, the abilities, habits, skills, and experience of the person, and the physical, geographical, cultural, and social aspects of the environment (Duncan 2006a, Moyers 2005). The occupations a person engages in are not static; they are dynamic and are influenced by the positive and negative experiences throughout the lifespan (Whiteford et al 2000). Whiteford et al (2000) go on to claim that as a basic human need, occupation is a source of choice, control, balance, and satisfaction, and a means of organising time, space, and materials.

Thibeault (2002, p. 199) suggests that engagement in occupation is also a means of creating social change. She states that, '[...] individual change results in due course in social change. Systemic social action starts with each citizen. The person who, because of us, embraces a healthier, more

Table 9.1 Definition of occupational problems (Kronenberg & Pollard 2005, Townsend et al 2007, Wilcock 1998b, 2003, 2005, Wilcock & Townsend 2000)

Occupational imbalance	Occurs when a person is unable to participate in occupations that enable him to use his physical, social and cognitive capabilities and capacities (e.g. a child with cerebral palsy may not be able to engage in school work effectively due to his increased muscle tone and athetoid movements)
Occupational deprivation	Occurs when a person is prevented from engaging in health-promoting occupations over a prolonged period of time, due to external forces (e.g. prisoners and refugees may lack the opportunities to do a variety of occupations due to the restrictions placed on them by their respective institution)
Occupational alienation	Occurs when there is a disconnection between the occupation a person engages in and his environment (e.g. a young adult with a brain injury may feel out of place and unable to engage in occupations he enjoys when residing in a nursing home primarily catering for older people)
Occupational injustice	Occurs when people are prevented from being engaged in doing what they decide to do, in a way that is most meaningful and purposeful for their situation (e.g. a person in need of a wheelchair and seating system to enable community mobility may be treated unjustly if the equipment that they are provided with through a government funding scheme is inadequate due to financial constraints of the funding scheme)
Occupational apartheid	Occurs when people are wilfully and politically restricted and segregated from participating in occupations based on race, colour, disability, nationality, age, gender, religion, political beliefs, status etc. (e.g. a child may be denied access to mainstream schools on the basis of his impairment, rather than academic ability).

peaceful life will exert a healthier, more peaceful influence around him'. Thibeault (2002, p. 200) goes on to say that occupation is the best approach to achieve social change because it 'confronts us with matter and clearly delineates our strengths and weaknesses, it has the power to refine self-knowledge and galvanize growth'.

The importance of occupation and its relationship with health and well-being, underpins the practice and focus of occupational therapy. As Crepeau (2003, p. 30) concisely stated, the job of the occupational therapist 'is ultimately to help people realise their humanity through occupational engagement'.

Complexity of occupational therapy practice

Occupational therapists assist individuals, groups and communities to identify practical options to adapt and overcome any occupational dysfunction, so that participation in all aspects of daily life is possible (Dickinson 2003). It is important to understand that occupational therapy is not about treating a disease or impairment; rather it is about focusing on developing the competency of people, assisting

them to find fulfilment through engagement in occupation (Watson 2006). This suggests that the meaning an individual finds during engagement in occupation is more important than the outcome or purpose (Hammell 2004). Hence, engagement in occupation becomes a synthesis of doing, being, becoming, and belonging (Hammell 2004, Lyons et al 2002, Rebeiro et al 2001, Wilcock 1998a, 1999) (Table 9.2). When occupational therapists talk of a balance among occupations, this does not necessarily refer to a balance between self-care, work and leisure occupations; rather it refers to a balance of affective experiences across all occupations that a person engages in – a balance of the meaning that these occupations hold for the person (Hammell 2004, Primeau 1996).

As a result of the focus on the 'doing, being, becoming and belonging' of occupations, the finding that 'occupation is health giving' (Wilcock 2005, p. 6), and the dynamic interaction that occurs between the person, occupation and environment, the skills and strategies that occupational therapists use have been defined as complex (Corr et al 2005, Creek 2003, Creek et al 2005). In addition to the focus on occupation, occupational therapy enabling skills and strategies are considered complex because the planning, implementation, and evaluation of

Table 9.2 Definition of doing, being, becoming and belonging (Hammell 2004, Lyons et al 2002, Rebeiro et al 2001, Wilcock 1998a, 1999)

Doing	Purposeful, goal-directed activities; provides a sense of purpose, fulfilment and affirms competence and self-worth
Being	Time taken to reflect and be introspective and contemplative; involves the realms of meaning, value and intentionality, perhaps providing the 'why' to what we do
Becoming	Envisioning one's future, developing ideas of who one wishes to become; denotes a process of change over time and of engaging in the choices we make in deciding which pathways to follow
Belonging	Sense of being included, of feeling valued by others; focuses on the importance of relationships and connectedness to the experience of meaning in everyday life

strategies are non-linear, and unpredictable, involving a continual shift of perspective that requires occupational therapists to engage scientific, ethical, and artistic thinking (Barnitt 1990, Butler 2004, Creek et al 2005, Royeen 2003). Hagedorn (2001, p. 34) referred to the complexity of occupational therapy practice when she explained that,

[occupational therapists'] core competencies and processes must somehow encompass the nebulous aspects of professional judgement and reasoning, problem solving and research, as well as the 'hands on' forms of therapeutic knowledge and skill.

Although occupational therapists use a range of complex and dynamic enabling skills and strategies when working with people to shape what matters most (Crabtree 2003, Thibeault 2006), there is no formula to follow when planning and designing enabling strategies. This means that occupational therapists have to consider more than just their scientific thinking; the evidence base for practice (Curtin & Fossey 2007, Hammell 2005, Whiteford 2005). This is not to suggest that occupational therapists should not seek out and, where appropriate, contribute to evidence for the strategies implemented. Rather, it is to suggest that occupational

therapists consider other forms of evidence, such as reflective experience, intuition, professional judgement, and expert opinion. This leads to the concept of 'wise practice' (Higgs & Titchen 2001, p. 13), which embraces the trilogy of scientific, ethical, and artistic elements of practice. Wise practice encapsulates the process that occupational therapists undergo when they are considering a multitude of information, including published research data and their reflections on practice, to develop effective and relevant enabling strategies (Paterson et al 2006). Hence, the concept of an evidence base for practice is broadened. Through the process of reflection, consideration of research evidence, and the outcome of consultations with others, the occupational therapist becomes a wise practitioner and is able to provide a clear, considered rationale for the enabling strategies that are developed and implemented.

In spite of there being no formula to follow when planning and designing enabling strategies, the focus or goal of the enabling strategies used by occupational therapists is clear and unequivocal. The overarching goal of occupational therapy is to enable people to engage in health and well-being promoting occupations (Moyers 2005, Stanley & Cheek 2003) – this is the core, the essence of occupational therapy enabling strategies and what makes the practice of occupational therapy different to the practice of other professions. Hence, this must be the focus and ultimate outcome of the work of occupational therapists.

Occupational therapists improve occupational performance and engagement, promote and maintain health, and prevent disease and impairment, through enabling engagement in occupations that are fulfilling, have personal meaning, and provide opportunity to develop and express one's identity (Moyers, 2005). Occupational therapists address occupational dysfunction, and assist people to regain competence and a positive occupational identity, by using a range of enabling skills and strategies that often include adapting the demands of the occupation, altering the physical or social environment, and teaching a person new skills or re-establishing lost skills (Duncan 2006a). Occupational therapists view people as occupational beings, and, as a result, use enabling skills and strategies to address occupational performance and engagement difficulties that, if not addressed, may lead to greater dependence, and/or a decline in health and well-being, and an associated reduced quality of life (Moyers, 2005).

When enabling skills and strategies are based on occupation, people should be able to see how engagement in therapy is connected to performance in an occupation that they find meaningful and purposeful; an occupation that is centred on their needs, interests and priorities (Crepeau et al 2003, Youngstrom & Brown 2005). Moyers (2005, p. 229) states that,

Occupations are chosen because of their potential to remediate impaired capabilities; to facilitate transfer of capabilities to multiple contexts; to enhance motivation to change and adapt; to promote self-exploration and development of identity; to match current capabilities; to provide opportunities to practise skills and develop habits; to provide feedback; to experience success, pleasure and other emotions; to interact with others.

The concept of enabling

To achieve the ultimate goal of occupational therapy, as identified by Crepeau et al (2003), occupational therapists need to embrace the concept of 'enabling' (Townsend et al 2007). Occupational therapists are considered to be enablers, as we enable people to engage in meaningful and health-promoting occupations. The Canadian Association of Occupational Therapists (1997, p. 50) defined enabling as 'facilitating, guiding, coaching, educating, prompting, listening, reflecting, encouraging, or otherwise collaborating with people'. In a more recent interpretation, Townsend et al (2007) state that enabling describes what occupational therapists actually do and consider it to be the core competency of occupational therapy. These authors go on to state that, 'enablement is the professional identity and trademark of occupational therapists who engage others through meaningful occupation to pursue goals for health, well-being and justice through occupation' (p. 91).

Townsend and Polatajko (2007, p. 367) suggest that the skills required to be enabling 'are value-based, collaborative, attentive to power equities and diversity, and charged with visions of possibility for individual and/or social change'. In being enablers, occupational therapists become critically reflective and attentive to inequities, differing perspectives, conflicts, diversity and issues of choice, risk and responsibilities.

In their exploration of 'enabling' Townsend et al (2007) propose some foundations to practising in this way. They suggest that working in an enabling way involves:

1. facilitating individual, group or community choice, involvement in just-right risk-taking, and an understanding of the responsibilities of the people occupational therapists work with and of the professional. This includes the acceptance of diversity amongst people, the delivery of services in an equitable manner, and recognition that all people have the right to be occupationally engaged.

2. collaborative person-centred practice that respects a person's rights by encouraging participation in all decisions related to his progress. Developing and implementing relevant and effective occupational therapy enabling strategies depends on the collaboration between the therapist and the people with whom they are working (Crepeau et al 2003, Duncan 2006a, Youngstrom & Brown 2005). This collaboration forms the basis of person-centred practice, in which it is essential that the therapist understands the person's world and context, including the person's family, friends, culture, economic status, etc. (Watson 2006). In being person-centred, occupational therapists aim to be aware of their own beliefs and values, and how these may influence their interactions with people. In addition, occupational therapists need to listen to people to facilitate their autonomy and engagement in their chosen occupations. Being person-centred means showing respect to and caring for the individual, and acknowledging that each person is a complex, capable and unique individual (Thibeault 2000). Commitment to working collaboratively also reinforces the development of a power-sharing partnership between people and therapists.

3. inspiring hope, confidence, and resilience to foster within people, the notion that change and transformation are possible. There needs to be an agreed understanding that change will take place and that people will be actively involved in effecting change. Occupational therapists need to envisage possible futures for the people they work with and encourage them to envisage possible futures for themselves (Fearing 2001, Townsend et al 2007). The focus of the collaboration between an individual and a

therapist is on assisting the individual to achieve the agreed vision of their future. As Fearing (2001, p. 213) states,

One of the arts of occupational therapy is in the occupations we choose to engage people in the present, to use what they have learned in the past, in order to create a future that makes life worth living. As occupational therapists we are in the business of assisting others to use their power to create their personal futures, which they carry within themselves [...] Once we know what we want our future to look like, we can make choices that will get us there.

Practice Scenario 9.1

Tilly had lived in a council house with her father, Bob, and younger brother, Matt. Her mother, Liz, had left the family when Tilly started primary school because she claimed that she could no longer cope, 'living with her two ungrateful children and a depressed husband who had turned to drink.' The family has had no contact with Liz since she left. Bob gave up drinking, and attends a drug and alcohol addiction support group each week. He does some casual labouring work, helping out a builder friend. However, he struggles to hold down a permanent job because of his depression, for which he was on medication. He found it difficult to be motivated to do things and, as a result, Tilly did most of the cooking and house cleaning. Tilly and her brother struggled academically at school. They both tried to do well but, partly as a result of their home life, they had little time to study and do homework.

When Tilly was 11 she was diagnosed with acute lymphoblastic leukaemia. Her medical treatment included intrathecal therapy, a therapeutic strategy for maintaining remission in people with this condition. Complications arose after her last dose of intrathecal therapy, leaving Tilly with a permanent complete C3 tetraplegia. This occurred when Tilly was 15 years old. As a result of the tetraplegia, Tilly is unable to move and requires 24-hour care for all her physical needs. She has limited neck, head and face movements, has difficulty swallowing and is only able to communicate in a whisper. She uses a respirator to assist her with breathing. This unexpected paralysis also left her emotionally vulnerable.

The hospital accepted fault for causing Tilly's tetraplegia and as a result Tilly was awarded significant financial compensation.

Enabling skills

In a radical re-think of how occupational therapists work, Townsend et al (2007) proposed ten skills that underpin all the strategies that therapists use to enable occupation. Although these skills are not exclusive to occupational therapists, the focus on using these skills to promote occupational engagement is unique to the profession. These 10 skills are also not exhaustive, but are an attempt to encapsulate the essence of occupational therapy practice and to identify what Duncan (2006b) would call, the core skills required for enablement. These skills would usually be used in combination with each other, rather than separately, as the complexity of working with people means that several skills may be required at any one time. In addition, the skills used will vary throughout the period of time that the therapist and person work together, corresponding to the changing emphasis of the strategies used to enable occupation. A brief overview of the skills is provided in Table 9.3, but reference should be made to Townsend et al (2007) for further details. An example of how each skill may be used is also provided in the table, based on Practice Scenario 9.1.

Enabling strategies

Strategies used by occupational therapists usually are placed in two major categories: top-down and bottom-up (Holm et al 2003, Weinstock-Zlotnick & Hinojosa 2004). Top-down strategies are generally considered to be more holistic, person-centred and more suited to the occupation-focus of occupational therapy. The focus of these strategies is on the social roles and responsibilities that define a person's participation both at home and in the community. These approaches usually start by focusing on a person's occupational roles and the meaning the person assigns to the occupations that are part of their roles; hence, occupational dysfunction or participation restriction is established first, and performance components, or a person's capabilities, are considered later. The rationale for this approach is that participation can be improved through adapted performance of occupations, even though impairments cannot be cured.

Bottom-up strategies generally focus on performance components and other foundational factors first, to obtain an understanding of a person's

Table 9.3 Enablement skills proposed by Townsend et al. (2007)

Enablement skill	Description of skill	Example of skill when working with Tilly
Adapt	Refers to the ability of the therapist to change existing environments or aspects of the task to meet a person's occupational performance needs. Part of this skill involves the breaking down of tasks into 'just-right challenges' (Townsend et al 2007, p. 117), problem-solving, reconfiguring an occupation or tailoring an occupation to the requirements of the person and/or environment in which the occupation is conducted (Dunn et al 1994, Holm et al 2003, Moyers 2005, Schell et al 2003, Townsend et al 2007, Youngstrom & Brown 2005)	*This skill required* when considering ways in which Tilly will have control over the things that people do for her – e.g. choice of clothes to wear; what and when to eat; deciding what to do during the day. As Tilly will be totally physically dependent on her father, brother, and paid carers, she will have to adapt considerably the way she would like things done, in addition to being able to inform people how she would like things done
Advocate	Refers to the ability of the therapist to act in a political manner, on behalf of people requiring their services, lobbying to ensure a person's needs are met. This strategy is political and can involve lobbying for policy change, when policies perpetuate inequities. This skill is key to addressing the concern occupational therapists have with 'health, well-being, inclusion, and justice for all in everyday occupations' (p. 117) (Townsend et al 2007)	*This skill required* to ensure that Tilly's choices and decisions are voiced and listened to by all those involved with her. This is especially the case as she is a teenager and most probably has not developed the skills required to be in control. This will include ensuring that she understands and has her say regarding issues such as housing (e.g. as she has a significant financial compensation she will be able to afford to have a house built to suit her needs, but as she has not ever been involved in designing a house, especially a house designed for a person with high tetraplegia, she will need an advocate to assist her to understand and make sound decisions); choice of carers (e.g. as she is going to work closely and intimately with the carers it is important that she is involved in their employment and training); and equipment preference (e.g. she may prefer to be pushed around in a manual wheelchair rather than use a powered wheelchair with an adapted controller)
Coach	Refers to the ability of the therapist to establish a partnership with a person, so as to encourage, guide, mentor and instruct that person on ways to achieve his occupational goals (Townsend et al 2007)	*This skill required* because Tilly will need guidance and encouragement in many areas as she learns to live with her impairment. This will mean working with her and her family to increase their understanding of tetraplegia and the implications, such as risk of pressure sores, bowel and bladder routines. It will also mean working with Tilly to encourage her to take just-right risks appropriate for a girl her age that she chooses to do, such as going out with her friends and having sleep overs. There may be specific occupations that Tilly wants to do that will require coaching and support, such as returning to school and completing her education and, when she is ready, investigating work options

(cont'd)

Table 9.3 Enablement skills proposed by Townsend et al. (2007)—cont'd

Enablement skill	Description of skill	Example of skill when working with Tilly
Collaborate	Refers to the ability of the therapist to develop a power-sharing, person-centred practice. The therapist and the person work together to plan and implement interventions to achieve the person's goals. In a collaborative relationship there is a mutual sharing of expertise and of respect for the skills the different partners have in the relationship. The skill of collaboration also refers to working together with other health and social welfare professionals for the benefit of the person. The skill of collaboration should be inherent in all interactions between occupational therapists and the people with whom they are working (Townsend et al 2007)	*This skill required* for all interactions with Tilly and her family. Tilly will probably feel little control of her situation initially, and the therapist will need to work with her to achieve a mutual power-sharing relationship. This will also be the case for Tilly's father and brother. In addition, many other health, social welfare, education, and legal professionals, in addition to builders and other trades people, and equipment suppliers, will be involved with Tilly. The therapist will need to collaborate with all of them to achieve Tilly's occupational goals
Consult	Refers to the ability of the therapist to provide information and advice to the individual and to others involved in the care of the individual. Consultation may occur with team members, government personnel, business representatives, special interest groups, etc. In the role of a consultant the occupational therapist must integrate, synthesise, and summarise multiple forms of data, and put forward recommendations that may reframe the problems, issues, challenges and opportunities, as a way of stimulating a course of action (Moyers 2005, Townsend et al 2007, Youngstrom & Brown 2005)	*This skill required* when providing information and advice to Tilly and her father and brother. In addition, the occupational therapist will need to liaise with a variety of people, mutually sharing expertise, to ensure Tilly's needs are being met. For example, the occupational therapist will need to provide information on the requirement for a powered wheelchair, and do this while consulting with the wheelchair supplier, the respiratory specialist about the ventilator, the physiotherapist regarding seating posture, the builder regarding use of the chair within the house, and the vehicle supplier to ensure the chair and Tilly can easily and safely be transported
Coordinate	Refers to the ability of the therapist to manage and pull together the multiple factors required to achieve a person's goals (including the involvement of other professionals) and to make the person's experience as seamless as possible. The aim is for everyone to be working towards the same purpose. Coordination also refers to the coordination of services for the effective running of departments and faculties (Townsend et al 2007)	*This skill required* to ensure that the multiple professionals and people involved in working with Tilly are working together. For example, arranging for all the people involved in building an appropriate house for Tilly and her father and brother, are linked in and talking with each other, and that the house is ready for when Tilly is discharged. Another example would bring together all the people involved in assisting Tilly and her father/brother to organise a care package and the employment of carers when Tilly is discharged home
Design/build	Refers to the ability of the therapist to accommodate the abilities of the person by changing or altering the physical environment (such as home modifications), providing of assistive technology or splints, and designing and implementation of programs and services. The term design is used to refer to the development of a plan or a strategy (Dunn et al 1994, Townsend et al 2007)	*This skill required* in the planning and design of a house to accommodate Tilly and her father/brother's needs. Also Tilly will require assistive technology such as a powered wheelchair and seating system for mobility, an environmental control system for controlling devices within the house (such as television, music system, lights), a vehicle to transport her while sitting in her wheelchair, and a computer system. This skill will also be evident in the plans developed for a safe discharge and re-integration into Tilly's community

Table 9.3 Enablement skills proposed by Townsend et al. (2007)—cont'd

Enablement skill	Description of skill	Example of skill when working with Tilly
Educate	Refers to the ability of the therapist to transfer specific knowledge in a meaningful and appropriate manner to the person, the person's family, other professionals and the general public. Therapists need to draw on relevant educational theories and apply these to their work in enabling occupations. There are many ways in which education can be done, such as demonstration, facilitating learning through doing, simulating, teaching, tutoring etc. This skill is also evident as part of the health-promotion strategies to prevent occupational dysfunction (Moyers 2005, Townsend et al 2007, Youngstrom & Brown 2005)	*This skill required* when informing Tilly and her family about her impairment. It is also required when exploring various equipment options (e.g. wheelchairs, beds, computer, environmental control system, etc.) to ensure Tilly and her father/brother understand the options, learn to use the equipment appropriately, and can instruct others how to use the equipment. Many interactions with Tilly and her family will involve some degree of education
Engage	Refers to the ability of the therapist to create opportunities and circumstances to promote optimal performance and engagement, related to the environment in which a person performs. This skill centres on involving and motivating a person in doing and participating, of engaging in occupation. The skill of engaging people in occupation is essential for health and well-being, and contradicts any notion of the person being a passive recipient of occupational therapy enabling strategies (Dunn et al 1994, Townsend et al 2007)	*This skill required* to motivate Tilly to engage in occupations that are meaningful to her and to envisage her future. This means encouraging Tilly to be involved in decisions that affect her and to develop strategies to enable her to do the things she wants to do. This will involve all the other nine enabling skills listed in this table to inspire hope, confidence and resilience
Specialise	This skill encompasses the many specific techniques that occupational therapists may use to achieve occupational goals. These techniques are usually developed through further training, related to an occupational therapist's area of practice. These techniques may be borrowed from other professionals and may not be occupational in nature, although they should be used to achieve occupational goals (Duncan 2006b, Townsend et al 2007)	*This skill required* when applying an understanding of spinal cord lesions and the impact this will have on Tilly's body. This will mean providing splints to prevent contractures, determining the most effective pressure-relieving cushion and seating support system when sitting in a wheelchair, moving and handing techniques to ensure safe transfers between wheelchair and bed, etc. This would also involve having specialised knowledge regarding the assistive technology that may be appropriate for Tilly

(NB: As proposed by Townsend et al. the skills are listed alphabetically to demonstrate that there is no prioritisation of the skills; all are considered to be equally important.)

abilities and limitations. The rationale behind this approach is that body structures and functions support occupational performance and engagement, so by improving a person's abilities, there will be a corresponding improvement in the performance and engagement of occupations; hence, if impaired physical, psychological and cognitive skills are remedied or compensated for, then it is possible for the person to re-engage in occupations.

Although neither strategy is considered to be better than the other, Holm et al (2003) state that top-down strategies are the most appropriate for occupational therapy practice. In contrast, Weinstock-Zlotnick and Hinojosa (2004) suggest that each type of strategy used in isolation is insufficient and ineffective. They propose that a combination of both types of strategies is essential to be effective. However, whether a strategy is top-down or bottom-up is irrelevant if the occupational therapist does not focus on promoting health, and preventing disease and impairment through facilitating engagement in occupations (Moyers 2005, Youngstrom & Brown 2005). Top-down and bottom-up strategies may be used interchangeably as long as the ultimate focus of the strategies selected is to enable occupation; as long as the focus is on the use of occupations, activities and tasks meaningful to the person in order to promote and maintain health and to improve occupational performance and engagement.

Drawing on both top-down and bottom-up strategies requires occupational therapists to be flexible in how they work with people and how they achieve the collaboratively considered occupational goals. This flexibility means that the occupational therapist must draw on a range of skills (Table 9.3) and strategies (Table 9.4). Moyers (2005) proposed that these strategies can include remediation, compensation, and education. Watson (2006) categorises these three strategies as 'therapy', the traditional strategies of therapists that tend to focus on working occupationally with individuals and small groups.

In addition to the 'therapy' strategies, Watson (2006) proposes three further strategies that occupational therapists are beginning to use more often, when working with communities and population: community development, transformation, and redistributive justice. These three strategies point towards a more political direction for occupational therapists, one in which they become social and political agents (Barros et al 2005). These strategies stress the importance of helping people to empower themselves (Galheigo 2005). The reason for a move to a more political agenda is strongly put forward by Pollard et al (2005, pp. 524–526):

Occupational therapists appear to be under increasing pressure to work towards genericism owing either to the influence of legislative and policy changes or to the profession's inability in some clinical areas to convince others of the scope of its skills or the need to be enabled in researching them. The core principles of occupation are being eroded, it seems, and the role of the occupational therapists is being limited to discharge agent or psychological technician. [...]

This reduction in professional horizons comes at a time of increasing occupational injustice through the global expansion of the gap between rich and poor. The clients whose discharge is facilitated by occupational therapists often return to a forbidding society. The interventions offered through the health and social care system are challenged by the rifts between the different socioeconomic groups, which produce wide divergences in life expectancy and quality. [...]

Some [...] argue for an occupational therapy that reconnects with the culturally and spiritually significant aspects of occupation in areas of poverty and conflict, where health and social care services often do not reach. These voices can inform practice where social and economic deprivation limit access to occupation, where population is ageing and where physical disabilities combined with low income are apparent. Here the effectiveness of health and social care technologies is limited by the conditions in which people live. [...]

Occupational therapy has the potential to benefit the wider society as well as helping the individual and can engage with marginalized people to make connections with excluded communities.

Clearly, these are important strategies for occupational therapists to use in their quest to create occupationally just societies for all community members.

A brief overview of each strategy is provided in Table 9.4. This includes an example of how each strategy may be used when working with Tilly (Practice Scenario 9.1).

Conclusion

Occupational therapy enabling skills and strategies are complex. When planning, implementing, and evaluating strategies, occupational therapists have to embrace and engage scientific, ethical, and artistic thinking to address the occupational goals of the person. As there is no formula to follow when working with people, occupational therapists need to become wise practitioners. Practising in this way ensures that occupational therapists become enablers, using their skills and strategies in an infinite variety of ways to promote and maintain the health and well-being of people, ultimately improving their occupational performance and engagement.

Table 9.4 Enabling strategies

Enabling strategy	Description of strategy	Example of strategy when working with Tilly
The following strategies are usually used when occupational therapists are working with an individual or small group		
Remediation	Strategies that focus on making changes in the person or population generally use approaches that remediate, restore or establish skills, refers to fixing the impairment; putting strategies in place for a person to recover lost skills or attain new skills; the focus is on identifying a person's skills and barriers to performance and then designing strategies that restore, maintain, develop and/or improve the person's abilities required for occupational performance and engagement. Pedretti & Early (2001) refer to these types of strategies as adjunctive methods, and see them as procedures that prepare people for occupational performance and engagement. These methods are preliminary to the use of meaningful activity, and may include exercises, facilitation and inhibition techniques, positioning, splints, etc. (Dunn et al 1994, Moyers 2005, Schell et al 2003, Youngstrom & Brown 2005)	*This type of strategy may include (NB: many remedial strategies will be carried out by other health professionals):* • Using hand splints and passive range of motion to prevent joint contractures • Awareness training to compensate for loss of sensation to body – increased use of auditory and visual senses • Cognitive strategies to develop problem-solving skills • Learning and study strategies to assist with education • Learning business skills to be involved in the employment of carers
Compensation	Strategies directed at adapting the environment or the task to match a person's abilities, are referred to as compensatory or adaptive strategies. These strategies also include those not focusing on changing the person or adapting the environment, but on making the best person–environment fit. In this case the focus is on matching the abilities of the person/population with the environment or task that is most enabling. The main focus of these strategies is to prevent or reduce occupational performance issues that may result from an impairment, to enable participation. When using compensation strategies changes may be made to the way the task is done, the tools required to do the task, and/or the environment (Holm & Rogers 1998, Moyers 2005, Youngstrom & Brown 2005)	*This type of strategy may include:* Change the task • Employ carers to perform everyday activities and to assist with hygiene needs • Inform family/carers what she wants to do and how she wants things done – this can include giving instructions for self-care activities, cooking food, outings, etc. • Head control or sip-puff control to manoeuvre a powered wheelchair, and operate an environmental control system and computer Change the tool/equipment • Computer for writing and communication • Environmental control system for controlling electrical appliances in the house, as well as for opening doors, windows, and using the telephone • Powered wheelchair and seating system for independent mobility • Adapted vehicle for safely transporting Tilly while sitting in her wheelchair Change the environment • Build a fully accessible house to accommodate her mobility needs – level floors, no steps, wide doorways, automatic opening doors, turning spaces, integrated environmental control system, ceiling hoists, etc.; the house needs to meet the needs of Tilly, as well as her father and brother, if they are to continue to live together • Work with students and teachers at Tilly's school to ensure they understand how to accommodate her needs • Work with local council to make local community services and shopping centres more accessible, where appropriate

(cont'd)

Table 9.4 Enabling strategies—cont'd

Enabling strategy	Description of strategy	Example of strategy when working with Tilly
Education	These strategies are used as part of everyday practice to empower individuals by imparting knowledge, to enable them to change their behaviour, attitude, beliefs, confidence, skills and decision making ability. When designing education strategies therapists need to incorporate theoretical principles and consider various factors such as content, delivery mode, and timing, to ensure that it is relevant to an individual's circumstances (Dunn et al 1994)	*This type of strategy may include:* • Informing Tilly, her father/brother, and carers about her impairment and the implications. • Demonstrate and train Tilly how to use the assistive technology devices, such as the powered wheelchair, computer, environmental control unit, adapted vehicle, and ventilator. • Inform teacher and students at Tilly's school about her needs • Produce a DVD to use with new carers to demonstrate how to move and handle Tilly correctly, and how to assist her with her self-care and hygiene • Explain requirements for the house design to architects and builders

The following strategies are *usually* used when occupational therapists are working with a community or population.

Enabling strategy	Description of strategy	Example of strategy when working with Tilly
Community development	These strategies are indicative of a move away from one-to-one therapy, towards a community based approach. Community development is a participatory approach that focuses on capacity building in which members of a community develop their own strategies to respond to the various local factors that impact on their occupational engagement. This may include working in community based rehabilitation and health promotion (Watson 2006)	*This type of strategy may include:* • Working with Tilly, her father and her brother, as a small community, to increase their capacity to accommodate her needs – where they become the experts • Establish support networks for the family – with friends, local service, charities, church groups, drug and alcohol addiction support group – to provide assistance if required and accommodate needs • Working with Tilly's school community to increase their capacity to ensure that her social and educational needs are accommodated
Transformation	These strategies involve the development of partnerships with groups who are marginalized, deprived and/or restricted, to develop services to meet their occupational needs. The aim of developing partnerships is ensure equity of service provision and opportunity. Occupational therapists need to change the way they work, being led by the groups they are partnering with rather than by their own expertise/employers. The partnerships have the ultimate goal of facilitating participation (Watson, 2006)	*This type of strategy may include:* • Working with local disability groups to ensure the implementation of policy that promotes the rights of people with disabilities – e.g. access to the school of choice, employment opportunities, accessible footpaths, availability of recreation and leisure facilities • Developing the advocacy and lobbying skills of people with disabilities to enable them to push for the rights • Listening to and collaborating with Tilly to ensure her needs are voiced and met; it may also be appropriate to introduce Tilly to a support group of people with disabilities so that her voice and needs can be considered as part of a collective
Redistributive justice	These strategies refer to taking on direct and indirect action and advocacy through political intervention and policy implementation to develop the occupational rights of all citizens. These strategies are for the wider society rather than just for a specific community (Watson, 2006)	*This type of strategy may include:* • Writing letters and personal lobbying to members of parliament, local councillors and other relevant community leaders to develop policies promoting equity of services for people with disabilities • When working with Tilly ensure the fair implementation of policies, such as may be to promote a fair equipment provision scheme, where she is not penalised from receiving essential assessment for and provision of equipment because she has significant financial compensation

References

Barnitt, R. (1990). Knowledge, skills and attitudes: What happened to thinking? *British Journal of Occupational Therapy*, 53(11), 450–456.

Barros, D. D., Ghirardi, M. i. G., Lopes, R. E., & Galheigo, S. M. (2005). Social occupational therapy: A socio-historical perspective. In: F. Kronenberg, S. S. Algado & N. Pollard (Eds.), *Occupational therapy without borders: Learning from the spirit of survivors* (pp. 140–151). Edinburgh, Elsevier Churchill Livingstone.

Baum, C. (2003). Participation: Its relationship to occupation and health. *OTJR: Occupation, Participation and Health*, 23(2), 46–47.

Butler, J. (2004). The Casson memorial lecture 2004: The fascination of the difficult. *British Journal of Occupational Therapy*, 67(7), 286–292.

Canadian Association of Occupational Therapists. (1997). *Enabling occupation: An occupational therapy perspective*. Ottawa: CAOT Publications ACE.

Christiansen, C. H. (1999). Defining lives: occupation as identity: an essay on competence, coherence and the creation of meaning. *American Journal of Occupational Therapy*, 53(6), 547–558.

Christiansen, C. H. (2006). Foreward. In S. Rodger & J. Zivianni (Eds.), *Occupational therapy with children: understanding children's occupations and enabling participation* (pp. ix–xi). Oxford, Blackwell Publishing.

Corr, S., Neill, G., & Turner, A. (2005). Comparing an occupational therapy definition and consumers' experiences: a Q methodology study. *British Journal of Occupational Therapy*, 68(8), 338–346.

Crabtree, J. (2003). On occupational performance. *Occupational Therapy in Health Care*, 17(2), 1–18.

Creek, J. (2003). *Occupational therapy defined as a complex intervention*. London, College of Occupational Therapists.

Creek, J., Ilott, I., Cook, S., & Munday, C. (2005). Valuing occupational therapy as a complex intervention. *British Journal of Occupational Therapy*, 68(6), 281–284.

Crepeau, E. B., Cohn, E. S., & Schell, B. A. (2003). Occupational therapy practice today. In: E. B. Crepeau, E. S. Cohn & B. A. Schell (Eds.), *Willard and Spackman's occupational therapy* (10th ed.) (pp. 27–30). Philadelphia, Lippincott, Williams and Wilkins.

Curtin, M., & Fossey, E. (2007). Appraising the trustworthiness of qualitative studies: Guidelines for occupational therapists. *Australian Occupational Therapy Journal*, 54(2), 88–94.

Dickinson, R. (2003). Occupational therapy: a hidden treasure. *Canadian Journal of Occupational Therapy*, 70(3), 133–135.

Duncan, E. A. (2006a). Introduction. In: E. A. Duncan (Ed.), *Foundations for practice in occupational therapy* (4th ed.) (pp. 3–9). Edinburgh, Elsevier Churchill Livingstone.

Duncan, E. A. (2006b). Skills and processes in occupational therapy. In: E. A. Duncan (Ed.), *Foundations for practice in occupational therapy* (4th ed.) (pp. 43–57). Edinburgh, Elsevier Churchill Livingstone.

Dunn, W., Brown, C., & McGuigan, M. (1994). The ecology of human performance: A framework for considering the effect of context. *American Journal of Occupational Therapy*, 47(7), 357–359.

Fearing, V. (2001). Change: Creating our own reality. *Canadian Journal of Occupational Therapy*, 68(4), 208–215.

Finlayson, M., & Edwards, J. (1997). Evolving health environments and occupational therapy: definitions, descriptions and opportunities. *British Journal of Occupational Therapy*, 60(10), 456–460.

Galheigo, S. M. (2005). Occupational therapy and the social field: clarifying concepts and ideas. In: F. Kronenberg, S. S. Algado & N. Pollard (Eds.), *Occupational*

therapy without borders: Learning from the spirit of survivors (pp. 87–98). Edinburgh, Elsevier Churchill Livingstone.

Hagedorn, R. (2001). *Foundations for practice in occupational therapy*. Edinburgh, Churchill Livingstone.

Hammell, K. W. (2004). Dimensions of meaning in the occupations of daily life. *Canadian Journal of Occupational Therapy*, 71(5), 296–305.

Hammell, K. W. (2005). Using qualitative evidence as a basis for evidence-based practice. In: K. Hammell & C. Carpenter (Eds.), *Qualitative research in evidence-based rehabilitation* (pp. 129–143). Edinburgh, Churchill Livingstone.

Higgs, J., & Titchen, A. (2001). *Professional practice in health, education and the creative arts*. Oxford, Blackwell Science.

Holm, M. B., & Rogers, J. C. (1998). Treatment of activities of daily living. In: M. Neistadt & E. B. Crepeau (Eds.), *Willard and Spackman's occupational therapy* (9th ed.) (pp. 340–341). Philadelphia, Lippincott.

Holm, M. B., Rogers, J. C., & Stone, R. G. (2003). Person–task–environment interventions: a decision-making guide. In: E. B. Crepeau, E. S. Cohn & B. A. Schell (Eds.), *Willard and Spackman's occupational therapy* (10th ed.) (pp. 460–490). Philadelphia, Lippincott, Williams and Wilkins.

Kronenberg, F., & Pollard, N. (2005). Introduction: A beginning … In: F. Kronenberg & S. S. Algado (Eds.), *Occupational therapy without borders: learning from the spirit of survivors* (pp. 1–13). Edinburgh, Elsevier Churchill Livingstone.

Lyons, M., Orozovic, N., Davis, J., & Newman, J. (2002). Doing-being-becoming: occupational experiences of persons with life-threatening illnesses. *American Journal of Occupational Therapy*, 56(3), 285–295.

Moyers, P. (2005). Introduction to occupation-based practice. In: C. H. Christiansen, C. Baum & J. Bass-Haugen (Eds.), *Occupational therapy: performance, participation and well-being* (3rd ed.) (pp. 221–234). Thorofare, NJ, Slack.

Paterson, M., Wilcox, S., & Higgs, J. (2006). Exploring dimensions of artistry in reflective practice. *Reflective practice*, 7(4), 455–468.

Pedretti, L. W., & Early, M. B. (2001). Occupational performance and models of practice for physical dysfunction. In: L. W. Pedretti & M. B. Early (Eds.), *Occupational therapy: Practice skills for physical dysfunction* (5th ed.) (pp. 3–12). St Louis, Mosby.

Peloquin, S. M. (2005). The 2005 Eleanor Clarke Slagle lecture: Embracing our ethos, reclaiming our heart. *American Journal of Occupational Therapy*, 59(6), 611–625.

Pollard, N., Alsop, A., & Kronenberg, F. (2005). Reconceptualising occupational therapy. *British Journal of Occupational Therapy*, 68(11), 524–526.

Primeau, L. (1996). Work and leisure: Transcending the dichotomy. *American Journal of Occupational Therapy*, 50(7), 569–577.

Rebeiro, K. L., Day, D., Semeniuk, B., O'Brien, M., & Wilson, B. (2001). Northern initiative for social action: An occupation-based mental health program. *American Journal of Occupational Therapy*, 55, 493–500.

Royeen, C. B. (2003). Chaotic occupational therapy: collective wisdom for a complex profession. *American Journal of Occupational Therapy*, 57(6), 609–624.

Schell, B. A., Crepeau, E. B., & Cohn, E. S. (2003). Occupational therapy interventions. In: B. A. Schell, E. B. Crepeau & E. S. Cohn (Eds.), *Willard and Spackman's occupational therapy* (10 ed.) (pp. 455–459). Philadelphia, Lippincott, Williams and Wilkins.

Schwartz, K. B. (2003). The history of occupational therapy. In: E. B. Crepeau, E. S. Cohn & B. A. Schell (Eds.), *Willard and Spackman's occupational therapy* (10th ed.)

(pp. 5–13). Philadelphia, Lippincott, Williams and Wilkins.

Stanley, M., & Cheek, J. (2003). Well-being and older people: a review of the literature. *Canadian Journal of Occupational Therapy*, 70(1), 51–59.

Thibeault, R. (2000). Magnum miraculum est homo. *Canadian Journal of Occupational Therapy*, 67(1), 3–6.

Thibeault, R. (2002). In praise of dissidence: Anne Lang–Etienne (1932–1991). *Canadian Journal of Occupational Therapy*, 69(4), 197–203.

Thibeault, R. (2006). Globalisation, universities and the future of occupational therapy: Dispatches for the majority world. *Australian Occupational Therapy Journal*, 53, 159–165.

Townsend, E., & Polatajko, H. (2007). *Enabling occupation II: Advancing an occupational therapy vision for health, well-being, and justice through occupation*. Ottawa, Canadian Association of Occupational Therapists.

Townsend, E., Beagan, B., Kumas-Tan, Z. et al. (2007). Enabling: Occupational therapy's core competency. In: E. Townsend & H. Polatajko (Eds.), *Enabling occupation II: Advancing an occupational therapy vision for health, well-being and justice through occupation* (pp. 87–135). Ottawa, Canadian Association of Occupational Therapists.

Turner, A. (2001). Occupation for therapy. In: A. Turner, M. Foster & S. E. Johnson (Eds.), *Occupational therapy and physical dysfunction: Principles, skills and practice* (5th ed.) (pp. 25–46). Edinburgh, Churchill Livingstone.

Watson, R. (2006). Being before doing: the cultural identity (essence) of occupational therapy. *Australian Occupational Therapy Journal*, 53, 151–158.

Weinstock-Zlotnick, G. & Hinojosa, J. (2004). Bottom–up or top–down

evaluation: is one better than the other? *American Journal of Occupational Therapy*, 58(5), 594–599.

Whiteford, G. (2005). Knowledge, power, evidence: a critical analysis of key issues in evidence based practice. In: G. Whiteford & V. Wright–St Clair (Eds.), *Occupation and practice in context* (pp. 34–50). Sydney, Elsevier.

Whiteford, G., Townsend, E., & Hocking, C. (2000). Reflections on a renaissance of occupation. *Canadian Journal of Occupational Therapy*, 67(1), 61–69.

Wilcock, A. A. (1998a). International perspective: Reflections on doing, being and becoming. *Canadian Journal of Occupational Therapy*, 65(5), 248–256.

Wilcock, A. A. (1998b). Occupation for health. *British Journal of Occupational Therapy*, 61, 340–345.

Wilcock, A. A. (1999). Reflections on doing, being and becoming. *Australian Occupational Therapy Journal*, 46(1), 1–11.

Wilcock, A. A. (2003). Population interventions focused on health for all. In: E. B. Crepeau, E. S. Cohn & B. A. Schell (Eds.), *Willard and Spackman's occupational therapy* (10th ed.) (pp. 30–45). Philadelphia, Lippincott, Williams and Wilkins.

Wilcock, A. A. (2005). Occupational science: Bridging occupation and health. *Canadian Journal of Occupational Therapy*, 72(1), 5–12.

Wilcock, A. A., & Townsend, E. (2000). Occupational justice: Occupational terminology interactive dialogue. *Journal of Occupational Science*, 7(2), 84–86.

Youngstrom, M. J., & Brown, C. (2005). Categories and principles of interventions. In: C. H. Christiansen, C. Baum & J. Bass-Haugen (Eds.), *Occupational therapy: performance, participation and well-being* (3rd ed.) (pp. 397–411). Thorofare, NJ: Slack.

Section **Three**

Essential foundations for occupational therapy

10

The art of person-centred practice

Thelma Sumsion

CHAPTER CONTENTS

Setting the scene 127

Defining a person-centred approach. 128

Issues in the implementation of
person-centred practice 129

Valuing uniqueness and autonomy of the
individual. 129

Respect and dignity 129

Enabling choice 130

Developing trust 130

Empowerment 130

Encouraging participation through
partnerships 131

Practical application 131

Conclusion. 132

SUMMARY

This chapter focuses on the art of person-centred practice in occupational therapy through a discussion of a variety of implementation issues that it is important to consider. A range of definitions of person-centred practice are presented initially to enable readers to find the definition that most closely relates to their work. The chapter then proceeds to present literature about implementation issues and reflections to facilitate the development of skills to promote person-centred practice. These issues include valuing the uniqueness and autonomy of the individual, respect and dignity, enabling choice, developing trust, empowerment, and encouraging participation through partnerships. Finally, these issues are connected to a practice example to provide clarity regarding the specifics of their implementation.

KEY POINTS

- When working with clients occupational therapists need to focus on the art of person-centred practice.
- It is important to value the uniqueness and autonomy of the individual.
- Respect and dignity are central concepts of person-centred practice.
- Choice must be enabled through the provision of adequate information.
- Trust is an important aspect of the relationship between occupational therapists and the people who require their services.
- The challenge in any relationship between an occupational therapist and a person is to empower the person.
- Occupational therapists must encourage participation by developing partnerships with people who require their services.

Setting the scene

Occupational therapy practice involves a complicated process that requires the therapist to employ a wide range of skills and strategies, and have the ability to apply these in the most effective way. The latter is the art of practice that combines knowledge with personal attributes; it is not just what you do, but how you do it. This art is particularly evident in the person-centred approach. To apply this approach you have to know yourself well, be comfortable enough to reflect on your personal values and open enough to understand the implications of that knowledge. Therefore, this chapter, through a focus on the art of person-centred practice, will outline some of the areas on which therapists need to reflect and truly value before this approach can be applied effectively. These are the things that no one can tell you exactly how to do. You need to understand your views on each of them and know yourself well enough to vary your approach as required within your personal comfort level. It is very difficult to be an effective person-centred therapist, but hopefully this chapter will move the reader along the continuum to success.

Defining a person-centred approach

The first step in the art of using a person-centred approach is to find and appreciate the definition that works for therapists and the people with whom they work. Fortunately, there are an emerging number of definitions within the health care literature from which to choose. The following will present a range of perspectives and act as a guide to finding the most appropriate one for your work. Please note that the word 'client' or 'patient' may appear in some definitions if a direct quote is being used, but for the purposes of this chapter 'person' has been equated with either of these terms.

Talerico et al (2003, p. 1) write in a nursing journal that 'person-centred care is an evidence based approach to care giving that uses care recipients' unique personal preferences and needs to guide providers as they customize health care'. Boise and White (2004, p. 1) state that this approach means 'individualizing care based on the personal needs, experiences, and routines that are meaningful to each resident'. Warner (1997, p. 7) raises the stakes by defining person-centred care as a 'concept that focuses on fulfilling patients' needs above and beyond their expectations'.

There are also several definitions within the occupational therapy literature. Three of these definitions have been chosen for use in this chapter as they relate to important concepts that will be highlighted in subsequent sections.

In 2002 the Canadian Association of Occupational Therapists (CAOT) proposed that client-centred practice entails:

Collaborative and partnership approaches used in enabling occupation with clients who may be individuals, groups, agencies, governments, corporations or others; client-centred occupational therapists demonstrate respect for clients, involve clients in decision making, advocate with and for clients' needs, and otherwise recognize clients' experience and knowledge

(CAOT 2002, p. 180).

The British College of Occupational Therapists (COT) does not appear to present a specific definition of person-centred practice, but the basic principles of this approach feature strongly in their Code of Ethics (College of Occupational Therapists 2005). There is a statement within this code indicating that services shall be 'client-centred and needs led' (p. 9). They state that 'the College is strongly committed to client-centred practice and the involvement of the client as a partner in all stages of the therapeutic process' (p. 5). Further support for this approach comes from the statement that 'occupational therapy personnel shall at all times recognize, respect and uphold the autonomy of clients and advocate client choice and partnership working in the therapeutic process. Clients have a right to make choices and decisions about their own healthcare and independence and information should be provided in a form and language that is understood by the client' (p. 6).

However, work on a relevant definition has occurred in the United Kingdom where Sumsion (2000, p. 308) involved a wide representation of therapists to create the following definition:

Client-centred occupational therapy is a partnership between the client and the therapist that empowers the client to engage in functional performance and fulfil his or her occupational roles in a variety of environments. The client participates actively in negotiating goals which are given priority and are at the centre of assessment, intervention, and evaluation. Throughout the process the therapist listens to and respects the client's values, adapts the interventions to meet the client's needs, and enables the client to make informed decisions.

These sample definitions contain many common elements that will be the focus of further discussion within this chapter.

Issues in the implementation of person-centred practice

There are many implementation issues to consider, including those outlined in the preceding definitions, when utilising a person-centred approach. This section will highlight some of the more important and challenging issues including uniqueness and autonomy, respect and dignity, choice, trust, empowerment, and participation. Within all of these elements the focus is on enabling the person to engage in occupation and fulfil occupational roles. However, the reader should not be lulled into thinking this is the complete picture. Each of these issues is very complex and requires a considerable amount of thought and consideration that goes well beyond the confines of this text. The picture becomes even more complex when the basic definitions are expanded beyond the individual to include groups or communities. Figure 10.1 outlines these issues and emphasises the fact that they are in constant motion. They will be discussed independently in the following sections, but in reality they are all interconnected.

Valuing uniqueness and autonomy of the individual

Before proceeding with any discussion about person-centred practice we need to review a basic premise underlying this approach. That premise is that you value the uniqueness and autonomy of the individual

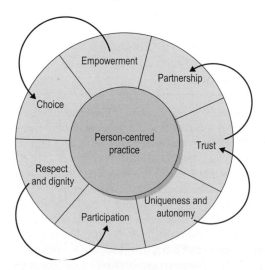

Figure 10.1 Wheel of person-centred practice

and you are willing to enact this belief. Rogers (1961) outlined these important components from the early days of this approach. You must believe that every individual is unique and thus will need a different approach, will have a different story to tell, and will need you to perform in a different way. That reality underpins the art in applying a person-centred approach. You also need to believe that people are individual, autonomous beings who can make their own decisions. Occupational therapists are fortunate to have models on which to base these two beliefs including the Canadian Model of Occupational Performance and Engagement (CMOP-E) (Polatajko et al 2007). There is also an interview-based outcome measure, the Canadian Occupational Performance Measure (COPM) (Law et al 2005). The latter provides a format within which to engage the person in a process; focusing on the person, enabling him to determine his priority areas for intervention to increase occupational engagement.

Respect and dignity

Respect and dignity are separate concepts, but they will be discussed together as they are so closely connected. These are very intricate and personal values that are linked to putting the other person first and treating the person as we would wish to be treated. It is about giving each person our undivided and dedicated attention to truly convey we are there for him or her. The Picker/Commonwealth Program for Patient-centred Care (Gertais et al 1993) conducted focus groups to determine the primary dimensions of this approach. The first one they identified was respect for the person's values, preferences and expressed needs. The reality of becoming an anonymous person in the hospital environment and worrying about the personal impact of illness, injury and impairment should be addressed through respecting each person's individuality (Edgman-Levitan 1997).

Respect is a central concept of the person-centred approach but requires some depth and clarity of thought to identify what it means. Falardeau and Durand (2002) conducted an extensive literature review in an attempt to address this challenge. They concluded that 'respecting the other means holding in high regard not just his opinions, choices and values, but also his capabilities, needs and limitations' (p. 137). This quote speaks to occupational therapists as all of these components are directly linked to our work.

Dignity refers to the individual 'maintaining self respect and being valued by others' (Lothian & Philp 2001, p. 2). It also relates to respecting the person's need for both physical and emotional privacy, showing respect and sensitivity to the person's cultural values, and treating people with kindness and respect (Gertais et al 1993). Dignity is shown to people by working with them as whole and unique human beings rather than as problems or diagnoses (Nelligan et al 2002).

The ability to truly operationalise respect and dignity brings the art of the person-centred approach to the foreground and exemplifies a therapist who can use this approach to its fullest.

Enabling choice

Choice is an important component of a person-centred approach and runs through the associated processes. In the early stages of working with people and explaining what a person-centred approach entails it is important to determine whether or not they want to make their own choices. Some people either because of feeling ill, their age, or cultural considerations would prefer that the health practitioner make all the decisions and simply tell them what to do (Say et al 2006). Even the decision to not make decisions cannot be made without the relevant information (Sumsion 2006). However, we should not assume that people do not want to have this responsibility without helping them to become familiar in the setting, and giving them enough information and knowledge to be confident in the decisions they are making (Waller 2002). This discussion should involve an objective review of that information, delivered in a way the person can understand with additional information from booklets, videos, and web sites, as necessary (Fallowfield 2001). In summary 'being person-centred means taking into account the person's desire for information and for sharing decision making and responding appropriately' (Stewart 2001, p. 445).

The range of issues over which people have choice is endless but from an intervention perspective may include care settings, large decisions that affect their lives (Eales et al 2001), strategies to use (Ford et al 2003) and what to eat (McKenzie et al 2001).

Enabling choice is very challenging and, to date, there are a limited number of studies to indicate that this makes a difference to the outcome of the intervention. However, Hsu et al (2003) conducted a study related to people's choice of their primary care provider. They found that giving people this choice resulted in higher overall satisfaction with the relationship and a greater likelihood of remaining with this health care professional.

There are of course challenges to enabling choice including the availability of resources from which to choose (Jones et al 2004) and recognising existing limitations (Hanman 2001). Who among us can have everything they want? There are limitations, both financial and personal, that have to be recognised when choices are being made.

Developing trust

It would be almost impossible to implement the components from the earlier definitions, such as using preferences and needs to guide the process, fulfilling needs, and enabling people to make informed decisions, if there was no trust in the relationship. By its very nature a person-centred approach requires people to work together in a close relationship that is doomed to failure if the partners do not trust each other.

If we are going to honestly bring people into the decision-making process, then they need to trust that our actions will follow our words. The process of developing trust includes working together to solve problems and ensuring open communication and effective collaboration, which can be accomplished in both short- and long-term settings (Ponte et al 2003). If time is limited then arriving on time, truly listening to the person's issues, clearly explaining the limitations of your involvement and following through on arrangements will go a long way toward establishing trust.

Empowerment

The Webster New Collegiate Dictionary (Woolf 1979, p. 370) – as well as many others that were consulted – defines empowerment as 'giving official authority or legal power'. However, Tones (1998) states that empowerment is an elusive, complex and multidimensional concept. This view is supported by Vander-Henst (1997) who found that there was no clear agreement on the definition of empowerment. This concept is also difficult to implement and measure (Tones 1998). So, now that the challenge of implementation has been established let us return to the positive elements and determine what can be done.

From a person-centred perspective empowerment is about moving the direction of care away from the professional and toward the person facing challenges. It is about implementing enabling strategies to promote occupational engagement. Frost (2001, p. 399) states this very well when she says that 'therapy is the recovery of dignity, systematically giving the patient his or her sense of self as the patient is taught how to have control and be responsible'. The role of the therapist is to work with people to develop the necessary skills to gain power so they can make decisions and take action in their lives (Dressler & MacRae 1998). However, it is important to remember that not everyone wishes to be empowered and may prefer to entrust their care and related decision-making to the health professionals (Lewin & Piper 2006).

There are some specific things that can be done to facilitate the empowerment process. These include setting personal goals, offering choices for intervention, respecting the person's choice, even if you do not agree with it, and referring people to requested agencies (Vander Henst 1997). Significant others, including community supports, can be included in meetings and case reviews (Opie 1998, Vander-Henst 1997) and services can be flexible enough to meet varied needs (Gaitskell 1998). Information is an extremely important part of empowerment and can, in fact, be equated to power (Honey 1999).

It must also be recognized that there are some barriers to truly empowering people within a well-established system. These barriers include rigid organisational power structures, the differences between the person's and the organisation's goals, concerns that people may not know what is best for themselves (Honey 1999) and fear of increasing people's expectations and putting more strain on an already overtaxed system (Poulton 1999).

Overall, it is important to begin activities related to empowerment in the person's comfort zone which is part of the initial stages of implementing a person-centred approach (Honey 1999). Within occupational therapy this empowerment is linked to occupation and enabling the individual to acquire the necessary skills to engage in their chosen occupation in a way that will work for them. The art of this process is in using and adapting the therapist's range of knowledge and skills to ensure that this occurs in each individual situation. This means not always providing the solutions but in helping people find the solutions that will work for them.

Encouraging participation through partnerships

Partnership is a crucial component of the person-centred process. It is important to understand up front that failure to accept the person as an equal partner in the process may result in an unsuccessful intervention (Weston 2001). There are different models to use when developing a partnership. These include the informed model that is based on a division of labour between the person and the health care professional. There is also the shared model in which the people involved share all stages of the decision-making process (Charles et al 1999). Obviously there are also many stages in between these two, but the important fact is for those involved in the partnership to clearly establish what this means and how it will work. Obviously the process takes on added complexity when partnerships are being formed with groups or organisations rather than individuals.

Several authors have addressed issues that impede the formation of a successful partnership. These include not truly implementing an individualised approach, lack of communication, lack of confidentiality, being a directive therapist and fostering inequality through not sharing information equally (Blank 2004). Other challenges are posed by the age of the person including the debate surrounding children's rights to form partnerships (Dixon-Woods et al 1999). Others have written about the challenges that arise when the therapist and partner have differing goals in the process (Brown & Bowen 1998, Sumsion & Smyth 2000).

Partnership is really a bottom-line issue in this entire process. It involves expert use of the other elements that have been discussed including respect, choice, trust, and empowerment. It is the process of truly understanding and enacting these concepts that will lead to the development of a successful partnership.

Practical application

The following practice example about Mr. George White (Practice Scenario 10.1) will be briefly linked to the issues discussed in this chapter and represented diagrammatically in Figure 10.1 to provide a concrete example of their implementation.

Practice Scenario 10.1
Mr George White

Mr. George White is a 69-year-old retired dairy farmer who was rushed to hospital when he collapsed at home after he experienced a myocardial infarct. He underwent a coronary artery bypass graft of 2 vessels 3 days later. Mr. White was referred to occupational therapy 5 days postoperatively to assist with discharge planning. He has been advised to follow the postoperative restrictions: no lifting of objects greater than 4.5 kilos; no pushing or pulling heavy objects, especially one-handed; and no driving for 6 to 12 weeks.

The occupational therapist finds Mr. White lying in bed gazing into space. She obtains his consent and asks him about his home situation, needs, and concerns related to discharge. She finds that Mr. White recently sold his farm and now lives with his 64-year-old wife in a two-storey condominium. This condominium has three steps at the entrance, bedrooms and full bathroom on the upper level, kitchen, living room, dining area and two-piece bath on the main level, and a family room, laundry room and workshop in the basement. His wife is in good health but does not drive. Although Mr. White is pleasant and cooperative throughout the discussion, his answers are brief and he occasionally has trouble finding the correct words. His affect is rather flat and he speaks quietly. When asked what he would be concerned about if he was to be discharged in the next few days, he states: 'I'm worried about my wife. It's a lot for her to deal with'. He is unable to identify specific issues. Mr. White tells the occupational therapist that he is too tired to try getting out of bed right now. They arrange to meet later that day.

In the afternoon, Mr. White is again lying in bed 'resting' but reluctantly agrees to get up. The occupational therapist observes that his transfers, range of motion and strength are reasonable, although his arm movements were slow and guarded due to sternum pain. While going through the assessment, the occupational therapist finds out that Mrs. White was responsible for all the household management tasks, although Mr. White occasionally helped. He also drove his wife to buy groceries and to church and social functions. The lawn and driveway maintenance were done by a private company. Mr. White enjoyed 'puttering in [his] workshop', fixing small appliances and building wooden toys and birdhouses for his grandchildren. When discussing these activities, Mr. White stated: 'I guess that's over. I won't be able to do any of that anymore'. When asked what his goals would be, Mr. White was only able to identify that he didn't want to be a burden on his family.

Practice Scenario prepared by occupational therapists at London Health Sciences Centre.

Mr. White's intervention occurred in an acute-care setting, so there was not a great deal of time to spend on developing a person-centred relationship. However, Mr. White's therapist showed she valued and respected him as an individual by listening to his story. She also began to develop a trusting relationship with him by returning at the agreed time and focusing on issues that were of concern to him. She continued this development as she engaged him in an 'activities of daily living programme' to increase his endurance, reinforce his abilities and teach him compensatory techniques and modified activities related to the applicable restrictions. She enabled his choices and began the process of empowerment by providing information about community resources that could assist with concerns, such as transportation, and discussing the possibility of a referral to community services that could review and assist with home accessibility. In addition she did not ignore the psychosocial issues, but helped him to identify these, ensured he had an understanding of his long-term prognosis and worked with him to develop plans so he could return to the occupations that were important to him. All of these actions and activities enabled them to work as partners to ensure both his immediate and long-term concerns were addressed.

Conclusion

The concepts and ideas outlined in this chapter are at the core of effective person-centred practice. The onus is on the therapist to face the challenge of bringing these concepts to life. Hopefully, the chapter has reinforced the concept outlined in the introduction that it is not what you do but how you do it. That is the art of practice that will ensure the success of the relevant intervention. Through reflection and the skilful application of principles related to valuing the person's uniqueness and autonomy, treating them with respect and dignity, enabling them to make choices, developing trust, empowering them to set and accept responsibility for their own goals, and encouraging the development of an effective partnership, a truly person-centred approach will emerge.

References

Blank, A. (2004). Clients' experience of partnership with occupational therapists in community mental health. *British Journal of Occupational Therapy*, 67(3), 118–124.

Boise, L. & White, D. (2004). The family role in person-centered care: practice considerations. *Journal of Psychosocial Nursing and Mental Health Services*, 42(5), 12–20.

Brown, C. & Bowen, R. E. (1998). Including the consumer and environment in occupational therapy treatment planning. *The Occupational Therapy Journal of Research*, 18(1), 46–63.

Canadian Association of Occupational Therapists (2002). *Enabling Occupation: an occupational therapy perspective*, (2nd ed). Ottawa, CAOT Publications ACE.

Charles, C., Whelan, T. & Gafni, A. (1999). What do we mean by partnership in making decisions about treatment? *British Medical Journal*, 319, 780–782.

College of Occupational Therapists (2005). *Code of Ethics and Professional Conduct*. Online. Available: http://www.cot.org.uk

Dressler, J. & MacRae, A. (1998). Advocacy, partnerships and client centered practice in California. *Occupational Therapy in Mental Health*, 14(1/2), 35–43.

Dixon-Woods, M., Young, B. & Heney, D. (1999). Partnership with children. *British Medical Journal*, 319(7212), 778–780.

Eales, J., Keating, N. & Damsma, A. (2001). Seniors' experiences of client-centred residential care. *Aging and Society*, 21, 279–296.

Edgman-Levitan, S. (1997). On the value of patient-centered care. *Journal of American Academy of Physician Assistants*, 10(3), 9–10.

Falardeau, M. & Durand, M. J. (2002). Negotiation-centred versus client-centred: which approach should be used? *Canadian Journal of Occupational Therapy*, 69(3), 135–142.

Fallowfield, L. (2001). Participation of patients in decisions about treatment for cancer. *British Medical Journal*, 323(7322), 1144.

Ford, S., Schofield, T. & Hope, T. (2003). What are the ingredients for a successful evidence-based patient choice consultation? A qualitative study. *Social Science and Medicine*, 56(3), 589–602.

Frost, M. (2001). The role of physical, occupational and speech therapy in hospice patient empowerment. *American Journal of Hospice & Palliative Care*, 18(6), 397–402.

Gaitskell, S. (1998). Professional accountability and service user empowerment: issues in community mental health. *British Journal of Occupational Therapy*, 61(5), 221–222.

Gertais, M., Levitan-Edgman, S., Daley, J., et al. (1993). *Medicine and health from the patient's perspective. Through the patient's eyes: understanding and promoting patient-centered care*. Jossey-Bass Publishers, San Francisco.

Hanman, D. (2001). Let's look outside the service system to give people a real choice. *Community Living*, 14(3), 12–13.

Honey, A. (1999). Empowerment versus power: consumer participation in mental health services. *Occupational Therapy International*, 6(4), 257–276.

Hsu, J., Schmittdiel, J., Krupat, E. et al. (2003). Patient choice: a randomized controlled trial of provider selection. *Journal of General Internal Medicine*, 18(5), 319–325.

Jones, I. R., Berney, L., Kelly, M. et al. (2004). Is patient involvement possible when decisions involve scarce resources? A qualitative study of decision-making in primary care. *Social Science & Medicine*, 59(1), 93–102.

Law, M., Baptiste, S., Carswell, A., McColl, M.A., Polatajko, H., Pollock, N. (2005). *Canadian Occupational Performance Measure*, (4th ed). Ottawa, Canadian Association of Occupational Therapists.

Lewin, D. & Piper, S. (2006). Patient empowerment within a coronary care unit: insights for health professionals drawn from a patient satisfaction survey. *Intensive and Critical Care Nursing* doi:10.1016/j.iccn

Lothian, K. & Philp, I. (2001). Maintaining the dignity and autonomy of older people in the healthcare setting. *British Medical Journal*, 322(7287), 668–670.

McKenzie, K., Matheson, E., Paxton, D. et al. (2001). Health and social care workers' knowledge and application of the concept of duty of care. *The Journal of Adult Protection*, 3(4), 29–37.

Nelligan, P., Grinspun, D., Jonas-Simpson, C. et al. (2002). Client-centred care: making the ideal real. *Hospital Quarterly*, 5(4), 70–76.

Opie, A. (1998). 'Nobody's asked me for my view': user empowerment by multidisciplinary health teams. *Qualitative Health Research*, 8(2), 188–206.

Polatajko, H., Davis, J., Stewart, D. et al. (2007). Specifying the domain of concern: Occupation as core. In: E. Townsend & H. Polatajko (Eds.), *Enabling occupation II: Advancing an occupational therapy vision for health, well-being and justice through occupation* (pp. 13–36). Ottawa, Canadian Association of Occupational Therapists.

Ponte, P. R., Conlin, G., Conway, J. B. et al. (2003). Making patient-centered care come alive: achieving full integration of the patient's perspective. *Journal of Nursing Administration*, 33(2), 82–90.

Poulton, B. C. (1999). User involvement in identifying health needs and shaping and evaluating services: is it being realised? *Journal of Advanced Nursing*, 30(6), 1289–1296.

Rogers, C. (1961). *On becoming a person*. Boston, Houghton Mifflin.

Say, R., Murtagh, M. & Thomson, R. (2006). Patients' preference for involvement in medical decision making: A narrative review. *Patient Education and Counseling*, 60(2), 102–114.

Stewart, M. (2001). Towards a global definition of patient centred care: the patient should be the judge of patient centred care. *British Medical Journal*, 322, 444–445.

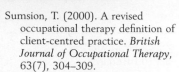
Sumsion, T. (2000). A revised occupational therapy definition of client-centred practice. *British Journal of Occupational Therapy*, 63(7), 304–309.

Sumsion, T. (2006). *Implementation Issues. Client-centred practice in Occupational Therapy: a guide to implementation*, (2nd ed). Edinburgh, Churchill Livingstone.

Sumsion, T. & Smyth, G. (2000). Barriers to client-centredness and their resolution. *Canadian Journal of Occupational Therapy*, 67(1), 15–21.

Talerico, K. A., O'Brien, J. A. & Swafford, K. L. (2003). Aging matters: Person-centered care: An important approach for 21st century health care. *Journal of Psychosocial Nursing & Mental Health Services*, 41(11), 12–16.

Tones, K. (1998). *Health education and the promotion of health: seeking wisely to empower. Health and empowerment research and practice*. London, Arnold.

Vander-Henst, J. A. (1997). Client empowerment: A nursing challenge. *Clinical Nurse Specialist*, 11(3), 96–99.

Waller, B. N. (2002). The psychological structure of patient autonomy. *Cambridge Quarterly of Healthcare Ethics*, 11(3), 257–265.

Warner, K. C. (1997). The core values of patient-centered care. *Aspen's Advisor for Nurse Executives*, 12(6), 7–8.

Weston, W. W. (2001). Informed and shared decision-making: the crux of patient-centred care. *Canadian Medical Association Journal*, 165(4), 438–439.

Woolf, H. (1979) (Ed) *Webster's new collegiate dictionary*. Thomas Allen & Sons Limited, Toronto.

Chapter **Eleven**

11

Occupation in context

Gail Elizabeth Whiteford

CHAPTER CONTENTS

Introduction 136

Context 1 – Family of origin: shaping the
emergent occupational persona 136

History and values. 136

Opportunities: the enabling or delimiting
impact of families on participation 137

Tempo and rhythm: families, time use
and occupation 138

Context 2 – Communities in which
we live 139

Physical and geographic characteristics
of communities and occupational
engagement 139

Naturally occurring geographic features . . 139

Built spaces 140

The sociocultural aspect of communities . . 141

Theme 1: culture influences norms and
forms of occupational performance and
engagement 142

Theme 2: cultural norms proscribe
acceptable occupational participants. 142

Theme 3: relationship between time and
occupation differs across cultural contexts . . 143

Theme 4: sociocultural influences on
places and spaces associated with
specific occupations 143

Differences between communities:
culture and occupation 143

Universality 144

Relationship between doing and being 144

Colonialisation 144

Context 3 – Political and economic
environments 145

Legislation, policy and occupational
participation 146

Conclusion. 147

SUMMARY

Individuals, families, communities and whole
populations engage continuously in a closely
bound, interdependent set of occupations on a
daily basis. One of the most significant and
universal aspects of these daily rounds of
occupations is that they always occur in several
contexts simultaneously. The relationship is a
dynamic one: occupational norms and forms and
patterns of engagement are shaped by these
contexts and to some extent, these contextual
forces in turn are influenced by the net impact of
occupations performed both over time and in
time. This chapter considers the familial,
geographic, socio-cultural and political contexts
in which occupations occur and the impact they
have.

KEY POINTS

- Occupation is always located and interpreted
  within a given context.
- There are multiple contextual forces that shape
  what, how and why people engage in
  occupations.
- There is a direct relationship between the
  contexts and the opportunities people have for
  occupational participation.

- Sociocultural values and norms influence what people choose to do and what they are obliged to do, and the ways in which they go about doing.
- Political systems, governments and the legislative and policy context impact on participation.
- Occupational therapists must understand the context if they are to fully enable participation.

Introduction

Occupation never takes place in a vacuum; it is always embedded within several distinct contexts simultaneously. However, the extent to which these contexts directly and indirectly influence the *norms and forms* of occupational engagement are not always immediately apparent. In this chapter, I will consider three distinct contexts that shape the occupations of individuals and groups on a daily basis, using illustrative narrative examples where possible.

The first context is that of the *family of origin*. In this section family as context will be the focus: the values, beliefs, histories, and aspirations of families and how its members may respond to these occupationally across the life course. The second context is that of the *communities in which we live*. The influence that communities have in shaping what we do every day will be explored from a *geographic/physical*, as well as a *social and cultural*, perspective. The third and final context that I will explore in this chapter is the *political and economic* environments that are a very real force shaping how populations of people are enabled or delimited in the occupational opportunities available to them.

As the reader can imagine, each of these contexts is very complex and difficult to do justice to in the space of this chapter. However, my aim is to provide readers with a basis for understanding three key conceptual points: first, occupation is always located and interpreted within a given context, second that a number of contextual forces dynamically shape how individuals and groups understand and experience occupations over time, and, finally, that there is a direct relationship between context and opportunities for occupational participation. One of the primary contexts in which most people experience occupation and participation is that of the family of origin. Because of its primacy and impact on the subsequent development of not only behaviours but also values and beliefs underpinning occupational engagement, it is discussed here first.

Context 1 – Family of origin: shaping the emergent occupational persona

Some years ago a colleague of mine (Alison Wicks) and I explored the concept of the occupational persona. At that time we defined the occupational persona as:

> *That dimension of self shaped by a myriad of factors both biological and sociocultural which is predisposed, as well as driven toward, engagement in certain types of occupations. Through the process of such engagement and the outcomes generated, the occupational persona is shaped, and to some extent, reinvented over time*
>
> (Whiteford & Wicks, 2000 p. 48)

One of the most obvious factors that impact upon a person's occupational persona is the family in which they are brought up. Whatever type of family it may be structurally, for example one with grandparents in primary caregiving roles or with same-sex parents or with adopted parents or any number of other variations, the impact of the family is very significant in an individual's occupational development (Llewellyn 1994). Of course, it is somewhat artificial to separate families from the dominate culture in which they are situated, because to some extent, the family's values and beliefs will mirror those of the prevailing sociocultural milieu. However, families per se are often overlooked in the occupation-focused literature, and I think they warrant special attention with respect to how they influence what people ultimately do in their lives.

History and values

All families have a history. Embedded in this history, and reinforced through the narrating of the history over time, are distinct themes of meaning. In particular, family histories are replete with stories about family members *doing*. Think about your own family; there's bound to be a story about a family member doing something brave, doing something important, doing something funny, responding heroically in the face of hardship, doing something caring or charitable, or maybe even doing something wrong. What is important is how the family interprets the actions and occupations of members over time within the rubric of the value and belief systems to which they adhere (Stagnitti 2005).

For example, the story of my grandfather holds significance as a lesson in hard work, commitment and social obligation in my extended family. As the oldest orphan in an institution during the Depression, he worked extremely hard to make sure that the routine of the orphanage ran smoothly every day, including the back-breaking work of chopping wood for stoves, doing laundry by hand and preparing food. As an adult, he worked hard to become a teacher and a primary-school principal, while always serving those less fortunate in society through a host of community roles. In his later years, he worked with orphaned and disadvantaged boys, and, after retirement until well into his 80s, became a volunteer teacher of English as a second language to migrant families. Over time and through the telling and re-telling of his story within the family, I was very much influenced by this history and the occupational values that were transmitted through it: achievements are based on hard work, make the world a better place through what you do every day and, finally, pay back your debt to society actively.

When working with families, then, it is important to spend time to try to understand the backgrounds, traditions, cultural orientation and themes that have, over time, shaped their value system with regard to occupations. Tuning into the history of a family requires time and a deeply narrative orientation in which occupational motifs can be uncovered (Clark & Richardson 1996, Wicks & Whiteford 2006). It is, however, an investment in ensuring that any interaction you have as an occupational therapist will be consistent with the deeply held values and beliefs of the people and families with whom you will work. A cogent story that captures this point comes from a book called 'Blokes and Sheds' in which people tell stories about the centrality of the 'shed' as a specific site of occupation:

> You can tell if a man has a shed. He's got a look about him. He knows he can create, can do things other men can't, there's a certain sort of confidence and pride. He doesn't run down to the shop to buy a new one, instead, its "give it here, I'll fix it." He wants to know how it works [...] how to make it work again. That was Dad. He knew the mechanics of the workings of life and it rubbed off on us all

(Thomson 2002, p.183)

Opportunities: the enabling or delimiting impact of families on participation

One of the most important ways through which a family influences its members is the way in which they respond to the opportunities available through which a member can develop skills and perhaps mastery in a chosen occupation. Of course this is also very context bound, as huge disparities exist between countries and societies (and between subgroups within societies) in terms of access to, and the availability of, things like education, leisure activities, recreational facilities, cultural spaces, and resources. Whilst for an affluent family the challenge may be in choosing between a number of possible occupational pursuits such as playing tennis, learning the guitar or horse riding, for families without financial resources the challenge often lies, not so much with *choosing between* occupational pursuits, as with having *access to* affordable options. In an era when leisure pursuits have become more expensive and commodified (Neumayer & Wilding 2005) this is increasingly the case for many.

The extent to which the family works to support extended occupational engagement over time has a very important impact on participation. The enactment of this commitment to and orchestration of children's activities and occupations has been termed *concerted cultivation* (Lareau 2003). In her landmark naturalistic study of the lives of American families with children aged 8 and 9 years old, Lareau uncovered the extent to which middle-class families cultivate the opportunities for their children and the numerous positive impact of this cultivation. These apparently include greater verbal abilities, enhanced understanding of abstract concepts and confidence in dealing with authority figures. The opposite of concerted cultivation, *accomplishment of natural growth* was identified as a more common approach in working-class families and describes an orientation of the parents in which children are basically more often left to both cope with school issues independently and facilitate their own leisure activities (Lareau 2003).

Clearly, there are a number of significant factors that influence such a difference in orientation. These are the same factors that contribute to social stratification such as education, financial status, parental working demands, transport, etc. From an occupational perspective the extent to which predictions can be made with respect to the attainment of mastery in selected occupations based on concerted cultivation or accomplishment of natural growth, may be limited. Consider for example the story of Australian Cathy Freeman. An Olympic gold medalist; Freeman comes from an indigenous family in which, as she says, many members had experienced racism at one time or another. In her biography, Freeman describes how hard her mother worked to support them as a sole parent:

With Dad gone, Mum found a job as a cleaner at the local high school to support us. Being a cleaner was the only thing Mum had ever been trained to do, but I never heard her complain about it. She'd had to leave school when she was fifteen because the laws in Australia wouldn't allow her to continue. No one thought it was important for aboriginal people to finish school or get a higher education in those days, even so, my mum is one of the wisest and smartest people I know. Every morning she'd get up at 6.30 to make our lunches then go and clean at North Mackay High School for a few hours…now that she was raising us on her own, Mum worked extra hard to make our lives as stable and normal as possible

(Freeman, 2007 pp. 18–19)

This is a powerful narrative in which the contribution of her mother to the creation of 'stable and normal' life provided a basis from which Freeman went on to achieve significantly at an international level. So, whilst in some contexts, a family's concerted cultivation of a child's numerous occupations may be a significant factor in the performance of the child subsequently, in other contexts the maintenance of a stable and safe environment in itself can be seen as a basis for achievement and mastery in selected occupations.

Tempo and rhythm: families, time use and occupation

It is not just what occupational beings do that impacts their health and wellbeing, but also the speed at which they do it.

(Clark 1997, p. 89).

Families do not just need to commit to and support the occupations of their members. They also need

to orchestrate, enfold (Bateson 1996), and manage their intersecting occupations in time. There are two main factors influencing families' time-use patterns: intra-familial factors and extra-familial factors. Within families, the ways in which numerous occupations are managed within time depends to some extent on the values and beliefs the family has towards things such as ritual events (birthdays, for example), routine, structured versus unstructured approaches to time use, spontaneity, and social and religious roles and responsibilities. You may have grown up in a family in which the ritual of a family meal time was strictly observed or one in which family members did their own thing at meal times. Some families socialise with other families and individuals a lot and have an open-house environment, whilst others maintain a more private space with less social contact. Indeed, some families spend a lot of time doing things together, whilst other families do not. There is no right or wrong in this regard, there are merely different ways of being and doing within families. The salient point is that the exposure we have as we are growing up to particular patterns and rhythms of time use alone and with others influences us significantly.

In a contemporary context, however, it does seem that all families, whatever approach they have to doing and being together, are finding it increasingly difficult to orchestrate their time in the face of increasing social and economic pressures (i.e. those extra-familial factors that to some extent shape all our lives on a daily basis). The overall tempo and rhythm of our lives have increased. One obvious factor impacting upon how much time families spend time together is the amount of time that the parents/breadwinners spend in employment. In Australia, for example, the trends are alarming but not dissimilar to many countries:

Fathers of children under 15 years who worked full-time in 2004–05 spent an average of 43 hours per week at work and one-third (33%) worked more than 50 hours per week […] Average weekly hours worked for full-time and part-time workers have increased over the last two decades. Full-time working hours for men increased by 1.9 hours per week to 43.2 hours between 1985 and 2005 and for women by 1.7 hours to 39.3 hours. More women are working, with 53% of women aged 15 years and over working in 2004, up from 40% in 1979. The growth in women's employment has been mainly in part-time work. In 2004, 24% of women aged 15 years and over were employed part-time, an increase from 14% in 1979

(Australian Bureau of Statistics 2006, p. 2).

Obviously, such trends impact on families in a range of ways, with the net result being less time spent in the family unit and more time engaged in occupations with others (non-family members). Although it is probably too early to determine just how families experience this shift in collective time use across many years, it most certainly will require a rethink of the availability of social structures and supports in everything from increased access to quality childcare to co-located educational and recreational facilities.

Context 2 – Communities in which we live

Physical and geographic characteristics of communities and occupational engagement

When people consider places that encourage them to engage in public places as part of the life of the community, they usually think of two aspects of place: first are the naturally occurring geographic features such as mountains or ocean beaches. The second is the constructed or built place such as entertainment centres [...] museums and parks

(Hamilton 2004, p. 186)

Naturally occurring geographic features

Following from the previous section on families, imagine how different your life may have been if you had grown up in a *different family in a different place*. Imagine, for example, that you grew up in sub-Saharan Africa. What would your life have been like? How would being in that space influence what you did every day, for example, preparing food, and the way you did it? Now consider what it may be like living in an Inuit community in Nunavut and preparing food there. Comparatively, if you changed geographic location, how many of your everyday occupations would change? How many would basically stay the same?

The physical characteristics of the environments that humans live in have influenced every aspect of daily life for eons, indeed, the interactions between humans and their geographies is a central motif of historical accounts of distinct cultures, civilisations, and societies. It has even been suggested recently that it is the physical conditions of countries that are implicated in the current inequality of wealth distribution globally (Diamond 1997). This is, however, a perspective with a complex causal argument, some of the ideas of which we will cover in the final section on the political and economic context of occupation.

As in the previous section, where we considered families distinct from society, it is a little artificial to separate the physical characteristics of environments from the cultural environments of the people who live in them. This is because there is an interactive effect, as noted in the landmark work by linguist Noam Chomsky (1986) on the relationship between the physical environment and language. His work allowed us to appreciate the fact that, for example, if you live in Iceland and are surrounded by snow, then you are more likely to have many ways of describing snow. Hence, the natural environment influences language which is the basis of the development of a system of shared meanings; in other words, culture. Language to some extent *is* culture, and it is this bound relationship that is the driving force of many distinct linguistic groups' attempts to preserve their unique language. A strong example of this is the development of the Kohanga Reo (literally 'language nest') movement in New Zealand, which exposes both Maori and non-Maori children to the indigenous, Maori, language at a pre-school level in order to create cultural learning through language development (Metge 1986).

So, physical environments, language and culture are inextricably linked it seems, but how do the characteristics of the geographic space impact on how people go about doing what they need and want to do every day? Essentially, there are two interconnected dimensions of the physical environment that shape forms of occupational performance and engagement; climate and topography. The impact these aspects of the physical environment have on the expectations of occupational behaviour was originally developed by Henry Murray (Hamilton 2004) as the theory of 'environmental press', but has been utilised theoretically in the occupational therapy literature in relationship to occupational engagement and competence (Rigby & Letts 2003).

In her study of the relationship between occupation, place and identity, Wiseman (2007) used a life history approach to understanding the issues for men retiring in rural Australia. The deep narratives of the men have illuminated just how complex the notion of environmental press is through uncovering how aspects of the Australian rural environment shaped the way the men went about doing things over the course of their lives. In the two extracts below, the first describes the relationship between distance and occupational form, and points to the constraints on participation experienced by one of the men as a young boy. The second is a poignant account of distance and hard terrain:

> *A lot of my life was involved with dad's job, the sale yards, and drovers and that sort of thing. As a twelve year old I rode as far as 25 miles with a drover, taking cattle away. When we got to where he was going he said OK that's it son, off you go and I had to ride home! He did buy me a lemon squash at the pub though. The other kids used to play football, and run around and stuff, I always had long pants on or even leggings because I used to ride the horse all the time. So I never thought I could really get out and kick the footy or anything. You can't just sort of lean your horse up against the fence and go and join in. The other thing is you'd be riding around town and if the other kids are riding a bike or walking it's hard to be sort of a companion if you aren't at the same level (George).*

> *A couple of years ago I saw a paddock for sale and I put my wife in the car and said there's a paddock out here I would like to buy as a little hobby farm for retirement, build a house on it even. We got to the edge of town and my wife looked at me and said "it's a long way out of town" and then I knew I was beaten. That has been our main difficulty. My wife hated being out on the farm and when we went out there the other day to visit a friend she remembered seeing me disappear over the steep dry brown hills in the landrover and wonder whether she was going to see me again, it was very steep country, not easy land to manage and I was always in the landrover or on a horse, no motorbikes in those days (Gerald).*

As is evident from the extracts above, distance, transport and occupational participation are closely linked. In fact as the first narrator above suggests, it is complex and multilayered, i.e. the fact that he had to ride a horse because he had to travel a vast distance meant that he was excluded from participation in things like 'footy' (football) not only because of his horse but because of the clothes he had to wear. So, whilst at a basic level 'transportation provides humans access to other people and places' (Hamilton 2004, p. 179), in and of itself, transportation can influence patterns of occupational participation and engagement; just picture your average urban train with commuters going to work and you see row upon row of people not interacting but listening to their iPods or working on laptops. Contextually, of course, transportation is a huge global issue as we face the decline of cheap available fossil fuels. This will mean that travel, in particular via individual means such as cars, will become increasingly restricted. This in turn will have significant impact on the lives and occupations of individuals and communities. Interestingly, whilst providing a thorough and disturbing critique of the decline of the fossil-fuel-based developed world, Howard Kunstler (2005, p. 304) concludes with the suggestion that:

> *…if there is to be a positive side to the stark changes coming our way, it may be in the benefits of closer communal relations of having to work intimately (and physically) with our neighbors, to be part of an enterprise that really matters, and be fully engaged in meaningful social enactments instead of merely being entertained to avoid boredom*

Built spaces

As well as the naturally occurring physical features of environments, characteristics of built environments also exert a strong influence on patterns of participation. One of the most significant areas that occupational therapists have historically been involved in is how built environments limit participation by persons with differential needs. This struck me during a visit to Turkey. At times, walking around the highly developed urban environment of Ankara, I found it hard going; steep steps, high curbs, and few cross walks. I tried imagining how a person in a wheelchair or someone using a walking frame would manage and decided that it would be extremely difficult if not impossible. It's not difficult to extrapolate from this scenario a causal chain of events: because of the barriers that much of the built environment represents, people with disabilities are not often out and about in public spaces, participating in everyday occupations. Because they are not participating to the same extent as others, they have low levels of visibility in society, and so, the disabling effect of the built environment is not readily apparent and attitudes remain unchanged. In this way then, the attitudes of the non-disabled can be just as much a part of the barrier to participation as the built environment itself (Hammell 2003).

One of the most significant developments in tackling the pressing need for the development of built environments in which diverse needs are catered for, has been that of universal design. Universal design has been described as an approach that:

> *… considers children, the elderly, people who are tall or short and those with various disabilities, it addresses the lifespan of human beings beyond the mythical average person […] universal design respects human diversity and promotes the inclusion of all people in all activities of life.*
>
> (Assistive Technology Network, cited in Ringaert 2003).

The places in which universal design should feature are of course those places in which people engage most often in a range of occupations in a given day or week: homes, schools, workplaces, transport, toilets, public, cultural built environments (e.g. sporting arenas and theatres), and places of worship. As has been pointed out, the nexus between occupation, the environment and the person and the impact this has on occupational performance is central to many occupational therapy models of practice (Rigby & Letts 2003) and occupational therapists have a potentially very important role to play in advocating at a range of levels for better built environments in conjunction with disabled people – as expert users (Hammell 2003). However, it is my contention that, with our expert knowledge of occupation and the meaning making dimension of occupational engagement *in place*, that we could be having a far greater and more expanded role in influencing the development of institutional and civic spaces.

As well as the physical characteristics of the built environment such as density, height, lighting, etc., there is another dimension that also affects occupational engagement: aesthetics. The extent to which built environments are *humanised* by features which make people feel more comfortable in them has been of greater interest to architects and institutional and civic planners in more recent times. Indeed, one of the principles of urban renewal has been to create spaces in which aesthetics are addressed directly based on a belief that this will influence patterns of social interaction and behaviour. There is some evidence that points to the saliency of this position. For example, a recent study found that factors such as colours, building height, street width, and visibility of the sky all impact on social sustainability and wellness (Porta & Renne 2005). The relationship between environmental aesthetics and occupational engagement is clearly an important dimension of how people live, work and 'be' in spaces that deserve our ongoing attention.

The sociocultural aspect of communities

The sociocultural context of occupation is arguably the most significant contextual force that shapes occupational behaviour. This is because, whilst the physical and built environments impact on what and how people do things, it is the cultural context through which people understand and ascribe *meaning* to what they do. In this respect, culture may be seen as a system of shared meanings (Geertz 1973) that enable survival in whatever environment communities of people live. Accordingly, it is the cultural context through which the richness and diversity of patterns and forms of occupational performance and engagement are revealed.

Consider the two extracts below. One is from the autobiography of Nobel Peace Prize winner Shirin Ebadi from Iran describing socialising at university in pre Khomeni days. The second is from a participant in Wiseman's (2007) study of older rural Australian men:

> *We didn't wear veils – in fact, the three veiled women in our class stood out – but neither did we date, in the Western sense of the word. We always gathered for coffees or weekend trips in*

mixed groups, and though the men and women studied together in the library, in class women occupied the front rows and men the back

(Ebadi 2006, p. 19)

Any adversity brings people together. We had a fire through there, and that involved everybody and everybody helped one another. People who might not have bothered to get to know one another found that it was important that you come together. We were involved with the church community, NSW Farmers and the Country Women's Association (wife). I don't know what they called it but there was also a strong group that used to get together at the pub every Saturday night {laughs}. It was a very good bonding experience. That was the strength, the pubs and the stores were the strength of the community. People get there together, sit down and have a yarn [chat], before poker machines came in. The whole family would be there. Kids would play something outside. It would be after tennis or cricket usually. I'm not advocating alcohol or anything like that, I wouldn't want you to think that, but it certainly helped to get people together. There was another thing, everybody would get their paper of a Saturday morning and stand around having a yarn. There's sort of the village aspect where people depend on one another and work together more. It's just one of those things that seems to belong to rural areas and it's hard to duplicate in town

(Hunter)

In these narratives, it is possible to glean several insights into the ways in which culture shapes occupation: culture influences norms and forms of occupational performance and engagement; cultural norms proscribe acceptable participants; relationship between time and occupation differs across cultural contexts; and sociocultural influences that associate places and spaces with occupations.

Theme 1: culture influences norms and forms of occupational performance and engagement

Although there may be some occupations that are common across national and cultural divides, for example parenting or dining, the ways in which people go about them may vary tremendously. That

is, the *form* of the occupation differs. A concept originally developed by Nelson (1988), occupational forms are '…sequences of action that are oriented to a purpose sustained in collective knowledge, culturally recognized and named' (Forsyth & Kielhofner 2006, p. 76). In the examples above, we first have descriptions of studying and socialising. Note that for studying, there are clear prescriptions with respect to the form: women at the front, men at the back. In the latter example, the form of socialising is a little more fluid (indeed the extent to which occupational forms are rule-bound varies across cultures) but it seems that the form is comprised of the elements of getting together, sitting down and 'yarning' (talking) – whilst the children play some sort of sport. Mostly we notice occupational forms in terms of how things are done when we find ourselves in a context or place where things are done very differently. For those who have never been in a market place in South East Asia, for example, bargaining as a specific form of the occupation of shopping can be a dramatically different experience.

Theme 2: cultural norms proscribe acceptable occupational participants

The most observable way in which cultural norms influence occupations and the ways people engage in them is through gender divisions. Participation in occupations by gender may be either covertly unacceptable (as in people may quietly disapprove, for example when they see a woman in a Western city drinking at a bar alone), or are explicitly unacceptable due to either legislative or religious sanctions, such as those seen in some Middle Eastern countries.

In Ebadi's biography for example, though it is not included here, she recounts the story of how she was stripped of her position as a judge when the change of leadership in Iran made it unacceptable for women to hold such positions under an interpretation of Sharia law. In most Western countries, the situation is a little different in that anti-discrimination legislation allows for (at least theoretically) equity of access to and participation in, occupations of choice. However, this doesn't mean that gender divisions in terms of who does what, still don't exist. Women still largely engage in the so-called 'second shift' of housework and parenting activities even when both parents work full-time (Bittman 2000, Primeau 2000).

Theme 3: relationship between time and occupation differs across cultural contexts

Occupations always take place in the stream of time (Christiansen & Baum 1997) and as Iwama (2005) rightly points out, there is a relationship between a sense of self, perceptions of time, and doing. Individuals as shaped by their sociocultural environments and histories perceive themselves *within* time in a particular way. Time tends to be apprehended by people as either a linear, unfolding phenomenon (associated with the Judeo-Christian tradition), or a cyclic, recurring one (associated with Buddhist tradition) (Hassard 1990). A fascinating treatment of the topic of how people understand, experience and respond to constructions of time, comes from Willis (2000) who suggests that the current pressure experienced in many Western countries with respect to time and what people need to *achieve* in time, has been influenced by the Christian notion of purgatory. She explains it as follows:

> One of the workplace tools of torture is time, both length of time and time intensity. Deadlines are one way of refining this discipline tool of work intensification. Attempting to meet a deadline causes "time induced anxiety." Achieving the deadline reduces anxiety, but only for a time, for in the modern world, deadlines follow the duration of hell […] the origin of this sadomasochism however, is not in hell, but the medieval invention of purgatory.
>
> (Willis 2000, p. 128).

Another important way in which cultural constructions of time influence occupation is through individual and community responses to *types of time*. By this I mean that there are specific times such as holiday time or time for ritual celebrations such as birthdays, weddings, etc. These types of time predicate certain occupations such as food preparation, for example, an excellent study of which has been conducted comparing the food-preparation rituals of women in New Zealand and the USA at Christmas time and those of women in Thailand at the time of the festival of Songkran (Wright St Clair et al 2004). As well as traditionally named times in a cultural calendar, there are also types of time that arise through unforeseen events, such as the bushfire described in the second extract at the beginning of this section. As the narrator says, *times of adversity bring people together*. And so, a time of adversity (as a type of time) is one which the cultural response is for people to join together in the face of threat and provide mutual support and comfort. Another type of time we have unfortunately seen more of in recent years is times of mass mourning in the wake of a tragic event. An increasingly common cultural expression in many Western countries at such times has been the spontaneous placement of flowers at significant sites – who, for example, can forget the unprecedented scenes at Kensington Palace following Diana's death? What people do, then, in different types of time can be seen as having an important role in unifying cultural communities and reinforcing a collective identity.

Theme 4: sociocultural influences on places and spaces associated with specific occupations

If you have ever had coffee in a coffee bar in Italy early in the morning, its likely to be crowded, people will be standing, they will mostly be men, and the coffee will be fantastic! People go to particular places to do particular things, and of course where you live is going to influence this dramatically. If we continue with the example of the ritual morning coffee, this could variously be in shops, cafes, tavernas, bars or streetside.

That the relationship between culture, occupation, place, and identity is a strong one is evident, as we both reflect on our own lives and observe the lives of others. Generally speaking, people will go to often extreme lengths to be in places where they experience meaningfully the connection between who they are through what they do every day. This can often be despite odds that militate against this. A striking example of this was when I was interviewing a woman who was a refugee from the Balkans conflict as part of a pilot study of refugee resettlement in regional Australia (Whiteford 2004). Despite the fact that she had been terribly unsafe in her former home in Bosnia, there was still a strong pull to be in a familiar geographic and cultural place, engaging in occupations in a familiar way. Indeed, for her, the life she lived in Australia was safe, but lonely and marginalising.

Differences between communities: culture and occupation

Whilst the discussion above relates to how culture can influence the how, who, when, and where of occupations, I have left till last this discussion of how culture influences what occupations are performed and, more importantly, what they mean. This is for two reasons; first, it is a complex issue, and, second, it is one of real importance to the profession now and as we move into a future in which we must embrace cultural diversity more fully than we currently do. There are three interrelated issues currently being discussed in the profession internationally with respect to culture and occupation: universality; the relationship between doing and being; and processes of colonisation and its impact on representations of occupation.

Universality

Based on some research findings from a study conducted in Aotearoa (New Zealand), I suggested in an article that occupational therapy practice and research should address the need to understand occupation (and independence) as a culturally relative construct (Whiteford & Wilcock 2000). The rationale for such a position was that, until relatively recently, occupation has been discussed and operationalised as though it were a universally understood and experienced phenomenon. Of course, this is not true. Rather, it is an inherently Eurocentric orientation towards, and construction of, occupation that has been promulgated (Darnell 2002, Iwama 2006, Watson 2006) through the literature to date. This is because, historically, the predominant voice has been a Western one; to date, most research and professional publications in the discipline of occupational therapy have come from North America, the United Kingdom and, latterly, Australia and South Africa, and have generally represented the prevailing values and norms of the dominant subgroups therein.

More recently, diverse voices are emerging which are interrogating the essentially individualistic orientation in the occupation-focused discourse (Bourke-Taylor & Hudson 2005, Dickie et al 2006, Kronenberg et al 2005, Lim & Iwama 2006, Odara 2005). In particular, Kondo (2004) presents an insightful discussion of how cultural values can have a strong influence on occupational choice with respect to obligation and responsibility which centralise the needs of others ahead of the individual. Using the Japanese notions of 'gimu' and 'sekinin', Kondo reflects on how familial and social relationships, and the attendant responsibilities embedded within these, have a profound influence on what people do; certainly personal choice based on individual needs and wants assumes a less prioritised position than it does in many Western sociocultural traditions.

Relationship between doing and being

Discussions of individualism vs. collectivism cannot take place outside of considerations of ontology, that is, how reality is understood and experienced by people, and clearly culture influences this in a profound way. You can be sitting next to someone on a bus, for example, and have a radically different construction of reality than they do based on who you are; your religious, ethnic and cultural background, age and gender, and your life experiences. In essence, your *being* is different. Whilst being has been discussed in philosophy for many years, in occupational therapy and occupational science discussion has focused around the relationship between being and doing, a focus led in part by the exploration of the relationship presented by Wilcock (1998).

Indeed, similar to the understanding that how occupation is popularly presented and understood has been inordinately influenced by Western philosophical traditions and values, so too has the discussion of the relationship between being and doing been skewed towards an emphasis on doing because of its centrality in contemporary Western life. Whilst Jensen (1998) explored the alternative, namely that *not* doing was of real importance and significance in traditional Aboriginal culture in Australia, most recently it has been argued that 'the being of the person must be recognized' (Watson 2006, p. 156) and that, inter alia, understandings of being per se must precede attempting to address doing. This is an important area for ongoing dialogue and theoretical development in the future, and needs to be informed by diverse voices and multiple perspectives. Indeed, exploring the existential and spiritual dimensions of who we are, what we do, and how we interact with the world around us, may in a global environmental context be seen as being of utmost importance in the future.

Colonialisation

If representations and discussions of doing and being have a Eurocentric cultural bias, this is no accident. Rather, it is because many cultures and traditions have been subsumed, silenced or annihilated through processes of colonisation. To date, discussions of indigenous perceptions of time (Whiteford & Barns

1999, Yalmambirra 2000), indigenous perceptions of identity (McKinley 2002), and processes of marginalization and occupational deprivation (Zeldynryk & Yalmambirra 2006) have been discussed relative to processes of colonization over time. Additionally, and of significance to the future of the profession, calls have been made to ensure that epistemological pluralism, inclusive practice and human rights underpin occupational therapy practice (Algado & Cardona 2005, Darnell 2002, Kronenberg & Pollard 2005). As such, these should be fundamental to a scenario in which occupational therapy may be most relevant, powerful and ethically focused, i.e. in close concert with the many cultural and contextual factors that shape it and ultimately contribute to it.

Context 3 – Political and economic environments

So far we have considered the familial, environmental and sociocultural contextual influences on occupation: form, meaning, performance and expectations. The next contextual layer that influences occupation individually and collectively is that of the economic and political environments in which we live. Comparatively, it is a context that is less visible and in some ways more complex than those previously discussed. It is, however, no less influential on the ways in which people go about doing the things they need and want to do in their everyday lives.

Economies and political systems are linked, and political systems are based on a framework of beliefs and values (ideologies) about how society should work, in particular, how resources are distributed. One of the most significant factors that affects people on a daily basis is the degree to which the ideology of the group in power affects control of the market. For example, in England, a participatory democracy with a capitalist economy, market forces determine availability, price and movement of consumer goods. Basically, this means that if I have money, I can buy what I want. By contrast, in Cuba, a socialist country with a heavily regulated economy, the market is restricted and this has an impact on the availability and choice of consumer items. So, even though I may have the money (harder when wages are low and commercial opportunities limited) I cannot necessarily get what I want. Although access to goods is something that many of us living in capitalist systems take for granted, it does have a

real impact on everyday life and patterns of occupational participation (Hocking 2006).

As well as accessing goods (and to some extent services), political systems and their corresponding economies influence access to *opportunities for occupational participation*. This is important because the extent to which groups of people, particularly those at risk of marginalisation, can access those opportunities which enable them to participate fully and equally in society, is a central concern in occupational therapy. An example of how the ideology and orientation of a government can influence access and participation can be found in my experiences of being involved in an intercultural fieldwork programme in Vietnam periodically for some years. The following is adapted from Whiteford, Occupational Deprivation: Understanding Limited Participation, in *Occupation, The art and science of living* (in press):

> *Vietnam is a liberal communist country. It is still resource poor but developing rapidly. Its policy environment is strongly influenced by communist ideals and values which put collective needs above those of individuals and prioritizes community development. In this context then I was not surprised to learn that the government recently started building massive internet access facilities, free for every citizen to use for several hours per week. This is based on a belief that all Vietnamese citizens need to be technologically literate so that they are not marginalised in the future. Hence, making real access to people on a massive scale (tens of millions) has created participation in technology and provided skills and opportunities for people now and into the future. Imagine what this has cost! In essence then, people who may have been disadvantaged in access to technology and the occupations associated with it have been enabled by the political and policy environment. They will not suffer from occupational deprivation as a result of not having adequate access to no or low cost technology.*

Lets take a different example now, but drawn from the same context. In the complex mix of culture, history and politics, disabled people are apparently not automatically given rights of citizenship in Vietnam. Again, in a political context in which the focus is on the collective, rather than the individual, the political environment does not support the mobilisation of (comparatively) high levels of resources to be made available to individuals. Accordingly, disabled people do not necessarily have access to an education which, whatever the degree of disability they may experience, does result in diminished opportunities for skills and knowledge development and, hence, occupational deprivation. If you don't have an education, it's difficult to participate in society: to work, socialise or even communicate effectively.

This is a powerful example of how people's lives can be impacted by governments in ways that affect inclusion and participation directly. Indeed, governments, based on their ideologies, create or delimit occupational opportunities for whole populations. Because this can have such a significant impact on what people are able to do on a daily basis, it is worth giving some consideration to the formal mechanisms through which this is enacted, and that is through the creation of legislation and policies.

Legislation, policy and occupational participation

Although terminology related to legislation and policy is constantly around us, especially in the media, it is worth starting with some definitions to clarify what each is and how it is created. When we talk about legislation, it is actually the term used to refer to the creation of laws by governments, and that these laws may be international, national or state. Table 11.1 provides examples of international, national and state laws which have relevancy for occupational therapists and the people that we may work with.

Although governments (and the ideologies they are based on as we have seen in the example drawn from Vietnam) and political systems vary, in principle, the legislative process is consistent. Essentially, it usually involves the making of laws through the presentation and discussion of a Bill and then voting by members of the government upon it. The final approval is made by the head of government and what was formerly a Bill now becomes a piece of legislation. This process is happening all the time and, to some extent, represents the business of government.

Interestingly, although we are pretty well 'swimming' in environments underpinned by policies – in everything from the places we work to the places in

Table 11.1

Level 1: International Law – The International Bill of Human Rights

"All human beings are born free and equal in dignity and rights. They are endowed with reason and conscience and should act towards one another in a spirit of brotherhood" From – the UNIVERSAL DECLARATION OF HUMAN RIGHTS (art. 1), adopted by General Assembly resolution 217 A (III) of 10 December 1948

The International Bill of Human Rights consists of the Universal Declaration of Human Rights, the International Covenant on Economic, Social and Cultural Rights, and the International Covenant on Civil and Political Rights and its two Optional Protocols (Fact Sheet). Both International Covenants on Human Rights, by which states accept a legal as well as a moral obligation to human rights, have been ratified by 132 countries including Australia, New Zealand, the United Kingdom and the United States of America. The Bill of Human Rights remains fundamental to the promotion and protection of human rights and freedom through the world

Level 2: Federal Law – The Australian Disability Discrimination Act 1992

This Australian Commonwealth Act was passed in 1992 to protect and promote the rights of people with disabilities in all facets of life. The Act's objectives are to eliminate discrimination on the grounds of disability in the areas of work, accommodation, education, access to premises and in the provision of goods and therapists. A therapist working in an education system supporting students with disabilities, or a therapist providing consultation on public access would be working within the guidelines of the Disability Discrimination Act

Level 3: State Law – The NSW Privacy and Personal Information Protection Act 1998

This Act introduces a set of privacy standards for the NSW public sector that regulate the way public sector agencies deal with personal information. It also provides a mechanism for complaints and investigations regarding breaches of the Act. The Act provides standards for the provision of personal information within and between agencies and a system to ensure permission and approval is provided for the sharing of personal information. For therapists working in the public sector the Act provides standards for discussing a person's details with other service providers, referring a person to another service provider and in the distribution of records or reports about a person

Adapted from Barbara & Whiteford (2005).

which we enjoy recreation, policy is a term that is harder to define than legislation. This is very probably because it is so ubiquitous and used fairly loosely. Generally speaking, a policy refers to a course of action adopted by a government, party or individual (The New Shorter Oxford English Dictionary of Historical Principles 1993). What is perhaps most confusing is that the use of the term varies, ranging from statements of intent through to a clear set of standing rules for action (Palmer & Short 2000). So, as well as impacting on whole societies of people in terms of occupational participation, we are also enabled and constrained professionally by the policy environment. Indeed, for us in occupational therapy, we are influenced and guided by policy at the highest level (i.e. that of the government, as well as at the grass roots level of the institution or organisation we are working within).

So, to summarise, governments create laws that get translated through the development and implementation of policies. These laws (pieces of legislation) affect access to resources and opportunities for participation in society. They also govern the actions of individuals, including professionals, at a national and institutional level. What is really important then, on a day-to-day basis, is how we in occupational therapy enact and influence those policies to enhance equity of opportunities for all people. However, this is not as straightforward as it may seem. This is because, although occupational therapists may believe in justice and equity, they may in actuality fall far short of doing so on an everyday basis, as was found in a study of occupational therapists working in institutional mental health settings (Townsend 1998). The reasons for this shortfall between belief and action are complex

and interconnected, but usually reflect an uncritical acceptance of institutional policies (Wilding & Whiteford 2008) even when they restrict the ability of the therapist to maximise the occupational opportunities of the person(s) they are working with. In essence, what we need to do is to ensure that we foreground the needs of those groups for whom occupational participation is difficult in different contexts – be it the physical, sociocultural or political contexts we have discussed so far – and maintain a critical and active stance in shaping and developing those policies which really count.

Conclusion

The history of occupation is as old as humankind. From doing elaborate paintings on cave walls through to skateboarding, people have enacted an innate pull towards active engagement with their environments – to *do* is essentially human. Indeed, so essential is this drive to know and understand the world not just passively but actively, we know now that situations in which people are restricted in or deprived of opportunities to engage in meaningful doing or occupations, that health and well-being can be severely compromised.

However, doing never occurs free of context. In this chapter we have considered some of the contextual forces that shape the occupations of individuals, families, communities, and societies and what impact they may have both overtly and covertly: geography, families, societies, cultures, and governments. In understanding the complexity of occupation relative to these contextual influences we are able to do a better job of enabling occupation for all people.

References

Algado, S., & Cardona, C.E. (2005). The return of the corn men. In: F. Kronenberg, S. Algado & N. Pollard (Eds.) *Occupational therapy without borders*. (pp. 336–350) London, Elsevier.

Australian Bureau of Statistics (2006). Living longer, working harder and using more energy. Retrieved 27/3/07 at http://www.abs.gov.au/Ausstats/abs/abs@nsf/Latest products/4102.0Media

Barbara, A., & Whiteford, G. (2005). Leisure as commodity. In: G. Whiteford & V. Wright St Clair

(Eds.) *Occupation and practice in context* (pp. 336–348). Sydney, Elsevier.

Bateson, M. (1996). Enfolded activity and the concept of occupation. In R. Zemke & F. Clark (Eds.) *Occupational science: The evolving discipline* (pp. 5–12). Philadelphia, Davis.

Bittman, M. (2000). Now its 2000: Trends in doing and being in the new millennium. *Journal of Occupational Science*, 7, 108–117.

Bourke-Taylor, H. & Hudson, D. (2005). Cultural differences: The

experience of establishing an occupational therapy service in a developing community. *Australian Occupational Therapy Journal*, 52, 188–198.

Chomsky, N. (1986). *Knowledge of language: It's nature, origin and use*. Westport, CT, Praeger/Greenwood.

Christiansen, C., & Baum, C. (1997). *Occupational therapy: Enabling function and wellbeing*. Thorofare, NJ, Slack.

Clark, F. (1997). Reflections on the human as an occupational being:

biological need, tempo and temporality. *Journal of Occupational Science*, 4(3), 86–92.

Clark, F., & Richardson, P. (1996). A grounded theory of techniques for occupational storytelling and occupational story making. In: R. Zemke & F. Clark (Eds.) *Occupational science: The evolving discipline* (pp. 373–392). Philadelphia, Davis.

Darnell, R. (2002). Occupation is not a cross cultural universal: Some reflections from an ethnographer. *Journal of Occupational Science*, 9, 5–11.

Diamond, J. (1997). *Guns, germs and steel*. New York, Norton.

Dickie, V., Cutchin, M., & Humphry, R. (2006). Occupation as a transactional experience. *Journal of Occupational Science*, 13, 83–93.

Ebadi, S. (2006). *Iran awakening*. London, Rider.

Forsyth, K., & Kielhofner, G. (2006). The model of human occupation: integrating theory into practice and practice into theory. In: E. Duncan (Ed.) *Foundations for practice in occupational therapy* (pp. 69–108). London, Elsevier.

Freeman, C. (2007). *Born to run: My story*. Camberwell, Vic, Puffin.

Geertz, C. (1973). *The interpretation of cultures*. New York, Basic Books.

Hamilton, T. (2004). Occupations and places. In: C. Christiansen & E. Townsend (Eds.) *Introduction to occupation: The art and science of living*. NJ, Prentice Hall.

Hammell, K. (2003). Changing institutional environments to enable occupation among people with severe impairments. In: L. Letts, P. Rigby & D. Stewart (Eds.) *Using environments to enable occupational performance* (pp. 35–54). Thorofare, NJ, Slack.

Hassard, J. (1990). *The sociology of time*. London, MacMillan.

Hocking, C. (2006). *The relationship between objects and identity in occupational therapy: A dynamic balance between rationalism and romanticism*. Unpublished doctoral thesis.

Iwama, M. (2005). Occupation as a cross cultural construct. In: G. Whiteford & V. Wright St Clair (Eds.) *Occupation and practice in context* (pp. 242–253). Sydney, Elsevier.

Iwama, M. (2006). *The kawa model. Culturally relevant occupational therapy*. London, Elsevier.

Jensen, H. (1998). Best practice for occupational therapy intenrvetion when working with Australian aboriginal people. *Proceedings from the 12th International Congress of the World Federation of Occupational Therapy Conference, Montreal*. Montreal, World Federation of Occupational Therapists.

Kondo, T. (2004). Cultural tensions in occupational therapy practice: Considerations from a Japanese vantage point. *American Journal of Occupational Therapy*, 58, 174–184.

Kroneneberg, F., & Pollard, N. (2005). Overcoming occupational apartheid. In: F. Kronenberg, S. Algado & N. Pollard (Eds.) *Occupational therapy without borders*. (pp. 58–86). London, Elsevier.

Kronenberg, F., Algado, S., & Pollard, N. (Eds.) (2005) *Occupational therapy without borders*. (pp. 58–86). London, Elsevier.

Kunstler, J. (2005). *The long emergency*. New York, Atlantic Monthly Press.

Lareau, C. (2003). *Unequal childhoods*. San Francisco, University of Southern California Press.

Lim, K.H.., & Iwama, M. (2006). Emerging models – an Asian perspective. In: E. Duncan (Ed.) *Foundations for practice in occupational therapy* (pp. 161–189). London, Elsevier.

Llewellyn, G. (1994). Parenting: A neglected human occupation. *Australian Occupational Therapy Journal*, 41, 173–176.

McKinley, E. (2002). Brown bodies in white coats: Maori women scientists and identity. *Journal of Occupational Science*, 9, 109–116.

Metge, J. (1986). *In and out of touch. Whakamaa in a cross cultural context*. Wellington, University of Victoria Press.

Nelson, D.L. (1988). Occupation: form and performance. *American Journal of Occupational Therapy*, 42, 633–641.

Neumayer, B., & Wilding, C. (2005). Leisure as commodity. In: G. Whiteford & V. Wright St Clair (Eds.) *Occupation and practice in context* (pp. 317–331). Sydney, Elsevier.

Odara, E. (2005). Cultural competency in occupational therapy. *American Journal of Occupational Therapy*, 59, 325–334.

Palmer, G.R., & Short, S.D. (2000). *Health care and public policy: An Australian analysis*. Melbourne, MacMillan.

Porta, S., & Renne, J. (2005). Linking urban design to sustainability. *Urban Design International*, 10, 51–64.

Primeau, L. (2000). Divisions of household work, routine and child care occupations in families. *Journal of Occupational Science*, 7, 19–28.

Rigby, P., & Letts, L. (2003). Environment and occupational performance. In: L. Letts, P. Rigby & D. Stewart (Eds.) *Using environments to enable occupational performance* (pp. 17–32). Thorofare, NJ, Slack.

Ringaert, L. (2003). Universal design of the built environment to enable occupational performance. In: L. Letts, P. Rigby & D. Stewart (Eds.) *Using environments to enable occupational performance* (pp. 97–116). Thorofare, NJ, Slack.

Stagnitti, K. (2005). The family as a unit in postmodern society. In: G. Whiteford & V. Wright St Clair (Eds.) *Occupation and practice in context* (pp. 213–229). Sydney, Elsevier.

The New Shorter Oxford English Dictionary on Historical Principles. (1993). Oxford: Clarendon Press.

Thomson, M. (2002). *Blokes & sheds*. Sydney, Angus & Robertson.

Townsend, E. (1998). *Good intentions overruled: A critique of empowerment in the routine organisation of mental health service*. Toronto, University of Toronto Press.

Watson, R. (2006). Being before doing: The cultural identity of occupational therapy. *Australian Occupational Therapy Journal*, 53, 151–158.

Whiteford, G. (2004). The occupational issues of refugees. In: M. Molineux (Ed.). *Occupation for occupational therapists* (pp. 183–199). London, Blackwell.

Whiteford, G. (in press). Occupational deprivation: Understanding Limited

Participation, in C. Christiansen & E. Townsend, (Eds.) *Occupation, The art and science of living* (2nd ed). NJ, Prentice Hall.

Whiteford, G., & Barns, M. (1999). Te Ao Hurihuri: The world turns. In: A. Harvey (Ed). *Time use methodologies in the social sciences*. New York, Plenum.

Whiteford, G., & Wicks, A. (2000). Doing, being, reflecting: An analytic review of the Journal of Occupational Science Profiles. Part 2. *Journal of Occupational Science*, 7, 48–57.

Whiteford, G., & Wilcock, A. (2000). Cultural relativism: Occupation and culture reconsidered. *Canadian Journal of Occupational Therapy*, 67(5), 324–336.

Wicks, A., & Whiteford, G. (2006). Use of life histories in occupation based research. *Scandinavian Journal of Occupational Therapy*, 54(2), 61–73.

Wilcock, A. (1998). Reflections on doing, being and becoming. *Canadian Journal of Occupational Therapy*, 65, 248–256.

Wilding, C. & Whiteford, G. (2008) Language, identity and representation: occupation and occupational therapy in acute settings. *Australian Occupational Therapy Journal*, 55(3), 180–187.

Willis, E. (2000). Deadlines and the purgatorial complex. *Journal of Occupational Science*, 7, 128–132.

Wiseman, L. (2007). *Occupation and identity: Understanding older rural men's experiences of retirement.* Unpublished Doctoral Thesis. Albury, Australia: Charles Sturt University.

Wright St Clair, V., Bunryarong, W., Vittayakorn, S., Rattakorn, P. & Hocking, C. (2004). Offerings: Food traditions of older Thai women at Songkran. *Journal of Occupational Science*, 11, 115–124.

Yalmambirra. (2000). Black time, white time, your time, my time. *Journal of Occupational Science*, 7, 133–137.

Zeldenryk, L., & Yalmambirra. (2006). Occupational deprivation: A consequence of Australia's policy of assimilation. *Australian Occupational Therapy Journal*, 53, 43–46.

12

Enabling communication in a person-centred, occupation-focused context

Sue Baptiste

CHAPTER CONTENTS

Introduction 152
   Person-centred practice. 152
   Occupation-based practice 152
   Personal autonomy 153
   Team-based practice 153
Strategies to enable communication. 153
Developing communication skills 154
   Empathy and sympathy 154
   Barriers to communication 155
   Assumptions. 155
Frameworks to guide the search for
understanding and establishing
relationships. 155
   The Calgary Cambridge Model of History
   Taking 155
   The Canadian Occupational Performance
   Measure 157
Conclusion. 159

SUMMARY

The complex context of the interview is centrally important to excellence in person-centred occupational therapy practice. This chapter overviews foundational concepts, frameworks and tools and enables an exploration of the complexities of communicating with people. The many facets of a person-centred approach to delivering occupational therapy services, and the importance of enhancing self-awareness in order to enable the process to unfold naturally are presented. Understanding people's stories, hearing their descriptions of what are the central meanings and purposes of their lives, is the essence of the occupational therapy philosophy. Fact-finding and interviewing are terms that connote a clear, firm process of establishing 'true' data in an ordered and systematic fashion. Such ventures as part of the therapeutic enterprise have their place, but not perhaps at the initial interface between therapist and person. At that first point of contact, the important thing is to create a context for respectful interaction, fertile ground for a solid basis for understanding and mutual problem-solving.

KEY POINTS

- Understanding individuals' stories, hearing their descriptions of the central meaning and purpose of their lives, is the essence of the occupational therapy philosophy.
- Common elements of person-centred practice include: respect, partnership, collaboration, and an entrenched belief that the person is central to the endeavour of delivering the needed services.
- The idea of practitioner personal empowerment is also one that translates well into person-centred practice, supporting the development of therapeutic partnerships with people requiring occupational therapy services and their families.
- Communication is the basis upon which health care delivery is predicated.
- Identification of occupational performance issues is the unique perspective that is offered by engagement in a person–therapist relationship within occupational therapy.

Introduction

The profession of occupational therapy has undergone many changes over the period of its almost one hundred year history, not the least of which is the most recent return to the foundational principles and pride in the occupational nature of practice. In concert with the notion of occupation being central to practice, is the intention to establish a partnership between individuals and therapists. Similarly, many countries in which occupational therapists practice have embraced a regulatory model for health professions that provides protection for the public related to the services they receive from regulated professions. This trend has necessitated that individual practitioners recognise the importance of lifelong learning in order to ensure ongoing competence, thus engendering expectations for a conscious and aware approach to practice, acceptance of professional autonomy and accountability. The complex nature of contemporary practice is even more complicated by the contexts in which occupational therapists work. Employers and workplaces have expectations that staff will work together in interprofessional teams with common goals focusing upon quality client care. At the same time, individual professionals strive to maintain their own professional mandate and philosophy. In order to create the context for a discussion about interviewing and information gathering, a review of foundational concepts would seem to be useful.

Through an exploration of foundational concepts, a ready appreciation can be gained regarding the complex nature of what occupational therapy practitioners do, as well as what is expected of them. Practice should be client-centred, occupation-based, acknowledge personal autonomy, and most often undertaken within a team-driven workplace, or at the least within a context where communication with colleagues is essential. Thus, there emerges an increased awareness of the critical importance of accurate information to enable the best care to be provided to the individuals who seek occupational therapy services.

Person-centred practice

The origins of the central concept of client-centred practice can be traced to the ground-breaking work of Carl Rogers which has formed a strong foundation for contemporary occupational therapy practice

(Law et al 1995). This approach to working with people revolves around the notion of partnership, mutual regard, the art of listening, and a commitment to identifying intervention priorities from the issues raised by each individual. It is from these principles that the use of 'client' was chosen, perhaps a word that creates some dis-ease for many, but which does suggest a service partnership rather than a hierarchical power-based relationship of expert and patient (Law 1998).

The emerging concept of person-centred care is similar to client-centred practice, but focuses centrally upon collaboration across all partners involved in the delivery of care to an individual or family. It also stresses the importance of seeing the professional as someone needing support and consideration in similar ways as the individuals receiving the service. Evidence would suggest that this multifaceted concept is showing a connection to positive health outcomes (Mead & Bower 2000, Tinney et al 2007) from the perspective of enhanced communication between patients and professionals as well as showing proof of the importance and relevance of education to enhance understanding of person-centred care.

Similarities between the two constructs are many, however, the additional term *patient-centred care* complicates the debate further. From an occupational therapy perspective, 'client' has become the adopted term since there was a concern that 'patient' tended to connote more of a passive relationship rather than a shared partnership. Conversely, concerns were also voiced that 'client' painted more of a picture of a business relationship, thus creating an imbalance in power and influence that may impact the therapeutic alliance in a negative fashion since 'the client is always right'. There are common elements of client-centred care to guide us forwards thus relinquishing the need to use the term patient. These common elements include: respect, partnership, collaboration, and an entrenched belief that the patient or client is central to the endeavour of delivering the needed services.

Occupation-based practice

The roots of occupational therapy stem from the careful attention to occupations that had meaning for those engaged in them and for the environment in which they were undertaken and performed. Somewhere over time, the way was lost and the profession struggled to define a niche in a world that was ever increasing in its reductionist stance and search for measurable 'truth'. In such a context, value and worth were best defined from observable and provable actions rather than reflective and subjective relational thought. However, since the 1980s a major practice shift has been occurring, within which a return to the original investment and belief in occupation has been realized. Component-based practice remains a viable option for care when part of an overarching occupation-based approach. Even in the most scientifically rooted practice context (such as a burns unit, hand clinic, acute care ward), there is a clear commitment to embracing person-centred practice and thus, a strong inclusion of concern for links to occupation for each person and his family.

Personal autonomy

Another element that is of key importance to communication within occupational therapy practice is the concept of personal autonomy. The central intent of personal autonomy is for an individual to possess personal rule over himself or herself while remaining free from controlling interference by others. The autonomous person acts with comfort in engaging with freely self-chosen plans and actions, the choices of which are guided by values, beliefs, knowledge and skills in the selection of those plans and actions. A person with reduced autonomy, on the other hand, can be controlled by others or feel incapable of deliberating or acting on the basis of his or her own personal choices or preferences for action. It is through the detailed and rigorous process of professional regulation that occupational therapy practitioners have a clear framework against which they can measure and assess their own practice, identifying learning gaps and areas for ongoing professional development. Many of these competencies are focused upon the individual's ability to practice in a person-centred, occupation-centred manner within an inter-professional context. This idea of personal empowerment is also one that translates well into person-centred practice, supporting the development of therapeutic partnership.

Team-based practice

Sound communication skills in teams are essential for supporting and advocating for the needs of each individual. Most health care professionals expect to work within a team or group within their workplace.

In order to be a successful and valued team participant, there is a need to articulate a ready definition of one's unique contribution to the overall enterprise. Functioning within hierarchies is becoming less obvious, and the incidence of sole representatives of individual disciplines covering a wide scope of service delivery is becoming more and more common. Therefore, the ability to recognise the value and worth of other team members while firmly providing one's own piece of the puzzle is an imperative of modern practice. Sound team relationships rely heavily on the abilities and willingness of members to value mutual respect and regard, honesty, and open communication which, in turn, will engender trust, thus facilitating excellence in care delivery. Therefore, the importance of sound information gathering through rapport building, interviewing and interpretation of information within a person-centred framework is a vital precursor to advocating well for patients and families when relating to colleagues in a team environment.

Strategies to enable communication

Given the four foundational concepts identified in the previous section, it would appear more appropriate to begin to talk about communicating rather than simply 'interviewing'. This allows us to address the intention of developing communication skills more broadly. It can be applied across all relationships within the therapeutic endeavour, from colleagues and peers to people requiring occupational therapy services, such as families, agencies, students, and others.

A discussion of and reflection upon the elements that constitute communication will help to establish a framework for the development of a personal approach to obtaining information through listening to people's stories. The central strategy for enabling communication involves the use and integration of several smaller strategies and the acquisition of skill sets related to enhanced self-awareness, enriched listening and hearing skills, and a conscious application of person-centred values such as respect, regard, and recognition of being in a mutual partnership, person, and professional (Chant et al 2002, Schirmer et al 2005).

Individuals, throughout their lives, have been 'trained' how to behave and what to expect when attending appointments with doctors and other professionals. Only in recent years has there been a move towards a consumer-based and consumer-influenced approach to health care delivery (Eysenbach & Hadad 2001), which dictates that we should be engaged together with the person providing the care in a mutual journey towards understanding the problem and what can be done about it. In order to be able to make that transition with relative ease, it is important that clinicians become aware of their own abilities, as professionals in their own right, to listen and then hear what their clients are telling them. The very nature of the occupational therapy profession is a narrative one; it is second nature to want to hear what is happening in the lives of people as told from their perspectives. It is only through this process that therapists can attempt to enter and understand people's lives to enable optimal outcomes and to ensure their engagement in occupations that are meaningful.

Therapists can begin to get a sense of the importance of understanding another person's perspective when they consider their own situation. Think of a time when you experienced particularly effective communication between yourself and someone else; a time when you were well attuned to each other; listening, supporting, and responding to each other, helping to bring out the best in each other; and resulting in a particularly good and meaningful outcome. To understand the complexity of this situation, consider the following questions: What made it such a good experience?; What did you bring – qualities, skills, capacities – that contributed to this positive experience?; What did the other person contribute that made it a successful and satisfying experience?; In what ways did the setting, context or situation contribute?; What lessons did you take from the experience?

Developing communication skills

A discussion of and reflection upon the elements that constitute communication will help in the development of a personal approach to obtaining information through listening to the stories of people who receive occupational therapy services. Communication is the basis upon which health care delivery is predicated. Currently, there is much attention being paid to the development of communication skills by many health professional groups (Chant et al 2002, Haidet & Paterniti 2003, Schirmer et al 2005). This attention stems from the importance of providing services that are relevant to individuals and their families, in a caring context of skilled professionals who listen well, respond with empathy and work collaboratively to ensure the best outcomes possible in the circumstance.

The following questions need to be considered in a conscious manner when establishing comfort and developing communication skills: What feeling is associated with the message being delivered?; What *is* the key message?; How does the manner in which the person tells the story impart the essence of it? Active listening is the desired state for anyone engaged in attending to a person's story. This is indicated by using direct eye contact as appropriate, with a welcoming, facilitative posture; facial expressions should reflect a state of attentiveness while remaining open and non-judgmental. Tone and volume of voice should be moderate, thus suggesting an understanding of the feelings and information being shared.

Perhaps one of the main difficulties in gaining awareness of personal practice skill levels relative to communication and relationship building is internalising the ability to reflect and act on the insights gained. This is particularly hard in the area of communication due to the complexity of the process and the number of potential influences on outcomes. Building any relationship is a process fraught with potential pitfalls; building a therapeutic partnership is no exception, necessitating enhanced levels of self-awareness in order to provide individuals with quality input and an investment in the partnership (Chant et al 2002).

Empathy and sympathy

Empathy and sympathy are similar constructs that can be confusing. Empathy is the process of developing rapport through the ability to be intuitive to another person's feelings and to be cognisant of non-verbal cues. Sympathy, on the other hand results in the one feeling sorry for the 'other'. Many people respond negatively to sympathy and to sensing a feeling of being pitied. When working within a person-centred context, the ability to have an empathic stance is essential to the maintenance of partnership. Although empathy and sympathy are used interchangeably in the context of practitioner–client relationships, there are subtle differences.

Barriers to communication

There can be many barriers to communication and they can reside in the environment within which the conversation or information-finding process is taking place. It is important to pay attention to the setting in which the interaction will take place, the manner in which the furniture is arranged and the comfort of the available seating. In addition, a positive communication environment is one within which there is a low noise level and more subtle lighting. The key to appreciating the impact of the immediate environment upon a conversation with a person is to be constantly aware and to check in with the person to ensure that comfort levels are such that the process can move forward in a positive fashion. It is also critical that language used to explore ideas with individuals is such that the use of forms, professional jargon or medical terminology is kept at a minimum while guarding against sounding pedantic or patronising.

Assumptions

The assumptions made based on particular agendas, perceptions, and observations can influence the manner in which talking with a person unfolds. Again, personal awareness by the practitioner of any previous history or knowledge is essential to ensure that this does not impinge upon the practitioner's ability to listen and hear new information. Similarly, working from a professional-centred framework, not a person-centred one, may influence the manner in which the person shares the information and how openly and naturally the story will unfold. Experiences are common where the person is asked, what seem like interminable, questions throughout which he begins to feel more of an automaton than a human being, a repository of data rather than an individual with rich life stories to tell.

Frameworks to guide the search for understanding and establishing relationships

For the purposes of the discussion here, the focus will be upon two tools that represent structures and processes to guide the understanding of a person's circumstance and provide a framework for develop-ing foci for intervention. These frameworks are the Calgary Cambridge Model of History Taking (CCMHT) (http://skillscascade.com 2007) and the Canadian Occupational Performance Measure (COPM) (Law et al 1990).

The Calgary Cambridge Model of History Taking

The CCMHT (Table 12.1) is a framework designed to clarify the steps and stages along the process of history taking in medicine (Haidet & Paterniti 2003, Kurtz et al 2005). While in occupational therapy we focus on building a story rather than taking a history, a brief overview of the defined steps can assist in understanding the core elements of the basic process.

This approach has been embraced widely by medical practice in many countries with some gratifying resulting trends. The literature indicates that better physician communication skills result in heightened client satisfaction and clinical outcomes, and, that such skills can be taught (Kurtz et al 2005, Susuki et al 2002).

The kinds of information that are of importance to occupational therapists are different from the core information needs of physicians, although there are some areas of commonality. Commonalities exist as both professions have similar needs to uncover what has caused the individual to seek help, to identify clear goals for intervention, to articulate a synopsis of the conversation with first steps in planning what will happen next. The main difference lies in the approach to gaining an understanding of the person's circumstances in order to guide the encounter. The physician is often focused, by perceived necessity and purpose, on understanding symptoms and starting immediately to frame a differential diagnostic picture in order to cure and/or care. The occupational therapist, again by necessity when guided by the central professional construct of 'occupation', is most interested in establishing a relationship that will enable conversations to ensue that inform the purpose and meaning of each person's life. From this understanding will stem a mutually agreed upon determination of priority issues of occupational performance and engagement to be addressed during the period of intervention.

The first essential task is to attend to the location chosen for the interaction as well as the comfort and

Table 12.1 Five stages of the Calgary Cambridge Model of History Taking (CCMHT)

Stage 1: Initiating the session	Make preparations for engaging in the session to ensure a comfortable environment, establishing initial rapport and clarifying the reason for being there.
Stage 2: Gathering information	Exploring the person's problems from an occupational perspective, against a backdrop of the person's environments, personal resources, strengths and areas requiring attention.
Stage 3: Providing structure	Make clear to the person the path being followed to paint a picture of the problem, while making sure that the conversation flows in a logical and comfortable manner.
Stage 4: Building the relationship	Pay attention to the moment and ensure that appropriate non-verbal behaviour and cues are utilised, involving the person in an open and honest manner and thus developing a deeper rapport. The explanation of the conversation and making plans for next steps incorporates the person's health and illness perspective, the provision of needed information, and explanations. This important part of the process ensures a shared understanding that will culminate in shared decision-making.
Stage 5: Closing the session	It is essential that the conversation ends in a timely and respectful fashion, incorporating a clear path for any further assessment as needed and plans for potential intervention as appropriate.

set-up in which the conversation will unfold. As mentioned previously, details concerning furniture type and placement, lighting, space, sound, and light levels must be considered. Setting the context also involves ensuring that the person understands who is there with them, why, what they can expect from participating in this conversation, and what the therapist is hoping to gain from the interaction. The person is then asked to give consent for the conversation and the relationship to continue.

The clearer these issues are at the outset, the more successful the outcome. However, there is also a need to be flexible and not to adhere totally to the expected conversational outline. If the person takes matters in a totally different direction, then this is where enhanced skills in listening and hearing are critical, as throwing away the plan might be the most valuable and appropriate response.

The body of the interview will differ depending on the purpose, the timing and the place of it within the person–therapist relationship. It is very important to be clear about the purpose of the interaction: is it to inform selection of a theoretical approach or an assessment tool, to develop an intervention plan, or to evaluate work completed and decide whether or not discharge is appropriate? Having clarity of purpose will help both partners in making the most of the time spent together.

Identification of occupational performance issues is the unique perspective that is offered by engagement in a person–therapist relationship within occupational therapy. This is the specific philosophical focus of the discipline and, as such, requires the use of a framework that supports the articulation by individuals of occupational performance issues of importance and meaning to them. It is here, within the body of the interview, that occupational performance issues can be identified and rapport consolidated, thus enabling a rich partnership to be forged. Most recently, an additional concept has been articulated as being a central piece of occupational therapy's unique contribution and that concept is occupational engagement. Townsend and Polatajko (2007) have proffered this construct as an addition to the original Canadian Model of Occupational Performance. They posit that the central construct of occupational therapy goes beyond occupational performance and embraces the essential notion of engagement. Occupational engagement suggests the broadest view of occupation that is recognised and addressed by occupational therapists (Townsend & Polatajko 2007).

Ending an interview/conversation within a framework of person-centred practice demands that there is a mutual agreement regarding what is hoped for in the interchanges, what was achieved and what will be the next steps. This approach supports a process that is fluid and flexible, and yet is contained within goals, targeted outcomes, and overarching mutually determined expectations.

The Canadian Occupational Performance Measure

The Canadian Occupational Performance Measure (COPM) is an outcome measure that was developed in response to the need for a measure that would support the practice process of Canadian occupational therapists. Since its debut, the COPM has been the subject of much research, resulting in an emerging picture of a tool that is reliable, valid, responsive, and with clinical utility (Carswell et al 2004, McColl et al 2006), and is now used around the world.

The COPM utilises a person-centred process to identify an individual's occupational performance issues that are of the highest priority from his perspective. This process also builds upon an occupation-centred expectation, thus illustrating a clear and transparent process of guiding occupational therapy assessment and intervention. This process does not replace specific assessment tools or approaches that are used by practitioners already and address particular areas such as neurological, sensory, cognitive, physical rehabilitative, socio-adaptive, and environmental. Rather, the COPM frames the identification of priorities for an intervention plan, based upon stated personal need and priority. This tool also offers the person and therapist the opportunity to use it as a focus for grounding partnerships rather than relying upon home-grown data collection options. The COPM process involves the following steps:

- The person identifies key occupational performance issues (OPI) in each of the domains of self care, productivity and leisure, through a wide ranging discussion facilitated by the occupational therapist.

- The person and therapist agree to concentrate on a maximum of five OPI for the first iteration of the intervention plan.

- The person rates (from 1 not at all important to 10 very important) the chosen OPI in terms of importance.

- The person rates (from 1 not at all satisfied to 10 totally satisfied) the chosen OPI for how he performs and how satisfied he is with how he performs the identified occupations.

After completing the COPM the person and therapist can discuss and agree on an intervention plan to be followed. After completion of intervention the person and therapist can complete the COPM again to compare ratings on the target occupational performance issues before and after intervention, and to identify if there are new issues to be addressed.

In short, the COPM enables individuals to participate in a meaningful way in the occupational therapy process through: identifying occupational performance issues; evaluating performance and satisfaction in problem areas; and measuring change in perceptions of occupational performance. The COPM asks individuals to report on occupational performance issues and does not seek to externally validate or substantiate self-reports. Through the use of the COPM, an issue is identified by a person because of unmet role expectations or environmental demands which interfere with successful completion of an occupation. The COPM can be applied to all people receiving occupational therapy services, although the approach to utilising the measure may need modification to accommodate some particular individual needs. This applies to people who have cognitive problems, those with pervasive mental illness, and those experiencing communication difficulties. Strategies to alleviate these barriers include the use of surrogate respondents and alternate symbols to rate importance, performance and satisfaction. This is a critical piece of any information-gathering experience, but is core to the successful application of a person-centred measure such as the COPM (Chesworth et al 2002, Law et al 1994, Trombly et al 2002).

The COPM addresses occupational performance issues and not the problems with individual components of occupational performance. Other assessments need to be completed in order to obtain a clear picture of impairment level of concerns to be addressed. Using the COPM does assist in clarifying the role of occupational therapy to the person, family, and other health professionals. Hence, through this process, it becomes easier to articulate why occupational therapists may not provide an intervention that would appear to be central to the perceived problems being experienced by the person. A sense of increased partnership with person and family is readily developed and intervention time becomes more efficient. Thus, through this process, purposeful activity, linked to occupations meaningful to the person, becomes inherent in therapy (Corr & Wilmer 2003, Donnelly et al 2004, Miller et al 2001, VanLeit & Crowe 2002).

Consideration of the structure provided by the CCMHT together with the occupation-centred approach of the COPM can provide a rich and informative framework within which to place the occupational therapy interview (Box 12.1).

Box 12.1

Excellence in person-centred communication

The following information aims to assist therapists to develop their own person-centred listening and learning styles.

A. Contextual considerations

Setting: it is imperative that the space in which the conversation is taking place be large enough to accommodate the participants with comfort, that the furniture and lighting are appropriate and that there are as few distractions as possible.

Professional presentation: at all times, it is very important to appear professional in dress and manner, to be punctual and unhurried in approaching the person. Dress codes differ depending on the type of practice setting but, regardless of the degree of formality/informality, tidiness and cleanliness are not negotiable!

Background knowledge and skill: reviewing the information available about the person is important prior to meeting in order to feel as prepared as possible. This will allow for the optimal use of possibly limited time which also shows respect for the person's time and priorities. It is also critical that a therapist feels prepared to understand and respond professionally to expectations for the conversation that may stem from the person's cultural background or other elements of why he is there and who he is.

Recording: it is important to advise the person at the beginning of the conversation if the preference is to take notes in order to remember the details of what occurred. Also, when completing the notes, report or letter to the referral source, the content should be organised using a person-centred, occupation-based framework that includes an honest and authentic representation of what the person said, followed by a clear accounting of the professional reasoning that led to the assessment and enabling strategies.

Confidentiality: all notes and personal information should be kept in a secure location. All practitioners must be aware of any ethical responsibilities around confidentiality that are expected by a regulatory college or any government legislation.

Individual, family or group interview: when there are several people or one person plus family and others, there are very different expectations of the therapist. It is more complex to manage an interview environment when there are many potential agendas and, therefore, it is important to be aware of personal skill levels in handling such a situation. If someone else being present would enhance the outcomes, then asking for another team member perhaps to join the conversation is an excellent strategy. In any case, it is essential that the existence and awareness of who is the primary person be maintained.

B. Non-verbal communication

The importance of non-verbal communication can never be underestimated.

Facial expression: facial expressions can telegraph a great deal of information, so it is important to be conscious of personal impact and to respond to feedback from others about impressions made. Projecting an authentic interest in the person can make a profound difference when establishing new relationships and reconfiguring existing ones. If you feel confused or uncertain, then it is important to talk about it rather than simply raise eyebrows or frown in a quizzical manner.

Eye contact: direct eye contact can project a sincere interest in and engagement with the conversation; however, it is important to ensure that such a direct gaze is not confrontational. In addition, eye contact can be culturally inappropriate so it is imperative that cultural sensitivity and awareness are applied at all times.

Posture: offering an open and welcoming stance either when seated or standing provides a positive beginning to any interaction. Mirroring the position of the other participant in the conversation can be seen as a message of comfort and engagement.

Box 12.1

Excellence in person-centred communication—cont'd

Movement/gestures: awareness of personal use of gestures and movement during conversations is an important skill to develop. Similarly, comfort with individuals who tend to be demonstrative is a valuable skill to include in your practice tool kit.

C. Verbal communication

Tone and inflections: sounding confident is desirable while verging on arrogant is not. Keeping the voice at a conversational level, controlling the speed with which the conversation unfolds and ensuring the tone is pleasantly heard are critical pieces of developing a helpful and productive interviewing style.

Reflecting understanding: an open and appreciative style of communicating will give the person a clear sense of what to expect and an appreciation of the therapist's authenticity.

Messages: at all times the language used should reflect empathy, positive engagement and authenticity. Being oneself is crucial to productive engagement with individuals.

D. Therapeutic conversations (interviews):

Introductions and clarification of purpose: when introducing yourself ensure that the person becomes familiar with your name and your perception of why the conversation is taking place. It is also essential that the role of an occupational therapist is made clear with particular emphasis being placed on the role in the context of the client's particular circumstances.

Building a history/story: it is essential to create a context within which the person will feel comfortable in telling his story on his own, letting the story unfold at its own pace providing words of assurance and interest to move the process along.

Identifying occupational performance issues from the perspective of the person: in the case of a true partnership, power and control are shared, with attention being paid to when the person's experiences and life knowledge are central to the conversation or when the therapist's skills and expertise take precedence. In fact, the person is the expert when addressing his life circumstances and identifying what is meaningful and a priority occupational performance issue.

E. Silence

Silence can be a powerful tool in reinforcing a partnership between therapist and person. Three to four seconds is a natural pause in a conversation, but may appear longer and rather threatening early on in the establishment of a relationship. A silence lasting up to ten seconds is reasonable and to be expected when someone is trying to share a story that is complex, disturbing and rich with personal meaning; however, gaining comfort with short silences is also a skill to be developed, together with a built-in ability to recognise when some interjection is required or deemed appropriate. At times, it can be a good strategy to share such discomfort with the person and, therefore, resolve it together.

Conclusion

Practice is becoming progressively more complex, with many emerging trends that are making the need for enhanced communication and information-seeking skills ever more critical. Organisational changes, from hierarchical to programme-based systems, have placed a very clear responsibility on the shoulders of individual practitioners to practice with a clear and readily identifiable mandate that easily illustrates each discipline's unique contribution. By engaging in a person-centred process of addressing occupational performance issues, occupational therapists are well placed to deliver this kind of service. Again, approaching the establishment of person–therapist partnerships from the perspective of learning about someone's story instead of developing a personal case data-base helps those with whom occupational therapists work to have a very clear understanding of the reasons for occupational therapy and the steps in the intervention process. Time is at a premium in systems that still claim to be sadly under-resourced, thus there is less time readily available in which to create supportive treatment environments – therefore, another reinforcement of the need to streamline rapport-building skills. A needed congruence between practice style and person-centred principles has emerged from the consumer movement, a societal expectation that is increasingly reinforced. Perhaps most critically, there is a deeply rooted need for occupational therapists to practice in a manner that is respectful and sensitive to cultural differences.

If occupational therapists embrace an approach to finding out about the occupational performance issues of the people who require their services, that was enriched by individual's stories, notions of 'taking a history' or 'completing an interview' could be relinquished in favour of allowing those stories to unfold, thus shaping the nature of occupational therapy assessments and interventions. This would become then a truly person-centred approach to practice.

References

Carswell A., McColl, M. A., Baptiste, S., Law, M., Polatajko, H. & Pollock, N. (2004). The Canadian Occupational Performance Measure: a research and clinical literature review. *Canadian Journal of Occupational Therapy*, 71(4), 210–222.

Chant, S., Jenkinson, T., Randle, J., Russell, G. & Webb, C. (2002). Communication skills training in health care; a review of the lliterature. *Nurse Education Today*, 22, 189–202.

Chesworth, C., Duffy, R., Hodnett, J. & Knight, A. (2002). Measuring clinical effectiveness in mental health: Is the Canadian Occupational Performance an appropriate measure? *British Journal of Occupational Therapy*, 65(1), 30–34.

Corr, S., & Wilmer, S. (2003). Returning to work after a stroke: An important but neglected area. *British Journal of Occupational Therapy*, 66(3), 186–192.

Donnelly, C., Eng, J. J., Hall, J., Alford, L., Giachino, R., Norton, K., & Kerr, D. S. (2004). Client-centred assessment and the identification of meaningful treatment goals for individuals with a spinal cord injury. *Spinal Cord*, 42, 302–307.

Eysenbach, G. & Hadad, A. (2001). Evidence-based patient choice and consumer health informatics in the Internet age. *Journal of Medical Internet Research* 3(2), e19.

Haidet, P. & Paterniti, D. A. (2003). 'Building' a history rather than 'taking' one. *Academic Medicine* 16(3), 1134–1140.

Kurtz, S. M., Silverman, J. & Draper, J. (2005). *Teaching and learning communication skills in medicine.* Oxford, Radcliffe.

Law, M., Baptiste, S., McColl, M. A., Opzoomer, A., Polatajko, H. & Pollock, N. (1990). The Canadian occupational performance measure for occupational therapy. *Canadian Journal of Occupational Therapy*, 57(2), 82–87.

Law, M., Polatajko, H., Pollock, N., McColl, M. A., Carswell, A., & Baptiste, S. (1994). Pilot testing of the Canadian Occupational Performance Measure: clinical and measurement issues. *Canadian Journal of Occupational Therapy* 61(4), 191–197.

Law, M., Baptiste, S. & Mills, J. (1995). Client-centred practice: what does it mean and does it make a difference? *Canadian Journal of Occupational Therapy*, 62(5), 298–301.

Law, M. (1998). *Client-centred occupational therapy.* Thorofare, NJ, Slack.

McColl, M.A., Carswell, A., Law, M., Baptiste, S., Pollock, N. & Polatajkp, H. (2006). *Research on the COPM: an annotated resource.* Ottawa, Canadian Association of Occupational Therapists.

Mead, N., & Bower, P. (2000). Patient-centredness: a conceptual framework and review of the empirical literature. *Social Science and Medicine*, 51(7), 1087–1110.

Miller, L. T., Polatajko, H. J., Missiuna, C., Mandich, A. D., & Macnab, J. J. (2001). A pilot trial of a cognitive treatment for children with developmental coordination disorder. *Human Movement Science*, 20(1–2), 183–210

Schirmer, J.M., Mauksch, L., Lang, F., Marvel, K., Zoppi, K., Epstein, R.M. & Brock, D. (2005). Assessing communication competence: a review of current tools. *Family Medicine*, 37, 184–192.

Susuki Laidlaw, T., MacLeod, H., Kaufman, D. M., Langille, D. B. & Sargeant, J. (2002) Implementing a communication skills programme in medical school: needs assessment and programme change. *Medical Education*, 36(2),115–124.

Tinney, J., Fearn, M., Hill, K., Dow, B., Haralambous, B., & Bremner, F. (2007). *Best practice in person-centred health care for older Victorians: report of phase 1. Report to sub-acute and transitional care services.* Washington, D.C., Department of Human Services, National Ageing Research Institute.

Townsend, L. & Polatajko, H. (2007). *Enabling occupation II: Advancing an occupational therapy vision for health, well-being and justice through occupation.* Ottawa, Canadian Association of Occupational Therapists.

Trombly, C. A., Radomski, M. V., Trexel, C., & Burnet-Smith, S. E. (2002). Occupational therapy and achievement of self-identified goals by adults with acquired brain injury: phase II. *American Journal of Occupational Therapy*, 56(5), 489–498.

VanLeit, B., & Crowe, T. K. (2002). Outcomes of an occupational therapy program for mothers of children with disabilities: Impact on satisfaction with time use and occupational performance. *American Journal of Occupational Therapy*, 56(4), 402–410.

Chapter Thirteen

13

Analysis of occupational performance

Gill Chard

CHAPTER CONTENTS

Introduction 162

What is analysis of occupational
performance? 162

Why is analysis of occupational
performance important? 165

Analysis of occupational performance. . . . 165

    Performance areas 166

    Performance skills 167

    Motor skills 167

    Process skills 167

    Communication/interaction skills 170

    Skills and capacities 173

    Performance patterns: Roles, habits and
routines 174

    Role 175

    Habits and routines 175

    Performance contexts 177

    Environments 177

    Activity demands 178

Person factors 178

Application of occupational performance
analysis 182

Conclusion 184

SUMMARY

This chapter focuses on the analysis of
occupational performance and provides guidance
on how to perform this core skill. Occupational
performance analysis is defined and described in
the context of the *doing* of a task. A distinction is
made between the whole task, steps of the task
and individual performance units (actions). A
rationale for the use of occupational performance
analysis is provided and the Occupational
Therapy Practice Framework (American
Occupational Therapy Association 2002, 2008) is
used to define and apply occupation terminology.
Occupation is explored from six broad
perspectives: performance areas, performance
skills, performance patterns, performance
contexts, activity demands, and person factors.
The analysis of occupational performance is
described and applied within a top-down (person-
focused) approach. The Assessment of Motor
and Process Skills (AMPS) is used in the context
of a practice scenario as the basis for the
application of occupational performance analysis
for persons with or without impairments.
Occupational performance analysis is explored as
a form of evaluation and how information gained
from this process can be used for intervention
planning including the adaptation and grading of
tasks and intervention review. Finally a
framework is explored for the analysis of actual
performance that focuses on the observations of
occupations as they are performed by the person.

KEY POINTS

- *Occupational performance analysis* is a
structured evaluation process that uses
observation of an individual to identify and
define factors that support or hinder
occupational performance and prevent that
person from being a full participant in life.
- Occupational performance analysis should
always be placed in the context of the
occupations that people want and need to
engage in or *do*. Occupation refers to the doing

of tasks; performance analysis is the observation of the smallest parts of the task referred to as *performance skills*.

- Performance skills include motor skills, process skills and communication/social/interaction skills. The way that individuals carry out their occupations are referred to as *performance patterns* and these include habits, routines, roles and rituals.
- Occupational performance analysis is the unique skill of occupational therapists. It enables them to identify strengths and limitations of occupational performance and draw conclusions about the needs of individuals with body structure limitations and activity or participation restrictions.
- Detailed information about strengths and limitations of performance can be used in collaboration with individuals and their families to clarify the cause of the problem and identify solutions in order to enable or enhance occupational performance.

Introduction

It is no accident that the early founders gave our profession the name of *occupational* therapy. They saw the need for individuals to be busy, or *occupied* with the ordinary and the necessary, the occupations and roles that were their everyday lives. The early founders were quick to note that when individuals were deprived of occupation their lives lacked purpose and meaning. By observing and analysing the skills required, occupations provided a therapeutic medium, either as 'therapy' or treatment in itself, or as a means to enable individuals to achieve independence by adapting or changing the way that occupations were performed. As the profession developed over the decades analysis of everyday occupations remained but the focus has shifted towards achieving or maintaining health and wellbeing and enhancing full participation in life.

This chapter defines and describes occupational performance analysis and explores how to apply it within occupational therapy practice. The Domains of Occupational Therapy, as defined and described in the Occupational Therapy Practice Framework (American Occupational Therapy Association 2002, 2008), are the underpinning theoretical framework and language used throughout this chapter. The Assessment of Motor and Process Skills (AMPS) (Fisher 2005) is used to demonstrate the application of occupational performance analysis in an individual context, and the Assessment of Communication and Interaction Skills (ACIS) (Forsyth et al 1997) is used to demonstrate application of occupational

performance analysis in a social context. The Evaluation of Social Interaction (ESI) (Fisher & Griswold 2008) is also introduced as an evaluation tool for analysis in a social context.

Broad categories of occupation are referred to as performance areas (American Occupational Therapy Association 2008) or performance issues (Canadian Association of Occupational Therapy 2002). The Canadian Association of Occupational Therapists describe these as everything that people do to take care of themselves (self-care), enjoy life (leisure), and contribute to the social and economic fabric of communities (productivity) (Law et al 1997, p.32). The American Occupational Therapy Association describes these as activities of daily living (ADL), rest and sleep, education, work, play, leisure, and social participation (2008).

While occupation refers to the *doing* of tasks, occupational performance analysis involves detailed observation of the smallest units of the task (including *performance skills*) in contexts (physical, social and cultural) relevant to the person. Performance skills include motor skills, process skills and communication and social interaction skills. The way that individuals carry out their occupations are referred to as *performance patterns* and these include habits, routines, roles and rituals. The places or environment in which individuals carry out their occupations are referred to as *performance contexts* and include cultural, personal, physical, social, temporal and virtual. The doing of occupations is influenced by two other factors: the person (their body functions and body structures; values, beliefs and spirituality) and the demands of the task (the process of the task, spaces and objects used and social interactions required).

The framework and terminology in this chapter used to describe occupational performance analysis can be found in Figure 13.1.

What is analysis of occupational performance?

Fisher (1998, 2005) describes occupation as the action of seizing or taking possession of, or occupying space or time, as well as a role or position that a person holds. In fact, occupations are everything that we do: it is the way we spend our time productively, in leisure pursuits and taking care of ourselves. The analysis of occupation (sometimes referred to as performance analysis) assists our understanding of:

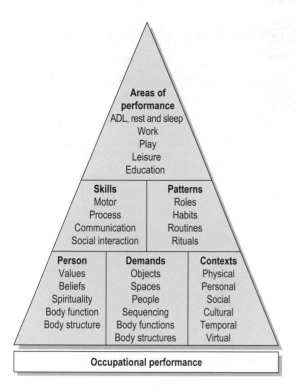

Figure 13.1 • Framework used to guide analysis of occupational performance. See also American Occupational Therapy Association 2002, 2008.

- the person (what an individual does, why an individual does what he/she does, how an individual does what he/she does)

- the places where an individual conducts their occupations: home, workplace, school or community

- how phenomena such as health, physical, social, societal, economic or political restrictions can disrupt an individual's roles and way of life.

Occupation is a process that unfolds over time; the doing of something towards a purpose, for example dressing oneself for work or walking the dog. It implies action, or as Fisher (2006) points out, the carrying out of actions – 'the *doing* of something and not what is done' (p.373). Fisher describes *what* is done as the task (to get dressed) whereas occupation implies action, either the global action of *dressing* oneself or the more specific actions of *grasping* the shirt and *manipulating* the button. Actions then are verbs: *doing* words, denoted by their *ing* ending – gras*ping*, reach*ing*, or ask*ing*. This is an important concept in understanding the breaking down of an occupation into smaller performance units.

Task analysis is analysis of what is done – to get dressed or to make a drink, in other words the demands of the *task* (bio-psychosocial and environmental) rather than the performance of skills by the person. Tasks consist of *shared concepts*: the making of a cup of tea is a concept understood by people from different communities, cultures, and countries. The process, tools and materials may vary with culture, age and ability but the task will result in the same end product (water that is heated, flavoured with leaves, with or without additions). All those who engage in this task will need to select and gather culturally specific tools and materials; move themselves and task objects from place to place, and make changes in their environment in order to proceed with and complete the task. The task (what is done) is composed of a number of steps and each step composed of a number of smaller units or actions. Each step is dependent on the development of skilled actions that have been practised on many occasions over time.

Occupational performance analysis is a structured, observational process used by occupational therapists to identify and define actions that support or limit a person's occupational performance and factors that prevent that person from being a full participant in home and community life. This can be illustrated in the description of Emily putting on her socks and shoes.

Emily is learning to put on her socks and shoes. She begins first by mastering a number of smaller actions such as gripping a sock, opening it up or spatially arranging it in order to place it over her toes, pulling it over her foot, etc. As she practises these actions over time, the individual performance skills become more precise and adept. These small discrete units or actions – organising the sock over the foot, pushing the foot into a shoe or manipulating shoelaces or fastening Velcro© also become more skilled. The actions are strung together one after another in an orderly sequence and grouped into logical steps; her sock must be put on before the shoe, her laces must be opened before attempting to put the shoe on her foot, and so on. Emily learns that there are easier and harder ways (patterns) of doing the steps and actions: that it is easier for her to adopt a sitting position rather than balance on one leg; that the heel of her sock must be placed under the foot otherwise it does not look or feel right;

her sock must be pulled right onto her foot before trying to pull it higher up her leg; and so on. The steps and actions of putting on socks and shoes are practised every day until Emily's occupational performance is skilled enough for her to complete the task efficiently, safely and without assistance. Eventually, the task becomes a skilled routine or habit that does not require full attention or thought.

Occupational performance analysis can be used to evaluate the quality and effectiveness of these small discrete steps and actions (the *process*) of performance rather than the outcome. The purpose is not just to see if Emily has a pair of socks and shoes on her feet at the end by the task, but to establish how competent she is in performing each action and step. Are there signs of increased physical effort or difficulty or clumsiness, or of performance being slow or delayed, either by inefficient use of time (it takes a long time to complete an action) or inefficient use of spaces (the steps or actions are organised in such a way that Emily has to constantly move from one space to another to complete the steps)? Emily might need assistance to complete some of the actions (pulling the laces tight enough) or steps (tying shoelaces). The steps and actions carried out by Emily in putting on her socks and shoes are summarized in Table 13.1.

Polatajko et al (2000) discuss two further performer prerequisites for optimal occupational performance: motivation and task knowledge. Motivation is an important factor that is known to influence a person's willingness to participate in and continue to the completion of tasks, especially under challenging conditions. There must be a desire or need on the part of individuals or an expectation by individuals (or their cultural group) that the tasks should be performed. Nelson & Thomas (2003) state that motivation, or human purpose, may be intrinsic or extrinsic. Intrinsic purpose involves doing something for its own sake, for the pleasure of doing it, while extrinsic purpose involves doing something for an external reason. For Emily the motivation is more like to be extrinsic: to put on her shoes and socks to please her mother or because she wants to be like her older sister. However, she might want to put her socks on simply because she likes the feel of them on her feet (intrinsic purpose). Whatever the reason, she would be more likely to initiate the task and persevere to completion if the purpose of the task was something that she wanted and desired to do for herself.

Table 13.1 Examples of steps and actions for Emily

Task	Steps	Actions
Putting on socks and shoes	Collect socks and shoes	Walking to storage place Finding shoes/socks Grasping shoes/socks Lifting shoes/socks Carrying shoes/socks Placing shoes/socks on floor
	Put sock 1 on foot	Reaching for sock Grasping sock Opening sock Arranging sock over toes
	Put sock 2 on foot	Pulling sock onto foot Arranging sock over heel Pulling sock up leg
	Repeat for sock 2	
	Put shoe 1 on foot	Reaching for shoe Grasping shoe Opening shoe Placing foot into shoe Organising tongue of shoe
	Repeat for shoe 2	
	Fasten laces	Grasping laces Pulling laces tight Asking for help Making a loop with the lace Manipulating laces with both hands Pulling loops tight

Fisher (2005, 2006) points out that task knowledge, or having an understanding of what is done, is also an important consideration. For Emily using her task knowledge in order to put on her shoes and socks is an important part of the process. She needs a basic understanding of what to do and some experience of how to do the task. This means having some experience of the task, having observed someone put her shoes and socks on and helped in parts of the process would be the very minimum. Emily is only 3 years old and is learning a new task. She needs to know how to get her toes into the sock, to grip it in such a way that she can pull it over her toes and then around her heel. As she pulls a sock over her foot she has discovered that it is easier to do this while sitting on the floor and so on. Such mastery is only achieved after much practise until knowledge of the task has become implicit.

Occupational performance analysis has been defined in many ways but always contains similar elements. Hersch et al (2005) describe a process that involves the analysis of the human and non-human components of an activity so that the activity can be used for a therapeutic purpose (as intervention). Hagedorn (2000, p. 307) defines it as:

An organised and structured process in which an activity is observed and described and broken down into its component parts in order to understand its structure, performance demands or therapeutic potential.

Trombly (2002) defines it as a process that involves determining what abilities, skills, and capacities are needed to do a specified occupation. In this chapter occupational performance analysis is considered as part of the evaluation process, where actual performance is observed in context, in order to identify factors that support performance or hinder performance (American Occupational Therapy Association 2008). It focuses on the abilities and skills of the person. Capacities are underlying body functions (musculoskeletal, neurologic, cardiovascular, etc.) and, together with contextual factors and activity demands (see Figure 13.1), are considered after an occupational performance analysis has been completed and are interpreted later as part of the demands of the task.

Why is analysis of occupational performance important?

We have considered so far how a child becomes skilled and adept at performing occupations. Skills can be described as: '… practised abilities that show deftness, dexterity and confidence in performance …' (Connelly & Dalgleish 1989, cited in Fisher 2005, p. 22)

As an adult we acquired many skills through repetition and practise; they form part of our habits and routines, often to the extent that we are not even aware of what we do or how we do it. Getting dressed in the morning is a good example of this. When we work with individuals whose occupations have been disrupted for example by age, illness, or trauma, we see the impact of body structure impairments on occupational performance. The frail elderly person who falls and fractures a hip is no longer able to use the same dextrous movement patterns in standing and sitting, and in reaching and

bending; the person who has had a stroke must adapt their performance skills and patterns in response to spasticity or muscle weakness in one side of his/her trunk and upper and/or lower limb of the same side; the person with a dementia is no longer able to remember where items are kept in the kitchen cupboards and either needs help to find them or to keep them visible on the countertop. Occupational therapists conduct occupational performance analysis in order to assess the extent to which the doing of occupations has been disrupted in order to identify those skills that are still intact, and those that inhibit competent occupational performance. Such detailed information about strengths and limitations of performance can be used in collaboration with individuals and their families to clarify the cause of the problem and identify solutions (an intervention plan) in order to enhance occupational performance. Fisher (1994) noted that the use of occupation as a tool for assessment and intervention provides a unique focus for occupational therapy. Using occupation as a therapeutic medium underpins occupational therapy (American Occupational Therapy Association 2002, 2008; Canadian Association of Occupational Therapists 2002, p. 40; College of Occupational Therapists 2006; Creek 2003). The ability to analyse and understand the demands of different kinds of occupations in order to use them as interventions is a unique skill of occupational therapists.

Occupational performance analysis should form part of the assessment process as it enables occupational therapists to gather information on the ability of the person to perform occupations competently and with satisfaction. Beginning with a focus on the person and their needs (rather than the underlying capacities or impairments) constitutes a top-down approach (Fisher 2006, Ideishi 2003, Trombly 1995, 2002). Ideishi (2003) recommends a top-down approach as occupations are then chosen by the person for their intrinsic meaning and purpose, and their perceived importance to life roles or social expectations of the culture, for example the need or desire to care for an elderly parent safely, competently, and with satisfaction.

Analysis of occupational performance

As we begin to define and use occupation terminology we can now apply it to the analysis of occupational performance. In this section we will examine performance analysis from six broad perspectives identified in Figure 13.1:

1. Performance areas

2. Performance skills

3. Performance patterns

4. Performance contexts

5. Activity demands

6. Person factors.

Performance areas

Areas of occupation are organised or categorised into caring for self (which includes personal and domestic activities of daily living), rest and sleep, education, productive work or employment, play, leisure activities, and social participation (AOTA 2008). When occupational therapists gather information in order to carry out a performance analysis it is important to consider occupations in all the categories that are important to the person. If a top-down approach is used then the occupational therapist will explore all the areas of performance that the person is concerned about. This usually involves defining what needs to be done on a daily or regular basis (caring for self, sleep and rest, productive or education areas) as well as the occupations that the person wants to do (playful, leisure, and social participation).

Fisher (2006) describes performance areas as a means of categorising daily life activities. Moreover, for occupational therapists activities should be described in terms of *actions* or the *doing* of occupations (dress*ing*, shopp*ing*, and play*ing*), rather than as a list of tasks (personal hygiene, sleep, and care of pets). Fisher (2006) maintains that this emphasis on doing is important as it gives a sense that something is happening and that the person is *doing* something or, at least, is an active participant. Occupational performance analysis is about observing an individual's active engagement in something. If nothing is being done or engaged in it is not possible for the occupational therapist to observe any actions, hence 'personal hygiene' has little meaning in terms of occupational performance analysis (there is no performance to observe or analyse), whereas 'combing' one's hair, or 'cleaning' one's teeth implies actions that can be observed and analysed. To gain a better understanding of performance areas work through Reflection 13.1.

Reflection 13.1

Performance areas

1. Make a list of all the occupations you carry out in a typical day. You might want to start with your morning routine and work through the day. Next, check this out against your actual routines, note what you have added or what you have forgotten (sometimes things that we do are so routine that we are not even aware of them). Do not forget rest and sleep, as well as periods of inactivity as these are still activities of *doing*. You might want to repeat the exercise over 2 or 3 days as some occupations may only be carried out once or twice a week but are still important to you.

2. Next categorise all of these occupations into one of the seven performance areas (self-care, rest and sleep, education, productivity, play, leisure, social participation). You might want to divide self care into personal ADL (care of self) and domestic ADL (care of others and maintenance of home environments). You might find that some occupations do not easily fall into one category and may need placing in more than one. Others, like cooking, may fall into different categories depending on the meaning (cooking for self after work – self-care; compared to preparing a meal to share with friends – leisure).

3. Finally, identify which of the occupations you *need* to perform and those you *want* to or enjoy performing. Remember to take particular note of your terminology and how you define tasks (what is done – study) and how you define your occupations (the things that you *do* – reading, writing, watching a DVD).

When carrying out an analysis of occupational performance it is important to talk to individuals about *all* of their areas of performance (regardless of whether you will address each one during intervention) not only is this a person-focused and top-down approach but it is the only way that you will get a real sense of who this person is and what is important to them. You can practice this with a study partner; interview each other, writing notes after each interview about the experience (as interviewer *and* interviewee). Share your experiences of what it felt like to be the therapist and client, and whether each of you felt that you had really understood what was wanted from the therapist about your occupations.

Performance skills

Skills are the abilities individuals demonstrate in the actions they perform (American Occupational Therapy Association 2002). In the context of occupational performance analysis, these small units are the observable actions that follow on, one from another, unfold over time and form a process that ends in the completion of the desired task – the doing of an occupation. These small units of performance (or skills) must be observable and goal-directed as they are actions carried out in order to complete a specific task for a functional purpose (Fisher 2006). If they are not observable they may relate to underlying body structure impairment such as cognition (remembering) or praxis (motor planning). For example, when you observe Robert make a telephone call you will observe that he is gripping the receiver, lifting it to his ear, articulating a message, listening to the responses and terminating the conversation. Occupational performance analysis involves observing the person perform these small units of the task, noting the quality of each, the context in which it takes place as it unfolds over time.

Performance skills are divided into three taxonomies: motor skills, process skills, and communication and social interaction skills (American Occupational Therapy Association 2002). Motor and process skills are derived from AMPS (Fisher 2005). Communication/interaction skills are derived from ACIS (Forsyth et al 1997, Forsyth, Lai & Keilhofner 1999). Social interaction skills are derived from the Evaluation of Social Interaction (ESI) (Fisher & Griswold 2008). These skills are listed in Tables 13.2, 13.3 and 13.4.[1]

Performance skills can be described and categorised in multiple ways (AOTA 2008). This chapter considers motor skills, process skills, communication and social interaction skills in the context of occupational performance analysis.

---

[1]In the second edition of the Occupational Therapy Practice Framework (American Occupational Therapy Association 2002) performance skills were modified to broaden skill categories to include sensory/perceptual, motor/praxis, emotional regulation and cognition. These categories relate more to body functions (motor, sensory, cognitive functions for example) and capacities (degree of grip strength, range of motion for example) than to observable performance skills and relate to language used in many generic standardised evaluations. As many of the items in these categories are not observable or goal directed they are not considered here as 'skills' in the context of occupational performance analysis.

Motor skills

Motor skills are described as the observable, goal-directed actions that a person carries out during the performance of a daily living task in order to move themselves or the task objects (Fisher 2005). These skills pertain to positioning, stabilising and aligning the body in relation to the task; obtaining and holding objects using one or more body parts in a way that supports task performance; moving the entire body or body part(s) in space or when interacting with task objects; and sustaining effort throughout the task performance (American Occupational Therapy Association 2002). Let us consider motor skills in the context of Sarah brushing her hair (motor skills in *italics* – see Table 13.2). We observe:

> Sarah *reaching* for and *gripping* the brush, *lifting* it to her hair, and *moving* the brush over her scalp. She also sits (or stands) without falling (*stabilises*) and *positions* herself in front of the mirror so that she can see. While *manipulating* the brush handle in her hand she brushes and using enough pressure – but not too much – she pulls the brush through her hair (*calibrates*) at the right speed (*paces*).

Process skills

Fisher (2005) states that process skills are described as the observable actions of performance a person does to:

a. logically sequence actions of task performance over time

b. select and use appropriate tools and materials

c. adapt performance when problems are encountered.

These skills pertain to sustaining effort and attention throughout task performance; seeking and using task-related knowledge; beginning, continuing, logically ordering and completing actions and steps; organising task spaces and objects; and anticipating, correcting and learning from the consequences of errors that arise during task performance (American Occupational Therapy Association 2002). Let us consider process skills in the context of Andrew cleaning his car (process skills in *italics* – see Table 13.2), we observe:

> Andrew *choosing* a bucket and sponge (or hose), *using* hot, soapy water to clean all the

Table 13.2 Performance skills: motor and process (Fisher 2005[1], Fisher 2006)

Motor skills

Body positions

Stabilises	Maintains an upright sitting or standing position while moving through the task environment or interacting with task objects such that there is no evidence of momentary propping or loss of balance that affects performance.
Aligns	Sustains an upright sitting or standing position, as required during the task performance, such that there is no evidence of persistent propping, leaning or loss of balance that affects the ongoing task performance.
Positions	Positions body, arms or wheelchair in relation to task objects (i.e. not too close or far away) as required for efficient arm movements during task performance.

Obtaining and holding objects

Reaches	Extends the arm, and when appropriate bends the trunk, to effectively place objects that are out of reach, includes skillfully using a reaching device to obtain task objects.
Bends	Actively flexes, rotates or twists the trunk in a manner and direction appropriate to the task, as when bending to pick up a task object from the floor or to sit down in a chair.
Grips	Pinches or grasps task objects such that the task object does not slip, e.g. from between the person's fingers, from between the teeth.
Manipulates	Uses dextrous grasp and release patterns, isolated finger movements, and coordinated in-hand manipulation patterns when interacting with small task objects, e.g. difficulty manipulating buttons when buttoning, difficulty manipulating a pencil when writing.
Coordinates	Uses two or more body parts together to stabilise and manipulate task objects during bilateral motor tasks, such as when holding a jar with one hand (or between the knees) and removing the lid with the other hand.

Moving self and objects

Moves	Pushes or pulls task objects along a supporting surface, pulls to open or pushes to close doors and drawers, or pushes on wheels to propel a wheelchair.
Lifts	Raises or lifts task objects, including lifting an object from one place to another, but without ambulating or moving from one place to another.
Walks	Ambulates on level surfaces and changes direction while walking without shuffling the feet, lurching, instability, propping or using assistive devices (cane, walker, wheelchair) during the task performance.
Transports	Carries task objects from one place to another while walking, seated in a wheelchair or using a walker.
Calibrates	Regulates or grades the force, speed and extent of movement when interacting with task objects, e.g. not too much and not too little, pushing a door with enough force to close it but not too much that it bounces open.
Flows	Uses smooth and fluid arm and wrist movements when interacting with task objects.

Energy

Endures	Persists and completes the task without obvious evidence of physical fatigue, pausing to rest, or stopping to *catch one's breath*.
Paces	Maintains a consistent and effective rate or tempo of performance throughout the performance of actions and steps of the entire task.

Table 13.2 Performance skills: motor and process (Fisher 2005[1], Fisher 2006)—cont'd

Process skills

Sustaining performance

Paces[2]	Maintains a consistent and effective rate or tempo of performance throughout the performance of actions and steps of the entire task.
Attends	Maintains focus on the task performance such that the person does not look away from what he or she is doing, thus interrupting the ongoing task progression.
Heeds	Uses goal-directed task actions that are focused towards carrying out and completing a specified task, e.g. the outcome originally agreed on – to make a cup of hot instant coffee for one person.

Applying task knowledge

Chooses	Selects necessary and appropriate type and number of tools and materials for the task, includes choosing the tools and materials that the person said they would choose prior to initiating the task.
Uses	Employs tools and materials as they are intended, e.g. uses a knife to cut and spread but not to stir food; and in a reasonable (including hygienic) fashion.
Handles	Supports, stabilises and holds tools and materials in an appropriate manner, protecting them from damage, slipping, moving or falling.
Inquires	Seeks needed verbal or written information by asking questions or reading directions or labels; does not ask for information where the person has a prior awareness of the answer.

Temporal organisation

Initiates	Starts or begins the next action or step without hesitation.
Continues	Performs single, sustained actions or action sequences without unnecessary interruptions or pauses so that once the action has started, e.g. filling the cup with water, the person continues on until the action or step is completed (the cup is filled).
Sequences	Performs steps in an effective or logical order for efficient use of time or energy and with an absence of randomness or lack of logic in the ordering of steps, or inappropriate repetition of steps (washing the same cup twice when it is already clean).
Terminates	Brings to completion single actions or single steps without inappropriate persistence (continuing to sweep the same piece of floor long after all the dirt has been swept up) or premature cessation (stopping sweeping the floor before all the dirt has been swept up).

Space and objects

Searches/ locates	Looks for and locates tools and materials in a logical manner, both within and beyond the immediate environment, including not asking where task objects are located before looking for them (provided the person was aware before beginning the task where tools and materials are located).
Gathers	Collects together needed or misplaced tools and materials in a logical manner including: collecting related tools and materials into the same workspace; collecting and replacing materials that have spilled, fallen or been misplaced.
Organises	Logically positions or spatially arranges tools and materials in an orderly fashion including: in a single workspace; between multiple appropriate workspaces, in order to facilitate ease of task performance, e.g. the workspace is not too crowded or too spread out.
Restores	Puts away tools and materials in appropriate places; closes or seals containers and covering where appropriate; restores immediate workspace(s) to original condition (including wiping up any spills or saving work on a computer before closing the program).
Navigates	Modifies the movement pattern of the arm, body or wheelchair to manoeuvre around obstacles that are encountered in the course of moving through space such that undesirable contact with obstacles (knocking over, bumping into) is avoided.

Table 13.2 Performance skills: motor and process (Fisher 2005[1], Fisher 2006)—cont'd

Adapting performance	
Notices/ responds	Responds appropriately to: i) non-verbal task related cues (task object rolling or falling, liquid dripping, appliances heating) that provide feedback regarding task progression; ii) the spatial arrangement of objects one to another (alignment of objects during stacking, edges of laundry during folding); iii) notices and responds to cupboard doors and drawers that have been left open during task performance.
Adjusts	Changes working environments in anticipation of, or in response to, problems that arise; anticipates or responds to problems effectively by making some change: between workspaces by moving to a new workspace or bringing in or removing tools and materials from the present workspace; or in an environmental condition (turning a tap on or off or a temperature up or down).
Accommodates	Modifies actions or the location of objects within the workspace, in anticipation of, or response to problems that might arise; anticipates or responds to problems effectively by changing the method with which one is performing an action sequence; changing the manner in which one interacts with or handles tools and materials already in the workspace; asking for assistance when appropriate or needed.
Benefits	Anticipates and prevents undesirable circumstances or problems from recurring or persisting; includes responding appropriately to verbal cues intended to lead to correction of errors.

[1]The ordering of Motor and Process skills is in line with Fisher's most recent publication (2005) and differs slightly from Table 2 in the Occupational Therapy Practice Framework (2002)

[2]Paces is both a motor skill and a process skill but only needs to be acknowledged once based on the person's overall rate or tempo of performance

bodywork without being distracted (*attends*), and *noticing/responding* to the dirt as he begins (*initiates*) washing the front of the car. He *continues* cleaning until all the dirt is removed in this area before moving to the next (adjacent) area as he logically (*sequences*) washes the whole car and stops (*terminates*) when each area is clean. When his bucket is empty he *notices* and makes an appropriate *response*, going to the tap (*adjusts*) and refilling the bucket (accommodates). His task is complete when the entire car is clean (heeds).

Communication/interaction skills

Communication and social interaction skills are observable operations used to communicate intentions and needs and coordinate social behaviour (Forsyth et al 1999). Fisher & Griswold (2008) define social interaction skills as *observable actions of social behaviour* that occur within the ongoing stream of performance that occurs within the context of engagement in an occupation that involves social interaction (i.e. a social exchange)(see Table 13.3). The *Evaluation of Social Interaction* (ESI) was designed to assess the quality of social interaction as

the person engages in *real* interactions, with intended purposes stated by the person and with social partners with whom the person would typically need or want to interact (Fisher & Griswold 2008). Communication and social interaction skills are listed in Table 13.4 and are likely to be an essential element of any occupational performance analysis where the person has difficulty with social interactions of any kind. Let us consider communication and social interaction skills in the context of Sarah purchasing a camera (communication/interaction skills in *italics* – see Table 13.4). We observe:

Sarah enters the store to purchase a digital camera (*manoeuvres*). She catches the eye of a salesperson (*gazes*) and seeks out assistance (*orients*). She says hello (*speaks*) and explains what she is looking for (*engage, articulates*). The salesperson moves towards the camera cabinet (*gestures*), and she follows (*postures*). She actively listens (*expresses*), discusses camera features (*converses, focuses*), and requests more information (*asks*) when she does not understand. Sometimes she does not engage in conversation but is fully present to what is happening (*respects*) while the salesperson

Table 13.3 Performance skills: Social interaction (Fisher & Griswold 2008)

Social interaction skills

Initiating and terminating social interaction

Approaches/starts:	greeting and/or initiating interaction
Concludes/disengages:	ending interaction

Producing social interaction

Produces speech:	communicating using speech, or signed/augmentative messages
Gesticulates:	using gestures to communicate
Speaks fluently:	speaking tempo

Physically supporting social interaction

Turns towards:	turning body and face towards social partner
Looks:	making eye contact
Places self:	keeping personal space and distance
Touches:	making physical contact with social partner
Regulates:	controlling impulses and behaviours

Shaping content of social interaction

Questions:	requesting information or opinion
Replies:	providing relevant response & detail to questions & comments
Discloses:	sharing personal information, opinions & feelings about oneself & others
Expresses emotion:	displaying affect and emotions
Disagrees:	disagreeing with social partner's stated suggestions or point of view
Thanks:	acknowledging information, compliments, help or material objects

Maintaining flow of social interaction

Transitions:	changing topic of conversation
Times response:	responding not too soon or not too late, interrupting
Times duration:	sending messages that are too long or too short
Takes turns:	dominating, being dominated

Verbally supporting social interaction

Matches language:	uses tone of voice, dialect, level of language appropriate to social partner
Clarifies:	making sure social partner follows conversation
Acknowledges/encourages:	responding to social partner, encouraging continued interaction
Empathises:	supporting social partner's feelings and experiences

Adapting social interaction

Heeds:	staying with the intended purpose of social interaction
Accommodates:	anticipating and preventing problems during social interaction
Benefits:	demonstrating social interaction skill problems that persist

Table 13.4 Performance skills: communication and interaction (Forsyth, Lai & Keilhofner 1999, Forsyth et al 1997, American Occupational Therapy Association 2002)

Physicality – pertains to using the physical body when communicating within an occupation

Contacts	Makes physical contact with others
Gazes	Uses eyes to communicate and interact with others
Gestures	Uses movements of the body to indicate, demonstrate or add emphasis
Manoeuvres	Moves one's body in relation to others
Orients	Directs one's body in relation to others and/or occupational forms
Postures	Assumes physical positions
Presents	Hygiene and dress

Information exchange – refers to giving and receiving information within an occupation

Articulates	Produces clear, understandable speech
Asserts	Directly expresses desires, refusals and requests
Asks	Requests factual or personal information
Converses	Talks so as to flow with interaction/conversation
Engages	Initiates interactions
Expresses	Displays affect/attitude
Modulates	Employs volume and inflection in speech
Shares	Gives out factual information or personal information
Speaks	Makes oneself understood through the use of words, phrases, sentences
Sustains	Keeps up social action or speech for appropriate durations

Relations – relates to maintaining appropriate relationships within an occupation

Collaborates	Coordinates one's actions with others towards a common end goal
Conforms	Follows implicit and explicit social norms
Focuses	Directs conversation and behaviour to ongoing social action
Relates	Assumes a manner of acting that tries to establish a rapport with others
Respects	Accommodates to other people's actions or requests

tries to meet her needs (*collaborates*) or receives cameras (*contacts*) to inspect (*respects*), and discusses more options (*shares, sustains*). Sometimes she distances herself from the salesperson by keeping her eyes downcast (*gazes*) and moving away from (orients) the camera cabinet. She makes her decision (*asserts*) and moves to the sales counter (*manoeuvres*) to pay. She takes out her purse (*presents*) and using her credit card (*collaborates*) completes the transaction

(*conforms*). At the end of the transaction she turns away from the counter (*orients*), says goodbye (*modulates*), and waves (*gestures*) as she leaves the store.

Fisher & Griswold (2008) point out that social interaction skills (like motor and process skills) should be observed and evaluated in the appropriate context (social interaction as it occurs during an occupation). In this way interactions that are difficult or problematic for the person will be observed in the naturalistic context (shopping or purchasing in the store). They also assert that this is what differentiates an occupational therapist's assessment from that of other professionals – the ability to observe the quality of the smallest units of performance (skills) as they unfold over time. If social interaction (and other) skills are assessed in contrived or 'test' situations using checklists of isolated components, than it is underlying body functions or person factors (articulation or vocalisation of sounds) that are recorded rather than social interaction *skills* during engagement in an occupation.

The unfolding of social interactions can be observed in a similar way to the unfolding of actions over time during the doing of a task. Fisher (2006) suggests a comparison of social interaction skills with the International Classification of Functioning Disability and Health (ICF) terminology and codes in the context of a communication exchange. In Sarah's interaction above we can also see links with the temporal organisation process skills: initiating, continuing, sequencing, and terminating the social interaction as a natural flow of steps or events:

- She initiates interactions using a range of appropriate strategies: eye contact, gestures, body language and speaking.

- She produces a variety of appropriate social interactions including speaking, expressing meaning, using body language and gestures appropriate to the social context.

- She maintains ongoing social interactions by looking at or turning towards or touching others appropriately, by placing herself at an appropriate distance and by controlling inappropriate behaviours.

- She shapes the content of the interaction by asking questions, providing answers, disclosing information, expressing emotion, difference of opinion and gratitude appropriately.

- She is able to maintain the flow of social interactions by sustaining conversations, changing topics, adding new ideas, and completing messages appropriately.

- She is able to time social interactions by responding and replying to messages without delays or hesitations, taking turns and timing responses with others.

- She is able to verbally support social interactions by using appropriate language,

clarifying or explaining messages, acknowledging responses, encouraging others, and demonstrating appreciation through verbal and physical responses.

- Finally she is able to terminate social interactions appropriately (Fisher 2006).

To gain a better understanding of performance skills work through Reflection 13.2.

Skills and capacities

When carrying out occupational performance analysis it is important to distinguish between performance skills (motor, process, and communication/social interaction skills) and underlying body functions (musculoskeletal, neurologic, cardiovascular, and cognitive) and body structures (muscles, joints, skin, eyes, voice, etc). Performance skills focus on what the person is doing, whereas body functions (capacities) focus on what the person's body is doing.

When we carry out occupational performance analysis we are able to observe motor skills (skills pertaining to moving oneself and tasks objects); process skills (skills pertaining to organising and sequencing events over time, and preventing/overcoming problems as they occur during the task performance); and, when interacting with others, communication/social interaction skills (skills pertaining to social interactions and intentions). We can observe Emily grasping her sock, searching for and locating her shoe and asking her mother for help when she cannot tie her laces, but we cannot see the functions of the brain – memory, cognition, emotions. These are related to the mind-brain-body performance sub system and cannot be and observed. When Emily is searching for and cannot find her shoe or cannot open her sock to arrange it on her foot we can only observe the outcome of these cognitive functions and motor planning not the actual body functions. This distinction is a very important one for occupational therapists.

An occupation-focused approach places the person and their chosen occupations at the centre of the analysis process. By observing an individual actually carrying out occupations (and social interactions) of choice, performance skills (motor, process and social interaction) are directly observed. Moreover, when the person is observed performing occupations in his/her preferred context (physical, social and cultural) the interaction of person, environment, and occupation can readily be seen. The

---

Reflection 13.2

Performance skills identification

Think about a short activity that you have performed today, for example making a drink, making a telephone call or using your computer. Use this task to identify the performance skills (motor, process, communication/social interaction) that you used to perform the activity:

1. List the steps of the task in the order that they occurred.

   Remember *a step* is a series of actions that follow one on from another that when put together form the entire task. For example when Emily was putting on her socks and shoes she had to find her sock, open it up, spatially arrange it over her foot, pull the sock onto her foot and so on (see Table 13.1).

2. Next select one of the steps and list all the actions (skills that relate to motor, process, social interaction) that were required for this step. Remember that an *action* is the smallest unit of occupational performance analysis and is discrete and purposeful. It is always a verb ... a 'doing' word (ending with *ing*) that describes what is happening now. Using your selected task, choose one of the steps and list all the skills (actions) you needed to perform that step. For example if brushing your teeth, one step might be to 'put toothpaste on the toothbrush' which requires the actions of gripp*ing* the toothpaste tube, manipulat*ing* the cap to remove it, squeez*ing* with sufficient force, notic*ing* the amount of

toothpaste, stopp*ing* when there is enough etc (see Table 13.1). (If you were alone there will be no social interaction skills observed for this step).

You may also need to distinguish between the task (to clean), the step of 'brush teeth' and the action of 'brush*ing*'. The step describes what is done (brush teeth) but the action denotes that something is happening and that you are an active participant (brushing).

Make your own list of actions first and then refer to the list of performance skills (motor, process, social interaction) in Tables 13.2, 13.3 and 13.4. You might want to add further actions that you had not thought about.

3. Using a study partner: observe them perform a very short and simple activity and make notes on what you observe. Do not be judgemental about what is done or how it is done; simply try to record everything that you see – actions over time. Sit down with your partner, list the major steps (try and limit these to 10) and then the actions for one or two selected steps. Using the performance skills in Tables 13.2, 13.3 and 13.4 might help. Remember to only discuss *what* was done and do not engage in conversation at this stage about *how* it was done – the order of the steps for example may be different to how you would order steps but we discuss this later (performance patterns).

---

person is central to the assessment process and the focus is on the doing of tasks.

When occupational performance analysis is based on actual performance in context there is rarely a need to assess the underlying body-function capacities. The occupational therapist is able to observe the quality of performance as well as challenges presented by physical, social, cultural and other environments. There is no need to make inferences (or guesses) about the person's strengths or limitations as they can be seen in context. Further, performance analysis (as opposed to activity analysis) does not rely on the identification of underlying capacities and deficits as it is focused on what is done. Most available assessment tools begin by focusing on body functions and body structures, including assessment of memory, behaviours, hand function or perception, are conducted by appropri-

ately trained professionals using specific standardised tests of impairment and incorporate a bottom-up approach. By conducting occupational performance analysis first in the context of what the client wants and needs to do, results that focus on performance issues can be used to plan and implement appropriate occupation-focused interventions.

Performance patterns: Roles, habits and routines

Having already considered performance areas and performance skills, next we need to consider how performance patterns might influence the doing of occupations. Performance patterns are the *way* that tasks are carried out and relate to activities that are habitual or routine (American Occupational Therapy

Association 2002). The performance of occupations takes place in context. What we do and why we do it is dependent on our personal, social, and societal roles and expectations.

Role

A role is defined as a set of behaviours expected by society and shaped by culture (American Occupational Therapy Association 2008) or the function or behaviour expected of a person occupying a particular position (Hagedorn 2000, p.311), for example, the formal role of a chairperson on a committee or the informal role of a parent within a family. Individuals participate in many different roles: student, worker, parent, child, homemaker, etc., and behave in different ways according to whom they are interacting with (behaviours with a friend are often different to behaviours with an employer) as well as societal and cultural expectations. Thus, particular roles may be internalised and associated with the behaviour expected by cultures or societies. An expectation of how one should behave: a parent's need to be a wage earner to provide for the family or a student may study diligently to pass an examination.

The roles that we assume say much about who we are and how we see ourselves, it is usual for us only to assume roles that we want and need to do and those that would be expected by the society and culture in which we live. These are important considerations when working with people. We have seen already that occupations have a purpose, but a person's role gives the occupations meaning. For example, the purpose of preparing a meal is to provide bodily sustenance. However, the meaning of meal preparation (and cooking) will vary depending on the role, for example, a working parent providing a meal for the family, or a single person cooking for him or herself or a host/hostess preparing food for a celebration dinner for friends. Although the outcome will be similar (a meal on the table), the intrinsic meaning (and enjoyment) of the occupation will vary depending on the role. The type of occupations we engage in will also be different depending on how we see our roles within a social, cultural and societal context. To gain a better understanding of performance roles work through Reflection 13.3.

Habits and routines

Habits involve learned ways of doing occupations that have developed through repeated experiences and unfold automatically (Keilhofner 1995), we do

Reflection 13.3

Performance of roles

1. Think about your life now and list all the roles that you currently do that are important to you. Next think about yourself as a child, list all the roles that were important to you then.

2. Compare your lists and note similarities and differences. What are the main differences and why? How have your roles changed over time and how might they change in the future as you begin to age?

3. Think about an older person you know quite well (it could be a grandparent), list the roles that they carry out on a regular basis and are important to them. Next, talk to this person and ask them about the roles that they value and try to find out why. How are their roles different to yours now and when you were a child? What do they do that you do not and why?

4. Select a role that you particularly enjoy and an occupation associated with that role and list ways that your behaviours may differ depending on who you are interacting with.

these things so frequently that we do not have to think about them. Routines are established sequences of occupations that provide a structure for daily life (AOTA 2008). Routines are *what* we do, whereas habits are the *way* we do them. Habits and routines are observable behaviours repeated at predicable intervals such as eating dinner, going to bed, and getting up. They are often organised by physical context such as day and night, sleep and wake, and provide stability in our lives, for example, our morning dressing routines or the route we drive to and from work each day. Keilhofner believes that habits guide our behaviour through repeated experience of them over time and within a context (or environment). Rituals are symbolic actions with spiritual, cultural or social meaning that shape the identity of an individual (AOTA 2008).

Segal (2004) described routines as patterned behaviours that have instrumental goals and rituals as a form of symbolic communication. She describes routines as giving life order and rituals giving it meaning, for example, mealtime rituals are not just about providing nourishment, but provide opportunities for socialisation, conflict resolution, and determination of power relationships. Segal (2004) interviewed 40 families about their daily routines and rituals. She found aspects of family organisation rich with symbolic and affective meaning imparting a sense of identity, belonging, and continuity across generations. Routines and rituals were so embedded in the fabric of family life that a simple intervention may require a whole family to change its routine thus also having to shift its identity. She asserts that even minor changes recommended to mundane family rituals is the most common reason for such interventions to fail.

This is also important when working with people as habits and routines may have been disrupted by illness or impairment and are often the first kinds of occupations that individuals want to re-establish, for example the morning routine of washing and dressing. A person who has recently lost roles or routines is familiar enough with them to understand what is wanted from them by an occupational therapist. Showing someone their clothes or taking them to the bathroom is a powerful means of communicating with them about a shared concept: their morning washing and dressing routine. Engaging people in familiar and regular occupations means connecting them with socially recognisable routines and roles. At times of change, especially disruption to habituation, individuals may feel confused or even disoriented without the familiar routines that shape the day, this is also a powerful tool for occupational therapists to be able to re-engage with them, provided of course that time has been taken to discover and understand these habits, roles and routines in the context of the person's life world. To gain a better understanding of performance patterns work through Reflection 13.4.

The occupational style that each of us uses is important only to ourselves; there is no right *way* to dress yourself, for example, only that clothes should be put on according to their purpose (underclothes go underneath outer clothes, socks go on feet, etc.). The method and ordering of steps each of us uses (process) may be different but the outcome will be the same. When working with people we often teach them new methods or make modifications to their environment without considering performance patterns and existing internalised routines and rituals. The older the person the harder it is to change these internalised routines. People with new impairments or cognitive decline will find it almost impossible to change and sometimes this difficulty is interpreted as stubbornness or 'non-compliance'. Understanding how hard it is for all of us to change the method of doing when we are often not even aware of our own

Reflection 13.4

Performance patterns – Habits and routines

1. Together with your study partner select and agree a familiar occupation or routine that you both perform regularly every day, for example making a cup or tea or coffee, getting in and out of the bathtub, etc. On your own perform this routine and make detailed notes of the order of the steps and the essential factors that must be done for the occupation to be completed with satisfaction – you may always warm the teapot, or put the milk in first (or last).

2. Next ask your study partner to observe you do this routine and make detailed notes of what he/she observes (a personal care task such as getting in and out of the bathtub can be carried out with clothes/underwear on). Compare your lists and note similarities and differences, what did your partner note that you did not. Change roles and observe your study partner's routine and discuss the outcome, you may discover that you have habits you are not even aware of.

3. Next perform the routine the way that your partner did and in accordance to your partner's performance patterns. Your partner can help and direct you when you tend to default to your own occupational style. Discuss the following:
   a. To do this activity I had to change…..
      (physical, cognitive and behavioural aspects)
   b. During this activity I felt. …
   c. During this activity I thought. …
   d. During this activity I remembered. …
   e. I learned from this activity that. …

4. If you cannot do the above activity with a study partner try this activity instead: select one of your routines, one that is very familiar and you do at least daily, every day of the year. Now carry out this routine in a different way, you might consider only using your non-dominant hand to carry out this routine or changing the order of the steps. Write reflections following completion of this activity answering the same questions as in 3 (above).

performance patterns and habits is essential if we are to engage in a person-focused approach. A key feature of occupational therapy is not to be prescriptive of the ordering of the steps, rather to work *within* the existing habits, routines and rituals (including the culture and traditions) of the person so that the person is less likely to experience disruption in enacting familiar occupations. First it is essential that *you* as a therapist familiarise yourself with the usual performance patterns, routines and rituals (traditions) of this person before attempting to introduce new, less effortful or more energy efficient ways of working. Changing the way individuals perform their usual routines can totally disrupt their way of life leading to disappointment and eventual failure.

Performance contexts

Environments

The term 'context' refers to the numerous and different environments in which individuals and their families or carers perform their occupations and roles. The importance of the interaction between persons and environments has long been recognised by occupational therapists, for example the Person-Environment-Occupation model (Law et al 1996); Occupational Therapy Intervention Process Model (OTIPM) (Fisher 2005, 2009); the Person-Environment-Occupation-Performance model (Christiansen & Baum 2005). Keilhofner (1995) suggests that environments may potentially support or limit performance by offering opportunities, resources, demands, and constraints, depending on the values, interests and performance capacities of the person. The performance context can be seen from six differing perspectives: the physical, cultural, social, personal, temporal and virtual contexts (American Occupational Therapy Association 2008):

- Physical (natural and built) environments includes the spaces, tools and materials that are normally found in that context, for example a kitchen would normally include a sink with running water, cupboard units, appliances such as cooker and refrigerator and tools needed to prepare, cook and serve food and clean up afterwards.

- Cultural context would take into consideration the customs, beliefs, rituals and behaviours that would apply to occupations conducted within this environment. For example it is normal in some cultures for additional facilities or appliances to be present, two sinks needed for preparation of different foods, or a washing machine in a kitchen because of the plumbing arrangements for water. In other cultures a washing machine might only be located in a separate laundry or utility area. The way that spaces are used and the kinds of tools and materials in the environment will also

be affected by the culture of the person and the societal in which they live. For example different tools and utensils would be found in a Western or European kitchen to an Asian or African kitchen as the kinds of foods that are prepared and the cooking methods are different. Similarly, the type of bed and kinds of bedding will differ according to cultures and sleeping rituals. Bed-making practices also differ according to climate (hot and cold) and sleeping rituals. Societal values and traditions are especially important where occupations include social interactions, for example shaking hands when being introduced or understanding what should or should not be said in education, employment or social circumstances. Familiarity with one's own cultural norms does not necessarily provide an insight into variations in cultural and geographical differences.

- Social contexts include social, societal and population expectations and behaviours that surround the occupation. For example, environments will differ according to their purpose (work, family, church, and leisure) and social expectations (such as dress, behaviours and rules). If specific rules or obligations apply then the context may have to accommodate these, a sports centre would have changing rooms with gender-specific facilities, a church would have spaces, objects and symbols necessary and appropriate for religious acts, etc.

- Personal contexts including age, gender, educational and socio-economic factors that enable engagement in age-appropriate or other occupations, for example a kindergarten would require spaces and objects for pre-school children that support their engagement in occupations of play, rest and sleep.

- Temporal contexts place the occupation in a timeframe that has a past, present and future. Occupations unfold over time and can provide temporal barriers or resources, the key feature here is to note how the temporal environment changes during the course of an occupation rather than what changes for the *person*.

- Virtual contexts become more important in our society as occupations involve the use of technology. For example communication that occurs by virtual means such as internet, wireless or satellite communications, chat rooms, email etc., where there is an absence of physical contact. Such environments can support performance as in a home teleworker using computer, internet, and telephone to conduct business, or inhibit performance as in the case of an older adult with dementia who can no longer grasp the concept of a wireless alarm, and thus refuses to carry the call device.

The spiritual context is seen to reside within the individual (rather than the context) and is considered under person factors.

Christiansen & Baum (2005) identify environmental factors as intrinsic and related to the person, influenced by physiological, psychological and spiritual factors; or extrinsic and related to the physical and social environments. The environment is the *context* of performance, which can dynamically influence the meaning and outcome of task performance (Christiansen & Baum 2005, Dunn et al 1994, 2003, Fisher 2005, Law 1991). Extrinsic factors such as natural and built environments, technology, space, and objects can positively or negatively influence outcomes. The physical environment of a kitchen can enable wheelchair users by allowing them to work, socialise and interact with task objects, people and spaces. The familiarity of a kitchen may support or limit how well an older person with memory loss is able to search for and locate needed items, sequence steps logically over time or even be able to complete the task. In general, we assume that individuals will perform occupations better in a familiar environment, but for some individuals the home environment can impede their performance. Park et al (1994) found that only 50% of community-living older adults demonstrated significantly better activities of daily living process ability in their homes than in a clinic. However, Nygård and colleagues (1994) found that eight out of 19 subjects with suspected dementia performed better in the home and three performed better in the clinic environment. It is important, therefore, not to make assumptions about settings in which evaluations of occupational performance take place, but to be aware that context can and does have an impact. If occupational therapists have concerns about the impact of the environment then they should work with individuals in that environment.

Activity demands

The expression 'activity demands' refers to the specific features of an activity that influence the type and amount of effort and efficiency required to perform the activity. This includes task objects, spaces and people (social aspects) in the task environment, as well as taking into account the process (ordering and timing of steps) of the activity and the body function demands (Figure 13.1) (American Occupational Therapy Association 2008). We have already discussed in the previous section how the environment (physical, social and cultural, etc.) and the task objects can support or limit occupational performance. If you were to make a hot drink or a snack in an unfamiliar kitchen, your performance would probably be less efficient as you took longer to search for and find task objects and materials, had some difficulty using unfamiliar electrical equipment such as the kettle, toaster or microwave and had to develop new performance patterns in spaces that were different to those that you are used to. If you were to send an email from an unfamiliar computer or from an electronic, handheld device (such as a Blackberry™) you may need assistance to complete the activity because of unfamiliarity with the task objects. This is an important point to remember when we bring clients to an unfamiliar kitchen in a hospital or clinic setting or observe social interactions in contrived contexts. The physical spaces, tools and materials that support performance are often referred to as 'naturalistic'. According to Fisher (2006, p. 380), naturalistic means that task performance occurs in an 'ecologically appropriate environment'. This usually means that it is the person's usual environment or is an environment in which they are familiar and are able to use tools and materials that they would typically use and be with the people that they would typically be with. A naturalistic environment, however, does not automatically support performance. Increasing age, frailty, or physical, sensory, mental or cognitive decline may also negatively increase the demands of familiar activities even in a naturalistic environment. To gain a better understanding of activity demands work through Reflection 13.5.

Person factors

While activity demands include external factors such as objects, spaces and people within the environment, person factors are internal and include specific abilities, characteristics and beliefs (American Occupational Therapy Association 2008). Person factors incorporate the values, beliefs

Reflection 13.5

Activity demands

1. First select a familiar task that you do on a regular (daily) basis: showering, walking the dog, sending an email, driving your car to work. Carry out this activity in your usual way and in the usual environment (your own bathroom, kitchen, office, car or route). Consider the following activity demands:
   - How does the size and arrangement of spaces and fixtures support or limit your performance of this task? (Space demands: size of the room [or car], available spaces [large park or small urban circle], worktops, light, ventilation, placement of shelves/storage units, accessibility and visibility of needed fixtures – sockets, switches, lights, mirrors, pedals, etc.).
   - How do the tools, materials and equipment support or limit the process of carrying out this activity? (Objects and their properties: position, weight/size, appropriate tools/utensils, equipment – electrical appliances, materials [food, cosmetics, cleaning], screen and keyboard, mirrors, fixtures, gates, posts, dog leash, etc.).
   - How are social and cultural interactions supported or limited? (Social structures, societal expectations, cultural rules, sharing, conversations, participation by others.) If this is a solitary activity how does the environment support or limit appropriate interaction (access, privacy, safety, etc.).
   - How does the environment support the task process (the way you carry out the task)? (sequencing/ordering of steps, route for driving/walking, time factor, personal/individual requirements, adaptability, etc.).
   - Are there any skills (motor, process, social interaction) that would be positively or negatively impacted? (positioning, reaching, bending, walking, enduring, sequencing, searching/locating, organising, navigating, answering a question, etc.).

2. Carry out the same activity using an unfamiliar environment or route (another kitchen/bathroom, a rental car or friend's car if appropriate) and carry out a similar analysis of the activity demands. Make notes on the factors that support or limit your own occupational performance in these spaces using these tools and materials. After carrying out the activity in an unfamiliar environment make notes on the following and share the outcome with your study partner:
   a. In the different environment I felt. …
   b. In the different environment I thought. …
   c. In the different environment I remembered. …
   d. I learned from conducting the activity in a different environment that. …

and spirituality of the person, together with body functions and body structures as defined by the International Classification of Functioning, Disability and Health [ICF] (World Health Organization 2001). While beliefs relate to cognitive content, values are principles, standards or qualities considered important by the person (American Occupational Therapy Association 2008) and might include personal integrity and commitment to the family for example. Spirituality includes a person's search for purpose of meaning in life (American Occupational Therapy Association 2008) and as such guides their actions towards a greater purpose beyond the personal. Like routines and rituals, values and beliefs can be so embedded in the fabric of the person's identity that a simple intervention may result in a disruption to their way of life that is so great that it is not possible for the person to change.

The ICF was developed to provide an international language and framework that can be used to describe and classify a person's capacities as well as their health condition (World Health Organization 2001). Codes that list activity and participation are used to classify nine areas that a person might engage in (performance areas). Codes that list functioning and impairment are used to classify eight body function areas and eight body structure areas. Each area can be influenced by contextual or environmental factors as well as personal factors (Table 13.5).

Body functions are the physiological functions of the body systems and include mental and sensory; neuro-musculoskeletal; cardiovascular, immunological, and respiratory; voice/speech; digestive, and endocrine; and genito-urinary and skin functions. Body structures include the anatomical parts of the body such as organs, limbs and their components that support body functions (World Health Organization 2001) (Table 13.6).

In terms of occupational performance analysis the ICF provides a useful classification of person factors in relation to impairment of body functions. While occupational performance analysis is unique to occupational therapy and relates to breaking down an occupation into its smallest component parts (performance skills), the ICF relates to the impairment of body functions and/or body structures and is a universal classification of impairments as they relate to activities and participation in general. This is an important distinction, as the overlap of terminology and language can be confusing especially if it is used interchangeably.

Table 13.5 Structure of the International Classification of Functioning, Disability and Health as it relates to the Occupational Therapy Practice Framework (www.who.int/classification/icf), reproduced with permission

Activities and participation	Functioning and disability		Contextual factors	
Activities and participation	Body functions	Body structures	Environmental factors	Personal factors
Learning and applying knowledge	Mental functions	Nervous system	Products and technology	Age, gender, race
General tasks and demands	Sensory functions and pain	Eyes, ears, tongue, nasal, sensation	Natural and man-made environments	Lifestyle
Communication	Voice and speech functions	Lips, tongue, pharynx, larynx		Habits
Mobility	Cardiovascular/ haematological immunological, respiratory	Cardiovascular and respiratory structures	Support and relationships	Social background
Self care				Education
Domestic life	Digestive, metabolic, endocrine	Digestive tract and related structures	Attitudes	Religion
Interpersonal interactions and relationships	Genito-urinary function	Genito-urinary and reproductive	Service systems policies	Life events
Major life areas (education and employment)	Neuro-musculoskeletal movement-related	Joints, muscle power, tone; structures of the head and neck; shoulder and upper limb; pelvis and lower limb; trunk		
Community, social, civic life	Skin and related functions	Skin, hair, nails		

Table 13.6 International Classification of Functioning, Disability & Health (ICF): Body Functions (www.who.int/classification/icf), reproduced with permission

Mental functions (including affective, cognitive and perceptual)

Consciousness	Level of consciousness, arousal
Orientation	To person, place, time, self and others
Intellectual	Retardation, dementia
Energy and drive functions	Motivation, impulse control, interests, values
Sleep	Quality, quantity, sleep patterns
Attention	Sustained and divided
Memory	Retrospective, prospective
Emotional functions	Appropriate range and regulation of emotions, self control
Perceptual functions	Visuospatial, body schema, sensory interpretation
Higher cognitive functions	Executive functions of judgment, concept formation, time management, problem solving, decision-making
Psychomotor functions	Experience of self, regulation of motor response to psychological events, motor planning
Language functions	Receive and express self through spoken/written/sign language
Calculation functions	Ability to calculate (add and subtract, etc.)

Table 13.6 International Classification of Functioning, Disability & Health (ICF): Body Functions (www.who.int/classification/icf), reproduced with permission—cont'd

Sensory functions and pain

Seeing functions	Visual acuity, visual field
Hearing functions	Responding to sounds, pitch and volume
Vestibular functions	Balance
Gustatory functions	Taste including smell
Touch functions	Sensitivity to touch, ability to discriminate
Proprioceptive functions	Kinaesthesia, joint position sense
Pain functions	Pain sensation – dull/stabbing/ache

Voice and speech functions

Voice functions	Articulate and produce sounds, words and communication

Functions of the cardiovascular, haematological, immunological, respiratory systems

Heart	Pulse rate, physical endurance, stamina, fatigue
Blood pressure	Hypotension, hypertension, postural hypotension
Haematological	Blood
Immunological	Allergies, hypersensitivity
Respiration	Breathing, rate, rhythm, depth

Functions of the digestive, metabolic and endocrine systems

Digestive/defecation	Food intake/output
Weight maintenance	Diet, obesity
Endocrine glands	Hormonal changes

Genito-urinary and reproductive functions

Urination functions	Fluid intake/output, micturition
Sexual functions	Libido, pregnancy, birth

Neuromusculoskeletal and movement related functions

Mobility of joint	Range of motion, postural alignment, joint stability/mobility
Muscle power	Strength, endurance
Muscle tone	Degree of tone, spasticity, flaccidity
Movement functions	Hand-eye/foot coordination, bilateral integration, walking patterns and gait
Involuntary movements	Motor reflexes, righting reactions, tics, tremors, motor perseveration

Functions of the skin and related structures

Skin functions	Presence/absence of wounds, cuts, abrasions; healing
Hair and nail functions	Protective, appearance

Application of occupational performance analysis

We have discussed thus far that the terminology and framework for occupational performance analysis are based on a number of factors including the Occupational Therapy Practice Framework (American Occupational Therapy Association 2002, 2008). In this context the person is placed at the centre of the process so that occupational performance analysis can support participation of the individual in his or her personal, social, and other appropriate life contexts. The occupation therapy process usually begins with an evaluation of the person's occupational needs in order to understand better his/her problems and concerns, in the context of his/her participation in a full and meaningful life. Problems and concerns are addressed in evaluation and intervention (American Occupational Therapy Association 2008), but the first part of the process is information gathering.

Thus, the first stage of the occupational performance analysis process usually begins with an interview between the therapist and the user of occupational therapy services. A range of information is exchanged relating to the person and his/her occupations in order to understand his/her skills and abilities, health and social status, personal and family circumstances, and participation in family and societal roles. Nelson & Thomas (2003) believe that gathering information involves two elements: verbal or self-reported information usually gathered by talking to the person or their care-givers (indirect assessment); and non-verbal information gathered through observation of a task (direct assessment). Nelson & Thomas state that what is said can be quite different to what is observed and, therefore, observation is essential. Throughout the information-gathering and observation processes the therapist begins to develop what Fisher (2005, 2009) refers to as therapeutic rapport, so that observations feel natural and appropriate.

The interview should begin with a brief occupational history as this information will guide thinking about the occupations, roles, daily life patterns, values, interests, and needs that are of importance to the person. According to the American Occupational Therapy Association (2008) an occupational profile is a summary of information that describes the person's occupational history and experiences, patterns of daily life, interests, values and needs. It is designed to gain an understanding of the background and perspective of the person. Questions that are useful might include: who is this person, what is important to them, what do they want and need to do, who are the important people in their life; and in what contexts do they live their personal, productive and playful lives? Hersch et al (2005) suggests preparing a brief occupational profile as this information can be used throughout all occupational therapy interactions to help maintain focus on the needs of the person. Clark (1993) noted that time spent listening to an individual's story is not only therapeutic for the person but reveals a depth of information about their lived experiences of health as well as illness. In the context of occupational therapy, both are important. While the reality of today's health care practice may preclude time spent in lengthy narratives with individuals, it is nonetheless important to put aside the time to listen and understand who this person is, their priorities and aspirations for the future.

The next step in the process is an observation of the person performing occupations that are meaningful and relevant to them. This evaluation can be formal or informal but should focus on actual performance of an occupation chosen by the person and performed in a context that is naturalistic and appropriate. An occupational performance analysis can be performed during this observation in order to identify assets, problems or potential limitations of occupational performance. Performance skills and patterns are observed, as well as the impact of activity demands and personal, physical and social contexts. The focus here is on occupational performance and the *doing* of the occupation and not the limitations of body functions or body structures. Formal, standardised occupation-focused assessments might include AMPS (Fisher 2005), the Assessment of Communication and Interactions Skills (ACIS) (Forsythe et al 1997) or the Evaluation of Social Interaction (ESI) (Fisher & Griswold 2008). These evaluation tools use direct observation of performance skills which can be recorded and documented in a structured and standardised manner. Performance skills include motor skills, process skills, communication and social interaction skills. Tables 13.2, 13.3 and 13.4 provide a description of the performance skills.

Following observations of the person performing meaningful occupations, the occupational therapist draws on his or her knowledge and experience of analysing occupation together with professional reasoning skills to perform an analysis of the observed performance. Crepeau (2003), states that practitioners analyse occupations using theoretical and practical knowledge and perspectives. Occupational performance analysis is a highly skilled and dynamic process that cannot be separated from the observation of the performance or the person who performed it, or his or her needs in a specific context. Highlighting strengths and limitations of performance skills and patterns, contexts, and activity demands are all integral to this process.

As strengths and limitations in performance skills, patterns, contexts, activity demands and person factors are identified, goals and outcomes then can be discussed and developed with the individual. This, in turn, leads to the development of an intervention plan which is implemented and evaluated, again using occupational performance analysis at a later date. At this stage the analysis of occupational performance is completed.

In Practice Scenario 13.1 we observe Mary (an occupational therapist) implementing a top-down approach with David, a newly referred user of the community occupational therapy stroke service.

Practice Scenario 13.1 David

Mary (occupational therapist) interviewed David at home, with his wife (Ellen) present. He is 66 years old and 6 weeks have passed since his cerebrovascular accident (CVA). Following 4 weeks of rehabilitation in the local stroke unit he has returned home to their small 2-bedroomed bungalow in which he and Ellen have lived for the past 8 years. He is able to carry out most personal-care tasks independently and safely but needs supervision with showering. He is not able to go outside unassisted. He has not yet attempted any domestic or meal-preparation tasks, but he would like to be able to make his own breakfast and other simple snacks, wash the dishes and help with laundry tasks. Before his stroke David helped with heavier household chores, and kept the garden neat and tidy. He would like to return to doing some of these tasks so as not to be a burden on Ellen.

After some discussion, Mary observed David make cereal and a glass of juice and handwash the dishes. She used the AMPS as her standardised assessment tool and was able to use information from the two AMPS evaluations (cereal and juice; handwashing the dishes) to analyse David's occupational performance. This provides the following information with regard to motor and process performance

skills. Definitions of these terms can be found in Table 13.2.

Performance skills

Body position: David had some difficulty maintaining an upright posture while standing at the sink, he propped on the counter top while standing and walking (*stabilises*). He also had some difficulty *positioning* his body effectively at the refrigerator and lower cupboard units so that he could obtain objects from the lower shelves.

Obtaining and holding objects: David was able to *reach* for and *bend* his trunk to obtain objects with minimal effort. He had weak grasp (*grips*) in his left hand making it difficult to hold and *manipulate* small objects such as cutlery, especially when he coordinated two hands together, as when opening the juice container and screwing the top back onto the milk container (*coordinates*).

Moving self and objects: David was able to open doors and drawers without undue effort (*moves*), but used two hands to *lift* heavier objects such as the milk container and teapot (when washing the dishes). He walked safely using one walking stick (*walks*), but this impeded his ability to *transport* items in the kitchen as he could not carry more than one object at once. Stiffness of movement of his left hand and wrist (*flows*) caused difficulty while washing dishes and his ability to grade the force of movement (*calibrates*) when placing objects on the countertops or dish drainer.

Sustaining performance (motor): David's performance slowed over time (*paces*) and, due to physical fatigue, he asked to sit down during the second task observation (*endures*).

Sustaining performance (process): David maintained focused attention (*attends*) throughout the task and completed both tasks as agreed (*heeds*).

Applying knowledge: David chose all needed tools and materials (*chooses*) and *used* them appropriately. He had difficulty supporting and stabilising larger objects (*handles*) such as the juice container during bilateral activities. He did not need to seek out additional information (*inquires*).

Temporal organisation: David was seen to hesitate before starting steps (*initiates*), he interrupted action sequences on a number of occasions (*continues*), ordered steps in a logical *sequence*) and spent a long time washing and washing some of the dishes (*terminates*). This led to steps taking longer to complete and performance being moderately inefficient.

Organising space and objects: David was able to *search and locate* all task objects and *gather* them into the workspace appropriately. However, his workspace at times was crowded (*organises*) resulting in him bumping into objects (*navigates*) and at other times he arranged tools and materials between two workspaces (*organises*) resulting in slowed and moderately inefficient performance. He *restored* all items at the end of both tasks.

Adapting performance: David was delayed in responding to water running out of the bowl (*notices/responds*) and he *adjusted* the taps constantly during the washing up task. He had limited ability to modify his actions (motor and process) in response to problems occurring (*accommodates*) and some problems (stabilising, positioning, manipulating, coordinating, transporting and handling) persisted through the task performances (*benefits*).

Social interaction and communication skills were not assessed at this time as these do not seem to impact negatively on task performance.

After the task observations Mary sat down with David and discussed with him the occupational performance analysis that she had carried out. The summary above describes the areas of difficulty that impacted most on David's occupational performance (with the motor and process skill items in italics). Next Mary discussed with David what he had found difficult and the reasons for this. A left-sided weakness following the stroke had resulted in a number of motor-sensory and perceptual body function impairments. The body-function and body-structure impairments that impacted negatively on performance can be found in Table 13.7. Activity and environmental demands can be found in Table 13.8.

Adaptation and grading

Mary implemented an intervention programme using adaptive occupation. David had already received 4 weeks of therapeutic occupation that focused on remediating muscle, sensory, and cognitive impairments (Table 13.6). Mary's decision to use adaptive occupation, an occupation-based intervention (Fisher 2006), was based on the results of her AMPS assessments and David's need to adapt his performance in the home because of neuromuscular body-function impairments (Table 13.7) and contextual and activity demands (Table 13.8). Enabling strategies focused on the:

- provision of assistive technology for use of one hand (e.g. non-slip mat, jar/bottle openers) and cardiovascular inefficiencies (e.g. perching stool)
- environmental modifications to the kitchen to make tools and materials more accessible and the environment less cluttered
- adapted methods of doing, including work simplification techniques to preserve levels of energy and take less time.

Mary also considered a number of ways that she could grade the intervention and increase David's tolerance:

- Increase tolerance by conducting the activity in sitting – washing dishes from a perching stool, positioning self at sink so that dishes are passed from weak side to strong side.
- Increase endurance by beginning with simple tasks – making a hot drink and building to more complex tasks – making a simple meal such as soup and crackers. Also by increasing the number of repetitions over time – washing a few dishes to washing all the dishes after every meal.
- Grading the difficulty of the activity – begin by activity in sitting to prevent poor posture or strengthen postural muscles, move to using a perching stool and finally to standing.
- Introducing techniques (methods) and tools (assistive technology) that will support performance, as performance improves these can be reduced or removed as performance becomes more dexterous and skilled.
- Increase social interactions by conducting the activity alone and without distractions, for example making one sandwich alone for self, and increasing this to include the presence of others in the room while making several sandwiches or a simple meal for others. This is particularly relevant for those with communication and social interaction skill deficits and could include promoting the handling of stress.

Finally, Mary re-assessed David at the end of her intervention using the AMPS as occupational performance analysis and to measure any change in performance and demonstrate outcomes of occupational therapy.

Conclusion

The purpose of this chapter has been to define and describe occupational performance analysis and discuss factors that affect how it is applied in

Table 13.7 Person Factors for David: including body functions from the ICF – motor and process skill (where equivalents exist) in italics

Person factors

Values	Values his role as a husband increases his sense of commitment and belonging
Beliefs	Expectation that he should contribute towards the household tasks and duties
Spiritual	High levels of motivation and personal investment in maintaining prior roles give meaning and purpose

Neuro-musculoskeletal movement-related functions

Mobility of joints	Range of motion and postural alignment (*aligns*) did not appear impaired
Muscle power	Weakness of left hand (*grips*) and arm impacted on ability to *lift* heavier items, tended to slide these (*moves*) Reduced postural control (balance) of left side of trunk (*stabilises*) and left lower limb weakness (*walks*)
Muscle tone	Increased muscle tone and spasticity in left wrist and hand affects smoothness of movement (*flows*); In the left trunk it impacts on *reaching* and *bending* into cupboards and *positioning* body at the units
Movement functions	Poor bilateral integration and hand/eye coordination were noted when manipulating small objects using two hands (or two body parts) together (*manipulates, coordinates, handles*) Reduced ability to control force of movement when using left hand (*calibrates*) Lurching gait and walking pattern (*walks*) cause some instability when transporting items (*transports*)
Involuntary movements	Occasional poor righting reactions were noted during standing and reaching resulting in transient loss of balance (*stabilises*) Slight tremor was noted in left hand when pouring (*flows*)

Cardiovascular functions

Heart	Poor physical endurance and stamina led to fatigue and a need to sit during the second task (*endures*)

Sensory functions

Seeing function	*Noticing/responding* to the water running from the tap and bowl may have been impacted by hemianopia
Touch/sensation	Mild loss of sensitivity to touch resulted in some fumbling of small objects with left hand (*manipulates*)
Proprioceptive function	Poor joint position sense of left side of body resulted in bumping into items (*navigates*)

Mental functions of perception and cognition

Energy	Maintained motivated to complete task but slowed as tasks progressed (*paces*)
Attention	Sustained focus attention (*attends*) and completed task (*heeds*)
Memory	Able to search for and find needed tools and materials (*searches/locates*) No need to ask for information or any need for verbal prompts (*inquires*) Completed the tasks without prompts (*heeds*) including putting everything away (*restores*)
Emotional functions	Appropriate range and regulation of emotions and self control (*respects from ACIS*)
Visuospatial functions	Reduced awareness of left side of space resulted in a tendency to bump into objects (*navigates*) and have items crowded on the right side of space (*organises*)
Time management	Gathering items to non-adjacent workspaces (*gathers*) delayed task progression Able to *sequence* steps in an efficient and appropriate order and without interruptions (*continues*)
Decision-making	Some hesitations or slow to begin (*initiates*) or end (*terminates*) actions – washing and washing dishes
Regulation of motor response to events	Turning off taps was delayed or sometimes random (*adjusts*) Delayed in responding to the water running out of the bowl (*notices/responds*)
Problem solving	Difficulty in anticipating and changing actions in response to problems encountered (*accommodates; benefits*)

Table 13.8 Contextual and activity demands for David	
Objects and their properties	Familiar objects support performance overall but impairment of left side (and left hand in particular) warrants the provision of different or adapted equipment for more efficient performance (non-slip mat, stabilising devices, etc.)
Physical spaces	Small kitchen area and cluttered worktops impede performance (*organises*)
Cultural	Familiar and naturalistic environment supports performance
Social	Presence of spouse supports performance and provides supervision/assistance if required
Sequence/timing	Previous habits and routines (rigid adherence to previous methods) slows performance (*paces*)

occupational therapy practice. Occupation terminology has been used within the Occupational Therapy Practice Framework (American Occupational Therapy Association 2002, 2008) and in particular how terminology used during the analysis of occupational performance can be applied in practice. The difference between performance skills (motor, process, and communication and social interaction) and body functions and structures (as described in the ICF) have been emphasised and in particular that occupational performance analysis refers to the analysis of performance skills and not body functions and structures. Following the implementation of occupational performance analysis and evaluation of performance skills, task analysis is used to evaluate the impact of body functions, body structures and activity demands. A top-down approach has been emphasised as this focuses first on the needs of the person and their unique occupational profile.

Occupation is the core of our profession and occupational therapists are experts in applying occupation as evaluation and as intervention. Learning to analyse occupational performance takes time, it is a complex and skilled process in itself and therapists should not expect to master it overnight. Practice and application to meaningful daily activities during practice placements and with other therapists will allow skills to develop and occupation terminology to become second nature.

References

American Occupational Therapy Association (2002). Occupational therapy practice framework: Domains and practice. *American Journal of Occupational Therapy*, 56(6), 609–639.

American Occupational Therapy Association (2008). Occupational therapy practice framework: Domains and practice, 2nd edition. *American Journal of Occupational Therapy*, 62(6), 625–664.

Canadian Association of Occupational Therapists (2002). *Enabling occupation: An occupational therapy perspective*. Ottawa, Ontario, Canadian Association of Occupational Therapists.

Christiansen, C. & Baum, C. (2005) *Occupational Therapy: Performance, participation and well-being*. Thorofare, NJ, Slack Inc.

Christiansen, C. & Baum, C. (1997) *Occupational Therapy: Enabling function and well-being*. Thorofare, NJ, Slack Inc.

Clark, F. (1993). Occupation embedded in a real life: Interweaving occupational science and occupational therapy. *American Journal of Occupational Therapy*, 47(12), 1067–1078.

College of Occupational Therapists (2006). *Definitions and core skills for occupational therapy*. London, College of Occupational Therapists.

Connelly, K. & Dalgleish M. (1989). The emergence of a tool-using skill in infancy. *Developmental Psychology*, 25, 894–912.

Creek, J. (2003). *Occupational therapy defined as a complex intervention*. London, College of Occupational Therapists.

Crepeau, E. B. (2003). Analyzing occupation and activity: A way of thinking about occupational performance. In: E. B. Crepeau,

E. S. Cohn, & B. A. B. Schell (Eds). *Willard & Spackman's Occupational Therapy, 10th ed*. Philadelphia, Lippincott Williams & Wilkins.

Dunn, W., Brown, C., McGuigan, A. (1994). The ecology of human performance: A framework for considering the effects of context. *American Journal of Occupational Therapy*, 48, 595–607.

Dunn, W., Brown, C. & Youngstrom M. J. (2003). Ecological model of occupation. In: P. Kramer, J. Hinojosa, & C. B. Royeen (Eds). *Perspectives in human occupation: Participation in Life*. Baltimore, MD, Lippincott Williams & Wilkins.

Fisher, A. G. (1994). Functional assessment and occupation: Critical issues for occupational therapy. *New Zealand Journal of Occupational Therapy*, 45(2), 13–19.

Fisher, A. G. (1998). Uniting practice and theory in an occupation framework: Eleanor Clarke Slagle Lecture. *American Journal of Occupational Therapy*, 52, 509–520.

Fisher, A. G. (2005). *Assessment of motor and process skills*, (6th edn). Fort Collins, Colorado, Three Star Press.

Fisher, A. G. (2006). Overview of performance skills and client factors, In: H. M. Pendleton & W. Schutlz-Krohn (Eds). *Pedretti's Occupational Therapy: Practice skills for physical dysfunction*, (6th ed) (pp. 372–402). St Loius, Missouri, Mosby.

Fisher, A. G. (2009). *Occupational therapy intervention process model: A model for planning and implementing top-down client-centred and occupation-based interventions*. Fort Collins, Three Star Press.

Fisher, A. G. & Griswold, L. A. (2008). *Evaluation of Social Interaction*. Fort Collins, Colorado, Three Star Press.

Forsyth, K., Salamy, M., Simon, S. & Keilhofner, G. (1997). *Assessment of Communication and Interaction Skills*. Chicago, University of Illinois.

Forsyth, K., Lai, J. S. & Keilhofner, G. (1999). The assessment of communication and interaction skills (ACIS): Measurement properties. *British Journal of Occupational Therapy*, 62(2), 69–74.

Hagedorn, R. (2000). *Tools for practice in occupational therapy: A structured approach to core skills and processes*. Edinburgh, Churchill Livingstone.

Hersch, G. I., Lamport, N. K. & Coffey, M. S. (2005). *Activity analysis: Application to occupation*. Thorofare, NJ: Slack Inc.

Ideishi, R. I. (2003). Influences of occupation on assessment and treatment, In: P. Kramer, J. Hinojosa, & C. B. Royeen (Eds). *Perspectives in humans occupation: Participation in life*. Baltimore, MD, Lippincott Williams & Wilkins.

Keilhofner, G. (1995) *A model of human occupation: Theory and application*, (2nd ed). Baltimore, MD, Williams & Wilkins.

Law, M., Cooper, B., Strong, S., Stewart, D., Rigby, P. & Letts, L. (1996). The Person-Environment-Occupation model: A transactive approach to occupational performance. *Canadian Journal of Occupational Therapy*, 63, 9–23.

Law, M., Polatajko, H., Baptiste, S., & Townsend, E. (1997), Core concepts in occupational therapy. In: E. Townsend (Ed.) *Enabling occupation: An occupational therapy perspective* (pp. 29–56). Ottawa, Ontario, Canadian Association of Occupational Therapists.

Law, M. (1991). The environment: A focus for occupational therapy. *Canadian Journal of Occupational Therapy*, 58, 171–179.

Nelson, D. & Thomas, J. J. (2003). Occupational form, occupational performance, and a conceptual framework for therapeutic occupation; In: P. Kramer, J. Hinojosa, C. B. Royeen (Eds). *Perspectives in human occupation: Participation in life*. Baltimore, MD, Lippincott Williams & Wilkins.

Nygård, L., Bernspång, B., Fisher, A. G. & Winblad, B. (1994). Comparing motor and process ability of persons with suspected dementia in home and clinic settings. *American Journal of Occupational Therapy*, 48, 689–696.

Park, S., Fisher, A. G. & Velozo, C. A. (1994). Using the Assessment of Motor and Process Skills to compare occupational performance between clinic and home settings. *American Journal of Occupational Therapy*, 48, 697–709.

Polatajko, H. J., Mandich, A. & Martini, R. (2000). Dynamic performance analysis: A framework for understanding occupational performance. *American Journal of Occupational Therapy*, 54, 65–72.

Segal, R. (2004). Family routines and rituals: A context for occupational therapy interventions. *American Journal of Occupational Therapy*, 59, 499–506.

Trombly, C. A. (1995). Occupation: Purposefulness and meaningfulness in therapeutic mechanisms: Eleanor Clarke Slagle Lecture. *American Journal of Occupational Therapy*, 49, 960–972.

Trombly, C. A. (2002). *Occupational therapy for physical dysfunction*, (5th edn). Baltimore, MD, Lippincott Williams & Wilkins.

World Health Organisation (2001). *International Classification of Functioning, Disability & Health (ICF)*. Geneva, Switzerland, World Health Organisation.

14

Psychosocial support

Jacqueline McKenna

CHAPTER CONTENTS

Introduction **190**

Holism 190

Adjustment to physical impairment 191

Psychosocial impairment 191

**Clarifying communication – concept and
purpose** **191**

The therapeutic relationship and
communication 192

**Effective communication within the
occupational therapy process** **192**

Training 193

Application of skills 193

**Skills for effective interpersonal
communication** **194**

Environment-creating skills 194

Relationship-building skills 195

Advanced communication skills. 196

**Personal awareness and the therapeutic
use of self** **199**

Psychosocial rehabilitation and support. . . **200**

Psychosocial enabling strategies **200**

Enabling adjustment – managing stress
and emotions 200

Emotional Intelligence 200

Aims of occupational therapy 201

Intervention 201

The application of psychosocial enabling
strategies 202

Summary. 206

Conclusion. **207**

SUMMARY

The focus of this chapter is on the need for
occupational therapists to provide psychosocial
support for individuals adjusting to physical injury
or impairment. Adapting to circumstance and
environment following physical injury or
impairment is a complex and demanding task,
not least in terms of emotional adjustment. The
provision of psychosocial support by the
occupational therapist is integral to the
application of holistic principles, ensuring the
psychological well-being of the individual is being
considered. In order to facilitate recovery via
person-centred, occupation-based enabling
strategies, the occupational therapist must
understand the perspective of the individual and
identify meaningful goals that accommodate
changes in self, role, and occupation. This
chapter will take a broad view of psychosocial
functioning and adjustment, acknowledging the
psychosocial needs of the individual and
discussing the role of an effective alliance that
supports individuals and their engagement in the
therapeutic process. The utilisation of skilled
interpersonal interaction within the provision of
this support will be specifically discussed, and
relevant concepts, principles, skills, issues, and
challenges considered. The support strategies
that occupational therapists might provide are
identified and illustrated by two practice
scenarios.

KEY POINTS

- Humanism, holism and occupational therapy are
  inextricably linked when providing person-
  centred support and intervention.
- The therapeutic alliance is of significant value
  within the process of occupational therapy.

- An understanding of the concept of communication and related skills underpins the development of skills required for the building of professional relationships.
- Skills for effective interpersonal communication include environment creating, relationship building, and advanced communication abilities.
- Personal awareness and the therapeutic use of self are essential to the dynamic process of an efficacious and collaborative relationship.
- Acceptance of impairment is broadly regarded as an adaptive outcome in the process of adjustment to physical impairment and will be achieved by the utilisation of enabling strategies by the occupational therapist.
- The utilisation of enabling strategies by the occupational therapist is potentiated by the application of efficacious communication skills.
- Emotional intelligence abilities can be enhanced and can have a positive impact upon adjustment and coping.
- The provision of psychosocial support requires a holistic, integrated, and collaborative approach.

Introduction

As I began to plan this chapter and consider the provision of holistic care, I recalled my own experiences in a large, hospital-based mental-health service. One referral made from the medical occupational therapy team to the mental health occupational therapy team resulted in my sitting by the bed of a young, immobile, man who had attempted suicide by jumping from a high structure. The referral said 'immobile, needs activity, is emotional and ?? depressed, please assess'. The prospect of a serious mental health issue was considered outside the remit of the medical team, who reported feeling unable to work with the individual's physical rehabilitation in any significant way, until the suicidal ideation, high expressed emotion, emotional needs, and motives were addressed. Similarly an elderly person with chronic obstructive pulmonary disease (COPD) was referred to the mental health service because her shortness of breath was making her anxious and she was having panic attacks. The individual was resistant to input from the mental health team, voicing concern at needing treatment from the 'psychiatrists'. Conversely, colleagues reported that an individual with an anxiety condition was referred to the medical team with a request for small kitchen appliances because of difficulties with fine motor control. Staff expressed concern that an anxious individual was having to wait for the referral to be picked up by the physical team and was being exposed to a new environment, potentially increasing her anxiety.

I introduce this anecdotal material not to imply any criticism, but to provoke consideration of those issues which might be raised when reflecting on the realities of holistic practice within our current roles and the contextual factors impacting upon that practice.

Holism

The humanistic philosophy of occupational therapy necessitates the application of holistic, person-centred principles and practice. Occupational therapy is concerned with performance of social roles. Factors fundamental to occupational engagement can be grouped into three areas; biological, cognitive and psychosocial (Atchison & Dirette 2007). The focus of enabling strategies will be determined by an individual's need and the occupational therapist must attend to both the biomedical aspects and the individual's experience of the situation, facilitating an empathic appreciation of the realities of living in an impaired or less able body (Crepeau 1991, Kendall & Buys 1998, Mattingley 1991).

Psychosocial adjustment to illness or impairment is conceptualised as a process which is complex and recurrent in nature, mediated by a wealth of individual and environmental factors. The occupational therapist must acknowledge the potential impact of these factors upon individuals in terms of their psychological health and coping skills, and upon therapeutic relationships, therapeutic engagement, and therapeutic efficacy.

An individual may give an indication of his or her emotional response to a situation and the therapist must be responsive and able to adjust her professional agenda in order to explore and address emotions and issues as necessary (Faulkner 1998). The creation and maintenance of space for emotional and psychological issues to be considered, and the provision of psychosocial support within the field of physical injury and impairment is absolutely vital in order to provide person-centred enabling strategies that match the holistic beliefs of the profession and meet the demands of the Code of Ethics and Professional Conduct (College of Occupational Therapists 2005).

Adjustment to physical impairment

Any individual attempting to deal with physical injury or impairment will require time and support not only to adapt to the resulting specific physical difficulties and the impact on occupational performance and engagement, but also to adjust to any psychosocial responses and ramifications. Yoshida (1993) suggested that individuals alternate between pre-impairment and post-impairment identities and that the occupational therapist may be working with those who are struggling with a range of responses including: fear, frustration, anxiety, anger, confusion, uncertainty, loss, despair, and depression. These responses can be experienced as the individual attempts to process events and adjust to the illness or impairment and the consequent impact upon their lives and that of others around them (Livneh et al 2004, Telford 2006). The experience of negative affectivity is noted as a prevalent reaction to chronic injury and impairment (Livneh et al 2004, World Health Organization 2002) and linked to poor psychosocial adaptation. According to Etherington (1990a), the majority of the problems encountered are related to emotional reactions, and emotional recovery is of equal importance in rehabilitation as the restoration of physical ability. Niemeier & Burnett (2001) claim that loss issues, emotional status, physical health, and coping are inextricably linked to the physical loss of ability and that they must be considered as such within the rehabilitation process.

Evidence supports that acceptance of impairment and the identification of realistic goals aids in adjustment. Conversely, denial of impairment is linked to poor psychosocial adjustment, poor illness management, and reports of mental health problems (Dangoor & Florian 1994, Telford et al 2006). Coping styles vary and the occupational therapist must remain cogent of the uniqueness of the individual experience and its impact upon adaptation. Empirical evidence suggests that optimism and tempered emotional responses have potential as an effective protection against mental health problems, assisting the individual in coping with stress or threatening situations in the short term (Niemeier & Burnett 2001, Olney et al 2004, Telford et al 2006). Ongoing psychosocial adjustment problems following acquired physical injury or impairment are linked conversely to successful rehabilitation outcomes (Browne et al 1990, Kendall & Buys 1998, Putnam & Adams 1992), and are also associated with extensive costs in terms of long-term utilisation of health and social care services.

Psychosocial impairment

Anxiety disorders and depression are the most prevalent non-psychotic disorders and are the most likely disorders to occur as part of the psychological sequelae of physical injury or impairment (World Health Organization 2002). Examination of the psychosocial concomitants of chronic physical illness or impairment, indicate clear links to poor psychosocial adaptation and reactions, including depression, anxiety, anger, and denial (Livneh et al 2004). Faulkner (1998) suggests that it is very difficult for most individuals to come to terms with a chronic and debilitating illness or impairment, and, as a result, depression is noted as a common response to a diagnosis of a serious illness, like cancer (Harrison et al 1994).

Depending upon the severity, any psychological disorder, including severe depression and/or anxiety, post traumatic stress disorder, or adjustment disorders, may need to be prioritised. This might necessitate that the occupational therapist employs specialist knowledge, skills and psychosocial rehabilitation techniques specific to the diagnosis, potentially necessitating a referral to specialist and/or mental health services. People tend to resist referral to mental health services as they do not perceive themselves as mentally ill, and they are often subsequently discouraged from seeking help based on concerns about this possibility (Etherington 1990b). The occupational therapist working within a physical setting must remain cogent of the fact that the emotional reactions and responses of the individual, and the efficacy of any support they receive, may influence the development of psychosocial dysfunction or ill health. To this end, monitoring of the person's psychosocial well-being is essential and specific assessment of psychosocial dysfunction may be required.

Clarifying communication – concept and purpose

The concept of communication is a complex one and much debate has occurred regarding formal definition and primary purpose. According to the Latin translation, the action of communicating means 'to share or make common'. Communication is a process within which messages are sent and received, the process is ongoing and dynamic, requires at least two communicators and is impacted by participant perception and the context and meaning in which it occurs (Hargie & Dickson 2004). Interpersonal communication is described as the exchange of feelings, meanings and information via verbal and non-verbal methods (Brooks 1971). It is direct and non-mediated, dyadic or in small groups, and is influenced by the personal qualities of the interactors (Alder et al 1998).

Hargie & Dickson (2004) postulate that there are six elements of skilled interpersonal interaction; attending to these elements can positively impact both the interaction itself and the well-being of the person receiving the intervention (Di Blasi et al 2001). These six elements are:

- The person situation context – personal baggage, including knowledge, attitudes, emotions, motivations and personality within the context of the environment, situation, age, gender, and culture
- Goals – desired end states impacted by persistence, appropriateness and selectivity
- Mediation – between goals, perceptions, emotions, and cognitions
- Response – plans and strategies
- Feedback – reactions to what is said
- Perception of feedback.

The therapeutic relationship and communication

The importance of a meaningful and collaborative relationship between the individual and the therapist is fundamental to individualised and culturally sensitive practice (Cole & McLean 2003). The therapist's use of unique abilities and characteristics as a tool within the relationship can empower participation of the individual, enrich enabling strategies and enhance outcomes (Rosa & Hasselkus 1996, Sumsion 2000). The individual's evaluation of the therapist's communication style relates directly to compliance and satisfaction ratings of the health care experience (Burgoon 1987). Tickle-Degnen (2002) and Lloyd & Mass (1992) linked therapeutic rapport and relationship, and, more specifically, attending skills, reading of non-verbal cues, and the ability to express emotions clearly and genuinely, to individual satisfaction, outcomes, and the perceived efficacy of the relationship.

The occupational therapist's use of self within therapy necessitates the use of both interactive

reasoning and communication skills (Whitcher & Tse 2004). These include: listening, questioning, working through and exploring skills (Burnard 2005). These techniques can be utilised in order to provide efficacious psychosocial support. Where an individual has impaired communication abilities, possibly as a result of a physical impairment, the therapist might tend toward adopting a more symptom-focused and pragmatic approach to professional reasoning (Tickle-Degnen 1995), this may result in less collaboration within the process of therapy. It is important to be mindful of communication difficulties and to ensure time, space and skills are utilised for the development of the relationship and the development of quality communication between the individual and the therapist. Working with people who have neurological deficits may result in issues with concentration, verbalisation, and fatigue, working in a surgical environment may present individuals dealing with phantom limb pain that impedes their ability to focus on therapeutic communication, and an elderly person recovering from a hip replacement may have sensory deficits impacting recognition of non-verbal cues. The therapist must be aware of any factors that might impact the collaborative alliance and the context of these factors within the impairment itself and the culture, gender, beliefs, values, experiences, and environment of the individual and the therapist (Hagedorn 1995).

Management of the needs of the individual in general terms will include the provision of psychosocial support requiring the occupational therapist to utilise interpersonal interaction skills in order to facilitate open and honest communication and self-expression. This will assist the individual with the exploration of feelings and expectations, and with the discussion of symptoms, adjustment, adaptive behaviour, coping strategies, and goals. Expression and exploration of issues relating to the individual's adjustment to illness or impairment, and the impact this has on occupational engagement, will enable the therapist to provide essential psychosocial support which will positively impact upon recovery.

Effective communication within the occupational therapy process

A true collaborative alliance does not happen by accident or by magic, and simply caring about an individual is not enough to develop an effective relationship. The efficacy of occupational therapy is impacted by the quality of the collaborative relationship. A balance of attitudes (caring), skills (communication) and values (professional, humanistic) are most likely to result in the development of a relationship that facilitates the occupational therapy process, enabling individuals to achieve health and well-being through occupational engagement (Lloyd & Maas 1991).

In order to enhance and develop the collaborative relationship the therapist will apply the principles of the person-centered approach (Rogers 1951), utilising mutual trust, collaboration and respect, negotiating goals and believing in the individual's potential for growth and change. These principles sit firmly within the humanistic philosophy of occupational therapy and are supported by the profession's Code of Ethics and Professional Conduct (College of Occupational Therapists 2005), which requires that we maintain respect and personal autonomy. The value of a partnership that is collaborative is supported by Sumsion (2000) and by Middlehurst (1991) who suggest that motivation for engagement in intervention is increased by involving the person in decision-making to ensure they perceive the intervention to be meaningful and purposeful.

True rapport and collaboration is possible only when communication is open and honest, and the therapist is charged with the responsibility of facilitating an effective two-way communication process. For the occupational therapist effective communication is an essential tool that supports holistic practice (College of Occupational Therapists 2005).

Training

The building of the relationship requires that the therapist has transferable knowledge and skills that should be established during training and developed in practice. Interpersonal skills and effective communication can be trained and are improved with practice. In order to achieve competence it is necessary to understand the skill, both conceptually and behaviourally, practice it, use it, and seek feedback on performance (Robbins & Hunsaker 1996). Over a number of years the author has facilitated advanced communication skills workshops for students using a combination of theoretical education and practice, including role and real play. Feedback and evaluation from students attests to the value of these skills

and their application within the practice setting. Their importance in supporting application of crucial elements of the occupational therapy process (engagement of the individual in therapy, interviewing, assessment, negotiated goal setting and collaborative problem solving) and the role of the occupational therapist as communicator and advocate (with colleagues, students, carers, external agencies, and the public) have been cited and reflect many of the core skills identified by the College of Occupational Therapists (2004). The need for training is supported by Pierce (2000) who suggests that interviewing skills are a necessity when attempting to draw out personal stories and narratives and argues that these are essential to the development of a competent occupational therapist. Therapists can utilise Rogerian principles not only to develop effective collaborative relationships but also to gather information and assess, identify and clarify problems, negotiate goals and help individuals deal with emotions and occupational engagement issues, ultimately facilitating change and adaptation (Middlehurst 1991, Whitcher & Tse 2004). The training of students in the efficacious application of communication skills is an essential component of undergraduate education (Bayne et al 1998, Burnard 2005, Dickson et al 1997, Jeffrey & Hicks 1997) and supports the College of Occupational Therapists Standards For Education (2002/2003) which aims to ensure training produces graduates who are fit for purpose and practice.

Application of skills

Effective communication skills are essential to ensure that the person is treated as an individual, is listened to and has his or her unique problems investigated and identified (Lapsley et al 2002). Couldrick (1997) supports the core values of restoring health and well-being through purposeful activity, and the use of interpersonal skills by the therapist to communicate effectively with the individual as a primary activity within an effective occupational therapy programme. The range of interpersonal skills an occupational therapist has are key, supporting the uniqueness of occupational therapy and its concept of 'doing with' rather than 'doing to' the person; facilitating engagement in a collaborative therapeutic process and, ultimately, enabling the individual to become independent (Lloyd & Maas 1992, Matheson 1998). Good communicators fashion their discussion in response to goals, emotions and motives, and a therapist mindful of this can acknowledge the needs and motivations of the people they are working with, and utilise communication activity to address these needs.

The application of advanced interpersonal skills by an occupational therapist working in the field of physical dysfunction can serve many purposes. According to Burnard (2005) these include:

- Enabling people to describe symptoms and the impact of their injury or impairment

- Exploring and handling emotion

- Exploring social and relationship issues

- Discussing pain, reactions to injury or impairment

- Identifying and developing coping strategies

- Identifying and clarifying needs, wants, goals, and motivators

- Coping with loss

- Conducting assessments.

Etherington (1990a) suggests that it is vital to facilitate the expression of feelings for people with physical injuries or impairments, in order that they might adjust and cope. Adjustment is impacted by sociocultural issues and Etherington (1990b) suggests that the occupational therapist could utilise their skills to change those attitudes that continue to assume that disabled people are incapable of making decisions. Providing a channel of communication will facilitate an active role in therapy and negotiation of occupational goals, enabling and empowering both the individual and the process of therapy.

Reflection 14.1 focuses on considering what factors are involved in making a relationship work well or that contribute to a relationship being a challenge.

Reflection 14.1

Factors that make a relationship work well

We cannot remove the therapist or the individual from the process of therapy; therefore, the therapy hinges on the interactions between the two.

One way to develop relationship-building skills is to reflect upon the relationships you have developed with people you have worked with as an occupational therapy student or occupational therapist.

Recall a relationship which was challenging

Identify the challenges in this relationship and the reasons this relationship was challenging. Consider the impact this had on therapy in terms of your own and the individual's engagement in the process; identify any negative impact. Consider your feelings about this relationship now and its influence on your practice. Identify the skills which could have been useful in dealing with these challenges and any changes you would make which could enhance the interaction.

Think of a relationship which worked well

Identify the skills you used to develop the relationship. Identify the evidence you have which tells you this relationship worked. Consider your feelings about this relationship now and its influence on your practice.

Skills for effective interpersonal communication

The occupational therapist will use a range of communication skills to establish and maintain effective working relationships, establishing a framework within which psychosocial support can be provided for the individual. The range of skills to be employed includes environment-creating skills, relationship-building skills, and advanced communication skills. Each of these will now be discussed in turn.

Environment-creating skills

Occupational therapists communicate with individuals in all kinds of contexts. In an ideal world an exploration of the individual's feelings following the loss of a limb would be aimed at providing structured psychosocial support and would be planned to take place in a private, neutral, safe, comfortable environment without distraction, and interruption. In reality, interactions happen wherever they arise, some planned, some unplanned, often on the hoof and sometimes triggered by questions, anxieties, responses and emotions, or during a scheduled assessment task or intervention activity.

Notwithstanding the realities of the working practice of an occupational therapist, attention should be paid where possible to basic comfort in terms of seating, lighting and temperature, privacy, personal safety, time resources, and boundaries. The therapist is responsible for making the environment conducive to interaction and adhering to the Code of Ethics and Professional Conduct (College of Occupational Therapists 2005), by preserving individual confidentiality, autonomy and dignity, assisting the person to set and use boundaries in terms of the content, time and scope of the interactions, and in terms of the relationship with the therapist.

Cultural issues and their impact upon any communication process are a contentious issue, focused around the relative importance of specific cultural knowledge versus adaptable communication expertise and personal awareness. Cultural differences should not be denied and might be an important factor within interpersonal interaction and therapeutic relationships in terms of norms and customs, communication behaviours, style, and interpretation. However, Burnard (2005) claims that misinterpretation occurs primarily due to assumptions of similarity, rather than due to problems communicating across and through different cultural orientations. The expression of emotion is a key issue for people dealing with physical injury or impairment and what is acceptable in terms of expression may be culturally driven and may influence what the person is willing or able to discuss with the therapist. Likewise the individual's experience of pain is another issue that may be linked to cultural expectation and norms.

Whilst the relevance of a person's background should be acknowledged and issues may be related to or compounded by issues of race, ethnicity, gender, religion and culture, therapists must not rely too heavily on these as explanations of the individual's problems. Emotional and psychological problems are universal and viewing each person as unique is most likely to result in a meaningful level of empathic understanding of the individual's perception and experience of injury or impairment. The confident and effective utilisation of a range of interpersonal skills will support trust development and ensure the therapist's credibility in the eyes of the person they are engaged with, facilitating them to communicate across and through sociocultural differences.

Relationship-building skills

Hinojosa et al (2003) suggest that occupational therapists must gain an understanding of each individual and his perspective before meaningful interventions can be negotiated and implemented. One aim of occupational therapy is to facilitate an individual's ability to find personal meaning (Bruce & Borg 1987) and the deployment of person-centred principles will facilitate autonomy and involvement in therapy (Burnard 2005, Kensit 2000, Rogers 1951). In order to operationalise these principles the therapist will need to employ attitudes and skills that will help to build the therapeutic relationship. Three key dimensions of relationship building have been identified by Carl Rogers (1951) and Lloyd & Mass (1991):

1. Respect – trust and unconditional positive regard

2. Empathic understanding

3. Genuineness – warmth and congruence.

Trust is integral to the relationship and is contingent upon an individual believing in and respecting the therapist (Hagedorn 1997). Building trust often requires patience and perseverance from both parties as boundaries are explored, eventually leading to the establishment of some degree of safety within the relationship (Bruce & Borg 1987, Hagedorn 2000). By demonstrating respect and commitment the occupational therapist will reflect a belief that a person has potential and is able to grow, change and solve their own problems. Warmth and genuineness will be demonstrated by the establishment of a genuine relationship facilitated by the therapist's approachability, consistency, congruence, and a willingness to be open, honest, non-defensive and spontaneous. This will support development of a trusting and productive relationship for both the individual and the therapist (Burnard 2005, Etherington 1990b, Hagedorn 2000), within which meaningful occupational goals can be established and addressed.

Unconditional positive regard is an essential skill in the building of the relationship (Rogers 1951), and means that the individual is viewed as a valued and worthwhile person with acceptance of and respect for the individual's unique subjective experience, regardless of whether this is reciprocal (Burnard 2005, Kensit 2000). According to Blank

(2004), therapeutic partnerships are fostered when the occupational therapist is non-judgemental and accepting. The occupational therapist can use unconditional positive regard to build trust and enable the person to freely express emotions knowing he will not be judged (Etherington 1990b). Suspending judgement can enhance listening skills and facilitate the process of empathic understanding. Empathic understanding is a core dimension of person-centred practice (Rogers 2001), and is vital to the development of a relationship within which the therapist aims to truly understand the person's subjective viewpoint and communicate this understanding to the individual (Burnard 2005, Kensit 2000, Lloyd & Maas 1992). Empathy is succinctly described by Kalisch (1971, p. 714) as, 'the ability to perceive accurately the feelings of another person and to communicate this understanding to him.'

Whilst it would be unrealistic to assume that all therapists are able to understand exactly how the experience of injury or impairment has impacted upon each individual, it is the therapist's ability to utilise verbal and non-verbal communication skills to communicate their understanding, which is paramount to the collaborative potential of the relationship. Empathy creates connections and respect for differences, facilitating a relationship through which both parties can be enriched (Cole & McLean 2003, Peloquin 1995).

Unconditional positive regard can be challenged by someone who may behave in a way that the therapist feels unable to accept. It can be hard to demonstrate this skill if an individual is behaving aggressively toward the therapist, or perhaps the therapist's and individual's values contradict each other significantly (Kensit 2000, Unsworth 2004). An individual may struggle to express warmth and, consequently, may have difficulty responding to the therapist and this could impact upon the development of the relationship and its potential as a therapeutic tool (Tickle-Degnen 1995). The realities of emotional commitment to every person with whom a therapist works must be noted and the therapist's capacity for true empathy cannot be presumed (Kensit 2000).

Genuineness requires mutuality and a balance of power that is difficult to achieve within the medical model structure of most of our health and social-care services. Despite National Health Service reforms and their focus on user involvement, health and social care provision in general terms largely remains paternalistic, safety focused, and resource constrained (Bayne et al 1998, Burnard 2005, Middlehurst 1991). The health care professional continues to be presented and perceived as an expert and the individual as a largely passive recipient of help. The influence of this power imbalance upon the therapeutic alliance must be monitored (Finlay 2001).

Advanced communication skills

Advanced communication skills are divided into listening, questioning, and working through or exploration skills (Burnard 2005). A range of advanced communication skills drawn broadly from a Rogerian model of person-centred therapy or counselling is presented in Table 14.1 (Rogers 1951, 2001). These skills are discussed by Burnard (2005), who claims they transfer well to the field of effective interpersonal communication for occupational therapists. Illustrative examples from the author's practice and classroom experience are included and applied to the context of physical injury or impairment, as appropriate.

Reflection 14.2 focuses on becoming aware of listening, exploring and working through skills.

Reflection 14.2

Skills of listening, exploring and working through

In order to develop the skills of listening, exploring or working through, analyse the use of these skills with an individual:

- Think about a situation when you have used listening, exploring or working through, identify which of these skills you used and your reason for utilising them. Recall what you actually said and the purpose of saying this.
- Summarise the interaction in terms of what worked and what did not.
- Identify what you would do differently if you were to repeat the situation.
- Identify any skills you need to become more confident in using.

Table 14.1 Advanced communication skills (Burnard 2005, Faulkner 1998, Hargie & Dickson 2004, Pollock & McColl 1998, Rogers 1951, Sviden & Saljo 1993)

Skill	Definition
Observation skills	Observation of people in terms of their presentation, verbal and non-verbal behaviour. Perceiving non-verbal cues and reactions can be indicators of mood, emotions and responses to the therapist and content of discussion that may not be verbally articulated – posture, eye contact, gestures and facial expression. Be aware of incongruence, discomfort and patterns. Remember the individual might be in pain

Listening skills

Skill	Definition
Active listening	Utilising non-verbal skills including body posture, facial expression, eye contact and gestures to demonstrate that the therapist is listening Asking relevant questions Paraphrasing information Summarising information Drawing out skills will maintain the flow, offer encouragement to the individual to talk (*'Tell me more about the pain you are in; go on, uh hmm, ok'*), nodding, smiling, and using eye contact and facial expressions to convey interest. Pollock & McColl (1998) discuss that the first stage of the process of problem identification is achieved by the therapist attending and responding to the individual's non-verbal communication during assessment

Questioning skills

Skill	Definition
Closed questions	Control of response is with the interviewer. Questions that will elicit a specific response used to check or clarify information, gain factual information useful during interviews and assessments *'Did you come by bus today?'* *'Do you understand what the doctor told you?'* *'So who lives with you?'* *'You say you don't like to be alone at night, is that why you live with your sister?'*
Open questions	The control of the response is with the respondent. Designed to help the individual explore and explain –'Who, Where, Why, What, How', questions, that encourage the expression of feelings Can be broad or focused Broad *'So what brings you to occupational therapy today?'* *'Tell me about your previous experiences with an occupational therapist?'* Focused *'So why did you refuse to let the occupational therapist into your house?'* *'How did you feel when the doctor gave you the diagnosis?'* *'What did you understand from the letter I sent you?'*

Working through/exploring/clarifying skills

Skill	Definition
Reflection	Rogers (1951) describes reflection as focusing on feelings, trying to identify the feelings the person has and asking them about this in a way that lets them confirm or reject the therapist's suggestion, which is drawn from conversation so far *'Would I be right in thinking you are very frustrated by this situation?'* *'It sounds to me like you felt humiliated by the lack of privacy?'* *'I'm wondering if you're feeling confused and overwhelmed by all the information'*
Paraphrasing	Mini summary, question or comment that uses the person's own words to show you are listening and draw out conversation Person: *'Last night I had a lot of pain again, and I feel very angry because the medication didn't help me'* Occupational therapist: *'So you're very angry because the medication didn't help your pain last night'*; *'You are very angry because the medication isn't working?'*

(cont'd)

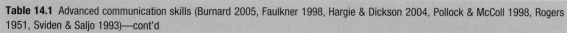

Table 14.1 Advanced communication skills (Burnard 2005, Faulkner 1998, Hargie & Dickson 2004, Pollock & McColl 1998, Rogers 1951, Sviden & Saljo 1993)—cont'd

Skill	Definition
Summarising	Useful at the beginning to recap what happened previously, at end to close conversation so both parties are clear, and during conversations when there is a change of theme or large amounts of information have been presented Summary should be presented back to the individual so the individual can agree or amend information 'So we have discussed having to ask for help to use the toilet and how difficult you are finding this. You feel frustrated by your inability to do this for yourself but can't bring yourself to ask your husband to help and can not see a way forward. Have I understood that right? Shall we start next time by focusing on talking to your husband about what is happening?'
Concreteness	Asking for examples to make sure both the therapist and the individual are clear about what the individual is saying Person: 'I always feel like I do it wrong when I try to explain to my kids what is going to happen to me – they get really upset' Occupational therapist: 'Give me an example of the last time you felt like you did something wrong'; 'Explain to me what happened the last time you tried to explain to your kids about your illness and it felt like you did it wrong' The therapist can also use concreteness to ensure dialogue is clear and unambiguous
Clarifying	Checking understanding of what the individual is saying: 'What do you mean when you say you are at the end of your tether?';'Can you help me understand what you mean when you say you just can't get over this illness?' Meanings are individual and relative to each person. The therapist should not assume what the individual means. Use the person's words, stay within their frame of reference and meaning. The therapist can also ask if the person has felt like this before, this may help understanding of the feelings, clarify them and revisit how and why the feeling occurs
Focusing	Helps the individual to focus on one issue or to identify which is the most pressing issue at present 'So you say your husband's attitude, your level of pain and the medication you are on are all getting you down – which of those is getting you down the most?'; 'So your husband, your pain and your medication are all really bothering you. It's important we talk about all of these issues, but, which of those do you feel it is important to discuss first?'
Confrontation	Can be used if it appears that something is being denied, or an issue is being avoided, patterns of behaviour are occurring or there is incongruence. Perhaps changing the subject, being evasive, avoiding answering questions. 'You say you are OK, that you are relaxed but I have noticed you are gripping the chair'; 'When I ask you about using a wheelchair you seem to change the subject'; 'When we meet, you appear unwilling to talk about how angry you are about how you were given this news until we are almost out of time'
Handling silence	Allowing time to think can be useful for both parties. Useful during interview when the individual has been asked a potentially difficult question, or if the therapist is delivering bad news. Silence can be very constructive; the individual could be making sense of thoughts and feelings, struggling to manage emotions, considering how much to tell the therapist or be unsure of how to answer the question. Be aware of the purpose of silences, the therapist must not let their own discomfort lead to filling the gaps or rushing in with another question. If there is a long silence the therapist can ask the individual what is going on: 'There has been a long silence, what are you thinking about?'; 'Do you need time to think?'; 'Do you feel able to pick up where we left off?' Silences can also provide time for the therapist to gather thoughts, check emotions, mentally recap and plan how to continue the interaction

Table 14.1 Advanced communication skills (Burnard 2005, Faulkner 1998, Hargie & Dickson 2004, Pollock & McColl 1998, Rogers 1951, Sviden & Saljo 1993)—cont'd

Skill	Definition
Handling strong emotion	Self-awareness and reflection will help the therapist handle her own emotions. All skills listed can be used. Use appropriate non-verbal behaviour – the therapist needs to be cautious with the use of touch; use touch for support if both parties are comfortable with it and it is culturally appropriate. Discomfort for either party will be obvious. Do not ignore the emotion, it is likely to be very important, allow time, then ask: 'Are you ok, do you want to carry on?'; 'You are obviously very angry/frightened/upset about this' If breaking bad news use a sandwich approach – prepare the individual, deliver the news, offer support. Prepare the individual: 'So you have had a stroke, as we discussed with the doctor this morning […] Deliver the news: It is very unlikely that the damage this has caused to the sight in your left eye can be corrected […] Offer support: This is very difficult […] it's a lot to take in […] It must be confusing/frightening/shocking […] I can try to help you get any information you need/answer any questions you might have […] We can spend some time talking about how this is affecting you […]'
Giving permission	Sometimes individuals struggle to express certain emotions, or consider them to be unacceptable or embarrassing. Giving permission can be very powerful in assisting with emotional expression 'It is ok to be upset and cry – this is a very difficult situation'; 'If you are angry about that it is ok – do you want to talk about it?'; 'It's normal to feel overwhelmed by this news' Giving permission may elicit strong emotion
Immediacy	Focusing on the here and now is especially good for the individual who finds it hard to express emotion. Step out of the content of the conversation and ask: 'How are you feeling right now, right this minute?'; 'What are you thinking about right now?'

Personal awareness and the therapeutic use of self

The therapeutic use of self is a dynamic process aimed at engaging the individual in a meaningful and effective affiliation (Bruce & Borg 1987, Lloyd & Maas 1993). The therapist utilises self-awareness, sensitivity, empathy and interpersonal skills to develop a collaborative therapeutic relationship drawing on the knowledge skills and experience gained during her professional education (Hagedorn 1995, 2000, Lloyd & Maas 1993). Person-centred practice aims to increase self-awareness and using genuineness will facilitate greater understanding of one's own strengths and limitations. As an occupational therapist it can be challenging to manage the professional reasoning skills we have developed as problem solvers in order to listen effectively, rather than thinking about the most suitable, obvious or practical solution to the problem. Self-awareness is vital to the process of effective communication and, consequently, to the provision of psychosocial support. According to Egan (1990), in order to be an effective helper it is important to understand how the interaction is impacted by the assumptions one makes and one's beliefs, values and standards, skills, weaknesses and idiosyncrasies. A person might challenge or contradict the therapist's worldview or values, making provision of support, development of the relationship and engagement in therapy more challenging. Developing self-awareness brings a greater understanding about oneself and one's ability to help constructively (Compton & Ashwin 2000). In addition, supervision should be utilised to deal with issues that arise, providing support, consultation, skill upgrading, and opportunities for further development of personal awareness for the therapist (Geldard & Geldard 2005).

The development of meaningful and useful collaborative relationships necessitates good self-awareness, empathy, communication skills and understanding. The emotionally intelligent occupational therapist will be warm, genuine, motivated, optimistic and persistent (Mayer & Cobb 2000); and will be able to understand and manage the emotions of self and others. These abilities are arguably essential within the climate of our current practice and are crucial to the development of effective, collaborative therapeutic relationships.

Reflection 14.3 focuses on acknowledging self-awareness.

Reflection 14.3

Self-awareness

In order to develop self-awareness, think about a practice situation when you were surprised by your emotional reaction to an individual.

Describe what happened. Identify the emotions you experienced. Summarise why this experience is a significant one for you. Describe what skills you utilised to help you make sense of and manage these emotions. Identify what you learned about yourself and how this experience has changed you and your practice.

Psychosocial rehabilitation and support

The process of psychosocial rehabilitation refers to the restoration of psychological and social functioning and is considered in general terms, a specialist area of occupational therapy practice that lies within mental health service provision. However, the biopsychosocial nature of physical injury or impairment and the consideration that an individual may resist referral to a mental health service, necessitate that the therapist working in a physical setting provide a holistic service that includes monitoring, assessment and basic treatment of those mental health disorders most likely to occur within the sequelae of physical injury and impairment. Evidence drawn from the field of liaison psychiatry suggests that the treatment of the psychological effects of physical dysfunction is a key area of practice and claims that interventions include physical (medical/nursing), psychological (psychotherapeutic interventions) and social (financial, housing and social assistance) (Guthrie 1996, Peveler et al 2000, Ruddy & House 2005).

Psychosocial enabling strategies

The current evidence base generally supports acceptance of impairment as an adaptive outcome for the adjustment process (Telford et al 2006), and the occupational therapist will enable this adaptation within the implementation of enabling strategies. Whilst the occupational therapist will play a key role in facilitating adjustment, person-centred practice necessitates that analysis of the efficacy of any coping strategies utilised by the individual consider not only the adjustment process, but also the context of adjustment in terms of the individual's values and beliefs, the realities of their limitations, and the social attitudes and reactions they experience (Hahn 1985, Olney et al 2004).

Enabling adjustment – managing stress and emotions

According to Schrever et al (2006, p. 201), 'severe physical disability is a long term stressor', and impairment-related stress is a key mediator in therapeutic engagement and in levels of self-esteem. Working with this stress in both the short and long term will be part of any rehabilitation and adjustment process, and the individual's own cognitive appraisal of injury or impairment is crucial (Schrever et al 2006), as it influences both emotional response *to* and the management *of* self. The perception, understanding and management of the emotions of self and others is essential for successful adaptation and adjustment to the change and trauma (Ciarrochi et al 2002), which might occur as a result of physical injury or impairment.

Giving prominence to an emotional agenda when working with individuals to deal with responses and adjustment to physical injury and impairment certainly has resonance with the wider cultural priorities of contemporary society. This might challenge the outcome-driven, resource-focused reality of occupational therapy service provision within medical settings (Hawkey 2006, Tickle-Degnen 1995, Turner et al 2003).

Emotional Intelligence

It is pertinent here to introduce the concept of emotional intelligence. This is a recently developed perspective in intelligence, developed from Gardener's (1983) key theory of multiple intelligences and specifically linked to his inter- and intrapersonal intelligences. Mayer & Salovey (1997) describe the emotionally intelligent person as better able to perceive, integrate and use emotions, understand their meanings, and manage the emotions of self and others to promote emotional and intellectual growth. It has been suggested by Olney et al (2004) and Telford et al (2006) that tempered emotional responses and a positive attitude have a role in:

- promoting of health

- protecting against psychological dysfunction

- assisting with management of stress

- coping with the difficult situations likely to be encountered in the adjustment process.

Goleman (1996) claims that emotional intelligence abilities can be developed and that competence enables resilience, survival, and self-protection alongside use of the following key emotional skills:

- Self-awareness

- Identifying, expressing and managing feelings

- Impulse control

- Delaying gratification

- Handling stress and anxiety.

The author suggests that the application of emotional intelligence principles to individuals dealing with the psychosocial challenges of adjustment to illness and impairment appears to have huge potential. It is suggested that the training and facilitation of emotional intelligence abilities can occur within an effective therapeutic relationship and by engagement in specific therapeutic activities within an occupational therapy programme.

Aims of occupational therapy

The occupational therapist will draw on primary frames of reference to inform practice and utilise applied frames of reference to focus the recovery process (Hagedorn 1997). It appears feasible to suggest that enabling strategies offered by the occupational therapist will focus on the provision of psychosocial support that aims to:

- engage the individual in an effective therapeutic process

- monitor and assess emotional status

- support self-esteem

- facilitate and develop emotional intelligence abilities including self/emotional expression and management of negative affect (anger and anxiety) and mood

- enable coping skills and strategies

- maintain motivation and control

- enable adjustment to physical dysfunction

- provide health education

- enable purposeful occupation.

Intervention

A variety of assessment and intervention strategies will be employed following negotiation with the individual in order to foster the collaborative relationship and enhance self expression and perceived personal control. Perceived personal control positively impacts upon health-related behaviours and supports psychosocial adjustment for people who may have a physical injury or impairment, such as a cardiac condition, cancer, diabetes, spinal cord injury or rheumatoid arthritis (Linveh et al 2006). Coping effectiveness and regulation of effect is also enhanced by control, meaning, purpose, and problem focusing (Linveh et al 2006, Taylor 1999), all of which can be facilitated by applying the principles of person-centred occupational therapy practice.

The efficacy of group interventions which provide education and support to the individual and/or their carers via group discussion and the sharing of feelings and information is well established (Finlay 1993). The utilisation and therapeutic value of support groups in the field of physical impairment is evidenced by numerous authors (Ashe et al 2005, Kendall & Buys 1998, McNulty 2004, Putnam & Adams 1992, Schrever 2006, Telford 2006), and supports their use in the context of adjustment and recovery.

Specific emotional difficulties can be addressed by utilising educational and cognitive behavioural techniques to manage anxiety, anger, and negative thinking, and to facilitate the development of basic coping strategies that are linked to adaptation and reduction of emotional distress. Psychosocial adjustment requires establishment of new cognitive schemas related to the post-impairment identity and experiences (Kendall & Buys 1998, Yoshida 1993) and will benefit from a cognitive behavioural approach and the application of specific cognitive behavioural techniques (Scott et al 1995, Stein & Cutler 2002). Such activities might include anxiety and anger management or assertiveness training that is focused on enabling coping and adaptation to physical dysfunction, and the independent functioning of any individual within their own environmental context.

The value of emotional self-management abilities is very relevant to the practice of the occupational therapist in this field. Emotional intelligence abilities can be facilitated both within a collaborative relationship, which supports honest communication, expression, trust and empowerment, and within specifically selected enabling strategies, which address development of the social, emotional and behavioural skills that are central to living in society (Hawkey 2006) and to occupational performance.

Examples of occupational therapy activity to develop emotional intelligence abilities include:

- Communication and emotion identification/emotion-sharing exercises

- Empathy development (understanding the feelings of others and impact of diagnosis)

- Role play/rehearsal of key conversations (e.g. giving family information about the diagnosis, explaining health needs to an employer)

- Modelling of effective skills and techniques

- Diary keeping and review/group discussion, sharing and support

- Impulse management skills

- Seminars and information giving.

Emotional intelligence skills facilitate adaptive problem solving, helping to frame problems and use creativity and flexibility in solution finding (Mayer & Salovey 1997), enhancing both the therapeutic outcomes and adjustment to disability.

Reflection 14.4 focuses on engaging a resistant individual in therapy.

| Reflection 14.4 |

Engaging resistant individuals in therapy

Engaging resistant individuals in therapy may be essential. Think about an individual who was reluctant to engage in occupational therapy:

- Identify why they were reluctant or resistant and how you discovered the reason for their reluctance.

- Identify the techniques used to try to engage them and the skills you employed.

- Identify the skills which worked and those which did not work.

- Summarise how the relationship you developed with this individual impacted his engagement in occupational therapy activity.

- Identify the skills you could have used to enhance the relationship further.

- Identify the positive impact these skills might have had on therapeutic engagement and/or outcomes.

- Consider if you learned anything about yourself when reflecting upon these relationships.

The application of psychosocial enabling strategies

The application of psychosocial enabling strategies is illustrated in the two Practice Scenarios.

Practice Scenario 14.1
Mrs. Dorothy Walters

Mrs. Walters is a 64-year-old woman who lives alone in the two-bedroom, terraced house which she has resided in for over 40 years. She worked part-time as a school dinner lady but gave up work over 25 years ago to care for her disabled son, which she did until his death 5 years ago. She has no contact with her husband who left the family home shortly after the birth of their son. Mrs. Walters had no other children.

Mrs. Walters was diagnosed with rheumatoid arthritis (RA) over 20 years ago. Her condition appears to have deteriorated recently. Previously, she has resisted any assistance from community services. However, she recently saw her general practitioner (GP) for a medication review, and was referred to the occupational therapist. Her referral read: '*RA advancing, lives alone, bereavement 5 yrs ago, anxious, isolated, difficulty accessing upper floors of house.*'

Establishing trust and boundaries

Chrissy, the occupational therapist, visited Mrs. Walters at her home. She finds that, although Mrs. Walters opens the door, she is reluctant to allow her into the house, stating that she only went to the GP for her medication, that she isn't going to have her bed downstairs or end up in a home and that she is fine. Chrissy recognised that Mrs. Walters was suspicious, unhappy and anxious about the visit, and used **reflection** to ensure that she understood these feelings, communicating to Mrs. Walters that her feelings are being heard and noted.

Chrissy was **genuine** and **respectful**, acknowledging that the purpose of the visit has not been explained effectively and suggesting that clearer information could be helpful. She provided factual and honest information relating to the GP's concerns but also reiterates that Mrs. Walters' views and opinions are paramount. Chrissy **summarises** the conversation thus far, **clarifying** and **validating** Mrs. Walters' feelings and demonstrating **empathy**.

During this conversation on the doorstep Chrissy explained that she would be interested to hear how Mrs. Walters found the RA was affecting her, and how she managed her pain, commenting that she might be able to offer useful information and advice. Chrissy also added that if Mrs. Walters didn't want to let her in or if it would be more convenient to call back, then that choice would be respected. Chrissy ensured here that Mrs. Walters was aware that any continuation of the visit was negotiable, and that she wished to collaborate with her to consider any difficulties, applying **person-centred** principles.

Building the relationship

Chrissy asked Mrs. Walters if she might come in for a limited period of time, allowing the client to control the time boundaries of the visit. She also made it clear that, although she might be able to suggest ways of making life a little easier, the choice to take any action was Mrs. Walters'. Chrissy was invited in and noted that Mrs. Walters' mobility was slow and laboured. Rather than embark on an occupation-based assessment, that Mrs Walters may have responded to with resistance at that point, Chrissy used **focusing** to help Mrs. Walters to identify what was bothering her most, rather than looking at what the therapist perceived to be most important.

Mrs. Walters reported that the pain in her hips and knees was 'a real nuisance' and that she felt more exhausted, but that as long as she could get upstairs she would be fine. She became agitated, stating that she managed, didn't want anyone tipping her house upside down and politely advised Chrissy to keep her wheelchairs and lifts for those who were 'more needy'. Chrissy **explored** who the 'more needy' might be using **summarising**, **clarification**, and **immediacy** and established that Mrs. Walters felt strongly that she would not tolerate strangers in her house, would not accept what she described as 'charity', was fiercely proud of her independence and of her ability to care for her son for so many years.

Chrissy explained a little about her role. She stated that she would be able to help Mrs. Walters understand more about RA and how to manage it. She **established** that Mrs. Walters had limited specific knowledge of her illness and it appeared that she did not want to know too much about it. This was Mrs. Walters' choice and it was respected by Chrissy, who recognised a need to work at a pace which suited Mrs. Walters. Chrissy invited Mrs. Walters to talk about her own roles and activities. She used some basic **drawing out** and **questioning** skills to engage Mrs. Walters in conversation, establish some facts, and begins to build up a relationship. Mrs. Walters reported that she didn't like to go out much or bother with people, and whilst this could suggest isolation and low mood, further discussion using **concreteness** in order to illustrate examples and patterns, suggested that Mrs. Walters had a routine within her home and viewed her role within the home as her most important activity, 'keeping it tidy' and 'keeping the rooms nice'. She reported having never really engaged in much activity outside the home and was glad to give up work to be with her son. Evidence suggested that RA can interfere with social roles and recreational activity (Wikstrom et al 2001), but Mrs. Walters reported having no desire to become involved with what she termed the 'elderly luncheon club'. She stated that, 'they just moan a lot' and added that she prefers her own company and that of one or two friends. She did comment that she has a neighbour round for coffee once a week, did a bit of baking and went to church.

Questioning, exploring and using empathy

Chrissy intended to approach the sensitive subject of getting up stairs, having already noted Mrs. Walters' earlier reaction to this subject. Chrissy prepared Mrs. Walters for a more difficult area of discussion, reminding her that if she didn't wish to answer any questions, didn't understand the question or wanted her to leave she just needed to say so. Chrissy indicated that she was concerned about Mrs. Walters using the stairs. When she enquired about getting upstairs, Mrs. Walters again became agitated, explaining that she was fine on the stairs and there was no need to fuss about it. She commented that a neighbour suggested she move into the lounge, and added that this was ridiculous.

Chrissy assumed that it must be painful to go upstairs and that it might be easier to avoid climbing them, remaining concerned that Mrs. Walters might injure herself. Rather than acting upon this assumption, she considered that Mrs. Walters' reaction to the subject suggested that going up stairs was very important, and used **reflection** and **focusing** to wonder about what matters most and why this matters so much to Mrs. Walters. Mrs. Walters explained that she goes upstairs to sit in her son's room, explaining that she goes in several times a day, 'it's peaceful and I enjoy it, just thinking …' stating that she keeps it just as it was. Chrissy used **reflection**, **clarification**, **focusing**, **giving permission**, and **concreteness** skills to establish how Mrs. Walters felt, establishing that she enjoyed sitting in the bedroom, reliving happy memories and that this activity had purpose and meaning for her. She understood that Mrs. Walters spent a lot of years caring for her son and was happy for him to continue to take up her time. Mrs. Walters' anxiety did not appear to be about isolation or grief but was about being unable to carry out this very important activity and continue her most significant life role of mother.

Assessing risk and dealing with emotions

Mrs. Walters disclosed her fear that as she had become more impaired, things had become more difficult and painful, and that she had been distressed by people saying she should leave the family home. Despite her impairment Mrs. Walters was adamant that her priority was maintaining her meaningful activity in the home and that she would go upstairs whether it 'hurts my knees or not'. This was Mrs. Walters' choice and, although Chrissy expressed concern, she acknowledged **respect** of this choice and verbalised this to Mrs. Walters, conveying **genuineness** and **empathy**. Mrs. Walters responded to this by demonstrating trust in Chrissy and agreed to show Chrissy her stair-climbing technique.

Chrissy was concerned about Mrs. Walters' safety and had some issues regarding joint preservation that she verbalised honestly. She used simple clear terms, avoiding technical language that might have negatively impacted upon the building relationship and the establishment of honest communication. Chrissy used **reflection**, **immediacy**, and **clarification** to establish the strength of Mrs. Walters' feelings and reflected that Mrs. Walters appeared unable to negotiate changing her behaviour at present because it was too anxiety-provoking to consider that she couldn't go upstairs. Chrissy verbalised her understanding of how vitally important getting upstairs was, acknowledging Mrs. Walters' fears, demonstrating **empathy**. Mrs. Walters became briefly tearful as she recognised that she was understood, agreeing that she 'couldn't bear it'. Chrissy stated that Mrs. Walters' safety was her priority and that activity might become

more difficult as the RA continued to affect her joints, demonstrating **honesty**, **respect**, and **genuineness,** and avoiding the temptation of false reassurance.

Mrs. Walters was **silent** and eventually Chrissy used **immediacy** to ask her what she was thinking. Mrs. Walters commented that she was scared about getting worse, but felt she had said too much, worrying that Chrissy's notes would say she had to go into a home. Chrissy asked Mrs Walters what she would be willing to consider, suggesting that making the stairs safer was a priority, again reinforcing that negotiated goals were the key to engagement in the therapeutic process. Chrissy also explained that looking after her joints was really important, and that looking at how she managed her household chores, in terms of how much she does each day, might help conserve energy, reduce pain, and leave her feeling less tired.

Setting goals and summarising

Chrissy wondered if Mrs. Walters felt ready to find out a little more about her condition, again allowing her to negotiate goals and work at her own pace. Mrs. Walters agreed to allow Chrissy to call again to talk about it and to look at the stairs, but added that she wasn't sure she'd 'have anything permanent'. Chrissy briefly **recapped** the discussion using **summarising** skills, arranged a second visit, **recapped** the purpose of it and thanked Mrs. Walters for her cooperation.

Practice scenario 14.2 Johnny Todd

Johnny Todd was 32 years old, he had two children aged 7 and 4 years, and lived in a bungalow with his wife. He was diagnosed with relapsing–remitting–non-progressive multiple sclerosis (MS) 4 years ago. He had experienced three exacerbations over the last 4 years, the most severe of which left him confined to a wheelchair for 2 months. Johnny had been admitted to the ward following an exacerbation that has resulted in blurred vision in his right eye, bilateral dysaesthesia, fatigue, and fine motor in-coordination. The referral was for an occupational therapy assessment, but included a note stating he was having panic attacks. Whilst the presenting problems were clear, the emotional well-being, occupational roles, environment, and social circumstances of Johnny needed to be explored by the therapist during the interview/assessment. Emma, the occupational therapist, saw Johnny on the ward.

Establishing trust

During the interview Johnny initially refused to engage in any assessment, stating he was exhausted from lack of sleep. He was hostile and aggressive with Emma, accusing her of keeping secrets and information from him. Emma used **clarification** and **immediacy**, asking Johnny what he meant by secrets and what he was thinking about when he talked about people keeping things from him. He stated that he was concerned that he had been mis-diagnosed and that he had a progressive form of the disorder and would not recover the neurological abilities that were currently compromised. Whilst medical evidence could have been used to challenge Johnny's perspective, Emma resisted the temptation to close down the conversation with technical information and demonstrated **respect** for his unique subjective experience, allowing his fears and feelings vital time and space (Kensit 2000). A range of communication skills were used to draw out the conversation, acknowledge Johnny's fear, anger, and frustration, and establish that he felt angry and resentful that he had this disease.

Focusing was used to identify that Johnny was bothered most by the 'panics' he had been having over the last year, he reported having 'sweats and palpitations' at night in bed and when out with the family in crowded places he felt sick and dizzy, and had to get home; which he reported as being 'very embarrassing'. He explained that these feelings had gotten worse and made him feel tired all the time; he felt 'ashamed' that he could not control them. Johnny's feelings were explored utilising **clarification**, **focusing**, **reflection**, and **concreteness**, and this highlighted his belief that some of the anxiety symptoms he described (numbness and pain in his arms and legs, headaches and poor concentration) must be related to the MS and must be mini attacks, confirming for him that his condition was changing and worsening. This had led to numerous visits to the general practitioner (GP) and a couple of trips to casualty, causing huge distress and disruption to the family.

When Emma asked about his roles within the family he became tearful stating that he was a father and a husband, but felt like a 'disabled burden', stating that he felt 'inadequate'. He described the importance of his roles as a freelance music teacher and carer to his two children, as his wife worked full time. He had played guitar all his life, describing this as having been his 'passion', and 'the thing he was best at'. Emma explored Johnny's self image, using **clarification**, **reflection**, and **silence**, to elicit feelings around his pre- and post-impairment self. Johnny reported having enjoyed playing in a locally successful band with his wife, which contributed more money to the household income. He felt that this was important. Recently, he had been unable to do these things and had avoided booking many music lessons and gigs over the past few months. He described feeling 'overwhelmed' by the tasks, worried about the quality of his playing, struggling with guitar chords and confidence, feeling tense and unable to concentrate. Emma recognised the impact this impairment was having upon his self-image and esteem, using **reflection**, **concreteness**, **confrontation**, and **focusing** to explore feelings and identify priorities with Johnny.

According to McNulty et al (2004), MS is a highly stressful and intrusive event and adaptation to it requires not only an initial adjustment, but the continuous effort of readjustment to its erratic, unpredictable symptoms. Johnny cited the unpredictable and uncertain nature of his illness and his increased dependence on his wife as something that was really bothering him, saying he felt it 'would only get worse' and that he 'felt guilty that his wife and kids were stuck with the consequences of his illness forever'. Emma used some emotion identification and sharing exercises to begin building emotional intelligence abilities and facilitate expression, exploration and understanding of feelings. Johnny stated that he was unable to discuss these feelings with his wife, suggesting that his moaning wouldn't help, and his wife had enough to deal with. **Clarification** was used to establish that his fear of discovering his wife's 'true' feelings was a constant worry, leaving him tense and anxious. Johnny reported feeling 'furious' with himself for 'putting on a brave face' for the last 2 years, which had left him exhausted. It also meant that he couldn't be himself and show how he felt because others now expected him to 'keep smiling and cope'.

Emma was aware of problems associated with MS in terms of fear of symptoms, fatigue, role strain, poor management of medical crises, and their impact on adjustment (McNulty et al 2004). Professional reasoning skills were used to establish priorities and recognise the immediate need to explore and manage Johnny's anxiety, which was manifesting itself in the form of generalised anxiety and panic attacks, and was impacting upon all areas of his occupational performance. Johnny had also identified the 'panics' as the most important problem, and the goal of addressing this issue was established collaboratively, motivating Johnny and supporting the alliance between himself and Emma. Johnny agreed to an assessment and the Stress Management Questionnaire (Stein 1987, cited in Stein & Cutler 2002) was administered.

Intervention techniques

Following this, Johnny's problems were conceptualised, helping him to link his thoughts, feelings and behaviours. Therapeutic goals were negotiated, supporting person-centred practice and empowerment. Johnny was offered a short, focused, anxiety-management programme utilising cognitive behavioural principles and strategies to assess and manage the behavioural and emotional components of the anxiety quickly, and to begin linking the anxiety to his fears about his wife's feelings and the suppression of his own feelings. The programme comprised five sessions focusing on increasing Johnny's knowledge and awareness of the nature, function and effect of stress and anxiety. In addition, Johnny was enabled to monitor his stress via diary keeping, and manage physical symptoms using relaxation and breathing techniques. Self-calming and regulation skills, including techniques to challenge negative automatic thinking and correction of faulty cognitive constructs, were also provided (Stein & Cutler 2002, Everett et al 2003, Scott et al 1995, Sheldon 1995). Follow-up intervention included consideration of an ongoing programme of group anxiety management in the community setting, enabling further application of cognitive behavioural techniques with a structured programme of around 12 weekly sessions. These interventions enabled acquisition of self-management skills and the support of self-efficacy and esteem.

Emotional intelligence training enabled Johnny to develop self-awareness, skills in identifying, expressing and managing feelings, communication skills, goal setting, impulse control, handling stress and anxiety, and the development of self-protection strategies (Goleman 1996, Mayer & Salovey 1997, Mckenna 2007). Specifically selected therapeutic activities were included in the occupational therapy programme on both a one-to-one and group basis, and included inter- and intra-personal social skills training which focused on issues and situations related to the impact of MS and the process of adjustment. These strategies enabled Johnny to enhance his emotional openness/adaptation, communication, problem-solving skills, and flexibility, which facilitated adaptive behaviour, accommodating changes in his engagement, performance, needs, and goals.

Summary

Practice Scenario 14.1 presents the application of communication skills to engage a resistant individual in the therapeutic process. By applying the principles of person-centred practice and utilising advanced communication skills, Mrs. Walters' needs were explored and the temptation to begin formulating solutions to problems based on obvious medical concerns and referral assumptions were avoided. The occupational therapist, Chrissy, utilised professional reasoning skills to explore stair mobility and safety. Only concentrating on this could have resulted in anxiety for Mrs. Walters. Emphasis on technical aspects of care and the provision of mobility aids (which at this stage were likely to be refused) would focus on pre-determined performance criteria, rather than exploring and understanding personal experience, perception, context and concerns (Cole & McLean 2003, Tickle-Degnen 1995). Chrissy also allowed her own potential preconceptions (suggested by the referral) concerning Mrs. Walters' grief and the potential suggestion that after 5 years it might be considered abnormal and need to be challenged. Chrissy explored Mrs. Walters' presentation, motivation, level of assertion, insight and positive attitude, and felt comfortable that her mental health was sound, although her mood was being impacted by pain and fatigue. Chrissy listened to Mrs. Walters during the visit, rather than trying to direct the conversation, exploring her perspective on events and discovering what was important to her, which contributed to the building of empathy (Finlay 2004). Chrissy utilised advanced communication skills to begin establishing a therapeutic relationship and, whilst time-consuming for a hard-pressed community occupational therapist with a long waiting list, this facilitated the engagement of a previously resistant person in the process of therapy, making the person accessible to the occupational therapist. By listening to Mrs. Walters' needs and establishing trust, collaborative occupational goals were set and Mrs. Walters was willing to allow Chrissy to make a series of return visits enabling further exploration and monitoring of psychosocial needs, assessment of self-care skills and risk issues, and the discussion of pain, fatigue and joint management, which will positively impact pain management, mood and the provision of accessible and accurate health education information pertinent to RA. Mrs. Walters was empowered and enabled to maintain roles and meaningful activity and to better manage, adjust to and adapt to impairment.

Practice Scenario 14.2 presents the facilitation of adjustment to physical impairment using specific enabling strategies (emotional intelligence training and cognitive behavioural intervention), that are applied specifically to the management of anxiety and emotional distress. For Johnny, the immediate management of his anxiety was necessary in order to provide psychosocial support and specifically address emotional needs. His engagement in any activity, including assessments, was likely to be mediated by his emotional state making accurate information inaccessible and potentially increasing his anxiety. Johnny's engagement in meaningful roles such as being a husband, father, musician and worker, were also being negatively impacted by the anxiety. Whilst Emma might be pressured into facilitating discharge quickly and efficiently, Price-Lackey & Cashman (1996) suggested that interventions driven by service protocols and pre-determined outcome goals, rather than a person's needs and goals, risk disregarding the adaptive capacities of the people who require our services and neglect the holistic principles of our practice.

In order to assist with adjustment and acceptance of impairment Emma applied advanced communication skills. These skills were essential in Johnny's therapy, building a trusting therapeutic relationship and enabling him to discuss his problems freely (Job et al 1997). Person-centred counselling principles are synchronous with the holistic practice of the occupational therapist (Lane 2000), itself a constituent part of theoretical models including the Canadian Model of Occupational Performance and Engagement (Townsend & Polatajko 2007) and enables the individual to become his own expert empowering his role in his own adaptation and recovery (Pierce 2000).

These strategies enabled Emma to offer psychosocial support and to specifically address some adjustment issues, including enabling emotional intelligence abilities, such as the expression and management of emotions in self and others. Johnny's issues included feelings of anger, fear, anxiety, uncertainty, loss, and dependence, which were complicated by the relapsing and remitting nature of the particular disease pattern, and required constant readjustment between the pre- and post-impairment self and its consequences (Yoshida 1993). Johnny was able to release feelings, address suppressed issues, and develop coping strategies using emotional intelligence training and cognitive behavioural techniques. The strategies employed here were coupled with health education related to the condition, and, specifically, management of pain and fatigue. He perceived that he had a limited purpose in life. Perception of a purpose is viewed as a major mediator of adjustment to impairment. The restoration of health through the use of purposeful activity and

meaningful occupation remain central to the occupational therapist's goals (Hagedorn 2000). Enabling Johnny's engagement in meaningful activities (specifically in playing music), which had spiritual significance in terms of his sense of self, was crucial in maintaining self-esteem and meaning. The re-establishment of occupational performance and roles within the family enhanced psychosocial well-being and facilitated adjustment and recovery.

Conclusion

Interpersonal interaction skills have a broad application within occupational therapy practice, not least in the establishment, development and maintenance of the therapeutic relationship. Subsequent engagement in the occupational therapy process and the effective application of assessment and enabling strategies is also impacted by the effective deployment of communication skills. Encouraging the participation of an anxious person in a group activity; ensuring an accurate kitchen assessment with a tearful person; providing information relating to disease prognosis in a form that the person is able and willing to understand; motivating a reluctant person to attend for splint refitting; and securing access to the home of a person in order to complete a risk assessment are all more likely if appropriate skills are utilised effectively to support the occupational therapy process.

Active listening skills are used to convey empathy. Effective questioning and working through skills facilitate open, honest communication, encouraging the description, exploration, emotional expression and clarification of the individual's issues. Whitcher & Tse (2004) describe communication skills as a therapeutic tool that enables interaction within a therapeutic relationship and also enables meaningful activity or occupation. The skilled therapist will invest time in the use of these skills. The therapist will aim to achieve interactions that support the individual alongside the process and content of the therapy in which they are engaged, contributing positively to meaningful engagement in efficacious occupational therapy treatment. The utilisation of interpersonal skills within a collaborative relationship aims to empower the individual, and the provision of integrated, holistic therapeutic interventions that meet the persons' psychosocial needs, will enable occupational functioning and well-being.

One of the major difficulties writing this chapter presented was in dealing with the overlap or division which exists between accepted provision of care by the occupational therapist working in physical and mental health services. I wonder at what point the therapist in a physical rehabilitation setting views an individual who is struggling to deal with a physical impairment and has become low in mood or anxious to be in need of treatment by a 'mental health' occupational therapist. I reiterate the empirical evidence we have suggesting that non-compliance and reluctance to engage with mental health services is significant within what Etherington (1990b) describes as the 'physical rehabilitation group'. I do not suggest that there is a simple answer and do not suggest that overstretched occupational therapists have the time to further extend their roles. However, as we are increasingly attempting to evidence our practice as a unique profession, this division, which Rigney (2000) asserts is one which we put there ourselves, may be restricting our professional identity and presenting a barrier to the holistic practice we claim to hold so dear.

Reflection 14.5 focuses on employing holistic principles in practice.

The occupational therapist considers the physical, psychological, and social elements of the individual, and our interventions rely upon our use of a range of skills to enable the individual to overcome, or learn to live with impairment. Our skills should be utilised to meet each individual's need and not rely on those skills we have most familiarity with, experience of, or confidence in (Rigney 2000). Whilst not intending to engage in the essential debate around resources and staffing, institutional structure, working practice and skill mix, and whilst also acknowledging that there are specialist areas of practice shaped by service development, skills training and client group, surely the occupational therapist must provide a basic level of holistic and integrated service to all.

Reflection 14.5

Employing holistic principles

Employing holistic principles is vital, think about two individuals you have worked with who might have been dealing with both physical and mental health issues:

- Consider if they were treated holistically and describe how this was operationalised or was not operationalised.
- Describe how the psychosocial and physical needs of each individual were met.
- Identify how has this experience has influenced your practice.

References

Alder, R., Rosenfield, L. & Proctor, R. (1998). *Interplay: the process of interpersonal communication*. (7th ed). Fort Worth, Harcourt Brace.

Ashe, B., Taylor, M. & Dobouloz, C. J. (2005). The process of change: listening to transformation in meaning perspectives of adults in arthritis health education groups. *Canadian Journal of Occupational Therapy*, 72(5), 280–288.

Atchison, B. & Dirette, D. (2007). *Conditions in occupational therapy – effect on occupational performance*. Baltimore, Lippincott Williams and Wilkins.

Bayne, R., Nicolson, P. & Horton, I. (1998). *Counselling and communication skills for medical and health practitioners*. Leicester, The British Psychological Society.

Blank, A. (2004) Clients' Experience of Partnership with Occupational Therapist in Community Mental Health. *British Journal of Occupational Therapy*, 67(3): 118–124.

Brooks, W. (1971). *Speech communication* Dubuque, IA, WC Brown.

Browne, G., Arpin, K., Corey, P., Fitch, M. & Gaffney, A. (1990). Individual correlates of health service utilisation. *Medical Care*, 28, 43–58.

Bruce, M. A. & Borg, B. (1987). *Frames of reference in psychosocial occupational therapy*. New Jersey, Slack.

Burgoon, J.K., Pfau, M., Parott, R., Birk, T., Coker, R., & Burgoon, M. (1987). Relational communication, satisfaction, compliance – gaining strategies, and compliance in communication between physicians and patients. *Communication Monographs*, 54, 307–324.

Burnard, P. (2005). *Counselling skills for health professionals*. (4th ed). Cheltenham, Nelson Thornes Ltd.

Ciarrochi, J., Deane, F. P. & Anderson, S. (2002). Emotional intelligence moderates the relationship between stress and mental health. *Personality and Individual Differences*, 32(2), 197–209.

Cole, M. B. & McLean, V. (2003). Therapeutic relationships re-defined. *Occupational Therapy in Mental Health*, 19(2), 33–51.

College of Occupational Therapists (2002/3). *Standards for education: pre registration education standards*. London, COT.

College of Occupational Therapists (2004). *Definitions and core skills for occupational therapy*. London, COT.

College of Occupational Therapists (2005). *College of Occupational Therapists: code of ethics and professional conduct*. London, COT.

Compton, A. & Ashwin, M. (2000). *Community care for health professionals*. Edinburgh, Butterworth Heinemann.

Couldrick, L. (1997). Counselling and counselling skills. *British Journal of Occupational Therapy*, 60(10), 463–464.

Crepeau, E. B. (1991). Achieving intersubjective understanding: examples from an occupational therapy treatment session. *American Journal Of Occupational Therapy*, 45(10), 1016–1025.

Dangoor, N. & Florian, V. (1994). Women with chronic physical disabilities: correlates of their long term psychosocial adaptation. *International Journal of Rehabilitation*, 17(2),159–168.

Di Blasi, Z. Harkness, E, Georgiou, A. & Kleijnedn, J. (2001). Influence of context effects on healthcare outcomes: a systematic review. *Lancet*, 357, 752–762.

Dickson, D., Hargie, O. & Morrow, N. (1997). *Communication skills training for health professionals*. (2nd ed). London, Chapman Hall.

Egan, G. (1990). *The skilled helper: a systematic approach to effective helping*. (5th ed). Monteray, CA. Brooks/Cole.

Etherington, K. (1990a). The Disabled Persons Act 1986: the need for counselling. *British Journal of Occupational Therapy*, 53(10), 430–432.

Etherington, K. (1990b). The occupational therapist as a counsellor towards attitude change in disability. *British Journal of Occupational Therapy*, 53(11), 463–466.

Everett, T., Donaghy, M. & Feaver, S. (2003). *Interventions for mental health*. Edinburgh, Butterworth Heinman.

Faulkner, A. (1998). *Effective interaction with patients*. London, Churchill Livingstone.

Finlay, L. (1993). *Groupwork in occupational therapy*. London, Chapman Hall.

Finlay, L. (2001) Holism in occupational therapy: elusive fiction and ambivalent struggle. *The American Journal of Occupational Therapy*, 55(3), 268–276.

Finlay, L. (2004). *The practice of psychosocial occupational therapy*. London, Nelson Thornes.

Gardner, H. (1993). *Multiple intelligences*. New York, Basic Books.

Geldard, K. & Geldard, D. (2005). *Practical counselling skills – an integrative approach*. New York, Palgrave Macmillan.

Goleman, D. (1996). *Emotional intelligence – why it can matter more than IQ*. London, Bloomsbury.

Guthrie, E. (1996). Emotional disorder in chronic illness: psychotherapeutic interventions. *British Journal of Psychiatry*, 168, 265–273.

Hagedorn, R. (1995). *Occupational therapy perspectives and processes*. Edinburgh, Churchill Livingstone.

Hagedorn, R. (1997). *Foundations for practice in occupational therapy*, (2nd ed). Edinburgh, Churchill Livingstone.

Hagedorn, R. (2000). *Tools for practice in occupational therapy: a structured approach to core skills and processes*. Edinburgh, Churchill Livingstone.

Hahn, H. (1985). Towards politics of disability: definitions, disciplines and policies. *Social Science Journal*, 22(4), 39–47.

Hargie, O. & Dickson, D. (2004). *Skilled interpersonal communication*. (4th ed). Hove, Routledge.

Harrison J., Maguire, P., Ibbotson T. & Macleod, R. (1994). Concerns, confiding and psychiatric disorder in newly diagnosed cancer patients: a descriptive study. *Psycho-Oncology*, 3(3), 173–179.

Hawkey, K. (2006). Emotional intelligence and mentoring in pre–service teacher education: A literature review. *Mentoring and Tutoring* 14(2), 137–147.

Hinojosa, J., Kramer, P., Royeen, C. B. & Luebben, A. J. (Eds) (2003). *Core concepts of occupation in perspectives in human occupation: participation in life*. Pennsylvania, Lippincott Williams & Wilkins.

Jeffrey, B. & Hicks, C. (1997). The impact of counselling skills training on the interpersonal skills of undergraduate occupational therapy students. *British Journal of Occupational Therapy*, 60(9), 395–400.

Job, T., Broom, W. & Habermehl, F. (1997). Coming out! time to acknowledge the importance of counselling skills in occupational therapy. *British Journal of Occupational Therapy*, 60(8), 357–358.

Kalisch, B. J. (1971). Strategies for developing nurse empathy. *Nursing Outlook*, 19(11), 714–717.

Kendall, E. & Buys, N. (1998). An integrated model of psychosocial adjustment following acquired disability. *Journal of Rehabilitation*, 64(3),16–21.

Kensit, D. A. (2000). Rogerian theory: a critique of the effectiveness of pure client-centred therapy. *Counselling Psychology Quarterly*, 13(4), 345–351.

Lane, L. (2000). Client-centred practice: is it compatible with early discharge hospital at home policies. *British Journal of Occupational Therapy*, 63(7), 310–315.

Lapsley, H., Nicora, L. W. & Black, R. (2002). *'Kia mauri tau' – narratives of recovery from disabling mental health problems*. Wellington, New Zealand, Mental Health Commission.

Livneh, H., Lott, S. M. & Antonak, R. F. (2004). Patterns of psychosocial adaptation to chronic illness and disability: a cluster analytic approach. *Psychology Health And Medicine*, 9(4), 411–430.

Livneh, H., Martz, F. & Bodner, T. (2006). Psychosocial adaptation to chronic illness and disability: A preliminary study of its factorial structure. *Journal of Clinical Psychology in Medical Settings*, 13(3), 50–260.

Lloyd, C. & Maas, F. (1991). The therapeutic relationship. *British Journal of Occupational Therapy*, 54(3), 111–113.

Lloyd, C. & Maas, F. (1992). Interpersonal skills and occupational therapy. *British Journal of Occupational Therapy*, 55(10), 379–382.

Lloyd, C. & Maas, F. (1993). The helping relationship: the application of Carkhuff's model. *Canadian Journal of Occupational Therapy*, 60(2), 83–88.

Matheson, L. N. (1998). 'Engaging the person in the process: planning together for occupational therapy intervention'. In: M. Law (Ed.). *Client-centred occupational therapy*. Thorofare, NJ, Slack Incorporated.

Mattingley, C. (1991). The narrative nature of clinical reasoning. *American Journal of Occupational Therapy*, 45, 998–1005.

Mayer, J. D. & Cobb, C. D. (2000). Educational policy on emotional intelligence – does it make sense.

Educational Psychology Review, 12(2), 163–183.

Mayer, J. D. & Salovey, P. (1997). What is emotional intelligence? In: P. Salovey, & D. Sluyter (Eds). *Emotional development and emotional intelligence: implications for educators.* New York. Basic Books, 3–29.

Mckenna, J. (2007). Emotional intelligence training in adjustment to physical disability and illness. *International Journal of Therapy and Rehabilitation*, 14(12), 551–556.

McNulty, K., Livneh, H. & Wilson, L. (2004). Perceived uncertainty, spiritual well being and psychosocial adaptation in individuals with multiple sclerosis. *Rehabilitation Psychology*, 49(2), 91–99.

Middlehurst, S. (1991). Counselling in occupational therapy. *Counselling*, 2(4), 135–136.

Niemeier, J. & Burnett, D. (2001). No such thing as 'uncomplicated bereavement' for patients in rehabilitation. *Disability and Rehabilitation*, 23(15), 645–653.

Olney, M., Brockelman, K. F., Kennedy, J. & Newsom, M. (2004). Do you have a disability? A population based test of denial and adjustment among adults with disabilities in the US. *Journal of Rehabilitation*, 70(il), 4–10.

Peloquin, S. (1995). The fullness of empathy: reflections and illustrations. *American Journal of Occupational Therapy*, 49(1), 24–31.

Peveler, R., Feldman, E. & Friedman, T. (2000). *Liaison psychiatry: planning services for specialist settings.* London, Gaskell.

Pierce, D. (2000). Occupation by design: dimensions, therapeutic power, and creative process. *American Journal of Occupational Therapy*, 55(3), 249–258.

Pollock, N. & McColl, M. A. (1998). Assessment in client-centred occupational therapy. In: M. Law (ed.). *Client-centred occupational therapy.* Thorofare, NJ, Slack Incorporated.

Price-Lackey, P. & Cashman, J. (1996). Jenny's story: reinventing oneself through occupation and narrative configuration. *American Journal of Occupational Therapy*, 50(4), 306–314.

Putnam, S. H. & Adams, K. M. (1992). Regression based prediction of long term outcome following multidisciplinary rehabilitation for traumatic brain injury. *The Clinical Neuropsychologist*, 6, 383–405.

Rigney, C. (2000). Physical or mental health: should we divide? *British Journal of Occupational Therapy*, 63(4), 177–178.

Robbins, S. & Hunsaker, P. (1996). *Training in interpersonal skills: tips for managing people at work.* (2nd ed.). New Jersey, Prentice Hall.

Rogers, C. R. (1951). *Client-centred therapy.* London, Constable & Robinson Ltd.

Rogers, C. (2001). *Client-centred therapy.* Suffolk, St. Emundsbury Press Ltd.

Rosa, S. A. & Hasselkus, B. R. (1996). Connecting with patients: the personal experience of professional helping. *Occupational Therapy Journal of Research*, 16(4), 245–260.

Ruddy, R. & House, A. (2005). Meta review of high quality systematic reviews of interventions in key areas of liaison psychiatry. *British Journal of Psychiatry*, 187, 109–120.

Schrever, N., Rimmerman, A. & Sachs, D. (2006). Adjustment to severe disability: constructing and examining a cognitive and occupational performance model. *International Journal of Rehabilitation Research*, 29, 201–207.

Scott, M.J., Stradling, S. & Dryden, W. (1995). *Developing cognitive behavioural counselling.* London, Sage Pubs.

Sheldon, B. (1995). *Cognitive behavioural therapy.* London, Routledge.

Stein, F. (1987). In Stein, F., & Cutler, S. (2002). *Psychosocial occupational therapy* (2nd ed). Australia, Delmar.

Stein, F. & Cutler, S. (2002). *Psychosocial occupational therapy.* (2nd ed.) Australia, Delmar.

Sumsion, T. (2000). A revised occupational therapy definition of client-centred practice. *British Journal of Occupational Therapy*, 63(7), 304–309.

Sviden, G. & Saljo, R. (1993). Perceiving patients and their non verbal reactions. *American Journal of Occupational Therapy*, 47(6), 491–497.

Taylor, S. E. (1999). *Health psychology.* (4th ed.) New York, McGraw-Hill.

Telford, K., Kralik, D. & Koch, T. (2006). Acceptance and denial: implications for people adapting to chronic illness: literature review. *Journal of Advanced Nursing*, 55(4), 457–464.

Tickle-Degnen, L. (1995). Therapeutic rapport. In: C. A. Trombly, (Ed) *Occupational therapy for physical dysfunction.* (pp. 299–308). Baltimore, Lippincott, Williams and Wilkins.

Tickle-Degnen, L. (2002). Client-centred practice, therapeutic relationship, and the use of research evidence. *American Journal of Occupational Therapy*, 56(4), 470–474.

Townsend, E. A. & Polatajko, H. J. (2007). *Enabling occupation ii: advancing an occupational therapy vision for health, well-being, and justice through occupation.* Ottawa, Canadian Association of Occupational Therapists.

Turner, A., Foster, M. & Johnson, S. (2003). *Occupational therapy and physical dysfunction, principles, skills and practice.* (5th ed.) China, Churchill Livingstone.

Unsworth, C. A. (2004). Clinical reasoning: how do pragmatic reasoning, worldview and client-centredness fit? *British Journal of Occupational Therapy*, 67(1), 10–19.

Whitcher, K. & Tse, S. (2004). Counselling skills in occupational therapy: a grounded theory approach to explain their use within mental health in New Zealand. *British Journal of Occupational Therapy*, 67(8), 361–368.

Wikstrom, I., Isacsson, A. & Jacobson, L. (2001). Leisure activities in rheumatoid arthritis: change after disease onset and associated factors. *British Journal of Occupational Therapy*, 64(2), 87–92.

World Health Organization (2002). *ICD–10 Classification of behavioural and mental disorders: Clinical descriptions and diagnostic guidelines.* Geneva, WHO.

Wright. B. A. (1983). *Physical disability – a psychosocial approach.* (2nd ed.). New York, Harper & Row.

Yoshida, K. K. (1993). Reshaping of self: a pendular reconstruction of self and identity among adults with traumatic spinal cord injury. *Sociology of Health and Illness*, 15(2), 217–245.

Chapter Fifteen

15

Advocating and lobbying

Valmae Rose, Kevin Cocks, and Lesley Chenoweth

CHAPTER CONTENTS

Introduction 212

Understanding and contextualising
models of disability 212

Models of disability 212

Vulnerable identities 213

Advocacy and lobbying in occupational
therapy. 214

Advocacy 214

Lobbying. 215

The occupational therapist as an agent of
change. 215

Strategies to effect change. 217

Managing the dilemmas and tensions
associated with advocacy and lobbying. . . 218

Conclusion. 219

SUMMARY

This chapter is designed to introduce the
concepts of advocacy and lobbying as they
pertain to the role of an occupational therapist.
As professionals with a broad theoretical
background and a comprehensive understanding
of the individuals with whom they work,
occupational therapists are in a unique position
to initiate, support, and implement change for
disabled people[1]. Advocacy and lobbying are
defined and contextualised through both real-
world examples and underpinning theoretical
frameworks; and the skills, knowledge and values
critical to developing occupational therapists as
agents of change are outlined. Finally, the
dilemmas and tensions that emerge when
venturing into advocacy and lobbying for change
are explored.

KEY POINTS

- Occupational therapists, by virtue of their skills, knowledge and value base, are well positioned to advocate and lobby for individuals striving for an ordinary (or extraordinary) life.
- Defining disability as either a personal tragedy (Moral Model) or in terms of deficit (Medical Model) locates disability within the individual and fails to address the issue of disabling environments.
- The Social Model proposes that society creates physical and attitudinal barriers that prevent or limit a person's full participation in the society.
- For professionals working with vulnerable people, advocacy can be understood as the act of directly representing or defending those people.
- Lobbying involves taking direct action to influence a political decision, policy or law.
- There are three strategies for influencing policy and effecting change: the rational-empirical, the normative re-education and the power-coercive strategies.
- Putting aside one's identity as a 'professional' or 'expert' to work *with* rather than *for* disabled people presents challenges for occupational therapists.

[1]The authors acknowledge the different nomenclature used in the disability sector. While in Australia the term 'people with disability' is the accepted term, we have used 'disabled people' in this chapter for coherency with overall text.

● Occupational therapists are in a position to extend the parameters of their practice moving beyond mere therapeutic strategies to consider the social barriers to people's enjoyment of a full and rich life.

It is individuals who change societies, who give birth to ideas, who, by standing out against the tide of opinion, change them.

Doris Lessing

Introduction

As occupational therapists, you are professionals who go about your work equipped with knowledge, skills and, ideally, a value base that is consistent with the goal of being of service directly to individuals, indirectly to their families, friends and ultimately to the community. You apply creative solutions to somewhat defined needs with the aim of supporting people to independently engage in the community with life roles they choose for themselves. You understand the value of meaningful relationships, you support people to be connected to their community and inspire them in the direction of their own personal vision for the future.

As an occupational therapist you have an understanding of the following:

● The complex factors involved in living and working in the community without hindrance.

● The importance of having valued roles and of experiencing the ordinary rhythms and routines of life.

● The ethical and moral right of all people to make and to experience the consequences of decisions about their own life; not just the everyday decisions, but the big ones – who to live with, where to live and how to define oneself.

● The importance of being defined by your own choices, desires and experiences, and not by your impairment or how you respond to services offered.

Occupational therapists, by virtue of their skills, knowledge, and value base, are well positioned to support individuals striving for an ordinary (or extraordinary) life, advocating on their behalf against injustice or lobbying for change at a range of levels. The occupational therapist knows the boundaries

and limitations of their learning and values, and, above all, their understanding of the lived experience of the people with whom they work. They do not pretend to understand the experience of the people they support and do not pass judgement. They trust the intuitive, self-determined actions and requests of people and comfortably work alongside those they support.

The purpose of this chapter is to introduce the concepts of advocacy and lobbying as they apply to the work of occupational therapists. While often part of the system or service that needs changing, the occupational therapist is in a unique position to initiate, support and implement change at a range of levels. This chapter will define and contextualise advocacy and lobbying for the occupational therapist, propose a range of skills, knowledge and values considered critical to effective advocacy and lobbying, and begin to explore the dilemmas and tensions that arise when venturing into advocacy and lobbying.

Understanding and contextualising models of disability

As occupational therapists, you will encounter a range of models that underpin your understanding of disability. These profoundly influence practice. Sometimes these models are implicit and, therefore, if left unexamined, can give rise to tensions and incoherence in practice. In this section, we explore a range of models that relate to disability and that can influence your practice.

Models of disability

Advocacy and lobbying are very different modes of practice for occupational therapists. You will be aware already that there are different models or perspectives on disability. Throughout history, disabled people have primarily been conceptualised and perceived as less than fully human, as evidenced by descriptors used in early literature and policy such as 'sub-normal' (see for example, Linton 1998). It is well recognised that our decision-making frameworks are significantly influenced by our personal values, belief systems, and commonly held assumptions about class, culture, race, gender, sexuality and, in particular, disability (Brehm et al 2002).

Disability activists and academics have identified two dominant paradigms or models in the history of oppression and the disempowerment of people with disability (the *Moral Model* and the *Medical Model*), with the emergence of a 'third way' (the *Social Model*) providing a viable way forward.

The *Moral Model* is the oldest paradigm for understanding disability. Based in religious mythology, it regarded disability as resulting from sin and shame, and led to the concealment and exclusion of individuals with impairments. Disabled people were primarily seen as objects of pity and charity (see for example Scheerenberger 1983). However, a positive outcome that emerges as a reaction to the moral model includes the formation of principles that have led to human rights and social justice for socially excluded and marginalised people.

The *Medical Model* of disability emerged as science took over from religion in the explanation of natural phenomena. The premise of the *Medical Model* is essentially that disability is the result of individual pathology, disease or injury; it is the problem of an impaired body or body function that requires attention (see for example, Bury 1996). When the cure is not forthcoming, issues relating to the disability are deemed to reside within the individual and to place no obligation on society in general. Support services tend to be limited and inadequate, and the lives of individuals with impairments are largely shaped by 'professionals' (Oliver 1990).

Occupational therapy has been strongly aligned with the medical model in the past, prior to the 'renaissance of occupation,' a term coined by Whiteford et al (2000). The interventions that stem from the medical model, therefore, are usually based on processes of assessment, therapeutic interventions and treatment of the individual (Kielhofner 2004).

It is also important to recognise that every level of legislation, policy and practice brings its own definitions of disability and a list of criteria by which people can be included (or excluded) as relevant. Defining disability as either a personal tragedy (individual/moral model) or in terms of deficit (medical model) both locate disability within the individual and fail to address the real issues – that of disabling environments (Chenoweth 2006).

Conversely, the *Social Model* comes from the perspective that disability is the result of social barriers and disabling environments. Here, the problem lies in a society which creates physical and attitudinal barriers that prevent or limit a person's full participation in the society (Ingstad & Whyte 1995). Thus, advocacy and lobbying are clearly located within the perspective of the social model (Craddock 1996).

Occupational therapists may incorporate both the medical and social models into their practice. Both have legitimacy and play an important role but it is important to understand and apply both perspectives appropriately. In acute settings, the *medical model* predominates and interventions need to address acute issues for an individual. However, beyond the acute stage, social forces and factors largely dictate what life will be like for a person with impairment. The occupational perspective on humans and health makes occupational therapists well placed to respond to these social forces and factors.

Vulnerable identities

It is widely acknowledged that throughout history and across cultures, disabled people have been visible but generally, their lives have largely been assigned to the margins of society (Norwich 2007). The following ode symbolises the reality of the lives often led by vulnerable and marginalised disabled people.

Ode to Vulnerable People's Lives

PINBALL LIVING

Balls in a pinball machine have no life of their own,

They are set into motion by someone else and

Then bounce from one place to another without any clear direction.

Sometimes even making big scores,

But then sinking into oblivion until someone sets them off again.

Anon

In general, society's beliefs and attitudes about disability are not mistaken in any simple way, as each assumption contains a kernel of experiential truth about encounters between those with authority and those with impairments. However, when tacit theories and untested assumptions like these underlie public policy and social relations, they severely limit the life opportunities of disabled people, their families and allies (Bury 1996). Table 15.1 lists several common negative assumptions

Table 15.1 Common negative assumptions about disabled people and the impact of these assumptions

Common negative assumptions that restrict and restrain disabled people

- Thinking of disabled people as partial, limited or lesser
- Putting disabled people on a pedestal
- Regarding disabled people as perfect objects of charity
- Seeing disability as a sickness to be fixed
- Stereotyping disabled people as a menace to themselves and society
- Attributing 'special' talents to disabled people
- Restricting the social circle of disabled people to other disabled people
- Locating the problem within the individual rather than in societal attitudes or in the built environment

Impact of negative assumptions on disabled people

- Rejection by family, neighbours, and even paid carers and services
- Isolation from non-disabled peers
- Restricted options for development, growth and enrichment
- Concentration of disabled people into social groupings of rejected people
- A very circumscribed set of role options
- Loss of control and autonomy
- Material poverty, impacting on health, housing and life expectancy
- Diminished sense of individuality and uniqueness
- Restricted social relationships, resulting in a lack of allies in times of need
- Neglect, damage and abuse

Adapted from Wolfensberger (1983) Social role valorization: a proposed new term for the principle of normalization. *Mental Retardation*, 21(6), 234–239.

about disabled people and the possible impact of these assumptions.

Historical and attitudinal factors have contributed to a failure of public policy dealing with disability in many jurisdictions. Services for disabled people have been primarily driven by economic and fiscal policy, rather than social policy, and human rights frameworks have largely taken a back seat. Demands for greater accountability for public funds, increasing requirements for legislative and regulatory compliance, and a long history of underinvestment in disability services has resulted in crisis-driven rather than needs-driven allocation of resources (Wills & Chenoweth 2005).

The failure of public policy for disabled people, particularly with regard to housing, personal care and support services, transport and law is well illustrated both in human rights reports and in anecdotal accounts of peoples' lived experience (Dennis & Chenoweth 2000, Kothari 2007). Disabled people have a much higher unemployment rate and a much lower workforce participation rate than their non-disabled peers. Disabled people are much more likely to be homeless, victims of crime (e.g. rates of sexual assault up to ten times those in the general population), under report crime and experience inadequate police follow-up (prosecution and conviction). In addition, incarceration rates of disabled people are up to 10 times greater than for people without impairment (Queensland Advocacy Inc 2007).

Advocacy and lobbying in occupational therapy

Advocacy

The concept of advocacy has primarily existed throughout recorded history as a concept in law, and is derived from the Latin *advocare*, which means *to be called to stand beside*. The right to legal representation dates from the system of law created by the Romans and this right has existed in British law since the 13th century. The concept of guardianship also evolved through Roman law to ensure the best interests of those with diminished decision-making capacity were upheld. Over the past 100 years or so, as notions of human rights have become more established, advocacy has become increasingly widespread and its conceptualisation further refined. Formal industrial advocacy has been provided by trade and labour unions for more than 100 years. The women's suffrage movement advocated strongly for the rights of women to vote. More recent social rights movements – the civil rights movement in America, the anti-apartheid movement in South Africa, and the Aboriginal land rights movement in Australia – have all helped to popularise ideas of rights.

Contemporary rights movements and protection regimes, such as those affecting children, older people and disabled people, have all led to the concept of advocacy for these groups. Early definitions of advocacy drew upon Wolfensberger's (1977) work, which has shaped the advocacy movement in many Western democracies. By the early 1990s in the human service arena, it was common practice to incorporate the word 'advocacy' into everyday language. In human service language, advocacy began to replace concepts such as lobbying, activism, community development, and good job performance. The word 'advocacy' almost seemed to have greater prestige for the user. Perhaps its usage reassured the practitioner that they were working within a social justice framework that validated their actions as being fair and ethical. Occupational therapists should take care not to use or practice the concept of advocacy loosely. A quote by an occupational therapist advocating for a disabled student in a mainstream setting reminds us of this:

> Remember that as an advocate you are there to help represent the views, wishes and best interests of the person you are advocating for. As an occupational therapist it can be tempting to slip into the role of mediator and take into account and give credence to both sides. This is not advocacy and will lessen the effectiveness of your advocacy. While it is desirable to resolve the tensions of the situation, as an advocate, you cannot compromise your position. It is important to make it clear to all parties before commencing, exactly what the role of an advocate is.
>
> Gretel, Occupational Therapist

Advocacy is a widely used term which has many meanings depending on the context. The online Oxford Dictionary defines an advocate as, (1) a person who publicly supports or recommends a particular cause or policy; and (2) a person who pleads a case on someone else's behalf.

This definition situates advocacy as a process of pleading or arguing about an idea or a cause. For professionals working with vulnerable people, advocacy can be understood as the act of directly representing or defending those people. Different professional groups define and interpret advocacy and the advocacy role according to their own principles, knowledge and skill base. For example, lawyers have a strict legal notion of advocacy while a social worker may see advocacy as including a broader range of activities. For occupational therapists, advocacy may be a relatively new idea but one which has increasing legitimacy when working with/for disabled people. Different ways to define advocacy are defined in Table 15.2.

Lobbying

As well as different forms of advocacy, occupational therapists and other allied-health professionals, such as social workers, are often engaged in other activities such as lobbying or activism. This might be as part of your paid role or it might be outside of work – something you engage with in a voluntary capacity as a concerned citizen.

Lobbying involves attempting to influence a political decision, policy or law. The exact origin of the word 'lobbying' is uncertain (Montpetit 2004). Lobbying usually takes a direct form – that is, directly to the government official, the politician or the leader with power to make decisions. Often we lobby such people to vote one way on a new law or policy – for example, on an anti-discrimination law or on a new funding programme for disabled people. We can also lobby more broadly – perhaps to the general public before a referendum on accessible transport or labour laws.

Lobbying needs to be differentiated from activism which refers to planned behaviour designed to achieve social or political objectives through activities such as consciousness raising, developing a coalition, political campaigning and producing publicity to influence social change. Activism is often undertaken as part of a bigger movement. For example, the Community Living Movement, an international social movement for supporting disabled people and their families to live in the community rather than in institutions, often employed activist tactics to get their message across and bring about social change. People in this movement have held street marches, gathered petitions, held media conferences and even made documentaries to get their message across. All these activities were well planned and coordinated and all involved significant publicity. Many occupational therapists were involved as activists alongside disabled people, families, and other professionals.

The occupational therapist as an agent of change

By definition, an occupational therapist working within the context of a human service organisation cannot be considered an independent advocate. They can, however, advocate or lobby internally or externally for change to an organisation, or on behalf of an individual or group.

Table 15.2 Different types of advocacy

Legal advocacy	Involves representation by legally qualified advocates, usually solicitors or lawyers
Formal advocacy	Sometimes called 'professional advocacy', usually refers to schemes run by voluntary groups employing salaried coordinators and paid staff
Citizen advocacy	A long-term, one-to-one partnership between user and advocate, usually as part of a coordinated scheme, with paid coordinator and volunteer partners
Self-advocacy	A term used to describe people speaking out for themselves. 'People first' organisations are an example
Peer advocacy	Defined as support from advocates who have themselves been service users
Social advocacy	Speaking, acting and writing with minimal conflict of interest on behalf of the sincerely perceived interests of a disadvantaged person or group to promote, protect and defend their welfare and justice by: • being on their side and no-one else's; • being primarily concerned with their fundamental needs; and • remaining loyal and accountable to them in a way that is emphatic and vigorous and which is, or is likely to be, costly to the advocate or advocacy group <div align="right">(Wolfensberger, 1998)</div>
Systems advocacy	Primarily concerned with influencing and changing the system (legislation, policy and practice) in ways that will benefit disadvantaged groups, particularly disabled people as a group within society. Systems advocates will encourage changes to the law, government and service policies and community attitudes. Usually systems advocacy agencies do not engage with individual advocacy. To do so can cause conflicts around the use of resources, focus and purpose. However, individual advocacy will highlight systems failure thus informing system advocates of emerging or existing areas requiring systemic reform
Individual advocacy	Refers to action taken to encourage and assist individuals with an impairment to achieve and maintain their rights as citizens and to achieve equity of access and participation in the community. Strategies may include speaking or standing up for the disabled person, supporting people to represent their own interests and making sure people know about the different ways they can have a say

Community service organisations often state advocacy as part of their organisational mission, but this is not to be confused with advocacy in its pure form (Community Services Code of Ethics 1994, as cited in Schissler Manning 2003). Specifically, these organisations refer to their role in educating the public and those who influence public policy about issues of concern to those the organisation serves.

Public policy (within a framework of legislation) reflects our beliefs, through government, about how resources should be allocated, to whom, and on what basis. In doing so, they determine the balance of power, choice and opportunity for people who are disadvantaged (Schissler Manning 2003).

In considering the respective roles of organisations and individual practitioners, with regard to influencing public policy (and ultimately outcomes for disabled people), it is important to understand the relationship between legislation, policy and practice. In simplest terms, legislation provides the foundation in law for public policy which in turn drives resource allocation for programmes and practice. The scenario is made more complex by the fact that the legislation, policy and practice that impacts on a person arises from a multitude of government departments, across multiple jurisdictions in an ever-changing political environment.

As well as recognising the implications of how disability is defined at a legislative and public policy level, the occupational therapy practitioner must also be discerning about the messages conveyed by the internal policy of their own organisation. To be effective, it is critical that the occupational therapist not view the organisation as the passive context in which they operate (Jones & May 1992). Irrespective of role, there will be many opportunities for the practitioner to constructively challenge and potentially reshape organisational policy. Table 15.3 provides suggestions for successful advocacy and lobbying.

Table 15.3 Tips for advocacy and lobbying

- Have a plan. Plan for incremental change to systems and policies that will result in sustainable change in people's lives
- Regularly check your own intentions. Sometimes, the personal agenda to influence can become bigger and more important than the goal
- Work to build credibility. Always be able to back up your argument with research and examples. Ensure your own behaviour reflects your arguments. Ensure all strategies are aligned with your stated goal and stated value base
- Work to demonstrate integrity in your lobbying. Respect confidentiality of information provided to you and keep all agendas on the table, that is, be transparent and communicate your intention clearly
- Manage the balance between gains for an individual versus gains for a group/community
- Manage the balance between short-term and long-term gains. Have a clear plan for your work and understand that compromise and patience will be required
- Avoid discouragement by celebrating small gains and staying focused on the goal
- Be prepared to be creative and flexible. If one strategy fails to deliver, be prepared to let it go and come up with another
- Avoid confrontation. Avoid setting people up to be outraged and unhappy when their energy could be guided towards creating a solution
- Build a network of supporters and actively support connections with and between them
- Ensure supporters are given all the information and are empowered to come to their own conclusions about the evidence (not just the evidence that supports your argument)
- Avoid exploiting people who are already vulnerable, in the interests of a short-term win

Strategies to effect change

Bennis et al (1976) describe three strategies for influencing policy and effecting change: the rational-empirical, the normative re-education and the power-coercive strategies. All three strategies involve the exercise of power, authority and influence in varying ways to effect change.

The *rational-empirical strategy*, which exerts influence to resist or promote change through the planning, research and evaluation of policy, will be relevant where occupational therapists have policy development roles or the opportunity to give feed-

back on policy through the agencies' continuous improvement processes. The following example illustrates this point:

The occupational therapist can significantly influence policy development by offering grounded examples, using real people and experiences, as evidence for why a particular policy direction will or won't work. A regular part of my work now is to gather disability service providers together to consider new government initiatives at an early stage. By giving service providers the chance to consider new initiatives early, they are able to give constructive feedback, using their current clients as evidence. Because the new policy is still in early draft stage and the feedback is given in the spirit of being helpful, government is usually happy to accommodate the recommended changes. The overall result is more grounded, useful policy, and a higher level of ownership by the agencies who will be implementing the policy.

Vanessa, Occupational Therapist

The *normative re-education strategy* focuses on the attitudes, values, skills and relationships within an organisation, and attempts to bring about change through education and training, as well as other organisation development techniques. This approach is a powerful and meaningful way for practitioners to inspire and implement change at a ground level. An example of how language can be a powerful strategy is found in the following quote:

When I started working for a non-government agency about four years ago, I noticed that many of my peers used language that promoted difference – an us and them attitude to government and to some of the other stakeholder groups we dealt with. I made a deliberate attempt to introduce new language such as working toward alignment rather than demanding change, and sharing/being open to a range of perspectives to refer to differences in opinion. This new language was used consistently, in a broad range of forums and publications, resulting in a significant reduction in adversarial interactions and better relationships over time

Vanessa, Occupational Therapist

The *power-coercive strategy* requires more direct use of power, influence and authority to effect change in policy and/or practice and may be less relevant to occupational therapists who operate at a ground level within the organisation.

Jones & May (1992) suggest the real point of influence for practitioners is at a practice level – the point at which policy is implemented. This is the point at which people gain access to services (and are supported to gain access to services). The practitioner, irrespective of their role, can use their discretion in applying rules and supporting people to make choices about the service they receive. It is at this point that the occupational therapist demonstrates congruity between their values and beliefs and their actions, as illustrated in Figure 15.1. Here Gretel reflects on this congruence:

Always remain assertive in the face of discrimination. I am always astounded by attempts to discriminate against disabled people, especially when this is masked by a smile and the assertion of care e.g. we are only concerned about his safety. This is a very insidious form of discrimination indeed.

This position was put to me when advocating for a family who wanted their son (with an intellectual impairment) to attend high school full-time. The principal stated that the student should only attend part-time so he would have a teacher-aide with him at all times. This decision was based on the possibility that the boy may use equipment in manual arts in an unsafe way. There had been no previous experience or evidence that this would be the case. Students without impairments don't need to prove they will be safe in all situations, yet apparently disabled students need to prove themselves before being afforded the same rights. Effective advocacy occurred and the school came to the realisation that their proposal was irrational and discriminatory.

Gretel, Occupational Therapist

Managing the dilemmas and tensions associated with advocacy and lobbying

Working to effect change as a practitioner within human service organisations can potentially give rise to a range of tensions and dilemmas. Not the least of these is the dilemma of trying to change a system of which you are also a participant. The incongruence associated with espousing social justice and equity as the basis of one's work yet failing to effect change is a potential source of frustration and discouragement for practitioners. Closely associated with this is the potential conflict between one's own values and aspirations and those of the organisation. Having to put aside one's identity as a 'professional' or 'expert' to work *with* rather than *for* disabled people may also present a challenge for the new therapist (Shields 1991).

Figure 15.1 • The knowledge, skill and value base for effecting change

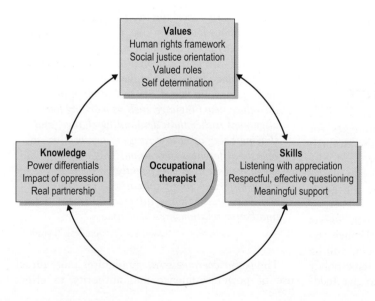

Conclusion

In this chapter we have outlined the elements of advocacy and lobbying and their relevance to work in the disability field. The vulnerability of disabled people and the failure of many policies and services to address their needs create situations and contexts where a broader change is required. As occupational therapists, you are in a position to extend the parameters of your practice to make a real difference. This means moving beyond mere therapeutic strategies to consider the social barriers to people's enjoyment

of a full and rich life. As Eric Dammann (1979) explains:

Belief in the values of the common people is our only hope. We cannot judge from how people behave under pressure of a society that forces them to compete for self interest or to be excluded. We must step out of our narrow social environment and learn to know the underprivileged who have never participated in our activities. When we have them with us, that will be real change from below.

References

Bennis, W. G., Benne, K. D., Chin, R. & Corey, K. E. (1976). *The planning of change*, (3rd ed). New York, Holt, Rinehart & Winston.

Brehm, S. S., Kassin, S. M., & Fein, S. (2002). *Social psychology*, (5th ed). Boston, Houghton Mifflin Company.

Bury, M. (1996). Defining and researching disability: challenges and responses. In: C. Barnes & G. Mercer (Eds). *Exploring the divide: illness and disability*, Leeds, The Disability Press.

Chenoweth, L. (2006). Disability. In: W. H. Chui & J. Wilson (Eds). *Social work and human services best practice*. Sydney, The Federation Press.

Craddock, J. (1996). Responses of the occupational therapy profession to the perspective of the diability movement. Part 2. *British Journal of Occupational Therapy*, 59(2), 73–78.

Dammann, E. (1979). *The future in our hands*. Oxford, Pergamon Press.

Dennis, R. & Chenoweth, L. (2000). *Moving out moving in: how 7 people with disability found their own home*. Brisbane, Octavia Group.

Ingstad, B. & Whyte, S. R. (Eds). (1995). *Disability and culture*. Berkeley, University of California Press.

Jones, A. & May, J. (1992). *Working in human service organisations: a critical introduction*. Melbourne, Australia, Longman Chesire.

Kielhofner, G. (2004). *Conceptual foundations of occupational therapy*, (3rd ed). Philadelphia, F. A. Davis.

Kothari, M. (2007). *Report of the special rapporteur on adequate housing as a component of the right to an adequate standard of living: mission to Australia*. Geneva, United Nations.

Linton, S. (1998). *Claiming disability: knowledge and identity*. New York, New York University Press.

Montpetit, E. (2004). Governance and interest group activities. In: J. Bickerton & A. G. Gagnon (Eds.). *Canadian politics*. Ontario, Broadview Press.

Norwich, B. (2007). *Dilemmas of difference, inclusion & disability*. Philadelphia, Taylor & Francis Group.

Oliver, M. (1990). *The politics of disablement*. London, The MacMillan Press Ltd.

Queensland Advocacy Inc (2007). *Disabled justice: the barriers to justice for persons with a disability in Queensland*.

Scheerenberger, R. (1983). *A history of mental retardation*. Baltimore, Brooks Publishing Co.

Schissler Manning, S. (2003). *Ethical leadership in human services: a multi-dimensional approach*. Boston, Allyn and Bacon.

Shields, K. (1991) *In the tiger's mouth: an empowerment guide for social action*. Newtown NSW, Millennium Books.

Whiteford, G., Townsend, E. & Hocking, C. (2000). Reflections on a renaissance of occupation. *Canadian Journal of Occupational Therapy*, 67(1), 61–69.

Wills, R. & Chenoweth, L. (2005). Support or compliance. In: P. O'Brien & M. Sullivan (Eds). *Allies in emancipation: shifting from providing services to being of support* (pp. 49–64). South Melbourne, Thomson Dunmore Press.

Wolfensberger, W. (1977). *A balanced multi component advocacy/ protection schema*. Downsview, Ontario, Canadian Association for the Mentally Retarded.

Wolfensberger, W. (1983). Social role valorization: a proposed new term for the principle of normalization. *Mental Retardation*, 21(6), 234–239.

Wolfensberger, W. (1998). *A brief introduction to social role valorization. A higher-order concept for addressing the plight of societally devalued people, and for structuring human services*. Syracuse, NY, Trinig Institute for Human Service Planning, Leadership and Change Agentry (Syracuse University).

Educational strategies

Tammy Hoffmann

CHAPTER CONTENTS

Introduction 222

Why do occupational therapists
educate? 222

Theories, models and principles that
guide the provision of educational
interventions 223

Adult learning theory 223

Health Belief Model 224

Self-efficacy theory 224

Transtheoretical Model 225

Partnerships between therapists and the
people with whom they work 225

Considerations when planning and
providing an educational intervention 227

Determine educational needs and
establish objectives 227

Decide on format for providing
education 228

Decide when to provide the
information 229

Consider impairments that may impact
on receiving and/or understanding
information 230

Consider health literacy 230

Content and design principles for effective
written health education materials 230

Evaluating the outcome of educational
interventions 231

Conclusion 233

SUMMARY

Occupational therapists provide education to
individuals as part of everyday practice. If
occupational therapists are to use education
effectively in their daily practice, they need to be
knowledgeable about relevant educational
theories and models, such as the Adult Learning
Theory, Health Belief Model, and Transtheoretical Model, which can provide therapists
with useful guidelines for planning educational
strategies. The concept of therapists working in a
collaborative partnership with individuals is also
an underpinning principle that should guide the
provision of education. In addition to
incorporating theoretical principles into the
design of educational strategies, therapists also
need to make considered decisions about the
content, format, timing, and evaluation of the
intervention as well as acknowledging and
accommodating individuals' health literacy and
any impairments they have that may impact on
the understanding of information. The aim of this
chapter is to provide guidelines and principles for
developing effective educational strategies for
use in occupational therapy practice.

KEY POINTS

- Education is a core component of all areas of
  occupational therapy practice and should be
  treated like any other strategy, with appropriate
  consideration given to its planning and
  evaluation.
- As well as imparting knowledge, education can
  also aim to alter individuals' behaviour, attitude,

beliefs, confidence, skills, and decision-making ability.

- Appropriate education empowers individuals and enables them to take responsibility for and participate in their health care.
- Educational theories, models and principles can serve as useful guides for therapists when they are planning educational strategies.
- When planning an educational strategy there are many decisions that therapists need to make and deliberation should be given to issues related to the content, format, timing, and evaluation of the strategy, as well as individuals' health literacy and any impairments that may impact on understanding information.

Introduction

Education is an indelible component of occupational therapy practice. Occupational therapists continuously use educational strategies in their day-to-day work with individuals. A survey of the intervention methods used by Australian occupational therapists who work with adults with physical impairment found that education and counselling were the most frequently used interventions, with three-quarters of participants indicating that they use these interventions often or most of the time (McEneany et al 2002). The widespread use of education was further confirmed by the finding that education and counselling were one of the top five intervention media used by participants from all caseloads except those working with older people, where they were rated sixth.

Despite the prevalence with which education is used by occupational therapists in their daily work with individuals, it is often not given the same thoughtful consideration as other interventions. While the reasons for this are not clear, according to McKenna & Tooth (2006a), there are a number of possible explanations for this, such as therapists:

- not perceiving education to be a specific type of intervention and considering it secondary to 'real' interventions that directly relate to the care and treatment of individuals

- lacking an understanding of educational theories and principles and the crucial role that education can have in empowering individuals

- considering education to be a basic and straightforward skill that does not require specialised planning or consideration.

However, the success of many occupational therapy interventions depends on the individual receiving effective education, and if occupational therapists are to use education effectively in their daily practice, they need to understand the theories of education and be knowledgeable about the practical considerations associated with providing education. The aim of this chapter is to provide guidelines and principles for developing effective educational strategies for use in practice.

Why do occupational therapists educate?

Education is far more than just imparting knowledge to individuals. In health fields, education has been defined as '…a planned learning experience using a combination of methods such as teaching, counselling, and behaviour modification techniques which influence [clients'] knowledge and health behaviour' (Bartlett 1985, p. 323). The definition continues and highlights that education is '…an interactive process which assists [clients] to participate actively in their health care' (Bartlett 1985, p. 323). From this definition it is clear that influencing both the knowledge and behaviour of individuals is at the centre of education. However, an educational intervention may also aim to build an individual's confidence, assist a person in making decisions related to their health, facilitate the acquisition of skills, or bring about some shift in attitudes or beliefs that will have a favourable effect on a person's health (Tones 2002, van der Borne 1998).

At various times, an occupational therapist will provide education for all of the above reasons. Consider the following examples of educational interventions that are commonly provided by occupational therapists:

- Teaching an individual who has had a stroke how to perform hand-strengthening exercises

- Educating a parent about activities to do with his/her child to help the development of fine motor coordination skills

- Demonstrating to an individual how to use newly prescribed assistive equipment

- Educating an individual about his chronic health condition and how to manage it

- Facilitating a person to incorporate movement precaution strategies into daily life following a total hip replacement

- Tutoring an individual with low back pain about strategies to use to cope with the pain and enable performance of everyday activities

- Educating an individual with diabetes about behaviours that they can take to prevent health problems and complications from developing.

Some of these educational interventions focus on influencing knowledge in the hope that this will also influence a specific behaviour, others aim to also facilitate skill development, while the intention of others is to additionally influence attitudes or beliefs and consequently lifestyle behaviours.

Education can take many forms. It can be incidental or planned, formal or informal. It is often a one-to-one interaction between just the therapist and the individual or it may take the form of a formal group education programme that the therapist is conducting for a number of individuals who have similar educational needs. There are also various formats that can be used to provide education, such as verbal, written, audio, video, computer-based or a combination of these. Considerations for the use of each of these formats are discussed later in the chapter. As well as providing education to individuals who they are working with, occupational therapists often need to provide education to each individual's family and friends as they also have informational needs. And, as with the individuals that the therapists work with, the educational needs of family members often extend beyond acquiring new knowledge and may, for example, require the learning of a new skill, such as how to assist with car transfers.

Theories, models and principles that guide the provision of educational interventions

As with other interventions, there are theories and models that can provide therapists with a broad framework for approaching and planning educational interventions. When planning an educational intervention, it is important that occupational therapists give appropriate consideration to the principles espoused by these theories and models. An overview of some of the theories and models to consider that are useful when planning educational interventions will be covered in the following section along with suggestions of the ways in which these can be practically applied.

Adult learning theory

Regardless of the goal of education, it is important that education aimed at adults is built upon the principles of adult learning. The central premise of this theory is that the learning process of adults differs to children and for successful adult learning, adherence to these principles is necessary. The key principles are described below, along with some of the implications for practice:

- Adults *need to know why they need to learn something before beginning to learn it* (Knowles et al 1998). Planning of an educational intervention should commence with an assessment of the needs of the individuals who are to receive the education. Education should meet the expressed needs of individuals and their families. Ironically though, individuals often are not aware of their need for information, and if they do not know that they are lacking information, they may not perceive a need for it (Buckland 1994). Consequently, to facilitate an individual's engagement in the learning process, therapists may need to initially educate an individual about the reasons for needing to learn and the benefits of it, prior to conducting a needs assessment.

- Adults need to be *actively involved in learning*, rather than passive recipients of information (Knowles 1980), with the goal of empowering learners and encouraging them to become self-directed and responsible for their learning (Wyatt 1999). This can be assisted by encouraging individuals to provide input into the design and delivery of educational experiences as much as possible and grading the goals and activities that are set so that confidence and success develop (Neufeld 2006).

- Adults have a *problem-centred orientation to learning* (Knowles 1980). It is important that the practical application of the concepts being learned is emphasised. This can be achieved by providing how-to information and opportunities for the practice of newly learnt skills.

- Adults enter the learning process with *prior experience* and it is important that learners' life experiences are acknowledged and utilised throughout the learning process (Knowles et al 1998). Therapists should identify individuals' prior health experiences and other life experiences and establish their existing knowledge, skills and attitudes, and plan educational interventions accordingly.

- Adults' *readiness to learn* will impact on the outcomes of their learning (Knowles 1980). Consequently, educational interventions should meet learners' expressed needs, be sequenced according to their readiness to learn, and appropriately target the learners' current confidence levels.

- Adults are most *motivated to learn when they see the content as relevant* (Knowles et al 1998). Providing education that meets individuals' expressed needs, explaining how the education they receive will help to achieve their goals, what practical steps they can take to implement the information that they are receiving, and providing feedback on their progress can all assist in enhancing individuals' motivation to learn.

Health Belief Model

The Health Belief Model was initially developed to explain the failure of people to participate in disease screening programmes (Rosenstock 1974), but today it is widely used as a theoretical framework for devising and implementing health education and health behaviour interventions. According to the Health Belief Model (Becker 1974, Glanz et al 2002), individuals are more likely to change their behaviour if they believe that:

- they are susceptible to the condition *(perceived susceptibility)*

- the condition is serious and if untreated will impinge on their lives *(perceived severity)*

- there are benefits of taking health action *(perceived benefits)*

- any negative aspects of the health action or barriers to undertaking it are outweighed by the benefits of the action *(perceived barriers)*.

Another component of the Health Belief Model is the concept of cues to action, which trigger the decision-making process that can ultimately lead to a change in behaviour (Becker et al 1974). The cues can be either internal or external. Internal cues such as symptoms may prompt an individual to seek assistance from a health professional, whereas examples of external cues are education provided by a health professional or media campaigns, such as those that encourage adults to exercise regularly and maintain a healthy weight (Janz & Becker 1984).

Therapists can provide information that specifically targets each of the four main components of this model. For example, in order to facilitate behaviour change in an individual who had experienced a stroke, the person needs to receive education that provides knowledge about the seriousness and life-altering consequences of stroke, his or her vulnerability to experiencing another stroke, and the powerful role that changes in behaviour can have in reducing the risk of a secondary stroke. The therapist should also provide the individual with an action plan that contains specific how-to information, discuss potential barriers to implementation of the action plan, and, together with the individual, brainstorm solutions to overcome or cope with these barriers. If the individual then decides that the benefits of taking action outweigh the tangible and psychological costs of not taking action, it is likely that the individual may undertake the desired behaviour change(s).

Self-efficacy theory

As the Health Belief Model became used with target groups where the focus was long-term changes in lifestyle behaviours, it was recognised that the concept of self-efficacy needed to be added to the model (Glanz et al 2002, Rosenstock 1988). Self-efficacy was first described by Bandura (1977) as a concept in social cognitive theory that is fundamental to behaviour change. Perceived self-efficacy refers to an individual's judgement of his or her ability to perform an action to reach a desired goal (Bandura 1986). According to self-efficacy theory, a person is more likely to perform a particular behaviour if engaging in that behaviour is expected to result in desired outcomes (Bandura 1986). Even if individuals recognise the value in changing their behaviour, they also need to develop the confidence to carry out the behaviour prior to attempting the behaviour (Bandura 1986).

Because one of the goals of health education is behaviour change, self-efficacy has an important role to play in health education. Self-efficacy has been found to be a major determinant in the initiation and maintenance of behavioural change (Bandura 1997, Strecher et al 1986). Self-efficacy influences the amount of effort that an individual will put into a task and the length of time that he or she will persevere with the task in the face of obstacles (Bandura 1977). According to self-efficacy theory, self-efficacy can influence the acquisition of new behaviours, inhibition of existing behaviours, and disinhibition of behaviours (Bandura 1977). It has been demonstrated that self-efficacy can be enhanced through education and that higher self-efficacy is related to successful attempts at behaviour change and improved health status (Clark et al 1992, Lorig et al 1989).

It is important to note that self-efficacy refers to specific behaviours in particular situations (Bandura 1977). It is not a global trait or personality characteristic. Unlike personality characteristics which are difficult to alter, self-efficacy is malleable and able to be altered (Lorig & Holman 1993). When a therapist is attempting to alter self-efficacy, using the strategies described later, it is important that the therapist is specific about the change sought, as self-efficacy is specific to each type of behaviour (Glanz et al 2002). For example, a therapist in a cardiac rehabilitation programme who was providing education to an individual about the need to make healthy lifestyle changes, would need to address a specific behaviour (such as regular exercise, quitting smoking, managing stress levels, and healthy eating) separately. Each type of behaviour would require separate discussion and action plans. There are a number of strategies that therapists can use to enhance an individual's self-efficacy (Prohaska & Lorig 2001, Strecher et al 1986), such as:

- *Performance accomplishment or skill mastery* – this strategy involves using incremental goal-setting, breaking the desired behaviour into smaller steps, and ensuring the individual achieves success in the performance of the easier steps before attempting the more difficult steps. An example of when a therapist may use this strategy would be when helping an individual with a lower-limb amputation learn to independently perform self-care tasks, such as dressing and showering. This strategy requires the therapist to use their skills in activity analysis and grading, which are core occupational therapy skills.

- *Modelling* – this strategy involves an individual observing other people who appear similar, such as peers, performing the desired behaviour. If written information is used as part of the educational intervention, it is important that the modelling strategy is also applied to the written material and that it contains illustrations of people similar to the individual in terms of characteristics such as age, body shape, and ethnicity.

- *Verbal persuasion* – in this strategy, therapists talk with individuals and emphasise the importance of the behaviour.

- *Reinterpreting signs and symptoms* – in this strategy, therapists clarify information with an individual, correct any myths or misconceptions that they may have, and aim to lessen any fear and anxiety about physiological signs and symptoms by explaining how to reinterpret them. For example, the therapist of an individual with an upper-limb burn who needs to perform frequent gentle stretching exercises to prevent contractures from developing, may need to explain to the person that feeling some pain or discomfort while doing the stretching is normal and that it is not harming, but helping, the burned area.

Transtheoretical Model

As highlighted earlier in this chapter, a characteristic goal of education is behaviour change. The Transtheoretical Model considers the transition points in behaviour change and the underlying factors that facilitate change from one stage to another (Prohaska & Lorig 2001). According to the Transtheoretical Model, change is a process that consists of six discrete stages and individuals move through these stages, although not necessarily in a linear fashion, as they adopt a behaviour (Prochaska et al 1992). Another element of this model is the process of change component, which states that there are specific activities that individuals use to progress through the stages (Prochaska et al 1992). The six stages, along with some strategies (Neufeld 2006, Prochaska et al 1992) that can be used to assist individuals to move through them, are described in Table 16.1.

Partnerships between therapists and the people with whom they work

The importance of adults actively participating in their learning has long been recognised by adult

Table 16.1 Stages of the Transtheorectical Model and strategies that can be used to assist individuals to move through the stages

Name of stage	Description of stage	Aim of strategies used in this stage
Precontemplation	The individual has no intention to change behaviour within the next 6 months	To increase awareness through activities such as providing information about the risk and the need for change
Contemplation	The individual has an awareness of a problem that needs action and intends to take action within the next 6 months	To increase the individual's confidence and motivation to change by reemphasising the benefits of change, discussing possible action plans along with potential barriers and solutions to coping with them, and where appropriate, incorporating the support of family and friends
Preparation	The individual intends to change behaviour within the next month and in the past year has taken significant action towards the desired behaviour	To initiate action, through strategies such as deciding on an action plan, breaking it into small steps and using goal setting to incrementally achieve each step
Action	The individual has made observable behaviour change, to a specified criterion that is sufficient to reduce risks to health, within the past 6 months	To help the individual commit to the change, by using strategies such as providing encouragement and support, discussing and problem-solving any difficulties that have arisen, enlisting the support of family and friends, and planning to prevent relapse
Maintenance	The individual has changed behaviour for more than 6 months and is striving to prevent relapse	To help the individual convert the new behaviour into a lifestyle habit, through activities such as joining self-help groups (if applicable), discussing and trialling coping strategies, and implementing steps to prevent relapse
Termination	The individual has total self-efficacy regarding the behaviour and regardless of the situation, does not revert to previous undesirable behaviour	Self-efficacy in this model refers to an individual's confidence to cope in high-risk situations and not revert to engaging in undesirable behaviours (Prochaska et al 2002)

learning theorists. However, in the health care setting, people have traditionally had a passive role where they have been provided with only the information that the health professional thinks they need to know (Coulter 1997). Over recent years there has been growing recognition of the need for people to be active partners in their own learning. The traditional model has been called a paternalistic model where it is assumed that the health professional knows best (Coulter 1997) and recipients of interventions do not need information or want to be involved in their care. Since then, various models of client–health professional relations that promote the active involvement of people in their care have been described, such as the active participation model (Roter 1987), patient-centred care model (Coulter 2002), the chronic care model (Bodenheimer et al 2002) and when the focus is on making decisions, the shared decision-making model (Coulter 2002).

Regardless of the titles of these models, the fundamental principle espoused by each – that of the active participation of people – is the same. Participation in health care and individuals having a collaborative partnership with their therapist is at the heart of person-centred practice (Law 1998), which is a guiding philosophy of modern occupational therapy practice.

Underpinning the concept of people as active partners in managing their health is individual empowerment and the ethical principle of autonomy (Coulter et al 1998). Paternalism can result in dependence on health professionals and erosion of an individual's self-confidence (Coulter & Magee 2003). It has been suggested that by increasing individuals' sense of control and participation in medical care, they may be more motivated to manage their illness and perform the desired healthy behaviours, which may in turn lead to better outcomes

(Greenfield et al 1988, Wyatt 1999). Effective communication between a health professional and an individual is essential to the development of the individual's self-confidence and motivation (Kaplan et al 1989).

To become empowered and active participants in their care, individuals need to be provided with information that they can use to manage their health. Without appropriate information, they cannot make informed decisions (Coulter 2002). However, actively involving individuals in their own care and establishing a partnership between the individual and therapist requires more than just the provision of education that is tailored to the individual's needs. It also involves a collaborative, two-way relationship between the therapist and individual, where the individual's beliefs, prior experiences, knowledge, and preferences for receiving education contribute to the relationship, in addition to the therapist's expertise (McKenna & Tooth 2006a). It is important to note that while the above section has focused on the importance of actively involving individuals in their own care, not all individuals may desire this level of involvement and some may prefer a more passive role. This is a legitimate choice that should be respected (Coulter 2002). However the opportunity to be actively involved should be available for all who want to take it (Tones & Tilford 1994). Therapists should be flexible and adapt their approach so that it meets individuals' preferences and needs.

Considerations when planning and providing an educational intervention

As well as using the theoretical considerations explained in the previous section of this chapter as the guiding principles when planning an educational intervention, for the education to be effective there are a number of other decisions that a therapist needs to make. An overview of some of the key steps and decisions that a therapist should take during the planning process will be covered in the following section.

Determine educational needs and establish objectives

For education to be person-centred, it must meet the needs of the individual. Generally, the most effective way to establish individuals' educational needs is by asking them (Lorig 2001). As well as establishing individuals' content needs, therapists also need to determine their preferences regarding the format and timing of the education. To determine content needs, therapists may also wish to use a checklist of topics as a prompt to ensure that topics are not overlooked. The topics listed on the checklist can be derived by the therapist's experience, previous groups or individuals involved and/or relevant scientific literature. For many conditions and situations, formal studies of individuals' informational needs have been undertaken and are readily available in the literature. Therapists may also wish to use a more formal means of establishing informational needs such as a knowledge test, attitude scale, or behaviour checklist. One advantage of using a formal assessment is that it can be used as baseline measurement and the assessment re-administered after the educational intervention has been provided, as a way of evaluating the educational intervention (see the section below on evaluating the outcomes of educational interventions).

The process of assessing individuals' educational needs is a continual one as needs change over time and depend on many factors, such as the nature and stage of their medical condition and their readiness to change. For example, an individual who has had heart surgery may initially be concerned about when they can return to self-care activities, whereas some weeks later, they may want to know about returning to driving.

After an individual's educational needs have been ascertained, therapists need to, in conjunction with the individual, set objectives for the educational intervention. Objectives typically describe the *behaviour or action* that is to be achieved, the *condition* under which the behaviour/action will be achieved, and the extent *(criterion)* to which the behaviour/action should occur to consider the objective achieved (McKenna & Tooth 2006b). The following example of an objective illustrates these three components: After reading the instruction sheet and also having it explained by the therapist *(condition)*, the individual will be able to explain the wearing regimen and care guidelines for his wrist splint *(behaviour/action)* without prompting from the therapist *(criterion)*. By setting guidelines such as this, at the conclusion of an educational intervention, therapists are able to impartially ascertain if the objective has been met.

Decide on format for providing education

There are many formats that therapists can use to provide education. When deciding which format to use, there are a number of factors that therapists should consider, such as the educational resources available to the therapist and the type of content being provided. Factors about the individual also need to be considered such as cognitive ability, educational level, vision, hearing, communication skills, preferred learning style (for example visual or auditory), cultural background and primary language. Therapists should also be aware that, where possible, using a combination of formats can often be more effective than using a single format (Theis & Johnson 1995). Education will be more effective when individuals have the opportunity to hear information, see it, have it repeated, and interact with it, than just, for example, hear it.

Verbal education is the most frequently used format, but one of the major problems with it is that individuals frequently forget the information that is provided to them (Kitching 1990), with estimations that most individuals remember less than one-quarter of what they have been told (Boundouki et al 2004). For this reason, written information is a particularly valuable format that should, ideally, be used to supplement or reinforce information that is presented verbally (Hill 1997), as this reinforcement can have a positive impact on the effectiveness of educational interventions (Theis & Johnson 1995). Written materials have the advantage of being available to refresh an individual's memory as needed (Ley 1988). Tang & Newcomb (1998) conducted a client focus group exploring education and found that individuals sought answers to their questions at the time they formulate their questions. This usually occurred after the individual had seen the health professional, not during the encounter. To some extent, written materials may be able to assist individuals in answering the questions that occur when they are not interacting with a health professional. Written materials have a number of advantages such as: message consistency, reusability, portability, flexibility of delivery, permanence of information, and they are economical to produce and update. A further benefit of written materials is that individuals can choose the level and amount of information that best suits them as their level of coping changes (Weinman 1990). Of course, prior

to deciding to use written materials with an individual, the therapist needs to consider the factors listed earlier, such as the individual's cognitive abilities, primary language, communication skills, vision, and reading ability. If a therapist chooses to proceed and use written materials with an individual, it is essential that appropriate attention is given to the design of the written materials. This issue is explained further in the 'Content and design principles for effective written health education materials' section later in this chapter.

Although verbal and written education are the two forms of education most commonly used by occupational therapists, there are other forms that therapists may find valuable in certain situations. The provision of information about some topics is particularly suited to a combination of verbal education, demonstration, and written information. For example, when educating individuals about exercises to perform, adaptations to activities, or how to use assistive equipment, demonstration is invaluable. Audio recordings can be a useful format when providing education to individuals who are unable to read, whether this is because of illiteracy, a visual or perceptual impairment, or some other reason. The use of videocassettes or digital video discs (DVD) that contain educational material can be useful, particularly when the education involves demonstrations, such as of movements, techniques, exercises, or activities. For example, a DVD that demonstrates how to carry out joint protection and energy-conservation techniques while performing self-care and household activities may be useful for a therapist to provide to individuals with arthritis, to reinforce information that has already been provided face-to-face by the therapist. By also providing a DVD, individuals can review the information when and as many times as needed. DVDs can also be useful when the topic being covered requires graphics to more effectively explain the content, such as explaining to individuals what happens in hip-replacement surgery so they can understand why movement precautions post-surgery are important. Video presentation of information caters to individuals with auditory learning styles, as well as those with visual learning styles and can assist individuals who have low functional health literacy or English as a second language to understand the content being conveyed. Audio, video and written materials all have the added advantage that individuals can share them with their family members, so that even if family were not present when the therapist was providing the information, they can still receive the information.

The use of computer-based materials, such as specifically designed programs and the Internet, as an educational format has grown in recent years. There are a number of ways in which computer programs can be used as an educational intervention, such as providing individuals with interactive information (see for example, Stromberg et al 2002), helping individuals to make health-related decisions (see for example, Hochlehnert et al 2006), or providing individuals with tailored printed information that is customised according to their informational and visual needs (see for example, Hoffmann et al 2004). Although it depends on the features of the software being used, there can be advantages of using computer programs to provide information, such as:

- they can enable individuals to interact with the information, view it at their own pace, and view only information that is relevant to them

- they often contain graphics that individuals can interact with and this can assist with understanding the information

- learning tools such as knowledge quizzes can be incorporated into them

- some computer programs enable individuals to print out the information that they have viewed on screen, providing them with a resource that they can refer back to at any time.

Computer programs should be designed so that they are user-friendly and able to be operated by individuals who do not have computer experience. A recent systematic review found that computer-based programs were effective in increasing individuals' knowledge and that they are generally well accepted by individuals (Beranova & Sykes 2007). Although computer-based education should not be a substitute for interaction with therapists, it can be useful for supplementing and/or reinforcing information that is provided by therapists.

As well as computer-based programs, the Internet can also be a valuable source of information for individuals and health information is one of the most frequently searched topics on the Internet (McMullan 2006). Individuals who wish to be active consumers of health information will have a need to seek out their own information either before and/or after they have seen their therapist (McMullan 2006). Therapists may find that individuals will come to them with information that they have found on the Internet and wish to discuss. Therapists need to be aware that 'Internet-informed' individuals will affect the traditional therapist–client relationship, and therapists should acknowledge individuals' search for information, answer questions they have about information that they have found, and assist individuals by directing them to reliable and accurate Internet sites (McMullan 2006).

Although most education is provided on a one-to-one basis, providing education in a group format can be a time-effective method for providing information to individuals who have similar educational needs, such as individuals scheduled to undergo hip-replacement surgery. The information that is provided in a group format is typically generic information and, therefore, group education should also be supplemented by one-to-one consultation(s) between each individual and the therapist to allow for provision of information that is specific to each individual's needs and situation. When deciding whether group education is appropriate for an individual, consideration of factors such as the individual's roles and responsibilities (such as full-time work), personality, and level of anxiety is important. Some individuals will benefit from the group process and being able to share and discuss issues with other group participants, others may not feel comfortable doing this. Although group education has advantages, this format also has potential disadvantages as it can be resource-intensive, involve significant preparation time for the therapists, and requires a therapist who has group leadership skills. Refer to the further reading section at the end of this chapter for citation details of a chapter by Lorig and Harris (2001) that provides details about the steps that health professionals should take when planning and conducting group education sessions.

Decide when to provide the information

Providing appropriate education to individuals at the appropriate time is critical and can greatly impact the effectiveness of the educational intervention. The extent of information that is provided at any point in time will vary according to many factors. When seriously ill, individuals may only want to receive brief information that is relevant to their immediate concerns. Later, individuals may want to receive more detailed information. Anxiety can prevent individuals from absorbing and processing information (Theis & Johnson 1995). Therapists should consider individuals' coping level and style each time that they provide information and be guided by individuals' readiness to digest information. There are no guidelines as to when the optimum time to provide information is, as this varies according to each individual, their circumstance and needs, and the type of information being provided. Therapists need to be sensitive to and guided by individuals' needs. To assist with the comprehension and recall of information, therapists should provide the information in more than one format (such as verbal and written), repeat information over time, and provide opportunities for reinforcement, clarification, and questions (Theis & Johnson 1995).

Consider impairments that may impact on receiving and/or understanding information

Individuals may have one or more impairments, such as a hearing, visual, cognitive, or speech and language impairment, that will impact how they are able to process information. These impairments may be pre-existing (such as hearing loss associated with ageing) or as a result of the health condition for which they are seeing the therapist (such as aphasia after a stroke). Therapists' choice of format(s) for providing information needs to consider any impairment(s) that individuals have. For example, the use of written information is not appropriate with an individual who has a severe visual impairment that can not be corrected (such as with corrective lenses) and information that is provided verbally should be supplemented by some other means, such as audio-taped information. There are a range of strategies that therapists can use to facilitate communication with individuals who have one or more of these impairments and further reading related to strategies specific to each impairment is recommended (refer to further reading section at the end of this chapter for details).

Consider health literacy

If written health education materials are used to provide information or supplement information that is provided verbally, the literacy level of the individuals receiving the information needs to be considered. The written material will not benefit individuals if they are unable to understand it. Health literacy refers to the '… cognitive and social skills which determine the motivation and ability of individuals to gain access to, understand and use information in ways which promote and maintain good health' (World Health Organization 1998, p. 10). Health professionals should be aware of the literacy skills of individuals so that they can alter the educational intervention accordingly (Weiss et al 1995). People with poor literacy often use a range of strategies to hide literacy problems (Weiss et al 1995) and are often reluctant to ask questions so as not to appear ignorant (Wilson & McLemore 1997). Although literacy levels can be influenced by education level, it has not been consistently found that reading skill is dependent on educational attainment (Weiss et al 1995). Therefore, in addition to obtaining information about an individual's level of educational attainment, it is recommended that therapists also assess an individual's reading ability (Weiss et al 1995, Wilson & McLemore 1997). There are a number of instruments that therapists can use to assess an individual's reading ability, such as the Rapid Estimate of Adult Literacy in Medicine (REALM) (Murphy et al 1993), the Test of Functional Health Literacy in Adults (TOFHLA) (Parker et al 1995), and the Medical Achievement Reading Test (MART) (Hanson-Divers 1997). These tests evaluate an individual's ability to understand medical terminology and language, and are quick and easy to administer. The principles for designing effective written health education materials are described below.

Content and design principles for effective written health education materials

When written health education materials are designed, there are a number of principles that should be followed in order to maximise their effectiveness. Put simply, for written information to be effective, it needs to be noticed, read, understood, believed, and remembered (Ley 1988). Studies have reported a mismatch between the reading level of written materials and the reading ability of the individuals who received the materials (Griffin et al

2006, Hoffmann & McKenna 2006a). The reading level, or readability, of a material refers to how easy it is to read. Written materials should be written simply, at the lowest level that conveys the information accurately (Hoffmann & Worrall 2004). If the reading level of the intended recipients of the material is known (see previous section for how to assess this), the reading level of the material should be two to four grades lower than the average reading level of recipients (Boyd 1987). If the reading level is unknown, a 5th–6th grade (typically equivalent to 10–11 years of age in the Australian education system) reading level is recommended (Doak et al 1996, Weiss et al 1998). There are a number of readability formulas that can be used to quickly and easily determine the readability of written material, such as the SMOG (McLaughlin 1969) or the Flesch Reading Ease formula (Flesch 1948). The latter is available through some word-processing programs such as Microsoft Word.

Although the readability of written materials is very important, there are many other features that contribute to the suitability of written materials and they can be grouped into the following categories: content, language, organisation, layout and typography, illustrations, and learning and motivation. After reviewing literature concerning the design of written health education materials, Hoffmann & Worrall (2004) compiled a list of recommended content and design features that should be followed when designing written materials. The principles are shown in Table 16.2. Checklists are available for therapists to use to evaluate the suitability of written materials they are considering using, whether self designed or from other sources. Two of these checklists are the Suitability of Assessment of Materials (SAM) (Doak et al 1996) and a checklist of content and design characteristics that was developed by Paul et al (1997).

Evaluating the outcome of educational interventions

Although therapists are accustomed to measuring outcomes and evaluating the effectiveness of the interventions that they provide, they often do not apply the same process to educational interventions. Therapists should evaluate the outcome of any educational intervention that they provide, as they would after providing any other intervention, to determine whether the education had the intended effect and whether the stated objectives have been met. This information enables the therapists to decide whether further education or reinforcement of the content is needed and whether the objectives, content, and/or delivery methods of subsequent educational interventions should be altered to improve effectiveness (Hoffmann & McKenna 2006b).

Evaluating the outcome of educational interventions can be done informally or formally and this usually depends on factors such as the objectives of the educational intervention, the purpose of the evaluation, and the time and resources available. Methods of informal evaluation include seeking feedback from individuals, ascertaining if they have understood the information that the therapist has provided to them, if their informational needs have been met, and if they have any unanswered questions. Individuals' satisfaction with the process of receiving education can also be assessed simply by asking them. Informal evaluation may be as simple as, for example, asking an individual who has had a stroke to correctly demonstrate to the therapist the adapted technique that he or she was taught to use when putting a shirt on. Even if formal methods of evaluation are used, informal questions relating to whether individuals have understood the information provided and if they have further informational needs should always be asked by the therapist.

Formal evaluation typically requires administration of formal outcome measures and therapists must decide which outcome(s) they will measure, which outcome measure(s) they will choose, and when and how the outcome measure will be administered. Any decisions regarding which outcome(s) to measure should be guided by the objectives of the educational intervention. For example, if the objective was to improve an individual's knowledge about the risk factors for coronary artery disease, then a knowledge test would be an appropriate outcome measure. However, if the objective of the intervention was to assist an individual to change their behaviour, for example, incorporating regular exercise into their week, then an outcome measure that assesses behaviour change would be needed.

Decisions about which outcome measures(s) to use will depend on whether there is an existing outcome measure that is appropriate for a therapist's needs. There are many published health-education measures (such as measures of knowledge

Table 16.2 Recommendations for designing effective written health education materials

Involve all key stakeholders, including patients, in the development and testing of the written material

Content

- Clearly state the purpose of the material
- Focus on providing information that is behaviour-focused (e.g. It is important that you do the exercises every day)
- Ensure that the content is accurate, up-to-date, evidence-based, and sources appropriately referenced
- Include the authors' names on the material and the publication date

Language

- Avoid judgemental or patronising language
- Aim for a 5th to 6th grade reading level
- Use short sentences, expressing only one idea per sentence
- Use short words, preferably one to two syllables, where possible
- Use common words wherever possible. Avoid the use of jargon or abbreviations. Include a glossary if jargon or unfamiliar words are necessary
- Write in the active voice and in a conversational style
- Write in the second person (e.g. 'you' rather than 'the patient')
- Structure sentences so that the context or old information is presented before new information. (e.g. 'To lower your risk of stroke {context}, you will need to make changes to what you eat' [new information])

Organisation

- Sequence the information so that the information that patients most want to know is at the beginning
- Use subheadings
- Present the information using bulleted lists where possible
- Group related information into lists, list no more than 5 points in each list, and label each list descriptively
- Keep paragraphs short and express only one idea per paragraph
- Summarise the main points, either at the end of sections or at the end of the material

Layout and typography

- Use a minimum 12 point font size
- Avoid the use of italics and all capitals
- Only use bold type to emphasise key words or phrases
- Ensure good contrast between the font colour (e.g. black) and the background (e.g. white)

Illustrations

- Only use illustrations if they will enhance the reader's understanding
- Use simple line drawings that are likely to be familiar to the reader
- Use an explanatory caption with each illustration

Learning and motivation

- Incorporate features that actively engage the reader (e.g. blank space to write questions down, short quiz, list 3 things that you should do)

From: Hoffmann, T. & Worrall, L. (2004). Designing effective written health education materials: considerations for health professionals. *Disability and Rehabilitation, 26,* 1166–1173, with permission from Taylor and Francis Journals. Available at: http://www.informaworld.com

for various conditions, satisfaction, self-efficacy, health behaviour, emotional health, and quality of life) and many of these are freely available. The Redman (2003) resource, which is listed in the further reading section at the end of this chapter, overviews many of the published health education measurement tools. However, for many of the educational interventions that are provided by occupational therapists, an existing outcome measure will not exist. In this case, therapists will need to adapt an existing outcome measure or create their own. There are some general guidelines to follow when adapting or creating outcome measures and these are described in the Hoffmann & McKenna (2006b) reference that is listed in the further reading section at the end of this chapter and summarised briefly below:

- Ensure that the outcome measure is kept as simple as possible and that there is no ambiguity or unnecessarily complex words or long sentences.

- Do not use biased or leading questions or items.

- Follow the guidelines in Table 16.2 to ensure that the measure is formatted in a 'user-friendly' manner.

- Obtain feedback on the measure from colleagues and alter as necessary.

- Pilot the measure with the type of individuals who it will be used with and alter as necessary.

After deciding which outcome measure(s) to use, therapists also need to decide when the measure(s) will be administered. Decisions about timing will be guided by the original objectives that were set for the educational intervention. For example, for educational interventions that have the objective of improving knowledge, it is appropriate to evaluate them shortly after the education has been provided, such as on the same day; however, it may be more appropriate to evaluate an educational intervention that aims to change behaviour over a longer period of time after a number of weeks has passed, so that individuals have had the chance to implement what they have learnt. An advantage of formal evaluation is that therapists can re-administer the same formal assessment that was used earlier when they were establishing individuals' educational needs, and then compare any changes in the individuals' performance (a pre-test post-test approach) that are likely

to have occurred as a result of their participation in the educational intervention. Because the same outcome measure may be used at both the beginning and end of an educational intervention, when initially planning an educational intervention, therapists should also plan how they are going to evaluate the intervention.

However, not all evaluation needs to be done before and after the intervention. Evaluating an educational intervention partway through its delivery can also be valuable, as this allows therapists to respond to individuals' feedback and progress, and adjust the remainder of the intervention accordingly. This applies to both individual interventions and group education sessions where, for example, a therapist may administer a brief questionnaire after two of the four scheduled classes have been held.

Before proceeding with the evaluation, therapists also need to decide how it will be administered. There are many available methods and choice will depend on factors such as the information sought, the individuals' needs and abilities, and the time and resources available (Hoffmann & McKenna 2006b). Use of a combination of methods is often most appropriate. Some of the most common methods of measuring outcomes include observation, interview, individual self-report, open-ended questioning, questionnaires, scales, tests, and diaries (Hoffmann & McKenna 2006b).

Conclusion

Education is an important component of all areas of occupational therapy practice and should be considered as a specific and valid intervention in its own right. As such, therapists should be knowledgeable about relevant educational theories, models and principles, and be guided by them when planning educational interventions. When planning and providing education, therapists also need to make many other decisions such as those related to the content, format, timing, and evaluation of the intervention. Practice Scenarios 16.1 and 16.2 illustrate the application of some of the principles that have been described in this chapter. With appropriate consideration of the principles and guidelines discussed in this chapter, therapists can aim to apply effective educational interventions to the individuals they work with, thus enabling them to participate fully in their own health care.

Practice Scenario 16.1
Mr. Williams

Mr. Williams is a 78-year-old man who was first seen by an occupational therapist 4 days after he had undergone total hip replacement surgery on his right hip. The occupational therapist conducted an initial interview with Mr. Williams to gather background information regarding his previous and current abilities, home environment, and understanding of hip movement precautions. The therapist also wished to obtain information about Mr Williams's priorities/goals while in rehabilitation. During the interview, the therapist learned that Mr. Williams was highly anxious about learning to do things 'exactly right' after surgery and was fearful of hip dislocation and any setbacks to his recovery. He reported that several friends had given him advice on what to do and what not to do, and he was confused about how he should go about doing daily tasks without risking the dislocation of his hip. The therapist also established that Mr. Williams had forgotten a lot of what he had been told prior to surgery about hip precautions and was not confident in his ability to manage his self-care tasks at home upon discharge.

Prior to his surgery, Mr. Williams lived alone and was independent in performing basic activities of daily living such as self-care tasks, most of his own domestic tasks such as cooking, doing the laundry, and light cleaning, and he enjoyed gardening and lawn bowls. Together, the therapist and Mr. Williams established that his goals prior to discharge were to be able to walk independently, get in and out of bed and chairs independently, and complete his own personal self-care tasks and light meal preparation. In this instance, the desired outcomes of education were for Mr. Williams to have:

a. sufficient knowledge of the necessary hip precautions following surgery
b. the skills and confidence to independently and safely complete his personal self-care tasks while also adhering to the relevant hip precautions.

The therapist chose to use a combination of educational materials with Mr. Williams. As she wanted to use written information, she quickly administered the REALM to Mr. Williams and established that he had approximately an 8th reading grade level (in the Australian education system, this is typically equivalent to approximately 13 years of age). Following this, she provided him with a well-designed information booklet ('Things you need to know about hip replacement surgery') that contained both written information and clear, useful illustrations. The booklet had previously been assessed using the SMOG readability formula and has a reading level of grade 6. The therapist used the information booklet as a teaching guide and explained the hip anatomy and the surgical procedure using the illustrations in the booklet to support the explanations. She then explained the practical implications of hip precautions using examples relevant to Mr. Williams' own personal circumstances and acknowledged the presence of his anxiety about dislocating his hip. At his bedside, the therapist demonstrated the use of long handled dressing and showering assistive devices to Mr. Williams, who then had the opportunity to practise using these devices, ask questions, and undertake practical problem-solving in relation to these tasks. The therapist provided Mr. Williams with feedback and encouragement as he practised using these assistive devices and Mr. Williams' confidence in his ability to undertake these tasks grew as he experienced success in performing them safely.

The following day, the therapist conducted an assessment of daily living activities with Mr. Williams and observed him perform showering, dressing, and transfer tasks while using the appropriate assistive devices. The therapist provided Mr. Williams with feedback about his adherence to movement precautions while performing the tasks. Over the following days, other members of the multidisciplinary rehabilitation team such as nurses and physiotherapists also provided Mr. Williams with consistent instruction and reinforcement of these same techniques. This contributed to Mr. Williams' mastery of transfers and daily-living skills, and also built his confidence in his ability to manage alone following discharge, thus reducing his anxiety.

A few days prior to discharge, the occupational therapist invited Mr. Williams to participate in a small group education session that was being held for people in hospital who had undergone hip surgery. Spouses/carers were also invited to attend the group. The group was led by the occupational therapist and used DVD-based movie images of scenarios to illustrate techniques for completing personal and domestic tasks at home following hip surgery. There was also some discussion about these issues and the group concluded with each participant completing a short quiz to gauge his/her level of understanding of, and ability to apply the information to practical daily life scenarios. Prior to his discharge, the therapist completed another assessment of daily living activities (this time it also included the preparation of a small meal) with Mr. Williams and observed that he was able to safely and independently perform self-care activities and light domestic tasks, adhered to movement precautions throughout all activities, and was confident in his ability to manage these tasks at home.

Practice Scenario 16.2 Luke

Luke is a 7-year-old boy living with his parents Maria and Anthony. Luke was referred to an occupational therapist by his paediatrician after his parents reported a 6-month history of faecal soiling. The referral letter indicated this was triggered by an episode when Luke was constipated and developed an anal fissure (a shallow tear in the skin at the opening of the anus) while passing a hard bowel motion. Through avoiding subsequent painful bowel motions Luke developed chronic constipation, and soiling became a daily occurrence. Physical examination and an abdominal X-ray revealed an impacted bowel, and Luke was treated medically with an enema to move the built up faecal matter. He was also prescribed a daily dose of stool softener; however, Luke was continuing to soil frequently at home and school, and reported being teased by his classmates.

Maria attended the first appointment with the therapist alone. The therapist used interview questions to gather a toileting history and elicit Maria's understanding of Luke's condition. Maria lacked knowledge of the physiological basis to Luke's continued soiling, and wondered whether it was a deliberate action. Maria had taken steps to help Luke cope with accidents at school (providing fresh underpants, meeting with the teacher) and felt this had helped reduce the teasing. As she had initiated contact with Luke's school, the therapist could see that Maria was moving into the 'action' stage of change. According to the Health Belief Model, Maria could perceive the benefits of taking further action for her son, but needed guidance on how to do this. However, her self-efficacy was diminished by the incorrect belief that Luke was deliberately soiling.

One formal educational session was held and attended by both parents. The therapist provided an illustrated brochure on childhood soiling and talked through each of the headings (e.g. What is constipation?), avoiding jargon. She emphasised that stretching of the large intestine can lead to problems sensing the presence of stool in the rectum, and that liquid stool often leaks past, passing into the child's underwear without the child feeling it. The therapist

explained that intervention involves re-establishing a toileting routine which, with the aid of stool softeners, appropriate diet, and exercise, allows the bowel to shrink down and the child to regain sensation over a period of weeks–months. By clarifying this information she was able to address Maria's misconceptions about soiling and help Luke's parents understand the expected timeframe for improvement. In conjunction with Luke's parents, the therapist generated goals for Luke, including: establishing toileting times, recording progress on a sticker chart, supporting Luke's use of more effective methods for emptying his bowels (posture and pushing techniques), and implementing a motivating reward system. At the end of the session, the therapist used a combination of closed and open-ended questions to ensure that Luke's parents had understood the information that she had provided and that they did not have any further questions. The information provided in the parent education session was reinforced in an informal manner by telephone and questions were encouraged at each of Luke's subsequent therapy appointments.

Maria accompanied Luke to his first appointment with the therapist. At this session, a fun quiz revealed that Luke was unaware of how his body worked and how lifestyle (e.g. diet) influenced his soiling. Over subsequent appointments, the therapist used large scale pull-apart models of a child's intestinal system (with and without an impacted bowel), colouring-in activities, and story books about children with soiling difficulties to increase Luke's understanding. She assessed the effectiveness of this intervention by asking Luke to make and describe a playdoh model of the intestinal system and draw a poster of healthy eating and exercise ideas. The therapist used a range of hands-on activities (e.g. blowing up balloons) to teach Luke an effective pushing technique to clear his bowel. When reviewed 4 weeks later, Luke's sticker chart demonstrated that he had adhered to his toileting routine, was eating healthier snacks, and was experiencing less frequent accidents. Educating Luke and his parents regarding both the physiology of soiling, and behaviours which return the bowel to its usual size, helped to motivate lifestyle change and reduce the frequency of Luke's soiling.

References

Bandura, A. (1977). Self-efficacy: Toward a unifying theory of behavioural change. *Psychological Review*, 84, 191–215.

Bandura. A, (1986). *Social foundations of thought and*

action: a social cognitive theory. Englewood Cliffs, NJ, Prentice Hall.

Bandura, A. (1997). *Self-efficacy: The exercise of control*. New York, W.H. Freeman.

Bartlett, E. (1985). At last, a definition. *Patient Education and Counselling*, 7, 323–324.

Becker, M. (1974). The Health Belief Model and personal health behaviour. *Health*

Education Monographs, 2, 324–508.

Becker, M., Drachman, R., Kirscht, J. (1974). A new approach to explaining sick-role behaviour in low-income populations. *American Journal of Public Health*, 64, 205–216.

Beranova, E. & Sykes, C. (2007). A systematic review of computer-based softwares for educating patients with coronary heart disease. *Patient Education and Counselling*, 66, 21–28.

Bodenheimer, T., Lorig, K., Holman, H. et al (2002). Patient self-management of chronic disease in primary care. *Journal of the American Medical Association*, 288, 2469–2475.

Boundouki, G., Humphris, G. & Field, A. (2004). Knowledge of oral cancer, distress and screening intentions: longer term effects of a patient information leaflet. *Patient Education and Counselling*, 53, 71–77.

Boyd, M. (1987). A guide to writing effective patient education materials. *Nursing Management*, 18, 56–57.

Buckland, S. (1994). Unmet needs for health information: a literature review. *Health Libraries Review*, 11, 82–95.

Clark, N., Janz, N., Dodge, J. et al (1992). Self-regulation of health behaviour: the 'take PRIDE' program. *Health Education Quarterly*, 19, 341–354.

Coulter, A. (1997). Partnerships with patients: the pros and cons of shared clinical decision making. *Journal of Health Services Research and Policy*, 2, 112–121.

Coulter, A. (2002). *The autonomous patient: ending paternalism in medical care*. London, The Nuffield Trust.

Coulter, A. & Magee, H. (2003). *The European patient of the future*. Philadelphia, Open University Press.

Coulter, A., Entwistle, V. & Gilbert, D. (1998). *Informing patients: an assessment of the quality of patient information materials*. London, King's Fund.

Doak, C., Doak, L. & Root, J. (1996). *Teaching patients with low literacy skills*, (2nd ed). Philadelphia, J.B. Lippincott.

Flesch, R. (1948) A new readability yardstick. *Journal of Applied Psychology*, 32, 221–233.

Glanz, K., Rimer, B. & Lewis, F. (2002). *Health behaviour and health education: theory, research and practice*, (3rd ed). San Francisco, Jossey-Bass.

Greenfield, S., Kaplan, S., Ware, J. et al (1988). Patients' participation in medical care: effects on blood sugar and control and quality of life in diabetes. *Journal of General Internal Medicine*, 3, 448–457.

Griffin, J., McKenna, K. & Tooth, L. (2006). Discrepancy between older clients' ability to read and comprehend and the reading level of written educational materials used by occupational therapists. *American Journal of Occupational Therapy*, 60, 70–80.

Hanson-Divers, E. (1997). Developing a medical achievement reading test to evaluate patient literacy skills: a preliminary study. *Journal of Health Care for the Poor and Underserved*, 8, 56–59.

Hill, J. (1997). A practical guide to patient education and information giving. *Baillieres Clinical Rheumatology*, 11, 109–127.

Hochlehnert, A., Richter, A., Bludau, H. et al (2006). A computer-based information tool for chronic pain patients: computerised information to support the process of shared decision-making. *Patient Education & Counselling*, 61, 92–98.

Hoffmann, T. & McKenna, K. (2006a). Analysis of stroke patients' and carers' reading ability and the content and design of written materials: recommendations for improving written stroke information. *Patient Education and Counselling*, 60, 286–293.

Hoffmann, T. & McKenna, K. (2006b). Evaluation of client education. In: K. McKenna & L. Tooth (eds) *Client education: a partnership approach for health professionals*. (pp. 159–182) Sydney, University of New South Wales Press.

Hoffmann, T. & Worrall, L. (2004). Designing effective written health education materials: Considerations for health professionals. *Disability and Rehabilitation*, 26, 1166–1173.

Hoffmann, T., Russell, T. & McKenna, K. (2004). Producing computer-generated tailored written information for stroke patients and their carers: system development and preliminary evaluation. *International Journal of Medical Informatics*, 73, 751–758.

Janz, N. & Becker, M. (1984). The Health Belief Model: a decade later. *Health Education Quarterly*, 11, 1–47.

Kaplan, S., Greenfield, S., Ware, J. et al 1989 Assessing the effects of physician–patient interactions on the outcomes of chronic disease. *Medical Care*, 27(Suppl 3), S110–S127.

Kitching, J. (1990). Patient information leaflets: the state of the art. *Journal of the Royal Society of Medicine*, 83, 298–300.

Knowles, M. (1980). *The modern practice of adult education*. New York, Cambridge.

Knowles, M., Holton, E. & Swanson, R. (1998). *The adult learner*, (5th ed). Houston, Gulf Publishing Company.

Law, M. & Mills, J. (1998). Client-centred occupational therapy. In: M. Law (Ed.) *Client-centred occupational therapy*, (pp. 1–18). Thorofare, NJ, Slack.

Ley, P. (1988). The use of written information. In: P. Ley (Ed.) *Communicating with patients*, (pp. 125–140). London, Chapman & Hall.

Lorig, K. (2001). *Patient education: a practical approach*, (3rd ed). California, SAGE Publications.

Lorig, K. & Holman, H. (1993). Arthritis self-management studies: A twelve-year review. *Health Education Quarterly*, 20, 17–28.

Lorig, K., Chastain, R., Ung, E. et al (1989). Development and evaluation of a scale to measure perceived self-efficacy in people with arthritis. *Arthritis and Rheumatism*, 32, 37–44.

McEneany, J., McKenna, K. & Summerville, P. (2002). Australian occupational therapists working in adult physical dysfunction settings: what treatment media do they use? *Australian Occupational Therapy Journal*, 49, 115–127.

McKenna, K. & Tooth, L. (2006a). Client education: an overview. In: K. McKenna & L. Tooth (Eds)

Client education: a partnership approach for health professionals, (pp. 1–12). Sydney, University of New South Wales Press.

McKenna, K. & Tooth, L. (2006b). Planning educational interventions. In: K. McKenna & L. Tooth (Eds) *Client education: a partnership approach for health professionals*, (pp. 112–127). Sydney, University of New South Wales Press.

McLaughlin, H. (1969). SMOG grading: a new readability formula. *Journal of Reading*, 12, 639–646.

McMullan, M. (2006). Patients using the Internet to obtain health information: how this affects the patient–health professional relationship. *Patient Education and Counselling*, 63, 24–28.

Murphy, P., Davis, T., Long, S. et al (1993). REALM: a quick reading test for patients. *Journal of Reading*, 37, 124–130.

Neufeld, P. (2006). The adult learner in client–practitioner partnerships. In: K. McKenna & L. Tooth (Eds) *Client education: a partnership approach for health professionals*, (pp. 57–87). Sydney, University of New South Wales Press.

Parker, R., Baker, D., Williams, M. et al (1995). The Test of Functional Health Literacy in Adults: a new instrument for measuring patients' literacy skills. *Journal of General and Internal Medicine*, 10, 537–541.

Paul, C., Redman, S. & Sanson-Fisher, R. (1997). The development of a checklist of content and design characteristics for printed health education materials. *Health Promotion Journal of Australia*, 7, 153–159.

Prohaska, T. & Lorig, K. (2001). What do we know about what works? The role of theory in patient education. In: K. Lorig (Ed.) *Patient education: a practical approach*, (pp. 21–55). California, SAGE publications.

Prochaska, J., Di Clemente, C. & Norcross, J. (1992). In search of how people change: applications to addictive behaviours. *American Psychologist*, 47, 1102–1114.

Prochaska, J., Redding, C. & Evers, K. (2002). The transtheorectical model and stages of change. In: K. Glanz, B. Rimer & F. Lewis (Eds) *Health behaviour and health education: theory, research and practice*. (pp. 99–120) San Francisco, Jossey-Bass.

Rosenstock, I. (1974). Historical origins of the Health Belief Model. *Health Education Monographs*, 2, 328–335.

Rosenstock, I., Strecher, V. & Becker, M. (1988). Social Learning Theory and the Health Belief Model. *Health Education Quarterly*, 15, 175–183.

Roter, D. (1987). An exploration of health education's responsibility for a partnership model of client–provider relations. *Patient Education and Counselling*, 9, 25–31.

Strecher, V., McEvoy, B., Becker, M. et al (1986). The role of self-efficacy in achieving health behaviour change. *Health Education Quarterly*, 13, 73–91.

Stromberg, A., Ahlen, H., Fridlund, B. et al (2002). Interactive education on CD-ROM: a new tool in the education of heart failure patients. *Patient Education and Counselling*, 46, 75–81.

Tang, P. & Newcomb, C. (1998). Informing patients: a guide for providing patient health information. *Journal of the American Medical Informatics Association*, 5, 563–570.

Theis, S. & Johnson, J. (1995). Strategies for teaching patients: a meta-analysis. *Clinical Nurse Specialist*, 9, 100–105.

Tones. K, (2002). Reveille for radicals! The paramount purpose of health education? *Health Education Research*, 17, 1–5.

Tones, K. & Tilford, S. (1994). *Health education: effectiveness, efficiency and equity*, (2nd ed). London, Chapman & Hall.

van den Borne, H. (1998). The patient from receiver of information to informed decision-maker. *Patient Education and Counselling*, 34, 89–102.

Weinman, J. (1990). Providing written information for patients: psychological considerations. *Journal of the Royal Society of Medicine*, 83, 303–305.

Weiss, B., Reed, R. & Kligman, E. (1995). Literacy skills and communication methods of low income older persons. *Patient Education and Counselling*, 25, 109–119.

Weiss, B., Coyne, C., Michielutte, R. et al (1998). Communicating with patients who have limited literacy skills: report of the National Work Group on Literacy and Health. *Journal of Family Practice*, 46, 168–175.

Wilson, F. & McLemore, R. (1997). Patient literacy levels: a consideration when designing patient education programs. *Rehabilitation Nursing*, 22, 311–317.

World Health Organisation (1998). *Health promotion glossary*. Geneva, Switzerland, World Health Organization.

Wyatt, T. (1999). Instructional technology and patient education: assimilating theory into practice. *The International Electronic Journal of Health Education*, 2, 85–93.

Further reading

Fleming, J. & Onsworth, T. (2006). Educational partnerships with clients who have cognitive impairment. In: K. McKenna & L. Tooth (Eds) *Client education: a partnership approach for health professionals*, (pp. 246–269). Sydney, University of New South Wales Press.

Hickson, L. (2006). Educational partnerships with clients who have hearing impairment. In: K. McKenna & L. Tooth (Eds) *Client education: a partnership approach for health professionals*, (pp. 226–245). Sydney, University of New South Wales Press.

Hoffmann, T. & McKenna, K. (2006). Evaluation of client education. In: K. McKenna & L. Tooth (Eds) *Client education: a partnership approach for health professionals*, (pp. 159–182). Sydney, University of New South Wales Press.

Lorig, K. & Harris, M. (2001). How do I get from a needs assessment to a program? Program planning and implementation. In: K, Lorig & Associates (eds.) *Patient education: a practical approach*, (pp. 85–142). California, Sage Publications.

McKenna, K. & Liddle, J. (2006). Educating older clients. In: K.

McKenna & L. Tooth (Eds) *Client education: a partnership approach for health professionals*, (pp. 183–205). Sydney, University of New South Wales Press.

Redman, B. (2003). *Measurement tools in patient education*. New York, Springer.

Worrall, L., Howe, T. & Rose, T. (2006). Educating clients with speech and language impairments. In: K. McKenna & L. Tooth (Eds) *Client education: a partnership approach for health professionals*, (pp. 206–225). Sydney, University of New South Wales Press.

Health promotion and occupational therapy

Rachael Dixey

CHAPTER CONTENTS

Introduction 240

Key ideas within health promotion 240

Approaches to health promotion 243

Naidoo and Wills' five approaches to
health promotion 243
Medical approach 244
Behavioural change 244
Educational approach 244
Empowerment approach 244
Social change approach 244
Beattie model of health promotion 244

Settings for health promotion 245

Evidence and evaluation 245

Occupational therapy and health
promotion 246

Education 247

Behaviour change 248

Conclusion 249

SUMMARY

The aims of this chapter are to introduce concepts of contemporary health promotion, to suggest ways in which occupational therapists can engage with health promotion, and to explore ways in which occupational therapy and health promotion have common aspects of practice philosophy. The chapter will provide a foundation in the skills, knowledge and values of health promotion, providing a sense of the toolkit that health promoters use, in terms of their orientation to the problem of helping people to improve their health. It will suggest that health promotion practice can be complex, with many and often competing ideas about the best way to 'do' health promotion. The chapter is not intended as a 'how to do' health promotion guide, but it will provide a foundation for the key principles and will hopefully show that health promotion is already part of the everyday work of occupational therapists.

KEY POINTS

- There are parallels between the development of health promotion and the occupational concerns of occupational therapy.
- Health promotion is the process of supporting people to increase control over the factors that influence their health and quality of life.
- Health promotion aims to facilitate individual, community and societal change.
- Key premises of health promotion are that the health of all individuals and groups *can* be improved, efforts to promote health need to be 'focused upstream', and health is open ended and positive.
- The Ottawa Charter proposed that for people to be healthy, the right kind of public policy needs to be in place, together with supportive environments that would address the environmental determinants of health.
- In order for health promotion to be effective, people need to be equal partners in all stages.
- Empowerment is *the* central task of health promotion; if people are empowered, they acquire increased power and control over their health.

Introduction

Certain parallels can be seen between the development of health promotion and the recent concerns of occupational therapy. Health promotion *is* concerned with those who have lost their health, but is more centrally concerned with whole, healthy populations, in order for all people to become as healthy as humanly possible. Health promotion then, *could* be used with individuals who have had a heart attack, in order for them to return to fitness, but aims primarily to work with healthy populations on *prevention* (healthy eating, exercise, etc.), and would also encourage the pursuit of ever-increasing levels of positive health as a 'good' in its own right. Likewise, occupational therapy has, in recent times, striven to assert its potential role with healthy individuals and communities to help them engage in life-enhancing occupations, rather than only playing a rehabilitation role with people who have become ill or unhealthy. The latter is clearly important and necessary, but there is also opportunity to work in more creative, proactive ways to prevent ill health occurring in the first place and also to enable healthy people to pursue the highest possible level of occupational well-being. Just as health promotion sees health as a human right, occupational therapy has begun to argue that the focus of occupational therapy should be 'on the right of all people to participate in meaningful occupations, and proposes allegiance to occupational rights: the right of all people to engage in meaningful occupations that contribute positively to their own well-being and the well-being of their communities' (Hammell 2008, p. 61).

Occupational therapy then, is inherently health promoting. To take this dimension of occupational therapy further, it is useful to consider recent developments in the field of health promotion and how they apply to occupational therapy. A range of allied health professions have entered discussions on what their distinctive contribution is to health promotion, including physiotherapy (French & Swain 2005), orthoptic practice (Rowe & Henshall 2005), and occupational health (Lisle 1996). Within occupational therapy, Wilcock's (2006) work stands out as fostering discussion about the ways in which occupational therapy promotes health and well-being. There are also many examples of how occupational therapy works to *prevent* ill health with healthy communities (Pereira & Stagnitti 2008) or to promote healthy ageing (Clark et al 1997, 2001).

The American Occupational Therapy Association (2007) has produced a useful position paper on health promotion which argues that the occupational therapist's role in health promotion is three-fold: to promote healthy lifestyles, to emphasise occupation as an essential element of health promotion strategies, and to provide interventions with individuals and populations.

Key ideas within health promotion

A reasonable starting point is to provide a model of health that suits the purposes of both health promotion and occupational therapy. In order to know what it is that we are promoting, it helps to have an understanding of 'health'. Labonte's model (adapted from Orme et al 2003) places well-being firmly at the centre with key aspects such as meaning and purpose also prominent (see Figure 17.1). This clearly goes beyond a medical model of health and illustrates how an occupational therapist could contribute to several of the dimensions that enable health as a 'by-product'. These include 'ability to do things one enjoys', 'good social relations' and 'control over life'. Control is a key notion that will be returned to below.

It is worth mentioning Antonovsky's (1979) salutogenic concept of health, which was developed to try to understand what makes people healthy, as opposed to what makes them unhealthy. Kobasa et al (1979) assert that *control* is one of three common factors in salutogenesis, the idea that an individual is able to influence the course of events. The other two factors are *commitment* – having a sense of curiosity for life and a sense of meaningfulness in life; and *challenge* – the expectation that life will change and that change is beneficial. Helping people to make appropriate changes is a key task of health promotion, and it aims to facilitate individual, community and societal change. Occupational therapy as a profession, through its professional influence and academic debate, can certainly effect societal change, but for the most part, individual occupational therapists are likely to work to encourage change with individual clients or patients, or with groups, and perhaps less frequently with whole communities.

A key premise of health promotion is that the health of all individuals and groups *can* be improved. Inequalities in health status are a constant feature of surveys in all countries. Why should there be

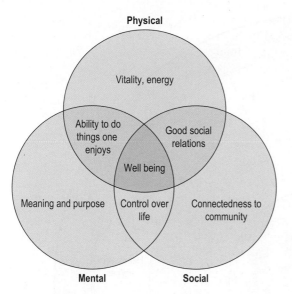

Figure 17.1 • Labonte's model (Orme et al 2003. Reproduced with kind permission of Open University Press. All rights reserved)

these differences? It is now incontrovertible that they are to do with the social and economic situation in which people live. Tackling inequalities is the starting point and the cornerstone of the value base of health promotion. Government attempts to reduce disparities in health have been tried in several developed countries, as in the USA's *Healthy People 2010* (US Dept of Health and Human Services 2000) or earlier in Australia (Nutbeam et al 1993), by setting targets. A series of reports in the United Kingdom show a rather gloomy picture in that inequalities in health are persistent and difficult to reduce, let alone eradicate (Acheson 1998, Marmot & Wilkinson 2006, Townsend 1988, Townsend & Davidson 1992).

A second key premise follows logically from the above concern with inequalities and with the poverty and deprivation on which these inequalities rest. That is, efforts to promote health need to be 'focused upstream'. This catch phrase has become common in public health circles and what it means is this: many attempts to improve health only occur after the damage has happened, i.e. they are focused on curative attempts to restore people to a state of health. McKinlay (1979) likened this to a person who is sitting on a riverbank, and finds that they are called to rescue an individual who is clearly struggling in the water. They haul that person out, and just as they reach the riverbank safely, they see another person struggling, and so on and so on. That

rescuer never has time to walk up the riverbank and find out who (or what) is pushing everyone in the river. The parallel with a doctor, nurse or other health professional that focuses on rescuing (curing) rather than on preventing is obvious. Health promoters try to focus their interventions on causes or determinants of ill health (whatever it is that makes people susceptible to illness in the first place), rather than on what might be happening 'downstream'. Of course, there will always be those who become ill, have accidents or develop illnesses about which little is known about prevention (such as multiple sclerosis, Alzheimer's disease, etc.), and so it is not the case that health professionals with a curative focus are not needed. However, the adage that 'prevention is better than cure' means that a cadre of workers is needed which focuses on just what is needed to prevent ill health before it occurs. This is what the health promotion profession can offer. Concern with determinants of health is central to that profession, and brings us back to a concern with health inequalities.

Health promotion also has as a key tenet that health is open-ended and positive. 'Health' is not simply about restoring a person to a 'normal' level of health or asserting that someone is well if they do not have an obvious disease or ailment. Health is about realising as much potential as possible, and going on to become *more* physically fit, *more* emotionally robust, *more* socially happy. The World Health Organization's (WHO 1986) well-known definition of health might be utopian, but it also suggests that, although this 'complete state' is difficult to achieve, as far as promoting health is concerned, the sky's the limit! The WHO (1986) has suggested that health is a resource for everyday life, not the objective of living, and Wilcock (2006, p. 315) follows by suggesting that an 'occupation-focused health promotion approach to wellbeing embraces a belief that the potential range of what people can do, be, and strive to become is the primary concern and … health is a by-product'. Health, then, is not to be focused on for the sake of it, but so that it can enable a person to live a full, meaningful life. It goes without saying that the model of health which health promotion adopts is a social model, not a medical one. The latter, with its disease focus, is narrow and does not enable illumination of the causes or determinants of health. Dahlgren and Whitehead's (1992) illustration (Figure 17.2) is often reproduced to indicate the range of factors which interplay to determine any one individual's state of health.

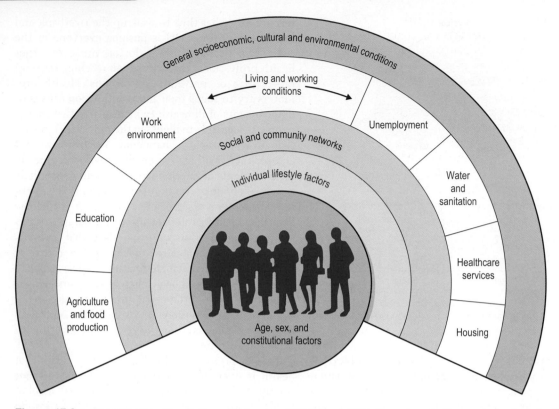

Figure 17.2 • Determinants of health (from Dahlgren and Whitehead 1992. Reproduced with permission from the World Health Organisation)

Health promotion is a relatively recent concept, having emerged in the 1980s in its current usage. The fact that it was possible to promote and increase people's health has, of course, been known for much longer than this, and can be seen in the attempts made by public health in most industrialised countries to promote health by better water and sanitation, housing laws, workplace legislation, assuring healthy diets, and so on. However, by the 1980s, these public health efforts to manage people's healthiness tended to take second place to the role of medicine, which had become spectacularly successful in many ways, but was increasingly seen as unlikely to cope with the rise of preventable 'lifestyle diseases', such as coronary heart disease, cancer, and stroke. Medical costs could be infinite. A second strategy to deal with making the population healthier was health education. Health education, it was argued, would enable people to become informed about how to prevent lifestyle illnesses and that once people understood, for example, the link between smoking and health, they would simply stop smoking, or if they knew the health benefits of

eating fresh fruit and vegetables, then they would eat them. Clearly this is a gross underestimation of the complexities of human behaviour and also can be victim blaming – if a family can not really afford fresh foods or does not know how to cook them then there is no point educating about this in the absence of providing that family with the means and/or skills to carry out the required behaviour.

So the emphasis on the role of medicine and on health education was seen as insufficient in dealing with the population's health. The landmark report that opened people's eyes to this fact was the Lalonde report (1974) on the Health of Canadians. This focused attention on to the social and economic determinants of people's health, and suggested that the key to improving health lies outside the health care sector (which is, on the whole, the illness or curing sector). Later, much of this thinking came together in the WHO conference held in Canada in 1986, which resulted in the Ottawa Charter on Health Promotion, which provides the foundation upon which the modern era of health promotion is built. The Charter shifted the main responsibility for improving health on to policy makers, arguing that for people to be healthy, the right kind of public policy needs to be in place, together with the supportive environments that would address the environmental determinants of health. This newer emphasis became known as 'health promotion' as opposed to a health education approach that represented a narrower focus on behavioural determinants of health – the idea that health is determined by individual behaviours and actions which can be addressed by health education.

The Ottawa Charter argues for action in five areas:

1. Building healthy public policy

2. Creating supportive environments

3. Strengthening community action

4. Developing personal skills

5. Reorientating health services.

The Ottawa Charter thus provided a broader base for promoting health, enabling it to move beyond merely being seen as encouraging individuals to change their behaviour, to place the responsibility on governments to make healthier public policy and to locate the *source* of health as outside the health care/illness sector. Canada continues to play a lead role in health promotion (Pederson et al 2005), but the overview of the value base of health promotion which will be presented here is from the Health Promotion Forum of New Zealand (2008):

- Health promotion:
  - works with people not on them
  - starts and ends with the local community
  - is directed to the underlying as well as immediate causes of health
  - balances concern with the individual and the environment
  - emphasises the positive dimensions of health
  - concerns and should involve all sectors of society and the environment.

- Health promotion is the process of supporting people to increase control over the factors that influence their health and quality of life. An important characteristic of health promotion is its focus on groups of people, either the whole population or specific subgroups. It places emphasis on changing the environment to enable behaviour to change. Health promotion draws upon principles of:
  - social change
  - physical change
  - policy development
  - empowerment
  - community participation
  - equity and health
  - accountability
  - building partnerships and alliances between groups.

- Health promotion draws on an explicit value base:
  - Individuals are treated with dignity and their innate self-worth, intelligence and capacity for choice are respected.
  - Individual liberties are respected, but priority is given to the common good when conflict arises.
  - Participation is supported on policy decision-making to identify what constitutes the common good.
  - Priority is given to people whose living conditions, especially a lack of wealth and power, place them at greater risk.
  - Social justice is pursued to prevent systemic discrimination and to reduce health inequities.
  - Health of the present generation is not purchased at the expense of future generations.

Approaches to health promotion

The New Zealand Forum summarises the philosophy and ethics of health promotion, while several writers have attempted to summarise the complexity of approaches to health promotion in practice, and two such attempts will be mentioned here: Naidoo and Wills' (2000) overview of approaches and Beattie's (cited in Scriven 2005) model of health promotion.

Naidoo and Wills' five approaches to health promotion

Naidoo and Wills (2000) provide a useful introduction to health promotion. They suggest that five main approaches to health promotion can be identified, differing in philosophy, aims, and means: medical, behavioural, educational, empowerment, and social change. In practice, the distinctions between these approaches might be somewhat blurred, and also elements of each might be needed to tackle a particular issue. However, the typology may be useful in distinguishing observed differences in opinion in the field about the 'best' way to carry out health promotion.

Medical approach

The medical approach is concerned with preventing disease and illness, tends to be 'top-down', and relies on giving information and trying to persuade the adoption of healthy behaviour. An example might be a general practitioner giving an overweight person a diet sheet, or a health visitor giving advice on weaning.

Behavioural change

The behavioural change approach is concerned with persuading people to think about their behaviours and, where necessary, to change them. An example might be a smoking cessation advice worker encouraging a pregnant woman to give up smoking.

Educational approach

The educational approach is concerned with providing learning opportunities for people so that they can understand the effects on their health, where to seek help, how to develop skills and so on, such that they can make informed decisions about their health. An example might be a youth worker educating a group of teenagers about sexually transmitted infections and how to avoid them.

Empowerment approach

The empowerment approach is concerned with working alongside people so that they can work out what health issues are important to them, and gain more power to influence the determinants of their health so they can take more control over their own lives. An example might be a community worker working with a disadvantaged community on how they can prioritise their health problems and then approach relevant authorities such as the housing authority (if they had problems, for example, with damp housing and asthma).

Social change approach

The social change approach is concerned with changing the social, economic, and political factors that affect health. An example might be a group of local councillors working with a Neighbourhood Action group to tackle antisocial behaviour and vandalism.

Beattie model of health promotion

There are many other writers who have attempted to conceptualise health promotion, but most suggest that health promotion is complex and is *more* than merely health education or attempts to change people's behaviour. Health promotion might have a bad press in that it is seen as attempting to *stop* people doing things, i.e. to reduce fat and sugar in their diet, consume less alcohol, give up smoking – but health promotion is far more than that – it is about creating the right conditions where people can live life to the full, realise their potential, maximise their health and not be held back by the risk of poor health. What is clear is that action is required in an organised and concerted fashion to tackle any particular issue. To use the example of childhood obesity, there is little point encouraging families to change their eating and exercise habits without governments also taking action to curb the advertising of 'unhealthy' foods, to attend to school curricula, to work with the food industry, and so on.

Beattie's model of health promotion (adapted from Beattie 1994) (Figure 17.3) has attempted to conceptualise this full range of activities necessary to bring about healthy change. The model suggests that activity is required in each of the four sectors in order to bring about change; again, using childhood obesity as an example, it might be that authoritative, top-down approaches which affect larger communities are needed to regulate the food industry, to ensure school meals meet certain standards, or to make transport planners consider child safety to a greater extent, so as to encourage walking and cycling. Authority figures, such as general practitioners/family physicians, might raise the issue with parents and caregivers on an individual basis. Using more negotiated approaches, a worker at a children's centre might work with groups of parents on aspects of healthy eating, starting a community garden to grow vegetables, or at an individual level, the school nurse or youth worker might work with individual young people on how to be less sedentary.

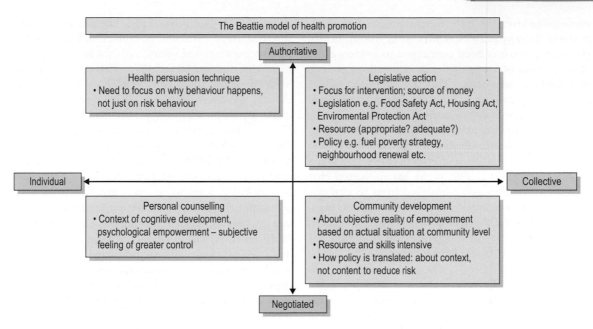

Figure 17.3 • Beattie's model of health promotion (from Bury, Calnan & Gabe (Eds), The sociology of the Health Service, 1994, published by Routledge, with permission)

This model can also be used to locate the positions of individual health workers. Many may work primarily with individuals rather than with whole communities and primarily in a top-down rather than bottom-up way – i.e. in a more authoritative style rather than in a negotiated way. Non-directive counsellors might work in the bottom left quadrant, which is where occupational therapists might also be located.

Settings for health promotion

The Ottawa Charter and the subsequent conferences and declarations that have elaborated on its ideas, suggest that health promotion is a set of broad activities operating at a number of different levels. One way of giving health promotion a sharper focus is the development of the 'settings approach' (see Dooris 2006, Whitelaw et al 2001), which suggests that it would be useful to look at a 'setting', such as the workplace, a village, a school, and so on, and to consider all the people whose lives are affected within that setting, and all the activities which take place within it, so as to consider how to make that setting healthier. The settings approach is now firmly in place within the health promotion field and has enabled the emergence of Health Promoting Schools and Colleges, Health Promoting Hospitals, Healthy Workplaces, a concern with Health in Prison, Healthier Islands, and the Healthy Cities movement. It can lead to 'joined up thinking' as it places health on the agenda of all policy makers and all staff within an organisation. It enables people to think about contradictions – for example, in a school where children are taught about healthy eating in class, they are not then confronted with unhealthy choices for school lunch, as the purpose of the settings approach is to ensure that all aspects are thought about in an holistic manner.

A major drawback of the settings approach is that individuals and groups existing outside settings will be excluded, such as children who are not in school, the unemployed, and so on. However, most public-health programmes in most countries also have initiatives designed to target 'hard-to-reach groups' or the 'socially excluded', in line with the concern with tackling health inequalities. This critique notwithstanding, the settings approach has added energy and systematic thinking to health promotion.

Evidence and evaluation

In keeping with the move towards evidence-based practice seen in a range of health and social care professions over the last 30 years, such as in occupational therapy (Cusick & McClusky 2000), health promotion too has been concerned to evidence the effectiveness of its activities and to adopt an evidence-based approach. This has brought about greater emphasis on *evaluating* health promotion interventions and also on *using* this evidence in the design and implementation of planned health promotion activities. Extensive debates about the best ways to provide evidence of effectiveness have taken place. The WHO (1998, p. 5) has suggested that 'the use of randomised controlled trials to evaluate health promotion initiatives is, in most cases, inappropriate, misleading and unnecessarily expensive', but not all agree with this perspective (see for example Rosen 2006). These debates will not be discussed in detail here. Suffice it to say, it is essential to evaluate the effectiveness of health promotion, to base interventions on sound theoretical underpinnings and with a clear understanding of the evidence base. Interventions in health promotion tend to be complex, to occur in community settings and are thus not conducive to the 'gold standard' randomised control trial. Green and South (2006) provide a comprehensive guide on how to evaluate health promotion interventions in the 'real world'.

Occupational therapy and health promotion

The outline of health promotion thus far is brief, and readers are encouraged to peruse both introductory texts (Ewles & Simnett 2003, Naidoo & Wills 2000), and more specialised texts (Tones & Green 2004, Tones & Tilford 2001) to gain more insight into the depth and breadth of health promotion. The aim of this section of the chapter is to consider the alignment of health promotion and occupational therapy, and, in so doing, to infer what health promotion can bring to the profession of occupational therapy, and also what insights occupational therapy can offer to health promotion. This section also considers some of the knowledge areas necessary for health promotion.

Scaffa and Brownson (2004, p. 485) note that 'community-level interventions are not as familiar to occupational therapy practitioners', but argue that they have an opportunity to 'respond to and help resolve the community health problems of the 21st century, including poverty, joblessness, inadequate

daycare and parenting skills, homelessness, substance abuse, mental illness, chronic disease and disability, unintentional injury, violence and abuse, and social discrimination' (p. 487). This opportunity to 'step outside of the box' of traditional occupational therapy (Withers & Shann 2008) was discussed earlier by Baum and Law (1998) and back in 1972 Finn offered a list of issues which occupational therapy needed to address for the profession to contribute successfully to community health, arguing that it had a unique perspective to do so. This 'wish list' included learning about communicating with communities, having a secure professional identity and embracing health promotion (Scaffa 2001). More recently, Fisher and Hotchkiss (2008) have discussed working with marginalized communities using a model of occupational empowerment in their work with women living in homeless shelters in the USA, illustrating that in some spheres at least, there is scope for occupational therapists to work at community level. The American Occupational Therapy Association (2007) suggests ways in which occupational therapists can contribute at community level, and these ideas are also explored in other chapters of this book. Health promoters, more often than not, work at community level, and there is scope for occupational therapists to join in existing teams.

The outline of the value base of health promotion provided above by the New Zealand Health Promotion Forum resonates with the client-centred practice base of occupational therapy, as described in *Enabling Occupation* (Townsend 2002). Client-centred practice features largely in the codes of ethics for occupational therapy (College of Occupational Therapists 2005) and also within attempts to align the occupational therapy and health promotion agendas, such as in *For the health of it: Occupational therapy within a therapy promotion framework* (Letts et al 1996). Sumsion (2005) suggests that client-centred occupational therapy practice hangs on the ideas of partnership, communication, choice, and power, and these resonate with key health promotion principles.

Within health promotion, the discourse around 'partnership' with communities and individuals is likely to be framed in terms of 'participation', 'collaboration', and 'involvement'. Peckham (2003, p. 70) argues that 'in adopting a more enlightened public health perspective, individuals and communities need to be seen as equal partners in promoting and producing health'. This equality of partnership implies a shift in the balance of power between lay people and professionals.

In order for health promotion to 'work', people need to be equal partners in all stages – top-down initiatives are likely to be resisted or ignored, and they are diametrically opposed to the key value of empowerment. A gradient of participation can be seen to increase empowerment (see Figure 17.4). A model which involves participation and empowerment clearly also involves the issue of choice, and emphasises the importance of voluntarism, i.e. of individuals not being coerced, but engaging willingly in activities which promote their health.

The issue of empowerment within health promotion has been explored by Laverack (2004) and it is becoming increasingly common to assert that it is *the* central task of health promotion. If people are empowered, they acquire increased power and control, which is at the heart of the most well-known definitions of health promotion, framed by the WHO (1986); 'the process of enabling people to increase control over, and to improve, their health'. This logically leads health workers such as occupational therapists into asking, what constitutes empowerment, and how can they facilitate the process of their clients becoming empowered? Scriven (2005) suggests that there are three important facets of personal development linked to empowerment:

1. Psychological perception involving enhancing self-esteem, self-efficacy, and internal locus of control.

2. Cognitive development involving increasing awareness of health information, and raising a 'critical consciousness'.

3. Life skills, including decision-making, assertiveness, and inter-personal skills.

Internal locus of control refers to the sense that individuals have of being in charge of their lives and is the opposite of being helpless or disempowered. (An external locus of control would imply that a person felt that their life was controlled by factors external to themselves, such as by fate or by other people.) Self-efficacy refers to the belief people have in their ability to achieve or to carry out what they want to – such as giving up smoking.

Harries (2005, p. 134) demonstrates how occupational therapy can help young people with eating disorders by 'building self-image, self-worth, communication skills, stress management skills and media awareness'. These ingredients are the 'standard fare' of many health promotion interventions, but linking these aspects to a 'return to valued occupational engagement' (Harries 2005, p. 131) is the occupational therapist's unique contribution.

Education

It can be inferred from the discussion above, that health education has gained a reputation for 'victim-blaming' and has been seen as a panacea when it could only ever be a partial solution to

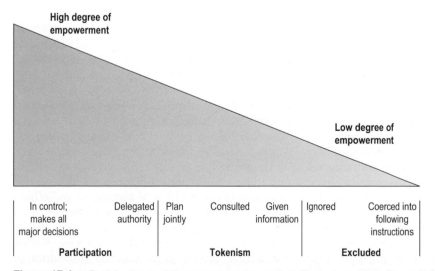

Figure 17.4 • Participation and the empowerment gradient (Reproduced from Tones & Green 2004 *Health Promotion: Planning and Strategies* with permission from SAGE Publications. © SAGE Publications Ltd. 2004)

improving health. Tones (1997, p. 37) has conceptualised health education as follows:

> Health education is any intentional activity which is designed to achieve health- or illness-related learning i.e. some relatively permanent change in an individual's capability or disposition. Effective health education may therefore produce changes in knowledge and understanding or ways of thinking. It may influence or clarify values; it may bring about some shift in belief or attitude; it may facilitate the acquisition of skills; it may even effect changes in behaviour or lifestyle.

A key weakness is apparent – the stress is on 'may' – but equally it 'may not' bring about required change, and the effect of increased knowledge on attitudes and behaviour is poorly understood and not especially straightforward. Clearly it is too simplistic to assume that if people are provided with correct information, they will act on it. Even if people are in the right environmental conditions to act upon advice and information, a complex series of psychological mechanisms can come into play which means that they do not act in the way the health educator would wish. Cognitive dissonance is one such psychological process, where new knowledge raises a sense of being uncomfortable with the status quo. An example might be where a person has their consciousness raised about their body mass index, perhaps through a healthy-eating course, and begins to ponder whether they need to lose weight. To reduce the dissonance, the individual either can dismiss the information, or decide to lose some weight. Once having made the decision of course, another series of complex processes come into play that will affect whether that person's intention is ever actually carried through!

The full complexity of the role of education in facilitating change will not be entered into here. The important point is that occupational therapists do not dismiss education, but rather, think carefully about its use and limitations. Most importantly, we need to consider how it can be used to good effect, because clearly there is a role for education, in providing information and skills to both patients and healthy individuals about their concerns. The adage 'knowledge is power' is still a powerful one.

In occupational therapy with people with rheumatoid arthritis, Adams and Pearce (2005, p. 145)

note that 'participatory self management education programmes will encourage the individual to change behaviour as well as improve their cognitive understanding of the disease'. They note that such programmes have been more effective in raising awareness than in creating long-term behaviour change, but a complete package of learning about psychological coping skills, practising skills to reduce physical symptoms as well as improving anatomical knowledge can result in more effective self-management.

Behaviour change

Behaviour change may be a key goal of health promotion, but as indicated above, the health promoter needs to be aware that people have differing socio-economic circumstances, presenting different obstacles to change. For a woman living in difficult circumstances, perhaps on a low income, a single parent and with small children, trying to give up smoking or reduce weight, where smoking might be a coping strategy and the nearest shops offering fresh fruit and vegetables are out of easy reach, it would clearly be necessary to tackle some of those living difficulties first before attempting to address healthier behaviours. A critique of the social psychological models that attempt to explain the processes of behaviour change is that they often pay scant attention to these wider determinants of health. However, they also offer useful insights into health behaviours, and potentially provide a theoretical basis for planning interventions.

Social cognition models such as the theory of reasoned action (Ajzen & Fishbein 1980), later developed into the theory of planned behaviour (Ajzen 1991), provide a theoretical account of how attitudes, subjective norms and behavioural intentions combine to predict behaviour. These are described as expectancy-value models, in that behaviour follows from what the individual expects will happen after following a particular action, e.g. 'If I work out at the gym I *expect* to get fitter'. According to the theory of planned action, intention to behave (a combination of motivation and effort) will be affected by subjective norms, or perceived pressure from significant others, and by attitudes, or salient beliefs about the health behaviour. Hobbis and Sutton (2005) point out the difficulties of using social cognition models to plan practical interventions or campaigns, but what these models perhaps help us to do is to consider all the factors which might lead to an individual being able to overcome the obstacles to making changes – or not. One useful model that attempts to understand the process of carrying out preventive health behaviours is Rosenstock's (1974) Health Belief Model. This basically asserts that in order for an individual to carry out the proposed behaviour, he or she needs to perceive that he or she is susceptible to the health threat, that the health threat is serious, that there are perceived benefits to the action, that there are minimal barriers or costs, and there needs to be some kind of 'cue to action' (Rosenstock 1974). The health promoter or occupational therapist can use these ideas to ascertain an individual's beliefs, and then work on the specific beliefs that hinder or help change. Rutter and Quine (2002) provide an in-depth discussion of the application of social cognition models to a range of health behaviours.

One behaviour change model which has been applied a great deal in practice is the stages of change model, also known as the transtheoretical model, developed by Prochaska et al (1992) (Figure 17.5). First used to help users of illegal drugs with their drug habit, this model has since been applied to helping people to stop behaviours, e.g. smoking cessation, and also to adopt behaviours, e.g. physical activity, condom use, and so on. The model can be used to assess readiness to change, and to tailor an intervention to the appropriate stage; someone who is motivated to change, for example, will need a very different intervention from the person who is unaware, or who is maintaining change and in need of support to do so. The idea is that people move through the stages, and the role of the therapist or health promoter is to facilitate successful movement through those stages. The model has been applied in a range of occupational therapy contexts, such as in mental health (Hawkes et al 2008, Lancaster & Chacksfield 2008) or in helping older people to undertake home safety modifications (McNulty et al 2004). The model has been subjected to a great deal of critique (see for example, Povey et al 1999), but it has been found to be useful in practice as a heuristic device.

Conclusion

This chapter has shown that concerted action is needed at all levels – national, community and individual – in order to promote health. Health promotion 'is equally and essentially concerned with creating the conditions necessary for health at individual, structural, social, and environmental levels through an understanding of the determinants of health: peace, shelter, education, food, income, a stable ecosystem, sustainable resources, social justice, and equity' (Trentham & Cockburn 2005, p. 441). We could also add 'occupation' to this list of the determinants of health. Occupational therapists have a clear and obvious contribution to make to health promotion, and it is appropriate to sum up in the words of the well-known academic occupational therapist, Thelma Sumsion (2005, p. 107):

There is a clear and positive link between client centred practice and health promotion. The concepts of partnership, communication, choice and power are foundational to both client centred practice and health promotion and must be implemented by occupational therapists committed to ensuring that clients have every chance of obtaining their health goals. The links between the two are strong, and when these two approaches are supported and clearly connected, the clients will be empowered to assume responsibility for their health, which is a unifying goal in both health promotion and client centred practice.

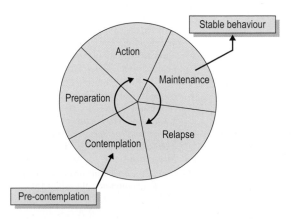

Figure 17.5 • States of change model (adapted from Prochaska & DiClemente (1992) In search of how people change: Applications to addictive behaviors. American Psychologist, 47, 1102–1114)

References

Acheson, D. (1998). *Independent Inquiry into Inequalities in Health Report*. London, The Stationery Office.

Adams, J., & Pearce, S. (2005) Occupational therapists and the promotion of psychological health in rheumatoid arthritis. In: A. Scriven (Ed.), *Health promoting practice; the contribution of nurses and allied health professionals* (pp. 138–151). Basingstoke, Palgrave MacMillan.

Ajzen, I. (1991). The theory of planned behaviour. *Organisational Behaviour and Human Decision Making Processes*, 50, 179–211.

Ajzen, I., & Fishbein, M. (Eds). (1980). *Understanding attitudes and predicting social behaviour*. Englewood Cliffs, NJ, Prentice Hall.

American Occupational Therapy Association. (2007). *Occupational therapy in the promotion of health and the prevention of disease and disability* [Electronic Version]. Retrieved December 12, 2007 from http://www.aota.org/Practitioners/Resources/Docs/Adopted/40983.aspx.

Antonovsky, A., (1979). *Health, stress, and coping: new perspectives on mental and physical well-being*. San Francisco, Jossey-Bass.

Baum, C., & Law, M. (1998). Community health: A responsibility, an opportunity, and a fit for occupational therapy. *American Journal of Occupational Therapy*, 52(1), 7–10.

Beattie, A. (1994). Knowledge and control in health promotion: a test case for social policy and social theory. In: J. Gabe, M. Calnan & M. Bury (Eds) *The sociology of the health service* (pp. 162–200). London, Routledge.

Clark, F., Azen, S., Zemke, R. et al (1997). Occupational therapy for independent–living older adults. *Journal of the American Medical Association*, 278(16), 1321–1326.

Clark, F., Azen, S., Carlson, M. et al (2001). Embedding health-promoting changes into the daily lives of independent-living older adults: Long-term follow-up of occupational therapy intervention.

Journal of Gerontology: Psychological Sciences, 56B(1), P60–P63.

College of Occupational Therapists. (2005). *College of Occupational Therapists Code of Ethics and Professional Conduct*. London, College of Occupational Therapists.

Cusick, A., & McClusky, A. (2000). Becoming an evidence-based practitioner through professional development. *Australian Occupational Therapy Journal*, 47(4), 159–170.

Dahlgren, G., & Whitehead, M. (1992). *Policies and strategies to promote equity in health*. Copenhagen, World Health Organisation.

Dooris, M. (2006). Health promoting settings: Future directions. *Promotion and Education*, 13(1), 2–4.

Ewles, L., & Simnett, I. (2003). *Promoting health: a practical guide*. Edinburgh, Balliere Tindall.

Finn, G. L. (1972). The occupational therapist in prevention programs. *American Journal of Occupational Therapy*, 26, 59–66.

Fisher, G. & Hotchkiss, A. (2008). A model of occupational empowerment for marginalised populations in community environments. *Occupational Therapy in Health Care*, 22(1), 55–71.

French, S., & Swain, J. (2005) The culture and context for promoting health through physiotherapy practice. In: A. Scriven (Ed.) *Health promoting practice; the contribution of nurses and allied health professionals* (pp. 155–167). Basingstoke, Palgrave MacMillan.

Green, J., & South, J. (2006). *Evaluation*. Milton Keynes: Open University Press.

Hammell, K. (2008). Reflections on... well-being and occupational rights. *Canadian Journal of Occupational Therapy*, 75(1), 61–64.

Harries, P. (2005) Health promotion in eating disorders: The contribution of occupational therapists. In: A. Scriven (Ed.), *Health promoting practice; the contribution of nurses and allied*

health professionals (pp. 127–137). Basingstoke, Palgrave MacMillan.

Hawkes, R., Johnstone, V., & Yarwood, L. (2008). Acute psychiatry. In: J. Creek & L. Lougher (Eds.). *Occupational therapy and mental health* (pp. 393–406). Edinburgh, Elsevier.

Health Promotion Forum of New Zealand, (2008). What is health promotion? Retrieved June 19, 2008, from http://www.hpforum.org.nz/page.php?7

Hobbis, I., & Sutton, S. (2005). Are techniques used in cognitive behaviour therapy applicable to behaviour change interventions based on the theory of planned behaviour? *Journal of Health Psychology*, 10(1), 7–18.

Kobasa, S., Hiker, R., & Maddi, S. (1979). Who stays healthy under stress? *Journal Occupational Medicine*, 21(9), 595–598.

Lalonde, M. (1974). *A new perspective on the health of Canadians: a working document*. Ottawa, Ministry of National Health and Welfare.

Lancaster, J. & Chacksfield, J. (2008). Substance misuse. In: J. Creek & L. Lougher (Eds.). *Occupational therapy and mental health* (pp. 535–556). Edinburgh, Elsevier.

Laverack, G. (2004). *Health promotion practice: power and empowerment*. London, Sage.

Letts, L., Fraser, B., Finlayson, M., & Walls, J. (1996). *For the health of it: occupational therapy within a health promotion framework*. Toronto, Canadian Association of Occupational Therapists.

Lisle, J. (1996). The role of occupational health services in promoting health. In: A. Scriven & J. Orme (Eds), *Health promotion: professional perspectives* (pp. 228–238). Basingstoke, Palgrave Macmillan.

Marmot, M., & Wilkinson, R. (2006). *Social determinants of health* (3rd ed). Oxford, Oxford University Press.

McKinlay, J. B. (1979) A case for refocusing upstream: the political economy of illness. In: Jaco, E. G. (Ed.) *Patients, physicians and illness* (pp. 9–25). New York, NY, The Free Press.

McNulty, M., Johnson, J. & Poole, J. (2004). Using the transtheoretical model of change to implement home safety modifications with community-dwelling older adults: An exploratory study. *Physical and Occupational Therapy in Geriatrics*, 21(4), 53–66.

Naidoo, J., & Wills, J. (2000). *Health promotion: foundations for practice*. London, Elsevier Health Sciences.

Nutbeam, D. & Harris, E. (2004). *Theory in a nutshell: a practical guide to health promotion theories* (2nd ed.). Sydney, McGraw Hill.

Nutbeam, D., Wise, M., Bauman, A., Harris, E., & Leeder, S. (1993). *Goals and targets for Australia's health in the year 2000 and beyond*. Canberra, AGPS.

Orme, J, Powell, J, Taylor, P, Harrison, T & Grey, M. (2003). *Public health for the 21st century*. Buckingham, Open University Press.

Peckham, S. (2003). Who are the partners in public health? In: J. Orme, J. Powell, P. Taylor, T. Harrison, & M. Grey (Eds) *Public health for the 21st century* (pp. 59–78). Buckingham, Open University Press.

Pederson, A., Rootman, I., & O'Neill, M. (2005). Health promotion in Canada: Back to the past or towards a promising future? In: A. Scriven & S. Garman (Eds) *Promoting health: global perspectives*. (pp. 255–262). Basingstoke, Palgrave MacMillan.

Pereira, R., & Stagnitti, K. (2008). The meaning of leisure for well-elderly Italians living in an Australian community: Implications for occupational therapy. *Australian Occupational Therapy Journal*, 55(1), 39–46.

Povey, R., Conner, M., Sparks, P., James, R., & Shepherd, R. (1999). A critical examination of the application of the Transtheoretical Model's stages of change to dietary behaviours. *Health Education Research*, 14(5), 641–651.

Prochaska, J.O., DiClemente, C.C. & Norcross, J.C. (1992). Measuring processes of how people change: Application to addictive behaviours. *American Psychologist*, 47, 1102–1114.

Rosen, L. (2006). In defense of the randomized controlled trial for health promotion research. *American Journal of Public Health*, 96(7), 1181–1186.

Rosenstsock, I. M. (1974). The Health Belief Model and preventive health behaviour. *Health Education Monographs*, 2, 354–386.

Rowe, F., & Henshall, V. (2005). Orthoptists and their scope for health promotion. In: A. Scriven (Ed.), *Health promoting practice; the contribution of nurses and allied health professionals*. (pp. 270–281). Basingstoke, Palgrave MacMillan.

Rutter, D., & Quine, L. (2002). *Changing health behaviour: intervention and research with social cognition models*. Milton Keynes, Open University Press.

Scaffa, M. (2001). Community-based practice: Occupation in context. In: M. Scaffa (Ed.), *Occupational therapy in community-based practice settings*. (pp. 3–18). Philadelphia, F.A. Davis Company.

Scaffa, M., & Brownson, C. (2004). Occupational therapy interventions: Community health approaches. In: C. Christiansen, C. Baum & J. Bass-Haugen (Eds.), *Occupational therapy: performance, participation, and well-being* (3rd ed) (pp. 477–492). Thorofare, NJ, Slack.

Scriven, A. (2005). Promoting health: Perspectives, policies, principles, practice. In: A. Scriven (Ed.) *Health promoting practice; the contribution of nurses and allied health professionals*. (pp. 1–16). Basingstoke, Palgrave MacMillan.

Scriven, A., & Garman, S. (2005). *Promoting health: global perspectives*. Basingstoke, Palgrave MacMillan.

Sumsion, T. (2005). Promoting health through client centred occupational therapy practice. In: A. Scriven (Ed.), *Health promoting practice; the contribution of nurses and allied health professionals*. (pp. 99–112). Basingstoke, Palgrave MacMillan.

Tones, K., (1997). Health education as empowerment. In: M. Siddell, L. Jones, J. Katz, & A. Peberdy (Eds), *Debates and dilemmas in promoting health: A reader*. (pp. 33–42). Milton Keynes, Open University Press.

Tones, K., & Green, J. (2004). *Health promotion: planning and strategies*. London, Sage.

Tones, K., & Tilford, S. (2001). *Health promotion: effectiveness, efficiency and equity*. (2nd ed). London, Chapman Hall.

Townsend, E. (Ed.). (2002). *Enabling occupation: an occupational therapy perspective*. (Revised ed). Ottawa, Canadian Association of Occupational Therapists.

Townsend, P. (Ed.). (1988). *Inequalities in health*. London, Penguin.

Townsend, P. & Davidson, N. (Eds). (1992). *Inequalities in health*. London, Penguin.

Trentham, B. & Cockburn, L. (2005). Participatory action research: Creating new knowledge and opportunities for occupational engagement. In: F. Kronenberg, S. Algado, & N. Pollard (Eds) *Occupational therapy without borders: learning from the spirit of survivors*. (pp. 440–453). Edinburgh, Churchill Livingstone.

US Dept of Health and Human Services (2000). *United States of America, Healthy people 2010: Improving Health and Objectives for Improving Health*. Washington DC: US Government Printing Office.

Whitelaw, S., Baxendale, A., Bryce, C., MacHardy, L., Young, I. & Witney, E. (2001). 'Settings' based health promotion: A review. *Health Promotion International*, 16(4), 339–353.

Wilcock, A. (2006). *An occupational perspective of health*. (2nd ed). Thorofare, NJ, Slack.

Withers, C. & Shann, S. (2008). Embracing opportunities: Stepping outside of the box. *British Journal of Occupational Therapy*, 71(3), 122–124.

World Health Organization (1986). *The Ottawa Charter for Health Promotion*. Geneva, World Health Organization.

World Health Organization (1998). *Health Promotion Evaluation: Recommendations to Policymakers. Report of the WHO European Working Group on Health Promotion Evaluation*. Copenhagen, World Health Organization.

Working with groups

Claire Craig and Linda Finlay

CHAPTER CONTENTS

Introduction 254

Valuing group work in physical
rehabilitation. 254

Types of group work 254

   Psycho-educational groups 255

   Occupational groups 255

The value of group work generally 256

   Sense of community connectedness 257

   Creative and/or productive
   opportunities. 257

   Evidence on the effectiveness of
   group work. 257

Planning a group 258

   Creating the group stage 258

   Recruiting stage 259

   Engaging stage 259

   Planning stage. 259

Managing the group. 259

   The beginning stages of a group 260

   The middle stages of a group. 261

   The ending stages of a group. 261

Conclusion. 261

SUMMARY

The primary aim of this chapter is to demonstrate
the value and range of group work associated
with working with people who have a physical
impairment. Psycho-educational and occupation-
focused groups – two main categories of groups
relevant to this group of people – are described
and illustrated by practice examples. The power
of using groups is their potential to foster a
sense of connectedness in which members share
experience and offer support for each other. In
addition, groups can provide opportunities for
members to be creative and/or productive which
has been shown to have positive impacts for
individuals. Practical guidelines for planning and
managing groups are covered, with the
application of these guidelines illustrated through
a practice scenario. Group work has a definite
role to play when working with people who have
a physical impairment, as involvement in a group
can enable members to not only share with and
learn from each other, but to engage in doing,
being and becoming.

KEY POINTS

- Group work has a role to play when working
  with people who have a physical impairment.
- Successful group work requires the creation of
  a supportive environment where individual
  members are able to give and take, express and
  listen, and offer and learn from each other, and
  engage in the process of doing, being and
  becoming.
- The most commonly employed groups tend to
  fall into two distinct, but overlapping, categories:
  psycho-educational groups and occupational
  groups.
- Psycho-educational groups either focus on
  teaching people skills to manage particular
  problems or take an information-giving health
  promotion approach.

- Occupational groups are the domain of occupational therapy given their focus on encouraging the development or maintenance of healthy leisure, work and self-care occupations.
- Groups have the potential to foster a sense of community connectedness through enabling mutual sharing, support and collective problem-solving.
- Occupationally focused groups provide opportunities for individuals to be creative and/ or productive.
- Preparatory work needs to occur before a group can start and this work can be divided into four pre-group stages: creating, recruiting, engaging, and planning.
- Groups need to be actively managed throughout all stages of the group, with each stage raising different challenges and responsibilities for the group leaders.

Introduction

At first glance you might be curious about why a chapter on group work is being included in a book focusing on physical rehabilitation. Group work has traditionally been viewed as an intervention used primarily in the mental health field. Does it – *should it* – have a role to play with people who have physical disabilities? Our answer to this question is a loud 'Yes!' While group work is not widely practised in physical settings, it still has a place in an occupational therapist's tool bag of interventions. It is all too easy to fall into the trap of seeing physical and mental health needs as being separate. Of course, they are not. Just think about the way physical, mental and social needs are intertwined when working with people with complex needs such as a person with neurological problems. To work with people with complex needs, occupational therapists need to draw on the full spectrum of intervention tools at their disposal.

Occupational therapists work with groups in many different ways both in institutions and the community. In order to enable service users to gain the most from their group work, occupational therapists need to have a clear idea about the role and potential of groups and how to ensure they are therapeutically focused rather than simply a social or recreational gathering. This is the focus of this chapter.

The primary aim of the chapter is to demonstrate the value and range of group work associated with physical rehabilitation and how it is practically applied in occupational therapy. First, the chapter outlines some of the types of groups available and discusses their value. The second section offers some practical guidelines for planning and running groups. The chapter also offers an exemplar practice scenario of the evolution of one particular group facilitated by the first author highlighting some of the processes and group dynamics.

Valuing group work in physical rehabilitation

While group work is not a commonly employed intervention in physical rehabilitation there are pockets of practice where it forms a key component. For instance, when working with older people and as part of interventions to do with modifying lifestyles (Jackson et al 1998).

When you think of group work in physical rehabilitation settings, what images come to mind? Perhaps the image is of a support group for people with chronic conditions and their relatives who meet once a month at the local hospital? Perhaps a 'rehab group' or 'hand therapy group' comes to mind with people sitting around a table and being seen by a therapist who goes round to each in turn? The parallel therapy being delivered in this way may be effective but, it is not really *group* work – or at least it is not exploiting the rich potential of group work. It is also not exploiting the benefits of using occupation.

Types of group work

A wide range of groups can be offered as part of a physical rehabilitation programme. The most commonly employed groups tend to fall into two distinct, but overlapping, categories: *psycho-educational groups* and *occupational groups*. Other types of group work seen in mental health settings, such as psychotherapy groups, are employed less frequently in physical rehabilitation. In practice, while there is often much overlap between these two broad categories, for example when focused on health promotion and Lifestyle Redesign™, they can be distinguished by their differences in aims and focus.

Psycho-educational groups

Psycho-educational groups either focus on teaching people skills to manage particular problems or take an information-giving health promotion approach. Typical examples of groups in this category would be those designed to manage problematic symptoms such as pain, or anxiety, and those focused on developing health and fitness. Psycho-educational groups tend to have a more generic focus which means that often they will be run by interdisciplinary team members and so occupational therapists may, or may not, be involved.

Two examples of different psycho-educational groups relevant to physical rehabilitation are presented here in Practice Scenarios 18.1 and 18.2.

Practice Scenario 18.1
Psycho-educational group –
Heart-y Living Group

The Heart-y Living Group promotes the health of cardiac patients. This is a weekly out-patients' group run by an occupational therapist and a physiotherapist in the gym at a local hospital. The aims of this group are:

- to teach the importance of exercise and diet in relation to coronary heart disease
- to promote new healthy exercise and diet behaviours
- to teach stress management techniques
- to provide emotional and social support helping participants to cope with the psychological consequences of experiencing a heart attack.

Individuals are referred to this closed eight-week group around the time they are discharged from hospital.

Practice Scenario 18.2
Psycho-educational group –
Coping with Pain Group

The *Coping with Pain Group* is for people experiencing chronic, severe pain. This is an open group held in the pain clinic on a fortnightly basis run by an occupational therapist and a clinical psychologist. Group members can access the group at any point during their attendance at the pain clinic. The aims of this group are to:

- help members to develop an understanding of the causes of chronic pain
- explore a number of recreational and psychosocial strategies that can be used to manage pain
- provide a supportive atmosphere to validate group members' experiences and reduce the isolation experienced by participants.

In the group, members have the opportunity to share their experiences of chronic pain while the co-leaders take the opportunity to begin to challenge some of the myths surrounding the relationship between activity and pain.

These examples of psycho-educational groups show an occupational therapist jointly leading the groups with a colleague from a different profession. Such collaborative group work models fit current practice where interdisciplinary and cross-agency working is valued and encouraged.

However, the focus on remediation and developing skills/knowledge rather than on occupation and practical *doing* does not sit entirely comfortably within the occupational paradigm (Molineux 2004). For those wishing to carve out a clearer occupational therapy role, psycho-educational groups could be included as part of a broader occupationally focused therapy programme. Here, for example, a service user might be encouraged to join an anxiety-management group as part of a wider occupational therapy programme focused on lifestyle management or participants attending an exercise group on the ward could be given the opportunity later to attend a similar group at a local leisure centre. For instance, with the Heart-y Living Group described above, initial sessions could take place in the gym but towards the end of the eight weeks emphasis could be placed on using community leisure facilities and family members could be invited to take part to increase their understanding. Placing the group aims in a broader life context overcomes the main drawback of many groups which do not exploit the full occupational potential of an activity and which consequently lack an occupational focus.

Occupational groups

Occupational groups could be viewed as being more specifically the domain of occupational therapy, given their focus on encouraging the development or maintenance of healthy leisure, work, and self-care occupations. Group work usually involves group members being actively involved and *doing*, for example, using arts or playing sports. Often the content of these groups is recreational and focused on encouraging social interaction. Usually group activities will have a community orientation and aim to provide opportunities for social networking and participation. As Wilcock notes, 'Social well-being will be enhanced if people are able to develop their potential through practice in a range of socially valued occupations' (1998, p. 104).

Occupational therapists preferring to work more explicitly within an occupational paradigm from the start see groups as a specific *environment* to be manipulated to facilitate and support 'occupations congruent with those individuals might normally perform' (Molineux & Whitford, 1999). Two examples of different occupational groups used to improve occupational function and enrichment are presented in Practice Scenarios 18.3 and 18.4.

Practice Scenario 18.3
Occupational group – *Genesis*

'Genesis' is the name of a community-based horticultural group for individuals who have experienced a stroke. This group is run by an occupational therapist and occupational therapy assistant. The aim of the group is:

- to provide opportunities for group members to engage in the health-promoting benefits of horticulture and gardening.

Participants are invited to work on a community allotment project. They are first asked to attend on a 'set day' while in hospital and immediately following discharge. However, as their rehabilitation progresses, they are able to attend the group on other days when it is facilitated by a group of volunteers and ex-clients.

Practice Scenario 18.4
Occupational group – *Living Well*

'Living well' is the name of an occupation-based preventive health programme aimed at meeting the needs of older people. This group, run by an occupational therapist and social care worker, aims to:

- enable participants to develop an understanding of the relationship between activity, health and well-being

- explore issues impacting on health and examine ways of addressing these
- consider how to incorporate health-promoting activities into existing routines.

This weekly group is held in a community resource centre. The group is advertised in the post office, local supermarket, and sheltered housing complex, and is publicised by community nurses. Prospective members meet with the occupational therapist and agree to attend for a set number of weeks.

It should be clear that these groups offer participants much more than opportunities for simple recreation and enjoyable diversion. The occupational focus of such groups is explicitly therapeutic as they are made relevant to group members' wider life contexts, lifestyles and physical/social needs. For instance, the participants in the *Genesis* group would benefit both physically and socially. In addition to building strength and stamina, and improving posture and balance, participants are likely to gain from the opportunity for social interaction and from the sharing of skills and resources. Rather than the therapist holding the locus of control, group members themselves could become the resource, modelling problem-solving techniques, sharing tips on ways to overcome challenges, validating experiences and within this, developing new roles which can be transferred to other situations.

The value of group work generally

The specific value of group work, whichever the variant, arises from the opportunities presented to engage multiple layers of relationships, beyond one-to-one interactions with the therapist. Specifically, this means that groups have the potential to foster a sense of *community connectedness* while enabling mutual sharing, support and collective problem-solving. Further, occupation focused groups provide opportunities for individuals to be *creative and/or productive* which, in turn, can enhance an individual's sense of well-being and esteem while developing skills and promoting change. All these values have been explored and solidly validated by research.

Sense of community connectedness

Examining the value of community connectedness, researchers have focused on how a sense of belonging can contribute to a positive sense of identity while encouraging new relationships and the formation of wide-ranging social support networks. Fieldhouse (2003), for example, found people attending a community horticultural group attached great importance to the social contact they gained helping them to feel part of a wider social network and a valued citizen within their community.

At a more immediate level, groups also allow members to share their experiences and learn from each other. Members can socialise and gain support from each other; they can model for and challenge each other. Groups can promote positive change in that they are powerful shapers of behaviour (which can be a positive or negative force) as group norms and pressures push us to respond to others' demands and expectations. Groups can also inspire and fulfil people's needs for human contact.

Evaluating the use of group work in palliative care, Firth (2000) demonstrated how groups offer mutual support and collective problem-solving strategies. They help 'people counter the view that dying is a private, personal experience. Through discussion of individual feelings and apprehensions, death…can be shared with others in the same boat' (Firth 2000, p. 27). To give another example, Laing (2007) describes her use of group therapy to improve communicative participation in people with dysarthria and multiple sclerosis. Group participants reported they had enjoyed the group and that it was satisfying working on their problems in a supportive environment which promoted the sharing of experiences.

Applying these ideas specifically to the context of physical rehabilitation, service users can gain much from sharing with, and relating to, others. They can gain support from sharing their experiences of pain and disability or the traumas of surgery, for example. They can also help encourage each other to 'keep doing the exercises' or they may be able to offer valuable tips for coping positively with ill health or disability. The value of such emotional, practical and social support should not be underestimated – particularly in the context of a busy unit where the therapist may not have the time to give this kind of attention to individuals. Group work can fill the gap by offering an enabling, supportive, structured environment for people to help each other and themselves. The therapist's role here is thus as much about facilitating this group support as it is providing hands-on individual teaching or therapy.

Creative and/or productive opportunities

Exploring the specific value of occupational groups in providing opportunities for individuals to be creative and/or productive, researchers have shown the positive impact occupational therapy and the use of meaningful activity can have. The specific combination of activity and group work employed by occupational therapists offers a 'unique and powerful tool to teach skills [and] promote change' (Finlay 2000, p. 40). Trace and Howell (1991), for example, applied Kaplan's (1988) ideas for the 'Directive Group' to working with older people. They found the set format of daily games, crafts and exercises improved both social interaction and task performance. Similarly, in occupational therapy Klyczek and Mann (1986) compared different treatment programmes at two psychiatric day centres. The programme was found to be significantly more effective for developing the use of leisure time, self-esteem, vocational adjustment and decision making.

The examples above notwithstanding, the overall evidence base validating group work is patchy. While there is a reasonable body of published accounts about the value of psychotherapy groups, there is limited literature on the value of activity-orientated and occupational therapy groups, and even less research on the use of group work in physical rehabilitation. Of the group work literature most relevant to occupational therapy, a distinction can be made between those studies using objective outcome measures and those focused on service users' subjective evaluations.

Evidence on the effectiveness of group work

Of the limited pool of studies using objective outcome measures, *The Well Elderly Study*, an experimental, randomised controlled research conducted by Clark et al (1997, 2001) in the United States of America, offers perhaps the most significant evidence in favour of group work and occupational therapy. It took over three years to complete the trial and involved 361 participants. The participants were randomly assigned to one of three groups: (1) a nine-month programme of group-based occupational therapy focused on Lifestyle Redesign™; (2) a control condition where participants engaged in group-based activities, which were non-professionally led; and (3) no intervention whatsoever. The results were powerfully consistent. In comparison with the two other conditions, the occupational therapy group produced clear benefits in numerous outcomes including physical and social performance, mental health and vitality (Clark et al 1997). Further, these benefits persisted over a six-month follow-up interval (Clark et al 2001). Interestingly, no difference was found between the group who received social activity and the no intervention group, suggesting that activity alone is not necessarily therapeutic. Similar results are reflected in other studies; for example, research by Okumiya et al (2005) showed the value of group work using music therapy and handicrafts for older people living in the community who had age-associated cognitive decline and/or mild depressive moods. Improvements were observed in mood, quality of life and cognitive function (though these were not sustained after the group work ended).

More evidence is available demonstrating the value of group work and occupational therapy using subjective measures. The work by Heather (2003) is notable. She evaluated the benefits of a group called 'Pro-motion' for people with severe and enduring mental health problems living in the community. People rated 'listening to others', 'sharing my views', 'being listened to' and 'sharing my needs' as being the most important benefits of being in their group. Other studies, such as that by Polimeni-Walker et al (1992), have shown that service users feel positive about their group experiences and that they enjoy the use of activities. Falk-Kessler et al (1991) carried out some research related to Yalom's (1975) often-cited 11 curative factors of group therapy. They found the experience of 'group cohesiveness', 'hope' and 'interpersonal learning' were perceived by both clients and therapists as being most valuable.

Sometimes group interventions are preferred to individual therapy assuming them to be a more economical option as more people are treated at one time. However, groups are only cost-effective if the intervention is effective as well. Sometimes service users' needs may be more simply and efficiently handled on an individual basis. It takes extra time and skills to manage a group. Sessions will last an hour or so whereas an individual consultation may only take minutes. Also group leaders need to set aside time to see group members individually to prepare them for the group and to monitor their progress. Then there is all the extra group preparation and post-group evaluation required.

A better argument might be to point to the evidence such as the Clark et al (1997) research which showed the value of the older people engaging in the occupational therapy intervention (which included both individual and group therapy). The researchers not only demonstrated that the health of the older people improved, they showed that the average savings in health care costs exceeded the cost of the occupational therapy itself.

Planning a group

Lots of preparatory work needs to occur before a group can start. This work can be divided into four pre-group stages: 'creating', 'recruiting', 'engaging' and 'planning'. When these pre-group stages have been completed and prospective members have made a positive commitment to attend, the therapist can concentrate on managing the group as it evolves.

Practice Scenario 18.5 illustrates some of these principles and describes the journey taken to establish a community group for older people called 'New Horizons'.

Creating the group stage

In the creating the group stage, the therapist first determines that there is a need for a group of this kind. Therapeutic groups involve more than simply getting people together. There needs to be an expectation that the outcome of the group will be an improvement in occupational performance, participation and well-being. Then specific decisions need to be made about the group *aims, format, proposed content* and *context*. The underlying rationale for all these questions should be concerned with what is going to make the group therapeutic and helpful. For example, group leaders may choose to run a particular kind of group such as one following the Functional Group Model, developed by Howe and Schwartzberg (1986). This group aims to enhance the occupational behaviour of members by encouraging them to engage in relevant occupational tasks in the context of group support.

Once the aims are clear, *group membership* needs to be established. Firstly, size of group needs to be planned bearing in mind the number of leaders needed or available. While six to nine people is thought to be the optimum number for psychotherapy groups, activity groups can run with more or less people providing there are enough staff available to attend to individuals. Secondly, the mix of group members needs to be considered. For their Functional Group, Howe and Schwartzberg (1986) suggest combining individuals who have similar goals, abilities and needs. They cite the example of how a recently admitted client following a stroke would not fit with a group of clients preparing for discharge. In contrast, two clients preparing for the homemaker role – one with joint inflammation and the other with an upper-extremity fracture – would be compatible. Referring to psychoeducational groups for children, Brown (1998) recommends that children need to be of similar ages and, if possible, in gender-specific groups.

Finally, there are *practical* decisions that need to be taken concerning where, when and for how long. Thinking about where the group should take place, are there particular hospital/community resources which can be usefully exploited? Thinking about when and how long the group should run for, consideration needs to be given to what is practical for members.

Recruiting stage

The recruiting stage involves getting referrals and then choosing the people for the group. Before this can happen, the group may need a campaign for advertising and marketing. Here the therapist may want to alert possible referral agents using letters and leaflets or perhaps use eye-catching posters to invite people to participate. The more professional and inviting the letters and posters look, the more likely it will be to get appropriate referrals which, in turn, will make the group more successful in the long run. So it is worth carefully planning this campaign in terms of timing and impact.

Engaging stage

Having recruited the group members, each member needs to be assessed and, if he or she is thought to be suitable for the group, time needs to be spent engaging them. The prospective group members need to know what they are signing up to and how the group is going to be helpful to them. They need to be inspired to attend and participate actively. The therapist in turn uses this opportunity to assess the individual's needs for planning future interventions and to be aware of factors which might stop the individual taking part. In effect, a contract to attend the group is established.

Planning stage

The final planning stage, which would usually occur as the group evolves over the weeks, is to identify aims/goals/objectives or outcomes for each group session. Linked to these aims the therapist has to choose the group activity to fit the needs and level of the group and what is going to be meaningful to the group members (Finlay 1993). Table 18.1 provides specific guidance on how to plan sessions. Then there are other practical planning decisions which need to be made to do with equipment/ resources needed, how members are going to get to the group and how the group environment will be set up. Care needs to be taken to consider any messages being given off, which can set up certain expectations. Placing chairs in rows, for example, might signal people are being invited to 'listen' while chairs in a circle suggests more active participation will be required. Creating a comfortable, welcoming area to greet members (e.g. offering coffee and biscuits) can help relax people at the start of the group.

Managing the group

Managing a group involves more than simply planning and running sessions. The complexity of what is involved should not be underestimated. Within the group context therapists need to be aware of the needs of individuals while also managing the dynamics and processes that occur when many personalities come together. It takes skill to learn to 'read' a group and understand what might be happening below the surface of what people are doing.

Groups continuously evolve as relationships develop over time; at different points members can be seen to come together working cooperatively while at other times they can seem to move apart through conflicts and tensions. Group leaders need

Table 18.1 Preparing for and facilitating a group session
The following list highlights key questions and issues for the group leader to be aware of when preparing for individual sessions. See Finlay (1993) for a more in-depth account of structuring a session

Introduction	How will members be greeted and introduced to the aims of the sessions?
	What can be done to make people feel welcomed into the group?
	Would it help, for example, to have some music playing or to invite people to help themselves to an initial drink?
Warm up activity	Depending on the nature of the group it can help to have an initial activity designed to bring the group together in the 'here-and-now'. Physical or stretching exercises might be appropriate to energise the group. Alternatively, each member could be invited to comment on their view of the day's topic or their progress from the week before and so forth
Main action phase	In this phase the main part of the session takes place where the activity/activities selected to achieve group aims are implemented
	What activity/activities are relevant?
	How should they be presented?
	What role should the group leader play during these activities?
Closing phase	It is important to offer a wind down period which can be used to draw any threads together. This might, for example, involve a question and answer slot or final exercise where everyone is asked to say 'one important lesson they have learned in the session'. Alternatively, the group might make some plans for the next meeting or use the final minutes to help clear up

to be able to understand what is happening and why as part of working towards enabling positive outcomes and they need to adapt their role accordingly.

The stages a group goes through have been described in various ways (Bion 1961, Tuckman 1965, Yalom 1985). Basically all groups have a beginning and ending stage and 'stuff' happens in between which may involve different degrees of both conflict and working effectively together. In each of these stages, group leaders face certain tasks, challenges and responsibilities. How they handle these could make the difference between the success or relative failure of the group.

Practice Scenario 18.5 illustrates some of these principles and describes the journey taken to establish a community group for older people called '*New Horizons*'.

The beginning stages of a group

During the beginning stages of a group, which usually includes the first few sessions, members will tend to feel uncertain, possibly even anxious, about what the group is going to involve. Depending on their level of experience and pre-group orientation, they

may be approaching the group with anticipation or dread. They may also feel shy about getting to know the others in the group.

The group leader's role at this stage is to help members settle into the group, making them feel as comfortable and welcome as possible. Simple interventions, such as providing housekeeping information and stating what is going to happen in the group and for how long, can help settle members (Lizzio & Wilson 2001a). Part of this job involves being clear about group roles, norms, expectations and ground rules so members know what they are supposed to be doing. Often the messages given early on can set the pattern for future sessions so it is important to get the tone right. For instance, a common trap leaders can fall into is to do too much talking in the very first session. This can put the group members in a passive role which may be counter-productive when the leader wants them to participate actively later. The other key part of the leader's job is to help facilitate group members getting to know and trusting each other. Activities which encourage members to share their experiences are useful here and it can help if the leader points out similarities in experiences between individual members.

The middle stages of a group

The middle stages of a group will vary depending on the group; though they will probably include times when the group is working well together and times when there are some conflicts. When a group is working well there is a feeling of cohesiveness as members cooperate and support each other. At these times, the leader might be well advised to step back and allow group members to take on more responsibility for the group. If conflict sets in and tensions erupt between members or against the leader, the leader might want to step in and take more control. The key here is to try to help keep the group members feeling safe (for example, by having clear boundaries of confidentiality and keeping to agreed 'group rules' such as accepting and respecting others' contributions). The decision about when to intervene or not is a hard one. The leader does not want to take over completely as this may disempower group members, yet there is a balance to be found as members should not be left to flounder in discomfort for too long. Too much floundering is likely to encourage members to vote with their feet and not come back to the group. How much direction to give or not is a decision that can only be made in the context of the specific group.

Research, for instance stemming from social identity theory (Tajfel & Turner 1979), has shown that group members can be helped to identify with their group and that this has clear implications for the group's effectiveness and how cooperative/competitive or involved members are likely to be (Tyler & Blader 2000, Yalom 1985). The leader can do two main things here: mark the emerging boundaries of the group and help each individual feel positively included in the group community (Lizzio & Wilson 2001b). Using language like 'us', 'we' and 'our group' can help, as can noting emerging themes such as saying, 'It seems that several of you are expressing this same point; who else feels the same?'

The ending stages of a group

During the ending stages of a group, whether this is the last few minutes of the final session or last few sessions, group members may well have mixed feelings that the group is ending including feeling sad, worried and angry. Some tensions and conflicts may creep back into the group dynamics. At the same time, some members may feel reluctant to acknowledge the group is finishing and try to find ways to prolong it. Depending on the type of group, the leader's responsibility is to find a gradual way to help members deal with the ending. The main aim should be to tie up loose ends and ensuring members do not leave with a sense of 'unfinished business'. Ideally, there should be some consideration given to following up any gains made. For instance, how might members manage the transition between attending the group and accessing groups in the future once they find themselves in the community?

One positive intervention the group leader can make as a group is finishing is to ask group members to evaluate the effectiveness of the group. Precisely how this evaluation is carried out will depend on the requirements of the service concerned and the type of group work involved. In some places, the main task may be simply to record individuals' progress. In other places, a record of the evolution of the group as a whole may be useful. Often both forms of evaluation are used in combination. For example, Heather (2002) describes the evaluation procedure for her group called *Pro-motion* for clients with severe and enduring mental-health problems living in the community. She asked her clients to rate (using a Likert-type scale) their overall evaluations of each session in terms of 'enjoyment', 'interest', and 'helpfulness'. By combining these results, she was able to audit the effectiveness of the group overall and she used this as a basis for further research.

Conclusion

This chapter has sought to demonstrate the value of the range of group work associated with physical rehabilitation and how it is practically applied in occupational therapy. Firstly, it considered the types of groups available and the value of occupationally connected group work. It then offered some practical guidelines for planning and running groups, and, finally, it gave an example of what can happen when a group is established, sharing a little of the journey that one group travelled.

Successful group work requires the therapist to create a space where individual members are able to give and take, to express and listen, and to offer and learn from each other in a mutually supportive environment, and, in doing so, to engage in the process of doing, being and becoming which is at the heart of occupational therapy practice. Facilitating groups in practice is challenging, exciting, sometimes frustrating, and will draw on your sensitivity, creativity, and ability to read and manage complex dynamics. This is a skill to be mastered. However, when group work is used appropriately it can lead to changes of mammoth proportions, and, as such, it deserves a place in occupational therapists' tool bag of interventions.

Practice Scenario 18.5
The 'New Horizons' Group

For the purposes of confidentiality all names and details have been changed to preserve anonymity.

Envisioning and planning the group

The impetus for the establishment of the group came from a small piece of unpublished research that the department had undertaken which examined the progress made by older people admitted to the hospital following a fall. It measured the physical gains sustained by clients six weeks following discharge. The findings showed that while individuals made good progress during rehabilitation in hospital, this was short lived. On discharge clients experienced severe loss of confidence and rarely left the confines of their home. Reduced exercise impacted on physical and psychological well-being leading to a vicious cycle of further loss of confidence and limited engagement in occupation.

Madhu and I (Claire) identified the need for a group that would form a bridge between discharge from hospital and return to the community. The aim was to engage group members in health-promoting activities and to provide opportunities to access leisure facilities. It was, therefore, decided to pilot a small 'closed' group (fixed membership) that would take place weekly over nine weeks.

Group members were referred via the ward-based occupational therapist. We met each person individually, describing the aims of the group and listening to what they felt the group could offer them. We used this time to undertake an initial assessment of the person's needs and discuss practicalities, such as transport and timing. Once we were clear that a group of this nature was appropriate, each person was invited to make a commitment to attend for a specified number of sessions, which was then formalised through the signing of a 'pre-group contract'. Individual needs were assessed using a number of occupational assessment tools. Where the group

was not appropriate for the person they were guided to other relevant facilities or services.

We undertook a needs assessment and from this the following overall goals were identified.

By taking part in this group, each participant would:

- understand the relationship between occupation, health and well-being
- engage in meaningful leisure pursuits to promote physical activity
- gain confidence in accessing community-based facilities
- identify factors that act as barriers in accessing leisure pursuits and develop strategies to overcome these.

Nine sessions were developed around the following themes:

1. Exploring occupation: understanding the relationship between what we do and how we feel
2. Occupation in the home and community: developing and maintaining occupational connectedness
3. Outing: identifying opportunities for occupation on the doorstep
4. Hobbies and pastimes
5. Transport
6. Outing: singing and Salsa
7. Managing pain
8. Home and community safety
9. Endings.

The location for the group was a local church hall, easily accessed via the main bus route. The venue had a kitchen and small seating area where group members could spend time chatting informally, make their own tea/coffee, and develop simple roles and build confidence in mobilising around the environment.

Managing the group

There were 12 group members in total: ten older people and two facilitators. We delivered the sessions using a model of didactic teaching, peer sharing, and active experimentation (Clark et al 1997).

Each meeting started with a period of reflection where members shared their experiences and described how they had taken forward any learning from the previous week. There was the opportunity to provide examples of occupations they had engaged in during that week, challenges faced and ways to these had been met.

As facilitators we would then share key information (for example the physiology of pain) before inviting the participants to relate this information to themselves through group discussion.

The highlight of the session was always the 'doing': engaging in active experimentation and putting theory into practice. Sessions ended with more discussion to evaluate what members had enjoyed and to make arrangements for the following week.

Every third session included an opportunity to contextualise these skills through a community outing. This would often involve using public transport, reading timetables, asking for information. This was perhaps the most powerful element of the delivery as group members shared that they gained great confidence from the group. What would otherwise have been a terrifying prospect was transformed into an 'exciting adventure' and with this new sense of confidence individuals were able to take further steps to generalise their skills more widely within the community.

We allocated two hours for the weekly group meeting. However, within this we varied the activities. This meant that while participants were not expected to concentrate for longer than 15–20 minutes at any one time they still had enough time to explore quite significant issues in depth if necessary.

Our group members always had time to *be*. The aim of the group was to enable participants to reflect on and utilise their skills and experiences. Over time individuals gradually assumed more of an active role within the overall facilitation of the sessions. This ensured that we were not creating an atmosphere of dependency.

Evaluation

Practicalities:

- For many of the group, transport was a practical barrier to attendance. We, therefore, arranged community transport for some participants. As the group progressed we addressed travel as a theme and, over time, responsibility was placed on group members to make their own arrangements, which they did with great success.
- We were careful to use resources that were inexpensive and facilities that were on the 'doorstep', making links with voluntary organisations and community services. These were the facilities that group members could access after the group had finished.
- Madhu and I worked closely together, planning the group, evaluating sessions and, above all giving each other support. We shared the facilitator's role and took turns leading group activities. This also ensured continuity so that

the group was not disrupted if either of us was away.

Challenges:

- We did not have a promising start and it took time for the group to develop an identity and to find its own atmosphere. There were ten members and our main challenge was balancing so many individual needs, helping participants to trust each other and the group process.
- There was friction at times. For example, during the session on pain the discussion spiralled out of control as Phyllis announced that women coped much better with pain than men and hinted that Ernest had not experienced what it was like to be in 'real pain'. In response Ernest stormed out. We had to work quickly to diffuse the situation and support Ernest and the group to move forward.
- When Madhu and I reflected on the session we questioned how attentive we had been to the building conflict, as we had been rather too focused on following our session plan. This was a good reminder that the art of being a good facilitator is to read the group, to pick up on non-verbal cues which denote whether someone is bored, tired, overwhelmed or angry, and to respond.

Transformations

- Over time the group assumed its own identity and group members began to draw strength from each other, sharing skills and resources, and engaging in the process of group problem-solving. The impact of this process on participants was transformative. For example:
  - Following an outing to the local leisure centre, Ernest began to bowl again and with encouragement from the group joined the local team. Between sessions, Jo would go along to offer him support and the two developed a strong friendship.
  - Kate was still very nervous when outdoors; however, the group outing did give her some confidence and she began to attend church again.
  - Flo still spent much of her day at home, but the strong social networks that were established meant that once a fortnight Kate, Eileen, and Phyllis would visit her and they would share a meal together.
  - June said that she felt that since her fall she had been 'asleep', but now she was a rosebud 'just waiting to bloom'.

- Follow-up assessments showed that group members were more physically active, less anxious, and successfully utilising community facilities. Through understanding the relationship between occupation, health and well-being our group were equipped to make informed choices and in doing so to experience significant life changes. These changes were a testimony to the group and to the group work process. As facilitators Madhu and I were privileged to be part of this and to recognise the incredible resources and resourcefulness individuals offered.

References

Bion, W. R. (1961). *Experiences in groups*. New York, Basic Books.

Brown, N. W. (1998). *Psycho-educational groups*. Philadelphia, Taylor & Francis.

Clark, F., Azen, S. P., Zemke, R. et al (1997). Occupational therapy for independent-living older adults: a randomized controlled trial. *Journal of the American Medical Association*, 278(16), 1321–1326.

Clark, F., Azen, S. P., Carlson, M. et al (2001). Embedding health-promoting changes into the daily lives of independent-living older adults: long-term follow-up of occupational therapy intervention. *Journal of Gerontology; Psychological Science*, 56B(1), 60–63.

Falk-Kessler, J., Momich, C. & Perel, S. (1991). Therapeutic factors in occupational therapy groups. *American Journal of Occupational Therapy*, 45, 59–66.

Fieldhouse, J. (2003). The impact of an allotment group on mental health clients' health, wellbeing and social networking. *British Journal of Occupational Therapy*, 66(7), 286–296.

Finlay, L. (2000). When actions speak louder: Group work in occupational therapy. In: O. Manor (Ed.). *Ripples: group work in different settings* (pp. 32–45). London, Whiting and Birch.

Firth, P. (2000). Picking up the pieces: group work in palliative care. *Group Work: An Interdisciplinary Journal for Working with Groups*, 12(1), 26–41.

Heather, F. (2003). Pro-motion: a positive way forward for clients with severe and enduring mental health problems living in the community, Part II. *The British Journal of Occupational Therapy*, 66(1), 25–30.

Howe, M. C. & Schwartzberg, S. L. (1986). *A functional approach to group work in occupational therapy*. Philadelphia, JP Lippincott.

Jackson, J., Carlson, M., Mandel, D., Zemke, R. & Clarke, F. (1998). Occupation in lifestyle redesign: the well elderly study occupational therapy programme. *American Journal of Occupational Therapy*, 52, 326–336.

Kaplan, K. (1988). *Directive group therapy*. Thorofare, NJ, Slack.

Klyczek, J. & Mann, W. (1986). Therapeutic modality comparisons in day treatment. *American Journal of Occupational Therapy*, 40, 606–611.

Laing, C. (2007). Group therapy to improve communicative participation in people living with multiple sclerosis and dysarthria. Online. Available http://www.mstrust.org.uk/publications/wayahead/1102(2007)._05.jsp 1 April, 2007.

Lizzio, A. & Wilson, K. (2001a). Facilitating group beginnings I: A practice model. *Group Work*, 13(1), 6–30.

Lizzio, A. & Wilson, K. (2001b). Facilitating group beginnings II: From basic to working engagement. *Group Work*, 13(1), 30–56.

Molineux, M. (2004). Occupation in occupational therapy: a labour in vain? In: M. Molineux (Ed.). *Occupation for occupational therapists* (pp. 1–14). Oxford, Blackwell Publishing.

Molineux, M. & Whiteford, G. (1999). Prisons: From occupational deprivation to occupational enrichment. *Journal of Occupational Science*, 6(3), 124–130.

Okumiya, K., Morita, Y., Nishinaga, M. et al (2005). Effects of group work programs on community-dwelling elderly people with age-associated cognitive decline and/or mild depressive moods: A Kahoku Longitudinal Ageing Study. *Geriatrics and Gerontology International*, 5(4), 267–275.

Polimeni-Walker, I., Wilson, K. & Jewens, R. (1992). Reasons for participating in occupational therapy groups: perceptions of adult psychiatric in-patients and occupational therapists. *Canadian Journal of Occupational Therapy*, 59, 240–247.

Tajfel, H. & Turner, J. C. (1979). An integrative theory of intergroup conflict. In: S. Worchel, W. G. Austin (Eds.). *The social psychology of intergroup relations*. (pp. 33–47). Monterey, CA, Brooks-Cole.

Trace, S. & Howell, T. (1991). Occupational therapy in geriatric mental health. *The American Journal of Occupational Therapy*. 45(9), 833–838.

Tuckman, B. W. (1965). Developmental sequences in small groups. *Psychological Bulletin*, 63, 384–389.

Tyler, T. R. & Blader, S. (2000). *Cooperation in groups: Procedural justice, social identity, and behavioral engagement*. Philadelphia, Psychology Press.

Wilcock, A. (1998). *An occupational perspective of health*. Thorofare, NJ, Slack.

Yalom, I. D. (1975). *The theory and practice of group psychotherapy*, (2nd ed). New York, Basic Books.

Yalom, I. D. (1985). *The theory and practice of group psychotherapy*, (3rd ed). New York, Basic Books.

Section **Four**

Working with and within communities

19

Community development

Nick Pollard, Dikaios Sakellariou, and Frank Kronenberg

CHAPTER CONTENTS

Introduction 268

What is community? 268

Why community development approaches
are necessary 271

Social opportunities and social capital . . . 272

   Is the community to be developed or is
   the community the vehicle for
   development? 273

Solutions. 274

   Arts and cultural action 274

   Environmental action 274

   Education and learning 275

   Social activism and disability 275

Conclusion. 276

SUMMARY

Community development refers to a collaborative
process of building social, economic, and human
capital. The combined effects of the demise of
social capital and the subsequent decline of
social opportunities, lack of education, and
poverty have led to deep community-based
restrictions in the occupational choices open to
people. Education or art-based community
interventions have the potential to construct a
sense of social cohesiveness and, through that, a
safe place that facilitates access to occupation.
In order for community development to respond
to local needs and be culturally appropriate, and,
thus, sustainable, local communities need to
have a central role in this process, actively
engaged in agenda setting and implementation.
In this process, occupational therapists can act
as catalysts encouraging participation.

KEY POINTS

- Community development refers to a process of
  capacity building, involving the people of a
  community in developing their own strategies to
  respond to the combined impact of social,
  economic, environmental, and political factors.
- Communities can be a source of inclusion and of
  exclusion – there are members and outsiders.
- Occupational therapists can be a catalysts to
  encourage groups to co-operate because of the
  working rapport they develop with people.
- Occupational therapists are being challenged
  to consider their role in addressing the
  occupational needs of people in their
  communities – to enable communities to create
  new ways to promote social cohesion, identify
  common goals and work together to achieve
  these.
- Occupational therapists in community
  development roles may find it difficult to
  negotiate the partnerships needed to establish
  positive outcomes across these differences –
  they need to avoid being drawn into disputes
  between groups which will compromise their
  ability to develop positive relationships with key
  stakeholders and produce results.
- The forms of community development depend
  on what can be locally negotiated – projects
  have to be within local capacities both in terms
  of the current availability of materials and
  infrastructure, and the resources needed to
  sustain them.

- Incremental development of the project ensures that the investment of resources in training facilities will not be wasted.
- Community development solutions cannot be developed by one person or one agency alone and require co-operation across the community.

Introduction

Community development refers to a process of capacity building which involves the people of a community in developing their own strategies to respond to the combined impact of social, economic, environmental and political factors. According to the Community Development Exchange (2007) such strategies are based on social justice and mutual respect, and aim to remove barriers to participation and sustainability. Despite these intentions, community-development initiatives are often the tools or products of government policy rather than local societies (Smith 2006a, 2006b). In the United Kingdom (UK) several government departments are working in concert on the changing health and social needs through rolling out a programme of workforce development and community change. Specific health aspects of these combined policies have been identified through *Choosing Health* (Department of Health 2004), the *National Service Frameworks* (e.g. Philp 2006) and *New Ways of Working* (Department of Health 2005), as well as the College of Occupational Therapists' (2006) paper on mental health needs, *Recovering Ordinary Lives*.

Such documents are generally reactions to demands from people with disabilities and their carers, but they are not generated by communities (Shakespeare & Watson 2002). As a consequence, the health and social care needs of clients, their carers and families are defined in terms that suit a policy agenda, but not in ways that describe their own experiences. Even when organisations like the College of Occupational Therapists or large charitable organisations issue documents on health and social needs, these reflect the position of the organisations and their need to maintain a political dialogue with government and other actors (Papadakis 2005). Thus, national policies may be reflected in local arrangements but these may still not meet specific community needs, for example, where communities within a particular administrative area are far apart or very different in their needs. Individual needs are forced to fit into these arrangements as well as they can, but once rules have been established it becomes difficult to make exceptions. Paraphrasing Hasselkus (2006, pp. 629–631) it is very easy to devalue the ordinary nature of everyday occupational experience. Sometimes local differences are recognised, but in other situations inflexibility can produce serious marginalisations (Kronenberg 2005, Smith 2005). One clear example of this is the position of asylum seekers and denied asylum seekers who are often unable to obtain basic needs (Davies 2008, Smith 2005). Accounts of community development do not always reflect these subtleties (Sakellariou et al 2006); perhaps for fear that negative accounts may damage ongoing relationships with funders and sponsors. One notorious example has been the response to a draft charities bill in Australia, proposing that charitable tax status be revoked if an organisation engages in debates about public policy (Maddison et al 2004, The Parliament of the Commonwealth of Australia 2003).

For a long time occupational therapists have been arguing for social changes to support occupational choice and meet the needs of communities (Hasselkus 2006, Townsend 1997). In several countries, particularly Brazil (Barros 2005, Galhiego et al 2005), South Africa (Lorenzo et al 2006, Watson et al 2004), Australia (Whiteford & Wright St Clair 2005) and Canada (Thibeault 2002), it has been suggested that there are long traditions of social activist engagement. In the UK community initiatives have recently been identified as an important direction in the development and survival of the profession (College of Occupational Therapists 2006). Through documents such as the World Federation of Occupational Therapists Position Papers on community-based rehabilitation and human rights (WFOT 2004, 2006), occupational therapists are being asked to reconsider their roles to address the occupational needs of people in their communities (Pollard et al 2005).

What is community?

The word 'community' has many benign connotations which suggest groups of people who live and work harmoniously (Williams 1976). It is a complex word which combines the sense of a group of people with common interests alongside that of a group of people with some historical association. Communities of interest can overlap with other communities formed around other interests or are composed of people who share a common history. It is possible to be a member of several communities simultaneously. However, an effect of modern urban development is that people often live in one community and commute to work in another (Putnam 2000). As a result people may come to know their work colleagues quite well since they share a history and common experience with this community, but never talk to the neighbours at home.

Many of the communities in the UK are diverse, representing not only migrant groups from other countries but from within the UK itself. As the word 'community' refers to many kinds of social groupings, it can mask the fact that people who live in the same geographical area may live in multiple, separate communities (Innes & Jones 2006, Somerville & Chan 2004, Williams 1976). Migrant communities may have more connection with people overseas than with their immediate neighbours, their community may not be defined simply by where they live (Putnam 2000). Perhaps it is because of these factors that communities are also the sources and the products of many forms of difference which impact on physical and mental health, such as noise, air pollution, levels of employment, crime and variances in overall wealth (Cagney et al 2005, Innes & Jones 2006, Lawrence 2004, Pintus et al 2006, Rimmington 2005, Shaw et al 2005).

Communities, because they are sources of inclusion, are also sources and places of exclusion: there are members and outsiders (Holmes 1991, Kirsh et al 2006, Sibley 1995). Social environments are rarely designed to accommodate the needs of disabled people who live in them.

Often the difference between care in institutions and care in community settings has been thought of as being simply about location and the idea that community settings are preferable (Sakellariou & Pollard 2006). In the context of health and social care the term 'community' has been associated with moves away from institutional care, particularly in mental health. However, it also applies to the wide range of interventions that are practised by occupational therapists, support workers and care assistants with the clients, in their own homes, who experience other forms of dysfunction.

Occupational therapists and other health professionals have not always appreciated the deeper complexities of working in community settings, and, in particular, whether they work **in** the community, **for** the community or **with** the community. The focus of community development is neither the locale of the project nor a philanthropic notion of 'doing good' for people who experience disabling situations. It is about 'doing good' **with** people. The difference might seem unimportant, but it is fundamental; community development is about assuming a role of facilitator, learning about the context and needs of a community and working with it towards relevant solutions (Community Development Exchange 2007, Smith 2006a).

Community policies have sometimes neglected to consider negotiation or involvement with the people they are intended to help in identifying adequate solutions (Kapasi 2006). Such approaches require a social activist role that was always at the base of occupational therapy intervention (Townsend 1997) and is highlighted in the recent discussion of occupational therapy's professional repositioning (Hasselkus 2006, Kronenberg & Pollard 2005a, 2005b, Pollard et al 2008). These interventions require synergistic approaches where community members are enabled to participate in all stages of programme planning and application in culturally appropriate ways as opposed to them being recipients of care. Practice Scenario 19.1 demonstrates how community interventions should be dictated by community needs.

Practice Scenario 19.1 Plenty Valley Therapeutic Community – a sustainable vision for community health care

Plenty Valley Community Health (PVCH) upholds a social model of health with a focus on increasing person-centred home- and community-based care. PVCH is located on the fringe of Melbourne, covering both urban and rural populations. It is a richly multicultural municipality, with 39% of residents born outside Australia. It is the fifth most disadvantaged local government area in the state of Victoria.

Greenwood

For the last 14 years PVCH has been running a Planned Activity Group (PAG) for adult men with an acquired brain injury (ABI). This 'Greenwood' programme is focused on nature and culture-based activities including horticultural therapy and creative art activities, such as mosaics, photography, art, and pottery. This programme is located in the main shopping strip in the rural town of Whittlesea. Evaluation has shown this activity-based group has provided opportunities for participants to develop new skills, social connection (both within the group and in community), a sense of belonging, the capacity to express their abilities and to share, and improve social skills.

Therapeutic community

In 2005, a potential new site at a farm location became available to PVCH and 'Greenwood'. This property offered an opportunity to explore how the programme developed at Greenwood could bring benefit to a broader range of people who received PVCH services. The need to respond to funding body criteria determined the direction of programme development, including initial groups. These included people with acquired brain injury (ABI), chronic illness, mental illness, and problems related to the ageing process, all of whom face the common challenges of occupational alienation, social isolation, and a lack of meaningful purpose in life.

Early in 2006 a proposal was put forward to PVCH Board of Management to form two consultative groups to develop ideas for the farm; a funding (management) group and a programme development (staff) group. One outcome of the multidisciplinary staff group (facilitated by occupational therapists) was a literature review, based on staff ideas, to develop an evidence-base for the therapeutic community concept. This document has proven a valuable tool to help to communicate and validate staff and participants' ideas both within PVCH, and to external parties, including government departments, funding bodies, and academic institutions.

By early 2007 the model of a Therapeutic Community was envisaged to include:

- the therapeutic activities of horticultural therapy, creative arts and community kitchens/ kitchen-gardens
- a safe and friendly environment that is inclusive of the broader community as a whole
- existing technologies of physiotherapy, occupational therapy, dietetics, nursing, disability, counseling, and health promotion applied through an activity platform in an integrated manner
- therapy that is person-focused, and provides meaningful integration back into the community through social and occupational engagement
- education and integration of the broader community and disabled people, people with chronic illness and older people, by providing a centre fostering community engagement

- a community consultation model of planning and development, considering the overall health service needs of the community in line with a vision of nature/culture-based activities.

It is anticipated that the centre will develop valuable links with community groups, organisations and industry. These links would encourage people to develop lasting social connections and interests so as to continue the work achieved while attending the centre. For example:

- developing projects with local schools using the kitchen-garden model could provide a platform for shared education and health promotion around healthy eating, including its relationship to dental care
- connection with local Parks Victoria, Landcare and local council could provide opportunity to grow plants for community re-vegetation programmes
- links with industry could provide opportunity for revenue for the programme, as well as valuable vocational options for PVCH participants
- local university students could have opportunity for projects engaging with the PVCH participants
- community artists could facilitate projects around social cohesion.

The value of this therapeutic community is its focus on community participation for healthy behaviours and the connections between people of all ages and abilities through nature and culture-based activities.

Organisational impact

In the process of developing the Therapeutic Community there have been several unintentional but fruitful lessons learnt. Meeting on a regular basis has resulted in:

- growth from a narrow discipline/diagnosis-specific focus to working collaboratively towards a greater whole
- an appreciation of common understandings
- increased capacity to work through potential challenges.

In particular, the process has resulted in an understanding of how discipline-specific practices can be applied through an occupational therapy occupation-based framework. Allowing the community of staff to come to these realisations and consequent decision, has strengthened and consolidated the vision for the site.

Finally, thinking about the practical implications of working in a Therapeutic Community has also facilitated the movement of PVCH health professionals towards person-driven practices, and allowed participants' input into the early development of ideas. Learning to work together across disciplines within the staff group has also given much insight into the nature of barriers and benefits of consultation, collaboration and developing community. It is recognised that consultation with participant groups will expand as the model develops, and the trust and rapport between PVCH and the community increases. In the meantime we recognise the important activist role staff can have in advocating for people. Empowerment of the staff, through the consultation process, in turn brings opportunity for participant empowerment.

Incremental development

The therapeutic community concept is being put into practice incrementally, in the context of organisational, funding and work demands at PVCH. A number of areas within PVCH have begun developing programmes that will have direct links with the site once it is completed. These include the introduction of the Clubhouse model to Greenwood; community kitchen projects at a number of sites; and consultation with local schools around the development of a school kitchen-garden programme. These developments are the result of growth in staff confidence and understanding of the concepts involved. Consequently, they have come to see how therapeutic community concepts could be applied to activities more widely in community health.

Plenty Valley Community Health, Victoria, Australia
Practice scenario provided by: Margaret Hogg, Tess Wilkinson, Susan Craddock (Occupational Therapists), Emma Hughes (Research Coordinator)

Why community development approaches are necessary

Sheffield, in South Yorkshire (UK), is a city with a wide variation in health due to a complex combination of economic, social and environmental conditions. Some areas of Sheffield, for example the suburbs of Dore under the foothills of the Peak District, have enjoyed considerable wealth. Others, only a few miles away, have experienced chronic impoverishment and heavy pollution from traffic and industry. There are substantial migrant communities, some well established over several generations. Average life expectancy in Sheffield is 88.8 (86.6 for men, 90.2 for women) in the Ecclesall neighbourhood and 70.9 (70.8 for men, 71.1 for

women) in Crookesmoor, a combined average difference of 17.9 years across the city (Sheffield PCT 2007). In two neighbourhoods it is less than might be expected in some far poorer countries than the UK, for example Algeria (72) Sri Lanka and Tunisia (both 74, all 2005 figures) (Unicef 2007), while several others have figures a few decimal points above 74. The average for England is 76.9 for men and 81.1 for women (epractice.eu 2007).

Some parts of Sheffield have experienced chronic and intergenerational unemployment that dates back to the decline of heavy industries in the 1980s and 1990s. Over time this unemployment has evolved into incapacity for work due to ill health (Ritchie et al 2005). Many people do not have easy access to fresh fruit and vegetables, and experience a less diverse and poorer diet than those in wealthier parts. Evidence suggests that people with lower incomes also have poorer education, smoke more cigarettes, drink more alcohol, exercise less, experience and fear crime more than their wealthier neighbours (Innes & Jones 2006, Pintus et al 2006, Rimmington 2006, Shaw et al 2005).

In addition to poor food, pollution and lack of exercise, a significant contributor to poor health for many people is reduced social opportunity; the means to facilitate occupational choices (Rebeiro 2000). The biggest underlying problem is lack of sustainable income. People who are living on basic wages or social security benefits often find themselves living in poor housing which is not properly insulated or heated. As energy costs are high people sometimes have to choose between buying adequate food and heating their homes (Lawrence 2004). They may keep one room in the house warm and let the rest stay cold, encouraging mildew and mould to form in the consequent condensation. An individual is less likely to leave a warm room to engage in other occupations. People are occupationally deprived when they are unable to make choices in what they do because of social disadvantages, inequalities or environmental constraints.

Areas of the UK which experience poverty generally have higher levels of crime, often related to factors of poor social cohesion which are made worse through social isolation (Green et al 2002, Howe & Crilly 2001, Innes & Jones 2006). The pattern of life in the UK has not only become more divergent in terms of wealth (Innes & Jones 2006, Shaw et al 2005). Communities have developed parallel lives with a separation that extends across many forms of social activity. Most people, including occupational therapists, have little experience of the diversity of the UK population at first hand (Smith 2005). Instead, people live and socialise in cultural- and age-related enclaves (Innes & Jones 2006). There are fewer play areas to provide social opportunities for young people (Kapasi 2006) whereas older people are more reluctant to go out for fear they may be mugged or that their homes will be burgled in their absence (Green et al 2002).

A third key problem associated with poverty and occupational deprivation is the lack of education. Poor literacy and numeracy contribute to intergenerational poverty. People who are unable to access information cannot effectively develop their skills, or use community resources and even health facilities. Even where leaflets are translated into community languages the intended audience is still often unable to read them (McPake & Johnston 2002). While those able to articulate their needs are more likely to obtain the services they want, others will go unheard unless they can find an advocate who is properly able to represent them, or they acquire the skills to do this themselves (Kapasi 2006). The job of the occupational therapist is to enable 'the societies in which we find ourselves to create new ways to promote social cohesion, identify common goals and working together to achieve these' (Kronenberg & Pollard 2006, p. 625).

Social opportunities and social capital

Lack of education and lack of opportunity produce a systemic situation of occupational apartheid and social alienation (Innes & Jones 2006, Kronenberg & Pollard 2005a, 2005b, Pintus et al 2006, Shaw et al 2005). Occupational apartheid occurs when groups of people are actively denied occupational choice through policies that exclude them. Social divisions have been actively reflected in local council policies for education provision or the development of facilities for particular communities within them, such as travellers' sites (Parry et al 2004). Some communities can develop a defensive insularity in which any individual's ambition is thwarted by the reduced expectations of others. For example, people who seek better education may be discouraged by their parents or friends (Sennet & Cobb 1972). They are advised that they will continue to be discriminated against despite the education they obtain, because

they cannot disguise their origins, and on the other hand they will be unable to fit in again if they return to their home community. When this happens, say Innes and Jones (2006), there are three options available: exit, loyalty to a community – which results in the exclusion of others – and effectively vocalising discontent in ways that will be acted upon by local authorities, perhaps through protest or riot.

These interlinked problems are produced by social division and exacerbate it. They increase anxiety and stress, and make it more difficult for people who experience disabling circumstances to manage their own lives effectively. Disabled people are often victimised because they are seen to be vulnerable, and incapable of offering resistance. For example, Sheffield has seen incidents where bins have been set on fire against the doors of disabled people's houses, resulting in serious injuries and death (Sheffield First 2006).

Most communities will already have some social networks. These may be informal groups of people who meet, for example, to sustain occupational roles through a fishing club, an allotment group or a neighbourhood watch scheme. They may be groups who organise activities around community needs they have identified, independently of local authority initiatives. These activities create 'social capital'. Social capital is based on the ability to use social connections and relationships to achieve individual or group goals (Putnam 2000). Individuals increase their social capital by interacting with others. People who are actively engaged in social networks are more likely to obtain help from others to do things such as maintain their home, garden or in childcare, remain in work, and stay healthy (College of Occupational Therapists 2006, Putnam 2000). However, not everyone can access social capital (Portes 1998), and those who are excluded become *more* excluded and experience less access to these opportunities.

Conditions management teams have been set up through the co-operation of the Department of Work and Pensions and National Health the Service to encourage people who are receiving incapacity benefits to improve their health by retraining for work (Bennie 2006, Department of Work and Pensions 2002). This *Pathways to Work* policy is aimed at reducing benefit dependency by identifying recipients who may be able to return to work, many of whom do not consider themselves to be impaired. The teams prioritise those with mental health, cardiovascular, and musculo-skeletal problems, working from both a professional perspective (which includes advice about healthy lifestyles), and by negotiating with employers.

Is the community to be developed or is the community the vehicle for development?

Whiteford (2005) discusses the development of Third Way politics, a form of political engagement with communities which turns away from top-down strategies. Instead the emphasis is on working with local organisations or 'actors' which arise from communities and are based around local need; an approach which is echoed in a recent government policy (Kearns 2004).

Putting this into effect is complicated both because of the diversity and separateness of many UK communities and because of the links some of them may have with others outside the UK. Many different kinds of agencies may be working in a community, from the statutory health and social care bodies such as primary care trusts and community health centres, care agencies under contract to social services, local and national charities and interest groups, local authority, private, and charitable housing groups. Some, but not all of these, may be run by groups of disabled people. Several voluntary associations are often managed by carers rather than service users who themselves could be actively involved.

The interests of each group may themselves be very diverse and even be a source of conflict. Historical differences may arise from local conditions and experiences or kind of care approaches being offered. Some agencies may pay their workers and others may be volunteer-based – the training and support to each can differ. Workers representing these bodies can be very helpful and positive, but they can also be obstructive, officious, and self-serving. They may be serving private interests, for example of those of a housing agency, rather than community interests (Somerville & Chan 2004). If occupational therapists are themselves employed in a community development role then it is worth reflecting carefully about the objectives of the organisation for which they work and how they fit with those across the spectrum of other actors in the community (Kronenberg & Pollard 2005b).

Occupational therapists in community development roles may find it difficult to negotiate the partnerships needed to establish positive outcomes across these differences, which Kronenberg and Pollard (2005b) have identified as conflict and co-operation situations. Occupational therapists often move around from one job to another, and so may not know the local community cultures. It may be difficult to appreciate what is going on in the interplay of committees, groups, and the political manoeuvres of individual members, or know whether it is appropriate to engage with these issues. On the other hand, being an outsider can enable therapists to present themselves as the kind of catalytic resource which facilitates people in helping themselves. This may come about through exploring and learning about the differences between the respective cultures of therapists and the communities with whom they are working (Dickie 2004).

These issues can be overwhelming and very time-consuming. Occupational therapists have to avoid being drawn into disputes between groups which will compromise their ability to develop positive relationships with key stakeholders and produce results. As professionals they have to prioritise how they will use their energies in determining appropriate solutions and also identify issues with which they cannot engage.

The forms of community development depend on what can be locally negotiated. The outcomes are often not those associated traditionally with occupational therapy in a health and social-care context. It is not a panacea for all problems but depends very much on local people and cultures, and how developments are perceived. As the Plenty Valley example shows (Practice Scenario 19.1), projects have to be within local capacities both in terms of the current availability of materials and infrastructure and the resources needed to sustain them. The project in which the occupational therapist is engaged will have to work alongside other priorities.

Solutions may have to be prioritised in terms of achievability, rather than what appears to be the most immediate need. For example, whereas people may really require security of income level, developing confidence in decision-making or learning new skills will ensure that increased incomes are sustainable over a longer term. The first strategies to be negotiated with the group may be exercises which enable people to realise their capacity for learning.

This incremental development of the project ensures that the investment of resources in training facilities will not be wasted. The confidence-raising exercise requires a lower economic commitment than those which follow. It underpins the subsequent work, engages community members in the conscious change needed to own the conceptual possibility of a facility in which they will be learning new skills, and makes it possible to enlist community members themselves to contribute resources to the larger project.

Community development solutions cannot be developed by one person or one agency alone and require co-operation across the community (Boyce & Lysack 2000, Fransen 2005). Occupational therapists can be a catalyst to encourage groups to co-operate because of the working rapport they develop with disabled people – especially since the inclusion of marginalized groups is a focus of many socially oriented policies.

Occupational therapists working in community development must also respond to the programmes which are being implemented with other groups. They need to avoid duplication and work out how different approaches can complement each other. Below are some examples of the kinds of community development actions that can be initiated to answer these needs. As yet the numbers of occupational therapists engaged in such projects are small, but practitioners need to be aware of typical activities if they are to engage with people in developing social action.

Solutions

Arts and cultural action

Arts-based and cultural activities have frequently been used to explore the experience of impairment (see Breines 2005), and the Plenty Valley example (Practice Scenario 19.1) gives a number of reasons for incorporating arts into their project. Occupational therapists have previously built links with community resources in adult education or local council arts bodies (Petridou et al 2005, Pollard 2002, 2003, 2008, Pollard & Smart 2005, Pollard & Steele 2002, Ryan & Pollard 2002, Schmid 2005). Adult educators, arts officers and people working in community facilities have not always been able to successfully reach marginalised groups, such as people with disabilities.

Activities can take the form of oral history, writers' workshops, painting or making traditional articles which express local traditions and experiences to affirm local cultures and the narrative of the community (Frank et al 2008, Pollard et al 2005b, Pollard, Schmid 2005). Story-telling, making songs and writing often do not require many material resources. Workshops can be a focus of exchange of ideas, and projects can be developed from the discussion that arises as a result of the narratives, for example publications, sound recordings and community performances (Algado & Burgman 2005, Algado & Cardona 2005, Kronenberg 2005, McNulty 2008, Schmid 2005). Some projects have focused on the need to educate other people about the experiences of impairment and caring for disabled people. In one example disabled people and carers developed a community publication in which they described issues such as the impact of disability on previously healthy lives, coping strategies they had found useful in managing and accessing the things they needed, and their hopes for their futures (Labelled Disabled 1991). Others have been purely about involvement in arts activities, for example mental-health users learning about literature, history and doing their own writing (Pollard 2002, Pollard & Steele 2002, Ryan & Pollard 2002) or acting in plays and film (Petridou et al, 2005). Although artistic activities can be a useful medium for exploring issues connected with disabilities, the key value for many of the participants is the opportunity to develop arts-related skills in their own right (Schmid 2005).

Environmental action

Many impoverished communities also experience environmental problems. Environmental action can be a way of positively engaging communities by encouraging them to take possession of neglected areas of land and work together to create community gardens, allotments, or playing fields (Steele 2005) and as described in Practice Scenario 19.1. Although some of these activities have been part of occupational therapy programmes from very early in the development of the profession, they have also become the focus of an emergent therapy, social and therapeutic horticulture (Fieldhouse & Sempik 2007). These actions can take the form of improving wasteland which has been scheduled for redevelopment, or claiming neglected allotment space. Often councils have allotments which have fallen into disuse and the potential green spaces these create can be lost to building programmes. Environmental action can often win the support of sponsor organisations, and are particularly useful forms of producing intergenerational and cross-cultural contact (Davies 2008, Sempik et al 2005). Gardens created in these spaces become a space which is owned by the people who have worked on them (Steele 2005) and in which, by focusing on the tasks associated with nurturing living things, can enable people to put aside their difficulties, at least for the time in which they are engaged (Davies 2008). Such facilities are also concrete evidence of the positive capacities of marginalised people. At the University of Vic in Catalonia, service users experiencing 'problems of social integration' have worked with students and university staff to develop a garden which serves as a resource for the whole community to use (Simo Algado et al 2007).

Education and learning

Disabled people can find it challenging to locate and access suitable educational opportunities, particularly in areas that have experienced poverty and deprivation. While the lack of literacy and numeracy skills can be found at all age groups in the community, the experience of education can often be a negative one, compounded by the fear of being made to look foolish (Smart 2005).

Occupational therapists can liaise with people working in adult education to develop ways of promoting learning, particularly through non-threatening educational opportunities focused around the needs of disabled people. Pecket Well College in Yorkshire is a co-operative college founded by adult learners with former adult education workers in response to funding cutbacks (Smart 2005). Students at the college attended classes in which disabled people were integrated with other people who wanted a second chance to learn. Students were encouraged to facilitate each others' education through the identification of their needs. For example, a person with vocabulary difficulties became a class 'word watcher' to monitor the teaching and demand explanation of difficult terms so that others could understand them.

A workers' education course for people at a Doncaster Sue Ryder home taught '2,000 years of Yorkshire History' by breaking down learning objectives into twenty-minute activities that could be achieved by people who had experienced head injury and had memory deficits. This used short practical activities, such as making plaster and applying it to a surface one week, and applying paint the following week, to learn about Roman wall decoration. Each activity produced a concrete artefact which could be used as a prompt and memory aid to facilitate the next week's activity.

As has already been identified under environmental action, education courses do not have to be about traditional subjects. They can be developed around issues of local interest such as local or regional history or reminiscence, hobby activities, learning about anything that a client group might want to find out about. They can be important ways of injecting skills into a community to meet local needs. An occupational therapist could enable a client group to negotiate directly with local Workers' Education Association tutors to identify how appropriate courses might be developed. An important outcome of such development is that those who receive education can be enabled to see themselves as having important skills to hand on, and another way in which education can be negotiated is for the community to identify its knowledge assets which can be traded against other learning (Algado & Cardona 2005).

Social activism and disability

Connecting people with opportunities within the communities in which they live can lead to various forms of social activism. Occupational therapists have complained that the genericism of health and social care often detracted from the occupation and person-centred work which had initially drawn them to the profession (Wilding & Whiteford 2006). Some of the recent 'rediscovery' of occupational therapy's relationship to social activism perhaps arose in response to a growing perception amongst professionals of the need to identify arenas for their skills in a changing marketplace (College of Occupational Therapists 2006, Frost 2006, Garner 2006, Healy 2006, Reel 2006). Social activism and community development opportunities often arise because people find themselves in adverse situations. Many disabled people occupy marginal situations in society, but these positions are also vantage points which can be used to question social values. Marx (1977) argued that the systematic rigidity of a society based on property rather than communal values fixes people in situations of disadvantage. Social action can be about reclaiming the power to pursue occupational choices through communal action.

Disability can be seen as a social phenomenon with a community-based solution. It is not so much the medical or physical condition which determines the experience of disability but the way the needs of disabled people are facilitated in the community (Murphy 1990, Sontag 1991). Even if someone receives treatment in hospital the success of their re-entry into the community depends very much on their circumstances and the level of support for their needs that they are able to obtain. To a large extent this can depend on the community concept of 'normality' and its construction of disability (Murphy 1990, Sontag 1991). If constructions of normality or disability are used to exclude people then this creates a problem for the whole community. Where do the criteria for 'normality' or 'disability' fall? The Plenty Valley example (Practice Scenario 19.1) sets out a number of opportunities to make and sustain community links around local resources.

The products of horticultural and arts-based interventions sometimes have the potential for development as co-operative or other forms of social enterprise or charitable trust (Schmid 2005). Each of these has its own advantages, and for some small groups it may be more feasible to operate as a co-operative rather than attempt to obtain charitable status. Co-operatives operate at all levels of business, but can be small enterprises established to provide community resources which are not otherwise available. By forming a co-operative it is possible to buy goods at trade prices and distribute them locally – for example, to grow and supply fresh fruit and vegetables or farm produce, sell art or craft products, or to provide a building and repair service. A co-operative may also be the basis for a local publication to celebrate community events or be a means of consciousness raising and confidence building. As they develop, small co-operatives can sometimes become social enterprises providing jobs, income and vocational training opportunities. Although the Plenty Valley example (Practice Scenario 19.1) does not describe the establishing of co-operatives it describes many projects which could easily be developed as enterprises. *Daily Bread*, based in Northampton, was set up in 1980. It is based on Christian principles, and employs people with a range of impairments in the supply of organic and wholefoods (Betts et al 2005).

Co-operatives and other forms of social enterprise have been a popular solution to local impoverishment and marginalisation in parts of Europe. They can be the means by which people can demonstrate their self sufficiency and communities their sustainability through occupation (Davister et al 2004, Grove 1999). The cause and effects of marginalisation are interlinked. Many impoverished communities lack not just income but a range of occupational resources (Hasselkus 2006, Wilcock 1998). People who because of their impairments may be regarded as commanding more to meet their needs may be expected by other community members to demand less. For example, if a person has to work in two part-time jobs they may not have the time to also give extra care to a disabled relative. Disability can be seen as a burden on the resources of other non-disabled family members. Furthermore, a family who has disabled members can be seen as burdensome by others in the community, perhaps because they require more spacious housing or can obtain help for their needs. Their access to assistance can seem unjust to their neighbours.

When people have fewer resources, one of the assets they can possess and have to defend is their difference, which may often lead to intolerance and social restrictions (Holmes 1991, Sennett & Cobb 1972, Sibley 1995). In climates of antagonism and resentment people have tried to avoid hostility by avoiding overt cultural displays which may draw attention (Holmes 1991). This can make it difficult to identify needs or establish a working rapport. The visits of occupational therapists and other professionals to a family home can make their needs conspicuous to other community members. Although professionals may take measures such as using unmarked vehicles and not wearing uniforms, other people can quickly identify that their neighbours are receiving support by other cues, such as the type of car or clothing worn by visitors, or the arrival of several people at a house at the same time. On the other hand, the development of a resource by disabled people can become a positive asset that is valued by other people in the community and establishes the basis for other forms of social capital.

Conclusion

Community development offers many challenges and opportunities for occupational therapists to negotiate their roles according to the needs of local populations. To be effective and to avoid being drawn into the conflicts associated with these issues, occupational therapists need to reflect carefully on their position and the acquisition of political skills (Kronenberg & Pollard 2005b). There are many difficulties and uncertainties, but a principal advantage they offer is that the central occupational objectives of such strategies and their many occupational spin

offs can be the basis for skills, cultural development and social capital which can last from generation to generation. These approaches can make significant improvements to the experience of disability, the quality of life and resilience to adversity.

References

Algado, S. S. & Burgman, I. (2005). Occupational therapy intervention with children survivors of war. In: F. Kronenberg, S. S. Algado & N. Pollard (Eds). *Occupational therapy without borders: learning from the spirit of survivors*. (pp. 253–268). Edinburgh, Elsevier/Churchill Livingstone.

Algado, S. S. & Cardona, C. E. (2005). The return of the corn men: an intervention project with a Mayan community of Guatamelan *retornos*. In: F. Kronenberg, S. S. Algado & N. Pollard (Eds). *Occupational therapy without borders: learning from the spirit of survivors*. (pp. 347–362). Edinburgh, Elsevier/Churchill Livingstone.

Barros, D. D. , Gihardi, M. I. G. & Lopes, R. E. (2005). Social occupational therapy: a socio–historical perspective. In: F. Kronenberg, S. S. Algado & N. Pollard (Eds). *Occupational therapy without borders: learning from the spirit of survivors*. (pp. 145–156). Edinburgh, Elsevier/Churchill Livingstone.

Bennie, N. (2006). Tinker, tailor, soldier, spy. *OT News*, 14(11), 25.

Betts, A., Owen, S., Hewitt, H. et al (2005). *An evaluation of three co-operative employment programmes for people with enduring mental health problems and their impact on the use of mental health services*. Nottingham: Shaw Trust/University of Nottingham. Available at www.shaw-trust.org.uk/file_uploads/Coop_final_report_TG_28_Jul_05.doc. Last accessed 2nd February 2007.

Boyce, W. & Lysack, C. (2000). Community participation: uncovering its meanings in community based rehabilitation. In: M Thomas, M. J. Thomas (Eds). *Selected readings in community

based rehabilitation*. (pp. 39–54). Newcastle Upon Tyne, Action For Disability.

Breines, E. B. (2005). *Occupational therapy: activities for practice and teaching*. London, Whurr.

Cagney, K. A., Browning, C. R. & Wen, M. (2005). Racial disparities in self-rated health at older ages: what difference does the neighbourhood make? *Journal of Gerontology*, 60B(4), 181–190.

College of Occupational Therapists (2006). *Recovering ordinary lives: the strategy for occupational therapy in mental health services 2007–2017, literature review. (Core)*. London, COT. Online. Available: www.cot.org.uk/membersweb/publications/categories/core/pdf/RecovOL-Lit_ft.pdf. Accessed 12th January 2007.

Community Development Exchange (2007). *What is community development?* Online. Available: http://www.cdx.org.uk/about/whatiscd.htm Accessed 2nd November 2007.

Davies, R. (2008). Working with refugees and asylum seekers: challenging occupational apartheid. In: N. Pollard, D. Sakellariou & F. Kronenberg (Eds). *A political practice of occupational therapy* (pp. 183–189). Edinburgh, Elsevier/Churchill Livingstone (in press).

Davister, C., Defourny, J. & Gregoire, O. (2004). *Work integration social enterprises in the European union, an overview of the existing model*. Liege, EMES European Research Network.

Department of Health (2004). *Choosing health: making health choices easier*. London, Department of Health.

Department of Health (2005). *New ways of working for psychiatrists: enhancing effective person-centred services through new ways of working in multidisciplinary and

multi-agency contexts*, London, Department of Health.

Department of Work and Pensions (2002). *Pathways to work: helping people into employment*, Norwich, HMSO.

Dickie, V. A. (2004). Culture is tricky: a commentary on culture emergent occupation. *American Journal of Occupational Therapy*, 58, 169–173.

epractice.eu (2007). *UK: improving life expectancy through the web*. Online. Available: http:// www.epractice.eu/document/3784. Accessed 12th November 2007.

Fieldhouse, J. & Sempik, J. (2007). 'Gardening without borders': reflections on the results of a survey of practitioners of an 'unstructured' profession. *British Journal of Occupational Therapy*, 70(10), 449–453.

Frank, G. & Kitching, H. J. (2008). Postcolonial practice in occupational therapy: the Tule River tribal history project. In: N. Pollard, D. Sakellariou & F. Kronenberg (Eds). *A political practice of occupational therapy* (pp. 223–235). Edinburgh, Elsevier/Churchill Livingstone (in press).

Fransen, H. (2005). Challenges for occupational therapy in community-based rehabilitation: Occupation in a community approach to handicap in development. In: F. Kronenberg, S. S. Algado & N. Pollard (Eds). *Occupational therapy without borders: learning from the spirit of survivors*. (pp. 166–182). Edinburgh, Elsevier/Churchill Livingstone.

Frost, P. (2006). New directions, challenges and choices. *OT News*, 14(12), 30.

Galhiego, S. (2005). Occupational therapy and the social field: clarifying concepts and ideas. In: F. Kronenberg, S. S. Algado & N. Pollard (Eds). *Occupational therapy without borders: learning from the spirit of survivors.* (pp. 89–100). Edinburgh, Elsevier/Churchill Livingstone.

Garner, T. (2006). Changing world, changing workplace, changing needs. *OT News*, 14(12), 31.

Green, G., Gilbertson, J. M. & Grimsley, M. F. J. (2002). Fear of crime and health in residential tower blocks, a case study in Liverpool, UK. *European Journal of Public Health*, 12, 10–15.

Grove, B. (1999). Mental health and employment: shaping a new agenda. *Journal of Mental Health*, 8(2), 131–140.

Hasselkus, B. R. (2006). The world of everyday occupation: real people, real lives. *American Journal of Occupational Therapy*, 60(6), 627–640.

Healy, J. (2006). Preparing OT students for new horizons. *OT News*, 14(11), 27.

Holmes, C. (1991). *A tolerant country? Immigrants, refugees and minorities in Britain.* London, Faber.

Howe, A. & Crilly, M. (2001). Deprivation and violence in the community: a perspective from a UK. *Accident and Emergency Department Injury*, 32(5), 349–351.

Innes, M. & Jones, V. (2006). *Neighbourhood security and urban change, risk, resilience and recovery.* York, Joseph Rowntree Foundation.

Kapasi, H. (2006). *Neighbourhood play and community action.* York, Joseph Rowntree Foundation.

Kearns, A. (2004). *Social capital, urban regeneration and urban policy*, CRN paper 15. www.bristol. ac.uk/sps/cnrspaperspdf/cnr15pap. pdf. Last accessed 24 December 2006.

Kirsch, B., Trentham, B. & Cole, S. (2006). Diversity in occupational therapy: Experiences of consumers who identify themselves as minority group members. *Australian Occupational Therapy Journal*, 53, 302–313.

Kronenberg, F. (2005). Occupational therapy with street children. In: F. Kronenberg, S. S. Algado & N. Pollard (Eds). *Occupational therapy without borders: learning from the*

spirit of survivors. (pp. 269–284). Edinburgh, Elsevier/Churchill Livingstone.

Kronenberg, F. & Pollard, N. (2005a). Introduction: a beginning. In: F. Kronenberg, S. S. Algado & N. Pollard (Eds). *Occupational therapy without borders: learning from the spirit of survivors.* (pp. 1–13). Edinburgh, Elsevier/Churchill Livingstone.

Kronenberg, F. & Pollard, N. (2005b). Overcoming occupational apartheid: a preliminary exploration of the political nature of occupational therapy. In: F. Kronenberg, S. S. Algado & N. Pollard (Eds). *Occupational therapy without borders: learning from the spirit of survivors.* (pp. 58–86). Edinburgh, Elsevier/Churchill Livingstone.

Kronenberg, F. & Pollard, N. (2006). Political dimensions of occupation and the roles of occupational therapy. *American Journal of Occupational Therapy*, 60(6), 617–625.

Labelled Disabled (1991). *People with disabilities talk about their lives.* Sheffield, The Labelled Disabled Collective.

Lawrence, R. J. (2004). Housing and health: from interdisciplinary principles to transdisciplinary research and practice. *Futures*, 36(4), 487–502.

Lorenzo, T., Duncan, M., Buchanan, H. & Alsop, A. (Eds.) (2006). *Practice and service learning in occupational therapy: enhancing potential in context.* Chichester, John Wiley.

McNulty, C. (2008). The Sleaford MACA group. In: N. Pollard, D. Sakellariou & F. Kronenberg (Eds). *A political practice of occupational therapy* (pp. 171–174). Edinburgh, Elsevier/Churchill Livingstone.

McPake, J. & Johnstone, R. (2002). *Translating, interpreting and communication support services across the public sector in Scotland.* Edinburgh, Scottish Executive Central Research Unit.

Maddison, S., Denniss, R. & Hamilton, C. (2004). *Silencing dissent, non-governmental organisations and Australian democracy.* The Australia Institute Discussion paper 65. Online. Available http://www.

tai.org.au/documents/dp_fulltext/ DP65.pdf. Accessed 10th November 2007.

Marx, K. (1977). The German ideology. In: D. McLellan (Ed.). *Karl Marx: selected writings.* (pp. 159–190). Oxford, Oxford University Press.

Murphy, R. (1990). *The body silent.* New York, W.W. Norton.

Papadakis, K. (2005). *Participatory governance and discourses of socially sustainable development: lessons from South Africa and the European Union.* Paper presented at the 8th Congress of the French Association of Political Science, Lyon 14–16 September. Online. Available: http://sites.univ-lyon2.fr/ congres-afsp/IMG/pdf/papadakis. pdf. Accessed 2nd November 2007.

The Parliament of the Commonwealth of Australia (2003). *Charities Bill (2003). Exposure draft.* Online. Available http://www.taxboard.gov. au/content/downloads/charities_ bill.pdf. Accessed 10th November 2007.

Parry, G., Van Cleemput, P., Peters, J. et al (2004). *The health status of gypsies and travellers in England, summary of a report to the Department of Health.* Sheffield, The University of Sheffield School of Health and Related Research.

Petridou, D., Pouliopolou, M., Kiriakoulis, A. et al (2005). Expanding occupational therapy intervention through the theatre and film. *Mental Health OT*, 10(3), 99–101.

Philp, I. (2006). *A new ambition for old age: Next steps in implementing the national service framework for older people.* London, Department of Health.

Pintus, S., Richardson, A. & McManus, C. (2006). *Basket of health inequalities indicators to monitor change and impact on health inequalities in Sheffield, (2005).* Monitoring Report, Sheffield, Sheffield Health Informatics Service.

Pollard, N. (2002). Doncaster–Dumfries, Part 1. *Federation*, 24, 13–15.

Pollard, N. (2003). Making adult learning fun. *OT News*, 11(3), 30.

Pollard, N. & Steele, A. (2002). From Doncaster to Dumfries. *OT News*, 10(11), 31.

Pollard, N. & Smart, P. (2005b). Voices talk and hands write. In: F. Kronenberg, S. S. Algado & N. Pollard (Eds). *Occupational therapy without borders: learning from the spirit of survivors.* (pp. 295–310). Edinburgh, Elsevier/Churchill Livingstone.

Pollard, N., Alsop, A. & Kronenberg, F. (2005). Reconceptualising occupational therapy. *British Journal of Occupational Therapy*, 68(11), 524–526.

Pollard, N., Kronenberg, F. & Sakellariou, D. (2008). A political practice of occupational therapy. In: N. Pollard, D. Sakellariou & F. Kronenberg (Eds). *The political practice of occupational therapy* (pp. 3–19). Edinburgh, Elsevier.

Pollard, N. (2008). Voices talk, hands write. In: E. Crepeau, E. Cohn & B. Boyt Schell (Eds). *Willard and Spackman's occupational therapy* (pp. 139–145) 11th ed. Philadelphia, Lipincott, Williams and Wilkins.

Portes, A. (1998). Social capital: its origins and applications in modern sociology. *Annual Review of Sociology*, 24, 1–24.

Putnam, R.D. (2000). *Bowling alone: The collapse and revival of American community*. New York, Simon and Schuster.

Rebeiro, K. (2000). Client perspectives on occupational therapy practice: Are we truly client centred? *Canadian Journal of Occupational Therapy*, 67(1), 7–14.

Reel, K. (2006). OTs just really seem to fit. *OT News*, 14(11), 26.

Rimmington, B. (2005). *Understanding local neighbourhoods using community researchers*. Sheffield, UK, East End Quality of Life Initiative.

Ritchie, H., Casebourne, J. & Rick, J. (2005). *Understanding workless people and communities: a literature review*. Norwich, Department for Work and Pensions.

Ryan, H. & Pollard, N. (2002). Poetry on the agenda for Scottish weekend. *Adults Learning*, January, 10–11.

Sakellariou, D. & Pollard, N. (2006). Rehabilitation: in the community or with the community. *British Journal of Occupational Therapy*, 69(12), 562–566.

Sakellariou, D., Pollard, N., Fransen, H. et al (2006). Reporting on the WFOT–CBR master project plan: the data collection subproject. *WFOT Bulletin*, 54, 37–45.

Schmid, T. (2005). Group projects: experiences and outcomes of creativity. In: T. Schmid (Ed.). *Promoting health through creativity.* (pp. 167–201). London, Whurr.

Sempik, J., Becker, S. & Alridge, J. (2005). *Growing together: a practical guide to promoting social inclusion through gardening and horticulture*. Bristol, Policy Press.

Sennett, R. & Cobb, J. (1972). *The hidden injuries of class*. Cambridge, Cambridge University Press.

Shakespeare, T. & Watson, N. (2002). The social model of disability: an outdated ideology? *Research in Social Science and Disability*, 2, 9–28.

Shaw, M., Smith, G. D. & Dorling, D. (2005). Health inequalities and new labour: how the promises compare with progress. *British Medical Journal*, 330, 1016–1021.

Sheffield First (2006). *Arson*. http://www.sheffieldfirstforsafety.net/asb_arson.htm. Last accessed 12th January 2007.

Sheffield PCT (2007). *Sheffield health and wellbeing atlas*. Online. Available http://www.sheffield.nhs.uk/healthdata/atlas/NHAreaProfile/atlas.html. Accessed 12th November 2007.

Sibley, D. (1995). *Geographies of exclusion*. London, Routledge.

Simo Algado, S. (2007). *Ciencia de l'Ocupacio*. Online. Available: http://www.uvic.cat/eucs/recerca/ca/ocupacio.html. Accessed 14th November 2007.

Smart, P. (2005). A beginner writer is not a beginner thinker. In: F. Kronenberg, S. S. Algado & N. Pollard (Eds). *Occupational therapy without borders: learning from the spirit of survivors.* (pp. 47–54). Edinburgh, Elsevier/Churchill Livingstone.

Smith, H. C. (2005). 'Feel the fear and do it anyway': meeting the occupational needs of refugees and people seeking asylum. *British Journal of Occupational Therapy*, 68 (10), 474–476.

Smith, M. K. (2006a). 'Community development', the encyclopaedia of informal education, www.infed.org/community/b-comdv.htm. Accessed: 15 December 2006.

Smith, M. K. (2006b). 'Community work', the encyclopaedia of informal education. www.infed.org/community/b-comwrk.htm. Accessed: 15 December 2006.

Somerville, P. & Chan, C. K. (2004). *Human dignity and the 'third way': the case of housing policy*. University of Lincoln, www.cf.ac.uk/cplan/conferences/hsa_sept01/somerville&chan.pdf. Accessed 24 December 2006.

Sontag, S. (1991). *Illness as metaphor and AIDS and its metaphors*. London, Penguin Books.

Steele, J. (2005). Bellbird garden. In: T. Schmid (Ed.). *Promoting health through creativity.* (pp. 180–182). London, Whurr.

Thibeault, R. (2002). In praise of dissidence: Anne Laing–Etienne 1932–1991. *Canadian Journal of Occupational Therapy*, 69, 3–10.

Townsend, E. (1997). Inclusivity: a community dimension of spirituality. *Canadian Journal of Occupational Therapy*, 64(3), 146–155.

Unicef (2007). *Information by country*. Online. Available: www.unicef.org/infobycountry.html. Accessed 5th November 2007.

Watson, R. & Swartz, L. (2004). (Eds). *Transformation through occupation*. London, Whurr.

Whiteford, G. (2005). Globalisation and the enabling state. In: G. Whiteford & V. Wright-St Clair (Eds). *Occupation and Practice in Context* (pp. 349–361). Sydney: Churchill Livingstone.

Whiteford, G., & Wright-St Clair, V. (Eds.). (2005). *Occupation and Practice in Context*. Sydney: Churchill Livingstone.

Wilcock, A. (1998). *An occupational perspective of health*, Thorofare, NJ, Slack.

Wilding, C. & Whiteford, G. (2006). Occupation and occupational therapy: knowledge paradigms and everyday practice. *Australian Occupational Therapy Journal*, 53, 1–9.

Williams, R. (1976). *Keywords*. London, Fontana.

World Federation of Occupational Therapists (2004). *Position paper on community based rehabilitation.* Forestfield, Western Australia, WFOT. Online. Available: www.wfot.org. Accessed 16th January 2007.

World Federation of Occupational Therapists (2006). *Position paper on human rights*. Forestfield, Western Australia, WFOT. Online. Available: www.wfot.org. Accessed 3rd March 2007.

Useful resources

Co-operatives: www.ica.coop

Social and therapeutic horticulture: www.thrive.org.uk

Stephanie Alexander Kitchen Garden Foundation: www. kitchengardenfoundation.org.au

Horticulture for all: www. horticultureforall.org.uk

The Disability Archive UK. www. leeds.ac.uk/disability-studies/ archiveuk/titles.html

Chapter Twenty

20

Developing partnerships to privilege participation

Roshan Galvaan, Peliwe Mdlokolo, and Robin Joubert

CHAPTER CONTENTS

Introduction 282

Marginalisation and barriers to
participation: occupational therapists
working with disabled people to eradicate
occupational injustice. 283

The United Nations' *Convention on the
Rights of Persons with Disabilities* as an
advocacy tool 284

A partnership approach: Five actions for
achieving participation and occupational
justice 288

   What can we learn from these two
   scenarios? 294

Conclusion. 295

SUMMARY

This chapter explores the impact of developing partnerships with disabled people and relevant stakeholders in occupational therapy practice. It is proposed that working in this manner has the potential to achieve occupational justice for disabled people. Five strategies for negotiating partnerships are suggested: collaboratively identifying needs; identifying policies that address the needs; working with service sectors to implement policies; lobbying and advocating for policy change; and working to develop key stakeholders' skills to meet the identified needs. The United Nations' *Convention on the Rights of Persons with Disabilities* is outlined as a key tool for advocating for the rights of disabled people when developing partnerships to bring about social change. This tool provides an understanding of how human rights and equal participation can be addressed while targeting specific areas during the implementation of services. Two practice scenarios are presented which illustrate how the strategies for developing partnerships are applied to occupational therapy practice in a community context.

KEY POINTS

- Disabled people face institutional, environmental, and social barriers to their inclusion and participation in mainstream society.
- Occupational justice is realised through understanding the contextual limits to peoples' participation and then advocating or working to provide the opportunities or resources to support peoples' participation in meaningful occupation.
- Occupational therapists must consider how they can privilege participation in order to promote the health and well-being of the people they serve.
- Emphasis is given to an occupational perspective of public health in discerning the ways in which occupational therapists should be working with disabled people and other marginalised groups to bring about sustained change.
- It is advocated that occupational therapists develop partnerships with disabled people and other relevant stakeholders to bring about sustained change.
- The United Nations' *Convention on the Rights of Persons with Disabilities* (United Nations 2006) is proposed as a key policy framework for ensuring the full participation of disabled people in society.

Introduction

This chapter invites occupational therapists to consider the implications of developing partnerships with disabled people and with relevant stakeholders when adopting an occupational perspective to public health. Disabled people and other marginalised groups may experience occupational injustice as a result of prevailing contextual determinants. Occupational therapists are challenged to consider how these occupational injustices may be addressed to the benefit of disabled people and society at large thereby promoting occupational justice[1].

Prevention and alleviation of occupational injustice for disabled people requires a shift in view from impairment in the individual to identifying the barriers in the environment. It implies that the prevalence and determinants of impairments and the barriers to participation experienced by disabled people be addressed. Public health's focus on the health of populations and the causes of ill-health has been criticised by Wilcock (1998) as being too disease-focused. Interventions in the field of public health have characteristically ignored the role of occupation in the mediation of peoples' health (Wilcock 1998). Taking an occupational perspective of public health is suggested as a means for understanding how occupational injustice may develop when working to eliminate its root causes. It is advocated that through partnering with disabled people to ensure equal participation, occupational injustices may be countered. This can be enacted through focused interventions that remove environmental barriers to participation.

The Standard Rules on the Equalisation of Opportunities for Persons with Disabilities were developed as part of the World Programme of Action concerning Disabled Persons (United Nations 1993). The World Programme of Action was adopted by the United Nations assembly in 1982 (United Nations 1982). The World Programme of Action's aims were focused on the prevention of disability, the provision of rehabilitation and the equalisation of opportunities for disabled people in order to ensure that they are able to fully participate in social and national arenas (United Nations 1982). Full participation of disabled people as a principal value in the World Programme of Action supported the recognition that occupation is fundamental to the health of disabled people, and that the environment plays a key role in this regard. Drawing on the United Nations Standard Rules and the World Programme of Action, United Nations developed the Convention on the Rights of Persons with Disabilities (United Nations 2006). The purpose of this Convention is to promote, protect and ensure the dignity and the full enjoyment of all human rights and fundamental freedoms by all disabled people (United Nations 2006). This Convention is both a human rights and development instrument and is cross-disability and cross-sectoral. Furthermore, it advocates that disabled people are capable of claiming their human rights as active members of society, rather than as recipients of medical care or welfare. Occupational therapists can identify with this perspective as the profession moves towards taking an occupational perspective of health.

Evidence has been given to suggest that the way people participate can serve to either promote or hinder the attainment of health and well-being (Cronin-Davis et al 2004, Wilcock 1998). The equalising of opportunities for disabled people to participate as citizens in local and global communities is, therefore, imperative if disabled people are to realise their own potential and experience health. The Convention on the Rights of Persons with Disabilities (United Nations 2006) provides key focus areas for the way in which disabled peoples' participation in daily life can be promoted. As a result it provides a guide for policy-making and practice and may be adopted as a key advocacy tool for use in occupational therapy practice. Presented in this chapter are ways in which occupational therapists can embrace the principles and strategies laid out in articles of the Convention on the Rights of Persons with Disabilities when working in partnership with disabled people for social change.

The application of ideas of participatory citizenship can assist occupational therapists to reorientate their thinking and practice to the health of populations (Townsend & Wilcock 2004). This developing perspective encourages occupational therapists to consider the influence of factors such as power, privilege and political action on people's ability to participate in daily life. Similarly, public health calls for the maintenance and improvement

---

[1]Occupational justice aims at equalising opportunities for participation by recognising difference (Townsend & Wilcock 2004). It enables different access to resources and opportunities because it recognises individual and group differences that may result biologically or through interaction with the surrounding environment.

of health of all people through collective and social action. This need for social action is based on a public service ethic, rather than a personal, professional work ethic. This public service ethic involves collaboration for the good of society and for social change. It requires fundamental principles of equity and equality in relationships distinct from traditional paternalistic health professional relationships. The way in which partnerships with disabled people are developed and maintained is, therefore, key to effective practice in different settings.

Occupational therapists must reposition themselves so that they appreciate a macro view. This will allow the profession to contribute to health promotion, the prevention of ill health and the prolonging of life, as well as enhancing the quality of life of disabled people.

Marginalisation and barriers to participation: occupational therapists working with disabled people to eradicate occupational injustice

Participation in daily life occurs through occupation (Wilcock & Hocking 2004). This means that the manner and patterns of people's participation in occupations is of relevance to health. The quality and characteristics of this participation have an impact on health for individuals, communities and populations (Wilcock 1998). Health, as a resource for everyday life, requires that efforts towards ensuring the physical, mental and social well-being of populations are considered (Wilcock 1998). Attention has to be given to improving the health of vulnerable groups. Groups of people may be rendered vulnerable as a result of contextual, socio-political and/or economic factors and, as a result, disabled people may be marginalised from participating in occupations despite progressive, inclusive policies.

Occupational injustices are said to exist when the participation of people is devalued, marginalised, segregated, restricted and/or exploited (Townsend & Whiteford 2005). Restriction in participation as a result of marginalisation and exclusion results in occupational injustice for disabled people. The impact of occupational injustice for disabled people

is vast, severe and direct. The costs, however, are shared by the rest of the population. For example, disabled people may have limited access to education and employment which leads to economic and social exclusion. Ban Kimoon's message for the International Day of Disabled Person's in 2007 indicated that according to estimates as many as half the number of disabled people in minority world countries and a greater proportion in majority world countries are not employed (Kimoon 2007). This means their rights to social, cultural and economic viability are compromised or denied such that decreased opportunities for participation in civil, political and social decisions may be experienced. Disabled people may then experience a negative social stigma which hinders their contribution to mainstream society.

The lack of opportunity for disabled people to contribute to decision-making, results in limited diversity of opinions and considerations which affects the development of communities at local and national levels. Silver & Koopman (2000) reinforce the fact that diversity is a major asset in the business world in terms of the economic development of companies where different people are employed. Decisions taken by non-disabled people in the absence of disabled people in various community structures and practices may favour the non-disabled group while further excluding disabled people. A study by the Community Agency for Social Enquiry for the Department of Health in South Africa indicated that disabled people who participated in this study felt marginalised and excluded (Silver & Koopman 2000). Due to disabled people's exclusion from the economy as productive citizens they often experience poverty as a factor that compounds their experience of physical impairment. Disabled people's human rights are often not realised (Office of the Deputy President of Republic of South Africa 1997) and they may carry a double burden. This means that not only do they carry the burden of impairment but also the burden of being excluded from mainstream society resulting in the inability to access their human rights.

The barriers to inclusion that disabled people face influence their ability to participate as citizens and take control of their own health through this participation. These barriers include: institutional (e.g. oppressive policies); environmental (e.g. physical inaccessibility) and social (e.g. discrimination and stigma). To illustrate how these barriers might be experienced in daily life let us take the example of a 7-year-old learner. Dean (pseudonym) was diagnosed with muscular dystrophy. He currently attends a mainstream school which he was initially able to access because the educators were unaware of his impairment. His educators now indicate that they find it difficult to teach him. Consequently he faces exclusion from this learning environment. The institutional policies held by the school limit the possibility of developing alternative teaching methods in the classroom that would ensure Dean's full participation. Furthermore, the educator's attitude towards Dean has been negative and one of reluctance to accommodate him in the classroom. This further compounded his experience of exclusion. As a result of this Dean became frustrated and expressed this in his behaviour, re-enforcing the educator's negative attitude towards him.

On a structural level, due to Dean's physical impairment, the school environment poses physical barriers to his participation: the only way of accessing his classrooms is via stairways; the playground is filled with obstacles which restrict his opportunities to participate in physical play with other learners. In addition, the attitudes of his peers in the playground may also further exclude him. The existence of these physical and attitudinal barriers contributes to the prevalence of occupational injustice. Although Dean is offered schooling at a mainstream school there is no understanding of what is required to ensure his inclusion in this environment. This causes him to be marginalised. Dean is not provided with what he needs to participate fully and his learning is severely compromised.

If occupational therapists espouse an occupational perspective of health it is imperative that they collaborate and form partnerships with various stakeholders in order to challenge these barriers. Townsend & Whiteford (2005) suggest that a participatory justice framework be negotiated in order to analyse occupational injustices. The outcome and process of working within this framework may mean that occupational therapists have to adopt a human development perspective, rather than a therapeutic one (Max-Neef 1991). This perspective facilitates a shift from working with health as the means and end in the process, to considering how to promote health using the most appropriate means. If participation in occupation is proposed as a key contributor to the health of individuals and populations (Wilcock 1998), then occupational therapists need to focus on promoting disabled peoples' participation in mainstream society to counter the mechanisms that

prevent their inclusion. This implies that stakeholders in collaboration with occupational therapists address underlying occupational determinants[2], such as restrictive national policies and social barriers, in order to promote individual and community development. This perspective is supported by Whalley Hammell (2006) when she encourages occupational therapists to work towards changing the environments that oppress disabled people through the formation of alliances with disabled people. This requires that the complexity of problems linked to contextual elements be considered so that solutions are designed to impact at a point where significant change can be generated.

Addressing occupational injustices stretches occupational therapists beyond the boundaries of the health sector and challenges them to consider different perspectives rather then simply resorting to the traditional therapeutic approach to which they have grown accustomed. In doing this, therapists become able to contribute towards mediating and advocating within contexts of relevance to groups, communities and populations.

The United Nations' *Convention on the Rights of Persons with Disabilities* as an advocacy tool

The application of the International Classification of Functioning, Disability and Heath (ICF) (World Health Organisation 2001) has been suggested as a way for occupational therapists to conceptualise their role in population health (Wilcock & Hocking 2004). While the ICF is useful in addressing the components impacting on participation restriction, it does not automatically allow for partnerships based on equal participation to be developed. This is because the ICF is fundamentally a classification system for impairment, rather than a tool for advocacy promoting social change. While it allows for the

---

[2]Occupational determinants have been described as those contextual elements that play a role in the way that participation happens for individuals and groups (Wilcock 1998). In her description of the occupational factors that lead to ill-health Wilcock (1998, p. 138) proposes that these determinants include underlying occupational factors, such as national policies and cultural values as well as the occupational institutions and activities that result from these underlying factors. Occupational institutions and activities could include factors, such as legislation, technology, education, health care systems, etc.

recording of the factors that impact on function and participation (World Health Organisation 2001) it does not provide the means to accurately and efficiently address the environmental challenges that disabled people face. To this end, it is viewed as limited in facilitating a participatory process for achieving occupational justice. In fact, Townsend & Whiteford (2005) suggest that the profession of occupational therapy must extend the notion of 'participation restrictions' as named in the ICF to mean something deeper and to include an environmental view that considers the influence of occupational injustice on the way people may or may not participate.

The United Nations' Convention on the Rights of Persons with Disabilities offers a framework for targeted strategies to promote participation. The way these strategies are outlined in the articles of the Convention indicate the very real need to critically examine the environmental barriers that disabled people face in terms of their participation. There are 50 articles that provide guidance on the State's responsibilities. The rules included in each of the preceding chapters are listed in Box 20.1.

Box 20.1

Summary of the United Nations Convention on the Rights of Persons with Disabilities

Article 1: Purpose of the Convention

To *promote, protect and ensure* the full and equal enjoyment of all human rights and fundamental freedoms by all disabled people, and to promote respect for their inherent dignity.

Article 2: Definitions

The Convention offers definitions for communication; language; discrimination on the basis of impairment; reasonable accommodation; and universal design.

Article 3: General Principles

Outlines the principles for the convention, these include:

- principles to promote non-discrimination
- full and effective participation and inclusion in society
- human diversity and humanity
- equality of opportunity
- accessibility
- equality between men and women
- respect for the evolving capacities of disabled children and respect for the right of disabled children to preserve their identities.

Article 4 General Obligations

Outlines the legal bind on state parties to honour the realisation of the rights and fundamental freedoms of all disabled people.

Article 5: Equality and Non-discrimination

The right to equality before the law without discrimination.

Article 6: Women with disabilities

In recognising that disabled women and girls are subject to multiple discriminations, appropriate measure will be taken to ensure the full development, advancement, and empowerment of women.

Article 7: Children with Disabilities

Necessary measures will be taken to ensure the full enjoyment by disabled children of all human rights and fundamental freedoms on an equal basis with other children.

Article 8: Awareness Raising

Effective and appropriate measures will be adopted to raise awareness throughout society, including at the family level, regarding disabled people, and to foster respect for the rights and dignity of disabled people; to combat stereotypes, prejudices, and harmful practices relating to disabled people, including those based on sex and age, in all areas of life.

Article 9: Accessibility

Appropriate measures will be taken to ensure disabled people's access, on an equal basis with others, to the physical environment, to transportation, to information and communications, including information and communications technologies and systems, and to other facilities and services open or provided to the public, both in urban and in rural areas.

Article 10: Right to Life

Reaffirmation that every human being has the inherent right to life and necessary measures will be

Box 20.1—cont'd

taken to ensure its effective enjoyment by disabled people on an equal basis with others.

Article 11: Situations of Risk and Humanitarian Emergencies

All necessary measures will be taken to ensure the protection and safety of disabled people in situations of risk, including situations of armed conflict, humanitarian emergencies and the occurrence of natural disasters.

Article 12: Equal Recognition before the Law

Reaffirmation that disabled people have the right to recognition as persons before the law.

Article 13: Access to Justice

Ensure effective access to justice for disabled people on an equal basis with others.

Article 14: Liberty and Security of Person

Ensure that disabled people enjoy the right to liberty and security of person.

Article 15: Freedom from Torture or Cruel, Inhuman or Degrading Treatment or Punishment

No one shall be subjected to torture or to cruel, inhuman or degrading treatment or punishment. In particular, no one shall be subjected without his or her free consent to medical or scientific experimentation.

Article 16: Freedom from Exploitation, Violence and Abuse

All appropriate legislative, administrative, social, educational, and other measures will be taken to protect disabled people, both within and outside the home, from all forms of exploitation, violence, and abuse, including their gender-based aspects.

Article 17: Protecting the Integrity of the Person

Every disabled person has a right to respect for his or her physical and mental integrity on an equal basis with others.

Article 18: Liberty of Movement and Nationality

Recognition of the rights of disabled people to liberty of movement, to freedom to choose their residence, and to a nationality, on an equal basis with others.

Article 19: Living Independently and being Included in the Community

Recognise and take effective and appropriate measures to facilitate the equal rights of all disabled people to live in the community, with choices equal to others.

Article 20: Personal Mobility

Effective measures will be taken to ensure personal mobility with the greatest possible independence for disabled people.

Article 21: Freedom of Expression and Opinion, and Access to Information

Appropriate measures will be taken to ensure that disabled people can exercise the right to freedom of expression and opinion, through all forms of communication of their choice.

Article 22: Respect for Privacy

Protection of the privacy of the personal, health, and rehabilitation information of disabled people on an equal basis with others.

Article 23: Respect for Home and the Family

Effective and appropriate measures will be taken to eliminate discrimination against disabled people in all matters relating to marriage, family, parenthood, and relationships, on an equal basis with others.

Article 24: Education

Ensure an inclusive education system at all levels as all disabled people have a right to education.

Article 25: Health

Appropriate measures will be taken to ensure access for disabled people to health services that are gender-sensitive, including health-related rehabilitation.

Article 26: Habilitation and Rehabilitation

Effective and appropriate measures will be taken to enable disabled people to attain and maintain maximum independence, full physical, mental, social and vocational ability, and full inclusion and participation in all aspects of life.

Article 27: Work and Employment

Recognition and promotion of the rights of disabled people to work on an equal basis with others and to gain a living by work freely chosen or accepted in a labour market and work environment that is open, inclusive and accessible to disabled people.

Box 20.1—cont'd

Article 28: Adequate Standard of Living and Social Protection

Recognition and promotion of the right of disabled people to an adequate standard of living for themselves and their families, and to the continuous improvement of living conditions.

Article 29: Participation in Political and Public Life

Guarantee of political right for all disabled people and the opportunity to enjoy these rights on an equal basis with others.

Article 30: Participation in Cultural Life, Recreation, Leisure and Sport

Recognition of the right of disabled people to take part on an equal basis with others in cultural life, and implementation of appropriate measures to enable disabled people to have the opportunity to develop and utilise their creative, artistic and intellectual potential, not only for their own benefit, but also for the enrichment of society.

Article 31: Statistics and Data Collection

Collection of appropriate information, including statistical and research data, to enable the formulation and implementation of policies to give effect to the present Convention.

Article 32: International Co-operation

Recognition and promotion of the importance of international co-operation, in support of national efforts for the realisation of the purpose and objectives of the present Convention.

Article 33: National Implementation and Monitoring

Designation of one or more focal points within government for matters relating to the implementation of the present Convention, giving due consideration to the establishment or designation of a coordination mechanism within government to facilitate related action in different sectors and at different levels.

Articles 34–50: International Monitoring Mechanisms

Article 34: Committee on the Rights of Persons with Disabilities
Article 35: Reports by States Parties
Article 36: Consideration of Reports
Article 37: Cooperation between States Parties and the Committee
Article 38: Relationship of the Committee with Other Bodies
Article 39: Report of the Committee
Article 40: Conference of States Parties
Article 41: Depositary
Article 42: Signature
Article 43: Consent to be Bound
Article 44: Regional Integration Organizations
Article 45: Entry into Force
Article 46: Reservations
Article 47: Amendments
Article 48: Denunciation
Article 49: Accessible Format
Article 50: Authentic Texts

The Convention on the Rights of Persons with Disabilities can be applied as a means of facilitating occupational engagement. The Convention legislates for full and effective participation and inclusion in society. Full partnership is embedded in the Convention as a general principle (Article 3); a general obligation (Article 4) and a right (Articles 29 and 30).

Occupational justice would prevail through meeting the obligations set out in the Convention, addressing the identified rights and target areas, and implementing and monitoring the cross-cutting measures. This would allow occupational therapists to address existing public health services and policy so that disability issues are integrated into practice rather than being addressed separately (Joubert et al 2006). For example, occupational therapists could collaborate with disabled people to raise awareness regarding the human rights and potential of disabled people. Advocacy and lobbying for policy changes that would result in improved participation would then be a key performance area in every occupational therapist's job, rather than something that is characteristically only included on occasion in traditional practice. Dyck & Jongbloed (2000) indicate that occupational therapists often experience barriers that prevent them from becoming involved in systemic advocacy. One of the barriers that they mention involves occupational therapists having limited knowledge of policies and legislation

(Dyck & Jongbloed 2000). While there is an appreciation of the difficulties involved in becoming advocates for change occupational therapists are invited to become familiar with policies of relevance and make a concerted effort to incorporate advocacy into everyday practice.

An occupational perspective on public health requires that the population's health needs are addressed in terms of participation (Wilcock 1998). This means that the manner in which the profession works with individuals, groups and communities, changes to incorporate a view of the desired outcome for the population. In order for the occupational therapy profession to accurately identify and target populations' health needs, its contribution would need to extend beyond simply conceptualising possibilities with reference to the interpretation of policies that produce change. Long-term, sustained change that brings about substantial health gains can only be achieved through entering into partnerships with communities and professionals across sectors. A partnership approach means that occupational therapists reposition themselves so that disabled people are able to assume power in matters that affect their participation in society. Striving towards this contribution would mean that occupational therapists scrutinise existing policies to identify the avenues that could be pursued in collaboration with disabled people. Occupational therapists should develop the skill of interpreting the implications of policy implementation and matching these to the expressed and identified needs of disabled people.

A partnership approach: Five actions for achieving participation and occupational justice

The authors of this chapter propose five actions that allow occupational therapists to work in partnership with disabled people in advocating for enhanced participation in occupation (Table 20.1). The five actions draw on the actions for health promotion outlined in the Ottawa Charter for Health Promotion (World Health Organisation 1986). In addition to this, the rights and obligations outlined in the United Nations' Convention on the Rights of Disabled Persons are used as a guiding framework for applying the intervention strategies for promoting disabled peoples' participation.

The processes associated with implementing these five actions are cyclical and do not follow in a linear order. Instead the earlier actions may be revisited in more depth as the process unfolds. Furthermore, more than one action may be applied concurrently. Given the iterative nature of this cycle, prolonged periods of engagement are necessary. This allows the needs to unfold and be re-defined.

Practice Scenarios 20.1 and 20.2 illustrate how occupational therapists can forge partnerships, foster participation and work towards occupational justice. They highlight the application of the five actions, and how the Convention on the Rights of Persons with Disabilities (United Nations 2006) can guide the occupational therapist to enable equity of opportunities through enhancing participation.

Practice Scenario 20.1 illustrates how Nolundi's participation was enabled through reflection on her occupations and the opportunity to participate in an organised group. Nolundi was involved in a collaborative process that helped identify her own needs. In this two-way learning process both Nolundi and the occupational therapists involved developed skills to advocate for other disabled people.

Practice Scenario 20.1 Regaining dignity through collective participation

Nolundi is a 55-year-old woman who is a single mother of a 20-year-old son. In 1992, she was knocked over by a bus. Her baby, whom she was carrying on her, died as a result of the accident. Nolundi sustained injuries resulting in complete paralysis of the left lower limb. She remained unconscious for about a week. The doctors insisted on amputating her left leg but she refused. At the time of the accident, she was employed as a domestic worker; a person who works within the employer's household.

Domestic workers are predominantly black women and get paid a minimal wage. They are responsible for home-management activities typically including domestic chores, such as *cooking*, *ironing*, *washing*, *cleaning* the house, buying foods and drinks, and accompanying and taking care of the children. Domestic workers in South Africa have experienced occupational injustice, particularly as a result of socio-political and economic factors, and so are often at risk of developing ill health as a consequence of their characteristic patterns of occupational engagement (Galvaan 2005).

Table 20.1 Five actions for achieving participation and occupational justice

Action 1: Collaboratively identify needs	Identifying needs in a collaborative way involves engaging in discussions with disabled people. The process and content of the discussions are equally important. The process should be one that facilitates open sharing and the emergence of diverse views. This allows for a range of needs to be expressed. Further discussions should then identify priority needs for the individuals and groups affected. To understand the complexity of problems occupational therapists must: become socially aware and responsive to emerging needs; analyse existing economic and social policies to identify how these restrict disabled people; collaborate to promote individuals to engage as social actors and agents; analyse the extent and particular opportunities that the environment represses or facilitates; and form partnerships with advocacy groups in order to collaborate towards facilitating social change
Action 2: Identify policies that address the identified needs	Once the priority needs have been identified, an analysis of the components of the needs should be conducted. This assists in focusing on the specific problem to be targeted so that particular policies can be identified
Action 3: Work with service sectors to ensure implementation of policies	If policies are in place, it becomes necessary to lobby for the implementation of these. The factors hindering service sectors from implementing the policies should be identified and possibilities for implementation should be explored
Action 4: Lobby and advocate with policy makers for the implementation and/or adaptation of policies	If policies remain unimplemented, then stakeholders must lobby and advocate for possible alternatives, compromises or plans. Change occurs with consistent lobbying
Action 5: Work with key stakeholders to develop the skills required to meet needs	The synchronisation of skill to work together and lobby becomes established through practice over time. Each person has their personal and professional strengths and can learn from the other. Occupational therapists and disabled persons need to be open to learning through implementing the above strategies

However, for Nolundi, being a domestic worker offered her an opportunity for productivity and an income. Prior to the accident, she was also involved in community activities, such as street committees and visiting those who had lost their loved ones. These valued roles were lost as a result of Nolundi's impairment from the accident.

Nolundi's life changed when she was approached by the community rehabilitation worker to attend a disabled women's support group that was organised by the South African Christian Leadership Assembly (SACLA). SACLA is a non-governmental organisation that works with disabled people in partnership with the University of Cape Town Division of Occupational Therapy and Disabled People South Africa (DPSA). Members of the disabled women's support group were involved in Participation Action Research (PAR) (Lorenzo 2005) facilitated by Dr Theresa Lorenzo and Peliwe Mdlokolo (occupational therapy staff members from the University of Cape Town). Peliwe Mdlokolo also worked on a community development entrepreneurship project that ran concurrently with the PAR.

The aim of the PAR was to address issues of social and economic development through a series of activities that included narrative action reflection (NAR) (Lorenzo 2005) workshops. It was anticipated that through story telling and sharing the women would be able to use their experiences to educate people about disability so as to remove barriers that they encountered in their communities.

Action 1: Collaboratively identify needs

Action 2: Identify policies to meet these needs

Nolundi noted that after the accident people in the community ignored her and would not invite her to any of the meetings that she used to attend. She would often sit alone and cry and did not know how to access resources. She did not receive any support from her family. Due to the social barriers, such as negative attitudes towards disabled people, she experienced difficulties in accessing the social development department for a disability pension. This continued despite the South African governments' progressive Integrated National Disability Strategy (Office of the Deputy President of Republic of South Africa 1997), which aimed to integrate disability issues, such as access to social welfare, social security, and community development into all government departmental strategies, planning and programmes. Nolundi felt that since people in the community ignored her she was denied the opportunity to contribute and participate as she did before. She thus experienced occupational injustice as a result of contextual elements. Her participation was limited because of the stigma attached to disabled people.

The NAR workshops (Lorenzo 2005) identified ways in which the disabled women's needs could be met. During Nolundi's participation in the NAR workshops she was given space to share her story and was able to identify all the challenges in her life. The importance of focusing on the needs of disabled women and allowing their voices to be heard is captured in the general principles and specifically in Article 6 of the United Nations' Convention on the Rights of Persons with Disabilities. Storytelling was a culturally relevant technique and promoted the sharing of their cultural lives (Article 30). It is indicated that disabled people should be allowed to share their intellectual capacity for the enrichment of themselves and their communities. She explored the challenges she faced at individual, family, and community levels. The importance of this opportunity was supported by the knowledge of the value associated with promoting a family life and personal integrity (Articles 19 and 23).

Identifying what she needed to change and manage in her family life enabled her to develop strategies for how to enhance this important aspect of her life. She was encouraged to explore the challenges that she perceived to be related to her physical impairment. The group process allowed Nolundi to be herself and explore opportunities that were available so as to bring meaning to her life. She indicated that she had to learn to be a friend to poverty as her opportunities to access resources as a black disabled woman were minimal. She indicated that she saw her impairment as an obstacle that stopped her from accessing resources and engaging in activities that were meaningful to her. This led her to stop engaging in activities that were meaningful in her life.

The storytelling process during the NAR workshops was viewed as a community development process and thus participation and ownership of issues was pivotal. This process focused on building the group and community's capacity to define and solve their problems. This participatory approach required that the occupational therapists recognised and managed the power usually associated with their professional status, such that it did not restrict the process of participation to evolve.

Action 3: Work with service sectors to ensure implementation of policies

Action 4: Lobby and advocate with policy makers for the implementation and/or adaptation of policies

Action 5: Working with key stakeholders to develop skills necessary to meet needs

The NAR workshops were a mechanism for promoting change through collaboratively identifying needs. Working together collectively in a group meant that it was easier to access resources like disability grants as experiences were shared amongst the group members. This is supported by the general obligations and Article 8 of the United Nations' Convention since it promotes that organisations of disabled people are able to identify needs and priorities, to contribute to public awareness and to advocate change.

Group members became self-reliant and used each other and the group as a resource for meeting their needs. The occupational therapist's role was to be part of the opportunity created through the group process and to share her skills or information if it matched the needs of the participants. This group process provided the members with the skills and the opportunity to be with others who shared similar experiences. Similarly, a study on the experiences of live-in domestic workers noted that sharing occupations with others was seen as more important for the experience of meaning than the occupations performed at the time (Luger et al 2003). The domestic workers placed the greatest value on sharing time with people who could relate to their experiences. Hence, occupational therapists need to consider the various forms in which meaning may be experienced. Valuing the variations in experience will allow occupational therapists to optimise the participation and outcomes being facilitated.

Concurrent with her participation in the NAR workshops, Nolundi participated in a community-development entrepreneurship project. This business development project involved both women and men with physical impairments. They aimed to develop skills related to sewing, leather work and cooking in order to successfully generate an income (van Niekerk et al 2006). This operationalised the target areas of education and employment (Articles 24 and 27). As Nolundi's skills developed and she understood different perspectives through the activities and storytelling in the NAR she was heard to say,

'This group has equipped me with a lot of skills and I no longer just sit and do nothing…Since I joined this group, I no longer sit and do nothing and bask in the sun. I have grown. I encourage other people, even those without disabilities.'

Nolundi began to encourage new members in the groups to get up and do whatever they could so as to gain experience and not feel sorry for themselves.

Final comment

This scenario has demonstrated the value of using a partnership approach whilst drawing on the United Nations' Convention as a policy framework. Through initially focusing on awareness raising through collaborative sharing, Nolundi was then able to work on the target areas of personal integrity, family life, education, and employment. This was achieved through accessing services (Action 3) and partnering with key stakeholders to develop necessary skills (Action 5). However, this was only possible after Nolundi had the opportunity to collaboratively identify needs (Action 1), which were interpreted in a policy framework (Action 2), and was able to work with others to lobby for change (Action 4). Nolundi regained her roles as a family member and active community member. Through the experience she gained from participating in both the disabled women's group and community-development entrepreneurship project facilitated by occupational therapists, she was able to participate in more personally meaningful community activities. As she stated,

'I am now a new person, I have regained my dignity and even those community members who used to ignore me invite me to their functions. I am not scared of being disabled. I always take over when I attend functions.'

Practice Scenario 20.2 identifies negative stereotypes towards disability as being one of the barriers to education for disabled children in the Ngcolosi community. This scenario describes how the need for disability awareness was defined and became better understood when the occupational therapist engaged with relevant service sectors. It provides insight into the fundamental necessity of using national policies to bring about change for disabled people.

Practice Scenario 20.2 Raising awareness for equal participation

Amarula is a community and tribal area that is found in the Valley of a Thousand Hills, in KwaZulu – Natal, South Africa. It is approximately 35 kilometres from the port city of Durban. In mid-2006 there were approximately 19,318 people living in Ngcolosi of which approximately 800 had a physical and/or mental impairment (Office of the Presidency of Republic of South Africa). These figures may be an underestimate because there is also a high prevalence of HIV and AIDS in the area with its concomitant neuropathies.

The majority of individuals living in Amarula live in relative poverty, with some people living in absolute poverty. Swanepoel & De Beer (2006) suggest that absolute poverty refers to a situation where the acquisition or not of the next meal may result in life or death. Relative poverty is an expression of one entity in relation to another that takes into account the deprivation of resources needed for survival and the inequality in society. This view of poverty recognises the multi-dimensional nature of poverty. The dimensions or indicators of poverty include various needs that are unmet or deprived. These include, amongst others, income and material deprivation; employment deprivation; health; education and living environment deprivation; human and social capital deprivation. According to Vavi (2004), unemployment in South Africa is approximately 54% and of those who are employed, 70% earn less than R1000 per month. The average salary is between R2000 and R4000 per month (Office of the Presidency of Republic of South Africa). This situation often results in the risk of occupational deprivation for those concerned and may also lead to crime and substance abuse (Joubert 2007). This means that people who live in this area experience occupational injustice. In addition, tertiary health care institutions and rehabilitation centres are far away in distance and expensive to access, costing approximately a hundred rand for a return trip.

Although there are some substantial homesteads built with brick, which have plumbing and electricity, a large proportion of the homes in Ngcolosi are built in the traditional fashion either in the form of the rondaval (a round structure with conical roof) or square wattle and daub home (Figure 20.1). These are built using poles and saplings woven in and out of each other, and then coated with a mixture of mud and cement, or sometimes even mud mixed with cow

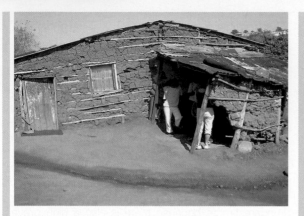

Figure 20.1 • Wattle and daub home

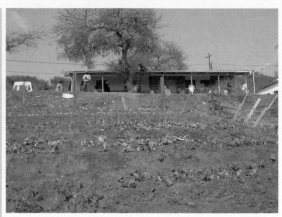

Figure 20.2 • Ngcolosi community outreach centre

dung which, when it dries, forms strong adhesive cement. The roofs are made of either thatched grass or corrugated iron. The population swells and ebbs by night and day or at weekends, because a large percentage of the young adults living there move out daily into the city and its suburbs to work and either return at night or over the weekend to rest and be with their families. There are schools, a clinic, a community outreach centre (Figure 20.2), and several church halls used for community activities such as meetings, weddings, and funerals.

Action 1: Collaboratively identify the needs

The Ngcolosi community outreach centre has been used for several years as a service learning centre by the occupational therapy, audiology, and speech pathology students at the University of KwaZulu – Natal. One of the projects in which the students are involved focuses on working together with disabled children and their caregivers. Community health workers identify and refer disabled children and their caregivers to the services offered by these students.

The age range of the children referred to in this project is between 6 months and 23 years. The children and adolescents experience difficulties in participation associated with cerebral palsy, visual and auditory impairment, intellectual impairments, congenital illnesses, and AIDS-related impairments. Article 7 of the Convention on the Rights of Persons with Disabilities encourages service providers to take the necessary measure to facilitate disabled children's participation. Services provided by the students include: developmental stimulation; correct positioning; accessing disability grants and schooling; as well as exploring solutions to specific needs.

This assists in establishing the pre-condition for equal participation for disabled persons by providing them with access to rehabilitation and support services (Article 26).

Over the years an analysis by the students of the local community's response to the disabled children and adolescents attending the community outreach centre indicated repeated problems in placing disabled children in the local schools. Feedback from caregivers indicated a lack of tolerance of disabled children by their peers as well as a lack of knowledge and skills of teachers in integrating and dealing with the different needs of disabled children. Subsequently, a project was initiated to raise awareness about disability at local primary and secondary schools. This project operationalised awareness raising (Article 8). Furthermore, the project aimed to equip the teachers with the necessary knowledge, skills and attitudes to accommodate the disabled children within the school environment (Article 30).

Action 2: Identify policies that address the identified needs

In 1996, shortly after the demise of apartheid, the Minister of Education of the new South African government appointed a commission to investigate 'special needs and support services in education and training'. It was instrumental in the formulation of the *White Paper 6: Special needs education – building an inclusive education and training system* (Department of Education 2001). The central objective of this paper was to extend policy foundations, frameworks and programmes of existing policy to address all bands of education and training. This would serve the purpose of recognising and accommodating the existing diverse range of training needs (Department of Education 2001). The focus being on the attainment of the learning potential of youth and adults through the provision of the necessary support; removing barriers from the education system to accommodate the diverse range of learning needs and to establish an inclusive education and training system (Philpott 2005).

In 2007 an attempt was made to facilitate collaboration between schools and the community outreach centre and to encourage teachers and school principles to engage more as agents of change. As a result of this a delegation of students together with occupational therapy lecturers from the University of KwaZulu – Natal arranged a meeting with the principal of the secondary school situated across the road from the community outreach centre. Their concern arose out of the fact that a large number of the older disabled children and adolescents who were attending the outreach centre had never been to school or had only attended school for a short while. This occurred as a result of the teachers' ignorance about disability together with learners being ostracised by their peers.

Action 3: Working with service sectors to ensure implementation of policies

The first phase of intervention implementation was to arrange a meeting with the school principal and teachers from the school across the road from the community outreach centre as a pilot study before implementing an awareness and training strategy in all schools in the area (Articles 4 and 8).

The aim of this meeting was to alert them to the identified problem and offer assistance in training the teachers to more effectively accommodate the needs of disabled children in their classes and also to become more able to identify children with possible learning needs. They were very enthusiastic about the possibilities of the project. The teachers were motivated to implement the Education White Paper 6 (Department of Education 2001). This policy aims to change education and training in South Africa so that it is responsive and sensitive to the diverse range of learning needs. It is an example of an implementation measure aiming to achieve full participation of disabled people, as stipulated in the Convention and specifically in school as in Article 24. However, the teachers felt that they lacked the skills to be able to implement this policy. This positive response on their part was indicative of their willingness to work with the role players in the community outreach centre and collaborate towards facilitating social change.

They also had difficulty dealing with the school-children who bullied the disabled children. The reason given for the bullying was the stigma attached to the disabled children since they were perceived to be different. The teachers acknowledged that bullying was prevalent at school, and that the disabled children were victimised. The teachers were unsure how to deal with this. They feared that this affirmed the negative stereotypes that the disabled children experienced. Mdlokolo and Joubert supervised the occupational therapy students. They all consulted with the provincial policy coordinator for the Education White Paper 6 (Department of Education 2001) to identify the province's strategy for implementing the policy. This consultation aimed to ensure that decisions regarding services were not taken unilaterally.

It was planned that the project would begin by addressing the barriers experienced by the adolescents at secondary schools before returning to those experienced by the primary school children (Article 9). This would not have been the occupational therapists' approach, since there was direct service being provided for the primary school learners. The openness to be guided by the provincial policy co-ordinator ensured that this, more contextually effective strategy was used. Thus, it was that after this meeting the project members were in a position to implement the second phase of their goal which was to bring about similar changes for the teachers and learners in other primary schools in the area and accordingly meetings have been arranged with a primary school nearby which has been identified as having a particularly large number of learners with special needs and impairments.

Occupational therapy students, who will help drive the process, will collaborate with occupational therapists, speech pathologists, remedial teachers and audiologists in designing workshops that meet the needs of orientating and training the teachers and learners in these schools. The occupational therapy students will also learn from the teachers and, therefore, this process will provide mutual learning experiences.

Action 4: Lobby and advocate with policy makers for the implementation and/or adaptation of policies

It is anticipated that once these two schools have undergone these awareness training workshops, which will be implemented by the rehabilitation professionals, community health workers, disabled children, and occupational therapy students, their implementation of the new knowledge and skills attained will be monitored and feedback from them will inform a more extensive programme, which may be extended to all schools in the area. This should result in far more disabled children accessing local schools and it is also possible that information obtained from this intervention may result in refinement of existing policy and planning within the White Paper 6.

The occupational therapists and students acted in accordance with Wilcock and Hocking's (2004) recommendations that population interventions by occupational therapists required that they work alongside others from diverse fields. They held a consultative meeting with the school principal and his deputy and the community health worker. They discussed the identified problem(s) at the school and after discussions amongst these group members it was indicated that the project would also involve the assessment of children identified as experiencing barriers to learning at the primary schools.

Action 5: Working with key stakeholders to develop skills in achieving the identified needs

Although this project is still in its infancy, it is planned that over the next few years a task team consisting of disabled people, teachers, parents, community health workers, and therapists will be established to monitor the progress of the integration of disabled children into schools in the area and to recommend in-service training when and where needs for this arise. Changes and adaptations to policy will also be recommended.

Final comment

Developing partnerships with schools, in areas such as Ngcolosi, allows for effective implementation of programmes to identify learners with learning and physical impairments. It also empowers teachers to more ably cope with such problems, thus reducing the need for costly therapeutic intervention. This in turn facilitates the implementation of White Paper 6 (South African Department of Education July 2001) and United Nations Convention on the Rights of Persons with Disabilities (United Nations 2006) ensuring that disabled children have access to education and that the necessary personnel training occurs to equip teachers to adequately implement appropriate learning strategies. It may also later impact upon the revision of existing policy.

What can we learn from these two scenarios?

- Interventions targeting appropriate needs and alleviating occupational injustices are possible

when occupational therapists work in partnership with disabled people and relevant stakeholders, such as disabled peoples' organisations. Participation in occupation that is meaningful and health-giving is a potential gain of interventions that privilege participation.

- The United Nations Convention on the Rights of Persons with Disabilities (United Nations 2006) has been proposed as an effective advocacy framework to discern the issues requiring consideration when working with disabled people. Both practice scenarios illustrated the value of this Convention as a means to bring about participation for change.

- Community-based interventions in areas where there are high levels of poverty and lack of resources requires innovative programmes that allow for sustainability by the people they serve. Similarly, work with marginalised groups, such as disabled people, in many contexts requires community-based interventions. It is not sufficient for change to happen only at an individual level. Change needs to happen at the level of the group and community in order for it to be meaningful.

- Change is more powerful and sustained when occupational therapists work collaboratively with groups as *facilitators* where people are enabled and encouraged to take their own initiative and control of the process.

- Goal sharing during participation in occupations at a group level enables people to make changes at an individual level because of the empowering nature of the group.

- The development of skills necessary for bringing about change was crucial to the outcomes of the process for the disabled people involved. All role players, including occupational therapists, need to develop the necessary skills to partner and advocate for change in order to more effectively address disability issues.

- Partnerships that resituate power with disabled people have tremendous potential to bring about change that is relevant for their lives. It is only through occupational therapists giving up the power that they hold in traditional occupational therapy practice that disabled people can be empowered to bring about changes that will promote occupational justice.

The development of partnerships implies that disabled people will be worked *with* rather than *for* in bringing about meaningful change.

• Occupational therapy can be progressive and meet the needs of the people it serves by taking a macro perspective, merging new approaches with old ones and by giving power back to the people who have been historically marginalised and disempowered by contextual factors.

Conclusion

Occupational therapists currently work with individuals, groups and communities. The profession has begun to charter what its services might look like if a public health perspective is taken. This chapter has suggested that forming collaborative partnerships where occupational therapists contribute as equal partners, not as expert leaders, is necessary if a public health perspective is to be embraced. Practice Scenario 20.1 illustrates how this may be facilitated

within a research context for individuals and groups. Practice Scenario 20.2 highlights how familiar occupational therapy services (working with children who experience barriers to learning) can be facilitated, parallel to services that create opportunities for equal participation. Both practice scenarios indicate that participation in meaningful occupations may reduce disabled people's experience of occupational injustice and marginalisation.

Partnerships between disabled people and relevant stakeholders (including occupational therapists) are a mechanism that allows for collective action. Disabled people can determine their destiny, such that change is sustainable and real, and not dependent on the continued involvement of professionals. Occupational therapists have an important contribution to make. Along with other stakeholders and through working as partners with individuals, groups and communities, the achievement of equal participation of marginalised groups can be strived for. Occupational therapists should be humble, but courageous in considering how they can assist disabled people to access equal participation.

References

Cronin-Davis, J., A. Lang, et al. (2004). Occupational Science: The forensic challenge. In: M. Molineux. *Occupation for occupational therapists*. Oxford, Blackwell Publishing Limited.

Department of Education. (2001). *Education white paper 6: Special needs education building an inclusive education and training system*. London, The Stationery Office.

Dyck, I. & Jongbloed, L. (2000). Women with multiple sclerosis and employment issues: A focus on social and institutional environments. *Canadian Journal of Occupational Therapy*, 67(5), 337–347.

Galvaan, R. (2005). Domestic workers' narratives: Transforming occupational therapy practice. In: F. Kronenberg, S. S. Algado & N. Pollard (Eds). *Occupational Therapy without borders: Learning from the spirit of survivors*. London, Elsevier Churchill Livingstone.

Hammell, K. W. (2006). *Perspectives on disability and rehabilitation*.

Edinburgh Churchill Livingstone, Elsevier.

Joubert, R. (2007 unpublished thesis). Indigenous Fruits from Exotic Roots: revisiting the occupational therapy curriculum. *Department of Education* Durban, University of KwaZulu Natal.

Joubert, R., Galvaan, R., Lorenzo, T. & Ramugondo, E. (2006). Reflecting on contexts of service learning. In: T. Lorenzo, M. Duncan, H. Buchanan & A. Alsop (Eds). *Practice and Service Learning in Occupational Therapy: Enhancing potential in context*. London, John Wiley and Sons Limited.

Kimoon, B. (2007). *International day of disabled person's*. Available online: http://www.un.org/News/Press/docs/2007/sgsm11305.doc.htm. Accessed 29 June 2008.

Lorenzo, T. (2005 unpublished thesis). We don't see ourselves as different: a web of possibilities for disabled women: how black disabled women in poor communities equalise opportunities for human development and social change.

Public Health. Cape Town, University of Cape Town.

Luger, R., Sherry, K., Vilikazi, B., Wonnacott, H. & Galvaan, R. (2003). A struggle for identity: domestic workers, ubuntu and time-off occupations. *South African Journal of Occupational Therapy*, 33(2), 11–14.

Max-Neef, M. A. (1991). Re-reading the Latin American situation: crisis and perplexity. In: M. A. Max-Neef (Ed.). *Human scale development: conception, applications and further reflections*. (pp. 1–12). London, The Apex Press.

Office of the Deputy President of Republic of South Africa (1997). *Integrated National Disability Strategy*. Pretoria, Office of the Deputy President, Rustica Press.

Office of the Presidency of Republic of South Africa (2006). *Development of indicators – mid term review*. Pretoria, Office of the Presidency of Republic of South Africa.

Philpott, S. (2005). *Policies relating to disabled people in South Africa. Notes prepared for the orientation* programme for occupational and speech and language therapy students. Howick, University of KwaZulu Natal, Disability Action Research Team (DART).

Silver, R. & Koopman, B. (2000). *Successfully employing people with disabilities. Business for good's focussed guide to employment equity*. Seapoint, INCE.

South African Department of Education (2001). *Education White Paper 6: Special needs education building an inclusive education and training system*. Pretoria, South African Department of Education.

Swanepoel, H. & d. Beer, F. (2006). *Community development – Breaking the cycle of poverty*. Lansdowne, Cape Town, Juta and Co.

Townsend, E. & Whiteford, G. (2005). A participatory occupational justice framework: Population based processes of practice. In: F. Kronenberg, S. S. Algado & N. Pollard (Eds). *Occupational therapy without borders: Learning from the spirit of survivors*. (pp. 110–116). London, Elsevier.

Townsend, E. A. & Wilcock, A. (2004). Occupational justice. In: C. H. Christiansen & E. Townsend (Eds), *Introduction to occupation: the art and science of living*. *Pearson* New Jersey, Education Inc, Prentice Hall.

United Nations (1982). *World Programme of action concerning disabled people*. Available online: http://www.un.org/esa/socdev/enable/diswpa00.htm. Accessed 29 June 2008.

United Nations (1993). *UN 22 Standard Rules on the Equalisation of Opportunities for People with Disabilities*. Vienna, United Nations.

United Nations (2006). *Convention on the rights of persons with disability and optional protocol*. Vienna, United Nations.

van Niekerk, L., Lorenzo, T. & Mdlokolo, P. (2006). Understanding partnerships in developing disabled entrepeneurs through participatory action research. *Disability and Rehabilitation*, 28(5), 323–331.

Vavi, Z. (2004). Labour and the tripartheid alliance. In: B. Bowes &

S. Pennington (Eds). *The story of our future: South Africa 2014*. Rivonia., The Good News (Pty) Ltd.

Wilcock, A. (1998). *An occupational perspective on health*. Thorofare, NJ, Slack.

Wilcock, A. & C. Hocking (2004). Occupation, population health and policy development. In: M. Molineux (Ed.). *Occupation for occupational therapists*. (pp. 219–230). Oxford, Blackwell Publishing Ltd.

World Health Organisation (1986). *Ottawa charter for health promotion*. Ottawa, Canada, World Health Organisation.

World Health Organisation (2001). *International classification of functioning, disability and health*. Geneva, World Health Organisation.

World Health Organisation. (2001). *International classification of functioning, disability and health*. Available online: http://www.who.int/classifications/icf/en/. Accessed 29 June 2008.

Chapter Twenty-One

21

Working towards inclusive communities

Hanneke van Bruggen

CHAPTER CONTENTS

Introduction 298

Poverty. 298

  Vulnerability 298

  Poverty and disability 299

Theoretical and policy overview 299

  Social and occupational (in)justice 299

  Occupational deprivation and
occupational apartheid 300

Social policies and participation
strategies 301

  Social cohesion 302

  Mainstreaming. 302

Occupational therapy contributing to
social reform. 302

  Practical implications 303

  Establishing partnerships 303

  Capacity building 306

  Facilitating inclusive education
(including attitudes) 308

  Managing and monitoring impact. 310

Conclusion. 311

SUMMARY

The development of occupational therapy collective approaches in which all individuals find their place is an essential step towards combating poverty and developing the concepts and practices necessary for an inclusive community.

The transformation of the so-called 'new' countries and the changing social reality in an enlarged Europe are causing a bigger gap between Europe's poorest and richest groups (Liddle & Lerais 2006). The development of occupational therapy education and practice in those regions is focusing on sustaining and reinforcing commitment to solidarity and occupational justice in order to strengthen inclusive communities. This is a rather new area of concern for occupational therapy and needs an understanding of the current debate about poverty, disability and community development, and mainstreaming policies. Occupational therapists in the 'new' countries, in close collaboration with the European Network in Occupational Therapy in Higher Education (ENOTHE), are developing community development strategies which contribute to social reform and an inclusive society. In this chapter three different practice scenarios demonstrate how occupational therapists apply community development strategies within their practice with groups of disabled people and disadvantaged groups and relate their work to national or international policies concerning disability. The potential role of the occupational therapist is to facilitate the poorest occupationally deprived groups to catch up and to enhance community development through engagement in education, employment, and leisure activities.

KEY POINTS

- Poverty and disability reinforce each other, contributing to increased vulnerability and exclusion for disabled individuals and their families.

- Disabled people are often at risk of marginalisation, social exclusion, or dependency; or in occupational terminology, occupational injustice, occupational deprivation, or occupational apartheid.
- Disabled people must be empowered by enhancing their rights to benefit from measures ensuring their independence, social integration and participation in the life of the community, and by making the environment more accessible through the elimination of technical, legal and attitudinal barriers.
- When occupational therapists promote occupational participation for all and consider the disabled person as a fully participative member of society, then the focus is on addressing the occupational needs, occupational rights and obligations of all citizens.
- One of the most important principles when working with occupationally deprived populations is that the people must have a voice and be full participants in the planning of their own programmes.
- When implementing community development programmes there are four strategies that occupational therapists may use: establishing partnerships, capacity building, environmental adaptation, and managing and monitoring impact.
- The role of occupational therapists needs to go beyond the traditional role of working with individuals with occupational needs in the health care sector to working with communities to facilitate inclusive environments.

Introduction

Most disabled people are likely to be disproportionately poor. Poverty and disability reinforce each other, contributing to increased vulnerability and exclusion for both disabled individuals and their families. In addition to this, poverty and social exclusion in their turn are interlinked, and, consequently, have the impact of reducing an individual's occupational opportunities.

Poverty

The most common way of assessing poverty is the economic, through indicators such as gross domestic product (GDP) and gross national product (GNP). GDP measures the financial value a country produces, through its own activities; however, it does not consider any activity where money is not exchanged, for example household activities. GNP is the value of all goods and services produced in a year by nationals of a country, including profits from outside the country.

The United Nations Human Development Index (HDI) overcomes the problem of addressing the complexities of poverty by including not only financial values, but also indicators for health, education, the environment, and mortality.

Caritas Europe is one of the biggest organisations in Europe, representing 48 organisations from 44 countries, which focuses its activities on poverty, migration, and social inequality. This organisation developed a definition of poverty as 'a multidimensional and multi-factorial phenomenon, deeply affecting human beings' identities and capabilities, not solely based on income, but including basic needs, basic human rights and such intangibles as vulnerability, risk, inequality, marginalisation, discrimination, exclusion, a feeling of powerlessness, and the circumscribing of options and choices' (Caritas Europe 2006, p. 16). Occupational therapists who enable people to fulfil their occupational needs (as one of the basic needs), advocate for occupational rights (as one of the human rights) and prevent or improve situations of occupational deprivation, are often involved in the process of poverty reduction and should be more aware of the factors causing it.

The reduction of poverty is a process which goes far beyond material and financial assistance. It needs to include strategies to diminish vulnerability and discrimination and to promote social inclusion or participation in all life areas. In order to adequately address the specific occupational needs of disabled people and vulnerable groups who are deprived from occupations, the strategy needs to be grounded in a comprehensive analysis of poverty issues. Watson & Swartz (2004) suggest that an occupational therapy response to the challenges posed by these complex situations requires promotive and preventive perspectives, where occupational opportunities are used to enhance the development of human potential, leading to health and well-being.

Vulnerability

There is no common definition of vulnerability. It may be associated with regional or economic factors, the local labour market, and individual and social characteristics. However, vulnerable groups are typically categorised in social terms according to age, sex, ethnicity, disability or family status. This obviously reflects the interaction between individual and social factors, such as discrimination and access to education, which affects employment prospects.

Poverty and disability

Social exclusion and social integration are terms with various meanings, but are often considered to be on two sides of one coin. This is in line with the official European Union (EU) view that precarious living conditions, such as long-term unemployment, poverty or multiple deprivations, imply a risk to social integration. It also follows the consensus that sufficient income, health, labour market attachment, social support and family back-up are important factors that contribute to a decent life for people. At the Lisbon summit in March 2000, building on a long-standing commitment to economic and social cohesion in the EU, the European Council declared that the number of people living below the poverty line and in social exclusion in the Union was unacceptable.

The European Commission (2005), in its report on social inclusion, notes that the actual living standards of those below the relative poverty line are strongly conditioned by a number of factors. These include house ownership, health conditions, security of work income and the need for extra care for elderly or disabled members of the household. Disability appears to have a strong correlation with poverty and exclusion. Poverty is estimated to be responsible for around 20% of disability. Poverty refers to more than just the absence of sufficient income and material wealth. It includes factors of social empowerment such as social exclusion, dependency and the ability to participate in society.

Statistics on disability are difficult to compare internationally as each country has a different definition of disability and a different degree of political will to publish such information. Many sources underestimate the number of people for whom a physical or mental impairment creates a substantial disadvantage when they seek employment or access to the wider benefits of citizenship. Some relevant facts and figures on disability are presented in Box 21.1.

According to the third report on poverty in Europe, migrants, and asylum seekers in particular, together with disabled people, are some of the most vulnerable groups of the EU population (Caritas Europe 2006). In the EU around 20 million people are *migrants*. They are defined as third-country nationals with temporary or permanent legal residence. The term migrant includes immigrants, refugees, persons under subsidiary forms of protection, asylum seekers, persons seeking other forms of protection, migrants in an irregular situation and repatriates. While some migrants come to the EU voluntarily, out of their free will, others are fleeing international economic turbulence, poverty, environmental decline, lack of peace and safety, human rights violations, and lack of democratic and judicial systems.

Theoretical and policy overview

The commonalities between all the previously mentioned groups is that they all experience, or are at risk of, marginalisation, social exclusion, dependency or in occupational terminology: *occupational injustice*, *occupational deprivation*, or *occupational apartheid*. The World Federation of Occupational Therapists (WFOT) is acknowledging the role of occupational therapists in facilitating the right of occupational participation for all and reducing occupational injustice, deprivation and apartheid (World Federation for Occupational Therapists 2004, 2006).

Social and occupational (in)justice

Social justice is a concept that recognises humans as social beings who engage in social relations and favours equitable access to opportunities and resources. Occupational justice is a concept to guide humans as occupational beings who need and want to participate in occupations in order to develop and thrive. The advocacy in this concept favours enablement of access to opportunities and resources (Christiansen & Townsend 2004).

Social injustice is perceived as the main driver of social exclusion. Within Eastern European countries, an absolute majority holds social injustice responsible for poverty. In all other countries at least 45% of the respondents identified social injustice as the primary cause of poverty. This sustains the idea that people are less likely to blame themselves for being excluded in countries where unemployment and economic hardship are widespread (Alber & Fahey 2004).

> ┃ Box 21.1

Some facts and figures related to disability

Disabled people

- Around 10% of the world's population, or 650 million people, live with an impairment. They are the world's largest minority (United Nations 2006).

- Impairment is estimated to affect 10–20% of every country's population, a percentage that is expected to grow because of poor health care and nutrition early in life, growing elderly populations and violent civil conflicts (United Nations 2006).

- Disabled people represent 50 million persons in the European Union (10% of the population) (Eurobarometer 2001).

Work, education, leisure and disability

- 6.8 million people of working age (or nearly 20% of the working age population) have an impairment, while in developing countries 80–90% of disabled people are unemployed compared to between 50 and 70% in developed countries (United Nations 2007).

- 38% of disabled people aged 16–34 across Europe have an earned income, compared to 64% of non-disabled people (Eurobarometer 2001).

- 41% of disabled people of working age have no educational qualifications in comparison to 18% of non-disabled people (Corporate Social Responsibility Europe 2006).

- One out of two disabled persons has never participated in leisure or sport activities in Europe (Eurobarometer 2001).

Economic and social exclusion

- A recent survey revealed that one in six (15%) young disabled persons said they had been turned down for a paid job, and told it was for a reason related to their impairment or health problem (Corporate Social Responsibility Europe).

- Incomes of households with at least one disabled person are 20–30% lower than the incomes of the average household (Corporate Social Responsibility Europe 2006).

Disability and poverty

- More than 1.3 billion people worldwide struggle to exist on less than $1 a day, and disabled people in their countries live at the bottom of the pile (Wolfensohn 2002).

- Unless disabled people are brought into the development mainstream, it will be impossible to cut poverty in half by 2015 or to give every girl and boy the chance to achieve a primary education by the same date – goals agreed to by more than 180 world leaders at the United Nations Millennium Summit in September 2000 (Albert & Harrison 2005).

- Poverty has a strong inter-relationship with disability. Poverty is estimated to be responsible for around 20% of disability (European Disability Forum 2002).

Justice is an implicit social vision in occupational therapy. The concept of occupational justice expresses ethical, moral, and civic concerns that participation in daily life should contribute to rather than undermine health, empowerment, and quality of life (Townsend & Whiteford 2005). Occupational injustices occur when participation in everyday occupations is: barred, trapped, confined, segregated, restricted, prohibited, undeveloped, disrupted, alienated, imbalanced, exploited, deprived, marginalised, or segregated. Occupational justice is a complementary extension, and more than a subcategory, of social justice. Social justice is necessary, but it is not sufficient to define the conditions required for an inclusion of all. Social justice overlooks injustices related to participation in daily life occupations – injustices related to doing.

Occupational deprivation and occupational apartheid

Occupational deprivation is defined as 'a state of prolonged preclusion of engagement in occupations of necessity and/or meaning due to factors *outside* the control of the individual' (Whiteford 2000, p. 201). The factors that produce occupational deprivation may be social, economic, environmental, geographic, historic, cultural or political in nature. Occupational deprivation is closely related to social exclusion insofar as the same risk factors may produce social exclusion and occupational deprivation. However, occupational deprivation focuses on the phenomena of being excluded from doing what you wish, want or need to do.

One of the categories of occupational deprivation mentioned by Whiteford (2000) is unemployment or underemployment. Europeans identify unemployment as a major driver of perceived lack of social integration. In particular, in the 'new' European countries, 21% of unemployed and 18% of retired persons report at least two symptoms of perceived lack of social integration. Unemployment is believed to be the most important reason for poverty.

In considering the impact of work on quality of life, it must be noted that work fulfils many positive economic and social functions. As a source of income and purchasing power, it empowers people and thus combats exclusion. As a source of income, status and social contacts, it serves as a basis of social recognition and self-esteem. It is an important mechanism of social integration. In terms of structuring people's daily lives and their life path it is also an important mechanism for social organisation (Alber & Fahey 2004). Finally, employment is assumed to have a central position in identity construction (Whiteford 2000). Unemployment is viewed here as one form of occupational deprivation.

Another term used within the framework of occupational justice is occupational apartheid, defined by Kronenberg et al (2005, p. 67) as 'the segregation of groups of people through the restriction or denial of access to dignified and meaningful participation in occupations of daily life on the basis of race, colour, disability, national origin, age, gender, sexual preference, religion, political beliefs, status in society, or other characteristics. Occasioned by political forces, its systematic and pervasive social, cultural, and economic consequences jeopardize health and wellbeing as experienced by individuals, communities and societies'.

Social policies and participation strategies

Shaping society in a fully inclusive way is one of the major objectives of the European social policy. It has become crucial to empower disabled people by enhancing their individual rights to benefit from measures ensuring their independence, social integration and participation in the life of the community and by making the environment more accessible through elimination of technical, legal and attitudinal barriers. Other objectives are a shift from long-term dependency on passive welfare benefits to active labour market measures, fostering social integration and fighting against marginalisation (social inclusion process), empowering and enhancing structures in society which sustain participation.

The European disability action plan (Council of Europe 2006) propose a broad-scope strategy that encompassed 15 key areas for disabled people (Box 21.2). The key objective of the Action Plan is to bring about the full participation of disabled people and disadvantaged groups in society, ultimately mainstreaming disability issues throughout all policy areas.

Box 21.2

Council of Europe Disability Action Plan (Council of Europe 2006, p. 3)

Action 1: Participation in political and public life	Action 2: Participation in cultural life	Action 3: Information and communication
Action 4: Education	Action 5: Employment, vocational guidance and training	Action 6: The built environment
Action 7: Transport	Action 8: Community living	Action 9: Health care
Action 10: Rehabilitation	Action 11: Social protection	Action 12: Legal protection
Action 13: Protection against violence and abuse	Action 14: Research and development	Action 15: Awareness raising

If occupational therapists promote occupational participation for all and consider the disabled person as a fully participative member of society, then the focus should be far wider than just health and rehabilitation. The focus should also be on addressing the occupational needs, occupational rights and obligations of all citizens.

Social cohesion

Within the framework of human rights the Council of Europe (2004) has developed a strategy of social cohesion that includes the commitment to making the rights of vulnerable people a reality. The Council defines social cohesion as the capacity of a society to ensure the welfare of all people, minimising disparities and avoiding polarisation. To ensure the welfare of all people the Council proposes that:

- the human rights of all people are respected, and all people are treated equally and without discrimination

- the dignity of each person and his/her abilities and contribution to society be recognised, fully respecting the diversity of cultures, opinions and religious beliefs

- each individual has the freedom to pursue his/her personal development throughout his/her life

- the possibility that each person can become an active and full member of society be recognised

- everyone needs to exercise responsibility in their use of social protection and social services.

Mainstreaming

Wolfensohn (2002) stated that unless disabled people are brought into the mainstream development it will not be possible to cut poverty in half by 2015. Mainstreaming disability is a strategy for making disabled people's concerns and experiences an integral dimension of the design, implementation, monitoring, and evaluation of policies and programmes in all political, economic and societal spheres. This is to ensure that disabled people benefit equally, and that inequality is not perpetuated (Miller & Albert 2005). As a consequence, disabled people should be included in all phases of any project and programme cycle. The goal is to create an inclusive society in which the needs of all

vulnerable and marginalised groups are taken into account. The basis of the concept of inclusion is the social model of disability and the rights-based approach, which demands a close exchange of views between different stakeholders. As the participation of disabled people is a central concern, capacity-building strategies for empowering disabled persons' organisations (DPOs) have become a fundamental issue.

Inclusive education is one example of a mainstream developmental approach seeking to address the learning needs of all children, youths, and adults with a specific focus on those who are vulnerable to marginalisation and exclusion (United Nations Education Scientific and Cultural Organization 2003). Inclusive education is at the basis of an inclusive society. Non-disabled as well as disabled children would equally benefit from being in the same educational environment. At the same time the fight against discrimination and prejudice can only be won by inclusion, and by educating children from their youngest age to respect human rights. Most disabled children can take part in mainstream education if they are provided with the necessary attitudinal support and any environmental barriers are removed.

Occupational therapy contributing to social reform

When contributing to social reform, occupational therapists must have a commitment to occupational justice. Appropriate occupational therapy practice can and should operate at the community and population level (Watson & Swartz 2004). This is particularly evident in the transitional countries of Europe, such as Romania, Bulgaria and Georgia, where an absolute majority holds social injustice as the main driver of social exclusion processes. In these countries issues of poverty and unemployment of migrants and disabled people cannot be resolved by individual solutions. They can be more effectively addressed through the use of a community-development approach. Community and population are used here interchangeably as 'a geographic or virtual connection between groups that engenders relationships based on proximity, interactions, or the development of shared values and experiences' (Christiansen & Townsend 2004, p. 275).

It is important to be aware that the word therapy is not very appropriate in this population approach. The community does not need 'therapy', but wants a fair engagement in occupations that should lead to a better quality of life. The occupational therapist plays a facilitating role and shares resources, limitations and risks within the group, and works towards a positive sustainable change through improved participation in occupations. Watson & Swartz (2004, p. 57) suggest that for community development to occur,

> [...] assistance from outside the community may be required; including assistance from occupational therapists, but this assistance must be delivered in a manner that respects the integrity, authority and customs of the people. Agents of change from outside the community must set out to work in partnership with the community so that internal and external change can occur.
>
> (Watson & Swartz 2004, p. 57).

Practical implications

One of the most important principles of occupational therapy with regard to occupationally deprived populations is that the people must have a voice and be fully participant in the planning of their own programmes. The following three practice scenarios taken from the community setting will describe the application of community-development strategies, from an occupational perspective.

Establishing partnerships

Partnership development is easy to talk about but quite hard to undertake. It requires courage, patience, commitment and determination over time. Partnerships enable different groups of people and agencies to collaborate, cooperate and coordinate in order to solve problems and to exchange resources. The relationship among partners can be temporary or permanent.

The Partnering Toolbook (Tennyson 2003) which has been developed particularly for community development, offers an overview of 12 phases for effective partnering and is outlined in Figure 21.1.

Partnerships take place at different levels (local, regional, national or international). Practice Scenario 21.1 provides an example of the development of partnerships by occupational therapists working with an internally displaced community in Georgia. As highlighted in this Practice Scenario, partnership involves acting on different levels.

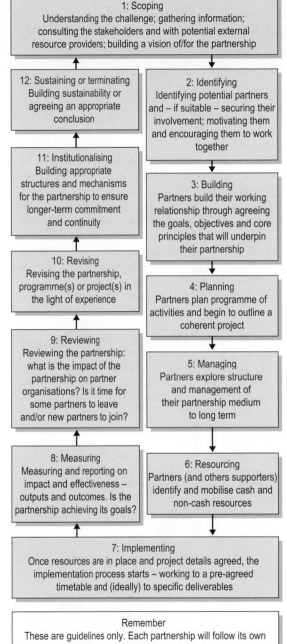

Figure 21.1 • The 12 Phases in the Partnering Process from Partnering Toolbook (reproduced with permission from Tennyson 2003 and the International Business Leaders Forum, 2003)

Practice Scenario 21.1 Developing partnerships to improve the living situation of internally displaced persons in Georgia

Background

Georgia is one of the post Soviet republics in South Caucasus. Nowadays the country has made a clear statement on the wish to join the European Union and North Atlantic Treaty Organisation. However, the whole situation of the country needs to be considered in the context of the difficult socio-economic challenges that Georgia, as a low–middle-income country, is still facing in spite of the impressive economic growth of the past years.

Following the break-up of the Soviet Union and the declaration of independence in 1991, Georgia had to confront two regions within its own borders demanding their own independence; Abkhazia and South Ossetia. The fighting that followed killed about 10,000 people and caused the displacement of some 300,000 people (United Nations Office for the Coordination of Humanitarian Affairs 2004).

Humanitarian agencies estimate that close to half of the displaced population live in collective centres, located in former hotels, schools, kindergartens, factories and hospitals. Of a total of 1,683 collective centres throughout the country, 70% do not meet minimum living standards, and are without adequate access to clean water, safe electricity systems and adequate insulation (Zoidze & Djibuti 2004).

The needs of the internally displaced persons (IDP) are context dependent and they are at risk of becoming occupationally deprived. The existing challenges are very similar to refugees, with the main difference being that IDP have never crossed the borders of their country and have remained so-called 'internal refugees' in their own motherland. According to Whiteford (2005, p. 85), 'The refugee experience can involve the permanent loss of life roles, drastic changes to others, and adoption of new roles by a sudden change in environment.'

Occupational therapy can address and respond to this phenomenon of occupational deprivation, by establishing partnerships with the aim of enabling participation in meaningful occupation in order to improve and maintain health and well-being. Occupational therapy in Georgia has been working with deprived communities since the profession emerged, with IDP being one of the largest groups of people receiving intervention and support from occupational therapists in Georgia.

Project: empowering IDP community in collective centre

The Norwegian Refugee Council (NRC) is one of the international humanitarian aid organisations that have worked with refugees and IDP in Georgia since 1994. It is with their help that contact has been obtained with one of the collective centres located in the Gori region of Georgia (near the conflict zone). This region of Georgia to which IDP from South Ossetia have been displaced, supporting the findings that most vulnerable people in Georgia are often found in conflict areas and in areas with a high concentration of IDP (United Nations Office for the Coordination of Humanitarian Affairs 2004).

The key issue related to IDP in Georgia is their multidimensional vulnerability (e.g. lack of capacities, poverty, substandard housing, unemployment, and exclusion). In such a period of personal crisis, such as being uprooted from their original home, individuals may have difficulties engaging in meaningful occupations, which will directly influence their health and well-being. Occupational therapy philosophy proposes that there is a dynamic relationship between engaging in occupation and health. Occupation is described as an important determinant of health and well-being that 'gives meaning to life'. Health is also strongly influenced by having choice and control in everyday occupation (Canadian Association of Occupational Therapists 1997, p. 31).

Using Tennyson's phases of the partnering process (Figure 21.1), the main goal of occupational therapy with IDP was to establish partnerships (Phase 1), to identify through participatory engagement their occupational needs and priorities (Phase 2), and to find joint problem-solving strategies (Phase 3).

The first phase of the project was to organise and run several community meetings in order to scope (Phase 1) and identify (Phase 2) the key partners and needs. Initially contact was obtained through the civil society representatives within different local non-governmental organisations (NGOs) working in the region for and with displaced people. This site visit and further meetings helped in the collection of the overall statistics in relation to the region and in the identification of the main challenges that IDP face in everyday life. These included uncertainty regarding housing, lack of social and human capital, limited access to valid information on the available benefits, health-care programmes, education, and other issues.

Following the initial meeting, several meetings were conducted at the Collective Centre with representatives from different age groups of community members to analyse the specific problems and outline the objectives. The meetings were planned together (Phase 4) and concentrated on facilitating creative group decision-making.

The occupational therapists had the task of uniting the IDP community, enabling them to name and prioritise their needs, and to identify and mobilise available resources (Phase 6) in order to implement a community project.

As a result of the meetings and mobilisation of the community, one of the most important issues identified as a priority was the lack of entertainment opportunities for the pre-school and school-aged children living in Collective Centres. The Collective Centre was quite far from the city centre; consequently, children lack opportunities to be integrated in mainstream life and take part in everyday occupations relevant to their developmental stage, age, culture, and ethnicity. There were no playgrounds, parks, sporting activities, or public kindergartens.

Based on these needs the community stated that there was a need to construct a playground for children in the Collective Centre.

The main strategy used in this project was the development of a partnership to enable community empowerment. With the support of an informal community leader (a person who guided the whole community in decision-making and problem-solving), the group of parents (mainly mothers) developed the project proposal for the local municipality (Phase 5). The meeting with the head of the municipal department of Gori ended with the handing over of construction materials for the playground (Phase 7). After this success the mothers started to identify internal local resources for a labour force, second-hand materials, and any kind of relevant contribution for the construction work (Phase 6).

Within 6 months the playground was constructed (Figures 21.2 to 21.6). Two comments capture the benefits that were felt by people as a result of the playground being constructed:

> You have made these children happier; they are at the playground from morning till evening.

(An elderly woman from the Collective Centre)

> I have no choice to take children for vacation elsewhere; the only place where they can have a rest in summer time is this playground.

(Mother of a five-year-old boy)

The Gori project in Georgia demonstrated that through the use of strategic partnerships with the key persons in the community (the parents, the Head of

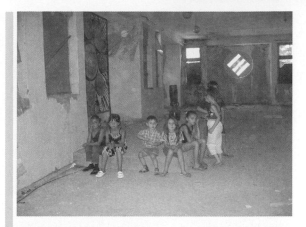

Figure 21.2 • An area where children played before the playground was constructed

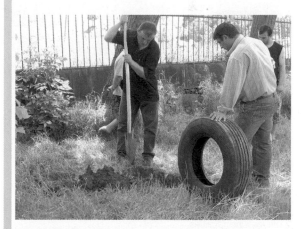

Figure 21.3 • Parents working on the playground

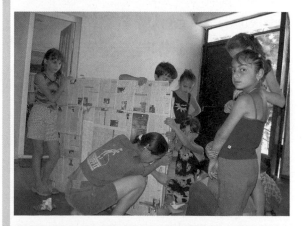

Figure 21.4 • Children helping with planning and development of the playground project

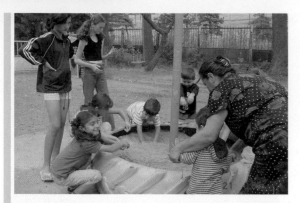

Figure 21.5 • Children and families enjoy the new play area

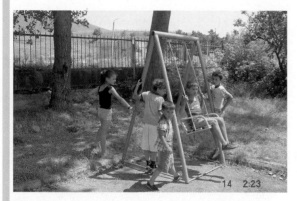

Figure 21.6 • The children enjoying their new playground facilities

the municipality and the occupational therapist), a common project was able to be completed and that through occupation (constructing the playground) the whole community was empowered. Based on this experience occupational therapists can claim to have a lot to offer deprived communities. Occupational therapists enable people to engage in meaningful activities and examples like this reinforce the value that occupational therapists have in such deprived communities.

This type of experience and the knowledge gained should lead to an increased understanding in occupational therapy of the occupational needs of displaced persons, and can serve as the basis for any population-based strategies in the future.

This Practice Scenario has been provided by Tamar Tavartkiladze.

One more efficient illustration of a partnership on a national level is that of the implementation of the state strategy on internally displaced persons (IDP) (2007) initiated by the government of Georgia, in response to the recommendations of the UN. The strategy aims to deal with all aspects of displacement, including education, health, housing, employability, social participation, and legal status. It aims to support the integration of IDP into Georgian society and facilitate their voluntary return to their homelands. The most significant part of the partnership process was the equal involvement of different representatives of civil society, IDP, and the international community alongside the governmental bodies; all agencies were lobbying and advocating for the target group in order to make IDP voices heard and well articulated in the policy output (Phases 11 and 12).

The knowledge and competency of the occupational therapist acquired during the implementation of this project with IDP was shared within the social thematic working group, covering education and health, on the basis of full membership.

The final result was a conceptual framework identifying the challenges faced by the displaced population in Georgia, and defining the goals and strategic directions to follow in order to improve the living conditions of IDP and enhance their quality of life for the future (Phase 12).

Capacity building

Another strategy identified within community development is capacity building. *Capacity* refers to the ability of individuals, institutions and societies to perform functions, solve problems, and set and achieve objectives. *Capacity building* is the process through which the ability to perform functions, solve problems, and set out and achieve objectives is obtained, strengthened, adapted, and maintained over time in a sustainable manner (United Nations Office for the Coordination of Humanitarian Affairs 2004). The capacity of the system forms, not only the procedural means for reaching results, but also the ultimate pre-condition for sustaining long-term actions within society. Morgan (2006) states that capacity can be defined as the emergent combination of attributes that enables a human system to create developmental value. He goes on to suggest that capacity can be conceptualised as being built on five core capabilities, which can be found in all organisations or systems: the capability to act, to

Table 21.1 Five core capabilities of capacity (Morgan 2006)

1. Capability to act	Degree to which decisions are implemented; degree and use of operational autonomy; action orientation within the system, integrity of the organisation, its leadership and staff; effective human institutional and financial mobilisation
2. Capability to generate results	Differentiate between building the capabilities of the organisation itself and the outcomes in the form of better quality of life or improved inclusive employment
3. Capability to relate to other actors and stakeholders	Networking and partnering are essential for capacity building to achieve goals and deliver programmes
4. Capability to adapt and self-renew	Ability of an organisation to master change and the adoption of new ideas
5. Capability to integrate or achieve coherence	Defining simple rules that govern operations, a leadership intent on achieving coherence and a shared vision of the intent of the organisation

generate developmental results, to relate, to adapt, and, finally, to integrate (Table 21.1). All five are necessary to ensure overall capacity.

Capacity building within occupational therapy must be holistic and involve participatory action, which implies that all critical sectors (such as the public sector, the private sector and civil society) and players (such as client groups with their families, employers, teachers, health professionals) should continue to be actively involved in helping to make choices and map out strategies. The occupationally deprived group should be facilitated to play a leading role in identifying their own needs and shaping innovative approaches to addressing those needs.

A holistic and participatory approach would generate gains if it were owned and implemented by all of the above stakeholders. This approach would pave the way for more sustainable actions and results.

To complement capacity building, resource mobilisation (e.g. local funding) must be a permanent feature in any programme. Resource mobilisation involves the active participation of all partners in the community, such as parents, employers, government, and donor organisations, who must all see it as their own responsibility and challenge. As sustainable human and institutional capacity building is a long-term process, it cannot be facilitated by a stop-and-go, unpredictable funding arrangement. Consequently, stakeholders and partners should consider and expedite efforts to develop and activate an orderly and predictable legal mechanism for replenishing the organisation's resources.

Practice Scenario 21.2 describes the capacity-building process of a group called NADI, in Georgia, who wanted to develop vocational and employment opportunities for disabled people.

Practice Scenario 21.2 Capacity building of 'NADI' in order to develop inclusive employment

One of the first actions to promote inclusive employment for disabled people in Georgia was to establish a union of parents and professionals. This organisation became known as 'NADI'. This organisation emerged out of the authentic *needs* of people, which is demonstrated by the following statement made at the end of their first meeting: 'We have to care for the future of our disabled children since we are still alive, we can't wait for our government for good'.

The establishment of NADI implied re-valuing and organising the existing capacities of disabled people and their families. NADI focused on taking control and on breaking down the stereotyped attitudes to disabled people, such as the belief that they were helpless. So rather than waiting and expecting others to take action on behalf of disabled people and their families, the organisation started to divide tasks, plan and act.

The first request made from the 'NADI' community to the occupational therapist involved in the organisation was to learn more about opportunities for employment for their disabled adolescents and to give an overview of inclusive employment and existing service opportunities in European countries.

Further capacity building took place in the form of adapting the Council of Europe Disability Action Plan (Box 21.2) to the Georgian reality. Responsibilities were undertaken for different areas including:

- Relating to other stakeholders (Table 21.1, point 3) and building a network between employers, vocational trainers, and representatives of the Ministry of Labour.
- Generating and disseminating results (Table 21.1, point 2); for example, promoting positive effects of inclusive employment and demonstrating best practice.
- Caring for sustainability, which involved fund raising and structural financial mobilisation (Table 21.1, point 1).

Each step in the process of capacity building was much more complex than simply following a linear project plan and achieving results. For instance, the step of raising money required much more than simply establishing partnerships with different donors. The donors in this situation do not receive any material benefit from their donation, neither is there any expectation of benefit in return. We knew that nobody would invest in the grand new initiative of establishing an inclusive employment firm (inclusive employment had never been organised before in Georgia), unless it had proved its value. Therefore, we could not rely on the conventional grant application processes, but had to think in a more creative way. Ultimately, we had to cut our ambitions of establishing a new inclusive work area and instead adapt already existing facilities (ordinary work-places in the mainstream).

In the conditions of non-existent state support or lack of economical subsidies for supporting the employment of disabled people, it was difficult to imagine being able to secure the involvement of commercial organisations. However, 'NADI', utilising personal networks with the business sector, investigated the values and the interests of commercial organisations, and tried to understand the economical and financial reasoning of the employers, as well as their public-relations policy (Table 21.1, point 3) as a way to encourage employers to employ disabled people.

The next step was to achieve the sustainability of the inclusive employment project. To do this, NADI targeted the state social protection programme. They chose the strategy of negotiation, rather than proving expertise and knowledge, when talking with representatives involved in this programme. The negotiations with representatives of the state social protection programme took 6 months. However, the result was the inclusion of paragraphs referring to inclusive employment within the state social protection programmes, sustained by budgetary calculations.

This project naturally acknowledged the need for inclusive vocational education for disabled people based on the competitive market economy requirements. The inclusion of the first disabled people in vocational education was made possible through the participation of a private vocational educational school. The success of this initiative resulted in another ministerial unit asking 'NADI' to expand the inclusive vocational education model to a state level.

Finally, the representatives of 'NADI' were invited to participate in the National Disability Group that was preparing the country's strategy for disabled people for approval by the parliament as the main policy document in the future.

This Practice Scenario has been provided by Ana Arganashvili.

In this Practice Scenario it is demonstrated that capacity building is not just the providing of some training and information. Capacity building requires the community to have an identity, a collective ability, and the desire to work together on a common project in spite of any barriers. In Practice Scenario 21.2 the public value of inclusive employment was developed, regardless of any instability and relative unpredictability intrinsic to the Georgian context.

Besides creating inclusive employment, inclusive education is widely seen as one of the most important gateways through which to escape poverty and exclusion. This in turn is why the promotion of inclusive education by occupational therapists is so vital for development in general and for disabled people in particular.

Facilitating inclusive education (including attitudes)

The United Nations Education Scientific and Cultural Organization (2005) proposed that inclusion is a dynamic approach of responding positively to student diversity. Furthermore, the United Nations Education Scientific and Cultural Organization suggests that individual differences should not be seen as a problem but as opportunities for enriched learning. Inclusive education is concerned with providing appropriate responses to the broad spectrum of learning needs in formal and non-formal educational settings. Rather than being a marginal theme on how some learners can be integrated in the mainstream education, inclusive education is an approach that looks at how to transform education systems in order to respond to the diversity of learners (United Nations Education Scientific and Cultural Organization 2003).

Tomasevski (2004) stated that inclusive education is a fundamental human right. No child should be forced to adapt to education, rather education should adapt to cater for the individual needs of each child. She proposed that a rights-based education approach, such as inclusive education is founded on three principles: access to free and compulsory education; equality, inclusion and non-discrimination; and the right to quality education, content and processes.

Facilitating inclusiveness is not only about putting in place inclusive policies that meet the needs of all learners, but also about changing the culture of classrooms, schools, city councils, and districts. It is important to note that the changes needed to successfully implement an inclusive education approach often begin on a small scale and involve overcoming obstacles, such as: existing attitudes and values; lack of knowledge and understanding; lack of necessary skills; limited resources and inaccessible environments; and inappropriate organisation.

Accepting change is really about learning. It means that schools should foster environments where teachers learn from experience in the same way that they expect their pupils should learn from the tasks and activities in which they are engaged (United Nations Education Scientific and Cultural Organization 2005).

Practice Scenario 21.3 illustrates how an occupational therapist can contribute towards facilitating an inclusive learning environment (including adapting and changing attitudes).

Practice Scenario 21.3
Occupational therapy taking part in the development of inclusive education

If basic education is for all and this can lead to learning to live together, as proposed by the United Nations Education Scientific and Cultural Organization (2001), then inclusive education is the key to creating equal opportunities for disabled people by assuring access to qualified education. Although the Bulgarian government recognised the rights of all

children to be valued equally (National Strategy 2003) prior to accession to the European Union, the practice of inclusion does not really exist. This is mainly as a result of the lack of adaptations and of supportive services in mainstream schools.

In 2004 a project promoting an occupational approach to developing inclusive education was initiated in Rousse, the biggest Bulgarian city on the Danube. Fortunately, at that moment, a number of actions were being undertaken at all levels to make the policies a reality. Children who would directly benefit from occupational therapy intervention were identified. Humanitas, a parents' non-governmental organisation, suggested a 6-year-old boy with cerebral palsy, whose family was determined that he should attend a mainstream school. The headmaster of the school close to their home agreed to accept him. The staff at the school agreed that for the inclusion of this boy at the school environment to work, they would have to adapt their capacity to ensure they could cater for the boy's needs. The United Nations Education Scientific and Cultural Organization (2003) states that inclusive education cannot be developed in isolation from overall school development and must be regarded as an approach to the development of the entire school system.

The needs assessment was based on the Person-Environment-Occupation Model (Law et al 1996). The Model guided the identification of environmental barriers and societal attitudes impeding the boy in the fulfillment of the student roles he would be expected to carry out (Baum & Law 1997). Strategies and resources to overcome these barriers were established.

Data were also gathered through a variety of assessment tools, such as interviews, observations, questionnaires, and the completion of the Canadian Occupational Performance Measure. Engagement of all participants in the analysis was considered a premise for increasing their adherence and satisfaction with the process, as well as for enabling them to solve future issues.

The assessment and analysis revealed a highly positive attitude and a high level of motivation in all participants. Despite this high motivation, it was also identified that the concepts of inclusion had not been fully clarified and this had resulted in a lack of appropriate interactions and collaboration amongst all participants. The teachers lacked information about the latest policies and the activities undertaken by local authorities and non-governmental organisations concerning inclusive education. The family was overwhelmed by doubts and by the ambiguity regarding the barriers their son would face. Therefore, strengthening the collaborative partnership of students, teachers, parents and community members was crucial for the inclusion process. The occupational therapist initiated a meeting, where the child's needs and necessary school adaptations were identified, and the expectations and demands of the child were clarified, thus leading to increased confidence of the family. A resource teacher was allocated to the school and opportunities for funding through new projects were established.

Occupational therapists have a substantial role to play in the implementation of inclusive education policies. By identifying issues to be addressed, providing evidence of successful strategies and improving relationship and cooperation, the school was empowered to build its own capacity in educating disabled children together with their healthy peers. Two years later the school proudly declared its leading position in inclusive education in Bulgaria.

Reforming systems to become inclusive is about not only putting in place recently developed inclusive policies that meet the needs of all citizens, but also changing the culture of classrooms, schools, communities, districts, etc.

This Practice Scenario was provided by Liliya Todorova.

Within this framework of occupational development by the community, the following section describes the final innovative approach for managing, monitoring and evaluating the impact of a project.

Managing and monitoring impact

There are increasing calls for new monitoring and evaluating approaches in community development projects that encourage learning and participation. The Managing for Impact Approach places monitoring and evaluating at the centre of learning and management processes (Pabari & Woodhill 2007). Unfortunately, top-down approaches to monitoring and evaluation which focus on the needs of experts, and public and private donors and are based on quantitative indicators, remain deeply entrenched in development projects. To implement learner-oriented practices, major investments in capacity building and engagement of all are needed. Furthermore, professionals and other stakeholders should be ready to learn, be open-minded and base their work on qualitative indicators to ensure high standards and facilitate further learning.

At the heart of the Managing for Impact Approach are people. This is in contrast with conventional Activity and Product Evaluation, where the main outcome of a project is measured on the quality of the product. The idea is that all those involved in a development initiative – communities, implementers, managers and donors – must be part of a learning alliance that seeks to achieve the greatest possible positive impact. In describing the Managing for Impact Approach, Pabari and Woodhill (2007) identify four clear interlinked tasks, which are briefly described in Table 21.2.

The success of this approach depends on the people involved ensuring that the necessary information is gathered, sound decisions are taken, and individuals take the initiative and perform to the best of their abilities. However, information is only useful if it is shared and discussed, enabling reflection and learning, so that good practice is disseminated.

Learning situations that can contribute to this process include partner meetings, informal discussions, participatory planning workshops and impact assessments, as well as performance appraisals and rewards for good performance. Pabari and Woodhill

Table 21.2 Four interlinked tasks of the Managing for Impact Approach (Pabari & Woodhill 2007)	
1. Guiding the strategy	Assessing whether an initiative is heading towards its goals (impacts) and, if not, quickly adjusting the strategy or even the objectives
2. Ensuring effective operations	Managing financial, physical and human resources to ensure that the outputs are achieved
3. Creating a learning environment	Establishing relationships with all involved in order to build trust, stimulate innovation, and foster commitment
4. Establishing information-gathering and management mechanisms	Ensuring systems are in place to provide the information needed, and encourage learning

(2007) state that to ensure that learning drives the developmental process it must be acknowledged that change is the result of coordination, integration and the commitment of all actors. As a result, the Managing for Impact Approach involves influencing relationships and the action of others to ensure the delivery of outputs.

Words such as 'learning', 'empowerment' and 'participation' are today common features of combating exclusion and occupational development strategies. At the heart of these strategies are people, relationships, and the ability to work together to learn and adapt to changing circumstances. This has implications for leadership, management, and the monitoring and evaluation of capacities, and includes the skills, knowledge and structures required for strategic, people-centred occupational development.

Conclusion

At the core of inclusive community development is the idea that participation is possible of all people.

The role of occupational therapists needs to go beyond the traditional role of working with individuals with occupational needs in the health care sector to facilitating inclusive communities (living situations, employment, education and leisure). This chapter has been an attempt to describe and illustrate community developmental theories, using Practice Scenarios from occupational therapists implementing appropriate strategies, working in the 'new' European member states. Four strategies inherent in implementing community development approaches have been presented: establishing partnerships, capacity building, facilitating inclusion, and managing for impact.

Working with communities implies that the individual is considered as a citizen within the community with rights as well as responsibilities and obligations. Working in this way will constantly challenge and confront occupational therapists. However, occupational therapists are encouraged to be proactive and become involved at all levels to ensure that community issues of marginalisation, poverty and mainstreaming are effectively tackled.

References

Alber, J. & Fahey, T. (2004). *Perceptions of living conditions in an enlarged Europe, European Foundation for the Improvement of Living and Working Conditions.* Luxembourg: Office for Official Publications of the European Communities.

Albert, B. & Harrison, M. (2005). *Messages from research: disability knowledge and research (KaR) Programme.* Department for International Development UK (available from www.disabilitykar.net).

Baum, C. & Law, M. (1997). Occupational therapy practice: focusing on occupational performance. *American Journal of Occupational Therapy, 51*(4), 278–288.

Canadian Association of Occupational Therapists (1997). *Enabling occupations: An occupational therapy perspective.* Ottawa, CAOT Publications ACE.

Caritas Europe (2006). *Migration: a journey into poverty.* 3rd report on poverty in Europe; available from http://www.caritas-europa.org/module/FileLib/Poverty2006ENWeb.pdf

Case-Smith J. (2001). Development of childhood occupations. In: J. Case-Smith (Ed.). *Occupational therapy for children.* (4th ed.), St Louis, Mosby.

Christiansen, C. H. & Townsend, E. A. (2004). *Introduction to occupational therapy; the art and science of living.* New Jersey, Prentice Hall.

Corporate Social Responsibility Europe (2006). *The European Business Network for CSR* (available from: www.csreurope.org)

Council of Europe (2004). *A new strategy for social cohesion: revised strategy for social cohesion.* Strasbourg: Council of Europe (available from: http://www.coe.int/t/dg3/socialpolicies/socialcohesiondev/source/RevisedStrategy_en.pdf)

Council of Europe (2006). *Council of Europe action plan to promote the rights of full participation of people with disabilities in society: Improving the quality of life of people with disabilities in Europe 2006–2015.* Strasbourg: Council of Europe (available from http://www.coe.int/t/e/social_cohesion/soc-sp/integration/02_council_of_europe_

disability_action_plan/Council_of_Europe_Disability_Action_Plan.asp)

European Commission (2005). *Draft joint report on social protection and social inclusion.* Brussels, European Commission.

European Disability Forum (2001), Facts and figures about disability (available from www.edf-feph.org)

European Disability Forum (EDF) (2002), *Policy Paper: development, cooperation and disability,* (available from: www.edf-feph.org)

Kronenberg, F., Simó Algado, S. & Pollard, N. (2005). *Occupational therapy without borders, learning from the spirit of survivors.* Edinburgh, Elsevier.

Law, M., Cooper, B., Strong, S., Steward, D., Rigby, P. & Lettis, L. (1996). The person-environment-occupation model: a transactive approach to occupational performance. *Canadian Journal of Occupational Therapy, 63,* 9–23.

Law, M., Haight, M., Milroy, B., Williams, D., Stewart, D. & Rosenbaum, P. (1999). Environmental factors affecting the occupations of children with physical disabilities. *Journal of Occupational Science,* 6(3), 102–110.

Liddle, R. & Lerais, F. (2006). A consultation paper from the bureau of European policy adviser Europe's social reality (available from: http://ec.europa.eu/citizens_agenda/social_reality_stocktaking/index_en.htm).

Miller, C. & Albert, B. (2005). Mainstreaming disability in development. In: B. Albert (Ed.). *Lesson from the disability knowledge and research (KaR) programme.* Department for International Development UK (available from http://www.disabilitykar.net/docs/gender.doc).

Ministry of Labour and Social Policy (2003). *National (Bulgarian) strategy for equal opportunities of disabled people.* Sofia, Ministry of Labour and Social Policy.

Ministry of Refugees and Accommodation of Georgia (2007). *State strategy on internally displaced persons in Georgia.* Tbilisi, Government of Georgia.

Morgan, P. (2006). *The concept of capacity; study on capacity, change and performance.* Maastricht, European Centre for Development Policy Management.

Pabari, M. & Woodhill, J. (2007), The managing for impact approach. *Capacity.org,* 31, *http://www.capacity.org/en.*

Tennyson, R. (2003). *Partnering toolbook.* London, The International Business Leaders Forum.

Tomasevski, K. (2004). *Manual on rights based education.* Paris, United Nations Education Scientific and Cultural Organization.

Townsend, E. (2003). *Ethical, moral and civic principles for an inclusive world.* European Network of Occupation Therapists in Higher Education Annual Meeting, Prague.

Townsend, E. & Whiteford, G. (2005). A participatory occupational justice framework. In: F. Kronenberg, S. A. Simo & N. Pollard. (Eds). *Occupational therapy without borders.* Edinburgh, Elsevier.

United Nations (2006). International Convention on the Rights of Persons with Disabilities, (available from www.un.org/disabilities/convention/pdfs/factsheet.pdf).

United Nations (2007). Enable fact sheet 1 (available from: http://www.un.org/disabilities/documents/toolaction/employmentfs.pdf).

United Nations Education Scientific and Cultural Organization (2001). *The first world* Terakoya Conference. United Nations Education Scientific and Cultural Organization available from http://portal.United Nations Education Sceintific and Cultural Organization.org/education/en/ev.php.

United Nations Education Scientific and Cultural Organization (2003). *Overcoming exclusion through inclusive approaches in education, conceptual paper, a challenge & a vision.* Paris, United Nations Education Scientific and Cultural Organization.

United Nations Education Scientific and Cultural Organization (2005). *Guidelines for Inclusion.* Paris, United Nations Education Scientific and Cultural Organization (available from http://unesdoc.United Nations Education Scientific and Cultural Organization.org/images/0014/001402/140224e.pdf).

United Nations Office for the Coordination of Humanitarian Affairs, *Situation report on Georgia for November, 2004.* United Nations Development Programme (available from http://iys.cidi.org/humanitarian//hsr/04b/ixl114.html).

Watson, D. (2006). *Monitoring and evaluation of capacity and capacity development.* Maastrict, European Centre for Development Policy Management.

Watson, R. & Swartz, L. (2004). *Transformation through occupation.* London, Whurr Publishers.

Whiteford, G. E. (2000). Occupational deprivation: Global challenge in the new millennium. *British Journal of Occupational Therapy,* 63(5), 200–204.

Whiteford, G. E. (2005). Understanding the occupational deprivation of refugees: A case study from Kosovo. *Canadian Journal of Occupational Therapy,* 72(2), 78–88.

Whiteford, G. E. (2006). *Occupation, participation, universities and communities: Towards a new ethic engagement.* 12th European Network of Occupational Therapist in Higher Education, Ankara.

Wolfensohn, J. D. (2002). *World Bank Statement,* Washington Post, December 3.

World Federation of Occupational Therapists (WFOT) (2004). Position Paper on Community Based Rehabilitation (CBR). Available from http://www.wfot.org/office_files/CBRposition%20Final%20CM2004%282%29.pdf.

World Federation of Occupational Therapists (WFOT) (2006). Position Statement on Human Rights. Available from http://www.wfot.org/office_files/Human%20Rights%20Position%20Statement%20Final%20NLH%281%29.pdf.

Zoidze, A. & Djibuti, M. (2004). *IDP health profile review in Georgia: new approach to IDP assistance initiative,* Tbilsi: United Nations Development Programme (available from http://www.undp.org.ge/Projects/new_approach.html).

Chapter Twenty-Two

22

Community-based rehabilitation: opportunities for occupational therapists in an evolving strategy

Kirsty M. Thompson, Christina L. Parasyn, and Beth Fuller

CHAPTER CONTENTS

Introduction 314

Understanding community-based
rehabilitation: an evolving strategy 315

Early community-based rehabilitation 315

Community-based rehabilitation
re-conceptualised: A community
development strategy 317

Occupational therapy and
community-based rehabilitation 321

Roles, skills and opportunities for
occupational therapists in
community-based rehabilitation 322

Transfer of rehabilitation knowledge
and skills 322

The provision of direct therapy 322

Referral services 322

Programme development and
implementation 323

Facilitating collaboration 323

Other roles 323

Conclusion 323

SUMMARY

Community-based rehabilitation (CBR) is a
strategy that promotes collaboration amongst
disabled people and their families, government
and non-government stakeholders to promote
an inclusive society that provides equal
opportunities for all. Originally designed as a
means of addressing the rehabilitation needs
of disabled people in the majority world, the
strategy has evolved from a medically framed
service delivery model to a community
development approach grounded in human
rights, empowerment, ownership, and
sustainability of a disability-inclusive community.
Despite this conceptual evolution, in practice
many CBR programmes continue with a
traditional rehabilitation emphasis. The World
Federation of Occupational Therapists (WFOT)
recognises the coherence of CBR and
occupational therapy approaches, promoting
CBR as a means of facilitating access to
occupation for all (World Federation of
Occupational Therapists 2004b). There are shared
beliefs in, for example, the importance of activity
and the right to participate, collaboration, and the
environment. Occupational therapists are well
positioned to contribute to the realisation of
quality CBR initiatives in many ways, including,
but not limited to, direct therapy, transfer of
knowledge to other stakeholders, as facilitators
of collaboration and contributors to advocacy,
policy, and evaluation of CBR.

KEY POINTS

- Community-based rehabilitation (CBR) is an
evolving strategy, moving from more medically
framed outreach services to a comprehensive
community development strategy.
- CBR seeks to improve the lives of disabled
persons by promoting human rights,
socio-economic development and an inclusive
society.
- CBR and occupational therapy are
philosophically aligned, with a shared emphasis
on for example, occupation, the environment,
collaborative relationships, and rights and
opportunities for meaningful participation for all.

- Occupational therapists' unique skills in enabling occupational engagement at an individual, community, and national level can play a crucial role in the realisation of CBR across multiple sectors, including, for example, health, education, and employment.
- The CBR strategy challenges occupational therapists to strengthen skills in facilitating knowledge and skills transfer, collaboration, and programme and policy development.
- Occupational therapists need to further develop research, policy, practice, and education initiatives concerning the role of occupational therapy in CBR.

Introduction

Sheona comes from a small village in the Philippines. She has spina bifida. As a young girl, it was generally considered in her community that she would need to be 'looked after' for the rest of her life, and that education and expensive rehabilitation services and equipment would be wasted on her. She had gone to primary school, but was withdrawn to 'provide what little help she could' in the family home, allowing her mother to earn much needed money by working in the fields. With limited mobility, she spent each day inside the home alone. This was her future – until a local community-based rehabilitation worker began working with Sheona and her family. Over time, Sheona accessed equipment to improve her mobility, small business training, and a US$100 loan to start a small general stall in her village. Today, she is an esteemed member of her family and community. She returned to school and finished her education; the shop has expanded and she now employs both her parents. The extra family income has been used to ensure her siblings continue in school instead of leaving early to work in the fields. Sheona is now at university studying to be a human rights lawyer. She wants to contribute to a better world for *all* disabled people.

Sheona's story reminds us what can be achieved through an investment and belief in the dignity and rights of all people to participate in everyday community life. Ideally, Sheona's story would be one of many amongst the estimated 10% of the world's population, or 650 million people, that live with an impairment (United Nations 2006b). Sadly though, it is estimated that only 2% of disabled people have

access to the rehabilitation services they need (Despouy 1993).

Community-based rehabilitation (CBR) emerged in the 1970s as an attempt to better meet the needs of the large population of disabled people in the developing world (World Health Organisation 1978). Since this time, the term CBR has been used to describe a wide range of services targeting disabled people in the community, including, for example, medical outreach services, self-help groups, vocational training, and health-promotion programmes. This led to confusion over what constitutes CBR. Recognising this, a joint position paper was issued by the International Labour Office, United Nations Educational Scientific and Cultural Organisation and World Health Organisation in 1994 and revised in 2004, clarifying the CBR strategy (International Labour Office et al 2004). In that paper CBR was defined as 'a strategy within general community development for the rehabilitation, equalisation of opportunities, poverty reduction and social inclusion of all people with disabilities. CBR is implemented through the combined efforts of people with disabilities themselves, their families, organisations and communities, and the relevant governmental and non-governmental health, education, vocational, social and other services' (p. 2).

CBR was founded in an attempt to meet the needs of disabled people, most of whom live in what have contentiously been termed 'third world' or 'developing' countries (Helander 2000, Thomas & Thomas 2002, World Health Organisation 1978). In this chapter, we employ the increasingly used term 'majority world' to describe this context. We do so for two key reasons. First, numerous so-called 'developing' countries in which CBR may be practiced, continue to slip further down the development index (United Nations 2005). Second, we believe 'majority world' highlights the fact that the vast majority of the world's population (including 80% of disabled people) live in this context (United Nations 2006b).

For the purpose of this chapter, we will focus on CBR in the context of the majority world. However, it is acknowledged that disabled people living in more 'developed' nations can also be subject to the conditions that CBR seeks to address, such as poverty, a lack of access to services, and compromises of basic human rights, including the inability to freely move about their community or access employment.

Understanding community-based rehabilitation: an evolving strategy

CBR is an evolving concept that seeks to promote the participation of disabled people in everyday community life. It continues to evolve from a medical, service-based orientation to a community development strategy grounded in the equalisation of opportunities for disabled people through collaborative programmes focused on human rights, poverty reduction and inclusion (International Labour Office et al 2004, Thomas & Thomas 2003).

In this section, we explore the origins and motivations for the early development of CBR. Despite the recent reconceptualisation of CBR, in practice, many CBR programmes continue to reflect traditional medically framed approaches (Disabled People's International 2005). Accordingly, occupational therapists may still encounter programmes reflecting these early approaches. For occupational therapists to play a continued role in the evolution and realisation of CBR, we must be able to identify and understand the different expressions of CBR in practice and the potential roles we can play.

Early community-based rehabilitation

Early CBR was conceptualised and evolved primarily as an extension of the primary health care system to inexpensively deliver services, particularly in areas in the majority world where there were inadequate resources for comprehensive institutional services (Helander 2000, Thomas & Thomas 2002, 2003, World Health Organisation 1978, 1989). Hospitals and rehabilitation centres were considered costly to establish and maintain, and were primarily located in large cities providing often prohibitively expensive services. Services remained inaccessible for poorer families, and those living in rural and remote areas. CBR covered a far wider geographical and socio-economic group at a reduced cost by shifting the responsibility of service delivery to minimally qualified 'non-professionals' including families and other volunteers from the community (Thomas & Thomas 2002). Geographical distances and costs meant that, wherever possible, local resources were used to make the required equipment. For example, buckets and sandbags may be used to make supportive seating and bamboo poles used to make parallel bars for practicing mobility exercises (Werner 1998).

Despite this shift in responsibility to the community, the role and location of professionals like occupational therapists did not change drastically with the advent of CBR. 'Community' was mostly understood to be a geographical location for service delivery that specialists like occupational therapists visit. Occupational therapists mostly continued to work from centres or institutions, 'reaching out' to communities to provide services such as basic training and support of CBR workers, or home-therapy programmes for parents and CBR workers to implement. Programmes were primarily initiated within communities by external agencies in what is known as a 'top-down approach' (Thomas & Thomas 2002).

A medical understanding of disability framed activities and goals of traditional CBR (Thomas & Thomas 2003). Accordingly, professionals remained the experts and so determined the needs of disabled persons. The programmes implemented by community workers were based on the assessments and recommendations of professionals. These programmes focused primarily on addressing impairments of the person's mind or body as a means of facilitating their participation in everyday community life. Therefore, interventions were mainly positioned within the health sector. The role of occupational therapists largely focused on prescription of direct therapy programmes and adaptive equipment, for implementation in homes, schools, and workplaces by local community workers.

In an international review of CBR that preceded the 2004 joint position paper, it was highlighted that most CBR programmes continued to primarily focus on health, and often exclusively on physical rehabilitation (World Health Organisation 2003). Though some CBR programmes were found to also focus on education and income generation, these activities were often run in isolation to health programmes. This vertical, individual sector approach was considered counter to addressing the multidimensional need for achieving well-being in all aspects of life. Furthermore, disabled persons themselves have highlighted that the continued medical focus ignored the human rights, and social and economic needs of disabled people and their families (Disabled People's International 2005). Occupational needs of individuals have been addressed in a variety of ways in CBR, by, for example, reducing impairments through rehabilitation, or facilitating access to vocational training and income-generation schemes. However, many CBR programmes focused on only a limited number of facets that affect occupation. In the context of disabling policies, systems, physical and sociocultural environments, many people continued to experience occupational marginalisation, including limited engagement in social events, leadership, politics and, importantly, decisions that impact on their lives (Wilcock & Townsend 2000). Realising this, many services, like NORFIL in Practice Scenario 22.1, have begun to reorient and broaden their CBR activities to more comprehensively support the well-being and development of disabled people and their wider community. This reflects the re-conceptualisation of CBR outlined below.

Practice Scenario 22.1 Evolution of CBR in Philippines

NORFIL Foundation Inc. is a non-profit, non-government organisation in the Philippines which has served disabled women, children and young people, their families and communities since 1983. NORFIL has a CBR team that comprises occupational therapists, social workers, physiotherapists, teachers, parents, and government employed day-care workers who volunteer time to identify disabled children in their communities.

Francis (10 years), the youngest boy in a poor family of nine children, lives in a farming village 14 kilometres from town. His father is a jeepney/taxi driver, whose daily earnings are the only source of livelihood. Francis has cerebral palsy with epilepsy, autistic-like behaviour and for many years lay in his bed all day.

Francis was referred by one of NORFIL's volunteers, and an occupational therapist and social worker visited him at home. An assessment was carried out and a home programme was developed and monitored by a NORFIL community worker. However, Francis' parents needed to work to provide for the family and pay for various medicines for Francis so their time at home was limited. Francis' slow motor-skill development caused his family to doubt the benefit of the home programme and, as a result, it was not regularly implemented.

NORFIL's staff realised that focusing on children, such as Francis, in isolation only partly improved their opportunities to be actively involved in the family or community. Therefore, NORFIL expanded their CBR programme to include building strong partnerships with local government units, support and educate parents and the community through counselling, rehabilitation training, community awareness, financial support, linkages to the existing support groups and also through supporting the capacity development of parent groups to advocate for their rights and the rights of their children.

With extra support such as education, counselling, regular follow-up home visits by the community worker, periodic visits by the therapist, and participation in the local parent support group programmes, Francis' family began to see him develop his motor skills. His mother began to implement the home therapy programme daily and his father worked with his neighbours to produce adaptive devices. These devices included a high-back wooden chair for supported sitting, and a pair of bamboo parallel bars for supported standing and walking. This partnership between Francis' father and his neighbours helped to raise awareness and challenge assumptions in the wider community about the value and rights of disabled people to be active members of their community. The commitment by Francis' parents to his occupational skill development resulted in the family becoming eligible to receive a medication subsidy by NORFIL. This subsidy alleviated the financial pressures felt by his parents.

Three and a half years on, Francis stands and walks with support, plays with objects, eats biscuits and drinks without assistance. His parents involve him in community events and are exploring options for Francis to gain an education. They now support and encourage the involvement of other parents of disabled children in community programmes. These positive changes in the community have contributed to local governments considering employing therapists to assist with developing disability policies and programmes in the Philippines.

The occupational therapist's role developed over the three and a half years of Francis' therapy programme. This role development reflects the evolution of CBR as outlined in Table 22.1. Initially, the therapist's role involved carrying out an assessment in the family home, explaining the problem areas to his parents, developing with them a home programme and educating Francis' parents and community volunteers on cerebral palsy, how to modify the home programme to develop occupational skills, and how to record their observations after each session. In line with the evolution of CBR and NORFIL's shift to a more comprehensive CBR programme, the therapist's approach to work shifted to become more community focused by:

- linking the family to the program and services of the local government unit

- linking Francis' parents to the existing parent support group
- identifying opportunities to alleviate the financial burdens faced by the family, such as the medication subsidy
- assisting the parent support group as requested through contributing technical knowledge and skills to the development and implementation of advocacy and education programmes.

This role shift enabled the therapist to be a resource for the wider community.

Community-based rehabilitation re-conceptualised: A community development strategy

The joint position paper on CBR identifies CBR as a *development strategy* that both improves the lives of disabled people as well as promotes the development of the community in which they live, thus also promoting an enabling environment for disabled people (International Labour Office et al 2004). Some key conceptual changes underlying this evolution are outlined below and summarised in Table 22.1.

CBR as a community development strategy suggests that the participation of disabled people is an issue for both disabled people and the wider community (Thomas & Thomas 2002). It thus broadens

from a focus on individuals to the broader community in which they live. It also promotes community participation and ownership of programmes and policies. Reflecting this, the key objectives of CBR are to (International Labour Office et al 2004, pp. 3–4):

1. ensure that disabled people are able to maximise their physical and mental abilities, to access regular services and opportunities, and to become active contributors to the community and society at large

2. activate communities to promote and protect the human rights of disabled people through changes within the community, for example, by removing barriers to participation.

Reflecting the World Health Organisation's (WHO) reorientation to disability as a social issue, CBR now frames disability within a social and rights-based model (International Labour Office et al 2004). This approach recognises that both medical impairment and social issues need to be considered in activities addressing disability (International Labour Office et al 2004, Nagata 2007, World Health Organisation 2001). This notion of disability is based on, and clearly explained in the International Classification of Functioning, Disability and Health (ICF), where the emphasis is on function, activity and environment (World Health Organisation 2001). In addition to factors of body structure and function, the ICF describes five environmental

Table 22.1 Evolution of community-based rehabilitation concepts

Concept	Traditional CBR	'New' CBR
Disability model	Medical	Social model; human rights
Rehabilitation concept	Primarily health sector; vertical sectors approach	Comprehensive, cross sector
Primary implementer	Individual project/organisation	Multi-sectoral programme; Networks between government and non-government stakeholders
Development approach	Needs based – identifying and meeting service needs	Rights based – identifying rights and empowerment of community to exercise and realise these rights; poverty reduction
Drivers/ownership	Professionals	Disabled people and wider community
Practice approach	Specialist and individual needs of disabled people	Inclusion through twin track – specialist and mainstream
Understanding of community	Geographical location for services	Wider community relationships are inclusive of disabled people (inclusive society)

factors that can limit activities or restrict participation: services, systems and policies; products and technology; natural environment and human-made changes to it; support and relationships; and attitudes (World Health Organisation 2001). Whilst the term 'occupation' is not used in these key WHO publications, the concept is clearly present.

CBR now recognises the importance of socioeconomic development and poverty alleviation to promote the social inclusion of disabled people. There is an irrefutable link between poverty and disability, with the World Bank estimating that 20% of the world's poorest people have an impairment (Elwan 1999) and there is a growing literature which explores this relationship (see for example Action on Disability and Development India 2001, Beresford 1996, Elwan 1999, Inclusion International 2006, International Labour Office et al 2004, Nagata 2007). If you live in poverty, you are more prone to be exposed to conditions that contribute to disability, such as poor nutrition and limited access to health services, poor housing and sanitation, and unsafe working and living conditions. Conversely, a person with a disability and their family face significant barriers to accessing rehabilitation, education, and employment that can reduce poverty.

CBR practitioners, including occupational therapists, can help ensure disabled people are included in mainstream development and poverty reduction initiatives through advocacy, strengthening partnerships with mainstream development initiatives, like education, health and leadership programmes, as well as participation in the development of national poverty reduction strategies and inclusive development policies and practices (Handicap International & Christoffel-Blindenmission 2006). They also play a role at the grass roots level through the implementation of, for example, quality health and livelihood activities in their community programmes.

Human rights are now emphasised as the central tenant of CBR. This is endorsed in the World Federation of Occupational Therapists position paper on CBR, which states that a core principle of occupational therapy is the right of all people to 'develop their capacity and power to construct their own destiny through occupation' (World Federation of Occupational Therapists 2004b, p. 1). CBR seeks to promote the right for disabled people to participate as equal citizens in all aspects of society (International Labour Office et al 2004).

CBR emphasises that both men and women have equal rights to participate in, for example, school,

work, social, economic, religious, and political activities. CBR seeks to advocate for and promote the application of these rights in government policies, and thus frames and supports the implementation of key international statements including the UN Standard Rules on Equalisation of Opportunities for Persons with a Disability (United Nations 1994) and, importantly, the United Nations' Convention on the Rights of Persons with Disabilities (United Nations 2006a).

Importantly, the 2003 review of CBR recognised the need to increase the participation of disabled people in CBR activities (World Health Organisation 2003). Specifically, disabled people must be present in decision-making bodies at all levels, including taking active roles in the political system as citizens and candidates. Disabled Peoples International (2005) has noted that despite these statements, disabled people have largely remained outside of decision-making processes. Practice Scenario 22.2 describes a disabled people's organisation that is adopting the CBR strategy and has disabled people at the core of development. Though initially focused on advice for individuals, this scenario highlights occupational therapists' increasing role in providing training and technical assistance in this organisation.

Practice Scenario 22.2 The role of disabled people's organisations in CBR

Bangladesh Protibandhi Kallyan Somity (BPKS), established in 1985, is a non-governmental organisation of disabled people. BPKS uses an approach it calls Persons with Disabilities' Self-Initiatives to Development (PSID). PSID creates opportunities for disabled people to design and implement their own initiatives which enable change in their lives and contribute to the overall development of the community. This approach reflects their integral role in applying the CBR strategy.

BPKS works to advance disabled people's organisations (DPO) from the grassroots to the national level. Organisations developed through PSID are owned and managed by disabled people and serve as the local focal point for service delivery, decision-making, training, and advocacy for disabled people in the area. These local DPO provide disabled people with much-needed basic services, such as therapy, health referrals, accessible sanitary facilities and assistive devices. They also establish and maintain mechanisms whereby disabled people implement and make decisions about the activities of the DPO. This provides disabled people with a voice and visibility in their community, which is a marked contrast to a society in which disabled people are largely confined to their homes and unable to participate.

Through PSID disabled people are now able to access vitally needed training in areas such as income-generation and economic management, and micro-credit loans, either from their DPO or through mainstream mechanisms to establish themselves as productive members of their families and communities. Advocacy at the national level has enabled disabled people to be central to the development and implementation of pro-disability legislation and services in Bangladesh, including areas such as employment, financial services, and an accessible infrastructure.

Occupational therapists have only been involved in BPKS since 2002. However, they are playing an increasing role in the organisation by providing substantial technical and occupational knowledge to assist programme implementation. Examples include:

- facilitating the increased occupation and, therefore, productivity of disabled individuals
- transferring therapy skills to local community workers to increase the coverage of therapy in the country
- providing technical advice to BPKS and other non-government organisations in the areas of accessibility, assistive devices, education, health and vocational opportunities for disabled people.

CBR now requires a multi-sectoral and multi-level collaboration in order to support the community, address the individual needs of disabled people, strengthen the role of disabled people's organisations and promote sustainability of CBR initiatives (International Labour Office et al 2004, Stineman 2002). This can include, for example, involvement of health, education, employment and labour, government and non-government, the media, sports and recreations groups, religious groups, and, centrally, disabled people's organisations (Disabled People's International 2005, International Labour Office et al 2004, Stineman 2002, World Health Organisation 2003, 2007a). Collaboration is needed from the national to the community levels of each sector to ensure consistent policy and practices, and appropriate referral services. Collaboration at each level

between the various ministries, non-government organisations and private sectors helps ensure an inclusive society is promoted in a comprehensive and coordinated way. Practice Scenario 22.3, describes a cross-sector and multi-level CBR initiative in Pakistan in which occupational therapists have been involved at various levels.

Practice Scenario 22.3 Multi-sector and multi-level engagement in CBR

In October 2005, an earthquake in the Karakorum Range of Northern Pakistan left 79,000 people dead, and thousands of people with physical injuries and trauma. Medical facilities were destroyed and people were evacuated to cities for medical and rehabilitative services. Limited existing services saw hundreds of injured people in vulnerable situations, cared for in makeshift centres and contracting secondary complications, including pressure sores and infections. Occupational therapists worked to train local volunteers in basic mobility and daily living skills, but this was not enough.

Rehabilitation workers, including occupational therapists, began to advocate for the inclusion of disabled people at all levels of society. Key stakeholders, including disabled people's organisations, allied health professionals, government organisations, non-government organisations, and community-based organisations, met for consultations to find ways to address the vulnerability and exclusion of disabled people. Stakeholders agreed that CBR was the most effective strategy to ensure the active participation of disabled people in community life. One such stakeholder, Handicap International, has developed CBR services in Northern Pakistan in partnership with the community, service providers and the Government of Pakistan.

Handicap International in partnership with community-based organisations, disabled people's organisations operate four 'Resource and Information Centres'. The aim of these centres is to:

- build capacity of community-level organisations to identify disabled people, provide basic therapy and coordinate referrals to rehabilitation services
- facilitate access to mainstream education and livelihood opportunities for disabled people
- provide technical advice for accessible construction of housing and public buildings

- raise awareness of communities regarding disability issues and the rights of disabled people
- build capacity of local disabled people to form self-help groups for advocacy, including provision of small grants
- offer a library of disability and development knowledge resources
- build partnerships between disabled people, civil society organisations and government for enhanced information flow and comprehensive service delivery.

Occupational therapists assist in the development, coordination, and continual improvement of information and resources. Facilitating community access to the centres and establishing links between community members and organisations is also a key role.

Partnerships with key rehabilitation services were formed and occupational therapists and other stakeholders facilitated curriculum development and training for community workers to assist social change and provide adequate services. Consequently, the capacity of service providers to deliver quality, comprehensive rehabilitation services has increased.

Handicap International and the government of Pakistan are strengthening the National Institute of Rehabilitation Medicine (a state-owned institute responsible for the provision of tertiary-level services, human resource development as well as development and implementation of national policies and strategies on disability) by:

- developing a strategy for the coordination, monitoring and evaluation of the CBR programme
- developing effective communication pathways which ensure the rights of disabled people are addressed within policy development
- promoting collaboration between all members of society.

Therapists' skills in networking, advocacy, and awareness raising, as well as service delivery are critical in this ongoing process.

The WHO 2003 CBR review recognised that guidelines were needed to ensure the realisation of this joint understanding of CBR in practice. Accordingly, WHO is working with key stakeholders to develop comprehensive guidelines for initiating a CBR programme and strengthening an existing CBR programme (World Health Organisation 2005, 2007a). These guidelines, in draft format at the time of writing this chapter, are scheduled for publication at the end of 2009. The guidelines highlight five key, overlapping and interdependent principles that inform and affect the development of CBR programmes: inclusion, participation, sustainability, empowerment, and self-advocacy (Table 22.2). These principles are outlined below, drawing on a World Health Organisation (2006) report outlining the preparation of the CBR guidelines.

These principles underpin the CBR matrix developed by WHO to illustrate the components that combine to form a CBR strategy, including health, education, livelihoods, empowerment and social components and their comprising elements (Figure 22.1). An effective CBR programme may contain these elements depending on local circumstances (World Health Organisation 2005). It is not sequential, but rather a series of options from which practitioners can select. Therefore, any one programme or practitioner will likely only address some of the components. A CBR programme may start with a particular element, gradually expanding to encompass other elements through programme expansion and networking. For example, in Practice Scenario 22.2, BPKS initially addressed vocational skills training for livelihood development and later expanded services to also provide financial and employment assistance to assist the income generation of the

Table 22.2 Principles that inform and affect the development of community-based rehabilitation programmes (World Health Organisation 2006)

Inclusion	Coverage of all types of impairments and to removing all kinds of disabling barriers, including environmental, physical, technological and attitudinal barriers that block access to mainstream political, social, cultural and economic activities
Participation	Active involvement of disabled people in all aspects of CBR programmes from policy to implementation and evaluation
Sustainability	Enduring benefits of the programme – in terms of future generations and independence from the initiating agencies
Empowerment	Local people, particularly disabled people make programme decisions and control resources. It requires capacity building of technical staff, managers and CBR workers
Self-advocacy	Collective notion that disabled people and their families consistently and centrally define the goals of the programme

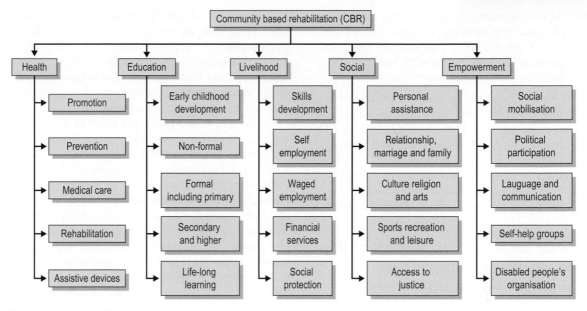

Figure 22.1 • The CBR matrix

disabled people's organisation members and their own members.

Though many programmes that align with the original concept of CBR still exist (i.e. focusing mainly on medical rehabilitation), others are moving to this more comprehensive CBR strategy. The compatibility of CBR and occupational therapy philosophies ideally positions occupational therapists to play an important role in the realisation of CBR in practice.

Occupational therapy and community-based rehabilitation

Many occupational therapists have noted the synergy between features of occupational therapy and CBR (Fransen 2005, Lysack 1995, Sakellariou et al 2006, Thomas & Thomas 1996, Twible & Henley 2000, World Federation of Occupational Therapists 2004b, Ying Yin Chui 1998):

1. 'Occupation' is at the centre of occupational therapy practice (World Federation of Occupational Therapists 2004a) and so it aligns strongly with CBR which is concerned with daily life and participation in activity.
2. Both occupational therapy and CBR emphasise the importance of the environment as it interacts with individuals to inform occupation (Imms 2006).

3. The right to occupation and opportunities, whilst respecting and valuing differing occupational capacities and meanings (Wilcock & Townsend 2000), is also fundamental to both occupational therapy and CBR (Clark et al 1991, Creek 1998). Indeed, the World Federation of Occupational Therapists (WFOT) promotes CBR as the strategy through which to facilitate access to occupation for all (Sakellariou et al 2006, World Federation of Occupational Therapists 2004b). While occupational therapy has historically had a medical intervention focus, there has been a conceptual revival of socially and rights-driven elements emerging in concepts like occupational justice (Jenkins 1998, Thibeault 2006, Townsend 1993, Townsend & Wilcock 2003).

4. Collaboration through enabling and empowering relationships is fundamental to successful CBR and occupational therapy practice. This includes sharing information and expertise and taking time to understand the story of the person or the wider community (Clark 1993). Both CBR and occupational therapy view the person or community as the central driver of this collaborative process, considering this is essential to a meaningful, purposeful, and sustainable impact (Jenkins 1998, Wittman & Velde 2001).

5. There is an emphasis on creatively adapting to the context in both occupational therapy and CBR (Fransen 2005). This includes designing programmes, which align with local priorities, needs and resources.

Overall, CBR could be said to reflect what occupational therapists have described as 'community-built' practice (Wittman & Velde 2001). That is: practice using collaborative and interactive approaches, based on principles of community empowerment, and addressing the individual, social and environmental factors affecting health and participation, in a person- and community-focused way.

Roles, skills and opportunities for occupational therapists in community-based rehabilitation

Fransen (2005) reviewed the literature to identify five current roles for occupational therapists working in CBR:

1. Transfer of rehabilitation knowledge and skills

2. The provision of direct therapy

3. Referral services

4. Programme development and implementation

5. Facilitating collaboration.

These and other roles are illustrated in the Practice Scenarios and explored in turn below.

Transfer of rehabilitation knowledge and skills

Occupational therapists are involved in the transfer of basic rehabilitation skills to community members, and the creation of positive attitudes through training, education and supervision (Fransen 2005). Occupational therapists' unique skills in facilitating occupational engagement could play a crucial role in the realisation of CBR. Sharing and transferring skills in addressing impairments, and adapting activities and environments to facilitate participation is vital. Transferring knowledge to others needs to be recognised by occupational therapists as a legitimate professional activity in its own right. Recent research by WFOT suggests that some occupational therapists have already identified this as a key role they play in CBR; however, the training they provided was primarily focused on addressing impairments

(Sakellariou et al 2006). Vanneste (1997) highlighted that with the re-conceptualisation of CBR as a community development strategy, it is important that traditional rehabilitation skills like these are still transferred, but that community development skills in, for example, advocacy and community motivation, are also developed and refined.

Occupational therapists will need to develop or improve the skills required to be competent in transferring their knowledge and skills. Though 'teaching a skill' is not unfamiliar to occupational therapists, competent transfer of skills will require occupational therapists to understand and apply concepts of adult learning, including how to train trainers, working with groups and populations, and the preparation and delivery of culturally appropriate training materials. Ensuring the application of this knowledge in the community will also require occupational therapists to have advanced skills in supervising, mentoring, and coaching (Fransen 2005, O'Toole & McConkey 1998, Thomas & Thomas 1996, Twible & Henley 2000).

The provision of direct therapy

Occupational therapists facilitate the participation of disabled people through the provision of direct therapy when it is needed. This therapy can include the provision of rehabilitative equipment, and the teaching of skills in advocacy and community awareness training (Fransen 2005). The WFOT research project into CBR noted that direct therapy was one of the key roles that occupational therapists were playing in CBR (Sakellariou et al 2006). This encompasses activities that seek to prevent impairment as well as promoting occupational engagement through the programmes designed. Though more consistent with traditional CBR, occupational therapists may still be called on to provide these services. However, this raises questions of sustainability if occupational therapists remain the sole providers of services without ensuring that their skills are transferred to the community.

Referral services

Occupational therapists are also involved in the provision of referral services and guidance to help people negotiate their way through and articulate their rights and needs within service systems (Fransen 2005). Within a multi-sector and multi-level CBR strategy, this requires occupational therapists to network with and have a good working knowledge of government and non-government providers across multiple sectors.

Programme development and implementation

Fransen (2005) noted occupational therapists in CBR can facilitate the establishment, development and implementation of programmes at government and community levels. Practice Scenario 22.3 strongly illustrates this. Significantly, CBR now challenges us to be directed by disabled people and their families in all stages of design, implementation and evaluation of CBR initiatives (Disabled People's International 2005, World Health Organisation 2006, 2007b). This requires a shift in approach from 'professional as expert' to one where we act as resources when invited (Bury 2005). It will require effective listening skills, and tools and practices for accessing and identifying community needs, priorities and resources (Jenkins 1998, Kumar 2002, Tjandrakusuma 1995).

Facilitating collaboration

Occupational therapists can also play a role in ensuring effective and efficient collaboration among the many stakeholders in CBR (Fransen 2005). This is a critical role occupational therapists can play within the multi-sectoral, multi-level CBR strategy and is illustrated in community Practice Scenario 22.3. The WFOT CBR data collection project, which surveyed many occupational therapists who have worked in CBR, raises some concerns about whether they are actually playing this collaborative role, given few people surveyed mentioned involvement with other stakeholders (Sakellariou et al 2006). This challenges us to identify, listen and learn from others involved in CBR (Hartley et al 2002).

Other roles

In addition to the five roles mentioned, occupational therapists can undertake roles in evaluating CBR and contributing to the evidence base about the impact of the CBR approach at individual, community and government levels (Bury 2005, Kenny 1999). The need to develop an evidence base through evaluation and research of CBR at policy and practice levels has been well recorded (see for example, Boyce & Ballantyne 2000, Disabled People's International 2005, Stineman 2002, Thomas & Thomas 2003, World

Health Organisation 2003). Despite this, little progress has been made in developing this evidence base (Hartley et al 2002). Research is also needed to better understand the role of occupational therapists themselves in CBR (Sakellariou et al 2006). Occupational therapists could be involved in research and evaluation, ideally employing participatory evaluation and research strategies that ensure disabled people, their families, and the wider community are involved (Cockburn & Trentham 2002, Guijt & Shah 1998, Hartley et al 2002, Schneider et al 2002, World Health Organisation 2003).

As demonstrated in all three Practice Scenarios in the Philippines, Pakistan and Bangladesh, occupational therapists play a role in advocacy both with and for the equal participation of disabled people. This includes lobbying government and organisations for more disability-inclusive policies and service systems, and, preferably, contributing to the development of both. Through their interactions with government and broader communities, occupational therapists in CBR are involved in shaping and developing, for example, health, education, and employment systems and policies that promote the sustainable and active participation of disabled people in all aspects of community life.

Conclusion

CBR and occupational therapy are philosophically aligned. Clearly some knowledge and skills required within the evolving CBR strategy are already part of occupational therapy. Other roles present challenges to occupational therapists to develop and foster new skills. Hartley and colleagues (2002) highlighted that professionals involved in CBR need to change their attitudes – to be more humble about their achievements, more respectful, acknowledging that they can learn from others, and more willing to share their knowledge and skills with others.

We began this chapter with Sheona's story. Realisation of the CBR strategy in practice can help facilitate a more inclusive society for all disabled people, working towards Sheona's story becoming common rather than exceptional. The concepts and skills underlying occupational therapy practice ensure we are ideally positioned to continue to play a significant role in the development and implementation of CBR, sharing our philosophy with communities to embed some of the principles of CBR discussed in this chapter.

References

Action on Disability and Development India (2001). *Building abilities: a handbook to work with people with disability*, (1st ed). Bangalore, Books for Change.

Beresford, P. (1996). Poverty and disabled people: challenging dominant debates and policies. *Disability and Society*, 11(4), 553–567.

Boyce, W. & Ballantyne, S. (2000). Developing CBR through evaluation. In: M. Thomas & M. J. Thomas (Eds) *Selected Readings in CBR: Series 1*. Bangalore, National Printing Press.

Bury, T. (2005). Primary health care and community based rehabilitation: implications for physical therapy. *Asia Pacific Disability Rehabilitation Journal*, 16(2), 29–65.

Clark, F. (1993). Occupation embedded in a real life: interweaving occupational science and occupational therapy – 1993. Eleanor Clarke Slagle Lecture. *American Journal of Occupational Therapy*, 47(12), 1067–1078.

Clark, F., Parham, D., Carlson, M. et al (1991). Occupational science: academic innovation in the service of occupational therapy's future. *American Journal of Occupational Therapy*, 45(4), 300–310.

Cockburn, L. & Trentham, B. (2002). Participatory action research: integrating community occupational therapy research and practice. *Canadian Journal of Occupational Therapy*, 69(1), 20–30.

Creek, J. (1998). Purposeful activity. In: J. Creek (Ed.). *Occupational therapy: new perspectives*. (pp. 16–28). London, Whurr Publishers.

Despouy, L. (1993). *Human rights and disabled persons*. Geneva, Centre for Human Rights and United Nations.

Disabled People's International (2005). *Disabled Peoples International position paper on community based rehabilitation (CBR)*. Online. Available: http://www.aifo.it/english/resources/online/books/cbr/reviewofcbr/DPI%20on%20CBR.pdf. Accessed 2 Aug 2007.

Elwan, A. (1999). *Poverty and disability: a background paper for the World Development Report*. World Bank.

Fransen, H. (2005). Challenges for occupational therapy in community based rehabilitation: occupation in a community development approach to handicap in development. In: F. Kronenberg, S. Simo'Algado & N. Pollard (Eds) *Occupational therapy without borders: Learning from the spirit of survivors*. (pp. 166–182). Sydney, Elsevier Churchill Livingstone.

Guijt, I. & Shah, M. K. (1998). Waking up to power, conflict and process. In: I. Guijt & M. K. Shah (Eds) *The myth of community: Gender issues in participatory development*. (pp. 1–23). London, Intermediate Technology Publications.

Handicap International, Christoffel-Blindenmission (2006). *Making Poverty reduction strategy papers (PRSP) inclusive*. Handicap International eV & Christoffel Blindenmission Deutschland eV, Germany.

Hartley, S., Kisanji, J. & Nganwa, A. (2002). Professionals participation in CBR programs. In: S. Hartley (Ed.) *CBR: A participatory strategy in Africa*. (pp. 72–85). London, The Centre for International Child Health.

Helander, E. (2000). Guest Editorial: 25 years of community based rehabilitation. *Asia Pacific Disability Rehabilitation Journal*, 11(1), 12–14.

Imms, C. (2006). The international classification of functioning, disability and health: they're talking our language. *Australian Occupational Therapy Journal*, 53, 65–66.

Inclusion International (2006). *Fact sheet on poverty and disability*. Online. Available: http://www.inclusion-international.org/site_uploads/11223821811255806183.pdf. Accessed 3 Jun 2007.

International Labour Office, United Nations Educational Scientific and Cultural Organisation, World Health Organisation (2004). *CBR: a strategy for rehabilitation, equalisation of opportunities, poverty reduction and social inclusion of disabled people* (position paper). Switzerland, World Health Organisation.

Jenkins, M. (1998). Shifting ground or sifting sand? In: J. Creek (Ed.). *Occupational therapy: new perspectives*. (pp. 29–46). London, Whurr Publishers.

Kenny, S. (1999). *Developing communities for the future*. Melbourne, Nelson ITP.

Kumar, S. (2002). *Methods for community participation: a complete guide for practitioners*. New Delhi, Vistaar Publications.

Lysack, C. L. (1995). Community participation and community based rehabilitation: an Indonesian case study. *Occupational Therapy International*, 2, 149–165.

Nagata, K. K. (2007). Perspectives on disability, poverty and development in the Asian region. *Asia Pacific Disability Rehabilitation Journal*, 18(1), 3–19.

O'Toole, B. & McConkey, R. (1998). A training strategy for personnel working in developing countries. *International Journal of Rehabilitation Research*, 21, 311–321.

Sakellariou, D., Pollard, N., Fransen, H. et al (2006). *Reporting on the WFOT–CBR Master Project Pan: the Data Collection subproject*. Online. Available: http://www.wfot.org.office_files/CBR%20Paper_301106%20Data%20Collection.pdf. Accessed 2 Aug 2007.

Schneider, M., Loeb, M., Mireembe, J. et al (2002). Collecting disability statistics: a participatory strategy. In: S. Hartley (Ed.). *CBR: a participatory strategy in Africa*. (pp. 172–184). London, Centre for International Child Health.

Stineman, M. G. (2002). Guiding principles for evaluating and reporting on worldwide community-based rehabilitation programs (report to inspire dialogue). Philadelphia, University of Pennsylvania.

Thibeault, R. (2006). Globalisation, universities and the future of occupational therapy: dispatches for the majority world. *Australian Occupational Therapy Journal*, 53, 159–165.

Thomas, M. & Thomas, M. (2002). Some controversies in community based rehabilitation. In: S. Hartley (Ed.). *CBR: a participatory strategy in Africa.* (pp. 13–25). London, Centre for International Child Health.

Thomas, M. & Thomas, M. J. (1996). *The value of physiotherapy and occupational therapy in community based rehabilitation: summary of discussion led by E Henley & R Twible.* Online. Available: http://www.dinf.ne.jp/doc/english/asia/resource/apdrj/z13fm0100/zl13fm0105.htm. Accessed 23 Jun 2007.

Thomas, M. & Thomas, M. J. (Eds) (2002). *Disability and rehabilitation issues in South Asia.* Bangalore, National Printing Press.

Thomas, M. & Thomas, M. J. (Eds) (2003). Manual for CBR planners. Bangalore, National Printing Press.

Tjandrakusuma, H. (1995). Participatory rural appraisal in community based rehabilitation: an experiment in central Java, Indonesia. *ActionAid Disability News,* 6(1), 6–10.

Townsend, E. (1993). Occupational therapy's social vision: Murial Driver Lecture. *Canadian Journal of Occupational Therapy,* 60(4), 174–184.

Townsend, E. & Wilcock, A. (2003). Occupational justice. In: C. Christiansen & E. Townsend (Eds). *Introduction to occupation: the art and science of living.* (pp. 243–273). Thorofare, NJ, Prentice Hall.

Twible, R. & Henley, E. (2000). Preparing occupational therapists and physiotherapists for community based rehabilitation. In: M. Thomas & M. J. Thomas (Eds) *Selected readings in CBR.* Bangalore, National Printing Press.

United Nations (1994). *The standard rules on the equalisation of opportunities for persons with disabilities.* New York, United Nations.

United Nations (2005). *Human development report 2005 – international cooperation at a crossroads: Aid, trade and security in an unequal world.* New York, United Nations.

United Nations (2006a). *Convention on the rights of persons with disabilities.* New York, United Nations.

United Nations (2006b). *Some facts about persons with disabilities.* Online. Available: http://www.un.org/disabilities/convention/pdfs/factsheet.pdf. Accessed 3 Jun 2007.

Vanneste, G. (1997). CBR in Africa: a critical review of the emerging issues. *Asia Pacific Disability Rehabilitation Journal,* 8(2), 34–37.

Werner, D. (1998). *Nothing about us without us: developing innovative technologies for, by and with disabled persons.* Palo Alto, Healthwrights.

Wilcock, A. & Townsend, E. (2000). Occupation terminology interactive dialogue: Occupational justice. *Journal of Occupational Science,* 7(2), 84–86.

Wittman, P. P. & Velde, B. P. (2001). Occupational therapy in the community: what, why and how? *Occupational Therapy in Health Care,* 13(3/4), 1–5.

World Federation of Occupational Therapists (2004a). *Definition of occupational therapy.* Online. Available: http://www.wfot.org.au/office_files/Definition%20of%20OT%20CM(2004).%20Final.pdf. Accessed 3 Aug 2007.

World Federation of Occupational Therapists (2004b). *WFOT position paper on community based rehabilitation.* Online. Available: http://www.wfot.org.au/officefiles/CBRposition%20Final.%20CM(2004).%281%29.pdf. Accessed 17 Mar 2007.

World Health Organisation (1978). *Declaration of Alma Ata.* Online. Available: http://www.aifo.it/ild_sito/cbr/Joint%20Position%20Paper%20Final%20Document.doc. Accessed 2 Jun 2007.

World Health Organisation (1989). *Training in the community for people with disabilities.* Geneva, World Health Organisation.

World Health Organisation (2001). *International classification of functioning, disability and health.* Online. Available: www.who.org.ch/icf. Accessed 26 Nov 2005.

World Health Organisation (2003). *International consultation to review community-based rehabilitation (CBR) (report on international consultation).* Geneva, World Health Organisation.

World Health Organisation (2005). *Meeting report on the development of guidelines for community based rehabilitation (CBR) programmes (meeting report).* Geneva, World Health Organisation.

World Health Organisation (2006). *Report on the 4th meeting on development of CBR guidelines.* Online. Available: http://www.who.org. Accessed 3 Aug 2007.

World Health Organisation (2007a). *Community based rehabilitation: United National agencies work with civil society to draw up guidelines for implementing community based rehabilitation programmes.* The WHO Newsletter on Disability and Rehabilitation 3 (May 2007). Geneva, World Health Organisation.

World Health Organisation (2007b). *Draft: WHO/ILO/UNESCO CBR Guidelines – Introduction.* Online. Available: http://www.dcdd.nl. Accessed 3 Aug 2007.

Ying Yin Chui, D. (1998). What is CBR? An implication of the roles of community OT in Hong Kong. *Occupational Therapy in Health Care,* 11(3), 79–97.

Chapter Twenty-Three

Entrepreneurial opportunities in the global community

Marilyn Pattison

CHAPTER CONTENTS

Global influences and directions for
occupational therapy 328

Entrepreneurial practice 329

Inspired by the pioneers of the
profession 329
Being entrepreneurial 331
Working entrepreneurially 332
Forward planning. 332
Strategic intent 332
Marketing. 332

Examples of innovation and
entrepreneurship. 333
Using technology in practice 333
Working as consultants. 334
Focusing on elderly people. 335
Reaching people through the use of
tele-health 335
Disaster preparedness and response. 336

Conclusion. 337

SUMMARY

Occupational therapists need to develop the capacity and power to construct their own destiny. The future of the profession is ours to make and in 20 years' or a hundred years' time our success will be the only reliable measure of how effectively we have taken hold of our vision. By joining together we can take the future, fold it back into the present and make that destiny a reality. An entrepreneurial approach to practice is about thinking outside of the box and finding increasingly innovative ways to deliver services and make a difference to people's lives, health and well-being. In order to do this as occupational therapists we need to challenge ourselves. The aim of this chapter is to provide encouragement and inspiration for therapists to create the future of the profession and direct their own destiny.

KEY POINTS

- Health care globally is undergoing sweeping reform and change.
- Occupational therapists need to be aware and keep up with the ever-changing health care market.
- International trends that will impact on occupational therapists include: demographic and societal change; rising expectations and consumerism; health informatics and telemedicine; new medical technologies; and increasing costs of health and social services provision.
- Occupational therapists need to be more pro-active and face the challenge of promoting their services and the profession to take their rightful place as specialists in health and social care.
- Occupational therapists' expertise lies in their ability to design creative solutions to complex problems, and the integration of multi-level variables into workable, effective and sustainable solutions.
- Occupational therapists need to have a more entrepreneurial approach to their work as entrepreneurship is about inspired creative individuals pursuing opportunities and taking 'calculated' risks.

- There are four types of identifiable entrepreneurs: strategic, calculative, reluctant, and repressed.
- To plan and implement strategies to change the way occupational therapists work they have to engage in strategic intent.
- Entrepreneurship involves a 'leap of faith' – and the commitment to make this leap.

Global influences and directions for occupational therapy

The World Federation of Occupational Therapists (WFOT) is the key international representative of occupational therapists and occupational therapy. The Federation believes that occupational therapy has a valuable contribution to make to the occupational engagement of people; as the engagement in occupation affects the health and well-being of people.

In 2006, the WFOT delegates met to consider and discuss what the future of the occupational therapy profession would be, bearing in mind the evolving nature of the health landscape. This discussion centred on the strong belief that occupational therapists need to understand what is impacting on the health landscape of the future and be ready to meet the changes. As a result of their discussions, the WFOT delegates saw that there would be:

- stronger links between research, education and practice

- broader roles for occupational therapists, including roles at policy levels to influence delivery models and political agendas

- a stronger move away from traditional health, further distancing occupational therapy from the medical model

- a diverse range of people requiring our services, including individuals, groups, communities and society, with occupational therapists working both with healthy, as well as ill, people through health promotion and preventative and rehabilitative healthcare models

- different service delivery models, with a greater emphasis on community-based models, and an increased use of technology, including the use of tele-care and virtual home visits via webcams

- wider and stronger liaison between occupational therapists and other professions outside of health, such as town planners, architects, engineers, and environmentalists, as new and emerging areas of practice continue to be developed.

It was proposed that in the future occupational therapists will become leading advocates for engagement in occupation, enabling people to achieve a good and decent human life.

Occupational therapy, like every other allied health profession, is impacted upon by the changing world and changing health environment. One major impact on the health landscape is the United Nations Millennium Development Goals (United Nations 2005).

The Millennium Development Goals (MDG) are the world's time-bound and quantified targets for addressing extreme poverty in its many dimensions – income poverty, hunger, disease, lack of adequate shelter, and exclusion – while promoting gender equality, education, and environmental sustainability. They reinforce basic human rights, such as the rights of each person on the planet to health, education, shelter, and security. Therapists are being challenged to work towards meeting the MDG. The MDG are listed in Box 23.1.

In addition to the MDG, occupational therapy practice was also influenced by the publication of *Towards a Common Language for Functioning, Disability and Health – International Classification of Functioning, Disability and Health (ICF)* (World Health Organisation 2002a). The ICF provides a

---

Box 23.1

United Nations Millennium Development Goals (United Nations 2005)

Goal 1: Eradicate extreme hunger and poverty

Goal 2: Achieve universal primary education

Goal 3: Promote gender equality and empower women

Goal 4: Reduce child mortality

Goal 5: Improve maternal health

Goal 6: Combat HIV/AIDS, malaria and other diseases

Goal 7: Ensure environmental sustainability

Goal 8: Develop a global partnership for development

standard language and framework for the description of health and health-related states. ICF emphasises health and functioning, rather than disability. Previously, disability began where health ended; once people became impaired, they were in a separate category. The World Health Organisation (WHO) wanted to move on from this kind of thinking and make the ICF a tool for measuring participation in society, no matter what the reason for a person's impairments.

The implications of the ICF for occupational therapy are in reinforcing the person-centred and community approaches that are already being implemented in many aspects of occupational therapy practice. From the occupational therapists' view, now reinforced by the ICF, the focus is on a person's occupations within their natural environment and on occupational routine for quality of life. The focus should be on the person's opportunity to make choices, set goals and better control circumstances to make life more meaningful (Sinclair 2004). It is about people engaging in activity and participating in occupation. It is also about equity of access to meaningful occupation. The ICF reinforces the philosophical underpinning of occupational therapy that all people are occupational beings; occupation and health are inseparable; and a profession known as occupational therapy should consciously work towards improving the occupational well-being of all people, not just those with impairment (Wilcock 2001).

Furthermore, occupational therapists are being challenged to respond to the following statement from the World Health Organisation (2002b, p. 9):

As a result of global economic adjustments, the health sector in many countries has undertaken reforms. Among the elements of the recent health reforms are a more substantial separation between the purchaser and provider functions, decentralization of the health system, increased consumer choice, an emphasis on clinical effectiveness and on health outcomes, the development of the private sector and the introduction of new delivery schemes such as managed care.

This statement underpins the global move towards change and healthcare reform, and occupational therapists need to consider what are the trends and drivers affecting the health and social services sector. The European Foundation for the Improvement of Living and Working Conditions (2003, p. 3) identified some of the trends and drivers as:

- demographic and societal change
- rising expectations and consumerism
- health informatics and telemedicine
- new medical technologies
- increasing costs of health and social services provision.

These trends and drivers underpin the strong calls for the traditional paradigm of the health workforce to be changed. Part of the problem is that the system is geared to deal with episodes of acute care rather than ongoing care of chronic conditions. The implications are that occupational therapists need to rethink how they deliver their services. Occupational therapists need to consider the development of different ways of working so that they can meet the needs of communities and populations, not just individuals. Occupational therapists need to overcome their fear of telling people what we do and learn to give direction about what needs to be done, in relation to obtaining occupational engagement for all people. If occupational therapists see people individually, they can see eight to ten people per day; if we take our role as consultants seriously we can impact on the lives of hundreds of people. If we are to be recognised by the community, we need to be in and participating within the community. We have valuable work to do in acute care settings, but we can also have a profound impact as consultants in the community. For occupational therapists to embrace change and promote the unique contribution that they make, they need to take a more entrepreneurial approach to their practice.

Entrepreneurial practice

Inspired by the pioneers of the profession

Sylvia Docker was an Australian who worked as a physiotherapist in World War I and, in 1935, after travelling widely, undertook her training as an occupational therapist at the London School of Occupational Therapy. She returned to Australia in 1938 where she pioneered the profession in Melbourne, Victoria, and subsequently commenced the first school of occupational therapy in New South Wales in 1942 (Wilcock 2002). Sylvia Docker MBE was a true pioneer of the profession and displayed 'O.T.' – *outstanding talent*.

In 1959, Sylvia Docker (Anderson & Bell 1988, p. 222) said,

> *In 1960 it will be 20 years since the first training in occupational therapy was started in Sydney, NSW, and I think we can be satisfied with the progress made in those 20 years. But the younger members of our profession must not be content – they must push on, extending the scope and value of the work, till we have quite left behind in antiquity the idea that occupational therapy is just giving some patients some craft work.*

Sylvia Docker, along with other pioneers of our profession, had lots of faith, and some proof, that what we do has an impact on the health and well-being of people and communities. When I ask occupational therapists about their work, they often say 'I am just a practitioner'. I would like to say that I *am* a practitioner – not *just* a practitioner. I practice my profession in the best way that I can and, from time to time, I feel frustrated that others don't always share my views on the value and contribution of occupational therapy. I tire of explaining what we do in much the same way as I am sure we all do. But as I start to explain, I always re-ignite my belief that as occupational therapists we make a significant impact on the lives of others, be they individuals, families or communities.

I want to celebrate the diversity of my profession. As a practitioner I want to feel confident that my education is supported by committed and scholarly academics, my practice is supported by evidence developed by top-class researchers and that occupational therapy services are managed by managers who are experienced and trained in management. As a practitioner I don't need to perform all of those other roles, I need to be supported by them. But as a practitioner I need to respect that the occupational therapists performing those other roles are still 'real' occupational therapists, even though they are not necessarily practitioners. As practitioners we need to recognise and support every aspect of our profession and appreciate that without it, we would not have moved forward from the notion that 'occupational therapy is just giving some patients some craft work' (Anderson & Bell 1988, p. 222).

The apparent lack of community awareness regarding occupational therapy is often put down to the fact that we are a young profession. The fact that sometimes we don't succeed with specific professional issues and standpoints is put down to the notion that we haven't been around very long. We often hear occupational therapists say that nobody knows what we do; or it is difficult to explain what we do because it is too complicated; or the trouble with occupational therapists is that there are so few of us. If occupational therapy is to move on from being the best kept secret, therapists will have to be more pro-active and face the challenge of promoting their services and the profession. In doing this occupational therapists can then take their rightful place in health and social care, and start behaving like the specialists they are, instead of pretending to be generalists.

In 1962, Dr. Mary Reilly inspired us to embrace the notion that occupational therapy can be one of the truly great ideas of 20th century medicine. She based her aspirations on what she unashamedly referred to as 'one of those great beliefs which has advanced civilisation'. This belief is none other than the hypothesis upon which our profession was founded (Lyons 1985, p. 45),

> *That man, through the use of his hands as they are energised by mind and will, can influence the state of this own health.*

Reilly (1962) said that a profession organised around this hypothesis had almost limitless potential. However, this potential needs to be harnessed and so we need to consider how we do this.

We continue to struggle to explain what it is that we do. Occupational therapists also seem to become disillusioned when we think others emulate what we do. Imitation of course is the sincerest form of flattery. However, because we work with daily activities we are inclined to believe the myth that what we do is common sense – if it is *common* why did we study for four years to get it whilst the rest of the general population somehow acquires this sense by osmosis? I think these issues that we grapple with make us question if what we do really does have an impact, or, worse still, we ourselves dismiss it as common sense.

In 1983 Robert Bing, President, American Occupational Therapy Association said (Anderson & Bell 1988, p. ix)

History can tell us that the seeming hardships, the self doubts of efficacy, the searching for our roots are actually precursors for establishing a new strategic vision and plan that could put us at the forefront of progress.

It is time for us to move on from these self-doubts of efficacy and this searching for our roots and to take our place at the forefront of progress. The fact is that if we keep doing the same thing in the same way then the same thing will happen – nothing will change unless we change it. The profession must evolve and practice should not remain static. For example, look in the kitchen gadget shops and see the items that are sold for all to buy – jar openers, fat-handled vegetable peelers, and non-slip mats. As a young occupational therapist I used to make them because they weren't commercially available. But we've gone beyond that now. We need to be at the forefront of change.

Being entrepreneurial

We need to strive to move beyond the traditional boundaries because that is what they are – boundaries. They fence us in and limit our practice. This doesn't mean walking away from our core skills, rather, it means applying those core skills in more and more sophisticated and, most importantly, effective ways. Our expertise lies in the design of creative solutions to complex problems. It is the integration of multi-level variables into workable, effective, and sustainable solutions that is the core of occupational therapy practice. We need to think entrepreneurially. Entrepreneurship involves innovation. An entrepreneur searches for change, responds to it and exploits it as an opportunity (Drucker 1985). There is no doubt we are operating in a changing health and social care market, and we need to be ready to seize the opportunities.

Reference to entrepreneurship in the occupational therapy context is limited. There is an increasing amount of literature on marketing and how to write business and/or marketing plans (Epstein 1992, Jacobs 1999); however, this tends to look at entrepreneurship in terms of owning a particular type of business.

Entrepreneurship is about inspired creative individuals pursuing opportunities and taking 'calculated' risks. Being self-employed or in a business does not necessarily mean that you are an entrepreneur.

Conversely not being self-employed or in a business does not exclude entrepreneurial practice. In fact, we are now seeing the word 'intrapreneurs' used to describe innovation within a business at any stage and on any scale. It is not necessary to have a world-changing idea or to create a totally new product; small changes are just as crucial (Kneale 2005, Pinchot & Company 2005). Entrepreneurial practice is not an area of practice like paediatrics, mental health or private business. It is an attitude of mind and is about seeing and seizing opportunities regardless of where we work. I think we can apply the principles of entrepreneurial practice allied with good marketing principles to any area of practice.

Foto (1998, p. 766) argues that the entrepreneurial approach requires 'not only traditional occupational therapy competencies, but also competencies of a corporate chief executive, a finance deal maker, a marketing strategist, a high powered sales person and a riverboat gambler'. If we segment these competencies we can start to reveal a willingness to develop a vision and take risks but in a strategic way. It is the implementation of that vision that adds the ultimate value. Foto (1998) describes entrepreneurial occupational therapy practitioners as those who tend to perceive themselves simply as allied health practitioners, who have discovered and seized opportunities for promulgating the practice of occupational therapy in new directions or, perhaps, moving into new venues.

Based on a number of discussions with colleagues around innovation and entrepreneurship the following list of general characteristics of entrepreneurs has been developed. Entrepreneurs:

- are opportunity focused: they don't wait for opportunities to arise but are always looking for opportunities
- are risk managers: this refers to calculated risk-taking not crazy, speculative gambles
- are creative: they think outside the box
- are innovative: they consider new uses for old ideas
- are high achievers: they have a high need to excel
- have a strong internal locus of control: they have a low belief that their life is controlled by others, rather they are the master of their own destiny
- are visionary: they aim to create the future, implementing strategic intent

- realise weaknesses and strengths, and will put together a team designed to work towards a vision

- have an ability to deal with uncertainty: they believe that there are no guarantees and that opportunities exist in uncertain environments; there is no such thing as failure, just an investment in experience.

How many of us have at least one or more of those qualities – of course we all do. Boyce and Shepherd (2000) explored entrepreneurship as a dimension of professional culture. Their research was undertaken across 19 allied health professional groups, including occupational therapy. They identified four types of entrepreneurs within the professions. These types are described in Table 23.1.

Entrepreneurship recognises and pursues new or existing opportunities in a market place. However, to do this successfully it is important to employ appropriate planning strategies that take into account these opportunities and how to maximise them.

Working entrepreneurially

In addition to marketing, there are at least two approaches used to move in new directions: forward planning and strategic intent.

Table 23.1 Types of entrepreneurs (Boyce & Shepherd 2000)

Types of entrepreneur	Description
Strategic	Engaged in purposeful externally focused and ambitious programmes of organisational and professional change – re-fashioning traditional concepts of professionalism
Calculative	Focus on the present, although aware of the future – invest effort in managing resources and issues that have a more medium-term operational dimension
Reluctant	Risk averse – 'we looked at it but it was too much work'
Repressed	Willing but unable group – often unable to participate in change because they have low status in the organisation

Forward planning

Forward planning is somewhat like trying to drive a car blindfolded and following directions given by a person who is looking out the back window. You are trying to work out where you are going based on where you have been. This approach attracts comments like, 'We tried that 20 years ago and it didn't work'. Plans can be thwarted before they are implemented because we are constantly looking back. This is not to say that we cannot learn from history, as history provides us with valuable experience and learning blocks. However, we need to consider plans within the current context, and note the variables that have changed; things are not the same as they were 20 years ago.

Strategic intent

Strategic intent is where we decide where we want to be and fold the future back into the present in order to make it happen; in essence forming a 'road map' for guidance. This is based on the ability to recognise the opportunities combined with a belief in our own ability to achieve; having a strong internal locus of control. In fact, some would argue that this is no different to formulating a plan for an occupational therapy programme. We know what our final goal is and we plan backwards to our starting point to identify the steps.

Marketing

Of course there is a risk involved, and we need to calculate that risk, but in my experience, occupational therapists are creative, innovative high achievers who can think outside of the box. What we are not so good at is communicating with others about how good we are at all of this – and that's where marketing comes in.

As professional practitioners we tend to regard marketing with some apprehension, even distaste. Many occupational therapists view marketing, selling and advertising as synonymous. However, marketing is a much broader concept than just advertising and selling. Marketing is the analysis, planning, implementation, and control of carefully formulated programmes (Kotler 1994). Again this is no different to the process we undertake when we plan an intervention programme. Marketing, in the true sense of the word, can provide the impetus and structure for the implementation of Reilly's (1962) hypothesis. If occupational therapy is to remain competitive well into the future, the design and implementation of marketing strategies is essential.

Occupational therapists need to stop looking to other professions to justify their existence. Why do we always feel grateful when a doctor sees the value of occupational therapy? Why do we feel so defeated when others don't agree with our opinions? We need to stand up for our opinions, not watch helplessly while other health professionals provide services that can be much better provided by occupational therapists. As an example of promoting my services, I preface my activities of daily living reports with the following comment:

> Occupational therapists are highly skilled in the assessment and treatment of individuals with difficulties in their activities of daily living.

Implicit in this statement is the message that occupational therapists are the best professionals to provide this service. We need to take responsibility for ourselves and the profession, and seize the opportunities, both as individuals and as a professional association, and continue to develop innovative occupational therapy services.

The following section illustrates how some occupational therapists are seizing opportunities, being innovative and working more entrepreneurially.

Examples of innovation and entrepreneurship

Using technology in practice

In its broadest sense technology is the technical means people use to improve their surroundings, involving the practical application of knowledge, especially in a particular area of expertise. There are a myriad of opportunities for therapists to apply technology, both information and non-information based.

Information and communication technologies (ICT) have arrived and therapists need to be innovative in how they participate. ICT is a collective term used to describe a wide range of technologies designed to facilitate communication and the flow of information. These technologies include personal computers, the Internet, email, videoconferencing, telehealth and mobile technologies. The use of this type of technology in practice is illustrated in Practice Scenario 23.1.

Practice Scenario 23.1 Information and communication technologies

The link between occupational therapists and information and communication technologies (ICT) seems a natural one. Occupational therapists have been using technology for as long as the profession has existed. We are masters at using and creating low- and high-tech devices to assist people to reach their full potential. ICT are just an extension of that – tools that we can use and manipulate to allow ourselves to be better therapists to help the people we work with reach their goals.

It is important to state that computers and other forms of ICT are tools only. The issues aren't really about the technology, but are about the people – the occupational therapists and the people with whom they work. As occupational therapists we focus on the person and we look at the context they are in and the various elements of their environment. This person-centred, holistic focus drives the way I approach e-health issues – the focus must always be on the person and their environment and ICT must be useful, meaningful or purposeful to the person for that tool to have value.

Our involvement in ICT will extend into the homes, workplaces, and the community. ICT will be used to enhance a person's ability to engage in a range of self-care, productive, and leisure occupations. Technology will increase its pervasiveness into the daily lives of our clients and we will need to help the people we work with resume or assume roles and occupations where ICT plays an integral part. For us to continue our roles as experts in occupation, we will need to ensure that we remain experts in ICT.

One of the common occupations we observe is the task of grocery shopping – can the individual put together a shopping list, physically go to the supermarket, choose the items needed, purchase them and return home. In the not too distant future, an individual is going to be referred to an occupational therapist for a similar assessment of their ability to live independently in the community. But instead of the 'standard' grocery store expedition, the occupational therapist is going to have to work with the person to make sure they have the cognitive skills needed to continue to use the Internet fridge in their kitchen. The person will have no need to physically visit the store but will attach meaning and purpose to being able to use the Internet fridge and to communicate with the family and the local GP via the telecare link in the laser television.

This Practice Scenario was provided by Louise Schaper, an Australian occupational therapist, a researcher and a self-proclaimed 'lobbyist' for the promotion and use of ICT within healthcare.

It is important to remember that application of technology does not have to be computer or engineering based. In many countries with low resources, low-technology solutions may be more appropriate. Practice Scenario 23.2 describes the use of appropriate paper technology (APT) as an example of low technology.

Practice Scenario 23.2 Appropriate paper technology

Appropriate paper technology (APT) (Packer 1995) originated in Zimbabwe in the late seventies; originally as part of low-cost art classes. APT is a way of making strong and useful articles from paper waste. All APT articles are designed to serve a useful purpose and cost virtually nothing to make.

I was first introduced to APT whilst working at the Occupational Therapy Training School in Uganda. In the late 1990s occupational therapy was a new profession in Uganda and resources were limited. Students at the occupational therapy education programme had to learn not only how adaptive equipment could help disabled people but also how to make the equipment they prescribed. Students learnt basic carpentry and needlework skills, and liaised closely with local craftsmen. However, wood and specialised skills were still costly and a low-cost alternative was needed.

APT uses waste paper and cardboard and glue made from local flour and water. In the dry season constructions can dry quickly enabling occupational therapists to make large pieces of equipment over a number of days/weeks. APT involves layering pasted paper strips to make a shape, sometimes cardboard is used to give larger constructions sturdiness; the paste dries clear and adds strength; all equipment can be painted and take on an individual theme. Finally a layer of varnish makes the product waterproof.

Students in Uganda are taught basic APT skills in their first year (i.e. how to use the basic APT principles and make commode stools, supportive seating, and

standing frames). Throughout their three-year occupational therapy education students build on basic skills and develop more complex structures to meet various people's needs (e.g. see-saw and slides to encourage play in children, splints to help maintain the positioning of wrists and ankles); thus developing the creativity and innovativeness of the students.

Ugandan occupational therapists also use APT as a therapeutic tool; the activity is a messy one and allows individuals a structure to work with whilst developing problem-solving and decision-making skills. People requiring occupational therapy services have been involved in making equipment for others and/or pieces that they themselves can use at home. Occasionally income-generating projects have been developed.

This Practice Scenario was provided by Samantha Shann, an occupational therapist and lecturer at the University of Northumbria, United Kingdom. Samantha worked in Uganda during the late 1990s and has taught appropriate paper technology (APT) to therapists in Fiji in 2006. She was also actively involved in the Executive Management Team of WFOT at the time of writing.

Working as consultants

There are a multitude of opportunities to put occupational therapy amongst the general population. A growing area of practice includes workplace-based programmes. This is not just about putting in place programmes for injured workers and assisting them to return to work, but, more importantly, working to promote health and well-being in the workplace. A facilitating environment characterised by trust and mature dependency, enables employee health and well-being, and contributes to the health of the organisation (French 2005). Practice Scenario 23.3 outlines one such consultancy service.

Practice Scenario 23.3 Private practice

When I first started the business, MPOT Pty Ltd, I had an administration office based in rural South Australia. All of the professional staff (consultants) worked from fully operational home offices with computers, faxes and internet, and were linked via a server and mobile phones. MPOT used a web-based business centre for consultants to download and upload information, such as training materials, reports, and billing information.

We bring small groups of staff together to work on specific projects linked to the company's strategic goals. We work on projects such as upgrading the way occupational assessments are undertaken, developing a range of daily-living packages, in conjunction with exploring options for speedier service delivery within a bureaucratically slowed system.

More than one consultant is allocated to each industry client wherever possible. The consultants also use the city-based office to catch up with each other and to have project meetings. We meet for a full-day staff meeting once per month. As part of the staff meetings we offer professional development sessions; however, consultants also have a professional development budget as part of their salary package.

MPOT provide services state-wide with consultants providing services on site in industry or in clients' homes. Occupation is used as an intervention media, and return to work and daily living programmes are developed with clear goals and measurable outcomes. The occupational therapists develop the return-to-work programmes and use company personnel or the rehabilitation consultant in the role of occupational therapy assistants to monitor the programmes at the worksite. Any changes to the programmes must be developed and authorised by the occupational therapists.

The market we operate within is impacted upon by the senior managers within the industries we deal with. Many of them are baby boomers and that demographic profile is one of instant gratification, with no effort; they want it, they want it now and they don't want to go to any trouble to get it – the perfect target market for the one stop shop. However, we can not offer all services, so MPOT has a number of strategic alliances in place with other companies who offer complimentary services and we combine with them for different contracts.

This Practice Scenario was provided by Marilyn Pattison who currently operates a private practice where she employs three other occupational therapists and three rehabilitation consultants (RCs). MPOT Pty Ltd offers services in injury management, injury prevention, and risk management in industry.

Focusing on elderly people

It is well documented that the population is ageing, particularly in minority world countries, and it is up to occupational therapists to make the links between occupation and health clear. Programmes aimed at maintaining the elderly and older people in the community, underpin a growing area of practice. One such programme is illustrated in Practice Scenario 23.4.

Practice Scenario 23.4 Resource centre for elderly people

The Elderly Resources Centre (ERC) was established by the Hong Kong Housing Society. This centre opened in July 2005, and defined a new type of facility for older people. It is a free, user-friendly, walk-in centre, providing education, interactive assessment, individual consultation, research studies and opportunities for referral to other community service agencies. The ERC bundles occupational therapy assessment with health and building-related information to provide a one-stop facility for older people.

Visitors take nine tests related to daily activities. Assessments include cognitive, vision, hearing, reaching, balance, and mobility. Using interactive computerised programs and virtual-reality games the assessment results are stored on smart cards; the assessment report is generated and given to the elderly citizens with recommendations for occupational therapy intervention, if required.

Visitors also increase their understanding of home safety by learning more about home hazards and safety facilities in its home simulation zone.

The central theme of the centre is environment as a focus for change to improve occupational performance. The Person-Environment-Occupation (PEO) model of practice is used to emphasise the many possibilities and opportunities for the reduction of environmental barriers and access to resources in order to optimise occupational performance.

The ERC offers services to caregivers, offering information and training to health professionals and family members. The centre also offers a display of assistive home products.

Further information about the Hong Kong Housing Society can be found at www.hkhs.com/.

Reaching people through the use of tele-health

If occupational therapists are to embrace community-based practice, we need to consider alternative ways to reach and collaborate with people who live away from major population centres. We need to consider ways in which our services can be effectively and efficiently taken to the people. One option that occupational therapists could incorporate into their practice is tele-health. This is illustrated in Practice Scenario 23.5.

Practice Scenario 23.5 Benefits of tele-consultations

The links between rural occupational therapists and experienced occupational therapists at the Royal Children's Hospital (RCH), a tertiary paediatric hospital in Melbourne, Australia, have recently been enhanced by the introduction of tele-consultations that can occur between therapists and their young clients with uncommon or complex conditions.

The advice and guidance provided to the rural occupational therapists has now been enhanced by the use of videoconferencing technology to enable them to include the child and parent in their consultation. The therapists can look at the child together, observe the child's performance, and discuss or demonstrate possible options for interventions. This enables the rural therapists to continue to provide the occupational therapy interventions in complex or uncommon cases without the need for families to travel to the tertiary paediatric hospital to be seen by experienced occupational therapists.

An example is 'Jamie', a healthy young baby born with a flexed and adducted 'clasp' thumb. His thumb needed to be managed by applying splints to correct the joint range and soft-tissue contracture and prevent recurrence. Early intervention was needed to gain rapid correction. Once the contractures were corrected, active use of the thumb needed to be facilitated and optimised with the progression of normal fine motor development.

Jamie's family lived in a coastal town, 400 km from the RCH. The local occupational therapist sought guidance from an RCH paediatric hand therapist in regards to Jamie when he was just a few months old. Information on the protocol was obtained and the local therapist fitted Jamie with splints. A few months later, after successful contracture reduction with splinting, further advice was sought regarding the next phase of management.

Jamie and his mother attended the local therapist's work place and, via a high-speed broadband digital network, a videoconference was held between them and the experienced paediatric hand therapist at the RCH. Issues raised included the need to balance the maintenance of night splinting with mobilising to facilitate the strengthening of his weak thumb muscles. Strategies were discussed which included functional splinting appropriate for Jamie's age and ongoing fine-motor and cognitive development.

The mother acknowledged the benefits of not needing to make a day trip to Melbourne for Jamie to be seen by an experienced therapist, noting the savings in travel costs, as well as minimising the impact on their family life, as she had other children to look after. She appreciated the opportunity to be able to ask questions of the therapists together and gain a greater understanding of the intervention strategies. The local therapist also acknowledged the benefit of extending her knowledge and skills without needing to travel.

This Practice Scenario was provided by Lin Oke, who at the time of writing was the Manager of the Occupational Therapy Department at the Royal Children's Hospital (RCH) in Melbourne, Australia.

Disaster preparedness and response

Sadly natural and manmade disasters are becoming an increasingly common occurrence. Traditionally, occupational therapists have not been automatically involved in disaster preparedness and response; however, through the WFOT Disaster Preparedness and Response (DP&R) (WFOT 2007) the opportunity to have occupational therapists further involved has been explored. There is a growing recognition and appreciation of the unique role of occupational therapy within the DP&R context (Work Smart with Heart 2005). WFOT through its DP&R project was able to work with local occupational therapists in Sri Lanka, Indonesia, Thailand and India following the devastating tsunami. Practice Scenario 23.6 briefly describes the issues that a group of Thai tsunami survivors identified when visited by a group of occupational therapists who were learning how to respond to people affected by disasters.

Practice Scenario 23.6 Reflections on meeting people affected by tsunami

As part of a workshop for local occupational therapists interested in working in complex emergency situations, a visit to an area affected by a tsunami was arranged. The occupational therapists met villagers who had been relocated to new areas. The occupational therapists reflected on their visit to the tsunami-affected areas of Thailand:

The village is 16 months post tsunami and until recently these survivors have been living in a camp. They have now been re-housed into a new village. They cannot go back to their original village; therefore, the new village is in a different location to their original village. The houses are very small and close together and the village is not close to the market, vocational centre or school. It is not easy to get around for disabled people. All of the houses are small, have steps and narrow doorways, and squat toilets.

The tsunami survivors were considered to be friendly and welcoming. They were willing to give information and answer questions. It initially appeared that they had adjusted to their situation. They said they had strong leadership and a lot of support both from non-government and government organisations. However, they also said they would like to be independent in earning their living. They described their situation as walking in the darkness and being unable to find the way out. The survivors identified a lot of problems that were very hard to deal with. There is sadness and depression among the survivors; they were free-floating, had nothing to do, no jobs and careers, no incomes – these issues all need to be dealt with. They also said they felt guilty that they couldn't help their relatives when the tsunami attacked, regretting that they had to let them pass away.

The villagers elaborated further and said they felt insecure and lived in an aimless, meaningless and incomplete community. They were grateful for the government assistance but they felt the organisations did not complete their work. For example: they have been trained in skills to make products but there was no market at which to sell their products and no assistance to create one. There had been no follow up regarding the results of implemented programmes. They had to be careful to live on the money they had and they felt they should be given assistance to go back to their original vocations. They don't believe the assistance has been given equitably and they are worried and frightened about their future.

A similar workshop was held in Indonesia in April 2006. One month later a major earthquake struck and occupational therapists and occupational therapy students were able to be involved almost immediately.

Conclusion

I would like to respond to the points that were raised earlier in this chapter:

- Nobody knows what we do: We are experts in the science of doing and living.

- I can't really tell you what we do because it's too complicated: We are performance improvers.

- The trouble with occupational therapists is that there are so few of us: We are a select and highly specialised group with a major contribution to make to the health and well-being of all people.

The future of the profession is ours to make and our success will be the only reliable measure of how effectively we have taken hold of our vision. I would like to think that we embrace the notion of strategic intent to enable us all to turn our visions into reality. By joining together we can take the future, fold it back into the present and make it happen right now. So the next time someone asks you what occupational therapy is – look them in the eye, raise an eyebrow and say incredulously – 'you mean you don't know?'

I have always subscribed to the philosophy that eventually science proves what faith has known for centuries. As said earlier in this chapter the pioneers of our profession had lots of faith and some proof that what we do has an impact on the health and well-being of people and communities. As the profession progresses we are gathering an increasing body of evidence to support our practice but moving into the future is still a 'leap of faith'. It is now important that we make that leap, so that when we do glimpse the future occupational therapy will be in it.

> *Come to the edge*
> *He said. They said 'We are afraid'*
> *Come to the edge*
> *He said. They came*
> *He pushed them and they flew.*
>
> (Apollinaire, Guillaume cited Hayward 1985)

My final challenge to you is to acknowledge that it is time for us all to walk to the edge and to take that leap of faith. It is time for us, as occupational therapists, to fly.

References

Anderson, B. & Bell, B. (1988). *Occupational therapy: it's place in Australia's history*. Sydney, NSW Association of Occupational Therapists.

Boyce, R. & Shepherd, N. (2000). *Entrepreneurship as a dimension of professional culture*. Sociological Sites/Sights The Australian Sociological Society 2000 Conference, Adelaide, Flinders University.

Drucker, P. F. (1985). *Innovation and entrepreneurship*. New York, Harper and Row.

Epstein, C. F. (1992). Marketing: A continuous process. In: E. Jaffe (Ed.). *Occupational therapy consultation: theory, principles and practice*. St. Louis, Mosby.

European Foundation for the Improvement of Living and Working Conditions (2003). *The Future of Health and Social Services in Europe*. Dublin, European Monitoring Centre on Change.

Foto, M. (1998). Competence and the occupational therapy entrepreneur. *American Journal of Occupational Therapy*, 52(9), 765–769.

French, G. (2005). The place of health in the health safety and environment culture of a manufacturing organisation: A case study. *Australian Journal of Occupational Therapy*, 52, 373–375.

Hayward, S. (1985). *A guide to the advanced soul*. Australia, In-Tune Books.

Jacobs, K. (1999). Marketing occupational therapy services. In: K. Jacobs & M. Logigian (Eds). *Functions of a manager in occupational therapy*. Thorofare, NJ, Slack.

Kneale, P. E. (2005). Higher education academy imaginative curriculum guide: Enterprise in the higher education curriculum: A companion guide for busy academics. Available online from http://www.heacademy.ac.uk. Accessed May 2006.

Kotler, P. (1994). *Marketing management analysis, planning, implementation and control*. (8th ed). New York, Prentice Hall International.

Lyons, M. (1985). Paradise lost! ... Paradise regained? Putting the promise of occupational therapy into practice. *Australian Occupational Therapy Journal*, 32(2), 45–53.

Packer, B (1995). Appropriate paper-based technology (APT) A Manual. London, Intermediate Technology Publications.

Pinchot and Company (2005). *Liberating the power of people*. Available online http://www.pinchot.com. Accessed May 2006.

Reilly, M. (1962). Occupational Therapy can be one of the great ideas of 20th century medicine. *American Journal of Occupational Therapy*, 16(1), 1–9.

Sinclair, K. (2004). International perspectives on occupation and participation. *World Federation of Occupational Therapists Bulletin*, 50, 5–8.

United Nations (2005). *The Millennium Development Goals Report, 2005*. http://www.unmillenniumproject.org/goals/index.htm.

Wilcock, A. (2001). *Occupation for health*, Vol 1. London, British Association and College of Occupational Therapists.

Wilcock, A. (2002). *Occupation for health*, Vol 2. London, British College of Occupational Therapists.

World Federation of Occupational Therapists (2004). CBR Position paper. Available from www.wfot.org.

World Federation of Occupational Therapists (2007). *Work smart with heart: Disaster preparedness and response project: Phase 2 report*. Perth, WFOT. Available from www.wfot.org.

World Health Organisation (2002a) *Towards a common language for functioning, disability and health – ICF*. Geneva, World Health Organisation.

World Health Organisation (2002b) *Human resources for health: developing policy options for change. Discussion paper (draft)*. Geneva, World Health Organisation.

Work Smart with Heart (2005). *Disaster Preparedness and Response Project: Phase 1 Report – Regional Post-Tsunami Action Planning and Capacity Building Workshop 11–16 December 2005 Sri Lanka*. Western Australia, WFOT.

Section Five

Working with the individual

Chapter Twenty-Four

24

Enabling engagement in self-care occupations

Helen van Huet, Tracey Parnell, Virginia Mitsch, and Annette McLeod-Boyle

CHAPTER CONTENTS

Defining self-care 342

Who one is. 343
Identity 343
Independence 343
Values and beliefs 344
Self-efficacy 344
Motivation 344
Choice 345
Meaning 345
Environment 346

Assessment 346

Purpose of assessment 346
Assessment decisions. 347
Assessment approaches to self-care 347
Developing an occupational profile 348
Interpreting assessment data 349
Establishing goals for engagement in
self-care 350

Strategies for enabling engagement in
self-care occupations. 351

Conclusion. 351

SUMMARY

Engagement in self-care occupations involves a complex interaction between the person, the occupation and the environment. By considering these three elements when working with a person who is experiencing a dysfunction in his self-care occupations, an occupational therapist can provide a person-centred approach to enabling engagement in self-care. The person elements that must be considered include an individual's identity, independence, self-efficacy, motivation, choice, and meaning. The environment is considered from a physical, social, cultural, and institutional perspective. The occupation element focuses on how the various self-care occupations are performed. The assessment of the performance of self-care occupations must take into account the purpose and rationale for the assessment, the most appropriate approach to use, the interpretation of the findings, and the establishment of collaborative goals based on the findings. A variety of strategies can then be used to remediate or compensate for a dysfunction in self-care occupations. Appropriate strategies need to be selected carefully and be in keeping with a person's identity and independence, values and beliefs, and the environmental context. Three practice scenarios are presented to illustrate how enabling strategies can be used in a person-centred way to address difficulties in self-care occupations.

KEY POINTS

- Engagement in self-care involves a complex interaction between the occupation itself; the person's identity, values and beliefs; and the physical, social, cultural and institutional environment in which the occupation is performed.

- The importance of person-centred assessment and enabling strategies are critical to enablement.

- Clarifying the purpose of self-care assessment will determine the method of assessment to be used and the type of data to be collected.

- Clear and collaboratively determined goals are crucial to planning and the selection of appropriate enabling strategies.

- The planning and implementation of enabling strategies should include consideration of the person's motivation, ability and desire to change and adapt, the personal importance of the self-care occupation, and the environments in which the occupation is performed.

- Independence in self-care may be the desired outcome for the therapist but not the individual.

Defining self-care

Self-care, both historically and in modern times, is ultimately influenced by the motivation of basic survival needs, managing one's health and being accepted by society. The terminology used when describing the occupation of self-care has included 'activities of daily living' (ADL) (James 2009) and 'self-maintenance' (Babola 2000). Activities of daily living have been described as personal activities of daily living (PADL); which includes "all activities of taking care of one's body" (p. 539), and instrumental activities of daily living; which involve the person interacting with his environment and have increased complexity. Self-maintenance has been stated as including everything from grooming, socialisation, and communication to emergency response and sexual expression (Babola 2000). In this chapter, self-care includes all the tasks necessary to ensure a person's health and well-being, and survival in society. This includes eating, toileting, personal hygiene, grooming and dressing; shopping for food and clothing; communicating with others; money management, travel, meal preparation, mobility, sleeping and sexual expression.

In the course of one chapter it is not possible to fully cover the range of issues related to self-care, the assessment of self-care, and the enabling strategies that may be facilitated by occupational therapists. Rather, the aim of this chapter is to provide

readers with a number of principles to guide assessment and intervention, in order to assist therapists to work collaboratively with people who have an occupational dysfunction affecting their self-care capabilities.

When considering what influences self-care it is important to consider who one is, a person's beliefs and values, and the environment in which the person lives. The elements pertaining to who one is, include the concepts of *identity* and *independence*. The elements pertaining to an individual's values and beliefs include the concepts of *self-efficacy*, *motivation*, *choice* and *meaning*. These elements, along with the *environment*, when considered together, influence the level of engagement in the occupation of self-care. Engagement in self-care has been seen as core to occupational therapy practice, but is often thought of as mundane, routine, or, as Hasselkus (2002, p. 628) states, as 'everyday occupations...seen but unnoticed'. However, it is this anonymity that grounds individuals in reality and actuality when engaging in the occupations that they do everyday. Although considered as mundane and routine, the actual doing of self-care is complex, and so the multiple elements that impact and enable this occupation must be considered. These elements will be further illustrated throughout this chapter by the three practice scenarios (Practice Scenarios 24.1, 24.2 and 24.3).

Practice Scenario 24.1 Max

Max is a 58-year-old male with a long-standing history of osteoarthritis. He is currently an inpatient at the local hospital having undergone an uncomplicated right total hip replacement 3 days ago. Prior to admission to hospital, Max was living at home with his supportive partner of five years, Steve, and was working as an accountant with the local council. The couple live in a modern, two-bedroom townhouse that is close to all amenities and the central business district. As required by the hospital protocols, prior to Max's planned surgery, the occupational therapist completed a home assessment, arranged minor modifications, and provided the standard equipment required by people following total hip replacement surgery. The occupational therapist was also required to assess Max's self-care status, and did this by conducting a shower assessment on day three post surgery.

Practice Scenario 24.2 Mark

Mark is a 19-year-old man who was a passenger in a high-speed motor vehicle accident in which he sustained a severe traumatic brain injury; the driver was killed. Mark was hospitalised for a period of 3 months at a metropolitan brain injury unit, before transferring to a transitional living unit (TLU) programme at a regional centre, 3 hours away from his place of residence. Prior to his accident, Mark was living in a rural town, completing his third year of a building apprenticeship. Though his parents and two younger siblings also live in the town, Mark lived with friends in a shared house situation.

Assessment information was obtained from the metropolitan brain injury unit before Mark commenced his four-week residential programme at the TLU. It was reported that Mark was displaying difficulty in initiating and completing a consistent routine of the self-care occupations of showering and dressing. In other self-care occupations, such as familiar meal preparation, Mark found it difficult to adequately plan what was required for the task, initiate the task and sequence it so as to complete the task, as well as to maintain concentration during the task. He is hoping to eventually complete his apprenticeship and become a builder.

Practice Scenario 24.3 Marjorie

Marjorie is a 42-year-old woman who has had chronic low back pain for 16 years. She is married and has one daughter who is living away from home. Marjorie's pain has become progressively worse. She is no longer working as a child-care assistant and has become house-bound.

Marjorie mostly stays in bed all day. She has been diagnosed with depression by her doctor and is currently taking medication for this. She cannot find the energy to get out of bed as she believes that this will aggravate her pain.

Marjorie is concerned about the burden she is putting on her husband who is doing most of the household tasks. She is also concerned about her ability to be intimate with him as a result of her pain.

Who one is

Identity

Christiansen (1999) constructs identity as a hierarchical framework of the self, self-concept and self-esteem in relation to a situation or environmental context. Of particular interest is self-concept, which is seen as the ideas people have about themselves, including their personality traits and idiosyncratic characteristics. Self-esteem is seen as the self-evaluative aspect of the self-concept, which is related to our perceived competency in performance of our occupations and life roles. A person's self-concept and self-esteem may evolve over time. Compare, for example, the way four-year-old children consider themselves within the world; to the view adults in their sixtieth year have of themselves. Consider how self-concept may change for either children or adults when their lives become disrupted by illness or impairment. It may be argued that a child will form a new self-concept over time, whilst an older person may find negotiating a changed identity to be more challenging.

How people evaluate their performance of self-care tasks may impact on how they view themselves within the social world. The impact of illness and impairment on identity must be considered when occupational therapists are engaging with people in self-care occupations. Studies have demonstrated the impact that ageing, chronic illness or impairment has on the identity of individuals (Guidetti et al 2007, Lysack & Seipke 2002, Magnus 2001, Satink et al 2004). For example, Guidetti et al (2007, p. 308) examined the experience of 'recapturing self-care' after a stroke or spinal cord injury and reported that, for some people, the inability to undertake self-care tasks made them reflect on '…how closely this aspect of their daily life was linked with their former identities….'

Independence

The concept of independence in occupation is one that has underpinned the practice of occupational therapy since its inception. Within Western society, independence is valued whereas dependence is not. Children strive for independence in their self-care through the use of practice and repetition until mastery is achieved. Hayase et al (2004, p. 192) have shown that 'the sharpest growth in self-care abilities occurs between the ages of 3–6 years' whilst independence in self-care once reached (around the age of 15), remains stable until about the age of 50, when deterioration begins to take place. Therefore, it cannot be expected that a 70-year-old person who has had a stroke will necessarily achieve the same level of independence as a younger person who has had a similar stroke.

As practitioners, occupational therapists base many of their interventions on promoting independence in self-care. The institutions that occupational therapists work within often demand independence as a requirement of completing care pathways and achieving discharge within set time frames. Hayase et al (2004) suggest that determining need for service should consider the implications of age-related ability rather than just outcomes of independence. This obviously has implications for our ageing population and the provision of community-support services.

Another factor to consider is the cultural fit of the concept of independence. Western societies are becoming increasingly multicultural, largely due to migration and the acceptance of refugees. The influx of different ethnic groups has meant a reconsideration of the concept of independence from a cultural perspective. Some cultures place greater value on interdependence. This sees individuals seeking support through the development of reciprocal relationships with families and available services. It centres on relationships, goals, and values, rather than on individual capabilities, and is based on reciprocity and respect (Beeber 2008). Whalley-Hammell (2006, p. 128) reflects that, although independence is considered 'the norm', interdependence is 'the usual'. In order to work effectively with people, occupational therapists need to explore what the concept of independence means to individuals, including a thorough examination of the person's culture, role demands and personal values. Consideration of independence beyond just physical independence is required; independence should also include the ability to make decisions, to be autonomous, and to have control over one's life.

Values and beliefs

Self-efficacy

Self-efficacy, according to Bandura (1977), is based on an individual's self-system that enables the person to exercise a measure of control over his thoughts, feelings, motivation and actions, in reference to some type of goal. A person's belief in his ability to perform a task has been linked to his actual successful performance (Carpenter et al 2001, van Huet & Williams 2007, Walsh et al 2004). When considering this in relation to self-care, a person's desire to engage, feelings around engagement, and belief in his capacity to engage, merit consideration. Indeed,

a person's belief (or perceived ability) in his capacity to perform the tasks and activities required for everyday living may be a more accurate predictor of day-to-day performance than actual ability (Sanford et al 2006).

Although there are measures of self-efficacy available, such as the Self-Efficacy Gauge (Gage et al 1994) and the Pain Self Efficacy Questionnaire (Nicholas 1988), a simple question of, 'Do you think you can do this?', may provide an indication of how the person is feeling in relation to performance of a self-care activity. Research demonstrates that people who experience occupational disruption due to illness or impairment report a reduced sense of being in control (Carpenter 1994, Guidetti et al 2007, Whalley-Hammell 2006). A person-centred approach to assessment, intervention and decision-making may assist in restoring a sense of control, thus enhancing self-efficacy (Hammel 1999).

Motivation

Motivational factors play a critical role in self-care. In order to consider motivation, an occupational perspective is required. By taking an occupational perspective of motivation towards engagement in self-care, consideration of choice and meaning can be examined (Christiansen & Townsend 2004).

Motivation is driven by both regulatory and purposeful factors. Regulatory or internal motivators include hunger (the drive to eat), pain (the avoidance of tasks that cause pain) and fatigue (the need to rest). These motivators are largely governed by nervous and endocrine systems in the body. Although their basis is physiological, the impact on engagement in activities and tasks can be significant.

Although distinct from regulatory motivators, purposeful motivators can influence activity and in some cases override regulatory motivators (e.g. a person can refuse to eat or ignore the pain). The idea that purposeful motivators influence task performance has its basis in the field of psychology, more specifically in the notions of conscious thought or cognitive process. The drive 'to do' may be seen as part of a person's personality characteristics and, therefore, be reflective of their identity. This motivational drive is also influenced by the personal goals that people make for themselves.

Motivation is, therefore, critical to enablement in self-care activities and tasks. If a person is not motivated towards a particular self-care task, the likelihood of engagement and successful completion is minimised. The lack of motivation requires the consideration of a range of factors, which include the person's interest in performing specific activities, how important self-care is perceived to be, and the person's sense of self-efficacy in completing the activity (Kielhofner 2008). It may be expected that it would be difficult to maintain motivation towards independence in dressing, if it took the person over one hour each day to complete this occupation. This may also be impacted if the person valued other occupations more highly (e.g. work or leisure occupations), and if the completion of the self-care task left the person fatigued and unable to participate in the self-chosen preferred activity.

Choice

Being able to make and have choices in what a person does is a fundamental human right. Townsend and Wilcock (2004, p. 260) see choice as 'the means by which humans decide what occupations are a priority and what occupations they consider the most useful and meaningful to them'. Choices may be determined by survival needs (e.g. the need to find food) or be culturally defined (e.g. the choice of clothing worn to a particular event). Ultimately, the concept of choice is one afforded to affluent societies where the value of choosing what one will do is nurtured and supported. Consider a situation when choice is removed or disregarded, such as in the health institutions in which occupational therapists often work. Providing people with choice within institutional settings is often a low priority when precedence is given to adherence to care pathways in relation to completion of self-care assessments and intervention. Promoting choice need not be difficult; for example, a therapist could ask a person if he prefers a shower or a bath. The therapist could also ask the person when he would normally have a shower or bath at home. By doing this, the therapist can enhance the person's feelings of control over a situation by providing choice.

Providing choice has the potential to bring both risk and responsibility to the therapist–person relationship. As a result, there is an ethical component to respecting people's views and allowing people to make choices which may carry inherent risks (Townsend et al 2007a). The right to take risks and to experience the consequences of the outcomes of these risks might be considered to be central to person-centred practice (Whalley-Hammell 2006). By collaborating with people in making decisions

and choices, occupational therapists should aim to gauge acceptable risk to promote 'just right' risk taking (Townsend et al 2007a, p. 101), and assist people in understanding the possible implications of their decisions.

Meaning

The meaning given to a particular occupation influences the importance of that occupation in a person's life. Kielhofner (2008) sees the importance of meaning as a primary factor that determines occupational engagement. Thus, the meaning attached to an activity acts as a motivator to actual performance of or engagement in that task. People derive enjoyment and satisfaction through participation in occupations of meaning. It is also important to note that the meaning attached to a certain occupation is individualistic; each person will perceive meaning differently depending on his perceived goals and beliefs, and the context of his environment.

Hasselkus (1997, p. 374) described the process of 'meaning making' through personal narrative or self-story. By asking people to tell their stories about how they see self-care and how illness or impairment impacts on this narrative, therapists can gain a level of understanding of the meaning of that experience. Indeed, in terms of engaging with people collaboratively in establishing priorities for intervention, it would appear paramount to have an appreciation of not only the meaning of a particular occupation, but also how this fits within the person's view of their own identity and future life.

The importance of identity, as previously discussed, is relevant here, as Christiansen (1999) proposed that our identity is shaped by our interactions with others and their reactions to us. Valuing a person's view of a situation and the meaning derived from engagement in an occupation can provide reaffirmation of a person's self-worth and provide opportunities to re-establish identities disrupted by illness or impairment.

In addition to being a motivating force behind engagement in occupations, meaning has also been described as an 'outcome of occupational engagement' (Polatajko et al 2007, p. 60). Successful performance and achievement can act as a reinforcer of the importance of that occupation for an individual and may have a positive influence on participation in other occupations (Rebiero 2000).

However, having said this, Whalley-Hammell (2004) challenged the need for all meaning to be related to purpose. There needs to be an awareness that people sometimes engage in occupations purely for the sense of belonging, or being human, in a social world, rather than achieving a set goal. As an example, do we expect that a person can learn to dress his upper body independently given the right environment, instruction and physical ability? How as therapists do we feel if the person asks for assistance or states that he would rather be doing something else? If we assist the person and enable him to then engage in another valued occupation, is this then not meaningful? As suggested by Hasselkus (2002), occupational therapists should embrace the value of being engaged in occupation for the experience this gives rather than just the outcome achieved.

Environment

The environment is the context within which occupational performance takes place and can be considered to include physical, social, cultural, and institutional factors (Polatajko et al 2007, p. 48). Law et al (1996) discuss the interactive, dynamic, and complex relationship between the person, the environment, and the occupation, and outline that the environment can have an enabling or constraining effect on an individual's performance of, and engagement in, occupations.

Occupational therapists have traditionally focused on the physical environment when working with people to enhance engagement in self-care activities (e.g. recommending and overseeing the completion of home modifications). However, it is useful to reflect on the social, cultural, and institutional environmental factors that may impact on a person's level of independence, their goals and future plans, and their motivation to engage. These factors have the potential to impact either directly or indirectly on the person's level of engagement in self-care. As an example, it is generally accepted that children are expected to gradually achieve independence in self-care activities; however, the cultural environment (including family traditions) and the social environment (including social class and economics) may influence the timing and acquisition of these skills (Guidetti & Soderback 2001).

Consider the following example where the occupational therapist did not fully consider the impact of a person's home environment. This person was deemed by hospital outcome measures to be 'independent' in showering (as assessed within the hospital setting), but was unable to maintain this level of independence when discharged. Review of the situation revealed that the person was, indeed, able to shower without assistance, but was unable to negotiate the 50-metre walk on uneven terrain from his caravan (where he lived) to the amenities block.

The use of relevant assessment and enabling strategies is important. These must be responsive to the needs of people and assist in achieving individual goals in self-care; this will require occupational therapists to consider each individual's environment in a comprehensive manner.

Assessment

Purpose of assessment

Assessment is recognised as an important part of the occupational therapy professional reasoning process (Boyt Schell 2009), so that the cause or nature of concerns relevant to occupational therapy can be analysed. For the purpose of this topic, assessment *could* be defined as the systematic collection of data and information (Reed & Sanderson 1999) for determining and understanding a person's capacity and capability to perform and/or engage in self-care activities. However, as demonstrated in the previous section, engagement in self-care encompasses a broader range of considerations beyond a simple understanding of a person's abilities. Assessment is only truly productive, therefore, if it provides relevant and reliable data and information that informs the full breadth of areas for consideration.

There are multiple reasons for undertaking assessment of self-care. From one perspective, it enables a better understanding of the effect of a medical diagnosis on engagement in self-care and daily living (Christiansen & Hammecker 2001), and promotes insight into how daily roles and routines may have changed for both the person who has been diagnosed, and those who are part of his social environment. Self-care routines may increase in complexity due to acquired illness or impairments (e.g. altered diet and fluid intake, adherence to medication) (Jaarsma et al 1999) and use of technology (e.g. glucometers and morphine pumps). These routines may also be affected by the availability of, or a change in, the level of social support (e.g. death of a spouse, reduction in support funding). For Mark (Practice Scenario 24.2), it involves understanding the long-term influence of a brain injury on his ability to perform self-care occupations; for Marjorie (Practice Scenario 24.3) this means understanding how low back pain has influenced her role as a partner, and what the changed circumstances mean for her husband, in terms of changed role demands or possible additional support.

Assessment can also identify current (Reed & Sanderson 1999) and potential levels of engagement (Christiansen & Hammecker 2001), and determine, in part, the ability to live independently and/or the degree and type of supports required. Max (Practice Scenario 24.1) has a supportive partner, and, therefore, he is confident in returning home, because he knows that his partner will provide the required assistance.

From another perspective, self-care assessment can achieve an understanding of what a person wants and/or needs to be able to 'do', and the factors that either enable or constrain occupational engagement in these activities (Hussey et al 2007). This may include exploration of past patterns of participation in self-care, as well as expected or anticipated future patterns (Hagedorn 2001). This may lead to an exploration of the person's current view of self and his aspired future self, leading to a greater understanding of 'who the individual is', and the individual's 'values and beliefs' (Neistadt 2000). Furthermore, it will highlight personal assets such as the person's knowledge and insight of his diagnosis or condition, learning ability, available support networks, the home environment, and difficulties being experienced.

Assessment of self-care occupations should be reflective of occupational therapy's beliefs and values – it should reflect an attitude of holism and person-centredness; an understanding of the dynamic relationship between people, occupations and environments; and recognise the uniqueness of both the individual and of performance (Klein et al 2008). Awareness of the personal and, in some instances, intimate nature of self-care is also essential. This can only be achieved with the establishment of a trusting, respectful and therapeutic relationship between practitioners, clients, client's families, carers, friends and/or nominated significant others. Marjorie (Practice Scenario 24.3), for example, expressed concern about her ability to be intimate with her husband. The therapist, through considered assessment, and a trusting relationship, would be able to understand the significance of this occupation in Marjorie's life and to her perception of herself, in her role as a partner.

Assessment decisions

Through the use of professional reasoning and in consultation with the person, occupational therapists will determine what is necessary to assess (i.e. the specific aspects of self-care to be targeted), and how this will be achieved (i.e. the type of assessments to be used). This is not always easily determined. In some settings, the therapist will need to choose a tool or method that will assess the relevant aspects of self-care most important to the person, and also meet the needs and criteria of the practice context (Letts & Bosch 2001) (e.g. some insurance companies may require objective, quantitative data, or rehabilitation facilities may have a standard set of assessments which all participants must complete on admission). In this situation, the institutional environment influences the assessment choices made. It may be that assessments solely done for this purpose will be incomplete and not take into account the full situation. For example, if, in order to satisfy the clinical pathway requirements of the hospital, the occupational therapist only completed a shower assessment in the ward bathroom with Max (Practice Scenario 24.1) on day three post surgery, the results would probably not be a true reflection of his ability to perform this task in his home environment.

Other considerations may include whether outcome measures are required, or whether a thorough understanding of the person's capabilities in particular aspects of self-care is required, so that a specific enabling strategy can be designed. It will also depend on whether the assessment is to be used for screening purposes, to determine, for example, whether a person may benefit from more intensive intervention, such as inpatient rehabilitation. An awareness of a person's abilities and the demands of completing self-care activities in specific environments are also crucial.

Assessment approaches to self-care

There are generally two approaches to evaluating the 'person' element of self-care. One approach involves the careful observation of the performance of self-care occupations in order to determine the individual's capacities to complete the selected tasks, the degree and nature of assistance required, and the need for support (both technological and human).

This can be achieved either informally (asking the person to perform selected tasks in as natural an environment as possible) or more formally, using established assessment tools. Using formal assessments will often yield a measure which can be used for later comparison (Reed & Sanderson 1999). However, informal observations may enable far more detailed data about the factors contributing to the performance of self-care occupations to be collected. Irrespective of the choice, it is necessary to evaluate baseline performance in order to plan appropriate intervention. Once initial assessment of self-care is completed, the need for further targeted assessment of areas of difficulty may be indicated. The causes of any activity limitations can then be explored in more depth (James 2009).

The second approach to self-care assessment involves collecting data that reflect the person's perceptions and perspectives of self-care. Self-reports will indicate what the individual believes is occurring during performance, and what is particularly problematic. In their study, Johansson et al (2007) discovered that people may request assistance with areas of perceived difficulty in performance, even when they may be able to complete activities. Therefore, the assessment should not just consider whether it can be done independently, but how easily it can be done. Furthermore, Petersson et al (2007) found that people's perceptions about their independence, and the level of difficulty and safety experienced when performing daily tasks, is important for supporting community living.

A tension may exist for practitioners who need to objectively observe performance and determine a level of independence (as dictated by the institution), but who also want to take into consideration an in-depth picture of self-care needs, choices, abilities, and desires. It may be that the latter proves to be more important to successful intervention than the former (Petersson et al 2007). However, using both of these approaches may also be useful, as it would allow for a comparison to be made, and a determination of the congruence between what is reported and what is observed, and, therefore, what is possible in terms of performance (Reed & Sanderson 1999). Areas of incongruence may require further investigation in order to determine whether there are other fears, concerns, or anxieties that need to be addressed. The decision of which assessment approach to follow should be flexible. This is illustrated by Max (Practice Scenario 24.1) who decided that he did not want or need to be indepen-

dent in showering and dressing prior to returning home as his partner, Steve, would assist him. By the use of a person-centred approach with Max and Steve, the therapist determined that the required self-care assessment could be directed towards safety, risk and responsibility, rather than independence.

Whatever the reason for assessment, making a suitable choice will require the practitioner to be familiar with the range of assessment tools available, content areas covered, the populations they were designed for, the type of information they will provide, and how data can be interpreted. The assessments conducted with Marjorie (Box 24.1) provide examples of self-care assessments that could be done; further examples can be found in the Further Reading list.

Thorough assessment of the self-care occupations demands that therapist pay attention to each of the elements which comprise the dynamic of occupational engagement: occupation, person and environment (Polatajko et al 2007).

Developing an occupational profile

Developing an occupational profile (Hussey et al 2007) may assist in determining priorities in self-care. Max, Mark and Marjorie (Practice Scenarios 24.1, 24.2 and 24.3), and their carers/partners/family, could be asked to describe what they do in a usual week, or month, perhaps using a planner if needed, so that usual occupations and routines can be identified. From this, self-care demands for each of them can be determined and targeted for assessment. This process can also assist people to identify their needs, interests and perceived difficulties (James 2009).

Adequate and accurate assessment of self-care occupations can only occur in the presence of a detailed understanding of the multiple components which make up each occupation. Careful analysis of each occupation will ensure that the degree of complexity embedded within it is recognised (Hagedorn 2001), and that all aspects of the occupation are considered during assessment, thus enabling identification of any performance limitations.

Physical, social and cultural environmental factors also need to be considered in relation to the roles and responsibilities of the person when analysing self-care occupations. Physical factors involve an awareness of the various contexts where self-care occupations will be performed and how these factors

Box 24.1

Shower assessment for Marjorie (Practice Scenario 24.3)

Marjorie indicated a desire to be out of bed, showered and dressed before lunchtime. The occupational therapist decided to assess Marjorie having a shower with the assistance of her husband. The steps involved in this, shared between Marjorie and her husband, were:

1. Getting out of bed and going to the bathroom
2. Obtaining all the items needed for having a shower and having her clothes laid out in the bathroom
3. Turning on taps and adjusting temperature of water
4. Getting into the shower
5. Standing or sitting for duration of time
6. Reaching for soap, shampoo, washer
7. Washing and rinsing self/hair (in the correct order)
8. Turning taps off
9. Getting out of the shower
10. Drying self
11. Dressing.

An informal assessment of this activity will enable various performance components to be observed. This will include:

Biomechanical: range of motion (e.g. reaching for taps), strength (e.g. opening and closing containers), endurance (e.g. standing for the duration of the shower), use of correct body mechanics (e.g. stepping around to adjust taps rather than twisting her back)

Sensory: pain tolerance, perception of temperature of water, tactile sensation to determine whether soap totally rinsed out of hair

Motor: balance and postural control when standing or sitting, controlled movement when pouring shampoo

Cognitive/perceptual: appropriate identification of products and their uses, remembering and completing tasks in the correct sequence.

In addition, the therapists will be able to assess the following aspects of the activity:

Intrapersonal: a sense of her standard of personal hygiene, choice of products used in the shower, timing of shower.

Interpersonal: working with husband to complete tasks involved in showering.

Environment: the size of bathroom, bathroom design and layout, availability and location of assistive devices, safety issues, lighting, and heating/cooling.

---

may impact on performance. Consider Mark (Practice Scenario 24.2); within the TLU environment he can perform basic meal preparation without assistance. In the shared house environment with multiple distractions, an assessment revealed that Mark experienced difficulties in this activity. Social and cultural factors influencing routines of self-care may take on greater significance (e.g. during special or religious celebrations) or may lead to the need to accommodate additional elements (e.g. the onset of menstruation or the wearing of particular clothes).

Interpreting assessment data

Information that has been gathered must be interpreted, if it is to be useful. On some occasions, interpretation will occur after the assessment process has been completed (e.g. if using a standardised test, results can only be understood once scores have been calculated and compared to independence criteria). In many situations, interpretation occurs during the assessment process and is recorded alongside the raw data. When this occurs, care needs to be taken that conclusions are not prematurely reached, and the assessment procedure compromised.

Practitioners need to use professional reasoning skills to interpret data regardless of the assessment used. The data may inform the therapist about levels of dependence/independence (Letts & Bosch 2001), or perceived difficulty (Johansson et al 2007) or perhaps perceived importance (Law et al 1998). Alternatively, it may give insight into the amount or quality of assistance needed, the use of assistive technology, the task elements that are difficult, or performance component deficits. Professional reasoning is also required to determine whether difficulty in some component areas might be generalised to other areas of performance (Letts & Bosch 2001). Insight and understanding gained from assessment then forms the basis on which goals are negotiated with people, and intervention options are considered and determined.

Establishing goals for engagement in self-care

A person's goals in relation to self-care will be influenced by the individual's self concept and the degree of competence he is hoping to achieve within a particular environment. As noted earlier, a person's perception of self may change when his life becomes disrupted by illness or impairment. A person's desire to engage in self-care and his beliefs about his ability to engage will influence goals for intervention. A person's goals need to focus on what the person sees as important for managing his whole life rather than the illness or impairment being the dominant consideration (Whalley-Hammell 2006). In order to achieve this, consideration needs to be given to formulating goals that outline the use of environments that best simulate the person's natural setting (Guidetti & Soderback 2001) in contrast to a purely clinical setting.

In acute-care settings, the establishment of goals may be influenced by the requirements of the institution that stipulate set protocols to promote consistency and outcomes that are deemed to be time- and cost-effective. In these situations, goal identification may occur concurrently with assessment to ensure effective and efficient service provision. Within the constraints of the institutional environment it is still possible for individual needs to be considered. For Max (Practice Scenario 24.1), his self-care goals would focus on safety rather than independence, which would still satisfy hospital criteria for timely discharge to the home environment. In response to this, the occupational therapist makes a note in Max's chart indicating his current level of independence (based on the assessment conducted) and his willingness to have his partner assist him in self-care on discharge. The mutually agreed goal centres on safety, which then becomes the focus of education and intervention with Max and Steve.

The collaborative partnership between the person and the therapist is reflective of goal identification that is person-centred.

The therapist needs to think about her own level of knowledge of a particular impairment and the impact of this on goal achievement. Here the therapist is using her understanding and knowledge of the illness or impairment to identify the steps required to facilitate engagement in self-care. The development of goals that can be achieved in the short term provides opportunities for the person to regain a sense of control over his own life and may provide the motivation for continued participation in ongoing goal setting and intervention. Guidetti & Tham (2002) state that, 'to be able to see and set goals in collaboration with the occupational therapist, [...] clients needed to realise the value of having self-control' (p. 265).

For Marjorie (Practice Scenario 24.3) goal setting was the initial step in regaining control over her life. Marjorie outlined what her goals were in regards to her pain and what she wanted to be able to do at home. Marjorie wanted her pain to go away, but didn't think that it would happen. She also wanted to be able to get out of bed, have a shower and get dressed. Marjorie and her therapist agreed on a goal for the following week; for Marjorie to get out of bed, shower and dress before midday. Marjorie really wanted to do this and believed that this was achievable if her husband provided some assistance.

The prominence and importance of self-care may not be acknowledged as significant if precedence is given to other occupations. Consider Mark (Practice Scenario 24.2) who has difficulty in understanding how his cognitive problems impact on him in his everyday life and wants to 'return to his apprenticeship as soon as possible'. The occupational therapist begins the process of goal identification with Mark by acknowledging his primary goal of returning to his apprenticeship. Mark is asked about the things he does to ensure he can do this apprenticeship (e.g. get up at a set time). Discussion with Mark is also centred on what he did everyday to look after himself to ensure he could do his apprenticeship (e.g. prepare breakfast, organise suitable clothing for the day and shop for groceries). From this discussion Mark and his occupational therapist were able to identify what steps needed to be achieved before Mark was ready to address going back to his apprenticeship. These then became short-term goals focused on self-care that linked to his overall goal of returning to his apprenticeship. This example demonstrates how the therapist's recognition of what the person hopes will ultimately be achieved can be the motivating factor in the ongoing development of collaborative goals.

Strategies for enabling engagement in self-care occupations

There is a broad range of strategies to enable engagement in self-care occupations. For example, Hussey et al (2007) list therapeutic use of self, therapeutic use of occupations and activities, consultation, and education as types of occupational therapy interventions to be considered. In contrast, Townsend et al (2007b) list a broad range of skills (including adapt, advocate, coach, educate and design/build) that occupational therapists can use in order to enable individual change, including change to facilitate engagement in self-care occupations. Other authors promote the use of remediation, compensation, and education strategies (Holm et al 1998). The strategies selected will be dependent on the person, the illness or impairment, the environment, and the agreed occupational goals.

For the purposes of this chapter, examples of strategies that can be used in relation to self-care will be given, in reference to the concepts discussed in the opening section of this chapter. Hence, examples of strategies that address who one is, a person's values and beliefs, and the environments that the occupation occurs in will be given. An illustration of how an occupational therapist might collaborate with a person to achieve an occupational goal, taking into account these concepts, is outlined for each of the three practice scenarios in Boxes 24.2–24.4.

Conclusion

Self-care occupations are an important focus of practice for occupational therapists. When working with people who have difficulties with their self-care occupations an occupational therapist must take into consideration the person's identity and concept of independence, values and beliefs, and the environments in which the self-care occupations are performed. These considerations will influence

Box 24.2

Example of education and assistive technology strategies for Max (Practice Scenario 24.1)

Goal
Max, given education regarding home safety, hip precautions and provision of assistive equipment; will be able to shower and dress in his home environment with assistance from Steve, within 10 days post surgery.

Who one is
Identity
Max sees himself as an equal partner in his relationship with Steve and understands that due to the relationship they have, he will be supported by Steve.

Independence
Although Max values being independent in many things he sees that the hip replacement will have a short-term impact; due to this he is comfortable with Steve assisting him to do some self-care activities.

Values and beliefs
Self-efficacy
Max believes he will become independent in self-care in the future without further intervention.

Motivation
Max's main motivation is to return home to live with Steve.

Choice, risk and responsibility
Max and Steve have made the choice that Max will be assisted by Steve with self-care occupations. Therefore, the therapist will educate Max and Steve to develop an understanding of the safety precautions related to his hip-replacement surgery and the issues related to safely returning to the home environment.

Meaning and independence
Being independent in self-care is not a priority for Max.

Environment
Adapting the physical environment
Adapt physical aspects of the home environment to enable Max to safely engage in self-care activities (e.g. installation of grab rails in the shower).

Social support networks
Ensure that Steve is able to take on the carer role and has the necessary skills and knowledge to fulfil this role.

Box 24.3

Example of compensation strategy for Mark (Practice Scenario 24.2)

Goal

Mark using his notebook and given a 20 minute time period will purchase five breakfast items in the supermarket, within 4 weeks.

Who one is

Identity

Mark sees himself as an adult who is independent from his family. He is friendly and likes living in a shared house environment. He also would like to complete his building apprenticeship.

Independence

Mark would like to be able to be independent in shopping for food and other essential items. He would eventually like to return to living in a shared house and knows that he will have to be able to do more for himself if he is to be able to do this successfully.

Values and beliefs

Self efficacy

Mark and the therapist believe that the goal is within Mark's current abilities.

Motivation

Using Mark's aim of completing his apprenticeship, the therapist and Mark identify the self-care goals necessary to achieve this. Being able to shop for and make breakfast is agreed on as a short-term goal. The therapist provides support and encouragement to Mark when he faces difficulties and setbacks in achieving this goal.

Choice

The therapist and Mark chose tools and strategies to achieve the goal. The success of the tools and strategies used are evaluated and refined.

Meaning

Mark can see that achieving this goal is a step towards obtaining his longer-term goal of completing his apprenticeship.

Environment

Physical, social and cultural

The therapist provides opportunities for Mark to practice remembering to use the notebook and refer to it during the shopping task. It is anticipated this practice will facilitate mastery and generalisation of the notebook into other tasks (e.g. steps to prepare breakfast). The notebook is used to list the items required to buy, with like items grouped together. Strategies for keeping on task include ticking off items on the list in the notebook and self-talk practice for when Mark becomes frustrated if items cannot be found.

Visual cues are also used within the physical environment, cueing the recall of the use of the notebook.

---

the assessments that an occupational therapist might perform to assist with the development of occupation-focused goals and person-centred enabling strategies. Whether the enabling strategies used involve remediation, compensation or education, or a combination of all three, it is important that the therapist collaborates with the person to ensure that they are working towards achieving a level of competence in self-care occupations that is ultimately satisfactory to the person.

Box 24.4

Example of education and compensation strategies for Marjorie (Practice Scenario 24.3)

Goal

Marjorie (provided that her husband lays her clothes out for her in the bathroom) will be able to get out of bed, be showered and dressed by midday, each day, within 3 weeks.

Who one is

Identity

By Marjorie achieving her set goal it is anticipated that over time she will regain a sense of control over her situation which will have a positive impact on her self concept and her ability to manage her pain.

Independence

Marjorie accepts that she will require assistance to complete self-care occupations.

Values and beliefs

Self-efficacy

Marjorie believes that if her husband lays out her clothes in the bathroom prior to showering, she will be able to complete the rest of the activity independently.

Motivate

By engaging with Marjorie to set realistic goals her motivation to perform showering and dressing tasks will be maintained. To achieve this goal, a graded approach to goal setting and attainment was used (e.g. Marjorie wanted to be up, showered and dressed twice in week one).

Choice

Marjorie has decided that it is important for her to be able to manage her showering and dressing within her pain limits. She has decided to focus on this activity rather than other household tasks.

Meaning

Being able to shower and dress by herself is important to Marjorie. The therapist provides strategies to enable showering and dressing, these include educating Marjorie on the following: the nature of chronic pain, energy conservation principles, use of correct body mechanics and use of deep breathing as a pain-management strategy during and after task completion.

Environment

Physical/social environment

By having her husband lay her clothes out for her and by sitting on a chair in the bathroom to dress, Marjorie will be able to complete the task by herself.

Physical environment

By ensuring that the bathroom is uncluttered Marjorie will have safe access to the shower.

Social environment

Marjorie, in consultation with her husband and the therapist, has decided to receive assistance with some household tasks in the short term. This decision will be reviewed after a three-month period.

References

Babola, K. T. (2000). Independent living strategies for adults with developmental disabilities. In: C. H. Christiansen (Ed.), *Ways of Living: Self-care strategies for special needs* (2nd ed.). Maryland, American Occupational Therapy Association.

Bandura, A. (1977). Self-efficacy: towards a unifying theory of behavioural change. *Psychological Review*, 84, 199–215.

Beeber, A. S. (2008). Interdependence: Building partnerships to continue older adults residence in the community.

Journal of Gerontological Nursing, 4(1), 19–25.

Boyt Schell, B. A. (2009). Professional reasoning in practice. In: E. B. Crepeau, E. S. Cohn & B. A. Boyt Schell (Eds.), *Willard and Spackman's occupational therapy* (11th ed.) (pp. 314–327). Philadelphia, Lippincott, Williams and Wilkins.

Carpenter, C. (1994). The experience of spinal cord injury: The individual's perspective – implications for rehabilitation practice. *Physical Therapy*, 74(7), 614–629.

Carpenter, L., Baker, G. A., & Tyldesley, B. (2001). The use of the Canadian Occupational Performance Measure as an outcome of a pain management programme. *Canadian Journal of Occupational Therapy*, 68(1), 16–22.

Christiansen, C. H. (1999). Defining Lives: Occupation as Identity: An essay on competence, coherence, and the creation of meaning, 1999 Eleanor Clarke Slagle Lecture. *The American Journal of Occupational Therapy*, 53(July), 547–558.

Christiansen, C. H. & Hammecker, C. L. (2001). Self-care. In: B. R. Bonder & M. B. Wagner (eds.), *Functional performance in older adults* (2nd ed), (pp. 155–178). Philadelphia, F.A. Davis Company.

Christiansen, C. & Townsend, E. (Eds). (2004). *Introduction to occupation – the art and science of living*. New Jersey, Prentice Hall.

Gage, M., Noh, S., Polatajko, H. & Kaspar, V. (1994). Measuring perceived self-efficacy in occupational therapy. *American Journal of Occupational Therapy*, 48(9), 783–790.

Guidetti, S., Asaba, E., & Tham, K. (2007). The lived experience of recapturing self-care. *American Journal of Occupational Therapy*, 61, 303–310.

Guidetti, S. & Soderback, I. (2001). Description of self-care training in occupational therapy: Case studies of five Kenyan children with cerebral palsy. *Occupational Therapy International*, 8(1), 34–48.

Guidetti, S. & Tham, K. (2002). Therapeutiv strategies used by occupational therapist in self-care training: A qualitative study. *Occupational Therapy International*, 9, 247–276.

Hagedorn, R. (2001). *Foundations for practice in occupational therapy* (3rd ed). Edinburgh, Churchill Livingstone.

Hammel, J. (1999). The life rope: A transactional approach to exploring worker and life role development. *Work*, 12, 47–60.

Hasselkus, B. (1997). Meaning and Occupation. In C. H. Christiansen & C. Baum *Occupational Therapy: Enabling function and well-being.* (2nd ed.). (pp. 374). Philadelphia, Slack.

Hasselkus, B. (2002). *The meaning of everyday occupation*. New Jersey, Slack.

Hayase, D., Mosenteen, D., Thimmaiah, D., Zemke, S., Atler, K., & Fisher, A. G. (2004). Age-related changes in activities of daily living ability. *Australian Journal of Occupational Therapy*, 51, 192–198.

Holm, M. B., Rogers, J. C. & James, A. B. (1998). Treatment of activities of daily living. In: M. E. Neistadt & E. B. Crepeau (Eds) *Willard & Spackman's occupational therapy* (9th ed.) (pp. 323–364). Philadelphia, Lippincott.

Hussey, S. M., Sabonis-Chafee, B., & O'Brien, J. C. (2007). *Introduction to occupational therapy* (3rd ed.). Missouri, Mosby Elsevier.

Jaarsma, T., Halfens, R., Huijer Abu-Saab, H., Dracup, K, Gorgels, T., van Ree, J., & Stappers, J. (1999). Effects of education and support on self-care and resource utilisation in patients with heart failure. *European Heart Journal*, 20, 623–682.

James, A. B. (2009). Activities of daily living and instrumental activities of daily living. In: E. B. Crepeau, E. S. Cohn & B. A. Boyt Schell (Eds.). *Willard and Spackman's occupational therapy* (11th ed.) (pp. 538–578). Philadelphia, Lippincott, Williams and Wilkins.

Johansson, K., Lilja, M., Petersson, I. & Borell, L. (2007). Performance of activities of daily living in a sample of applicants for home modification services. *Scandinavian Journal of Occupational Therapy*, 14, 44–53.

Kielhofner, G. (2008). Volition. In: G. Keilhofner (Ed.), *Model of human occupation: Theory and application* (4th ed.). Philadelphia, Lippincott, Williams & Wilkins.

Klein, S., Barlow, I. & Hollis, V. (2008). Evaluating ADL measures from an occupational therapy perspective. *Canadian Journal of Occupational Therapy*, 75(2), 69–81.

Law. M., Cooper, B., Strong, S., Stewart, D., Rigby, P. & Letts, L. (1996). The person-environment-occupation model: A transactive approach to occupational performance. *Canadian Journal of Occupational Therapy*, 58, 186–192.

Law, M., Baptiste, S., Carswell, A., McColl, M.A., Polatajko, H., & Pollock, N. (1998). *Canadian occupational performance measure*. Ontario, CAOT Publications ACE.

Letts, L. & Bosch, J. (2001). Measuring occupational performance in basic activities of daily living. In: M. Law, C. Baum & W. Dunn (Eds.), *Measuring occupational performance: Supporting best practice in occupational therapy.* (pp. 121–159). Thorofare, NJ, Slack, Inc.

Lysack, C. L., & Seipke, H. L. (2002). Communication the occupational self: A qualitative study of oldest-old American women. *Scandinavian Journal of Occupational Therapy*, 9, 130–139.

Magnus, E. (2001). Everyday occupations and the process of redefinition: A study of how meaning in occupation influences redefinition of identity in women with a disability. *Scandinavian Journal of Occupational Therapy*, 8, 115–124.

Neistadt, M.E. (2000). *Occupational therapy evaluation for adults: A pocket guide*. Baltimore, Lippincott, Williams and Wilkins.

Nicholas, M. K. (1988). Pain self-efficacy questionnaire – Unpublished tool.

Petersson, I., Fisher, A.G., Hemmingsson, H., & Lilja, M. (2007). The Client-Clinician Assessment Protocol (C–CAP): Evaluation of its psychometric properties for use with people ageing with disabilities in need of home modifications. *Occupational Therapy Journal of Research: Occupation, Participation and Health*, 27(4), 140–148.

Polatajko, H.J., Davis, J., Stewart, D., Cantin, N., Amoroso, B., Purdie, L., & Zimmerman, D. (2007). In: E.A. Townsend & H.J. Politajko (eds.), *Enabling occupation II: Advancing an occupational therapy vision of health, well-being and justice through occupation.* (pp. 13–36). Ottawa, CAOT Publications ACE.

Rebeiro, K. L. (2000). Client perspectives on occupational therapy practice: Are we truly client-centred? *Canadian Journal of Occupational Therapy*, 67(1), 7–14.

Reed, K.L & Sanderson, S.N. (1999). *Concepts of occupational therapy.* (4th ed.) Philadelphia, Lippincott, Williams and Wilkins.

Sanford, J., Griffiths, P., Richardson, P., Hargraves, K., Butterfield, T. & Hoenig, H. (2006). The effects of in-home rehabilitation on task self-efficacy in mobility impaired adults: A randomized clinical trial. *Journal of American Geriatrics Society*, 54 (11), 1641–1648.

Satink, T., Winding, K., & Jonsson, H. (2004). Daily occupations with or without pain: Dilemmas in occupational performance. *OTJR: Occupation, Participation and Health*, 24(4), 144–150.

Townsend, E.A., Beagan, B., Kumas–Tan, Z., Versnel, J., Iwama, M., Landry, J., Stewart, D. & Brown, J. (2007a). Enabling: Occupational therapy's core competency. In: E.A. Townsend & H.J. Polatajko (Eds.) *Enabling occupation II: Advancing an occupational therapy vision for health, well-being & justice through occupation.* (pp. 87–133). Ottawa, CAOT Publications.

Townsend, E.A., Trentham, B., Clark, J., Dubouloz-Wilner, C., Pentland, W., Doble, S. & Rudman, D.

(2007b). Enabling individual change. In: E.A. Townsend & H.J. Polatajko (Eds.) *Enabling occupation II: Advancing an occupational therapy vision for health, well-being & justice through occupation.* (pp. 135–151).Ottawa, CAOT Publications.

Townsend, E.A. & Wilcock, A.A. (2004). Occupational justice and client-centred practice: A dialogue in progress. *The Canadian Journal of Occupational Therapy* 71(2), 75–88.

van Huet, H. & Williams, D. (2007). Self-beliefs about pain and occupational performance: A comparison of two measures used in a pain management program.

OTJR, Occupation, Participation and Health, 27(1), 4–12.

Walsh, D., Kelly, S., Johnson, P., Rajkumar, S. & Bennetts, K. (2004). Performance problems of patients with chronic low-back pain and the measurement of patient-centred outcome. *Spine*, 29(1), 87–93.

Whalley-Hammell, K. (2004). Dimensions of meaning in the occupations of daily life. *Canadian Journal of Occupational Therapy*, 71(5), 296–305.

Whalley-Hammell, K. (2006). *Perspectives on disability and rehabilitation: contesting assumptions; challenging practice.* Edinburgh, Elsevier.

Further reading

James, A. B. (2009). Activities of daily living and instrumental activities of daily living. In: E. B. Crepeau, E. S. Cohn & B. A. B. Schell (Eds.) *Willard and Spackman's occupational therapy* (11th ed, pp. 538–578). Philadelphia: Lippincott, Williams and Wilkins.

Law, M., Baum, C. & Dunn, W. (2001). *Measuring occupational performance: Supporting best*

practice in occupational therapy. Thorofare: Slack Inc.

Mulligan, S. (2003). *Occupational therapy evaluation for children: A pocket guide.* Philadelphia: Lippincott, Williams and Wilkins.

Neistadt, M. E. (2000). *Occupational therapy evaluation for adults: A pocket guide.* Baltimore: Lippincott, Williams and Wilkins.

Rodger, S. & Brown, G. T. (2006). Developing, promoting and managing self-care needs. In: S. Rodger & J. Ziviani (Eds.) *Occupational therapy with children: Understanding children's occupations and enabling participation.* (pp. 200–221). Carlton: Blackwell Publishing.

Chapter Twenty-Five

25

Leisure

Ben Sellar and Mandy Stanley

CHAPTER CONTENTS

Introduction 358

What is leisure? 358

Leisure as residual time 358

Leisure as activity 359

Leisure as experience 359

The leisure experience 360

Perceived freedom. 360

A sense of intrinsic reward 360

Enjoyment or pleasure. 360

Relaxation 360

Temporality and flow 360

Leisure and recreation 361

Relationship to health. 361

Application to practice 362

Leisure assessment tools. 364

Measurement of time 364

Leisure as activity 365

Critique of tools 365

Leisure as experience 366

Ways of enabling participation in leisure . . 366

Temporal aspects 367

Adaptation of the environment and/or occupation. 367

Occupational substitution 367

Leisure as means 367

Conclusion. 368

SUMMARY

This chapter discusses a range of theoretical perspectives around leisure and how each impacts on assessment and intervention in occupational therapy. Though traditionally conceived of as discrete activities or non-work time, the focus here is instead placed on leisure as a subjective experience, a perspective capable of acknowledging the dynamic nature of leisure in the complex lives of people. The significance of leisure experiences is discussed, justifying the call for more emphasis to be placed on this important aspect of people's lives. A range of possible assessment tools is provided, as well as a discussion of how to use these as a preliminary stage in a process aimed at rich and detailed analysis of the individual leisure experiences of people and groups. Such depth of analysis ensures that new or modified occupations retain the key determinants of the individual's idiosyncratic leisure experience.

KEY POINTS

- Multiple theoretical perspectives of leisure have been proposed including leisure as free time, discrete activity or subjective experience.
- Conceptualisations of leisure as a subjective experience defined by the individual are capable of transcending boundaries of activity and time and acknowledge the dynamic interaction of person, environment and occupation.
- Leisure is a significant occupational category for people contributing to identity, life satisfaction and occupational balance.
- The tools used to assess, and methods used to incorporate leisure in occupational therapy

programmes are dictated by the theoretical perspective taken by the therapist.

- Leisure may be incorporated into interventions with individuals, groups or communities to achieve therapeutic ends.
- Despite the availability of assessment tools, occupational therapists need to undertake in-depth, critical analysis of individual leisure experiences to effectively match new or modified occupations with the idiosyncratic needs of the individual.

Introduction

Although leisure is discussed as distinct from play this distinction is not so clear in reality. Leisure is often playful and play is often leisurely. Distinction between the two concepts is frequently made based on the age of participants such that adults engage in leisure while children in play. But at what age is this transition made and how does the play of adults with children fit into this dichotomy? The following discussion of leisure and how it may be conceptualised or employed within occupational therapy contexts is intended to relate to people from any age, but the examples throughout reflect work with adults.

The chapter first outlines the key theories and dilemmas surrounding the concept of leisure by exploring the difficulty with definition and how leisure may contribute to health. This is followed by an exploration of when and how leisure may be assessed and employed in a therapeutic context with individuals and groups to bring about meaningful individual outcomes.

What is leisure?

For many people leisure is a central and highly valued part of life. It helps us to reduce stress, develop and express our identity, as well as achieve occupational balance and well-being (Di Bona 2000, Iso-Ahola 1997, Lee et al 1994, Neulinger 1974). Unfortunately, within Western, work-oriented cultures, leisure is often given less importance than work and has historically been viewed as indulgent, unproductive and even sinful (Dare et al 1987). To some extent occupational therapists have also been guilty of emphasising the importance of work over leisure by focusing on assessments and interventions around productive and self-care occupations (Specht

et al 2002, Suto 1998). This has resulted in leisure receiving less attention than it deserves and, subsequently, confusion over what the term even means.

Though used commonly in everyday language, leisure is a difficult concept to clearly define. There has been considerable debate in many fields about how to describe leisure, though no universally accepted definition has yet been achieved (Primeau 1996, Sellar & Boshoff 2006). This ongoing debate has highlighted three common approaches to defining leisure as: time, activity or experience.

Leisure as residual time

Residual or free time is perhaps the most common-sense understanding of leisure. From this perspective leisure is defined simply as any time spent free from the necessities and constraints imposed by vocational or domestic labour (Kelly & Freysinger 2000, Primeau 1996, Suto 1998). It is assumed that this time is discretionary, allowing us to freely choose the occupations in which we wish to engage. Of prime significance for this approach is the choice that free time affords and little, if any, attention is given to what the person actually chooses to do, so long as it occurs outside of work time. The residual time approach lends itself well to measurement as time can be easily quantified and enables comparisons between different groups based on age, sex, gender, vocation, nation of origin or disability status (Kelly & Freysinger 2000). Comparisons can also be made across the life course, exploring changes in time use from childhood through to old age.

Residual time definitions of leisure are succinct and easily understood but are significantly limited. The first difficulty is that they assume that time can be clearly divided into either work or non-work and that only one occupation can be undertaken at any one time. In fact it is rare that occupations fit discretely into leisure, productivity or self care, instead being more often embedded (Christiansen & Townsend 2004). Reading while commuting to work or listening to music while washing the dishes are common examples of how people can nest occupations to save time and incorporate leisure into obligatory occupations.

A further critique of residual time definitions of leisure targets the assumption that free time will be filled with freely chosen activities, but this is not always possible (Parry & Shinew 2004, Russell

& Stage 1996). For individuals without access to transport, finance, community resources or social networks, free time can be anything but leisurely. Displaced or marginalised groups such as those seeking employment, disabled people or people seeking refuge are often faced with an excess of free time (Russell & Stage 1996). Russell and Stage's (1996, p. 118) study of Sudanese women in a Kenyan refugee camp found that, faced with 'an abundance of meaningless free time, a thwarting of traditional role activities, and a dependency on others', leisure was in fact viewed as a burden. Instead of providing an opportunity for self-fulfillment and expression through engagement with occupations of personal and cultural meaning, free time was filled with inactivity, potentially leading to leisure boredom (Iso-Ahola 1997). Simply having a great deal of free time did not mean it was filled with meaningful activity. Therefore, while time is an important factor in understanding leisure, consideration must also be given to the occupations in which people wish, and are able to engage.

Leisure as activity

Like residual time definitions, views of leisure as observable behaviours or activities are common within both general society and occupational therapy theory and practice (Suto 1998). Proponents of this view suggest that leisure can be described as a list of those occupations defined as leisurely by any individual, community or even a society. Such a view again lends itself well to measurement as lists of leisure interests can be quickly generated and complemented by a measure of participation frequency (Kelly & Freysinger 2000).

However, as with most attempts to succinctly define leisure, this approach also suffers from limitations. Like residual time definitions, activity approaches assume a clear distinction between work and leisure. Beyond the issues already discussed, these two leisure definitions raise further difficulties.

Ideas of leisure as non-work are supported by and validate the cultural overvaluing of vocational and productive occupations. Western societies, informed by the Protestant work ethic and individualised consumer culture, have traditionally placed a high value on economic status, capital accumulation and a sound work ethic (Iso-Ahola

1997, Rojek 2004). Such influences have led to leisure being seen as frivolous, meaningless and even sinful (Dare et al 1987), having value only in enabling people to enjoy rest and relaxation (Iso-Ahola 1997) or invest in tourism and leisure economies (Kelly & Freysinger 2000). Activity and time definitions fail to explore the unique qualities of the occupation or time that actually makes it leisurely for the individual. Instead, they construct leisure as the lack of something, proposing no unique identifying characteristics outside the context of work. As we shall see later this deficit construction is in part responsible for leisure being associated with recreation or relaxation.

A major difficulty with viewing leisure as a form of activity or time is that they each fail to account for the environmental and psychosocial factors that influence how we feel while engaging in an occupation. These views assume that what constitutes work time and activity are consistent and static across individuals, times and contexts, yet variations in these factors can significantly change the meaning associated with the occupation. Attending a social gathering on a weekend with friends whose company you enjoy may certainly be described as leisure. On the other hand, attending a social gathering out of obligation to a friend or family member might be anything but leisurely, and yet it could hardly be described as work. Instead it might be termed productivity as the purpose of the occupation is to maintain social and family networks.

Leisure as experience

To overcome the difficulties with the previous two understandings many authors have explored the idea of leisure as experience (Iso-Ahola 1997, Lee et al 1994, Neulinger 1974, Sellar & Boshoff 2006, Tinsley et al 1993). From this viewpoint leisure is embedded within the consciousness of the individual (Kelly & Freysinger 2000). The form of the activity and the time in which it is done are relatively meaningless, with the primary concern instead placed on the meaning that the individual attributes to the experience of engagement. Leisure can, therefore, be experienced anywhere, at any time, during any occupation so long as the individual subjectively defines the experience as leisure. Though such an understanding overcomes certain limitations, it raises the question, how do we know when we are experiencing leisure?

The leisure experience

Surely we need to know *what* something is before we can say we are experiencing it. The exact nature of the leisure experience is highly personalised but studies have shown that several characteristics might serve as markers of leisure experiences. Many studies have sought to explore or describe specific characteristics and have highlighted more than thirty (Iso-Ahola 1997, Lee et al 1994, Sellar & Boshoff 2006, Tinsley et al 1993). These can be grouped into five key themes that frequently recur throughout the literature.

Perceived freedom

Perhaps the primary aspect of the leisure experience is that we feel free from obligations, thus allowing us to make choices about which occupations we engage in and how we perform them. Constraints are often thought of as extrinsic, such as vocational and domestic duties which for many are significant, consistent and consuming obligations limiting the time and energy that individuals have for engagement in leisure. However, constraints can be intrinsic and more subtle. In a study of older people's leisure experiences, Sellar and Boshoff (2006) found that for the experience to emerge people needed to feel free from a perceived obligation to maintain an occupational identity as an efficacious and contributing member of society. People may feel guilty when participating in leisure if they feel they have not 'earned' it or if it is perceived as 'unproductive' (Lee et al 1994, Sellar & Boshoff 2006). Discriminatory policies, institutions or community values that marginalise individuals on the basis of disability status, financial status, sexuality, gender or country of origin may also impose constraints.

A sense of intrinsic reward

Leisure experiences are rewarding in and of themselves. For many, engagement in vocational occupations is rewarded only by extrinsic social status or financial benefits and the subsequent lifestyle opportunities these afford. However, such engagement, done '*in order to*' may lose degrees of perceived freedom discussed earlier (Neulinger 1974, p. 17). Instead leisure occupations reward participants with an experience that is intrinsically valued as well as,

or instead of the outcome produced. Outcomes such as artwork, a healthier body or increased knowledge may result from engagement in painting, jogging or reading respectively, but these are not the primary motivations for engagement. Instead, the experience of the process is given more value by the participant and it is this focus on process that constitutes the third unique and defining quality of the leisure experience.

Enjoyment or pleasure

Leisure experiences are typically described as enjoyable (Lee et al 1994, Specht et al 2002). Indeed, why would we freely choose to spend our time doing things we did not take pleasure in? This is not to say that leisure is entirely pleasant, as often strenuous activities that require a great deal of physical, emotional and/or spiritual effort may only retrospectively be defined as enjoyable (Lee et al 1994).

Relaxation

Relaxation is commonly cited as a key benefit of leisure both in theory and common conversation. Though frequently associated with physically inactive occupations, such as reading or watching television, many people find relaxation in more strenuous pursuits, such as rock climbing, artistic pursuits or woodworking (Kelly & Freysinger 2000). Relaxation is an important potential outcome of the leisure experience but should not be overstated or positioned as the primary goal of leisure engagement. If immersion in the experience is secondary to a relaxing outcome then the intrinsic value of the occupation is diminished and engagement becomes focused on recreation, rather than self-actualisation (Tinsley et al 1993).

Temporality and flow

During leisure experiences people often report a decreased awareness of the passage of time to the point where they feel that time has flown by or disappeared (Sellar & Boshoff 2006, Tinsley et al 1993). This is a familiar experience for many and usually emerges when the challenge of an activity and the skills of the individual are matched such that success is experienced but without boredom emerging.

A decreased awareness of time is central to Csik-szentmihalyi's (1991) concept of flow which has strongly influenced our present understanding of leisure experiences. Flow is a subjective psychological state that occurs when someone is completely immersed in an occupation (Emerson 1998). Many would be familiar with the experience of 'losing time', looking at a clock to find that an hour or maybe two has just elapsed in what might feel like five minutes. Csikszentmihalyi and Mei-Ha Wong (1991) suggest that flow is an optimal psychological state and represents the highest level of well-being. Flow is said to occur when engaged in occupations that (Emerson 1998):

- provide a clear sense of control over one's actions
- are rewarding in and of themselves
- have clearly defined goals
- provide immediate and clear feedback
- achieve an outcome that is perceived as meaningful.

If these characteristics are present in an occupation people generally feel happier, stronger, more creative and satisfied (Csikszentmihalyi 1991). Though flow appears to give some answers to the nature of leisure experiences it also raises some challenges.

We have already stated that the view of leisure as experience means that it can occur anywhere and anytime, which means it could also occur during vocational occupations. This is supported by Lefevre (1988) who showed that people experience flow 54% of the time at work and only 17% of the time during leisure. Further, participants experienced apathy during 52% of their leisure time and 16% of their work time (Lefevre 1988). Despite these results people were more motivated to be at leisure than at work. So why were people motivated towards times and activities that fostered the experience of apathy? One theory is that being in flow is highly demanding, requiring physical and mental energy (Lefevre 1988). Therefore, people in their non-work time may seek out occupations such as sleeping, watching television or hanging out with friends that enable them to recreate and restore energy levels.

Leisure and recreation

As the name implies recreational occupations are those that are aimed at re-creating or restoring mental, physical and spiritual energy sources drained by prior activity (Howell & Pierce 2000). People may achieve recreation through sleeping, napping, watching television, quilting or any other occupation specifically aimed at re-energising themselves (Howell & Pierce 2000). Recreation and restoration are often used interchangeably and share many common characteristics and functions, but both are quite distinct from leisure. Both refer to processes in which people prepare themselves to re-engage with demanding occupations emerging from vocational, social, familial or civic responsibilities. Recreation could be described as 'organized [sic] activity with the purposes of the restoration of the wholeness of mind, body and spirit' (Kelly & Freysinger 2000, p. 18). But is recreation the same as leisure?

Earlier we discussed some characteristics of the leisure experience including relaxation and intrinsic reward or value. Recreational occupations certainly fit the first characteristic as their primary goal is to relax the body and mind. However, these occupations do not provide an intrinsic reward and it could be argued, are not free. Instead these are obligatory occupations in which the demands of the body force us to engage in occupations that serve it. While leisure experiences emerge as a result of the intrinsic occupational process, restorative occupations are defined by the extrinsic occupational outcome, namely recovery from prior exertion and preparation for future effort. Though leisure may certainly be relaxing, this is a secondary effect of engagement and the intrinsic reward is the motivating element.

Relationship to health

Having explored some key concepts and dilemmas associated with leisure, it is important to now explore the connection between leisure and health. Leisure has been shown to have broad positive effects on well-being, coping with a wide range of stressors, as well as reducing the impacts of physical dysfunction.

As we have explored, leisure serves as a unique medium of self-expression and identity formation which are both important to perceptions of well-being. For many, the inability to maintain previous patterns of leisure engagement due to the loss of physical, cognitive or social capacities can result in a 'fracturing of the self and a sense of uncertainty about the future' (Kleiber et al 1995, p. 291). Hutchinson et al (2003, p. 154) showed that leisure can be a very effective tool in maintaining a 'sense of competence, independence, and continuity of self', vital to the individual's well-being.

Leisure also has a commonsense and evidence-based relationship to reducing stress. Kleiber and colleagues (2002) describe leisure engagement as having self-protective, restorative and transformative potential for those coping with stresses from work, life role changes or illness. The friendships and social supports developed through leisure engagement help to buffer the effects of stress on physical and mental health (Coleman & Iso-Ahola 1993, Kleiber et al 2002). These positive effects have been explored with individuals experiencing transitions associated with physical dysfunction, such as spinal cord injury and multiple sclerosis (Hutchinson et al 2003).

While issues of maintaining a sense of self and relieving stress might not seem directly related to physical dysfunction, they have been shown to potentially provide hope and optimism (Hutchinson et al 2003). More directly, the physical benefits such as those described by Drummond and Walker (1996) may also emerge from engagement in leisure, as they found that engagement in a leisure programme following stroke increased people's mobility and physical energy levels.

Application to practice

Having begun this chapter exploring leisure definitions, we still have not arrived at a clear and succinct conceptualisation. Indeed, what is clear is that no such definition exists and would, in fact, be paradoxical, as the nature of leisure is variable across times, contexts and people (Neumayer & Wilding 2005). Leisure cannot be defined as a discrete list of activities, distinct times or exact feelings. It is a subjective assessment of an experience emerging from the dynamic interplay of time, activity and environment. Fundamentally, elements of this experience include perceived freedom from obligations and intrinsic motivation to engage (Iso-Ahola 1997). In this way leisure can be an extremely powerful occupational tool for therapists providing a range of potential outcomes and benefits.

It is, thus, important to now explore the use of leisure in occupational therapy interventions. After exploring when leisure might be used in therapy, we will discuss the tools that are used by occupational therapists when discussing leisure with people and,

finally, how occupational therapists might work with individuals or groups to improve engagement in leisure occupations. Two Practice Scenarios are provided to illustrate key points (Practice Scenarios 25.1 and 25.2).

Practice Scenario 25.1 Marko

Anna, an occupational therapist working at a rehabilitation unit specialising in brain injury, has been asked to see Marko. Marko is 43 and had a head injury two months ago. He has made significant progress in his rehabilitation and is now attending on an outpatient basis. He walks slowly because of a left-sided hemiparesis, has a wide-based gait and poor balance, but prefers not to use a walking aid. Marko is somewhat impulsive and has some persisting problems with judgement.

Anna completed the Canadian Occupational Performance Measure with Marko during which he named fishing as a leisure occupation he is currently unable to do, and which was the top priority for him to work on. In an Occupational Performance History Interview Marko identified that he has always enjoyed fishing from a small dinghy, as it is something that he did as a small boy with his father. He has always enjoyed being able to bring home the catch to contribute to the family as well as the relaxing nature of fishing, where he is able to get away from the hustle and bustle of life and just sit quietly waiting to catch a fish. Socialising with the other fishing and boating enthusiasts was also important. Marko's partner does not want Marko to return to fishing as he thinks it is too risky with Marko's poor balance and problems with judgement.

Anna sat with Marko and explored the options for working towards the goal of participating in fishing as a leisure occupation. Together they considered the following:
- Person – *Marko* – what were his strengths and limitations?
- Occupation – *fishing* – using Marko's knowledge of the occupation, what occupational performance components are involved?
- Environment – *a small boat on the water* – they analysed the affordances and the barriers to engagement in fishing within the environment.

Together using Marko's expert knowledge from many years of fishing and Anna's knowledge of occupational analysis they worked on matching Marko's capacities with the demands of going fishing. They developed a range of strategies and Marko agreed to try the following:

- Change the environment to a more stable one – fishing from the pier rather than a small boat after practicing by the side of a small pond in the grounds of the rehabilitation centre.
- Using a fishing harness to hold the fishing rod leaving Marko's right hand free to do the work.
- Adapting a market shopping trolley to hold all the fishing gear, fishing rod and a small folding seat so that Marko does not have to carry gear and can concentrate on walking.

Marko's partner agreed to the plan as long as Anna accompanied Marko on the first trip. Marko's partner was still a little anxious about him going fishing and the risk of falling, but accepted that the plan was much safer than having Marko fishing from a boat. In addition, it was important to both of them that Marko was able to get out and participate in some occupations on his own. The adaptations altered the occupational form of fishing, however, they retained the elements that Marko enjoyed and, thus, maintained the leisure experience within the context of his reduced capacities.

Practice Scenario 25.2 Older people living in the community

Occupational therapy students Phillipa and Amanda agreed to complete a project as part of their studies with a large provider of residential and community aged-care services. The agency had identified a need for a wider range of leisure occupations for older people beyond the stereotypical occupations, such as bingo and sing-alongs. Whilst a number of older people do enjoy those occupations, it was thought that a wider range was needed that help to promote a positive view of ageing.

The aim of the project was to provide an opportunity for members of the community over the age of 65 to engage in adventurous and challenging activities in an outdoor environment. Participants were recruited through circulating letters to community fitness and social groups for older people. The students also visited some groups and gave a presentation on the project.

They began by holding a focus group with a small group of people to explore the leisure occupations that people were involved in, and the factors that contributed to their participation. They also explored the occupations they had not tried and reasons why. It appears that the older people were concerned

about potentially injuring themselves attempting activities beyond their capacities, and wanted to learn about new activities at a pace that accommodated their abilities and limitations. Lastly the focus group sought opinions and ideas about occupations that the older people would like to try. From the information gained they developed a list of possible occupations and surveyed participants. By a democratic process the majority selected orienteering.

The students then had to educate themselves about orienteering and how to run groups. Orienteering is the sport of finding one's way through the countryside with the aid of a map and/or compass. It can be a competitive sport involving a high level of fitness and skills in map reading, or an enjoyable non-competitive challenge. To assist them, the students solicited the voluntary assistance of an experienced orienteer.

In the first group session the participants were introduced to basic map reading and orienteering skills before completing a 2.5 km course in a National Park. The next two sessions were in the parklands on the outskirts of the central business district and were graded in terms of the demands of the course length and heights of climb and the number of control points to be visited. The fourth and final session was held in the botanical gardens and participants competed in a timed challenge to see how many control points they could visit in one hour. The session was completed with a feedback discussion about the whole programme. The week following the completion of the project the group met independently and held an orienteering event.

Feedback from participants highlighted the perceived benefits, which included the stimulation from new learning, an increase in health from walking, socialising with others, and that it made them feel good. Interest grew as the programme progressed and new participants joined in. Groups of older people out in public spaces promote a positive message about growing older and keeping engaged in active leisure occupations. The programme highlighted that older people will try adventurous leisure occupations if introduced gradually in a graded supportive manner that takes account of individual capacities and limitations.

Despite leisure being a highly valued part of life it appears that occupational therapists have given more attention to paid work and self-care occupations. Surveys of occupational therapy practice in Australia (McEneany et al 2002), the United States

(Turner et al 2000) and the United Kingdom (Craik et al 1998) all suggest that leisure receives less attention by occupational therapists in the acute physical setting compared to the psychosocial practice setting where it appears that leisure is more valued and, thus, incorporated into practice. If occupational therapists are to be true to the philosophical and theoretical foundations of the profession, then they would typically explore leisure occupations with anyone who has experienced or is experiencing a major occupational transition. Transitions may be gradual and progressive, or sudden, and require people to renegotiate or re-orchestrate their daily occupations, change routines and generally re-examine their time use.

A significant transition occurs for people who retire from paid employment and find themselves with an abundance of un-obligated time to fill with occupations that are meaningful and satisfying, and that provide many of the benefits of vocational occupations (e.g. social aspects, routine, a sense of contributing to the social and economic fabric of society). Other transitions could include a disabled person becoming a parent, or someone becoming the parent of a disabled child, which places unique demands on the family. Larson (2006) found that for mothers of children with autism, the child's preference for routine made the orchestration of family occupations particularly stressful and impacted the mother's ability to engage in leisure occupations. Both the transition to retirement and parenthood reflect changes in role and time, but not necessarily physical capacity.

Changes in physical capacity are common and can be either sudden or gradual. Sudden transitions occur, for example, as a result of a cerebrovascular accident, a head injury, a work accident, or a spinal-cord injury where a distinct event causes a change in physical capacity. More gradual transitions as a result of changing physical capacity are experienced by people who live with chronic pain or limited joint range of movement from rheumatoid arthritis, as well as breathlessness and reduced endurance from cardiac problems. People on long-term oxygen therapy have reported significantly lower levels of life satisfaction in general, and with leisure participation when compared to people with chronic obstructive pulmonary disease and those without lung disease (Sturesson & Branholm 2000). It has also been found that following a diagnosis of multiple sclerosis people changed the number of leisure occupations they engaged in, often giving up

two-thirds of their leisure interests, with significant correlations between pain and morning stiffness and change in leisure occupations (Wikstrom et al 2001).

For older people, fear of falling can lead to a change in participation in leisure occupations. In a Dutch study (Delbaere et al 2004) of over 200 older people living in the community it was found that older people who experienced falls and developed a fear of falling tended to restrict their occupations, particularly those outside of the home in unfamiliar surroundings. This reduction in occupational repertoire then led to a reduction in physical capacities, which also increased the likelihood of further falls. Given the information about barriers to participation in daily occupations following falls it could be hypothesised that leisure occupations are the most likely to be eliminated from the occupational repertoire. Participation in a full range of occupations including leisure appears to be important for maintaining health and mobility in old age.

Though therapists may only meet a person for the first time at the point of such transitions, a thorough assessment is required to develop an understanding of those leisure occupations and experiences that are meaningful for the individual and situate them within an historical context, such that re-engagement can be effectively enabled.

Leisure assessment tools

Leisure assessments present many dilemmas as the chosen tools reflect a number of assumptions regarding the nature of leisure. As discussed previously, universal agreement on the nature of leisure does not exist, so the therapist must think carefully about which assessment is chosen and why. It is, therefore, important to discuss common tools that relate to the first two definitions offered in the first section of this chapter, that is leisure as time, and leisure as activity. Further, a critique of available tools and consideration of more qualitative approaches to accessing information about leisure participation and experience is useful in acknowledging the significance of this aspect of leisure.

Measurement of time

This approach aims to measure the frequency of participation in leisure occupations and the type of participation. Tools such as time diaries can be used, requiring people to record over a typical week all the times they spend in occupations they would describe as leisure. This reveals quite a lot of information about the temporal aspects of participation including; what days, what time of day, how often, how much time, what is the routine? Time diaries can also be used to include extra information about the context, such as where and with whom the occupation is performed.

A simple alternative to the time diary is to present the person with a circle and ask them to think of the circle as a pie representing 100% of their time. The person is then asked to divide the circle into segments that represent the percentage of time spent in occupations related to productivity, sleep, personal care, and leisure. This gives a visual representation of time use that can be quite powerful as a first step towards creating change. Despite strategies like time diaries and pie diagrams appearing to be closely aligned with views of leisure as residual time, people are given the opportunity to define their leisure times, and, thus, there is some acknowledgement of the experiential element.

Leisure as activity

Ideas of leisure as activity might suggest the use of an interest checklist, which, as the name suggests, involves the use of a comprehensive list of leisure occupations. The person is asked to indicate which of the occupations on the list they have done in the past, currently do, or would like to do in the future. As is fairly evident, the therapist gains information about the sorts of leisure occupations that the person might be interested in incorporating into the intervention plan. If therapists utilise occupations that are of interest to the person, they are more likely to engage the person in the therapy programme. The checklist most widely used by occupational therapists is the Interest Checklist first developed by Matsutsuyu (1969) and further developed by Rogers et al (1978). Other checklists include the Leisure Interest Profile for Adolescents (Henry 1998) and for Seniors (Henry 1997) as well as the Activity Index (Gregory 1983).

Interest checklists are limited in several ways. The range of occupations to choose from is inherently limited as a comprehensive list of all possible choices could not feasibly be collated. Also, checklists are culturally biased and may not be appropriate for people whose country of origin is different to that for which the tool is validated. Interest checklists for people who reside in cooler climates may not be suitable for people who live in tropical climates or vice versa. Some activities are also specific to the opportunities that the geographic location provides so that, for example, considering water-based activities in an inland location with no close bodies of water is not feasible. Some leisure occupations may not be available for all people because of socio-cultural values and expectations. In some cultures it is not considered appropriate for men and women to be doing the same leisure activities, or the appropriate attire for the activity may not be congruent with the values of the cultural group. Activities may also be quite age specific, for example, nightclubbing may not be an activity that is participated in and enjoyed across the life span.

The Activity Card sort (Baum 1995) is an instrument for assessing older people's participation in occupational performance of leisure activities as well as other instrumental, socio-cultural activities. It consists of a set of picture cards that depict adults performing activities and the person is asked to sort the cards into those that they currently engage in and those in which they have participated previously. The tool has been developed and adapted for various cultural groups including North American, Australian, Hong Kong and Israeli (Katz et al 2003) overcoming the issue with cultural relevance.

Occupational therapists have also developed tools to assess leisure relevant to a specific group. One such example is the Nottingham Leisure Questionnaire developed for use with people who have had a stroke (Drummond & Walker 1994). The questionnaire asks about leisure activities participated in during the previous year and the frequency of participation. The assessment has acceptable test–re-test reliability and inter-rater reliability and is suitable for self-administration (Drummond et al 2001).

Critique of tools

Thus far, we have discussed a range of tools that can be used to assess various aspects of leisure. These tools have their place in therapy and research as ways of collecting objective information about leisure participation so that change can be measured and monitored to establish the effect of a transition or the impact of an intervention. Measurement tools are, however, restricted in what they can evaluate and the degree to which they can truly access the affective dimension of experience. It could also be argued that since many of the tools have been developed there have been significant changes in the way we lead our lives, particularly in the use of technology, and thus ideas about leisure in the 21st century may be different from those at the time of development.

One attempt to measure the affective element of leisure participation is by measuring satisfaction with leisure with tools such as the Leisure Satisfaction Scale (Beard & Ragheb 1980). Di Bona (2000) recommended occupational therapists use a modified version of the leisure satisfaction scale and reported it to be a valid measure of leisure satisfaction. This scale and many others that are available to occupational therapists come from the discipline of leisure science rather than occupational therapy. Whilst occupational therapists often borrow knowledge from other disciplines, and, indeed, we share common knowledge (for example, knowledge of human anatomy) it must be remembered that the philosophical underpinnings of that tool may not be congruent with the tenants of occupational therapy. Suto (1998) argued that as the concept of leisure is further developed within occupational therapy there is a need for a concurrent development of assessments, which reflect a person-centred occupational perspective.

The Meaningfulness of Activity Scale (Gregory 1983) which has been used alongside the Activity Index is a scale that has been used within occupational therapy research. It is a Likert-type scale that derives a score for three dimensions of meaningfulness; enjoyment, autonomy and competence. The measure of autonomy asks the person whether they want to do the activity or have to do it. This measure of autonomy appears to come close to the notion that we have promoted earlier in this chapter of freedom of choice that denotes a leisure experience.

The tools discussed thus far have limitations but they do provide a valuable beginning point for discussions with people about leisure that can lead to more in-depth conversations about its subjective meaning.

Leisure as experience

Practitioners may need to use more qualitative interview approaches to access information about leisure experience. A compromise between purely quantitative or qualitative approaches is offered by assessment tools such as the Canadian Occupational Performance Measure (COPM) (Law et al 1998) or the Occupational Performance History Interview (OPHI) (Kielhofner & Henry 1988), which provide a structured framework for eliciting information about leisure occupations that people have performed and are having difficulty with currently. The COPM provides a score for satisfaction with performance and one for importance, as well as information about the value to the person in terms of priority.

Assessments such as the COPM are commonly used by occupational therapists when beginning to work with a person to help establish the individual's needs and priorities (Dedding et al 2004). These types of assessments include much more than leisure, but by using such an assessment the therapist can be efficient in collecting information about all areas of a person's life. Instead of using a more global assessment a therapist can always choose to focus purely on leisure and in particular leisure experience. This can be done by having an in-depth conversation with the person to gather rich qualitative data.

Building rapport with people through showing interest in them as an individual and listening to their values and priorities will be very important to accessing more in-depth information about leisure experience. The therapist can ask open-ended questions about leisure occupations to try to find out more about the meaning of the experience of any given occupation. Questions such as how does doing *this particular activity* make you feel? What do you like about it? What do you get from participating in *this particular activity*? What would it mean if you could no longer engage in *this particular activity*?

Once a therapist has explored leisure participation and leisure experience with a person or group it is the therapist's role to collaboratively address the identified occupational issues and enable engagement in occupations that promote leisure experiences.

Ways of enabling participation in leisure

The approaches to intervention generally used by occupational therapists can be grouped into four broad categories. These approaches all assume an underpinning of person-centred practice. We turn now to explore briefly each of the categories.

Temporal aspects

This involves close examination of how a person uses their time and makes time for leisure. A close examination of time use will enable the person to begin the re-orchestration of time often necessitated by occupational transitions. For some people it may be exploring what they do and where leisure would fit in. For people experiencing fatigue as a result of multiple sclerosis or a heart condition the therapist may help them to prioritise what is important, and educate them about energy conservation so that they can do the things they have to do and the things they want to do. It could also include examination of habits and routines. Following Ludwig's (1997) study of the importance of routine to the well-being of older women she suggested that occupational therapists give much greater consideration to the use of routine. If people incorporate leisure occupations into their routine it is much more likely to happen and thus they are more likely to achieve a healthful balance of occupations.

Adaptation of the environment and/or occupation

Traditionally, occupational therapists are known for their use of adaptive equipment and their skills in environmental modification in order to allow participation. This can be applied to participation in leisure occupations by adapting the occupation and/or environment when the demands of the occupation and the capacities of the person are not well matched. Occupational therapists can use existing commercially available adaptive equipment or design new devices.

The utilisation of adapted equipment or environmental modifications has to be carefully considered. The therapist always needs to consider if there is a simple alternative strategy before prescribing adaptive equipment. It is important that the adaptation should not interfere with the individual meaning of the occupation. For example, if the meaning of participating in a leisure occupation is about being independent and doing things for oneself, then having to rely on another person for assistance with adaptive equipment or to modify the environment each time

will alter the meaning derived from the leisure occupation. Therapists should employ only those adaptive strategies that facilitate engagement in the occupation in such a way that the original meaning is maintained.

Occupational substitution

If the person can no longer participate in a leisure occupation that they find meaningful or enjoyable and it is not possible to consider adapting the occupation or the environment it may be necessary to explore alternative occupations. This is often when checklists are used as a starting point to help the person explore where their interests might lie when searching for alternative occupations. Another way of substituting occupation is through exploring the leisure experience that was gained from the original occupation and searching for leisure occupations that might give that same experience, but be within the capacities of the person. The occupational therapist would ask questions such as:

- what was it about that occupation that was enjoyable?
- what did they get from it?
- what alternatives might give them the same or similar experience?

Once an alternative occupation has been identified the occupational therapist can work with the person to identify their learning needs, and work out a graded programme to exploring the new occupation, aimed at developing competence and then mastery.

Leisure as means

Occupational therapists work on developing a person's capacities and abilities to participate in daily occupations by developing occupational performance components. Leisure occupations are often used in this way as the means in therapy rather than the end (Primeau 2003). The purpose is not necessarily to enable participation in that occupation, but to use the leisure as a vehicle for developing the underlying occupational performance components. If the person experiences an increase in any of the occupational performance components they may be enabled to participate in a whole range of occupations necessary for daily life. Use of a leisure occupation to remediate occupational performance components is likely to be interesting and enjoyable, and will contribute to the person being motivated to participate in the therapy programme. The intrinsic motivation provided by leisure means that engagement in the therapy programme may be maintained despite slow improvement or setbacks. Use of leisure within a remedial approach is referred to as a 'bottom-up' approach to improving underlying occupational performance components; however, there is a question about whether skills taught in this way are generalised to occupational performance. Further, Neumayer and Wilding (2005) argue that there is a philosophical debate about the use of leisure to achieve therapeutic goals rather than for the benefits of engaging in leisure as an occupation that occupational therapists have not engaged in or resolved. They question whether the intrinsic benefits of leisure will be lost if leisure is used to achieve other goals. Though other therapists argue for a top-down approach rather than a bottom-up, it is beyond the scope of this chapter to fully articulate this debate.

Conclusion

Leisure is a very challenging concept. It operates as a subjective personal experience situated in the context of time and occupation and can mean different things to different people based on their culture, disability status or age amongst other factors. Such fluidity necessitates that therapists use assessment strategies that acknowledge the person's individual experience, avoid imposition of their own values, or limit the person's expression through the use of tools with an overly narrow focus. Further, whether seeking to use leisure as ends or means, strategies need to enable engagement by adapting only those elements of the environment, person or occupation that will not impinge on the leisure experience. If the therapist is able to achieve this, leisure can be an extremely powerful tool in therapy, providing intrinsic motivation to engage in occupations that may have secondary physically therapeutic benefits, thus facilitating an effective partnership in developing and implementing intervention plans.

References

Baum, C. (1995). The contribution of occupation to function in persons with Alzheimer's disease. *Journal of Occupational Science: Australia*, 2(2), 59–67.

Beard, J. & Ragheb, M. (1980). The leisure satisfaction measure. *Journal of Leisure Research*, 12(1), 20–33.

Christiansen, C. & Townsend, E. (2004). An introduction to occupation. In C. Christiansen & E. Townsend (Eds.), *Introduction to occupation: The art and science of living* (pp. 1–27). Upper Saddle River: Prentice Hall.

Coleman, D. & Iso-Ahola, S. E. (1993). Leisure and health: The role of social support and self-determination. *Journal of Leisure Research*, 25(2), 111–128.

Craik, C., Chacksfield, J. & Richards, G. (1998). A survey of occupational therapy practitioners in mental health. *British Journal of Occupational Therapy*, 61(5), 227–234.

Csikszentmihalyi, M. (1991). *Flow: The psychology of optimal experience*. New York, Harper & Collins.

Csikszentmihalyi, M. & Mei-Ha Wong, M. (1991). The situational and personal correlates of happiness: A cross-national comparison. In: F. Strack, M. Argyle & N. Schwartz (Eds). *Subjective well-being*. (pp. 193–212). Toronto, Pergammon Press.

Dare, B., Welton, G. & Coe, W. (1987). *Concepts of leisure in Western thought*. Dubuque, Kendall/Hunt.

Dedding, C., Cardol, M., Eyssen, I. et al. (2004). Validity of the Canadian Occupational Performance Measure: A client-centred outcome measurement. *Clinical Rehabilitation*, 18(6), 660–667.

Delbaere, K., Crombes, G., Vanderstraaten, G. et al. (2004). Fear-related avoidance of activities, falls and physical frailty: A prospective community based cohort study. *Age & Aging*, 33(4), 368–373.

Di Bona, L. (2000). What are the benefits of leisure? An exploration using the leisure satisfaction scale. *British Journal of Occupational Therapy*, 63(2), 50–58.

Drummond, A. E. R. & Walker, M. F. (1994). The Nottingham leisure questionnaire for stroke patients. *British Journal of Occupational Therapy*, 57(11), 414–418.

Drummond, A. & Walker, M. (1996). Generalisation of the effects of leisure rehabilitation for stroke patients. *British Journal of Occupational Therapy*, 59(7), 330–334.

Drummond, A. E. R., Parker, C. J., Gladman, J. R. F. et al. (2001). Development and validation of the Nottingham Leisure Questionnaire (NLQ). *Clinical Rehabilitation*, 15, 647–656.

Emerson, H. (1998). Flow and occupation: A review of the literature. *Canadian Journal of Occupational Therapy*, 65(1), 37–44.

Gregory, M. (1983). Occupational behavior and life satisfaction among retirees. *American Journal of Occupational Therapy*, 37(8), 548–553.

Henry, A. (1997). *Leisure interest profile for seniors* (research version 2.0). Boston, University of Massachusetts.

Henry, A. (1998). Development of a measure of adolescent leisure interests. *American Journal of Occupational Therapy*, 52(7), 531–539.

Howell, D. & Pierce, D. (2000). Exploring the forgotten restorative dimension of occupation: Quilting and quilt use. *Journal of Occupational Science*, 7(2), 68–72.

Hutchinson, S., Loy, D., Kleiber, D. et al. (2003). Leisure as a coping resource: Variations in coping with traumatic illness and injury. *Leisure Sciences*, 25(2), 143–161.

Iso-Ahola, S. E. (1997). A psychological analysis of leisure and health. In: J. Haworth (Ed.) *Work, leisure and well-being*. (pp. 131–144) London, Routledge.

Katz, N., Karpin, H., Lak, A. et al. (2003). Participation in occupational performance: Reliability and validity of the activity card sort. *OTJR: Occupation, Participation and Health*, 23(1), 10–17.

Kelly, J. & Freysinger, V. (2000). *21st century leisure: Current issues.* Boston, Allyn & Bacon.

Kielhofner, G. & Henry, A. (1988). Development and investigation of the occupational performance history interview. *American Journal of Occupational Therapy*, 42(8), 489–498.

Kleiber, D., Brock, S., Lee, Y. et al. (1995). The relevance of leisure in an illness experience: Realities of spinal cord injury. *Journal of Leisure Research*, 27(3), 283–299.

Kleiber, D., Hutchinson, S. & Williams, R. (2002). Leisure as a resource in transcending negative life events: Self-protection, self-restoration, and personal transformation. *Leisure Sciences*, 24(2), 219–235.

Larson, E. (2006). Caregiving and autism: How does children's propensity for routinization influence participation in family

activities? *OTJR: Occupation, Participation and Health*, 26(2), 69–79.

Law, M., Baptiste, S., Carswell, A. et al. (1998). *Canadian occupational performance measure*, (2nd ed). Ottawa, CAOT.

Lee, Y., Dattilo, J. & Howard, D. (1994). The complex and dynamic nature of leisure experience. *Journal of Leisure Research*, 26(3), 195–211.

Lefevre, J. (1988). Flow and the quality of experience during work and leisure. In: M. Csikszentmihalyi & I. Csikszentmihalyi (Eds) *Optimal experience: psychological studies of flow in consciousness*. (pp. 307–318). Cambridge, Cambridge University Press.

Ludwig, F. (1997). How routine facilitates well-being in older women. *Occupational Therapy International*, 4(3), 213–228.

Matsutsuyu, J. (1969). The interest checklist. *The American Journal of Occupational Therapy* 23(4), 323–328.

McEneany, J., McKenna, K. & Summerville, P. (2002). Australian occupational therapists working in adult physical dysfunction settings: What treatment media do they use? *Australian Occupational Therapy Journal*, 49(3), 115–127.

Neulinger, J. (1974). *The psychology of leisure*, (2nd ed). Illinois, Charles C Thomas.

Neumayer, B. & Wilding, C. (2005). Leisure as commodity. In: G. Whiteford & V. Wright-St Clair (Eds) *Occupation and practice in context*. (pp. 317–331). Sydney, Elsevier.

Parry, D. C. & Shinew, K. J. (2004). The constraining impact of infertility on women's leisure. *Leisure Sciences*, 26(3), 295–308.

Primeau, L. (1996). Work and leisure: Transcending the dichotomy. *The American Journal of Occupational Therapy*, 50(7), 569–577.

Primeau, L. (2003). Play and leisure. In: E. Crepeau, E. Cohn & B.

Schell (Eds) *Willard and Spackman's occupational therapy*. (pp. 354–363). Philadelphia, Lippincott Williams & Wilkins.

Rogers, J., Weinstein, J. & Figone, J. (1978). The interest checklist: An empirical assessment. *American Journal of Occupational Therapy*, 32(10), 628–630.

Rojek, C. (2004). Postmodern work and leisure. In: J. Haworth & A. Veal (Eds) *Work and leisure*. (pp. 51–66). London, Routledge.

Russell, R. & Stage, F. (1996). Leisure as burden: Sudanese refugee women. *Journal of Leisure Research*, 28(2), 108–121.

Sellar, B. & Boshoff, K. (2006). Subjective leisure experiences of older Australians. *Australian Occupational Therapy Journal*, 53(3), 211–219.

Specht, J., King, G., Brown, E. et al. (2002). The importance of leisure in the lives of persons with congenital physical disabilities. *The American Journal of Occupational Therapy*, 56(4), 436–445.

Sturesson, M. & Branholm, I. (2000). Life satisfaction in subjects with chronic obstructive pulmonary disease. *Work*, 14(2), 77–82.

Suto, M. (1998). Leisure in occupational therapy. *Canadian Journal of Occupational Therapy*, 65(5), 271–278.

Tinsley, H., Hinson, J., Tinsley, D. et al. (1993). Attributes of leisure and work experiences. *Journal of Counseling Psychology*, 40(4), 447–455.

Turner, H., Chapman, S., McSherry, A. et al. (2000). Leisure assessment in occupational therapy: An exploratory study. *Occupational Therapy in Health Care*, 12(2/3), 73–85.

Wikstrom, I., Isacsson, A. & Jacobsson, T. (2001). Leisure activities in rheumatoid arthritis: Change after disease onset and associated factors. *British Journal of Occupational Therapy*, 64(2), 87–92.

Chapter Twenty-Six

26

Play

Karen Stagnitti

CHAPTER CONTENTS

What is play? 372

Theories of play 372

Play development 373

Types of play 373

An occupational perspective on play 373

The value of play 377

    Long-term health and well-being 377

    Pretend play and language 378

    Literacy and learning 378

    Pretend play and narrative competence . . 378

    Social interaction and competence 379

    Creativity and problem-solving 379

'Play as means' or 'play as ends' in
occupational therapy 379

    'Play as a means' in therapy 379

    'Play as an ends' in therapy. 383

Conclusion 387

SUMMARY

Children's play reflects their development, their inner world, their social understanding and the essence of who they are. In occupational therapy, play is used as a means to engage children in assessment and intervention. When play is used 'as a means' the therapist is focused on specific skills and uses play to engage the child. In this situation, not only does the child demonstrate to the therapist the 'doing' of a particular skill, but the child also engages in the 'being' of play – the enjoyment of play. More recently within the profession, a better understanding of the importance of play in and of itself has resulted in the development of new approaches to play assessments and play interventions. These developments have assisted in the understanding of 'play as an ends'. When the play ability of the child is assessed, the therapist is less directive in his or her assessment, and observations are made regarding the 'doing' of play as well as the child's enjoyment of play (the 'being' of play). Intervention to build the child's play ability is monitored by the therapist with the aim of the child 'becoming' a player. When children become players they are able to self-initiate ideas in play, participate with peers, and enjoy the play for longer. Evidence of the benefits of becoming a player have shown enhancement in the health and well-being of children.

KEY POINTS

- Play is one of the most complex of the behaviours of childhood.
- Understanding of the 'doing' and 'being' of play helps understand the 'becoming' and 'belonging' of the person.
- In order to play, a child requires developmental ability in the areas of language, motor skill, sensory awareness, social skills, emotional awareness, and cognition.
- Understand play and you engage the child in therapy.
- Parents, guardians and professionals may need to learn how to play.
- The environment includes toys, unstructured objects, peers, adults, and space.
- Play is an ends, not only a means.

What is play?

In this chapter, play is considered only in the context of childhood. This does not negate adult play (represented, for example, as rest or leisure in various occupational therapy models) but rather defines the boundaries for the discussion in this chapter. Play is the 'most essential and meaningful occupation' of children (Algado & Burgman 2005, p. 251). It is the language of children (Algado & Burgman) because children can express in play what they cannot express with verbal language. Play has been deemed to be important for all aspects of physical, emotional, sensory, perceptual, and cognitive development (Canadian Association of Occupational Therapists 1996).

Difficulties in defining play have had implications for the assessment of play (Bundy 2005, Lautamo et al 2005). In essence, because play has been difficult to define, it has not always been used in assessment in paediatric occupational therapy (see Couch et al 1997, Reid 1987, Rodger 1994) and this has had implications for working with children. Since the 1990s, attempts have been made by occupational therapy and other researchers to associate some behaviours with play (Bracegirdle 1992, Goodman 1994, Parham & Primeau 1997, Stewart et al 1991, Sturgess 2003). Hence play is considered to be:

- more internally than externally motivated
- able to transcend reality as well as reflect reality
- controlled by the player
- more focused on the process than product
- usually safe, fun, unpredictable, and pleasurable
- spontaneous and involves non-obligatory active engagement
- non-literal
- opportunistic and episodic
- imaginative
- creative.

More broadly, play has also been defined as exploratory in nature, consisting of a variety of activities that involve movement and manipulation in relation to the environment, and encompassing motor, sensory, and cognitive/perceptual skills (Anderson et al 1987, Pierce 1997, Robinson 1977, Sutton-Smith 1967).

Stagnitti and Unsworth (2000) stated that pretend play is a uniquely identifiable and essential play type. Pretend play is synonymous with the following terms: imaginative play, fantasy play, thematic fantastic play, representational play, and make-believe play. Stagnitti and Unsworth suggested that pretend play not only includes many of the play behaviours noted above, but also consists of two play types: symbolic play and conventional-imaginative play. Symbolic play includes three key behaviours (Leslie 1987, Lewis et al 1992): use of an object as something else (e.g. a box is used as a car), attribution of a property to an object (e.g. the box 'car' is fast), and reference to an absent object (e.g. the box car stops at the 'station'). Conventional-imaginative play is play with commercial toys (for example, dolls and trucks) and occurs when the child pretends a toy is something else (e.g. a train carriage is a boat), attributes a property to a toy (e.g. the doll is asleep), or refers to an absent object (e.g. a sweep of the arm indicates a door to a house). Conventional-imaginative play is in contrast to functional play. In functional play children play with commercial toys by functionally relating the objects together without the element of pretend (Casby 1992, Lewis et al 1992).

When engaging in pretend play it is assumed that children play with two different types of play materials: conventional toys and unstructured objects. The term 'conventional toys' has also been referred to as highly structured toys (Pulaski 1973), high realism toys (Phillips 1945), realistic toys (Jeffree & McConkey 1976), and miniatures (Clifford & Bundy 1989). Unstructured play materials have been referred to as low realism toys (Phillips 1945), junk material (Jeffree & McConkey 1976), or unstructured toys (Pulaski 1973).

Theories of play

Theories of play have been categorised into the classical theories of play, modern theories of play and socio-cultural theories of play (for further details see Mellou 1994, Parham & Primeau 1997). Classical theories include the surplus energy, the relaxation (or recreation), the pre-exercise and the recapitulation theories of play. Modern theories include the arousal modulation, the psychodynamic, and the cognitive developmental theories of play. Socio-cultural theories of play include the play as socialisation and the meta-communicative theories. Through time, the main protagonists of these theories have been either influenced by prevailing views (e.g. the Pre-exercise theory and Recapitulation theory are influenced by Darwinian theory) (Parham & Primeau 1997) or introduced new concepts (e.g. Freud is a key author of the psychodynamic theories). These theories present the varying concepts of play held over the past two centuries and show the value ascribed to play in child development over time (Stagnitti 2004a). While the earlier theories of play argued there was no inherent value in play, the theories from the pre-exercise to modern theories argued, to various degrees, the value of play to child development. The next section takes a closer look at play within child development.

Play development

In the first year of life, play development revolves around the development of large muscle movements, sensory motor awareness, social awareness, and manipulation and exploration of objects. In the second year of life emotional attachments to important figures strengthen, the child begins to play imaginatively, starts to use objects as symbols, and words begin to be uttered. By the third year of life (i.e. 24–36 months), the child's play becomes complex with logical sequential actions, increased awareness of their social environment, and increased use of symbols in play. The development of large and small muscles, sensory, social, cognitive, language, and emotional understanding, and manipulation and exploration of objects continues, along with increasing complexity in pretend play. By 5 years of age, the child can play with groups of peers using characterisations, role play, and abstract symbols, and can create social situations where emotions can be contained within the play. The doll (or other object with life-like features) has a life of its own in parallel with the child. Table 26.1 presents more detailed information on the development of play in children from 0 to 5 years.

Types of play

There are several different types of play. Table 26.2 lists types of play, a description, the assumed benefits and examples of activities that would be associated with the specific type of play. Please note that the term 'assumed benefits' has been used

deliberately as there is only limited evidence to support the benefits of play. The types of play outlined in Table 26.2 could also be construed as different skills grouped together as types of play. The unique feature of play is that 'it is in the eye of the beholder' (Stagnitti 2004a, p. 5) and so what could be regarded as play by one, is regarded as skills by another. The purpose of Table 26.2 is to demonstrate that play is an all-encompassing occupation and to suggest a structure for understanding this complex occupation.

An occupational perspective on play

In occupational therapy, play is considered to be extremely important to child development and viewed as being important in itself (Parham & Primeau 1997, Rodger & Ziviani 1999). In the following section, this view is explained in terms of 'doing', 'being', 'becoming', and 'belonging' (Wilcock 1999, 2006).

The 'doing' of play is what children do in terms of play skills (e.g. the technique of throwing a ball) and abilities (e.g. the capacity to throw a ball to another), and their developmental level of play. 'Purposeful doing' (Wilcock 1999) in play is when children play ('do') at their developmental level in a play activity that is culturally, socially, and personally meaningful to them. Wilcock noted that 'doing or not doing are powerful determinants of well being or disease' (1999, p. 3). When children do not play, they are at risk of ill health, poor developmental outcomes and social isolation (Taneja et al 2002, Walker et al 2005). When children play (do), they are stimulated, practising skills, exploring the world, showing curiosity, and increasing their well-being (Taneja et al 2002, Walker et al 2005).

The 'being' of play is connected to the doing of play. Wilcock (1999) says that ' "Being" is about being true to ourselves, to our nature, to our essence and to what is distinctive about us to bring to other as part of our relationships and to what we do' (p. 5). She goes on to suggest that being or 'to be' requires time to discover who we are, time to think, reflect, and exist (Wilcock 1999). 'To be' a player requires time to play, time to discover, time to explore, and to be curious, and time to just enjoy playing. By being a player, children can experience creativity in occupation because they are solving problems of daily life and engaged in intellectual,

Table 26.1 The development of play

Age	Play development
0–6 months	Children spend a lot of energy developing large muscles so that they can move against gravity. They learn to hold up their head while leaning on their forearms, rolling over from back to stomach, and they begin to sit up. Their eye–hand co-ordination develops as primitive reflexes integrate. Children begin to co-ordinate eye and hand and hand-to-hand. They experiment with objects, manipulate objects and transfer objects from hand to hand. They repeat actions so as to integrate information, they respond to voice, touch, and visual cues
7–18 months	During this period the child begins to crawl and then walks independently pushing large toys. Bilateral arm use continues to develop. Children can roll a ball to an adult, listen selectively, and look at a picture book. From 12 months, they can hold a crayon and scribble and use two hands in play. During play, children use trial and error in problem solving. Experimentation and manipulation of objects predominates play with pretend play beginning to develop. From 13 to 18 months, pretend play begins with children's play themes centred on the body, such as pretending to have a drink or going to sleep. Children use one pretend action during play (e.g. pretending to put the doll to bed). Children understand the functional use of objects, such as a spoon goes with a cup and money goes in a purse. Children imitate others around them and carry out actions previously seen (e.g. feeding the doll)
18–24 months	During this period children's play actions move from illogical (e.g. pushing a truck, then putting in the items) to logical (e.g. putting items in a truck, then pushing the truck). Play themes reflect life in the home. Play actions can be repetitive as the child learns and understands new concepts. A child begins to use an object as something else (e.g. a block as a mobile phone), although this may be observed earlier in children who are developing well. Children now understand that others may like the same things as them and so they show others their favourite book or point out items of interest, such as when passing a bus. Children begin to be able to throw and kick a ball, and jump on two feet. They can turn pages of a book and string beads
2 years	Children's play themes reflect their own experience and develop from those reflected in the home (e.g. wanting to undertake domestic chores) to themes outside the home (e.g. shopping, visiting relatives.) By 24 months, the child has logical sequential actions in play. Play is short and there is no planned storyline. Children begin to use one object as something else, starting with a physically similar object, such as a box for a bed. By 30–36 months, the child can use the same object for several functions (e.g. the box can be a car, bed, hat, container or table). Children enjoy playing beside others and increasingly take note of what other children are playing. The children now understand that the doll is separate to them and they can wait for the doll to 'wake up' or have a drink. Children begin to hop and ride a trike and manipulate a toy with moving parts
3 years	Play themes now include fantasy themes with characters from television, books, and various media being incorporated into play. By 42 to 48 months, the child shows evidence of a play strategy. That is, the child thinks of what to play then finds the items needed to play that scenario. The child can use body parts in play (e.g. fingers can be a comb). Children play in association with others and in doll play, the child begins to designate characteristics to the doll
4 years	Children's play themes now contain two stories because they create problems to solve in the play story. For example, playing in home corner the 'mother' may have a sick baby, or may have no 'food'. Children begin to use abstract problem solving. Children begin to play in groups, co-operating, negotiating, arguing, and fighting. Play is pre-planned with a storyline, although the storyline in the play may evolve over several days. Children now use any object in substitution, for example, a shoe can be used as a telephone. In role play, a child may have several roles in the same play session. Children can skip, hop, copy diagonal lines, complete a 10-piece puzzle, and play games with language (e.g. saying similar-sounding nonsense words to real words)
5 years	Children can now play any theme and can now make up a completely fictional story. The same play theme may be played out over several weeks. They use language to embellish object play and to explain the use of creations they have made. Play in groups continues to develop with co-operation, negotiation and arguments. When playing a role, the child is now expected by peers to maintain the same role throughout the play. The doll has its own life and has possibly been married, has a career, and has its own adventures. In their play, children begin to be more realistic and less fantastic in their play compared to 4-year-olds. Five-year-olds can participate in organised games with rules

Table 26.2 Types of play

Type of play	Description and assumed benefits	Sample of activities
Gross motor play	Description Large muscle movement Assumed benefits Balance, strength, stability, posture, self-esteem	Running, climbing, rolling, ball catching, skipping, jumping, balancing, large block play
Fine motor play	Description Small muscle movement Mainly concerned with hand function – finger movement, in-hand manipulation, also wrist, shoulder, trunk movement Assumed benefits Hand control, hand and finger strength, ability to achieve in school tasks involving hand skills, fine motor skill development, handwriting, self-esteem	Threading, drawing, tracing, play dough, small block play, pegboard, scissors, manipulation of small objects
Visual-perceptual play	Description Visual skills and visual perception skills Assumed benefits Recognition of shapes and letters, recognition of colours, memory improvement, reading, self-esteem	Puzzles, shape-matching games, colour-matching games, visual and auditory memory games
Auditory play	Description Hearing and listening skills, auditory discrimination, auditory figure-ground Assumed benefits Concentration, attention, listening	Auditory memory games, I spy, play with sounds of words, listening games, match that sound games
Sensory motor play	Description Tactile, vestibular, proprioceptive, kinaesthetic, gustatory, olfactory abilities Assumed benefits Leads to sensory integration, sensory-motor competence, increased co-ordination, increased balance, self-esteem	Swinging, touching different textures, mud play, water play, rolling in a blanket, scooter board play, guessing games, sand play
Pretend play	Description Symbolic play and conventional-imaginative play Behaviours include: use of object for something else; attribution of a property to an object, reference to an absent object Behaviour that occurs when there is imposed meaning Assumed benefits Divergent and convergent problem solving, social awareness, social and emotional integration, ability to symbolise, increase in language utterances, greater understanding of story	Role play, home corner play, dressing up, play when there is imposed meaning such as swimming in the ocean but children are lying on the ground moving their arms and legs, playing transport vehicles in the sand pit

playful activity (Russ 2003, Wilcock 2006). 'To be' players, children require time, space, and props. Occupational therapists are often quick to intervene and 'do', but appreciating the 'being of play' means that therapists may need to stop 'doing'. For therapists to understand the 'being' of play, it is appropriate that they observe the play, the child's attitude towards playing and whether the child is engaged in the play.

'Doing' and 'being' compliment each other. If a child cannot do, then it is difficult for that child 'to be' when it comes to play. For example, during data collection for some play research I was involved in several years ago, I came across a child, who, during a child-initiated play assessment kept looking at this toy watch and saying that 'he had to go'. When I mentioned we had more time to play, he held one of the toys, put it down and then repeated that 'he had to go because [his friend] would be at kinder now'. He also admitted that while he had similar toys at home he didn't know what to do with them – he didn't know how to play with them. After five more minutes and several suggestions from himself that he should be going, the session finished. This child could not 'be' and did not enjoy playing because he could not 'do' play. On further examination, his play was restricted and limited to adult-directed activities, gross motor play activities, such as football or bike riding, or peer-led activities.

The 'becoming' of play is the potential for growth (emotionally, physically, and cognitively), of transformation into a participating member of society, and self-actualisation of who one is (Wilcock 1999). Through play, children can become players who can self-initiate play ideas and contribute these ideas when playing with peers, friends, and siblings. They can become people who are able to grow to their full potential and contribute to society. By becoming, children can 'belong' and participate. They can belong to their peer group, their class group, and their family group. 'Belonging' means that they are accepted by their peers, family group, and community.

Doing, being, becoming and belonging give a sense of spirituality or meaning to play as a purposeful occupation in childhood. Play as a purposeful occupation is seen as a basic human need which is linked with a child's health and well-being (Wilcock 2006). Play reflects 'the essence of self' (that is, the spiritual aspect of occupation) (Canadian Association of Occupational Therapists 1999) and is valued by and is meaningful to children when they choose play (Canadian Association of Occupational Therapists, 1999). The ability to choose play is most easily seen when children can self-initiate play, and so have control and choice over what they play (Ferland 2005, Missuna & Pollock 1991). The boy in the previous example could not self-initiate play and had restricted choice over what he played as he was dependent on adult and peer support. Through the occupation of play, children 'do', they enjoy 'being' in the moment, and they 'become' players who can initiate play ideas and contribute to peer play.

Many children who are seen by an occupational therapist cannot play, or their play development has been disrupted. To assist children to value play and

find it meaningful, the occupational therapist must also value play as a meaningful occupation. By understanding the 'doing' of play (e.g. play development, skills and abilities), the 'being' (e.g. the enjoyment of and time to play), and the 'becoming' and 'belonging' (e.g. joining with peers as a player) that play brings to the life of a child, the therapist can engage with children and assist them to play.

Another way to frame how a therapist can assist a child to play is to take into account the occupation of play in conjunction with the person of the child and the child's environment. The occupation of play incorporates the 'doing', 'being', 'becoming' and 'belonging' of play, and while the person and the child's environment are embedded within Wilcock's framework, the three components of person, environment, and the occupation of play also reflect the values of the person, environment, occupation, and performance (PEOP) theoretical model (Baum & Christiansen 2005). The person and environment components of working with children to develop their play skills are covered in more detail below.

The child is central to the person component. The child's development in play, including affective, cognitive, social and physical performance components, along with the child's diagnosis, gender and age, are all considered by the therapist. The therapist will also need to deal with people involved in the child's life, including the parents/carers, siblings, extended family, and foster carers. For example, the abilities of the parent (or foster parent or guardian) to play and the attitudes of the parent towards play are considerations that will impact on therapy. Siblings and extended family are part of the child's social environment, but there are times when they impact on the person component, for example, siblings may be included in play sessions or the values of extended family may impact such that discussion with extended family about the child's therapy may need to be scheduled. When the person component represents the therapist, consideration is given to the therapist's values, skills and philosophical orientation and how these will impact on interactions with the child.

'To be' in play requires time, space, and materials. Other aspects of the environment that impact on play include: the socio-economic status (SES) of the child's family, the family's access to services, toys and play materials in the environment, early childhood settings and facilities, culture of the family and society, geographical location of the child (e.g. rural, urban, remote), access to transport, parental health and attitudes, siblings, peers, presence of extended family, health professionals, and policies of the health service and government in relation to children. As children's play reflects the culture and society in which they live (Factor 2005), considerations could also be made to the effect societal change has on play. For example, Sturgess (2003) voiced concern about changes that are occurring in Australian society that could damage healthy play and noted an increase in adult-directed activities for children and less time spent in child-directed play. Simmond's (2005) gave an account of her experiences in Vietnam using communal play groups to challenge the cultural norm of leaving children in their cots all day.

The experience of children in being able to engage in play within their environment can be facilitated by the therapist when a therapist understands and values the doing, being, becoming, and belonging of play within the child's context. An analysis of a child's occupational engagement in play may result in the identification of:

- poor occupational engagement due to a lack of inherent play ability in the child (e.g. difficulty in 'doing' play through developmental delay in play ability)

- poor occupational engagement due to a lack of time, space, or play materials, such that 'being' in play is severely affected (occupational deprivation)

- poor occupational engagement due to lack of access to space and play materials, attitudes of parents/carers, cultural restrictions, which can lead to play deficits in doing, being, becoming, and belonging (occupational injustice)

- occupational imbalance due to lack of play experience because of excess time spent in a wheelchair, or in other occupations such as self-care. Occupational imbalance could also occur due to avoidance of types of play because of lack of ability in that play (e.g. spending excess time playing with electronic games, watching TV, videos and DVDs because of an inability to self-initiate play ideas). Occupational imbalance has implications for doing, being, becoming and belonging in play.

- occupational alienation due to ability to play with only one type of play material (e.g. play consists of spinning wheels on a car). When such restricted 'doing' in play occurs, 'becoming' and 'belonging' are severely affected.

The value of play

Children develop skills when they play (the 'doing' of play), they spend time in the enjoyment of play (the 'being' of play) and through play they become socially connected with their siblings, peers, and carers, and their intellect and physical and emotional well-being is stimulated and enhanced (the 'becoming' of play to be a player and 'belonging' to a group). The recognition of value and importance of play is shared by many other professions (for example, see Bruner et al 1976, Sutton-Smith 1997, Westby 1991). Below are some of the studies which provide evidence for the value of play to child development.

Long-term health and well-being

Evidence of the value of play in the long-term health and well-being of individuals is beginning to appear in the literature. Walker et al (2005) followed-up children in Jamaica over a 19-year period. They were concerned with early childhood stunting and its effect on long-term development. Over the 19-year period, they tracked children who were stunted in their growth. They systematically assigned 129 children to one of four groups. These groups were: control, supplementation, stimulation, and stimulation and supplementation. The supplementation group comprised a 1 kg milk-based formula per week and the stimulation group comprised a weekly visit to the home by a community health worker who encouraged interactions through play to improve mother–child interactions. Thirty-two children who were not stunted were matched to the control group. When the children were followed-up at 17–18 years of age, they found that the stunted children who received the home-based stimulation in early childhood sustained cognitive and educational benefits at 17–18 years of age compared to those who did not receive stimulation (Walker et al 2005).

The Early Years Study in Canada (Norrie McCain & Fraser-Mustard 1999) highlighted the fact that brain development in early childhood is rapid and that early stimulation and positive interactions between children and adults, is extremely important for brain development and consequent skills and abilities throughout life. They highlighted that stimulation in the first three years of life was critical to a child's long-term development (Norrie McCain & Fraser-Mustard 1999).

Pretend play and language

The emergence of pretend play in children has been linked to the emergence of true language (Westby 1980, 1991) because the ability to use language and the ability to pretend play require mental representation (Westby 1980). Mental representation presupposes the ability to symbolise and language is the use of words as symbols and pretend play includes the use of objects as symbols (e.g. the box symbolises a car). McCune (1995) found that pretend play development came before language development and Lyytinen et al (1999) found that pretend play and vocabulary production of 14-month-old toddlers uniquely contributed to their language skills at 2 years of age. Furthermore, pretend play development in the second year of life coincides with two-word utterances (Greenspan & Lieberman 1994, Lewis et al 1992, Lowe 1975, Lunzer 1959, McCune Nicolich 1981, Piaget 1962, Sleigh 1980, Whittaker 1982, Wing et al 1977). For example, Lowe (1975) noted that decentration (that is, the ability to use an object as real, outside of self, such as doll play) occurred at the same time children began putting words together.

Literacy and learning

Much of the work researching the connection between pretend play and literacy has concerned language-literacy tasks such as oral language, narrative competence, and decontextualised language (Nourot & Van Hoorn 1991, Pellegrini & Galda 1993, Roskos 1991, Schrader 1990, Westby 1991). Narrative competence is the ability to generate a story and this occurs when children act out scenes in their play, such as mothers and fathers. Decontextualised language is the use of words or actions in a context that is not dependent on context (Pellegrini 1985). Decontextualised language is thought to be the common base between pretend play and language-literacy because when children pretend play they use decontextualised language. When a child uses decontextualised language in play, the child is required to use language to explain to others the meaning of the play (e.g. the storyline of the play) as well as the meanings of objects used in play. In a study of 65 school-aged children, Pellegrini (1980) found that a child's level of pretend play was a significant predictor of achievement performance in reading and writing in the first year of school. Inability to use decontextualised language (e.g. talking about flying to the moon when you are at school) has been associated with lack of academic success in children with learning disabilities (Westby 1991). The quality of a child's pretend play has been found to discriminate between preschoolers who are typically developing and preschoolers who have been identified as being at risk for pre-academic problems (Stagnitti et al 2000).

Pretend play and narrative competence

Narrative is also referred to as storytelling, and it is the type of language that children and adults engage in when relating stories. Narrative competence involves the child's ability to form mental representations of a story structure (Pellegrini 1985). To understand a narrative a child must understand character-appropriate language and behaviour, such as a character's actions, motives, and goals that are consistent with a particular story (Pellegrini 1985, Westby 1991). Narrative competence assists with 'forward thinking' because as a child reads a story, they start to predict what may be coming, how characters will behave, and what they will say (Westby 1991). The ability of a child to recognise and use these aspects of narrative has been identified developmentally in children's pretend play. For example, Pellegrini (1985) noted that 3-year-old children used language to enact characters and 4-year-old children used language to attribute motives and feelings to characters.

Re-enacting stories has been found to aid story comprehension of preschool children and improve the story comprehension of older primary school children who have reading comprehension levels below their age level (Christie 1994, Pellegrini & Galda 1993). Pretend play appears to serve a developmental function related to narrative competence during the preschool period. Nicolopoulou (2005) put forward the suggestion that play and narrative are on a continuum, with play being at one end involving the enactment of the narrative and discursive exposition of narrative being at the other end.

Social interaction and competence

Children who have higher developmental levels of pretend play have been found to be more socially competent, and have a greater understanding of emotions. For example, Howes and Matheson (1992) studied the social play of children aged between 10 and 59 months. They found that children who showed more complex play were more pro-social, less aggressive, and less withdrawn than the children with lower developmental levels of play. Lindsey & Colwell (2003) found that children who demonstrated higher developmental levels of social pretend play had a greater understanding of emotions than children with lower levels of pretend play. They also found that boys who engaged in physical play had a greater understanding of emotions than boys who did not.

Baron-Cohen (1996) and Leslie (1987), among others, have linked theory of mind (a theory of how people perceive or 'read' social situations) with pretend play. Baron-Cohen (1996) explained that when pretend play development begins, children also begin to understand that others can have different beliefs to themselves.

Creativity and problem-solving

Sandra Russ's work has examined the association of pretend play with the development of creative problem-solving (Russ 1998). She followed up 31 early primary school children over a 4-year period to investigate if their pretend play ability, when they were in first and second grade, predicted their divergent thinking and problem-solving when they were in grade five or six (Russ et al 1999). The study results showed that the quality of the children's pretend play when they were younger predicted their divergent problem-solving over time, independent of their intelligence quotient (IQ). This study added evidence to the concept that cognitive and emotional processes in pretend play are stable over time. A study by Wyver & Spence (1995) found a reciprocal relationship between pretend play and divergent problem-solving, with preschool children who displayed higher developmental levels of pretend play having better problem-solving ability

than preschool children who displayed lower developmental levels of pretend play.

'Play as means' or 'play as ends' in occupational therapy

In this section, the practical applications and issues for working with children in occupational therapy are discussed. These applications and issues are presented under the following two main headings: 'play as a means' and 'play as an end' in therapy. These headings are not to be confused with definitions of play where a characteristic of play is 'a means not an ends' (e.g. see Sturgess 2003). When play is considered 'a means not an ends', the meaning is that play is often enjoyed because of the process (the 'being') of play and that there is no product produced. For example, when children play 'mothers and fathers', they enjoy the role play, the characterisations, and 'being' of play. The child's enjoyment of 'being' in the play does not have a visible product at the end of the day when they have finished playing.

The terms 'play as a means' and 'play as an ends' in this section refer to the occupational therapist's use of play in assessment and intervention with children. When play is used 'as a means' in therapy, play is not the focus of the assessment or the intervention. Another skill (e.g. motor skill) is the focus and play is the means to engage the child in the activity so the motor skill can be practised. When play is used 'as an end' in therapy, play is the focus of the assessment and intervention.

Table 26.3 summarises occupational therapy theory when play is used as a means in therapy and when it is used as an ends in therapy.

'Play as a means' in therapy

Rodger and Zivianni (1999) noted that using play as a means in therapy is a valid use of play. In much of the therapy assessment and intervention in paediatric occupational therapy using play as a means is often called 'the art of therapy' (see Bundy 1991). Play as a means in assessment is integral to many assessments for children with items presented to children as games. Miller (1988, 2006) uses games as play in her assessments of the pre-academic skills and assessment of functional activities to engage children in the assessment tasks. For example, the

Table 26.3 Occupational therapy theory applied to play as a means and play as an ends

Occupational therapy framework		Play as a means	Play as an ends
Assessment			
Doing	What can the child do	Understanding of broad concept of play, understanding of play through engagement of child for motor, sensory, visual-perceptual and auditory tasks. The following skills are assessed using play to engage the child either through games or activities: • Motor skills (gross and fine motor) • Sensory skills • Visual-perceptual skills • Auditory skills • Sensory-motor skills • Cognitive skills • Social skills • Self-help skills	The child's play itself is assessed using a play assessment Play skills, abilities, and developmental level are assessed Play is central to a child's health and well-being. Play itself is meaningful and purposeful for the child
Being	Does the child enjoy play, sustain play, spend time playing and exploring and being curious	Play is not the focus so 'being' in play is only considered as a way to engage the child so the therapist can assess the child. The therapist is directive throughout assessment	Therapist is passive in assessment, lets the child lead in assessment, notes if child can sustain play. Therapist gives the child time to play, to 'be' in the play
Becoming	What is the potential for this child: participation in society, with peers, in family as a sibling	Based on child's skills, in context with family setting, therapist decides on level of intervention to assist child to reach maximum potential	Based on the child's ability to self-initiate play and engage with peers, family, therapist decides on level of intervention to assist child to reach maximum potential and 'become' a player
Person	Who is the child, parent, and therapist	Child: diagnosis, age, sex, position in family, history, development Parent: concerns, attitude to child, attitude to therapy, marital status Therapist: experience, priorities in treatment, knowledge, ability to engage the child through play	Child: diagnosis, age, sex, position in family, history, play developmental level Parent: concerns, attitude to child, attitude to therapy, marital status, ability to engage with play with their child Therapist: experience, treatment approach through play, ability to engage the child through play, ability to give child the power through play
Environment	Cultural, institutional, societal, any context outside of the person	Consideration of child's opportunity to engage in motor activities, sensory, cognitive, visual-perceptual and auditory tasks. School environment, family circumstances, and peers	Consideration of child's access to play materials, space, and time to play Consideration of family attitude to play, school performance, social connectedness

Table 26.3 Occupational therapy theory applied to play as a means and play as an ends—cont'd

Occupational therapy framework		Play as a means	Play as an ends
Intervention			
Doing	The doing in treatment	Therapist prepares tasks or activities for child to complete either during clinic sessions or home programme. Tasks based on child's motor, cognitive, sensory, visual-perceptual or auditory needs. Child engages in motor, sensory, cognitive, visual-perceptual, and auditory activities through games and activities designed for the child	Therapist prepares play materials and play scene ideas for child and as child leads and responds to play scene, the therapist adjusts activity level to child. Child engages in play sessions with consideration of play theme, developmental level of play, ability to sequence play actions, object substitutions, role play, social interaction, use of doll/teddy in play, consideration of the type of play materials
Being	The enjoyment of the child, and engagement of the child during therapy	Therapist focused on completion of activities. Therapist engages child in each activity by using play or games	During play sessions, therapist waits for child to respond. Therapist paces the session to the child's level of play understanding. Therapist encourages exploration of play materials and curiosity
Becoming	Potential for growth, self-actualisation. Potential for this child: participation in society, with peers, in family as a sibling	Therapist provides opportunities for the child to be challenged so that skills can be developed for maximum potential	Therapist adjusts challenging, waiting, responding, and extending child's play skills so that the child is able to self-initiate play ideas and engage with others, so child 'becomes' a player
Person	Child, parent/carer, therapist	Child: skill level and developmental levels considered in preparation for intervention programme. Parent/carer: parent skills, attitude and concerns considered in preparation for intervention programme. Therapist: Intervention offered is dependent on case load, policy of workplace, equipment, and space for treating	Child: play ability and play developmental levels considered in preparation for intervention programme. Parent/carer: parent play skills, attitude, ability to engage child, and concerns considered in preparation for intervention programme. Therapist: intervention offered is dependent on case load, policy of workplace, available play materials, and space for treating
Environment	Socio-economic status of family, access to services, objects in environment, value of play placed by parents, parent ability to play, peers, children in family, early childhood settings and facilities, culture	Family access to transport, educational and health services and social supports considered in therapy plan. Therapy plan also considers equipment, space, and time of family. Therapy activities take into account cultural and societal meanings to the child and family	Family access to transport, educational and health services and social supports considered in therapy plan. Therapy plan also considers available play materials, space, and time of family. Play scenes planned for therapy take into account cultural and societal meanings to the child and family

fine-motor activities in the Miller Function and Participation Scales are 'make a fish' and 'penny bank' (Miller 2006). Developmental assessments of children also present activities to children such as blocks, ball, textas and paper in the form of play to engage them, so that through the child's play with these materials, the therapist can ascertain the child's developmental level (Stagnitti et al 2000). In these instances, play is the means to assess motor, functional, and developmental levels of the children. The playfulness of the therapist during these assessments also contributes to the child's enjoyment and engagement of the activities (Bundy 1991). In the analysis of the assessment results, the therapist would consider the child's ability to perform specific skills, such as gross motor skills, fine motor skills, sensory, and visual perceptual skills, and so on. In this case, the therapist is assessing the 'doing' components of play.

When implementing interventions, play is used to engage the child in activities. Ayres used play to engage children in sensory integration therapy (Ayres 1972). For example, the therapist or child may suggest that the bolster swing is a wild, bucking bull (Bundy 1991) so that the emphasis to the child is on being able to stay on the 'bucking bull', but the therapist is really interested in providing vestibular input to the child to improve balance. In designing developmental programmes for children, activities are chosen to match each child's developmental needs and these activities are presented to the child as games or play. Gray (1998) noted that using activities as 'doing' to treat the components of performance (e.g. physical, cognitive, and psychosocial skills) was using occupation as a means. She argued that using occupation as a means meant that the therapist also chose activities that were personally meaningful, culturally and developmentally relevant, and goal directed for the person involved.

An example of using play as a means is outlined in the following section. On a visit to a local preschool, the therapist was asked to provide suggestions on how to encourage a child with a progressive neurological condition to engage in gross motor activities. The child was 5 years' old and was becoming aware that she was different to the other children. She used a walker to walk and found it difficult to keep up with the gross motor activities of her peers. As a result she was reluctant to engage in such activities. After spending some time with her, the therapist ascertained that she was developmentally advanced in her cognitive, language, and pretend-play

abilities. An obstacle course was set up, which the child ignored as she continued with the finishing touches to a drawing of a teddy. She continued to ignore the obstacle course until the therapist realised that the obstacle course could be a jungle with dangerous animals in it, such as snakes. The child immediately engaged with the play idea, stood up, went to the obstacle course and began to negotiate a balance beam and various other pieces of equipment. As the child used the equipment, the therapist lay on the ground and pretended her hands were snakes that were trying to reach the child. The child continued to negotiate the 'bridge in the jungle' until she reached the end of the balance beam. This is an example of using play as a means to engage a child in an activity. For the child, the enjoyment was 'being' in the play, for the therapist the emphasis was on the gross motor skill, not the play skill.

The use of play as a means to engage children in assessment or treatment assumes that play is a broad concept, an all-encompassing occupation. It includes motor skills, visual skills, sensory skills, auditory skills, and cognitive skills. When play is used as a means, play itself is not being assessed nor is it being treated. Play (in the broadest sense of the word) is used as a means by the therapist to engage the child, while the therapist's focus is on particular skills. 'Play as means' in therapy is further illustrated in Practice Scenario 26.1.

Practice Scenario 26.1 Play as means

Children between 6 and 7 years with a physical impairment participated in a group programme that was designed to promote posture and muscle tone control, reach and grasp, finger isolation, pronation and supination, wrist extension, shoulder range of motion, crossing the midline, visual tracking and sensory awareness, tolerance and exploration. The aim of the group programme was to improve the hand skills of each child. The long-term occupational goal was for these children to be able to engage in the occupations of self-care, eating, brushing teeth, and manipulating objects in play, etc.

Hand skills were chosen as the aim because the various hand skills practiced in the group were key components to achieve these occupations in the lives of these children. Most of the children who participated had fluctuating tone; low when resting and high tone when initiating movement. They also had sensory integration issues, including gravitational insecurity and tactile defensiveness. One session of this group is briefly described below as an example of 'play as means' in therapy.

The session began with music to increase the arousal level of the children. This music was selected with the music therapist to be upbeat, but not over-stimulating. While the music was playing proprioceptive input was provided into the shoulders, pelvis and knees to help the children know where their bodies were in space. Then the children moved onto large rolls to play a game of 'Row row row your boat'. The children with gravitational insecurities were set up with blocks under their feet so that they were in contact with the ground at all times. During the song the children were rocked from side to side to break some of their extensor tone patterns.

After transferring into class chairs action songs were sung that incorporated actions to encourage upper-limb stretches (e.g. 'Bend It, Stretch It', 'Open Shut Them'). The children chose which action song to sing. They then pretended to climb a beanstalk. When climbing the beanstalk the songs were adapted to create rhythmical intention for the children to complete the stretching activities.

Moving on from stretches the children chose between finger puppets and play dough. The children were allowed to freely play with the play dough or finger puppets, but because of sensory issues as well as their high tone most of the children needed co-active assistance to do this. Again, action songs were used to encourage hand and finger movements. For example, 'Pat-a-Cake' might be sung when playing with play dough to make different shapes.

Messy play followed play dough/finger puppets. The chosen materials for messy play (such as paint or strawberry topping) were placed in a position that required the child to access different planes to encourage reach, grasp, and crossing the midline. The children were encouraged to explore the messy materials. Each child was encouraged to reach their individual goals of finger extension, pronation, and supination, and to reach and grasp using paint brushes, rollers, etc.

The session ended with some relaxation and visual tracking practice. The children often chose to watch bubbles while listening to calming music. This was considered a great way for the children to relax and organise their bodies before lunch.

This Practice Scenario has been provided by Catherine Reilly, an occupational therapist who at the time of writing worked at Glenallen, in Melbourne, Australia. Glenallen is a special school for children with physical and/or health impairments. The age range of the students is 4.8–18 years. Catherine worked with students of all ages, who had a range of impairments.

'Play as an ends' in therapy

When play is used as an ends, play itself is considered an important goal and becomes the focus of the assessment and the intervention. The 'doing', 'being', 'becoming' and 'belonging' of play are all considered by the therapist. The therapist is interested in restoring the child's occupational life (Gray 1998) as a player. When play is used as an ends, the therapist has a clear idea or definition of what play is and is sensitive to the fact that play provides an insight into the child's inner world and is a window into a child's development (Eisert & Lamorey 1996). In the section above on what is play, definitions of play included the terms: non-literal, creative, suspension of reality, and transcends reality. These terms refer to the element of pretend, of imposing a meaning onto a situation. For example, when using a box as a bed for a doll the child uses the box in a non-literal way (it is a bed not a box). Play as an ends implies that play is unique in and of itself. Play is identifiable – it can be measured – and, while it incorporates motor skills, auditory skills, sensory skills, and visual skills, it is more than specific skills. Pretend play is characterised by being non-literal and involving the suspension and transcending of reality, and if you note in Table 26.2, the assumed benefits of pretend play are unique compared to other play types.

Assessment of play as an end in itself requires measurement of: a child's ability to initiate and develop play ideas, engage with a variety of play materials, and sustain and enjoy play. That is, the 'doing' and 'being' of play. In Table 26.4, play assessments used and devised by occupational therapists are listed. The Knox Preschool Play Scale (Knox 1997) assesses play in a broad sense (i.e. motor skills are included with dramatisation skills). The Play History (Takata 1974) assesses play, in a broad sense also, through an interview of the child's carer. The Test of Playfulness (Bundy 2005) assesses the attitude a child brings to a situation. The Symbolic and Imaginative Play Developmental Checklist (Stagnitti 1998) assesses the developmental level of a child's pretend play and the Child-Initiated Pretend Play Assessment (Stagnitti 2007) assesses a child's ability to spontaneously initiate and sustain pretend play. The Play Assessment in Group Setting (PAGS) (Lautamo et al 2005) assesses a child's play in a social setting and the Assessment of Ludic Behaviours (Ferland 2005) assesses the play attitudes of children with a physical impairment.

Table 26.4 Play assessments

Assessment name	What is measured	Time, space and materials required
Knox Preschool Play Scale (Knox 1997)	Categories of play: gross motor, exploration, manipulation, construction, imitation, imagination, dramatisation, music, books, territory, interest, purpose, attention, co-operation and language Dimensions of play: space management, material management, imitation, participation	***Time required:*** 2 × 30 minute observations ***Space:*** observations of free play in indoor and outdoor familiar environments ***Materials:*** materials and toys for the KPPS are found within the child's own environment ***Age:*** 0–6 years
Play History (Takata 1974)	Past and present play experiences in terms of: epochs of play – sensorimotor, symbolic and simple constructive, dramatic and complex constructive and pre-game, games, recreational Elements of each epoch – materials (what), action (how), people (with whom), setting (where)	***Time required:*** Not given ***Space:*** semi-structured interview with a parent or carer. Setting not given ***Materials:*** interview so materials are paper and pen for examiner ***Age:*** not specified
Test of Playfulness (version 4) (ToP) (Bundy 2005)	The ToP assesses intrinsic motivation, internal locus of control, freedom to suspend reality, and framing (i.e. how the child maintains the play scenario and understands social cues within the play context). These attributes are scored under the headings of extent, intensity, and skilfulness	***Time required:*** 2 × 15–20 minutes ***Space:*** observation of free play in an indoor and outdoor familiar environment ***Materials:*** materials are within the environment ***Age:*** 3 months –18 years
Symbolic and Imaginative Play Developmental Checklist (SIP-DC) (Stagnitti 1998)	Play themes, sequences of play action, object substitutions, role play, social interaction, doll/teddy play	***Time required:*** not given but allow 30 minutes ***Space:*** usually indoor area within the child's home, preschool, or playgroup setting ***Materials:*** found within the child's environment. Suggested materials are: teddy, spoon, cup, box, cloth for younger children under 3 years and a toy kit such as a doctor's kit or doll's house for children 3 years and over ***Age:*** 0–5 years
Child-Initiated Pretend Play Assessment (ChIPPA) (Stagnitti 2007)	Elaborateness of a child' pretend play Child's ability to use symbols in play Child's ability to self-initiate play	***Time required:*** 18 or 30 minutes, depending on age of child ***Space:*** room for a sheet to be thrown over two adult chairs to make a cubby so therapist and child can sit on floor in front of the cubby ***Materials:*** supplied with the kit ***Age:*** 3–7 years
Assessment of Ludic Behaviours (Ferland 2005)	The areas of ludic interests, abilities, and attitude are assessed on this assessment Ludic is a French word meaning playful, jesting	***Time required:*** 1 hour for observation and 1 hour for interview ***Space:*** space within a clinical setting ***Materials:*** available in Ferland's book

Table 26.4 Play assessments—cont'd

Assessment name	What is measured	Time, space and materials required
Play Assessment in Group Setting (PAGS) (Lautamo et al 2005)	Natural social contexts of play are considered: expressing a playful attitude, creating and engaging in play stories. 54 items reflect meaningful doing and playful attitude, mindful doing, organisation, and social imaginative play behaviour	**Time required:** not specified **Space:** play performance in natural day-care context **Materials:** within the environment **Age:** 2–8 years
Pediatric Volitional Questionnaire (Geist & Kielhofner 1998)	Not strictly a play assessment but elements are observed during children's play. Gives a measure of volition, based on the Model of Human Occupation Questionnaire on a child's motivational strengths and weaknesses in various environments. 15 items	**Time required:** not given **Space:** observations made by therapists in several environments **Materials:** within the environment **Age:** 2–6 years

Excluding the Play History, all these assessments are observational or non-directive. This is in contrast to assessments which use play as a means where the therapist is directive and asks the child to complete certain tasks (or games).

When play is assessed as an ends, the therapist is passive in the assessment process. The therapist observes what a child can do (the 'doing'), how the child engages (the 'doing' and 'being'), if the child can sustain a play idea and enjoy play (the 'being'). The therapist understands the implications of deficits in play for 'becoming' a player and 'belonging' to a group.

When play has been assessed, the therapist then prepares an appropriate intervention programme based on the child's play ability. Pretend play has been used in interventions in medical settings for decades and been shown to be effective in preventing and reducing anxiety and distress (Moore & Russ 2006). Empirical literature on the topic is sparse (Moore & Russ 2006). One programme which uses pretend play as the intervention is the Learn to Play programme (Stagnitti 1998). This programme is designed to treat the child's play deficits so that the child can begin to self-initiate play ideas and sustain play by playing out pretend play scenarios. In this programme, it is the child's ability to self-initiate play and become a player that is the focus. Figure 26.1 gives an overview of the Learn to Play treatment programme.

To use play as an end in itself as intervention, the therapist is required to understand developmental levels of play and key behaviours that are required for a child to play (the 'doing'), engage the child in the enjoyment ('being') of play with the aim that the child becomes a player ('becoming') with peers in play ('belonging'). For pretend play, children require the ability to self-initiate and sequence play actions in a logical way, use objects as symbols in play, use dolls/teddies or a character in play, engage in role play (using themselves in character), socially interact with peers, and engage in a play scenario or play theme.

The Learn to Play programme uses several techniques to engage the child in play, such as, the therapist gets the child's attention, models the play action/s, talks about the play (e.g. the teddy is hungry and needs something to eat), repeats the play action/s, may help the child manipulate the objects, uses emotions in play (e.g. the therapist uses voice, facial expression, body language), and uses various play ideas around a similar play ability. For the latter this requires the therapist to know the aspect of play ability being engaged with and to use this ability in other play scenarios. For example, the play ability to use one object for two different substitutions during play may mean that the therapist uses a box as a car, then a bed; and then for the next play scene, use a block as soap, and then as food for a cow to 'eat'. Stagnitti (2004b) reported that through the Learn to Play programme, a child with autism became a player (the 'becoming'). That is, the child was able to engage in play in unstructured situations (e.g. a sand-pit play), engage with peers

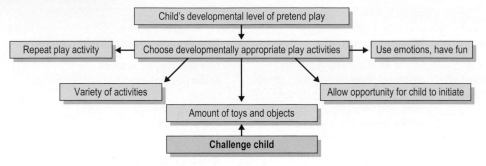

Figure 26.1 • The Learn to Play treatment model

through play, became more socially aware, ceased in destroying other children's play scenes, and communicated with peers using more language.

When working on the ability to play, the therapist is teaching the child to take control of the situation, to initiate play ideas and to lead the play. The therapist gives control to the child, so that the child can 'be' and 'become' a player.

Other techniques which use play as an end in itself for the health and well-being of children are: child-centred therapy (Axline 1969, Wilson & Ryan 2005), narrative play therapy (Cattanach 2003, 2006), filial therapy (Landreth & Bratton 2006), dynamic play family therapy (Harvey 2006), and psychodynamic play therapy (Erikson 1985). The techniques which use play as being an end in itself for the improved health and well-being of children have traditionally been used in situations where children have been traumatised, neglected, abused, or distressed. Often, in these situations, the play of these children is chaotic and, as they heal, their play becomes more organised and complex.

Wolfberg's work on Integrated Play Groups (Wolfberg & Schuler 1993, 1999) focuses on developing social play skills in children who have been diagnosed with autism-spectrum disorders. In her technique, typically developing peers are taught to play with peers with autism. Scaffolding is used as a technique by the adults involved building the play skills of children. Ferland (2005) focused her work on children with physical impairment and developed the Ludic Model as an intervention to develop play skills for these children. Her model considers the interest of the child, the attitude, and actions of the child so that the therapist can develop within the child an enjoyment in play ('being') and increase

the capacity of the child to act ('doing'), so that the child develops a sense of autonomy and well-being ('becoming').

An example of play as an ends is illustrated in Practice Scenario 26.2.

Practice Scenario 26.2 Play as an ends

Chris was a 4-year-old boy with a diagnosis of autism. He would sometimes play with television character dolls, such as 'Fireman Sam' or 'Buzz Lightyear'; however, his imaginative play dialogue and actions came straight from the television programmes or movies, and he rarely deviated from these. Although adults were impressed with his memory, it affected his interaction with his peers at kindergarten. Typically, he would get upset when other children entered his play and used phrases which weren't part of his learned repertoire. Chris would run off, unable to integrate their ideas into his play. This had the negative effect of further isolating him.

Chris attended a block of 6 weeks' therapy where the focus was imaginative play, with the goal of increasing flexibility in play scenarios. The session began with toys relating to familiar scripts and the therapist would name the dolls/teddies as characters from familiar television shows or videos which Chris knew. She would let him act out familiar scripts at the beginning of the session. Then she would gently interrupt his script, adding new actions and phrases. Wilbur from 'Charlotte's Web' was a character which

Chris used a lot, so the therapist would introduce another farm animal to the scene and playfully add conversation, such as 'I don't want to do that, I'm hungry, could we have some biscuits please?' The therapist would then model the animal eating a biscuit (where the biscuit would be a wooden block). Chris would often return immediately to his script. However, the therapist would model the alternative sequence of actions several times during the session in between Chris' returns to the script.

The next session the therapist would again model the interruption and often Chris would cope with this, because he had become familiar with this new script and in effect it had become part of his repertoire of actions. After four sessions, Chris would occasionally add a little more to the script spontaneously, such as '...and we could give him a drink'. When this happened the therapist would enthusiastically go with his idea and say affirmations such as, 'I like your new idea; that makes me want to play more'. At each consequent session the therapist would say comments like 'what's a new thing we can do in this story?', so that Chris got the idea that he had to generate a new action or phrase in the sequence. She would also make sure there were some blocks, paper, pipe-cleaners, boxes and other random materials, so that there were things which could easily be adapted for the play scene.

At the conclusion of this block of therapy, the therapist asked kindergarten staff to support Chris during play at kinder and assist him accepting other children's ideas during interactive imaginative play. She explained to the staff the method by which she had introduced new ideas, and encouraged them to use the same type of language when convincing him to try a new action. So, if a kindergarten friend started to deviate from Chris' familiar script, the staff would immediately say comments such as, 'That's Bobbie's new idea for this story, isn't that a great idea Chris? Now let's practise that again'. The staff would then repeat whatever the other child had introduced to the scene. Chris would need this support to change his behaviour, and tolerate some additions, although too many new ideas would still challenge him.

This Practice Scenario has been provided by Rachel Peters, a paediatric occupational therapist working with children with impairments and delays for many years in community-based settings. At the time of writing she was working with a multi-disciplinary team in South-West Victoria, Australia.

Conclusion

When play is used as a means, the occupational engagement in play is understood and explained in terms of a child's motor, cognitive, sensory, visual-perceptual, and auditory abilities. The child assessment information, together with information from parents/carers, teachers, concerned others, and environmental factors surrounding the child and family (such as cultural considerations, social supports, geographical location, financial situation, and access to space and equipment) are all considered by the therapist for each child. The therapist can then identify possible reasons for occupational engagement being below expected levels for the child or, alternatively, if there are any occupational engagement concerns. Action is then taken either to develop the child's skills through activities and home programmes, or to modify the environment, or to bring in alternative supports for the child and/or family. Actions of the therapist are designed to assist the child to 'become' by concentrating primarily on the 'doing' of play.

When play is used as an end, occupational engagement in play is assessed through play assessments and observations of the child's play. Insight is gained into the child's inner world and play abilities are identified. Occupational engagement in play for the child is dependent on many factors. A play assessment will help the therapist to understand the play ability of the child. This information, together with information from the family, teachers, and concerned others is considered in conjunction with knowledge of the child's environment (such as family circumstances, geographical location, access to services, cultural considerations, social supports, and access to play materials and equipment). Decisions are then made as to the occupational engagement and priorities for the child to become a player. All decisions of the therapist must consider the child's potential to develop. The therapist creates circumstances to encourage, monitor and give the child control of the play so that the child becomes a player. The 'becoming' of the child, is the long-term goal of occupational therapy.

References

Algado, S. S., & Burgman, I. (2005). Occupational therapy intervention with children survivors of war. In: F. Kronenberg, S. S. Algado & N. Pollard (Eds). *Occupational therapy without borders*. (pp. 245–260). London, Elsevier, Churchill Livingstone.

Anderson, J., Hinojosa, J., & Strauch, C. (1987). Integrating play in neurodevelopmental treatment. *American Journal of Occupational Therapy*, 41, 421–426.

Axline, Virginia M. (1969). *Play therapy*. New York, Ballantine Books.

Ayres, A. J. (1972). *Southern Californian Sensory Integration Tests*. Los Angeles, Western Psychological Services.

Baron-Cohen, S. (1996) *Mindblindness. An essay on autism and theory of mind*. London, MIT Press.

Baum, C. M. & Christiansen, C. H. (2005). Person-environment-occupation performance: an occupational-based framework for practice. In C. H. Christiansen, C.M. Baum & J. Bass-Haugen (Eds). *Occupational therapy: performance, participation and well-being* (3rd ed.). (pp. 244–259). Thorofare, NJ, Slack Incorporated.

Bracegirdle, H. (1992). The use of play in occupational therapy for children: what is play? *British Journal of Occupational Therapy*, 55, 107–108.

Bruner, J., Jolly, A. & Sylva, K. (Eds). (1976). *Play, its role in development and evolution*. New York, Penguin Books.

Bundy, A. (1991). Play theory and sensory integration. In A. Fisher, E. Murray & A. Bundy (Eds), *Sensory Integration. Theory and practice*. (pp. 46–68). Philadelphia, F. A. Davis.

Bundy, A. (2005). Measuring play performance. In: M. Law, C. Baum, & W. Dunn (Eds). *Measuring occupational performance. Supporting best practice in occupational therapy*. (2nd ed) (pp. 128–149). Thorofare, NJ, Slack.

Canadian Association of Occupational Therapists. (1996). Position Paper: Occupational therapy and children's play. *Canadian Journal of Occupational Therapy*, 63(2) Insert.

Canadian Association of Occupational Therapists, (1999). *Enabling occupation: An occupational therapy perspective*. Ottawa, CAOT Publications ACE.

Casby, M. W. (1992). Symbolic play: development and assessment considerations. *Infants and Young Children*, 4, 343–348.

Cattanach, A. (2003). *Introduction to play therapy*. London, Psychology Press.

Cattanach, A. (2006). Narrative play therapy. In: C. Schaefer & H. Kaduson (Eds.). *Contemporary play therapy: theory research and practice*. (pp. 82–101). Guildford, Guildford Press.

Christie, J. (1994). Academic play. In: J. Hellendoorn, R. Van der Kooij & B. Sutton–Smith (Eds.), *Play and intervention* (pp. 203–213). Albany, SUNY Press.

Clifford, J. & Bundy, A. (1989). Play preference and play performance in normal boys and boys with sensory integrative dysfunction. *Occupational Therapy Journal of Research*, 9(4), 202–217.

Couch, K. J., Deitz, J. C. & Kanny, E. M. (1997). The role of play in pediatric occupational therapy. *American Journal of Occupational Therapy*, 52, 111–117.

Eisert, D. & Lamorey, S. (1996). Play as a window on child development: the relationship between play and other developmental domains. *Early Education and Development*, 7, 221–235.

Erikson, E. H. (1985). Play and actuality. In: J. Bruner, A. Jolly & K. Sylva (Eds.), *Play, its role in development and evolution* (pp. 688–704). New York, Penguin Books.

Factor, J. (2005). *The Australian Children's Folklore Collection: The Encyclopedia of Melbourne*. Cambridge University Press: Cambridge.

Ferland, F. (2005). *The Ludic Model. Play, children with physical disabilities and occupational therapy*. (2nd ed.), Ottawa, Canadian Association of Occupational Therapists.

Geist, R. & Kielhofner, G. (1998). *A user's guide to the Pediatric Volitional Questionnaire*. Chicago, Model of Human Occupation Clearinghouse, University of Illinois.

Goodman, J. F. (1994). 'Work' versus 'play' and early childhood care. *Early Childhood Care*, 23, 177–196.

Gray, J. (1998). Putting occupation into practice. Occupation as ends, occupation as means. *American Journal of Occupational Therapy*, 52(5), 354–364.

Greenspan, S. I. & Lieberman, A. (1994). Representational elaboration and differentiation: a clinical-quantitative approach to clinical assessment of 2- to 4-year-olds. In: A. W. Slade & D. Wolf (Eds.), *Children at play* (pp. 3–32). New York, Oxford University Press.

Harvey, S. (2006). Dynamic play therapy. In: C. Schaefer & H. Kaduson (Eds.). *Contemporary play therapy: theory research and practice*. (pp. 55–81). Guildford, Guildford Press.

Howes, C. & Matheson, C. C. (1992). Sequences in the development of competent play with peers: Social and social pretend play. *Developmental Psychology*, 28(5), 961–974.

Jeffree, D. M. & McConkey, R. (1976). An observation scheme for recording children's imaginative doll play. *Journal of Child Psychology*, 17, 189–197.

Knox, S. H. (1997). Development and current use of the Knox Preschool Play Scale. In: L. D. Parham & L. S. Fazio (Eds.), *Play in occupational therapy for children*. (pp. 35–51). St. Louis, Mosby.

Landreth, G. & Bratton, S. (2006). *Child parent relationship therapy (CPRT): a 10-session filial therapy model*. New York, Routledge.

Lautamo, T., Kottorp, A. & Salminen, A–L. (2005). Play assessment for group settings: a pilot study to construct an assessment tool. *Scandinavian Journal of Occupational Therapy*, 12, 136–144.

Leslie, A. (1987). Pretense and representation: the origins of 'theory of mind.' *Psychological Review*, 94, 412–426.

Lewis, V., Boucher, J. & Astell, A. (1992). The assessment of symbolic play in young children: a prototype test. *European Journal of Disorders of Communications*, 27, 231–245.

Lindsey, E. W., & Colwell, M. J. (2003). Preschoolers emotional competence: links to pretend play and physical play. *Child Study Journal*, 33, 39–52.

Lowe, M. (1975). Trends in the development of representational play in infants from one to three years – an observational study. *Child Psychology Psychiatry*, 16, 33–47.

Lunzer, E. A. (1959). Intellectual development in the play of young children. *Educational Review*, 11, 205–224.

Lyytinen, P., Laakso, M-L., Poikkeus, A-M. & Rita, N. (1999). The development and predictive relations of play and language across the second year. *Scandinavian Journal of Psychology*, 40, 177–186.

McCune, L. (1995). A normative study of representational play at the transition to language. *Child Development*, 31, 198–206.

McCune Nicolich, L. (1981). Toward symbolic functioning: structure of early pretend games and potential parallels with language. *Child Development*, 52, 785–797.

Mellou, E. (1994). Play theories: a contemporary review. *Early Child Development and Care*, 102, 91–100.

Miller, L. J. (1988). *The Miller Assessment for Preschoolers. Manual*. New York, Psychological Corporation.

Miller, L. J. (2006). *The Miller Function and Participation Scales*. New York, Harcourt Assessment.

Missuna, C., & Pollock, N. (1991). Play deprivation in children with physical disabilities: The role of the occupational therapist in preventing secondary disability. *American Journal of Occupational Therapy*, 45, 882–889.

Moore, M. & Russ, S. W. (2006). Pretend play as a resource for children: implications for

pediatricians and health professionals. *Journal of Developmental and Behavioural Peditrics*, 27(3), 237–248.

Nicolopoulou, A. (2005). Play and narrative in the process of development: commonalities, differences, and interrelations. *Cognitive Development*, 20(4), 495–502.

Norrie McCain, M & Fraser-Mustard, J 1999, '*Reversing the real brain drain: Early years study*', (pp. 1–207). Toronto, Children's Secretariat.

Nourot, P. M., & Van Hoorn, J. L. (1991). Symbolic play in preschool and primary settings. *Young Children*, 46, 40–50.

Parham, L. D., & Primeau, L. A. (1997). Play and occupational therapy. In: L. D. Parham & L. S. Fazio (Eds.), *Play in occupational therapy for children* (pp. 2–21). St. Louis, Mosby.

Pellegrini, A. D. (1980). The relationship between kindergartner's play and achievement in prereading, language and writing. *Psychology in the Schools*, 17, 530–535.

Pellegrini, A. D. (1985). The relations between symbolic play and literate behavior: a review and critique of the empirical literature. *Review of Educational Research*, 55, 107–121.

Pellegrini, A. D. & Galda, L. (1993). Ten years after: a reexamination of symbolic play and literacy research. *Reading Research Quarterly*, 28, 162–175.

Phillips, R. (1945). Doll play as a function of the realism of the materials and the length of the experimental session. *Child Development*, 16, 123–143.

Piaget, J. (1962). *Play, dreams and imitation in childhood*. New York, W. W. Norton & Company.

Pierce, D. (1997). The power of object play for infants and toddlers at risk for developmental delay. In: L. Parham & L. S. Fazio (Eds.), *Play in occupational therapy for children* (pp. 86–111). St. Louis, Mosby.

Pulaski, M. A. (1973). Toys and imaginative play. In: J. Singer (Ed.). *Child's world of make believe*. (pp. 74–101). New York, Academic Press.

Reid, D. (1987). Occupational therapist's assessment practices with handicapped children in Ontario. *Canadian Journal of Occupational Therapy*, 54, 181–187.

Robinson, A. L. (1977). Play: the arena for acquisition of rules for competent behavior. *American Journal of Occupational Therapy*, 31, 248–253.

Rodger, S. (1994). A survey of assessments used by paediatric occupational therapists. *Australian Occupational Therapy Journal*, 41, 137–142.

Rodger, S. & Ziviani, J. (1999). Play-based occupational therapy. *International Journal of Disability, Development and Education*, 46, 337–365.

Roskos, K. (1991). An inventory of literate behavior in the pretend play episodes of eight preschoolers. *Reading Research and Instruction*, 30, 39–52.

Russ, S. (1998). Play, creativity, and adaptive functioning: implications for play interventions. *Journal of Clinical Child Psychology*, 27, 469–480.

Russ, S. (2003). Play and creativity: developmental issues. *Scandinavian Journal of Educational Research*, 47, 291–303.

Russ, S. W., Robins, A. L. & Christiano, B. A. (1999). Pretend play: Longitudinal prediction of creativity and affect in fantasy in children. *Creativity Research Journal*, 12, 129–139.

Schrader, C. T. (1990). Symbolic play as a curricular tool for early literacy development. *Early Childhood Research Quarterly*, 5, 79–103.

Simmond, M. (2005). To practice to learn: Occupational therapy with the children of Vietnam. In: F. Kronenberg, S. S. Algado & N. Pollard (Eds.) *Occupational therapy without borders. Learning from the spirit of survivors*. (pp. 277–286). Oxford, Elsevier Churchill Livingstone.

Sleigh, G. (1980). A study of some symbolic processes in young children. *British Journal of Disorders of Communication*, 15, 163–175.

Stagnitti, K. (1998). *Learn to play. A practical program to develop a child's imaginative play*. Melbourne, Co-ordinates Publications.

Stagnitti, K. (2004a). Understanding play: implications for play assessment. *Australian Occupational Therapy Journal*, 51, 3–12.

Stagnitti, K. (2004b). Occupational performance in pretend play; implications for practice. In: M. Mollineux (Ed.) *Occupation for occupational therapists*. (pp. 103–121). Oxford, Blackwell Science.

Stagnitti, K. (2007). *The Child-Initiated Pretend Play Assessment manual and kit*. Melbourne, Co-ordinates Therapy Services.

Stagnitti, K. & Unsworth, C. (2000). The importance of pretend play to child development: An occupational therapy perspective. *British Journal of Occupational Therapy*, 63, 121–127.

Stagnitti, K., Unsworth, C. A. & Rodger, S. (2000). Development of an assessment to identify play behaviours that discriminate between the play of typical preschoolers and preschoolers with pre-academic problems. *Canadian Journal of Occupational Therapy*, 67, 291–303.

Stewart, D., Harvey, S., Sahagian, S., Toal, C., Pollock, N. & Law, M. (1991) *Play: the occupation of childhood*. Research Report No. 91–93. Hamilton, Ontario, Neurodevelopmental Clinical Research Unit, The Ontario Ministry of Health.

Sturgess, J. (2003). A model describing play as a child-chosen activity: Is

this still valid in contemporary Australia? *Australian Occupational Therapy Journal*, 50, 104–108.

Sutton-Smith, B. (1967). The role of play in cognitive development. *Young Children*, September, 361–369.

Takata, N. (1974). Play as a prescription. In: M. Reilly (Ed.), *Play as exploratory learning. Studies in curiosity behaviour* (pp. 209–246). Beverley Hills, Sage Publications.

Taneja, V., Sriram, S., Beri, R.S., Sreenivas, V., Aggarwal, R., Kaur, R. & Puliyel, J. M. (2002). 'Not by bread alone': impact of a structured 90-minute play session on development of children in an orphanage. *Child: Care, Health & Development*, 28, 95–100.

Walker, S. P., Chang, S. M., Powell, C. A., & Grantham-McGregor, S. M. (2005). Effects of early childhood psychosocial stimulation and nutritional supplementation on cognitive and education in growth-stunted Jamaican children: prospective cohort study. *The Lancet*, 366, 1804–1807.

Westby, C. (1980). Assessment of cognitive and language abilities through play. *Language, Speech, and Hearing Services in Schools*, 11, 154–168.

Westby, C. (1991). A scale for assessing children's pretend play. In: C. Schaefer, K. Gitlin & A. Sandrund (Eds.), *Play diagnosis and assessment*. (pp. 131–161). New York, John Wiley & Sons Inc.

Whittaker, C. A. (1982). *Relational play and the emergence of mental representation in hospitalized profoundly retarded children*. Washington D. C., Paper presented to the American Academy of Child Psychiatry.

Wilcock, A. (1999). Reflections of doing, being and becoming. *Australian Occupational Therapy Journal*, 46, 1–11.

Wilcock, A. (2006). *An occupational perspective of health*. (2nd ed). Thorofare, NJ, Slack.

Wilson, K. & Ryan, V. (2005). *Play therapy: a non-directive approach for children and adolescents*. (2nd ed). London, Elsevier Science.

Wing, L., Gould, J., Yeates, S. R. & Brierley, L. M. (1977). Symbolic play in severely mentally retarded and in autistic children. *Journal of Child Psychology Psychiatry*, 18, 167–178.

Wolfberg, P. J. & Schuler, A. L. (1993). Integrated play groups: A model for promoting the social and cognitive dimensions of play in children with autism. *Journal of Autism and Developmental Disorders*, 23(3), 467–489.

Wolfberg, P. J. & Schuler, A. L. (1999). Fostering peer interaction, imaginative play and spontaneous language in children with autism. *Child Language Teaching and Therapy*, 15(1), 41–52.

Wyver, S. & Spence, S. (1995). Cognitive and social play of Australian preschoolers. *Australian Journal of Early Childhood*, 20, 42–46.

Chapter Twenty-Seven

27

Work rehabilitation

Catherine Cook and Sue Lukersmith

CHAPTER CONTENTS

Introduction 392

Work occupations. 392

The meaning of work 392

Occupational therapy and work 393

Work rehabilitation 394

The work rehabilitation process 395

Phase one: assessment 401
Assessment of the worker 401
Assessment of the workplace 402

Phase two: professional reasoning –
matching worker and work tasks 403

Phase three: goal setting and outcome
measurement 403

Phase four: therapeutic interventions 404
Return-to-work programme 404
Modifications of the environment, tasks,
tools or equipment 405
Education or training 405
Other interventions 405

Phase five: implement interventions,
monitor and review 407

Conclusion. 407

SUMMARY

Work is an important occupation for many people, not only providing financial rewards, but also contributing to the individual's self-esteem, fulfillment, identity, social interaction and status within the community. Occupational therapists become involved when an individual's participation in work activities is affected by injury, impairment or illness. There is increasing evidence that work rehabilitation programmes developed to facilitate return to work as soon as possible following injury or illness are cost-effective and beneficial to the worker. This chapter outlines the features of successful work rehabilitation programmes. A work rehabilitation process consisting of five phases is outlined and the role of the occupational therapist in each of the phases described. Although the work rehabilitation process presented is operational in a number of countries, the process described will vary depending on legislative frameworks and workers' compensation and insurance systems.

KEY POINTS

- Work rehabilitation is a dynamic process requiring the occupational therapist to adopt a biopsychosocial approach in which physical, psychological, social, cultural and environmental factors are considered.
- Successful work rehabilitation programmes involve an early referral; rehabilitation situated in the workplace; provision of modified work options; communication between all stakeholders; establishment of clear goals, timeframes and outcomes; and ongoing monitoring of progress.
- Occupational therapists, with their focus on the analysis of occupations have a unique role in work rehabilitation.
- There are five key interconnected phases of work rehabilitation: assessment, professional reasoning, establishing short- and long-term goals, develop interventions, and implementation.

- A thorough assessment needs to be conducted that includes the worker, his job, and environmental and personal contexts.
- Professional reasoning skills are used to match the demands of the job with the capacity of the worker and to establish goals and develop a well-reasoned therapeutic intervention programme.
- Implementation of interventions includes monitoring and reviewing the progress of the worker.
- Facilitating communication between all stakeholders throughout the work rehabilitation programme is essential.

Introduction

As work is integral to the lives of most individuals seen by occupational therapists, it is important that we understand why people work and the meaning ascribed to work by both the individual and society. In this chapter the term 'work' will refer to the productive occupations performed within an employment setting.

Occupational therapists become involved when an individual's participation in work occupations is affected by illness or injury. Although work has always been a core concern of occupational therapy, increasing numbers of occupational therapists are employed in the specialist area of work rehabilitation. The primary focus in this practice area is return to work following injury, illness or disease. Hence, *work rehabilitation* as described in this chapter will relate to those individuals who have acquired injury, illness or disease whilst employed. The injury, illness or disease may or may not be work related and may be of a physical and/or psychological basis.

A number of terms are used with respect to the rehabilitation of injured workers. The terms occupational rehabilitation (used in Australia) and disability management (used in North America) are terms that are often used interchangeably (International Labor Organisation 2002, National Occupational Health Safety Commission 1995). Generally, these terms are applied when the worker has a pre-existing relationship with an employer. Common to all of these is the focus on the return of the injured worker to the workplace, generally occurring within a workers' compensation system (O'Halloran & Innes 2005). Vocational rehabilitation encompasses a wider group of individuals who may be working, have never worked or who have become unem-

ployed due to a health condition (Department Work Pensions 2004). This chapter will focus on 'workers' – that is those individuals who have an existing relationship with an employer, as their needs differ from those who are not in active employment. As terms and definitions vary throughout the literature, working definitions of key terms can be found in Table 27.1.

Work occupations

For many people, work is an important occupation and can be described as activity performed to produce goods or services of value to others. It involves mental or physical effort directed to achievement of a goal. In the broadest sense, work is goal-directed activity (Szymanski 2003). Although work is required to maintain life and meet basic needs, an individual's occupational role as a worker contributes to their self-esteem, fulfilment, identity, social interaction and status within the community (Harpaz & Fu 2002).

In the general community, work equates with paid employment. However, within the occupational therapy literature, definitions of work encompass both paid and unpaid productive occupations (Hagedorn 2001, Kielhofner et al 1999). The value of work occupations was recognised by the founders of occupational therapy who believed that the structure provided by working could help cure people with mental illnesses (Baker & Jacobs 2003). Since these early times work occupations have been used as a therapeutic medium within many areas of occupational therapy practice (Sandqvist & Henriksson 2004).

The meaning of work

In most Western societies, there is an expectation that most individuals will engage in paid or unpaid work. The type of work in which people participate is influenced by the societal and cultural standards of their community (Brown et al 2001).

A number of valued outcomes have been associated with work. Work can provide a sense of belonging in a community, enabling the individual to contribute to the needs of others in society (Baker & Jacobs 2003; Brown et al 2001; Sager & James 2005). Individuals are also evaluated and identified within society in terms of various roles and functions

Table 27.1 Definitions of key terms related to work rehabilitation

Worker	A person who experiences an injury or illness whilst employed, resulting in restrictions to participation in work
Usual duties	The duties undertaken by the worker in their place of work prior to or at the time of their injury or illness
Work rehabilitation	A structured, well-reasoned therapeutic programme to facilitate a return to work for workers whose participation in work has been affected by a temporary or permanent injury or illness. The injury or illness may or may not be work related
Ergonomics	The scientific discipline concerned with the understanding of interactions among humans and other elements of a system. Ergonomists contribute to the design and evaluation of tasks, jobs, products, environments and systems in order to make them compatible with the needs, abilities and limitations of people (International Ergonomics Association 2000)
Therapeutic return to work programme	Hours, duties and/or performance expectations of the job are gradually increased until the worker is able to return to full duty (Krause 1998). This is also known as graded work
Suitable duties	Short-term work duties to assist the injured worker's rehabilitation which may include parts of the usual duties, or alternate duties. Must be meaningful and productive work
Light duties	Temporary or permanent activity less than regular or full duties which enables the worker to perform a job according to a set of conditions prescribed by a health worker. These duties range from adaptation of pre injury job to an entirely different job and tend not to be productive or valued within the workplace (Krause 1998)
Interventions	Treatment by other health professionals or by the occupational therapist. Examples include physical therapies to increase fitness, strength or endurance, cognitive behavioural therapy, pain management programmes, adjustment to disability counselling
Capacity	An individual's ability to execute a task or action, aims to indicate the highest probable level of functioning that a person may reach (Australian Institute of Health and Welfare 2003)
Stakeholders	Any participants involved in and impacting on the work rehabilitation process. This includes the worker, employer, other health professionals and the payer (insurer or funding body)

that they perform. This may be related to their profession, their role within the organisation or the tasks that they perform (Harpaz & Fu 2002). The worker role contributes to a person's identity, and provides a source of meaning and satisfaction in life. Satisfaction with work is more likely to be high if the values and attitudes of the employee match those of the employer (Brown 2001).

Injury, illness or disease can result in either temporary or permanent loss or change to the person's work roles. Absence from work due to injury, illness or disease results in significant costs, in both economic and human terms, to the individual, the employer and society. Adverse effects to the worker include depression, decreased participation in activities of daily living, psychological distress and negative impact on family and social relationships (Kirsch & McKee 2003).

Occupational therapy and work

Occupational therapists can become involved when an individual's work participation is restricted by injury, illness or disease. Although occupational therapists have a long history in the rehabilitation of individuals who have experienced work-related injuries, it is only recently that occupational therapists have become involved in the workplace, assisting people to return to work, or remain in work, following injury, illness or disease (Deen Gibson & Strong 2002). Successful return to work is a complex process involving many factors. The biopsychosocial model that considers the physical, psychological and social-cultural factors which influence a person's capacity has been adopted in occupational therapy practice since the early 1960s (Sandqvist & Henriksson 2004). This approach enables the occupational therapist to take into account all factors which will impact on the person's ability to participate in life and work occupations.

Occupational therapists use the principles of ergonomics during the work rehabilitation process to assess the tasks and jobs of the worker, and to identify risk factors within the workplace. Ergonomic principles are applied when making recommendations for changes to work tasks, tools, equipment or the working environment. If complex redesign or modification to tools or equipment is required, the occupational therapist will need to seek the assistance of appropriately qualified professionals, such as ergonomists, engineers or designers. In addition to the rehabilitation of individual workers, occupational therapists may be involved in the provision of other services, such as injury-prevention programmes (Jundt & King 1999).

Occupational therapists work within a larger system of occupational rehabilitation or disability management, the aim of which is to facilitate a workers' return to work following injury, illness or disease. The process of rehabilitation will vary between countries due to legislative frameworks, and workers' compensation and insurance systems. Over the past few years, the International Labour Organisation (ILO) has developed a number of codes of practice regarding disability and work, the most recent being a Convention on the Rights of Persons with Disabilities, which was ratified by the United Nations (United Nations 2007). The Convention represents a major change in that it prohibits discrimination on the basis of disability in all forms of employment.

Work rehabilitation

Work rehabilitation is a dynamic process involving multiple phases and encompassing a range of actions (Young et al 2005a). The occupational therapist is required to synthesise and analyse significant amounts of information gathered from the workplace, the individual worker and other health professionals. The therapist must then use professional reasoning skills to determine the most appropriate therapeutic programme to facilitate the worker's return to work. This programme must identify and

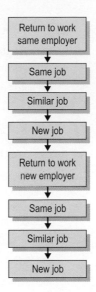

Figure 27.1 • Return to work hierarchy

address any mismatch between the worker's work capacity and their usual work tasks.

The primary aim of work rehabilitation is to safely return the worker to work as soon as possible following injury, illness or disease. Secondary aims are to provide a safer work environment, reduce health care costs, decrease lost work days and to increase worker satisfaction and productivity (Williams & Westmorland 2002). Ideally, the worker will return to their own job, in their own workplace. If they are unable to return to their previous workplace, a hierarchy for return to work has been recommended (Figure 27.1) (National Occupational Health and Safety Commission 1995).

Whilst there is the potential for return to work outcomes to have a significant impact on the individual, employers, and system payers (e.g. insurer or funding organisation), the process is as important as the outcome (Young et al 2005b). There are a number of features which contribute to a successful work rehabilitation programme:

- *Early referral for work rehabilitation following injury or illness.* The goal of early referral is to maintain the individual at work or return them to meaningful work as soon as possible. Contact between the worker and workplace should occur soon after injury or illness (Franche et al 2005).

- *Rehabilitation is workplace based.* Rehabilitation is implemented in close connection with the worker's usual or proposed job, in realistic work environments, involving real tasks, with the workplace site as the centre of the work rehabilitation process (Durand & Loisel 2001, Loisel et al 2003, Sandqvist & Henriksson 2004).

- *Provision of appropriate modified work.* Workers offered modified work are twice as likely to return to work as those who are not, and lose half the number of work days (Krause et al 1998).

- *Communication* is a key element in determining the success of work rehabilitation (Kirsh & McKee 2003, Loisel et al 2003, Sager & James 2005). The research evidence confirms that providing information to the key stakeholders on their role, responsibility, expectations, legislation, costs (as appropriate), and the details of the programme ensures commitment and co-operation (Kirsh & McKee 2003, Sager & James 2005, Westmorland et al 2002, Williams & Westmorland 2002).

- *The work rehabilitation programme should be well reasoned with clear goals, time frames and outcomes.* Workplace interventions should be linked and combined with other interventions (Durand & Loisel 2001, Loisel et al 2003). These interventions may be concurrent but have complimentary goals. The programme should include an educational component for the worker (Sager & James 2005) and the workplace supervisor/manager (Franche et al 2005).

- *Workers should receive ongoing monitoring of their progress throughout the rehabilitation process* (National Occupational Health and Safety Commission 1995, Russo & Innes 2002, Westmorland et al 2005, Williams & Westmorland 2002).

The work rehabilitation process

Work rehabilitation is indicated when an individual's injury or illness impacts on their occupational performance at work. The World Health Organisation's (WHO) International Classification of Functioning (ICF) (World Health Organisation 2002) has been adopted as a useful framework for work assessment in occupational therapy (Gibson & Strong 2003, Sandqvist & Henriksson 2004).

The ICF recognises a person's functioning as a dynamic interaction between health conditions, the environment and personal factors (World Health Organisation 2002). The worker's injury or illness (health condition) affects the body structures and function resulting in activity limitations thereby restricting their participation in work. Contextual factors, such as the physical, social and attitudinal environment of the workplace and the person's community environment can be either a barrier or facilitator to the work rehabilitation process. Personal factors, such as a person's age, education, coping styles, social and cultural background, and previous life and work experiences will also impact on rehabilitation. These factors can influence the assessment, interventions, timing and outcome of work rehabilitation and need to be considered throughout the work rehabilitation process. Figure 27.2 outlines a proposed framework for work rehabilitation.

The work rehabilitation process consists of five key phases:

- Phase 1: *Assessment* of the worker, their usual work and the contextual factors (personal and environmental) which impact on their return to work.

- Phase 2: *Professional reasoning* to determine whether a match exists between the worker and their usual work.

- Phase 3: *Establishing of short-term and long-term goals.*

- Phase 4: *Developing interventions* – a therapeutic return to work programme and interventions.

- Phase 5: *Implementing* the programme, monitoring, measuring outcomes and reviewing.

Adjustments may be made to goals or interventions following unexpected events such as surgery, or physical or psychological illness. This may require the therapist to move through the five stages again in the context of new information.

Each phase involved in a work rehabilitation programme is described below. Practice Scenarios 27.1 and 27.2 will be used to illustrate the five key phases.

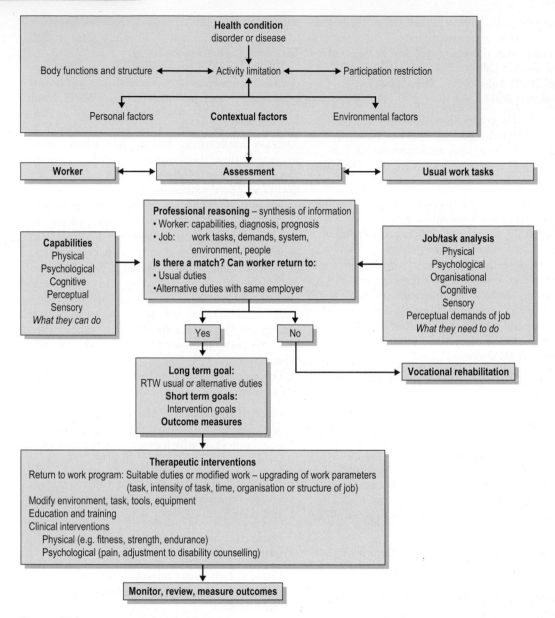

Figure 27.2 • Work rehabilitation process

Practice Scenario 27.1 Matthew: Therapeutic Work Rehabilitation Programme

Matthew is 42 years old. He lives with his wife and two children. He enjoys playing football and coaching his son's football team. As this is his second episode of low back pain (LBP) he is concerned about his ability to resume full-time work.

Work profile

Matthew has worked as a machine operator for 5 years with the same company, a metal fabrication and manufacturing company. His work history involves a range of semi- and unskilled machine operation and process work. He has had no formal training and holds no educational qualifications.

Phase 1 and 2: Assessment and professional reasoning

Medical history, diagnosis and prognosis

Matthew has experienced non-specific low back pain since he twisted and bent his back whilst operating a machine at work 4 months ago. Scans have not identified any specific pathology. He had a previous incident of LBP 1 year ago after playing football. The pain from this incident resolved in 2 months.

Body function and structure

Matthew reports experiencing pain and numbness in the sacro-iliac area. He rates his pain on a visual analogue scale (VAS) to be 4–6/10, worse at the beginning of the day. He takes two doses of analgesic medication per day. Range of motion is marginally reduced in the lumbar spine in forward flexion and right rotation. All other movements and muscle strength are within normal limits.

Activity and participation

Mobility and tolerances Standing and walking tolerance is limited to one and a half hours and sitting to one hour before an increase in pain. His balance is good and there is no alteration to gait.

Self-care activities He is independent with all self-care activities.

Home duties He performs limited pre-injury domestic duties (e.g. taking out the garbage bins, mowing his small level lawn, washing up). He no longer completes the shopping, and he has suspended his home renovations and redecorating plans. He has stopped coaching and playing football. His score on the Oswestry Low Back Pain Disability Questionnaire was 54%, indicating severe disability (Fairbank et al 1980).

Contextual factors His wife is becoming less tolerant of his complaints of pain.

Workplace assessment – Matthew's usual work tasks

Matthew is a machine operator which involves him rotating between up to four workstations per day depending on production. All tasks are repetitive, requiring bilateral upper-extremity strength and fine hand function.

Workstation 1 (powder coating machine) Prolonged walking, periodic stationary standing for three and a half hours before a rest break, and repetitive reaching between chest and shoulder height (Figure 27.3).

Workstation 2 (metal punch machine) Repetitive bending and reaching to hip height (25 times per hour) (Figure 27.4).

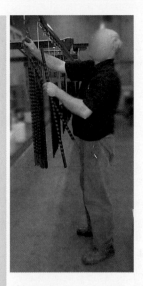

Figure 27.3 • Powder coating machine

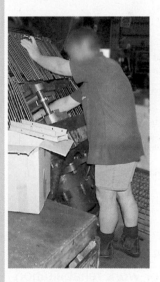

Figure 27.4 • Metal punching machine

Workstation 3 (packing aluminium lengths) Repetitive lifting aluminium lengths from the machine to the pallet on the floor (30 times/hour). Weight 2 kg per length (Figure 27.5).

Workstation 4 (metal drilling machine) Prolonged sitting to drill for most of the 3½ hours. Occasional standing and bending to floor level three times in 1 hour to pick up the metal section from the floor (Figure 27.6).

Environment Concrete floor, the building is cold in the early mornings. Each machine requires some knowledge and skill gained through on-the-job

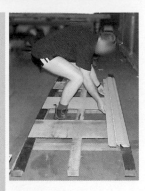

Figure 27.5 • Packing aluminium lengths

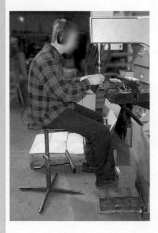

Figure 27.6 • Metal drilling machine

training. The machine operator is required to meet production demands, and there is a bonus system per individual (not team).

Phase 3: Goals for work rehabilitation programme

Long-term goal

Matthew will return to usual full-time work duties as a machine operator working on any of the four workstations within 6 weeks.

Short-term goal

1. Matthew to increase standing/walking tolerance to 4 hours in 4 weeks.
2. Matthew to perceive less pain each day after working on usual work tasks and hours.
3. Matthew to resume all usual home tasks within 4 weeks and home decorating in 6 weeks.

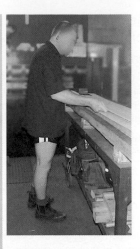

Figure 27.7 • Packing aluminium lengths workstation modified

Phases 4 and 5: Develop and implement work rehabilitation programme

Intervention

Matthew agreed to modify his early-morning routine to minimise lumbar flexion during the first hours after he is out of bed. He placed his work clothes and shoes on a chair in the evening to avoid bending, stood to have his breakfast rather than sat and stood while waiting for and catching the train to work. He performed stretching and strengthening exercises in the afternoon after work. Over 6 weeks he upgraded his home activities, commencing on cleaning roof gutters in week 4, to painting the walls of one room (week 5) and then shopping (on Saturday afternoon – week 6).

Relevant research evidence to this case study

Snook (1998)[1] in a randomised control trial, concluded that the control of forward and lateral lumbar flexion for at least 2 hours in the early morning may reduce the intensity and number of days in pain for individuals with chronic, non-specific low-back pain. The bottom line is that to exclude or minimise activities or exercise that involve lumbar flexion for at least 2 hours after rising is a form of self-care to minimise low-back pain.

[1]The information is provided in this section as an example of how the evidence can be applied to an occupational therapy intervention. The cited study has some methodological limitations (RCT Phase 1 preliminary OTSeeker score 6/10, RCT Phase 1 & 2: PEDro score 4/10) and was for a specific client group: chronic, non-specific low-back pain. Prior to implementation of such strategies, therapists should refer to the original cited publication to determine if the research is applicable to their individual client.

Workstation modification

Packing workstation modified so that the packing pallet is placed on a bench eliminating bending (Figure 27.7).

Return to work programme

Grading of tasks requiring lumbar flexion (bending) to reduce pressure on the disc and thus reduce pain, so that standing and bending tolerance can be gradually increased over time:

Week 1–2 (5 hours per day): At the beginning of the shift work for 3 hours on Workstation 1 (powder coating) where no lumbar flexion is required, followed by 2 hours on Workstation 2 (metal punch), where some lumbar flexion is required.

Week 3–4 (6 hours per day): As per weeks 1–2, in addition work one hour on Workstation 3 (modified packing) at the end of the day. Lifting is from waist to waist height, carried over 2 m.

Week 5–6 (8 hours per day): As per weeks 3–4, in addition work on Workstation 4 (metal drilling) for the last 2 hours of the day.

Matthew was monitored for durability of work tasks for a further 4 weeks.

Outcomes

At the end of the programme Matthew:

* could tolerate standing/walking for up to 4 hours
* used all machines
* worked 7½ hours per day
* did all his home tasks
* perceived pain was reduced to VAS 1–2/10
* has an Oswestry Low Back Pain Disability Questionnaire score of 20% indicating minimal disability
* was not taking any analgesic medication.

This practice scenario was provided by Sue Lukersmith.

Practice Scenario 27.2
Celeste: Therapeutic Work Rehabilitation Programme

Celeste is 32 and engaged to be married. She plays competition netball. She is concerned about the lack of improvement in her pain. She is extremely anxious about returning to work as her immediate supervisor has intimated that Celeste's injury is not genuine and that she is just seeking time off work to organise her wedding.

Work profile

Celeste has worked as a legal secretary for 8 years. She is secretary to a senior partner and two other part-time lawyers.

Phases 1 and 2: Assessment and Professional Reasoning

Medical history, diagnosis and prognosis

Celeste began experiencing pain in her right (dominant) wrist and forearm 6 weeks ago following working 18 additional hours per week overtime for 3 weeks. X-rays and nerve conduction studies were normal. An ultrasound indicated that she had an inflammation of extensor carpi ulnaris and anconeus. Her doctor prescribed anti-inflammatory medication, analgesia and referred her to a hand therapist.

Body function and structure

Pain Celeste reports experiencing pain on the right (ulnar) side of her wrist and in her forearm. She describes her pain as constant but varying in intensity. Typing rapidly increased pain from a level of 5/10 on a Visual Analogue Scale (VAS) to a 9/10 after 4 minutes. She takes three doses of analgesic medication per day.

Range of motion Celeste has no reduction in movement, but experiences pain at the end of range for ulnar deviation and wrist extension in her right wrist. It was noted that there was a reduction in the strength of her extensor carpi ulnaris.

Activity and participation

Dexterity and tolerances Her fine motor activity in her right hand was limited to 4 minutes before experiencing an increase in pain levels. Her right-hand grip strength was reduced by 10–15% when compared to normative data. She was limited to being able to carry objects of no more than 3 kg and to be able to do this only on an occasional basis.

Self-care activities She was independent with all self-care activities but reported experiencing pain when styling her hair.

Home duties She was independent in doing household tasks but did experience pain when preparing meals (chopping, slicing, peeling, and stirring) and carrying loads in her right hand (groceries shopping, garbage bins, and laundry basket).

Leisure Celeste was unable to play netball due to her pain.

Contextual factors Her fiancée has provided some assistance. Celeste is frustrated that she cannot play netball and is expressing concern that she is putting on weight prior to her wedding due to inactivity.

Workplace assessment – Celeste's usual work tasks

As a legal secretary Celeste did various clerical tasks, some self paced and some subject to deadlines. All tasks require bi- or unilateral (right) hand/arm activity and many tasks involve repetitive fine motor activity. Some upper-limb strength is required to handle files (up to 2 kg), ledgers and urn (up to 4 kg), meal trays (5 kg), and archive boxes (up to 16 kg).

Telephone work When answering inbound calls Celeste uses a telephone headset.

Typing Celeste types letters and reports for approximately 70% of her working week; she will type for up to 45 minutes without a break. It was observed that when typing and using a mouse she had an ulnar deviation of her hand at her wrist. She also had sustained wrist extension during keyboard and mouse work.

Paralegal work This type of work involved Celeste using the telephone, obtaining documents, conducting research via the internet, lodging papers with courts/offices, and meeting clients for documentation signage. It was estimated that she spent 20% of her time doing these activities.

General office work Part of her role also involved the organisation of the board room for meetings, organising and collecting and catering, filing documents, and dealing with the mail. It was estimated that she spent 10% of her time doing these activities.

Environment Celeste works in an open-plan office, with good lighting, and has a fixed height desk, with a right side return. She uses a standard computer, monitor, keyboard and mouse (all operated with her right hand), and a telephone with headset. She has an adjustable office chair which has been set too low, a document holder to the right of her monitor, and a number of large filing cabinets.

Phase 3: Goals for work rehabilitation programme

Long-term goal

Celeste will return to her usual work duties as a full-time legal secretary within 12 weeks.

Short-term goal

1. Celeste to increase fine motor activity with right hand to 20-minute intervals without increase of pain within 3 weeks.
4. Celeste to resume home duties and leisure (netball) tasks within 10 weeks.

Phases 4 and 5: Develop and implement work rehabilitation programme

Return-to-work programme

Education was provided to the immediate supervisor regarding the nature of Celeste's injury, her physical restrictions and the return-to-work process:

Weeks 1 and 2 (4 hours per day): 5 minutes typing continuously every 30 minutes, alternated with telephone, paralegal work and filing. No lifting of archive boxes or catering trays for first 10 weeks.

Weeks 3 and 4 (4 hour per day): Typing increased to 10 minutes every 30 minutes alternated with other tasks as above.

Weeks 5 and 6 (6 hours per day): 10 minutes typing alternated with other tasks as above.

Weeks 7 and 8 (6 hours per day): typing increased to 20 minutes every 30 minutes alternated with other tasks as above.

Weeks 9 and 10 (full pre-injury hours): 20 minutes typing continuously every 30 minutes, alternated with other tasks as above.

Weeks 11 and 12 (as above): Commence lifting of archive boxes, catering trays.

Other intervention

Celeste to take part in a 10-week hand-therapy programme that aims to reduce tendon inflammation and strengthen muscles. She also needs to carry out an exercise programme which should be performed three times a day (before work, after lunch, and evening).

Environmental modifications

Celeste will use an alternative mouse/input device to reduce extreme wrist postures. Her chair is adjusted to reduce shoulder elevation and wrist extension. Additional 'macros' are designed along with keystroke alternatives for use instead of mouse movements. The telephone was relocated to the left-hand side to reduce workload on her right hand.

Training

Facilitate Celeste to use her mouse in both her right and left hands and to be aware of how to adjust her workstation.

Outcomes

At end of the programme Celeste:
- had a reduction in her resting pain with a score of 0/10 on the Visual Analogue Scale

- had an occasional increase in her pain levels related to specific tasks, as noted by her score of 3/10 on the Visual Analogue Scale; however, the pain did not usually last for more than 15 minutes
- reduced her intake of analgesic medication to approximately twice weekly
- resumed full-time work
- could type for 30 minutes continuously without any increase in pain
- was able to obtain her pre-injury typing speed
- was able to perform all her pre-injury clerical duties
- resumed playing netball.

This Practice Scenario was provided by Sandina Bailey, an occupational therapist working with people with injuries returning to work. At the time of writing she was working with the Commonwealth Rehabilitation Service in Sydney, Australia.

Phase one: assessment

Phase one involves the assessment of the worker, the requirements of their job, and the personal, environmental and contextual factors which impact on their return to work. A range of assessments are conducted using objective measures where possible, some of which may also be used as outcome measures for the interventions and return-to-work programme. The information necessary to the work rehabilitation programme varies between individual workers, workplaces, tasks, systems, cultures, and countries. Below is a typical range of information required for carrying out workplace rehabilitation. It is not intended to be an exhaustive list of all the information and assessments potentially performed in this area.

Assessment of the worker

An assessment is made of the current status of the worker to determine the impact of their health condition on their ability to participate in the workplace. The range of information that may be obtained is listed below, grouped into the ICF domains for a health condition/disorder or disease occurring whilst at work.

Diagnostic and prognostic information

Diagnostic and prognostic information is obtained through general and specialist medical practitioners, test results, consultation with other health professionals (e.g. treating physiotherapist), and, for some, information is provided by the worker. The informa-tion relates to the *body function/structure* components of the ICF and includes:

1. Medical diagnosis
2. Planned medical intervention (e.g. operation)
3. Anticipated long-term recovery (medical prognosis)
4. Previous medical and therapeutic interventions (nature, timing)
5. Outcomes of current or previous therapies (beneficial or not)
6. Progress to date (improved or stabilised).

Interview with the worker

The worker is interviewed to establish his current and previous capabilities at work, and his activities of daily living at home. His perception of the impact of the injury or illness on his work, lifestyle, leisure, family life, and domestic responsibilities is discussed. Workers are asked about their usual daily routine since ceasing work, their ability to use transport, their symptoms, and their medication use. This addresses the *activity limitations and participation restrictions* components of the ICF.

Information regarding the worker's subjective view of his work and his support systems is sought during the interview. These include social support network, responsibilities, and relationships (family or work colleagues), his interests, values and roles outside of work (Keogh & Fisher 2001). Any cultural influences, family attitudes or personal circumstances that may impact on the return to work process are established.

The worker's skills, experience and the meaning of work to the individual are explored with respect to career stage. The therapist also aims to establish the worker's attitude to their current work, workplace and their role in the organisation (Fisher 1999). Attitudes and compliance with past medical and other interventions, the reasons for poor compliance (where relevant) are discussed with the worker and objectively assessed (where possible). This addresses the *personal and environmental contextual factors* components of the ICF.

Assessment of the worker's capacity

The individual's capacity for work is assessed. Assessments used can include on-the-job evaluations, workplace-based assessments, work simulations, physical capacity evaluations or functional capacity evaluations (FCE) (Innes & Straker 2002). FCE can provide information on the worker's capacity to perform a broad range of demands related to work, or may be specific to a particular job. FCE assists in a prediction of the timing of return to work, the level of work, and sometimes the content of the work tasks (short to long term) (Innes & Straker 1999, Schonstein & Kenny 2001). FCE allows the therapist to match the residual work capacity of the individual with the work demands, rather than measuring impairment only (Gibson & Strong 2003).

The range of information obtained from FCE includes:

- Body function and structure:
  - Muscle strength relevant to the work tasks
  - Range of movement relevant to the tasks
  - Patterns (changes) to muscle use
  - Identification of sensory system impairment (sensation, vision, hearing)
  - Cognitive and perceptual function relative to work tasks.

- Activity limitations and participation restrictions:
  - Hand function (grasp, strength, dexterity)
  - Lifting and carrying capacity
  - Mobility and postural tolerances (sitting, standing, walking, reaching, climbing, squatting, push/pull)
  - Materials handling technique
  - Endurance/basic level of fitness/response to sustained activity
  - Appropriate speed of activity completion (productivity)
  - Perceived pain (level and body area)
  - Pain management strategies and their impact on perceived pain.

- Contextual factors – personal and environment:
  - Lifting technique
  - Features of work clothing (including personal protective equipment, shoes).

The functional capacity evaluation may be conducted within the workplace using the worker's usual duties, or in a clinic-based setting. A functional capacity evaluation conducted at the workplace better measures the actual demands of the job when compared to a standardised functional capacity evaluation. However, the results are specific to the usual work duties and are less able to be generalised to other work tasks (Gibson & Strong 2003, Innes & Straker 2002).

Assessment of the workplace

Three main methods of data collection are used to assess duties and tasks within a workplace: interviews, observation, and measurement.

Manager/supervisor interviews

The aim of the interview is to determine the employer's understanding of work rehabilitation, to confirm the exact nature of the worker's usual duties and to establish the range of suitable duties available at the workplace. In particular, the occupational therapist needs to establish:

- the employer's awareness and understanding of work rehabilitation (worker and workplace benefits, procedures, past experience of work rehabilitation)

- responsiveness of the employer to a potential on-site return-to-work programme

- potential support for worker throughout the programme

- flexibility/options for suitable tasks to be incorporated in the return-to-work programme

- workplace attitude and perceptions of the worker (legitimacy of the injury, work performance)

- workplace attitude and perceptions of the worker's role within the organisation, work content (complexity, productivity demands)

- relationship with co-workers including the impact of worker's injury on other team members

- perception of identified suitable duties as productive, valued duties within the workplace

- the legislative context (occupational health and safety and workers' compensation legislation) and the workplace systems, policies and practices to comply with this legislation

- availability of funding for interventions, work rehabilitation programme or new workplace equipment costs

- current or proposed restructure, retrenchments or expansion of workforce, market or government policy changes which may impact on the organisation (Australian Institute of Health and Welfare 2003).

Workplace assessment – job analysis

The aim of the workplace assessment is to assess the physical, cognitive, psychosocial and environmental demands of the worker's usual duties and/or potential suitable duties with the same employer.

A job analysis involves making a detailed list of the tasks involved and the skills required. This analysis provides information on what the worker has to do, how to do it, why he does it and what skill is involved in doing it (International Labour Organisation 2007). The information is obtained through observation, measurement, timing of tasks/cycles and documentation (e.g. job or position descriptions, safe operating procedures). Additional sources of generic occupational information are through job classifications systems such as the Australian Classification of Occupations (ASCO) (Australian Bureau of Statistics 1997), or O*NET (National Center for O*NET Development 2007).

The following are assessed:

- *Physical demands*: sitting, standing, walking, climbing, lifting, carrying
- *Risk factors*: awkward postures, static postures repetition (cycle time and repetition per hour/day); loads (nature of coupling and load dimensions) and load handling (weight, distances/height, distance from body, acceleration of movement)
- *Cognitive requirements:* critical thinking, information acquisition and processing, mental planning and scheduling, learning, communicating, comprehending, translating knowledge, perceiving and interpreting interpersonal information, and using intuition (Shaw & Lysaght 2008)
- *Behavioural demands*: social relationships, worker and management responsibilities, general competencies, and accountabilities (Shaw & Lysaght 2008)
- *Organisational demands*: work patterns – days/hours/shifts worked (includes shift cycle/rotation), peak work demands, staff levels, bonus systems, team-based work, job rotation, and training
- *Environmental demands:*
  - Work-area design: physical terrain, layout of equipment/machines, presence of ramps/stairs/lifts, and obstructions in walkways/circulations, space
  - Work tools and equipment
  - Risk factors: factors which potentially impact on the return-to-work programme or place the worker at risk, such as working outside, extreme temperatures, air quality, noise, floor surfaces, vibration (hand/arm), or contact stress. Specific measurement of these factors, if required, should be performed by appropriately qualified professionals.
- Psycho-social issues:
  - Job control, support at work, job satisfaction, team morale, team work, job security, responsibility for others, and opportunities for career progression (Australian Institute of Health and Welfare 2003, Workplace Health & Safety 1999).

Phase two: professional reasoning – matching worker and work tasks

Reasoning is used throughout the work rehabilitation programme. It is not an isolated process, but occurs simultaneously within the activities performed by the occupational therapist in each phase of the programme. A work rehabilitation programme involves a complex bio-psychosocial matching process. This involves comparing the capabilities of the worker and the demands of the work tasks (Sandqvist & Henriksson 2004). Matching requires the occupational therapist to reason so that the work rehabilitation programme is effective. Reasoning also assists the occupational therapist to identify barriers and, where possible, strategies to minimise these barriers.

Phase three: goal setting and outcome measurement

The occupational therapist uses professional reasoning to predict the likely long-term work-capacity goals and the interventions needed to achieve a return to work. At the completion of the assessment phase, the long-term goal of either return to usual work duties or return to permanent alternative duties with the same employer is established. This goal, which includes the time frame for return to work, is determined with consultation and agreement from the worker, the doctor, the employer, and, where relevant, the insurer or funding body.

Following consultation with his employer, Roger returns to work on part-time administrative duties in another department, which involves him working in the office completing photocopying and filing tasks. He is sitting all day except for when he is photocopying. Roger is unhappy being placed on 'made-up' duties – tasks temporarily transferred from another worker. He also does not think the duties utilise his machine operation skills. He finds them boring and he lacks motivation to attend work. Roger dislikes being separated from the manufacturing floor of the company. He takes 8 weeks to build up to full-time hours in the administration department before resuming full-time work on his usual duties.

Discussion

In this example, whilst the outcome was positive, the time taken for the worker to return to full-time usual duties (11 weeks) may have been several weeks longer than necessary. The research suggests that there are potential harmful effects of prolonged bed rest for low-back pain (Hilde et al 2001). Resting after a low-back injury is inconsistent with research evidence, which recommends a gradual resumption of usual activities and a graded exercise programme for non-specific low-back pain (Hayden et al 2005, Hilde et al 2001, Maher et al 1999). After 2 weeks of rest, the worker's physical tolerances may have reduced further with sedentary duties for 8 weeks. It is likely that the worker would become further de-conditioned with key physical tolerances required of him in his usual duties (e.g. standing tolerance). The risk of re-injury when he returns to his usual duties may also be higher subsequent to the de-conditioning. Other factors influencing the programme are the fact that the duties are not 'value added' or productive for the employer, but rather taking tasks from one worker to give to another. Furthermore, the injured worker dislikes the tasks and would prefer to be with his co-workers in manufacturing. Work rehabilitation programmes that involve injured workers in meaningful productive work where they are contributing to and are valued at the workplace, provide a sense or personal self-worth are more likely to be accepted and succeed.

Practice Scenario 27.4
Sally: Time-waster Interventions

Sally is a registered nurse of 13 years' experience. She injures her shoulder whilst assisting a patient to transfer from the bed to a wheelchair. The diagnosis is a significant partial-thickness tear involving the rotator cuff tendons (supraspinatus and infraspinatus) of her non-dominant left shoulder. She works on the male orthopaedic ward of a large district hospital. Her doctor states that it will take 18 months for the injury to resolve. She is referred to physiotherapy and undergoes 12 weeks of manual therapy before a return to work is considered. The therapist devises a return-to-work programme, which involves a goal of returning to work in alternative duties with the same employer, although the type of duties is not specified.

On her return to work Sally is transferred to work in the stores section, processing orders from the various wards and departments. Her permanent substantive position remains a nurse in the orthopaedic ward. A further 12 weeks pass with Sally remaining on the tasks in stores section, working full-time hours (7.30–4 pm rather than afternoon shift as she did when working on the ward). The different hours for work complicate her childcare arrangements before school. After 6 months, the Nursing Manager seeks clarification on Sally's capacity to return to the orthopaedic ward. The orthopaedic ward has been short-staffed for 6 months since Sally's injury. Sally's long-term return-to-work goal is discussed. Sally will have physical restrictions for a further 12 months (lifting and carrying). The hospital decides to terminate her employment. Seven months after her injury, Sally is no longer employed.

Discussion

In this example, Sally could have returned to work on suitable alternative duties within her physical capacity, but more closely related to her nursing skills. One of the key concerns with Sally's time-waster programme above is the delay in establishing Sally's long-term return-to-work goal. The long-term goal should have been resolved as soon as possible, in less than 6 months post injury and before she commenced her return-to-work programme. After assessment of all factors relating to her health condition (including the prognosis, physical capacity and psycho-social factors), consideration should have been given to return-to-work on similar, less physically demanding nursing duties with the same employer (e.g. venepuncture) (Figure 27.1). A therapeutic return-to-work programme utilising her nursing training and skills would enable her early return to work whilst undertaking interventions such as physiotherapy. Her return-to-work programme would also likely involve commencing on reduced hours with a graded return to usual hours of work. This therapeutic programme has the potential to impact on Sally's psycho-social well-being as well as reduce inefficiencies at the workplace.

Phase five: implement interventions, monitor and review

The program is implemented with regular reviews undertaken to monitor the worker's progress toward the short- and long-term goals. At times, short-term and, sometimes, long-term goals have to be adjusted (e.g. as a result of a change in diagnosis). Additional secondary outcomes may also occur (e.g. decreased use of pain medication, higher job satisfaction, better sleep pattern). Finally, monitoring of the worker's capacity to maintain work over a realistic period is also important (e.g. durability of return to work programme). This may involve brief contact with the worker and employer for a month after programme completion.

Conclusion

Work is an important occupation for most individuals of working age. Occupational therapists become involved when an individual's participation in work occupations is restricted through injury, impairment or illness. Work rehabilitation is a dynamic process requiring thorough assessment of the worker's abilities and the physical, environmental, psychosocial, and cognitive and behavioural demands of work. A carefully reasoned programme which aims to match worker abilities with job demands is developed in conjunction with the worker, employer and other health professionals. Features of successful work rehabilitation programmes include: the provision of appropriate suitable work duties; intervention strategies to address specific physical or psychosocial issues; good communication between all stakeholders, and careful monitoring and support of the worker during the return-to-work process. Occupational therapists, with their focus on the analysis of occupations have a unique role in work rehabilitation. This chapter has outlined a process for work rehabilitation which involves five phases. The role of the occupational therapist in each of the phases has been described.

References

Australian Bureau of Statistics (ABS) (1997). *ASCO – Australian Standard Classification of Occupations (No. 1220.0)*. Canberra, ABS.

Australian Institute of Health and Welfare (AIHW) (2003). *I.C.F. Australian User Guide*. Canberra, AIHW.

Australian Institute of Health and Welfare (AIHW) (2003). *I.C.F. Australian user guide* (Version 1.0. Disability Series ed., Vol. AIHW Cat DIS 33): Canberra: AIHW.

Baker, N. & Jacobs, K. (2003). The nature of working in the United States: An occupational therapy perspective. *Work*, 20, 53–61.

Brown, A., Kitchell, M., O'Neil, T., Lockliear, J., Vosler, A., Kubek, D. & Dale, L. (2001). Identifying meaning and perceived level of satisfaction in the context of work. *Work*, 16, 219–226.

Cohn, E. S. (2003). A way of thinking about occupational performance. In: E. B. Crepeau, E. S. Cohn & B. A. Boyt Schell (Ed.) *Willard & Spackman's Occupational Therapy* (10th ed., pp. 131–138). Philadelphia: Lippincott Williams & Wilkins.

Cook, C., McCluskey, A. & Bowman, J. (2006). *Increasing the use of outcome measures by occupational therapists*. Retrieved April 20, 2007, from http://www.maa.nsw.gov.au/default.aspx?MenuID=188#174.

Deen, M., Gibson, L. & Strong, J. (2002). A survey of occupational therapy in Australian work practice. *Work*, 19, 219–230.

Department Work Pensions (DWP) (2004). *Building capacity for work: A UK framework for vocational rehabilitation*. Retrieved Feb 6, 2007, from http://www.dwp.gov.uk/publications/vrframework/dwp_vocational_rehabilitation.pdf.

Durand, M. & Loisel, P. (2001). Therapeutic return to work: rehabilitation in the workplace. *Work*, 17, 57–63.

Fairbank, J. C., Couper, J., Davies, J. B. & O'Brien, J. P. (1980). The Oswestry Low Back Pain Disability Questionnaire. *Physiotherapy*, 66, 271–273.

Finch, E., Brooks, D., Stratford, P. & Mayo, N. (2002). *Physical rehabilitation outcome measures: a guide to enhanced clinical decision making*. Hamilton: Canadian Physiotherapy Association.

Fisher, G. S. (1999). Administration and application of the worker role interview; looking beyond functional capacity. *Work*, 12, 13–24.

Franche, R., Cullen, K., Clarke, J., Irvin, E., Sinclair, S., Frank, J., and the Insititute for Work and Health (2005). Workplace based return to work interventions: a systematic review of the quantitative literature. *Journal of Occupational Rehabilitation*, 15(4), 607–631.

Gibson, L. & Strong, J. (2003). A conceptual framework of functional capacity evaluation for occupational therapy in work rehabilitation. *Australian Occupational Therapy Journal*, 50, 64–71.

Hagedorn, R. (2001). *Foundations for practice in occupational therapy* (3rd ed.). Edinburgh: Churchill Livingstone.

Harpaz, I. & Fu, X. (2002). The structure and meaning of work: A relative stability amidst change. *Human Relations*, 55(6), 639–667.

Hayden, J., van Tulder, M. W., Malmivaara, A. & Koes, B. W. (2005). Exercise therapy for treatment of non-specific low back pain (Cochrane review consumer summary). *Cochrane Database of Systematic Reviews* (3).

Hilde, G., Hagen, G., Jamtvedt, G. & Winnem, M. (2001). Advice to stay active as a single treatment for low back pain and sciatica (Cochrane Review). *The Cochrane Database of Systematic Reviews* (4), Pages Art. No:CD003632. DOI:003610.001002/14651858. CD14003632.

Innes, E. & Straker, L. (1999). Validity of work related assessments. *Work*, 13, 125–152.

Innes, E. & Straker, L. (2002). Workplace assessments and functional capacity evaluations: Current practices of therapists in Australia. *Work*, 18, 51–66.

International Ergonomics Association (IEA). (2000). What is ergonomics? Retrieved May, 2007, from http://www.iea.cc/browse. php?contID=what_is_ergonomics.

International Labor Organisation (ILO) (2002). Managing disability in the workplace. Retrieved 14th March, 2007, from http://laborsta.ilo.org/

ILO (2007). Managing disability in the workplace. Available online: http://laborsta.ilo.org. Accessed 14th March 2007.

Jundt, J. & King, P. M. (1999). Work rehabilitation programs: A 1997 survey. *Work*, 12(2), 139–144.

Keough, J. L. & Fisher, T. F. (2001). Occupational-psychosocial perceptions influencing return to work and functional performance of injured workers. *Work*, 16, 101–110.

Kielhofner, G., Braveman, B., Baron, K., Fisher, G., Hammel, J. & Littleton, M. (1999). The model of human occupation: Understanding the worker who is injured or disabled. *Work*, 12, 37–45.

Kirsh, B. & McKee, P. (2003). The needs and experience of injured workers: A participatory research study. *Work*, 21, 221–231.

Krause, N., Dasinger, L.K. & Neuhauser, F. (1998). Modified work and return to work: A review of the literature. *Journal of Occupational Rehabilitation*, 8(2), 113–139.

Law, M. (2005). *All about outcomes: an educational program to help you understand, evaluate, and choose adult outcome measures* (2nd ed.). Thorofare: Slack Inc.

Loisel, P., Durand, M., Diallo, B., Vachon, B., Charpentier, N. &

Labelle, J. (2003). From evidence to community practice in work rehabilitation: The Quebec experience. *The Clinical Journal of Pain*, 19, 105–113.

Maher, C., Latimer, J. & Refshauge, K. (1999). Prescription of activity for low back pain: What works? A systematic review. *Australian Journal of Physiotherapy*, 45(2), 121–132.

National Center for O*NET Development (2007). *O*NET OnLine*. Retrieved May 2nd, 2007, from http://online.onetcenter.org/find/.

National Occupational Health and Safety Commission (NOHSC) (1995). *Guidance Note for Best Practice Rehabilitation Management of Occupational Injuries and Disease*. Retrieved March 23, 2007, from http://www.ascc.gov.au/NR/rdonlyres/9E42BB45-FD0D-474B-8DDA-3D30239C66D0/0/BestPracticeRehabilitation Management.pdf.

O'Halloran, D. & Innes, E. (2005). Understanding work in society. In: G. Whiteford & W.-S. Clair (Eds.) *Occupation & Practice in Context*. Sydney: Elsevier.

Russo, D. & Innes, E. (2002). An organisational case study of the case manager's role in a client's return-to-work programme in Australia. *Occupational Therapy International*, 9(1), 57–75.

Sager, L. & James, C. (2005). Injured workers perspectives of their rehabilitation process under the New South Wales workers compensation system. *Australian Occupational Therapy Journal* 52, 127–135.

Sandqvist, J. L. & Henriksson, C. M. (2004). Work functioning: A conceptual framework. *Work*, 23, 147–157.

Schonstein, E. & Kenny, D. T. (2001). The value of functional and work place assessment in achieving a timely return to work for workers with back pain. *Work*, 16, 31–38.

Shaw, L. & Lysaght, R. (2008). Cognitive and behavioral demands of work. In: K. Jacobs (Ed.) *Ergonomics for therapists*. Missouri: Mosby Elsevier.

Snook, S. (1998). Self-care guidelines for the management of nonspecific low

back pain. *Journal of Occupational Rehabilitation*, 14(4), 243–253.

Szymanski, E. & Parker, R. (Eds.). (2003). *Work and disability* (2nd ed.). Austin, Texas: Pro-ed.

United Nations (2007). *Convention on the rights of persons with disabilities*. Retrieved 30th April, 2007, from http://www.un.org/disabilities/convention/conventionfull.shtml.

Westmorland, M. G., Williams, R., Strong, S. & Arnold, E. (2002). Perspectives on work (re) entry for persons with disabilities: Implications for clinicians. *Work*, 18, 29–40.

Westmorland, M. G., Williams, R, Amick, B., Shannon, H. & Rasheed, F. (2005). Disability management practices in Ontario workplaces: Employees' perceptions. *Disability and Rehabilitation*, 27(14), 825–835.

Williams, R. & Westmorland, M. (2002). Perspectives on workplace disability management: A review of the literature. *Work*, 19, 87–93.

WorkCover NSW (2000). *Workplace assessment*. Retrieved June 2, 2008, from http://www.workcover.nsw.gov.au/NR/rdonlyres/F7F41C21-02AE-47BE-9811-9A66F1E13A07/0/guide_or03_4130.pdf.

Workplace Health and Safety, Queensland Government (1999). *Manual Tasks Advisory Standard 2000*. Retrieved February 8, 2005, from http://www.whs.qld.gov.au/advisory/adv028.pdf.

World Health Organisation (2002). *Towards a common language for functioning, disability and health: ICF*. Retrieved Feb 15, 2007, from http://www3.who.int/icf/beginners/bg.pdf.

Young, A. E., Roessler, R.T., Wasiak, R., McPherson, K.M., van Poppel, M.N. & Anema, J.R. (2005). A developmental conceptualization of return to work. *Journal of Occupational Rehabilitation*, 15(4), 557–568.

Young, A. E., Wasiak, R., Roessler, R. T., McPerson, K. M., Anema, J. R. & van Poppel, M. N. (2005). Return to work outcomes following work disability: stakeholder motivations, interests and concerns. *Journal of Occupational Rehabilitation*, 15(4), 543–556.

Chapter Twenty-Eight

28

Home modification: occupation as the basis for an effective practice

Catherine Bridge

CHAPTER CONTENTS

Introduction 410

Home as a design product for purchase
or rental 410

Home affordability and home-modification
funding. 411

Home as an emotional place 412

Legislation relevant to home-modification
practice 413

Occupational basis for modification
reasoning 414

Occupational basis for modification
knowledge. 415

Home-modification assessment 416

Home visiting and clarity of assessment
purpose 417

Home-modification intervention 420

Communication skills in home-modification
practice 423

Modification recommendations. 426

Conclusion. 427

SUMMARY

This chapter explores the importance of home
modifications for people with occupational
performance difficulties, and ways in which
housing interventions can influence occupational
performance, making the conduct of meaningful
activities safer, easier, and less painful. The
house or home that we dwell in can have major
consequences for access to economic and health
resources, social participation, functioning and
well-being. Evidence that supports the
effectiveness of home-modification interventions
is presented and barriers that occupational
therapists need to address for individuals are
explored. Also explored are some of the factors
that need to be considered in regard to deciding
to implement home modifications. Modification
reasoning is explained, and practice scenarios
are used to explore some of the professional
reasoning processes typically employed.

KEY POINTS

- For home modifications to be valued and useful
  for the individuals concerned it is important to
  explore what the home and the objects within it
  mean to each individual, especially to their sense
  of self.
- Understanding and relating an individual's
  occupational performance activities, like
  entering, passing through, listening, viewing, and
  applauding, etc., to home-modification
  intervention is critical in ensuring intervention
  effectiveness.
- The majority of existing housing stock is likely to
  require renovation and modification in order to
  meet the changing requirements of users over
  their lifespan.
- When the existing home design becomes
  problematic for a user, relocating to a new home
  with a more appropriate design may be the
  simplest and most economical option.
- The dimensional information required is
  determined by the nature of the tasks that the
  person wants and/or needs to be able to
  perform and the current environmental fit

between the person and their home environment.

- Access standards and building codes while useful for general guidance cannot account for individual need, as they do not account for individual occupational habits and preferences, and generally assume standardised mobility device usage and/or full upper-limb reach ranges.

Introduction

The term *home modification* is a composite of two words: home and modification. *Home* is a place where a person lives; nevertheless, the concept of home is broader than a physical dwelling as it affords stability, privacy and intimacy in an otherwise hostile universe (Bachelard 1994). Home is central to one's life and thus what it affords or limits impacts on both health and well-being. *Modification* has been defined synonymously with other terms such as adaptation, adjustment, maintenance, reconstruction, remodelling, redesign, and renovation. As a term, it is associated with the process of change and correction, and is generally thought of as time delimited, with clear start and stop points. In other words, for each home-modification occasion the start point is the referral and the stop point is satisfactory sign off of the building work prior to making the final payment to the building contractor.

Home modification is closely associated with the notion of home renovation or remodeling, but can be distinguished on the basis of scale (modifications are typically thought of as less extensive) and purpose. Remodelling is typically lifestyle or activity driven, such as, adding on a rumpus room for growing children, whereas the term modification, implicitly de-emphasises fashion, aesthetic or stylistic concerns that are inherent in the notion of remodelling. More formally, in a programmatic or funding sense the term *home modification* refers to structural changes to a person's home so they can continue to live and move, or be moved, safely. It typically encompasses the fitting of rails, ramps, alarms or other safety and mobility aids (NSW Department of Aging 2007). In some circumstances it may also include bedroom, bathroom and kitchen alterations and additions. Generally, home modification does not include general repairs to the house, but does include explicit changes to improve occupational performance, safety or accessibility.

Occupational concerns within the home are associated with how valued occupations are performed and where issues are evident how corrections and alterations of living spaces might resolve them. Thus, the domain of home modification practice specifically addresses aspects of health, disability, and safety for individuals when valued activities are compromised. Indeed, 'assessment of need and the subsequent provision of equipment and adaptations is the greatest part of an occupational therapist's job' (Maczka 1990, p. ix). The fact that home modifications is core to occupational therapy practice should be unsurprising, as the relationship between people, their housing, and the objects within them, is critical to their sense of safety, efficacy, and well-being (Burridge & Ormandy 1993, Conway 1995, Ineichen 1993, Krieger & Higgins 2002, Lowe 2002, National Housing Federation 1998, Smith & Alexander 1997, Thomson et al 2002, Wilkinson 1999, Young & Mollins 1996). Feeling safe at home increases confidence in performing valued tasks (Rogers et al 1997).

Previous research has established the effectiveness of home modifications for carers, older people, and people with dementia, sensory loss and cognitive problems. While there are a relatively few random control trials, there is a growing body of research evidence that indicates home modification can:

- reduce institutionalisation and promote participation and community inclusion (Iwarsson et al 1998)

- significantly reduce the number of falls in older people (Campbell et al 2005, Cumming et al 1999, Thompson 1996)

- delay performance loss and dependency (Gitlin 2003, Lawton 1977, Wahl & Weisman 2003)

- reduce the overall cost of care by decreasing the risk of injury and hospitalisation or institutionalisation (Gibson et al 2001, Mann et al 1999).

Home as a design product for purchase or rental

Home ownership affords homeowners security of tenure and makes the process of home modification simpler. However, to purchase a home is often out of reach for many, particularly those on low incomes, with or without impairments. Homeowner-occupation levels above 75% are exceeded only by a very small number of countries such as Australia, Portugal, Greece, Iceland, Slovenia, Lithuania and Hungary (Scanlon & Whitehead 2004). While a homeowner is free to choose to make modifications if required, tenants and strata-title[1] holders depend on agreement from the body corporate[2], an owners' corporation or landlord. If permission is received for a tenant to modify a dwelling, it is generally the responsibility of the tenant to organise and pay for it. Further tenants may be required to remove the modifications and make good the dwelling when their tenancy ends. Additionally, the condition or structure of a dwelling may make modification impossible or prohibitively expensive. For instance, structural changes to a bathroom in a high-rise unit could impact the structural stability of the building as a whole.

The reason home modifications are so common for older and disabled persons is the fact that residential housing generally assumes average adult dimensions and reach ranges as a design baseline based on healthy and fit adults (Imrie 1996). As a consequence, inaccessibility in the form of stairs, doors, corridors, bathroom, etc., renders remaining in the community without substantial and costly retrofitting problematic (Stark 2001). Thus, the majority of our housing stock is likely to require renovation and modification in order to meet the requirements of its human occupants and their occupational preferences over time.

Universal design is a recent response to this inertia. Universal design means design for people of all ages and abilities to the greatest extent possible without the need for adaptation or specialised design (Connell et al 1997). Thus, universally designed housing is intended to better cater for the range of physical dimensions and capacities as people move through the life course. Universal housing is designed to improve housing sustainability by increasing durability of the home over the lifespan, hence 'lifetime housing', 'barrier-free', 'accessible', 'visitable' or 'adaptable' home designs are other terms often used interchangeably to mean much the same thing,

albeit with narrower or broader inclusions as the case might be.

When the fit between the person and their home becomes problematic, relocating to a new home with a more appropriate design may be the simplest and most economical option (Jung et al 2008). However, finding a home that has appropriate design features may be difficult, as humans and their occupations are so diverse it is inevitable that even in the best case modifications will still be required. For instance, a ventilator-dependant person with tetraplegia might require unobstructed clear spaces and facilities unavailable in a visitable or standard universally designed house. Additionally, new housing construction is relatively low. In Australia, for instance, even with high housing demand and reasonable land availability new build has remained relatively stable at only 2–2.5% of the total housing stock (Australian Bureau of Statistics 1998). This means that even if laws such as the 1998 UK Home Visitability legislation (Imrie 2003, Milner & Madigan 2001) were to be introduced, the majority of housing stock will remain inaccessible. In time, however, there should be greater choice with many more homes having the potential to be easily and more cheaply modified.

Home affordability and home-modification funding

One of the most constraining factors in housing decision will be a person's financial capability. Better homes and better neighbourhoods are likely to be more expensive due to high demand (Wiseman 1980). As financial concerns are a barrier to home purchase, modification, and maintenance, there are programmes in most countries that support home purchase and/or fund home-modification services. However, the provision of this support varies greatly between counties and even within countries, which highlights the implication of national funding structures on access and equity to both homeownership and to home-modification programmes. For instance, injury-related compensation generally includes home modification costs when needed. Furthermore, individuals may be eligible for home-modification support under a range of programme auspices such as:

- veteran's programmes

- disability services

---

[1] Strata title is a form of ownership devised for multi-level apartment blocks, which have apartments at different levels or 'strata'. Strata title exists in Australia, Canada, Singapore, South Africa, Indonesia, Malaysia, Fiji and the Philippines.

[2] In Australia, the term 'body corporate' refers to a home owners' association charged with the administration of one or more housing units. Owners pay a monthly fee to provide for common maintenance and help cover future repair.

- community housing co-operatives
- social housing programmes
- Aging in Place initiatives, etc.

Financial assistance for private home modifications can also be applied for through local charity and community service groups, such as the Multiple Sclerosis Society, Lions, Apex and Rotary, etc. Unfortunately, many potential consumers are unaware of available funding programmes. In Australia, as in many countries, there is a general lack of 'help lines' or cross-service information outlining loan schemes and other funding sources, and their associated eligibility criteria, which typically vary from region to region and in some cases are quite varied and numerous.

Home as an emotional place

Choosing a home, as already suggested, has pragmatic and financial ramifications, but, in addition, it can be an important spiritual and emotional place. Understanding and valuing people's emotional attachments to physical environments and the objects within them is critical in understanding individuals themselves and their place in the world (Hocking 1997). For home modifications to be valued and useful for each individual it is important to explore what the home and the objects within it mean to each person and their sense of self. For instance, a home fulfils many needs for people who reside within them, including a place of self-expression, a vessel of memories and a place of refuge from the outside world (Marcus-Cooper 1997).

Home-modification service providers typically place the highest priority on performance outcomes, but failure to factor in meaning and personalisation of the spaces and the objects within them may lead people to reject home-modification interventions (Bridge 1999, Clemson et al 1999a). Failure to explore the significance of objects and home itself to the occupiers is a failure to address the personalisation of space. Indeed, personal objects evoke memories of people and places in the past and in so doing make us feel connected and rooted.

A systematic review of the literature on barriers to home modifications indicated that the most commonly mentioned were psychological (i.e. concern about stigma, lack of social support, perception of them not being needed or denial of disability) and practical (i.e., cost, aesthetics/desirability, lack of

secure tenure, lack of home-modification knowledge) (Bridge et al 2008). Further, there is some evidence that persons who are depressed and/or cognitively impaired are less likely to value environmental changes (Mann et al 1996).

The prevalence of psychological resistance to home-modification interventions highlights the need to properly address emotional and psychological factors. This is especially so as 30% of those participants sampled about their attitudes to home modifications and who may have benefited from home modification had some form of cognitive impairment, either alone or with a physical impairment of some sort (Bridge et al 2008). Further, Wylde (1998) found that general home-modification knowledge and acceptance of the formal service system was a better predictor of home-modification uptake than were the demographics associated with measurement of performance capacity. Clemson et al (1999) identified a number of factors that emerged from in-depth interviews on decision-making outcomes including:

- knowledge of environmental risks
- having an injury history
- personal perspective (i.e. preventative versus immediate functional outcome)
- acceptance of risk
- attachment to objects (i.e. symbolic meaning and vessel of memories)
- exploration of alternatives
- valuing the recommended change
- feasibility (i.e. ability and opportunity) for change
- beliefs (i.e. that risk could be effectively averted via behavioural change alone)
- degree of perceived personal freedom in decision-making affecting the home.

They went on to conclude that the need for 'ownership of ideas and exerting control within the context of an individual's environment' was critical to 'successfully addressing barriers to environmental change' (p. 9). Hence, educational efforts, related to home-modification services, need to meet the consumer on his terms and in his preferred language. Thus, time spent in education and/or in identifying an individual's personal risk perceptions and beliefs is central to ensuring effective home-modification outcomes.

Legislation relevant to home-modification practice

Occupational therapists, who work in the area of home modifications, must have knowledge of basic accessibility guidelines, local and national building codes, and other relevant legislation (i.e. negligence, product liability, trespass, etc.) (Lamport 1993). This is because, when planning to modify a home, it must be compliant with all necessary building codes, standards and regulations. Environmental legislation and regulations need to be checked (Bridge & Kendig 2005), especially as zoning laws and/or development legislation may directly impact on home modification options. Generally, building codes stipulate the minimum necessary standards (e.g. health, safety, amenity, and sustainability of the buildings), while accessibility standards provide guidance on aspects of physical accessibility relevant to design outcomes.

The degree to which legislation is implemented depends on national and local governments and involves consumers and access consultants. However, the degree to which accessibility standards are implemented depends on whether they are called up in legislation or regulation (Bridge & Simoff 2000). Nearly all countries have disability standards. In the United States the Americans with Disabilities Act and the Fair Housing laws have worked to provide more adaptable and accessible public and private dwellings (Watson 1990). This has been echoed more recently and forcefully in the UK which became the first nation in the world to mandate basic disability access in every new home by passing the Visitable Homes Act in 1998 (Stewart 1999). This Act requires that every new home must have an entrance without steps, a downstairs bathroom, sufficiently wide halls, all doorways passable by wheelchairs, and other elements of universal design. Standards are typically written by expert committees set up and supported by government. They are under continuous review, being updated regularly to take account of changing technology, industry practices, and community expectations.

In addition to laws and regulations governing construction, most countries now have rights-based disability discrimination legislation that covers access to premises. While legislation varies from country to country and region to region, there are typically a number of requirements, which apply everywhere.

Table 28.1 Hierarchy of building administration control

Concept	Explanation
What (constitutes building)	The regional *Building Act* (maybe incorporated into a Development Planning Act) regulates all new building and renovating existing buildings
Who (may undertake building)	Any *Building Licensing Act* controls licensing of builders and allied trades
Where and when (accessibility is required)	The relevant *Building Act* sets out 'where and when' any national accessibility provisions must be considered
Way (modification is provided)	This sets out the process for compliance with *Building Acts*, i.e. deemed to satisfy compliances with dimensional minima in codes/ standards or performance appraisal
Why (modification must be provided)	The relevant *Disability Discrimination Act* can be used to ensure that tenants and those in less secure housing are not discriminated against

Table 28.1 summarises the hierarchy of legislation and its relevance to modification outcomes.

It is important to understand that most access standards are concerned with public buildings, so are typically not mandatory for design or modification to private homes. However, access standards do provide guidance as to the features that need to be considered in a residential setting, as they set out the minimum dimensions for circulation spaces and provide dimensional minimum for the placement of structures, fittings and fixings. The underlying assumption in their development being that attention to wheelchair footprints (i.e. the amount of vertical and horizontal space occupied by a standard wheelchair) and wheelchair frame flexibility will benefit all. Access standards are continually reviewed and as part of this review process there is ongoing pressure to include a greater range of disability concerns and environmental settings.

Public access standards while useful for general guidance cannot account for individual need as they do not account for users' transfer preferences and generally assume full upper-limb reach ranges. In addition it is important to be aware when reading access standards that design solutions are often the result of compromises resulting from requirement conflicts. A requirement conflict occurs when a standard solution for one type of impairment does not work for another type. For instance, elimination of kerbs and/or edges to improve wheelchair circulation may pose hazards for individuals with severe vision loss unless additional tactile or auditory orientation cues are provided. This is because while a kerb poses a barrier to wheeled mobility it provides a mobility cue for those with visual loss. Thus the addition of tactile ground indicators in conjunction with a kerb ramp is the preferred public-access solution. Another well-known design conflict is between those with ambulatory impairments and wheelchair users. Ambulatory users (i.e. those individuals who prefer to walk) generally prefer a situation in which they can support themselves using their upper limbs and too large an unobstructed circulation space without rails may leave them more vulnerable to falls.

Occupational basis for modification reasoning

A number of professions including architecture, environmental psychology, and environmental gerontology have a stake in home-modification knowledge, and thus contribute to our understandings and thinking about home-modification problems. Design is what is taught in architectural education and builds from a set of idealised specifications towards specific construction goals that result in a particular form and structure. However, 'design' per se, apart from not being a skill belonging in an entry-level occupational therapy curriculum, is not what is required in home-modification practice.

Home-modification reasoning unlike design reasoning commences with a home that already exists so already has a particular form and function. All homes are composed of a set of building components and the process of home modification, therefore, involves repositioning, replacing, and/or adding components in order to resolve a particular person–environment mismatch. For instance, modification of a shower-hob commences with the evaluation of an existing product. This means that in order to modify the shower-hob it needs to be understood in terms of its design function (i.e. water containment) and structures (i.e. height, width, etc.). Further, this needs to be assessed from the perspective of a particular set of valued activity patterns belonging to a

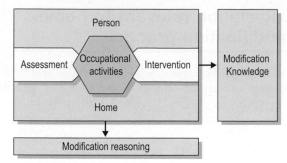

Figure 28.1 • Home modification reasoning

particular individual or set of individuals. Hence, the focus is not just a particular shower area or a particular health condition, instead both *person-* and *home*-based *modification knowledge* is integrated via knowledge of relevant *occupationally based activities*.

Of equal importance to modification knowledge in assessment and intervention are the *reasoning abilities* of modification practitioners. In *modification reasoning* the most crucial but difficult areas are *assessment* and *intervention*. Figure 28.1 illustrates these two stages and indicates how they relate to modification problems. Both the terms assessment and intervention relate to a practitioner's interactions and reflections on what they observe. Both terms are interrelated and, although presented in a linear form, in real everyday reasoning, follow so fast on each other that they are difficult to separate. Assessment is an active process that requires selective attention and assists human reasoners to make sense of complex and sometimes contradictory data. The development of the ability to *notice* and attend to *cues* appropriately in the home-modification scenario is crucial in learning discrimination. In intervention, the focus shifts to overt action in extending and testing understanding. Observing and/or measuring humans and their physical environment in terms of features and their component attributes provide the data needed for occupationally successful outcomes.

Occupational reasoning means that the shower-hob's water-containment structures need to be evaluated in terms of their location, height, surface and shape; not because of form or aesthetics, but because of anticipated or real changes in user requirements (i.e. a user's difficulty with walking, stepping and/or balance). Thus, evaluation of a building problem from a home-modification perspective judges the qualities of all relevant components by their features relative to the intervention goal. Modification may be motivated by desire to improve safety by reducing or eliminating the building components that require good dynamic balance. Following the assessment phase, a number of modification alternatives may be considered. For instance, alternatives that may be considered may include removal of the shower hob or a ramp with a shower floor in-fill.

However, consideration of alternatives requires a wider analysis. In the case of the shower-hob replacement this would involve consideration of the impact on available circulation space, existing wall support structures and existing floor treatments. Thus, modification reasoning requires movement from a specific building component out to its wider contextual situation. This enables a better understanding of the dependencies and interrelationships between components. Consideration of the wider implications allows a better understanding of the problem and makes possible a more explicit statement of modification goals. The feasibility of modification as an activity depends on being able to evaluate and appropriately communicate the extent and scope of the changes required. For instance, as mentioned previously, there will be situations where deciding to relocate may be the best option.

Occupational basis for modification knowledge

Occupational therapy knowledge is used to design interventions to remediate and/or compensate for the physical, psychological, and social impact of impairments. Home assessment relies on trained observation and current practice is predominantly assessment by interview and observation. Indeed, observations of activity or task performance are the norm for measuring accessibility and usability, and are generally attributed a high level of face validity (Steinfeld & Danford 1999). Nevertheless, skilled observation of the person and/or the environment in regard to the person–environment fit is extremely complex, as many factors need to be noted, related and evaluated. For instance, when considering the location of a fitting as simple as a rail to assist independence in transferring on and off the toilet, an experienced occupational therapist typically consid-

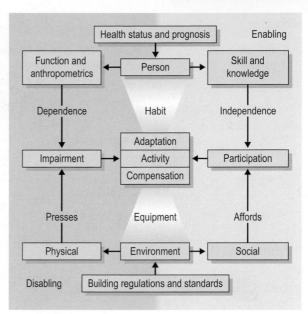

Figure 28.2 • Activity centric dynamic between the person and the environment (Bridge 2005)

ers at least 13 variables and their relationships to each other (see Table 28.2).

A framework for associating personal attributes and environmental attributes is illustrated in Figure 28.2; this illustration places occupations at the doing or *activity* level at its centre because it is the set of actions performed by a person (the minutiae of occupational performance) that set-off the dynamic nature of person–environment fit. For instance, it is activities like entering, passing through, listening, viewing, and applauding, etc., which underpin occupational performance and in conjunction with the presence of impairment determine the level of independent participation. Individuals carrying out occupations have a human body with particular performance potentials and human measurements (i.e. anthropometrics) in conjunction with socially acquired activity-relevant skill and knowledge. An individual's ability to perform is shaped, on the one hand, by their health status and their performance of preferred habit/routines; while on the other hand, an environmental setting shapes the occupations afforded by defining the activity spaces and the equipment available. It is the interaction between individuals and their environmental setting that enables the development, practice and fulfilment of personally valued activities (Schkade & McClung 2001).

Table 28.2 Complexity of decisions associated with toilet rail placement

Toilet grab rail attributes	Number and type of typical values to be considered	Relationship to person attributes
Length (end to end)	Minimum length is 300 mm and increments are usually in 150 mm units	Person's height and height of any co-habitants, persons ability to flex and extend hips and knees and consistency of this ability
Profile	Circular, square, oval	Person's hand size, degree of muscle tone and dynamic grip strength
Diameter	Minimum is 20 mm but can go up to 50 mm	Person's hand size, degree of muscle tone and dynamic grip strength
Shape	Straight, angled, curved	Number of persons utilising a grab rail and their ability to shift centre of balance in a normal sit-to-stand manoeuvre
Location of fixings	Wall, ceiling, floor	Person's upper-limb segment length and preferred transfer procedure
Distance from pan to proximal projection point	Can vary widely	Person's arm segment length
Distance from floor to distal projection point	Can vary widely	Person's height and limb segment lengths
Material	Wood, plastic, galvanised iron, chrome, aluminium, brass	Person's ability to exert dynamic grasp, torso and upper-limb muscle strength and the possibility of contact with water
Fixings	Screws, loxins, dynabolt	Persons weight, wall fabric
Surface texture	Degree of slip resistance	Possibility of contact with water, excessive sweating in hands or contaminants such as soap
Angle of insertion	Vertical, horizontal, variety of angles in between	Number and height of all users utilising the same rail, person's stated transfer method
Projection from wall surface	Can vary, minimum is considered to be 25 mm	Size of hand and chance of arm becoming entrapped should a slip occur
Obstructions and protrusions that might prevent usage	Pipes, wires, toilet roll holders	Ability of an individual to gain grip purchase

Home-modification assessment

Home-modification assessment requires considerable skill and knowledge (Barnes 1991). Occupational therapy education is designed to assist occupational therapists to assess performance abilities and risks associated with carrying out meaningful occupations (i.e. self-carer, homemaker, handyman, etc.), activities (i.e. toileting, bathing, etc.) and tasks (i.e. getting up/down from a seated position, opening a door, carrying hot liquid, etc.).

According to Cooper et al (1991), the knowledge and skills that occupational therapists acquire from their entry-level education that equips them to effectively determine the fit between individuals and their home environments include:

- a health care perspective
- assessment of performance
- knowledge of modification interventions and assistive technology
- knowledge of specific diseases and disability
- knowledge of life span development.

Experienced occupational therapists can usually quickly identify competing explanations from observations and can thus provide the most appropriate interventions. For example, difficulty in moving from sitting to standing could be due to one or all of the following: stiff joints, poor endurance, unsuitable footwear, or slippery/unstable surfaces. Therefore, being able to identify what to measure and being confident about the reliability and accuracy of measurements is essential in communicating and defending decisions and producing best practice outcomes. Additionally, occupational therapists are expected to be knowledgeable about the different types of equipment that will allow a person to live safely and independently (Davis & Sterling 1993).

However, while some agreement about basic skill and knowledge exists, all entry-level courses differ slightly and good home-modification assessment outcomes depend on consistency and reliability of observations. Therefore, in order to try to ensure more common outcomes for individuals seeking home-modification assistance, practitioners are typically encouraged to select and apply a range of standardised assessment tools or *attention-directing* observational frameworks. Using a standardised assessment can improve an occupational therapist's ability to observe, communicate and document home-modification problems. Having a formal set of attributes to observe or check-off facilitates need identification and assists practitioners to sift through data in order to better identify and prioritise the key issues.

Problem definitions are crucial to human observations. For instance, the identification of *hazards* requires clarity about what a hazard is, and reflection on what might be considered hazardous under what circumstances, etc. For instance, poor night lighting in pathways to toilets or difficulty responding to a telephone call is commonly associated with falls in the elderly (Clemson 1997). The point is that in order to accurately assess a construct-like *hazard* one has to be knowledgeable about what constitutes hazards and be able to clearly identify them in a uniform manner. Unfortunately, few therapists have the time to measure everything in the home and about the person, so it is critical to know what to measure and when to do so.

Table 28.3 overviews the four most researched and commonly applied home-modification assessment tools which include the SAFER (Oliver et al 1993), Westmead Home Safety Inventory (Clemson 1997, Clemson et al 1992, 1996, 1999, HOMEFAST

(Mackenzie 2002) and the 'Home Enabler' (Iwarsson & Slaug 2001, Iwarsson & Isacsson 1993, Iwarsson et al 1998). However, these tools vary significantly in purpose, comprehensiveness of coverage and theoretical basis. Thus, each tool has particular strengths and weaknesses. While standardised home assessment tools all provide forms that are clearly set out and of comparable time to use, there are some fundamental differences regarding the population being assessed, scoring type, features highlighted and stated purpose across the tools reviewed.

Home visiting and clarity of assessment purpose

In order to use time most efficiently it is essential that there is clarity about the intended purpose of your home visit. This is particularly so, as arrangements must be made in advance regarding personnel, equipment and transportation, so the actual home visit runs as smoothly as possible. Unfortunately, it is not always possible to predict what you will encounter while home visiting, so ensuring that you have emergency procedures and plans in place prior to the visit is also essential. In planning for your visit you need to:

- contact the person and any relevant others to ensure coordination

- decide what to take and ensure it is in working order and available

- get yourself, your equipment and if necessary the person to the home address

- ensure that you are covered for all contingencies (i.e. insurance, accidents and emergencies).

Being clear about the purpose of assessment is critical as how the problem is framed determines what aspects of the environment and the person need to be observed and/or measured. Defining significant dimensional information is determined by the nature of the tasks that the person wants/needs to be able to perform and the current environmental fit between the person and their home environment. For instance, as illustrated in Table 28.4, the purpose of the assessment defines what is considered problematic and indicates what aspects of the person and the home needs to be observed and/or measured.

Anthropometry (or person-related data) concerns the study of the range of human physical dimensions: such as height, weight, reach, range, and

Table 28.3 Summary of four standardised home assessment tools

SAFER	Westmead Home Safety Inventory	HOMEFAST	Home Enabler
Stated purpose			
Home assessment by occupational therapists	Home hazard identification by occupational therapists	Home hazard utility screening of older people	Home accessibility assessment by occupational therapists, and as a social participation and planning tool
Number of items			
97 items in total	56 items in total. Summary form also available for experienced practitioners	25 items in total	198 items in full version (also shorter version possible). Four parts, outdoor environment, entrances, indoor environment and communication
Theoretical basis			
Based on IADL categorisation (i.e. mobility, medication, etc.) with inclusion of aspects of living situation (trip hazards) and fire hazards. Little or no theoretical base and associated issues with content and construct validity	Limited to housing environmental data associated with falls and successful fall-related interventions	Includes data about function and environment. Little or no theoretical base and associated issues with content and construct validity	Includes data about functional limitations and environment. Based on the enabler model developed from a 1979 review of the literature on accessibility
Scoring			
Paper-based checklist with triparted scoring, addressed/ not addressed and problem with space for comments. Total score may be summed and compared to 95th and 99th percentile data from Canada	Paper-based checklist with triparted scoring (i.e. hazard/ no hazard and not relevant). Most are based on occupational therapist observation with patient, self-report option being used for lighting alone	Paper-based checklist with primarily dichotomous scoring (i.e. yes/no). However, 13 items have a 'not applicable' option. Scores can be summed, fallers had a higher mean hazard score but this was non-significant	Computer application that creates functional and environmental profiles. Designed to run on a personal computer running Windows. Primarily dichotomous scoring (i.e. yes/no). Computes weighted scores based on linking between functional and environmental profiles
Characteristics of person and the environment identified			
Evolved out of occupational therapy home visit proforma's currently in use in Canada. Concept of person and environment unclear	Evolved out of international environmental review of fall factors. Concept of environment related to environmental settings. Concept of person unclear	Evolved out of NSW Home falls safety checklist. Concept of person and environment unclear	Evolved out of the enabler accessibility matrix and Swedish handicap codes. Concept of person similar to WHO impairment levels. Concept of environment related to environmental settings

Table 28.3 Summary of four standardised home assessment tools—cont'd

SAFER	Westmead Home Safety Inventory	HOMEFAST	Home Enabler
Interaction between person and environment			
Unclear, behaviours implicit with exception of cognitive impairment markers such as wandering	Unclear, scoring is based on environmental hazards. The relationship to diagnosis, mobility, fall history and anthropometric dimensions implicit	Unclear, scoring is based on observation of a combination of environmental factors and human performance in environment factors	Relationships are predetermined and weighted according to observed severity of impairment generally
Relation to home modification			
Manual contains suggestions for modification interventions	Free text space for problem summary and action plan	Allows problem identification but no explicit ink to modification	Problems are summarised across the four sections but no explicit link to modification
Strengths			
• Familiar and commonsensical • No prior training required if used by an occupational therapist • Logical layout • Problem identification linked directly to helpful hints about potential solutions • Evidence of psychometric review particularly in terms of reliability	• Excellent training tool • Comprehensive • Evidence of psychometric review (i.e. attention paid to issues of reliability and validity) • Designed to be used in conjunction with the inventory prompt thus not bulky or difficult to apply	• No prior training required • Evidence of psychometric review of inter-rater reliability and content validity • Good reliability for showering and bathing • Evolved out of NSW Home falls safety checklist • Intended for rural application • Designed for speed of administration	• Having two separate profiles increases flexibility allowing one functional profile to be compared across several environmental profiles and vice versa • Evidence of psychometric review including content and external validity based on Swedish handicap codes. Inter-rater reliability good • Predictive environmental score is based on presence and severity of functional impairments
Weaknesses			
• Limited information on sample sizes, selection methods and population demographics • No cautions or limitations listed • Summary score based on ordinal level data • Insufficient space to record recommendations	• Takes considerable time to process manual and integrate concepts • Some aspects not always valid for the environment of concern • No detail provided about potential solutions • Insufficient space to record recommendations	• Reliability assessed with occupational therapists, occupational therapy assistants and a social worker • Significant reliability difference with expertise • Poor reliability for outdoor paths	• Does not address hazards per se (i.e. omits smoke detectors and fire egress) • Requires education and training to apply appropriately • Consensus about functional limitations and degree of dependency on equipment unstable

Table 28.4 The nature of the occupational activity being assessed determines the characteristics of the home and person that need to be measured

Purpose of assessment	Person	Home
To assess transfer hazards (i.e. inability to move from lying to sitting unassisted)	Bed transfer performance Head height Weight	Type and size of bed Bed height Area of unobstructed circulation space in bedroom Circulation space around and under bed Condition of ceilings
To assess most appropriate wheeled mobility aid for home use (i.e. hoist assessment)	Dynamic balance performance Seat width Seat height Seated eye height Seated range of movement Weight	Changes in level Height and width of steps/stairs Width of corridors Width of doorways Obstructions to circulation space Loose rugs/mats Position of power points Type and height of storage Type and height of windows
To assess usability of shelving (i.e. inability to hang clothes)	Reach range (active range of movement) Hand function Muscle strength	Toe clearance Shelving height Shelving depth Position in relation to other fixtures (net unobstructed area surrounding opening) Method of opening (i.e. door type, direction of swing, type of latch, etc.)

the circulation space needs of humans. Person-related data assist in informed decision-making that will optimise the best fit between humans and their physical environments. Unfortunately, anthropometry is not an exact science; it uses bony landmarks and is complicated by the fact that body size varies with age, sex, race, socio-economics (nutrition), and even occupational choice (i.e. policemen and fireman tend to be both larger and stronger than average). Other variables include whether data are recorded with shoes on or off and, in the case of people with mobility aids, the height of the wheelchair seat is crucial in determining such things as reach range.

Human body dimensions that impact on the physical environment are of two basic types (Panero & Zelnik 1979):

1. Structural – these are measurements of height, weight and body segments in static positions.

2. Performance – these are measurements associated with dynamic tasks, such as reach ranges, and are much more difficult to obtain accurately (partly because of the body's wobbly bits and partly because these are no universally agreed protocols for this sort of measurement).

Anthropometric data are often presented in graphic form as in the 'Human Scale' charts (Diffrient et al 1990) and in the 'Designing for the Disabled' anthropometric diagrams used by Goldsmith (1984). When anthropometric charts are unsuitable, calculation of individual data for each person is needed. The selections of both anthropometric and environmental measurements that need to be gathered are based on the nature of the particular task characteristics under consideration. What may be optimal for a particular individual may not be for others in the same physical environment and compromises or adjustability of objects will need to be factored in. If this is so, you need to determine whose and/or what dimensions are most critical and be able to rationalise your position.

Home-modification intervention

Occupational knowledge is used to design interventions to remediate or compensate for the physical, psychological, and social aspects of impairments.

Home modification requires considerable skill and knowledge, and entry-level occupational therapy training is designed to assist occupational therapists to assess performance abilities and risks associated with carrying out meaningful occupations (i.e. self carer, homemaker, handyman, etc.), activities (i.e. toileting, bathing, etc.) and tasks (i.e. getting up/down from a seated position, opening a door, carrying hot liquid, etc.).

Differences in human shapes and abilities, in combination with physical, social and cultural environments, mean that many, if not all, built environments require modification to meet their users' activity needs over their lifespan. Housing that can accommodate changes in people's capacities over the lifespan can enable them to live and remain in their homes as long as possible. Housing design features, such as ramps and handrails, can facilitate independence in daily living. Understanding human performance in a range of occupational contexts is something that as a profession we pride ourselves on, particularly from the standpoint of impairment and the variability of human ability. But consideration of human ability has not been the prime organising principle of either homes (as mentioned previously) or product design (i.e. furniture, fittings and tools of daily life). As a result much of what is currently available in the form of intervention solutions (often sold as assistive devices), has been created for small niche markets and, therefore, may not come in a range of colours or styles. Indeed, they often look unattractive or, even worse, carry connotations of hospitals, institutions or disability, so are likely to confront the potential user with their disability status.

Further, knowledge concerning human abilities in the context of particular residential environments derives from phenomena that are inherently complex and dynamically indivisible. Thus, no generalisable stock solution exists for the full range of individual, geographic, and cultural phenomena that shape housing need, instead what constitutes a good solution must be interpreted in context (Harrison & Parker 1998). Worse, Stark (2001) laments the fact that much previous home-modification research effort has been confined to enumeration and quantification of existing environmental barriers, which is fine for establishing change in performance, but fails to shed light on individual occupational patterns, particularly those that include multiple intervention strategies (home modification, assistive devices, and care support).

All intervention solutions have certain dimensional specifications that make them more or less suitable. Thus, despite using standardised assessment tools, it is critical to fully assess and document a particular situation as measurements of the person (i.e. their height, weight, reach range, etc.) and their home environment (i.e. height of steps, unobstructed circulation space, etc.) will be needed. For instance, failure to specify the start and stop point of a rail can impact costs and can delay modifications being contracted. In the worse-case scenario it may lead to damage to property or inappropriate modifications, both of which have legal implications in the form of product liability and negligence. Therefore, the occupational therapist must be careful not to make assumptions about these factors, leading to incorrect interventions. Practice Scenario 28.1 illustrates the importance of considering fully the user's activities and bodily structures before recommending intervention solutions.

Practice Scenario 28.1
Considering the person's activities and bodily structures during home modifications: A salutary lesson

Jack a 55-year-old medically retired accountant returned home from hospital after an acute episode of multiple sclerosis. While in hospital and prior to discharge an occupational therapy assessment was requested as Jack reported that he lived alone in his own home and that he was having trouble managing his showering independently due to experiencing dynamic balance problems and muscle weakness. In Jack's file his therapist noted that there was 'no history of recent falls' and she recommended replacement of Jack's existing towel rails and replacement with a 'modular rail' in a colour designed to blend with the bathroom décor. Following the occupational therapy assessment, the rail was installed by the local home modification service. Unfortunately, several weeks later, Jack was having more difficulty than normal when he lost his balance and started to fall, he already had his hand on the rail, but as his feet slipped out from under him his arm slipped under the rail effectively entrapping his upper arm. Jack was too weak and in too much pain to free himself and so the rail suspended him for 10 hours prior to his readmission to emergency care with resultant severe shoulder injuries further hampering his ability to care for himself at home.

For the occupational therapist concerned to avoid a charge of negligence, what should they have done differently? This requires a more careful look at Jack's story and, while the notes do not clarify the particulars of the modular rail prescribed, it would have most likely complied with the relevant national standards, which specify the clearance between the rail and the adjacent wall surface (Standards Australia 1998). Fabrication or manufacture of products such as the rail to standards is intended to ensure that the rail will enable a power grip (Oram et al 2006). Thus, we have to infer that Jack must have had substantial wasting of his upper limb muscles and may, in addition, have been of a slight build prior to the onset of any impairment. However, we only know this in hindsight, as the occupational therapist concerned made no mention anywhere in Jack's case files of this being noted or of any measurements of Jack's body being made.

Best intervention practice is always based on anthropometrics (e.g. human measurements) and observation of actual activities (e.g. Jack's grasp and rail usage) possibly with a temporary clamp-on or suction rail. The therapist concerned should have presented an alternative non-standard solution with an appropriate rationale based on these observations. Unfortunately, a non-standard solution would have required one-off manufacture but might have prevented Jack's injuries and better protected the occupational therapist concerned from a charge of negligence.

In order to accommodate as many people as possible it is important to identify all potential users of a particular space and then to reflect on the critical dimensions which will inform appropriate placement of fixtures and fittings to accommodate their human height, mass, reach, and range dimensions (anthropometrics). It is unusual for occupational therapists to take measurements of things such as ceiling height, unless of course an overhead track hoist or monkey bar suspended from the ceiling are being considered.

Introducing a degree of individual adjustability or adaptability is often the only way large differences in occupational preference and anthropometric dimensions can be accommodated. Where differences in anthropometric dimensions are greater than can be dealt with by adjustability, another solution is to duplicate fittings and locate them in relation to minimum and maximum ranges. Practice Scenario 28.2 further illustrates the modification reasoning

process in moving from assessment to intervention and back again.

Practice Scenario 28.2 Modification reasoning as an iteration between person and home knowledge

Julie is a 44-year-old secondary school mathematics teacher and lives in her own home with her partner of 16 years. Her neurologist referred her for occupational therapy assessment of her personal care tasks following an acute episode of Meniere's disease. A Meniere's episode generally involves severe vertigo (spinning), imbalance, nausea, and vomiting. The average attack lasts from 2 to 4 hours. Following a severe attack most people find that they are exhausted and must sleep for several hours. There is a large amount of variability in the duration of symptoms and Julie had reported a general unsteadiness that worsened when she was feeling tired or stressed.

Prior to meeting with Julie, the occupational therapist reflected on the referral information in order to prepare for the assessment (Table 28.5). This reflective process is structured in order to enable the therapist to plan for the assessment appropriately and to select any tools and/or equipment needed for the home visit. The reflective process steps used are based on the professional reasoning process ideas outlined by Bridge & Twible (1997). During the modification reasoning, additional key words and concepts are added as they occur, to ensure a thorough understanding of the knowledge base required for good assessment and intervention outcomes.

The occupational therapy initial assessment and home-environment analysis included a general assessment of Julie's activities of daily living, with Julie responding to questions posed by the occupational therapist about her daily routine and her perception of her own performance in those tasks. Julie's level of satisfaction with her performance was also discussed. Julie identified a number of areas that she was not satisfied with regarding her performance *post discharge*. These included: ascent and descent of the front steps, preparing a simple meal using the microwave or stove, attending work, toileting (especially at night), and showering.

Julie identified toileting and showering as the tasks that she was most concerned about and wanted the occupational therapist to suggest techniques and/or modifications to improve her performance and safety in these areas. As part of the collaborative process,

Table 28.5 Use of a reflective framework for problem sensing with Julie

Key words	Source and level of knowledge	Related knowledge	Implications for redesign
Meniere's	Medical dictionaries and other specialised texts	Dizziness Poor balance Fatigue	Safety implications should Julie fall during an attack Consider reduced upper limb and lower limb strength when undertaking sit–stand transfers Consider proprioceptive deficits that may impact on mobility
Fatigue	Personal experience and knowledge of normative measurement practices	Physiological and psychological implications Often measured on a uni-dimensional severity scale or via gauge of metabolic work intensity	Performance will fluctuate depending on time of day and recency of last attack
Female perineal hygiene	Knowledge of female anatomy and knowledge of normative cultural practices	Aspects of female perineal hygiene and associated activities Difference in toileting task performance between day and night	Impact of 'straining' on blood pressure/light-headedness

the occupational therapist also recommended that stair safety also be reviewed. Julie was agreeable to this.

An activity analysis of toileting was carried out at both task and skill level (Table 28.6). It was relevant that Julie had suffered a Meniere's attack the day prior to the assessment and was still experiencing follow-on fatigue. She reported she was also feeling stressed and guilty as she had taken 2 days off work and felt she was letting her fellow teachers down. An activity analysis for each area identified by Julie and the occupational therapist was also carried out. From the assessment and analyses the problems listed in Table 28.6 were identified for the task of toileting.

The task assessment, observation, and measurement of Julie and her home environment are needed to test the hypotheses regarding potential interventions. Figure 28.1 highlights where the assessment and intervention meet in the context of Julie's ability and her environment. This model has been used to develop Table 28.7 which illustrates a small sample of the intervention reflection framework employed in Julie's case.

This Practice Scenario has been provided by Lyndal Millikan. At the time of writing she was working with The Centre for Health Assets Australasia, in Sydney, Australia.

The occupational therapist needs to be certain she has thoroughly understood the person in the context of their home environment and has sufficient measurements to communicate the implications of this. Once this occurs the occupational therapist moves on to communicating options to the individual, or individuals, concerned. While the occupational therapist may be responsible for recommending a particular set of options, those people who live with the modifications must make decisions about which modifications will best satisfy their situation and whether to go ahead or not with the modifications.

Communication skills in home-modification practice

There can be a relatively large number of people involved in the home modification, ranging from the person for whom the modification is intended to architects, builders, tradespersons and funders. Thus, good communication is critical to ensure acceptable home-modification outcomes. This is because each stage of the construction process is dependent on particular skills and each contribution must be timed appropriately for the work to proceed smoothly. The size of the job will, to some extent, determine the stakeholders or actors. For instance, installation of a toilet grabrail in the bathroom may only involve the disabled person, the homeowner, the occupational therapist, and a builder. It is the role of the occupational therapist to provide enough

Table 28.6 An activity analysis of toileting

Task	Skill	Performance level	Comment
Toileting – bladder and/or bowel use	Enter toilet	Independent	
	Turn on light (when applicable)	Independent	
	Turn/pivot 180° so Julie is facing away from toilet	Need some help	Uses right hand to stabilise self on wall
	Undo and lower trousers/underpants	Independent	
	Stand to sit	Independent	Uses right hand to stabilise self on wall
	Stabilise self on toilet seat	Independent	Reports that she will lean against the wall on the left side if feels dizzy
	Use toilet	Independent	
	Reach for, unroll and tear off appropriate amount of toilet paper	Independent	
	Manage perineal hygiene	Need some help	Uses left hand to stabilise self on wall
	Prepare clothing for stand	Independent	
	Sit to stand	Independent	
	Re-adjust clothing	Independent	
	Pivot 180° to face toilet	Need some help	Uses right hand to stabilise self on wall
	Flush toilet	Independent	
	Turn/pivot 180° so Julie is facing away from toilet	Independent	
	Turn off light	Independent	

documentation for the builder to make cost estimation and to contract and carry out the work (Bridge 1999).

If your assessment and communications with the person and relevant others reveal that the home is amenable to modification, the occupational therapist will discuss alterations and adaptations with the person. At this stage the person may:

- disagree
- agree and want to organise a family member or friend to complete the work
- agree and contract a builder and/or architect to complete the work
- agree but be unable to self-finance the desired work.

If the person disagrees, the occupational therapist should document the problem, the proposed intervention, rationale for the intervention, potential funding sources and give the person a copy of the report prior to discharge.

Some individuals have a family member or friend who is skilled enough to carry out simple modifications. Other people will need to call in a builder and/or architect to carry out the work. In both of these cases it is the responsibility of the occupational therapist to adequately brief the person who will be carrying out the work. This involves communicating exactly what is proposed and providing enough detail so the work can be carried out satisfactorily. What is required in terms of drawings and specifications will vary depending on whether or not external funding is being sought. Some individuals will not have adequate financial resources to independently undertake large-scale modifications and will, therefore, need to apply for assistance.

In more complex modification works, where walls are being removed or repositioned, new rooms added or new structures created, the number of

Table 28.7 Framework for intervening with Julie

Problem identified	Need	Actual problem	Other considerations
Instability/dizziness during sit-to-stand transfers at toilet increasing risk of falls	To attend to toileting tasks independently	Yes	The toilet is not in the centre of the room; it is closer to the left wall (if seated). A rail would not fit comfortably between Julie and the wall on this side of the room
			The height of the toilet from the finished floor to the top of the seat is 420 mm. Julie states this is a comfortable height for her to stand from and sit to
			Julie's partner also uses this toilet room
Instability/dizziness during overhead reaching activity increasing risk of falls	To independently reach required items such as toilet paper and feminine hygiene products	Yes	There is shelving above the toilet used to store extra toilet paper, feminine hygiene products, air freshener, a few magazines and some ornaments
Instability/dizziness during shower transfers increasing risk of falls	Likelihood of personal injury should Julie fall into the glass or overbalance during the transfer	Yes	Currently using static glass piece of shower screen for support in transfers
Instability/dizziness during showering tasks increasing risk of falls	Likelihood of personal injury should Julie fall into the glass or overbalance during showering tasks	Yes	Currently leans against the wall for support during showering

people involved can increase dramatically. The primary role of an architect is manipulation of form and space in development of a design and then oversight of the construction process or design management (Lawson 1997). An architect typically organises specialist consultants, structural engineers, and draftsmen, and coordinates design documentation and communication with local government authorities and road-traffic authorities, as required. The builder on the other hand is the person usually responsible for costing and actually carrying out building works. They are responsible for coordinating and managing the tradespeople on site on a daily basis. It is this person who books the tradespeople (e.g. plumber, electrician) and who ensures that building supplies and workflow are on time.

Different countries and regions have differing laws and regulations, but it is quite common for a building contract to be required when the cost of works exceeds a set price. When a building contract is required it is typically entered into between the homeowner and the builder based on drawings and specifications that set out the cost and scope of works. The contract is what guarantees a certain quality of product by a certain date and any changes or variations to this contract will both increase cost and the amount of time taken. It is, therefore, critical that the occupational therapy drawings and documentation are included in the building contract as this is the only tool that can ensure that they are appropriately considered.

Therefore, it is critical that all design documentation and understandings be based on sound communication between all those involved. It is essential that documentation and verbal communication are sufficient to ensure an appropriate cost and time estimate that will lead to the desired end product. If design documentation is sound, but something goes wrong in the construction process, it will be rectified at the builder's expense. Most stakeholders or actors from the building and construction world have had little or no experience with impairment; what they are most familiar with is in the form of standards and codes. In building and construction like any complex activity there are a range of assumptions that underpin the design and construction process. Inappropriate assumptions can, unfortunately, lead to significant problems if

KEY POINTS

- Universal design is based on the premise that it is possible to design products, buildings and exterior spaces to be usable by all and hence facilitate the social integration of all people, regardless of size, age, or any condition affecting sight, hearing, cognition, or physical ability.

- Universal design can be applied to housing, transportation, places of employment, education, and parks and recreation facilities to maximise the number of people who can do things independently in a particular environment.

- There are seven principles of universal design: equitable use, flexibility in use, simple and intuitive use, perceptible information, tolerance for error, low physical effort, and size and space for approach and use.

- Within the home, entrances, kitchens, and bathrooms are considered the most critical areas in which principles of universal design could be applied.

- The universal design approach to solution development applied in the home environment can be extended into the workplace to support the needs and desires of people wishing to remain active and independent regardless of age, physical or sensory circumstance.

- Occupational therapists can play a major role in environmental adaptation resulting in the person being more independent and in control.

Introduction[1]

The recent development of the design concept *universal design* is gaining worldwide recognition and offers significant benefit to the occupational therapy profession. Universal design is a broad conceptual revision to traditional design practice where much of the environment and products contained therein were designed to the specifications of an 'average male' in the prime of life. A new paradigm has emerged that suggests it is possible to design products, buildings and exterior spaces to be usable by all, but acknowledging that in specific cases some

people will still need specialised accommodations. The ultimate goal of universal design is the social integration of all people, regardless of size, age, or any condition affecting sight, hearing, cognition, or physical ability. A related concept is found in the United Kingdom, known as *inclusive design* with a similar goal and framework.

The ultimate goal of universal design becomes more and more relevant for all as it is recognised that as people go through life some will acquire a change in abilities as a result of accident or illness, while others experience similar changes as part of the aging process. Globally, the vast numbers of people reaching retirement age, people remaining in the workforce longer, and people with and without impairment now living well into their 70s and beyond, suggests a strong market for supportive and *age-friendly environments*. Public policy research indicates that governments are beginning to implement policies to support the delivery of health care in community settings in order to reduce spending on hospital and nursing home care. As most people prefer to avoid institutional living, wishing instead to remain in their homes or age in place, there will be an increasing demand for *in-home services*, including the services of occupational therapists.

Universal design should be the leading premise driving all new building and product design since the environment can be either a powerful barrier to or a facilitator of equal opportunities for people with unique abilities. Additionally, it is now recognised that incorporating the needs of a range of human conditions creates better design for the population at large.

This chapter focuses on how universal design can be incorporated into housing and product selection, specifically addressing key elements and features that provide the greatest usability. Design features and suggestions are illustrated that can be used to meet the needs of a specific individual, while at the same time create an environment comfortable for other family members. When universal features are well integrated, they are invisible. A feature may provide a base line of accessibility for a person with an impairment but be designed in such a way as to provide a more universal outcome for all. This chapter is written for occupational therapists as they help people throughout their lifespan accomplish living tasks, learn new skills, adapt to permanent losses, and participate fully in life. As a result universal design can offer a broad new perspective; it can be applied to home modifications and product

---

[1]This information is provided by The Center for Universal Design, College of Design at North Carolina State University, Raleigh, NC, USA. A national research, training, and technical assistance centre, the Center evaluates, develops, and promotes accessible and universal design in housing, buildings, outdoor and urban environments and related products. The Center's work manifests the belief that all new environments and products, to the greatest extent possible, should be usable by everyone regardless of their age, ability, or circumstance. More information is available by contacting the Center or visiting the website at http://www.design.ncsu.edu/cud/.

selections to enhance the lives of the individual, family members, visitors, friends, personal care assistants, and in-home health care providers. Occupational therapy practitioners make excellent modification consultants because they are trained to assess a person's mobility, sensory and cognitive limitations and potential obstacles.

Principles of universal design

In the United States, the universal design concept is defined by seven principles (Table 29.1):

1. Equitable use
2. Flexibility in use
3. Simple and intuitive use
4. Perceptible information
5. Tolerance for error
6. Low physical effort
7. Size and space for approach and use

Table 29.1 The Principles of Universal Design (*Version 2.0 – 4/1/97*)

1. Equitable use

The design is useful and marketable to people with diverse abilities.
- Provide the same means of use for all users: identical whenever possible; equivalent when not
- Avoid segregating or stigmatizing any users
- Provisions for privacy, security, and safety should be equally available to all users
- Make the design appealing to all users.

2. Flexibility in use

The design accommodates a wide range of individual preferences and abilities.
- Provide choice in methods of use
- Accommodate right- or left-handed access and use
- Facilitate the user's accuracy and precision
- Provide adaptability to the user's pace.

3. Simple and intuitive use

Use of the design is easy to understand, regardless of the user's experience, knowledge, language skills, or current concentration level.
- Eliminate unnecessary complexity
- Be consistent with user expectations and intuition
- Accommodate a wide range of literacy and language skills
- Arrange information consistent with its importance
- Provide effective prompting and feedback during and after task completion.

4. Perceptible information

The design communicates necessary information effectively to the user, regardless of ambient conditions or the user's sensory abilities.
- Use different modes (pictorial, verbal, tactile) for redundant presentation of essential information
- Provide adequate contrast between essential information and its surroundings
- Maximize 'legibility' of essential information
- Differentiate elements in ways that can be described (i.e. make it easy to give instructions or directions)
- Provide compatibility with a variety of techniques or devices used by people with sensory limitations.

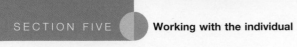
Table 29.1 The Principles of Universal Design (*Version 2.0 – 4/1/97*)—cont'd

5. Tolerance for error

The design minimizes hazards and the adverse consequences of accidental or unintended actions.
- Arrange elements to minimize hazards and errors: most used elements, most accessible; hazardous elements eliminated, isolated, or shielded
- Provide warnings of hazards and errors
- Provide fail safe features
- Discourage unconscious action in tasks that require vigilance.

6. Low physical effort

The design can be used efficiently and comfortably and with a minimum of fatigue.
- Allow user to maintain a neutral body position
- Use reasonable operating forces
- Minimize repetitive actions
- Minimize sustained physical effort.

7. Size and space for approach and use

Appropriate size and space is provided for approach, reach, manipulation, and use regardless of user's body size, posture, or mobility.
- Provide a clear line of sight to important elements for any seated or standing user
- Make reach to all components comfortable for any seated or standing user
- Accommodate variations in hand and grip size
- Provide adequate space for the use of assistive devices or personal assistance.

© Copyright 1997 North Carolina State University – Center for Universal Design, College of Design.

Design of entrances, kitchens and bathrooms

The design of entrances, kitchens, and bathrooms – the most critical areas of a dwelling unit – are the key areas addressed in this chapter. Elements and features presented here are not exhaustive, but they are included to provide a framework and increase the understanding and application of universal design.

Universal entrances

There are common barriers to gaining entry into many dwellings. Uneven ground, sloping landscapes, stairs, inadequately sized porches, thresholds and narrow doorways impede an individual's ability to unlock, open, enter and close the entry door (Figure 29.1). The solutions critical to a person with a temporary or permanent impairment, an older adult, or a person with a gait impairment, also benefit the young professional with a rolling briefcase, luggage, or bags of groceries, children with overstuffed book bags and sporting equipment, mothers with strollers, and movers delivering heavy appliances.

A universal entrance is comprised of many features that allow use by a person with impairment, including a walkway up to a porch or entryway at the same level as the dwelling unit. Additional elements include parking close to dwelling units, a gently sloping walk without steps from parking to the unit entrance, a minimum 1.52 m × 1.52 m manoeuvring space at the entrance, and a door with a minimum clear width of 86.5 cm to 91.5 cm. Additional features, when incorporated, result in a truly universal entrance providing safe and *equitable use* by all people. Examples of additional features include a cover over the entrance to protect from the outdoor environments, a package shelf near the door to rest personal items, a movement/motion sensor to automatically turn on the porch light when someone approaches, a sidelight or peephole at 107 cm and 152.5 cm above the floor, ambient and focused lighting at the keyhole, and high-visibility numbers (Figure 29.2).

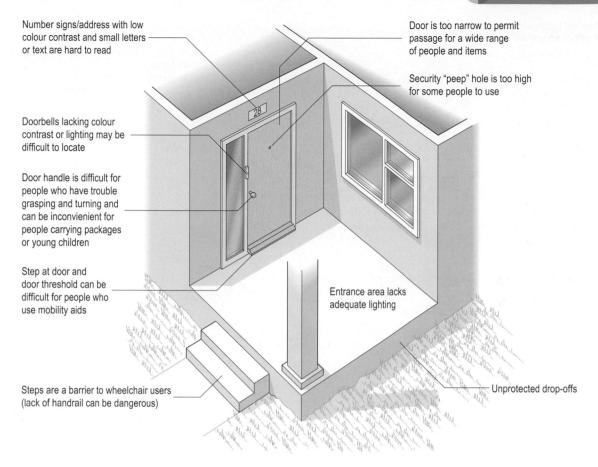

Number signs/address with low colour contrast and small letters or text are hard to read

Door is too narrow to permit passage for a wide range of people and items

Security "peep" hole is too high for some people to use

Doorbells lacking colour contrast or lighting may be difficult to locate

Door handle is difficult for people who have trouble grasping and turning and can be inconvienient for people carrying packages or young children

Step at door and door threshold can be difficult for people who use mobility aids

Entrance area lacks adequate lighting

Steps are a barrier to wheelchair users (lack of handrail can be dangerous)

Unprotected drop-offs

Figure 29.1 • Common barriers at entrances

An ideal entrance would allow a person with a walker, cane, wheelchair or other mobility device enough room to manoeuvre while opening the door. Reducing the threshold minimises tripping hazards and is an advantage to small children, people with vision loss, older adults who may have difficulty walking, and others. The space just inside the door should be uncluttered, have a bench to sit and rest or change shoes, as well as a shelf to place heavy packages. In addition to providing a place to rest objects while closing and locking the door after entering, this will provide a similar staging area when leaving the home. In residential modifications the typical factors of style, characteristics of the building site, and type of construction cannot be as easily manipulated as they can in new construction. When modifying an existing entrance, options to create a stepless entrance include ramps, vertical platform lifts and landscaping. An overlooked solution, provided land is available, is to reposition the entrance as shown in Figure 29.3. The advantages and disadvantages for each option must be carefully considered.

Ramps

Ramps are the most familiar residential accessibility modification (Figures 29.4 and 29.5). They can be built relatively quickly and inexpensively. Ramps accommodating rises above 70 cm require extensive construction, may be very long and quite expensive and require maintenance. Ramps should be thoughtfully planned so they are constructed in a style compatible with the dwelling. Some residents consider ramps stigmatising and are concerned that they label the occupant as weak or vulnerable.

Platform lifts

Platform lifts take up less than 2.8 m² of space. An electrically operated vertical platform wheelchair

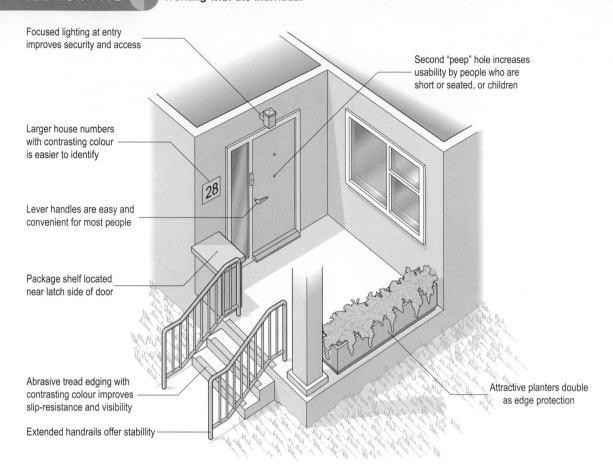

Focused lighting at entry improves security and access

Second "peep" hole increases usability by people who are short or seated, or children

Larger house numbers with contrasting colour is easier to identify

Lever handles are easy and convenient for most people

Package shelf located near latch side of door

Abrasive tread edging with contrasting colour improves slip-resistance and visibility

Extended handrails offer stabillity

Attractive planters double as edge protection

Figure 29.2 • Remodelled entrance (with stairs)

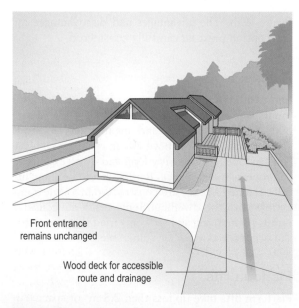

Front entrance remains unchanged

Wood deck for accessible route and drainage

Figure 29.3 • Repositioned entrance with a ramp

lift can avoid the space problems of long ramps. Lifts should be located under cover for weather protection (Figure 29.6). One advantage of lifts is they may be installed for temporary use, removed and installed elsewhere.

Site conditions

Site conditions may offer an opportunity to use landscaped earth pathways for a more natural and blended solution than other options. This approach may include a retaining wall, an earth berm, and sometimes a bridge to an entrance. A safe path with a gentle slope of 1:20 (rise to length) can be built without railings (unless there are abrupt drop-offs on either side or users need them), thereby avoiding the cost and intrusive appearance of railings. Landscaped options may be more expensive than a functionally equivalent ramp solution, but usually have a longer lifespan and require less maintenance. Depending on the site, relocating the entrance can

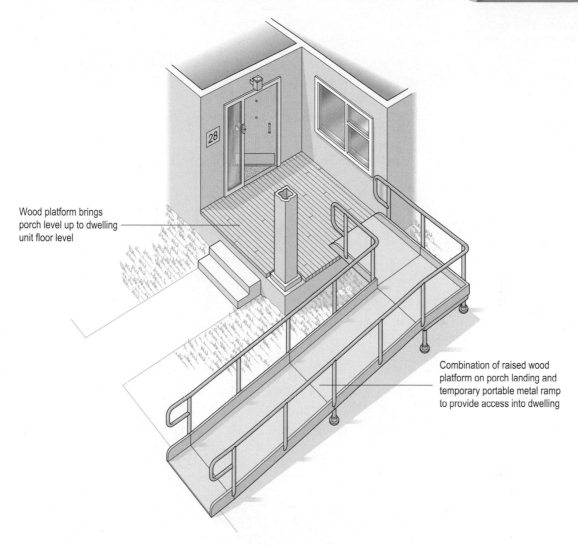

Wood platform brings
porch level up to dwelling
unit floor level

Combination of raised wood
platform on porch landing and
temporary portable metal ramp
to provide access into dwelling

Figure 29.4 • Combination of raised platform and temporary ramp

also be a solution. Integrated site solutions are generally more aesthetic and usually generate a more universally designed solution (Figures 29.7 and 29.8).

Universal kitchens

When considering home modifications for a person, their needs, desires, and future level of ability, combined with the kitchen's current condition, creates a potential problem for which there may seem to be no easy answer. However, features found in a universally designed kitchen can often simplify the solution. Figure 29.9 illustrates what, in the United States, would be considered a modest kitchen with universal features installed and identified.

It may be difficult to modify an entire kitchen. But evaluating the room, and assessing a person's needs, will point toward certain features that will support individual requirements and promote active participation alongside other family members in food preparation and clean-up, as well as the informal activities critical in family life. Counters at different heights may provide space for all household members to use in the kitchen. Countertops with knee-space below, and/or sinks with knee-space, allow a person in a standard dining chair, stool, or wheelchair to more easily work at the countertop in a seated position.

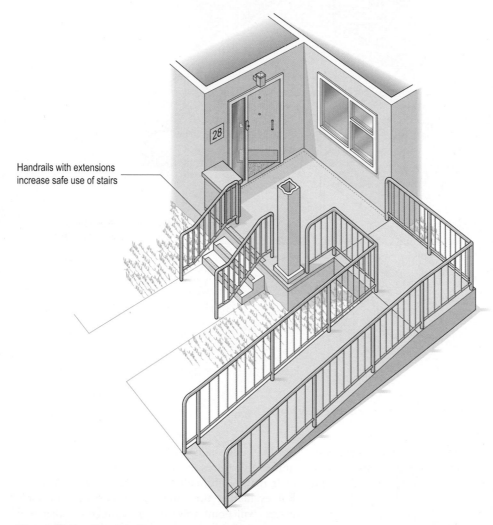

Handrails with extensions
increase safe use of stairs

Figure 29.5 • Permanent ramp

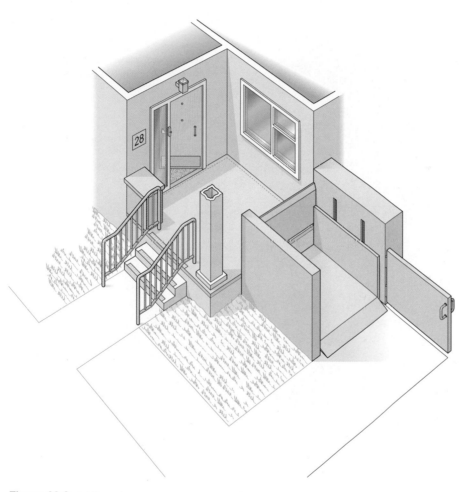

Figure 29.6 • Lift

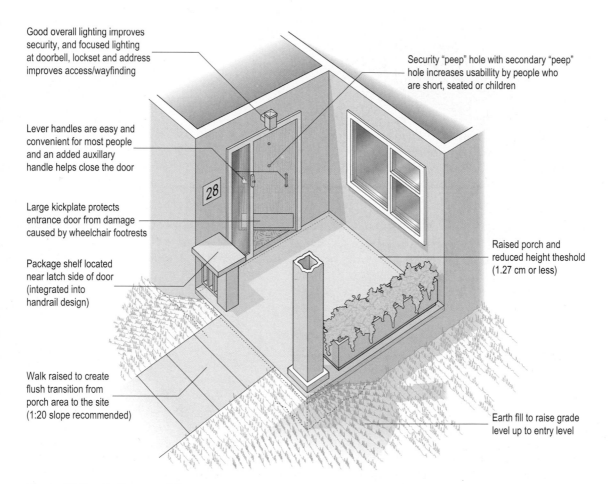

Good overall lighting improves security, and focused lighting at doorbell, lockset and address improves access/wayfinding

Security "peep" hole with secondary "peep" hole increases usabillity by people who are short, seated or children

Lever handles are easy and convenient for most people and an added auxillary handle helps close the door

Large kickplate protects entrance door from damage caused by wheelchair footrests

Raised porch and reduced height thesthold (1.27 cm or less)

Package shelf located near latch side of door (integrated into handrail design)

Walk raised to create flush transition from porch area to the site (1:20 slope recommended)

Earth fill to raise grade level up to entry level

Figure 29.7 • Earth, cut and fill at entrance

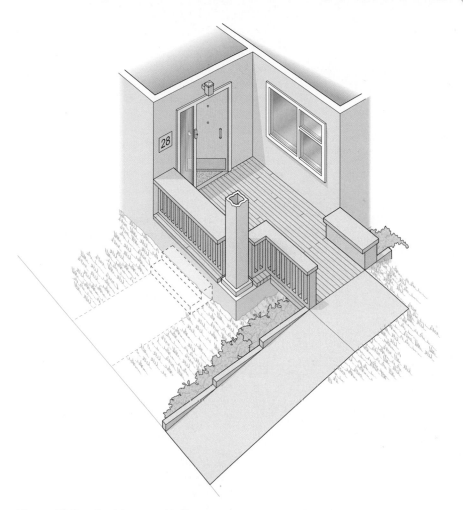

Figure 29.8 • Earth berm and bridge

Examples of universal features to consider are counters/work surfaces at different heights, convenient for cooks of varied statures. Food, pot/pan, and dish storage at a range of heights is helpful for everyone, but especially those with reaching, stooping, kneeling, and/or lifting limitations.

Refrigerated storage

Refrigerated storage presents similar reach concerns, as do other types of storage. Side-by-side refrigerators are usually easiest for most people to use because the frozen food section and the cold storage are vertical, with some area of each reachable by all. Models with the freezer over fresh food storage are frequently difficult for people with limited reaching ability. If the freezer over the fresh food storage is the only option, models with the bottom of the freezer located no more than 111.7 cm to 121.9 cm above the floor are best. A model with the freezer underneath the fresh food may be an option except for those for whom bending and stooping is troublesome. A more universal solution, currently on the market, is designed with drawers located under-the-counter. These models have separate compartments for fresh and frozen food.

Lowered work surfaces

The opportunity to sit while performing tasks is important for people who cannot stand more than a few minutes, especially older adults. To provide sitting space at the sink (or counter/work surface) for a person using a stool or wheelchair, consider having an adaptable cabinet fabricated. The removable options, shown in Figure 29.10, allow the

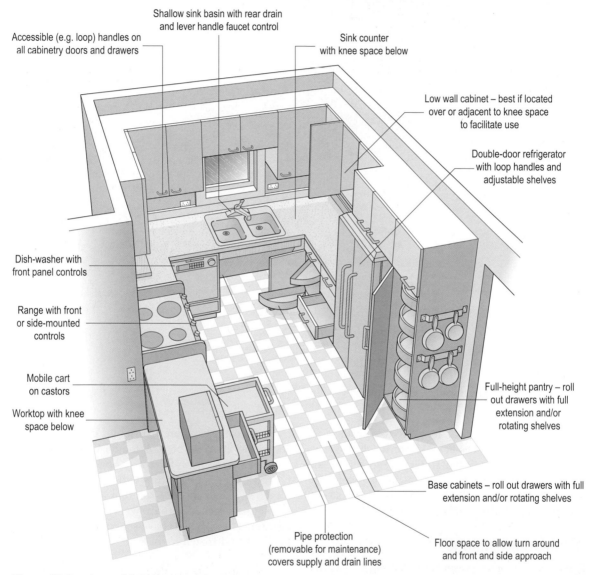

Shallow sink basin with rear drain
and lever handle faucet control

Accessible (e.g. loop) handles on
all cabinetry doors and drawers

Sink counter
with knee space below

Low wall cabinet – best if located
over or adjacent to knee space
to facilitate use

Double-door refrigerator
with loop handles and
adjustable shelves

Dish-washer with
front panel controls

Range with front
or side-mounted
controls

Mobile cart
on castors

Worktop with knee
space below

Full-height pantry – roll
out drawers with full
extension and/or
rotating shelves

Base cabinets – roll out drawers with full
extension and/or rotating shelves

Pipe protection
(removable for maintenance)
covers supply and drain lines

Floor space to allow turn around
and front and side approach

Figure 29.9 • Accessible kitchen

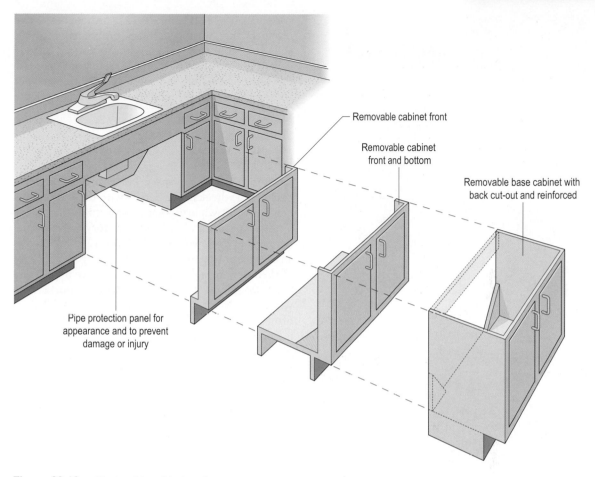

- Removable cabinet front
- Removable cabinet front and bottom
- Removable base cabinet with back cut-out and reinforced

Pipe protection panel for appearance and to prevent damage or injury

Figure 29.10 • Removable cabinet options

kitchen to have a traditional appearance and function while acknowledging the future need for knee-space. A more immediate method for concealing knee-space, while maintaining the traditional appearance, includes using self-storing retractable door hardware, where the doors open and slide along the inside walls of the cabinet interior (Figure 29.11). The best solutions provide a shallow basin with a rear located drain to ensure adequate knee-space.

To provide a truly universal sink, the sink counter should be adjustable through a range from 71 cm to 107 cm with the high end of the range accommodating tall people. Challenging the conventional fixed plumbing mentality is a significant hurdle for this solution. Although not yet commonly available, it is anticipated that such universal adjustable cabinetry will be on the market in the near future.

Controls

For people with reduced sensory acuity, appropriate signals and controls that give auditory, visual, and tactile feedback are critical. As outlined in Table 29.1 the principles *simple and intuitive use, perceptible information, tolerance for error*, and *low physical effort* are all critical attributes for controls and signals. Incorporating the principles makes the function of the controls and signals more easily understood by a person distracted by children, a foreign guest, a child, an older adult, or a person with a cognitive impairment.

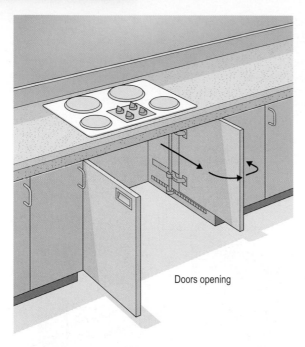

Doors opening

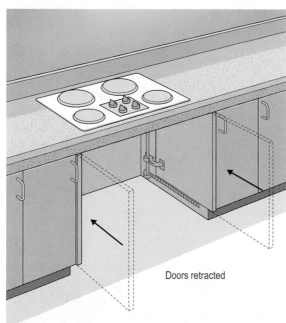

Doors retracted

Figure 29.11 • Use of self-storage doors

Universal bathrooms

The bathroom is one of the most complex and dangerous rooms in a home. Surfaces are hard, often wet, and generally lack sufficient handholds or

gripping surfaces (Figure 29.12). Although assistive products that solve temporary problems are available, and often necessary, modifications that include permanent, aesthetic, and universal features increase the safe, successful, and more independent use of all typical fixtures found in a bathroom (Figure 29.13).

Lavatories

Lavatories with knee-space below are useful for a person in a wheelchair, a person with limited stamina needing to sit while grooming, or a child standing on a step stool to get close to the lavatory to brush his/her teeth. Often wall-hung lavatories are installed as an expedient way to provide the knee-space. Because of their design, wall-hung lavatories have little if any shelf space and, therefore, provide no surface on which to place toiletry and personal items. This is often problematic for anyone with difficulty reaching up into wall cabinets or bending over to retrieve items that inevitably fall off a wall-hung lavatory. Countertop lavatories with base cabinets similar to those shown in the kitchen (Figure 29.10) provide a traditional bathroom appearance with greater *flexibility in use*. A more recent lavatory design with 45-cm-deep counter space, mounted on a shallow-base cabinet or wall hung works well in many residential applications and provides a universal outcome.

Toilets

Traditionally many modest residential bathrooms are designed with all plumbing fixtures installed along a common wall, leaving little room for manoeuvring if using a mobility device. Design standards for accessibility contain many details describing toilet height, clear floor space, distance from a wall or adjacent fixture, and location of flush valve, etc. One of the key features for designing a universally usable bathroom is adequate clear floor space for *approach and use* of the toilet. A modest change in the wall at the back of the toilet combined with additional space to the side of the toilet greatly increases the independent, as well as assisted, use of the fixture. Offsetting the toilet wall 25.4 cm to 30.5 cm provides extra space for the user to position the wheelchair seat parallel to the toilet seat. A safer and easier parallel transfer can then be made (Figure 29.14).

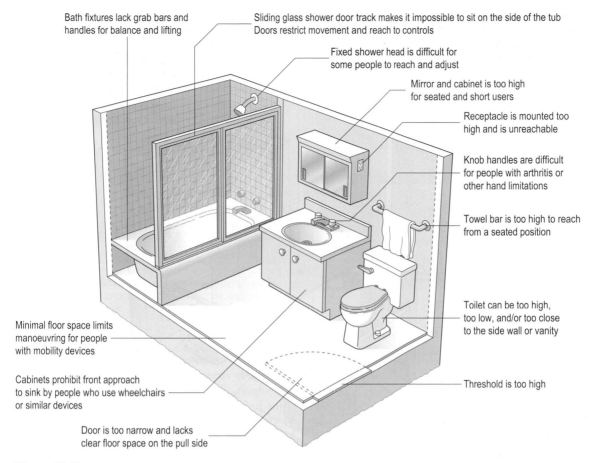

Bath fixtures lack grab bars and handles for balance and lifting

Sliding glass shower door track makes it impossible to sit on the side of the tub
Doors restrict movement and reach to controls

Fixed shower head is difficult for some people to reach and adjust

Mirror and cabinet is too high for seated and short users

Receptacle is mounted too high and is unreachable

Knob handles are difficult for people with arthritis or other hand limitations

Towel bar is too high to reach from a seated position

Toilet can be too high, too low, and/or too close to the side wall or vanity

Threshold is too high

Minimal floor space limits manoeuvring for people with mobility devices

Cabinets prohibit front approach to sink by people who use wheelchairs or similar devices

Door is too narrow and lacks clear floor space on the pull side

Figure 29.12 • Common barriers in bathrooms

Bathing fixtures

Traditionally in the United States, many dwellings have a combination bathtub/shower fixture, giving the user the option of standing to shower or sitting in the bathtub. Climbing in and out of a bathtub can be difficult and dangerous for people whose balance, strength, or mobility may be temporarily or permanently limited. Some people who use a wheelchair find bathtubs with showers completely unusable.

A relatively new fixture design in the United States, the curbless shower, is extremely versatile and can be considered universal. These showers feature a very low or no threshold at all so users may easily walk or roll into the unit. Curbless showers also may have a built-in seat, a hand-held shower, and appropriately placed grab bars for support, though can still be used in a traditional manner where the bather stands to shower. The only bathing option that a curbless shower does not offer is the opportunity to soak.

A more innovative concept, the universal or three-way bathing area, incorporates several bathing fixtures in a single small space. The floor space devoted to the bathtub approach doubles as the curbless shower. A soaking tub is added, along with a bench seat that runs along the back of the shower and extends behind the head of the bathtub. Some of the possible bathing options include: standing to shower, sitting on a portable chair or in a shower-wheelchair, soaking in the tub, and sitting on the shower bench (Figure 29.15). The design, usable by just about everyone, generates a truly universal outcome.

Offset controls

A simple adjustment in installation practices, offsetting bathtub and shower controls toward the outside of the fixture, allows users to set and test water temperature before entering the fixture. If installed as part of a modification, some re-plumbing and

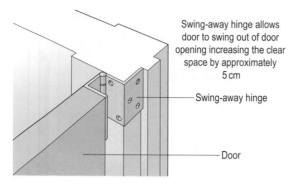

Figure 29.16 • Swing-away hinges

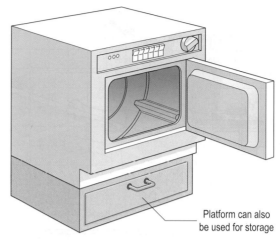

Figure 29.17 • Raised appliances

Widening doors with swing-away hinges

In many instances, doorways are not wide enough for an individual assisting another person whilst walking or using a mobility device. Installing swing-away hinges (Figure 29.16) on a door will increase the clear opening of a narrow doorway, allowing furniture to be more easily moved and large parcels to be carried without struggling.

This hinge style allows a door leaf to swing entirely out of the opening while minimizing structural changes. It is important to provide as close to an 81.5 cm clear opening as possible. Sometimes reversing the swing or opening direction will increase manoeuvring space on the latch-side of the door, making it possible for people using mobility devices to enter independently. An adequately sized door providing a 81.5 cm clear width (usually accomplished with a 86 cm or 91.5 cm door) is more universal, meeting the principles of *equitable use, flexibility in use, and clear space for approach and use*.

Washing-machine height

The most easily used washing-machines (and dryers if available) are front-loading machines with front-mounted controls. If the appliances (either in the dwelling unit or in a shared common laundry area) are installed on an elevated platform, reaching inside is more comfortable and easier for most people including those who are short, pregnant, or have back problems. Bending, stooping, and reaching increase in difficulty the older a person gets. Recognising this, several companies worldwide are now manufacturing washers and dryers elevated on an integral base (Figure 29.17).

Closet storage

An adjustable rod and shelf provide the greatest degree of flexibility in storage since they can be moved to the most convenient arrangement for an individual at any time, meeting the principles of *equitable use, flexibility in use, and low physical effort*. Modestly priced as well as more expensive systems using shelving standards and wire frame shelves are available which provide an infinite range of storage and hanging heights (Figure 29.18).

Application to practice

The universal design approach to solution development applied in the home environment can be extended into the workplace to support the needs and desires of people wishing to remain active and independent regardless of age or physical or sensory circumstance. Where an individual of 60 years old was once expected to begin retirement, today they often are starting second careers or downsizing and buying second homes. Universal design solutions afford the ability to participate in activities of daily living at home and to continue to contribute in the workplace without stigma. Practice Scenarios 29.1, 29.2 and 29.3 highlight how universal design can be used to solve specific changes in ability.

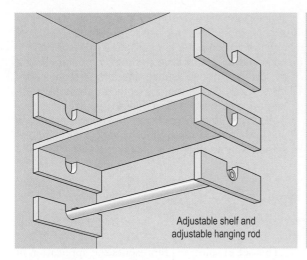 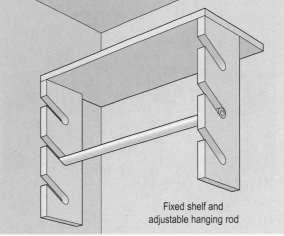

Adjustable shelf and adjustable hanging rod

Fixed shelf and adjustable hanging rod

Figure 29.18 • Adjustable storage

Practice Scenario 29.1 Mae

Mae is 81 years old and is recently widowed. She loves to cook and firmly refuses to acquiesce to her grandchildren's request to move out of her family home. Last winter Mae slipped and fell on the icy steps outside her home. She broke the radius and ulna in her left arm and dislocated her shoulder, limiting her strength and range of motion. If the house had been modified to include the universal features noted in the *Universal Entrances* section, this accident may have never happened.

Problem

Mae's age-related decrease in physical strength interacting with the injuries limit her ability to perform activities of daily living such as cooking and retrieving moderate-to-large objects from overhead shelves. Her cooking is made additionally challenging by the heavy cast iron cookware she uses.

Solution

Her original cookware was replaced with a lightweight universal cookware with a light-coloured interior to improve visibility of contents. The pots and pans all have a circular bottom gradually shaping into a square at the top. The two corners of each pot or pan create natural pouring spouts and the handles on the alternate two corners interlock with the lid handles. The double-handled design provides better leverage when transporting and pouring than single-handle cookware. The recessed lids have an integral steam vent for safe and easy straining and draining, but more importantly the recessed lid and vent prevent dangerous 'boil-overs'.

A table slightly higher than desk height with locking castors was provided so Mae could sit on a tall chair to prepare food. The rolling table is wide enough not to tip and tall enough to allow her to more easily move a full pot to and from the sink, the stove or cooktop and the kitchen counter. Easy-to-turn castors make pushing and steering effortless. Anti-slip hot pads are used to steady the pots while being moved. Additional features, as shown in Figure 29.9, could also be included to further improve the kitchen for Mae's use.

Practice Scenario 29.2 Carla

Carla is 32 years old, lives in a mid-sized city and has been working as a childcare provider for seven years. She owns her own childcare business, a licensed high-quality facility. Though she is dedicated to excellence in providing her service she usually avoids technology. Carla currently has several three-year-old children in nappies which she frequently changes. Although not overweight, the children are tall (95th to 98th percentile in height) and, therefore, heavy to lift.

Problem

Carla's upper and lower back and left elbow have been hurting to the point where she feels that she may have to give up her daycare business.

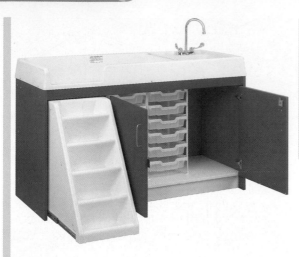

Figure 29.19 ● Unique nappy-changing cart. Photo courtesy of Tot-Mate

Solution

A unique nappy-changing cart was purchased for Carla (Figure 29.19). The cart was designed with the work surface at standing elbow height to promote an upright posture, reducing stress on the low back. It has pull-out steps, safety rails, an integrated work sink, nappy disposal and under-cabinet storage. The steps allow Carla to guide the children up and into position, rather than bending, lifting and lowering them onto the table.

Practice Scenario 29.3 Steve

Steve is a 47-year-old professor at a major university and has recently been named as the department head. He consults for a California company to keep his examples in the class current and skills relevant. Steve works on his computer 4–6 hours a day, is an avid golfer and embraces technology.

Problem

Steve has begun to forget appointments and develop headaches, and he has cut back on golf citing neck pain.

Solution

Four changes were suggested for Steve to reduce his stress and to work in a neutral neck posture. The suggestions were unobtrusive and relatively easy to accomplish. Steve replaced his bifocals and cell phone with computer glasses and a palm pilot/phone combination. He repositioned his computer monitor by lowering his adjustable *(flexibility in use)* height table, made use of the computer's accessibility features and is making an effort to reduce his stress through planning and exercise. The computer glasses and lower monitor allow Steve to look at his computer screen with his neck in a neutral posture.

This set of solutions represents the application of the principles of universal design. The pots, pans and cart are used easily by Mae and all members of her extended family and friends. The nappy-changing cart is used by Carla and her staff and provides ease and comfort for the parents and grandparents of the toddlers. Steve, needing to lower the height of his computer monitor quickly was able to do so by using the adjustable-height feature of the table.

Conclusion

Universal design is an evolving strategy being used to create liveable, marketable environments for everyone. It is an inclusionary design that applies to housing, transportation, places of employment, education, and parks and recreation facilities to maximize the number of people who can do things independently in a particular environment. It also applies to how services and programmes are provided and how communication is offered to a person who may have a condition affecting sight, hearing, or cognition. Likewise, products created with a universal design approach have features which make them useful to a wider range of people.

From the occupational therapist's perspective, services can be more easily provided in facilities equipped with universal features and products. When the environment is adapted through building modifications, installations, and/or product selections resulting in the person being more independent and in control, a healthy interdependent emotional connection with family and friends can be maintained (see Box 29.1 for additional tips).

Box 29.1

Identifying opportunities for universal design solutions

- Identify the obstacles to the person by performing a walk through of their day (preferably with them). The occupational therapists should ask themselves about how well the person can:
  - get out of bed, dress, and get to the bathroom
  - move from the bathroom to the kitchen, prepare meals and eat
  - perform activities of personal hygiene
  - clean the house, and wash the dishes and laundry
  - interact with family, friends and care assistants.
- Consider the equitable and ease of use philosophy incorporated in the principles of universal design when visualising or observing the task being performed:
  - During each daily activity, is the person forced to exert extra effort or are they limited by the products, fixtures or structures around them?
  - Ask questions pertaining to the principles such as:
    - Does the person have to reach or stretch to accomplish a task?
    - Can the person see and understand the information in the environment?

- Is text large enough, in the correct language, in an easy-to-understand word choice?
- Is there adequate lighting and good contrast?
- Are redundant channels of feedback available, such as auditory or tactile feedback?
- Consider the context in which the activity is normally performed. In addition to the simple activities such as turning a door knob, look at the person's ability to perform an entire sequence of tasks such as entering or exiting the house:
  - Can the person enter the house with groceries or enter quickly and safely, avoiding being a target for conflict?
  - Does the solution scream 'here lives someone with a disability' or does if afford most users a similar experience?
  - Can activities of daily living be improved significantly by the design of the built environment, not relying exclusively on adaptive aids?
  - Is this solution going to make someone feel an enhanced sense of competence?

Additional resources

Ambrose, I. (1997) *Lifetime homes in Europe and the UK.* York, UK, Joseph Rowntree Foundation.

Barrier Free Environment Inc. (1991). *The accessible housing design file,* New York, Van Nostrand Reinhold.

Beecher, V. & Paquet, V. for the Building Research Institute, Hoersholm, Denmark (1997). Survey instrument for the universal design of consumer products. *Applied Ergonomics* 36(3), 363–372.

Brewerton, J. & Darton, D. (1997). *Designing lifetime homes.* York, UK, Joseph Rowntree Foundation.

Carlson, J., Taira, L. & Dunleavey, E. (Eds), (1999). *Aging in place: designing, adapting, and enhancing the home environment.* York, UK, Joseph Rowntree Foundation.

Carroll, C., Cowans, J. & Darton, D. (1999). *Meeting Part M of the Building Regulations and designing lifetime homes.* York, UK, Joseph Rowntree Foundation.

Christophersen, J. (1995) *The growth of good housing, the Norwegian State Housing Band.* Oslo, HB-3061.

Danford, G. S. & Tauke, B. (Eds). (2001). *City of New York, M.s.O.f.P.w.D., ed. Universal Design New York. 2001.* New York City, Center for Inclusive Design and Environment Access.

Demirbilek, O., Demirkan, O. & Halime, H. (2004). Professional Architecture. Universal product design involving elderly users: a participatory design model. *Applied Ergonomics,* 35, 361–370.

Department of Environment (1992). *Building Regulations (England), Section M.* London, UK, Department of Environment, Transport and the Regions.

Dittmar, S. & Gresham, G. (Eds.) (1997). *Functional assessment and outcome measures for the rehabilitation health professional.* Gaithersburg, MD, Aspen Publishers, Inc.

Dobkin, I. & Peterson, M. J. (1999). *Gracious spaces: Universal interiors by design.* New York, McGraw Hill.

Haigh, R. (1993). The ageing process: a challenge for design. *Applied Ergonomics,* 24(1), 9–14.

Hitchcock, D. R., Luckyer, S., Cook, S. & Quigley, C. (2001). Third age usability and safety – an ergonomics contribution to design. *International Journal of Human-Computer Studies,* 55(4), 635–643.

Imrie, R. (2006). Independent lives and the relevance of lifetime homes. *Disability and Society,* 21(4), 15.

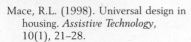

Mace, R.L. (1998). Universal design in housing. *Assistive Technology*, 10(1), 21–28.

Pirkl, J. (1994). *Transgenerational design*. New York, Van Nostrand Reinhold.

Preiser, W. F. E. & Ostroff, E. (Eds). (2001). *Universal design handbook*. New York, McGraw-Hill.

Steven Winters Associates (1997). *Minimum requirements for housing corporation grants. Accessible housing by design: Universal design principles in practice*. New York, McGraw-Hill.

Story, M. & Mueller, J. (2003). *A guide to evaluating the universal design performance of products*. Raleigh, NC, Center for Universal Design, College of Design, NC State University.

Story, M., Mace, R. & Mueller, J. (1998). *The universal design file: Designing for people of all ages and abilities*. Raleigh, NC, Center for Universal Design, NC State University.

The Housing Corporation (1993). *Scheme development standards*. *Revised 1995*. London, The Housing Corporation.

Wyche, S. (2005). *Designing speculative household cleaning products for older adults. Proceedings of the 2005 conference on Designing for User eXperience*. San Francisco, California, American Institute of Graphic Arts.

Wylde, M., A. Baron-Robbins, & Clark, S. (1994). *Building for a lifetime: The design and construction of fully accessible homes*. Newtown, CT, The Taunton Press.

Assistive devices for enabling occupations

Helen Pain and Sue Pengelly

CHAPTER CONTENTS

Introduction 454

Enabling occupations with assistive
devices. 454

Design of assistive devices. 455

Policy context 456

History of assistive device provision in
occupational therapy 456

Problem solving and reasoning 457

   Problem-solving process 459
   Step 1: Assessment 459
   Step 2: Planning 460
   Step 3: Intervention. 464
   Step 4: Evaluation 465

Conclusion. 466

SUMMARY

This chapter presents the theory, values and problem-solving process available for occupational therapists to use in relation to assistive devices. The knowledge required includes understanding the inter-relationship between person, environment and occupation, and the role assistive devices can play in achieving a good fit between the three. The essential skills are: *active listening* – to understand occupational problems and goals; *research* – to explore the range of assistive devices available; *effective communication* – to provide clear information about options, and fourthly, *problem solving and creative thinking* – to generate and compare options, and determine satisfactory solutions. The value base presented is person-centred where choice, respect for individuality, and partnership working are all emphasised. It also draws on the social perspective of health and disability to encourage occupational therapists to act as a resource for people requiring assistive devices rather than as experts prescribing equipment.

KEY POINTS

- Assistive technology is a term used to refer to any product or service designed to enable independence for disabled or older people. Within this general category, assistive devices refer specifically to products.
- Assistive devices have great potential to be used to enable self care, leisure and productive occupations.
- There has been a historical shift within occupational therapy from the prescription of equipment aimed to overcome dysfunction, towards partnership working in the selection of assistive devices to enable occupations.
- Person-centred working and effective communication are essential to promote autonomy, choice and informed decision-making.
- A problem-solving process model is used to guide the selection of assistive devices.
- Professional reasoning, drawing on theory-based, meaning-based and pragmatic reasoning, are combined through reflective practice to explain and justify decisions made.

Introduction

As occupational therapists our key role is to '... enable people to achieve health, well being and life satisfaction through participation in occupation.' (College of Occupational Therapists 2004, p. 1).

While other chapters in this book explore a variety of ways to reach this aim, this chapter will examine the use of assistive devices. The provision of equipment for mobility and activities of daily living has long been an established element of practice within occupational therapy. The rapid development of technology and design, alongside the increasing proportion of older and disabled people within the population, has expanded the options available and focused attention on assistive technology (AT) as an increasingly important area of practice.

The term disability equipment has been widely replaced by that of assistive devices. This is a component of assistive technology which has been defined as, 'any product or service designed to enable independence for disabled or older people' (Foundation for Assistive Technology 2007). This definition was agreed in the United Kingdom (UK) during a King's Fund consultation meeting in 2001 as it provides a clear person-centred focus and identifies the outcome as maximising independence. This remains a broad definition which comprises products, services and newly emerging technologies. Assistive devices refer specifically to products and will be used in this chapter to include both products specially designed to assist disabled and older people, and well-designed mainstream products which achieve that aim. Examples of assistive devices that may be used in different settings can be found in Table 30.1. Table 30.2 provides examples of assistive devices that may be used to assist a person with particular impairments.

Enabling occupations with assistive devices

Occupational therapists recognise that there is a dynamic inter-relationship between individuals and their environment as they engage in occupations (Canadian Association of Occupational Therapists 2002). An alteration in any component part of the system will have an impact on occupational engagement, which is maximised when there is a

Table 30.1 Examples of assistive devices in different locations

Home	Smart homes[1], smart technology[2], environmental control systems[3], stair-lifts, adjustable height sinks, rails, raised toilet seats, accessible showers, fall detector, dressing devices, video door bell, smoke alarm, profiling bed, wheelchair with integrated technology, reminders to prevent wandering/turn off cooker, software for screen magnification, screen access through speech and braille, talking watch/microwave, flashing door bell, vibrating alarm clock
School	Computers, reading services, communication aids, software for screen magnification, screen access through speech and braille
Work	Computer software, telephone accessories, voice control of computer, ergonomic design of office space, software for screen magnification, screen access through speech and braille
Leisure and recreation	Sports wheelchairs, loop systems, computer games for partially sighted children, audio-books, page turners, environmental control systems, adapted sport equipment
Health and social care	Telecare[4] and telehealth[5]

[1] *Smart homes* are new houses which incorporate a single network to connect a multitude of devices, including home security, entertainment, monitoring, communication and environmental controls.

[2] *Smart technology* includes movement detectors and lifestyle monitoring sensors which are available to install in existing houses to enable telecare monitoring service to take place.

[3] *Environmental control systems* allow independent control of electrically powered devices through a single control system.

[4] *Telecare* refers to any service that brings health and social care directly to a user, generally in their own homes, supported by information and communication technology (Audit Commission 2004). This involves data being collected through sensors and sent electronically to a monitoring centre. Basic units include community alarms, with more advanced intelligent systems being available to monitor activity levels.

[5] *Telehealth* systems allow the remote monitoring of vital signs and specific conditions, virtual consultations, health information and advice to be available at home.

Table 30.2 Examples of assistive devices that may be used to assist a person with particular impairments

Person with a change in their health or at risk of accident	Self-care equipment (e.g. dressing devices), falls detector, telehealth
Older person living alone requiring reassurance	Community alarm, video door bell, smoke alarm
Person with degenerative condition	Wheelchair with integrated technology, smart technology, adapted home
Person requiring palliative care	Environmental control system, profiling bed, manual handling equipment
Older person with dementia or person with learning difficulties	Telecare, monitors to check bed/room occupancy, use of fridge and reminders to prevent wandering/turn off cooker, etc.
Person who is partially sighted	Software for screen magnification, screen access through speech and Braille, talking watch/microwave
Person who is deaf	Flashing door bell, vibrating alarm clock, loop system
Disabled person in employment	Full ergonomic design of office space, voice control of computer
Person with dyslexia	Language support, voice recognition and planning software, dictaphone

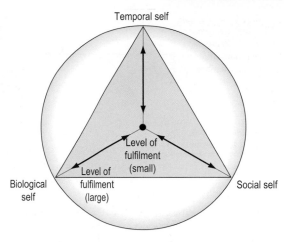

Figure 30.1 • Schematic expression of three-dimensional model of self, with kind permission of Tamako Miyamae, WFOT presentation 1998

without being expected to change the native functioning of the individual' (Anson 2006, p. 351).

Design of assistive devices

The approach to designing assistive devices has gradually become more person-centred and focuses on achieving a good fit with all aspects of the user's self. Rather than continuing to design for the 'average person', there has been greater attention paid to ergonomics and inclusive design. Stephen Pheasant (1996) was influential in promoting a practical ergonomic approach which places the person at the centre of the design process by orientating it around detailed anthropometric data. This seeks to fit the product to the users, rather than the other way around, aiming for the majority (95%) of the target population to be able to use the final product. Universal or inclusive design (Design for all 2007) which aims to consider everybody's needs is particularly important to occupational therapists because it is based on sound ergonomic and anti-discriminatory principles (O'Brien 2006). Helen Hamblyn Research Centre (2007) promotes design using those principles. The shift toward mainstream inclusive design is evident in everyday life, including velcro fixing for shoes, accessible storage in kitchens and websites designed to accessibility standards (WAI 2007). However, the proportion of the population able to use a product will seldom reach 100% and there remain occasions when people with severe impairments need bespoke products.

good fit between the individual and their environment. The model presented in Figure 30.1 represents a person who has achieved a balance between all aspects of self and the environment, enabling optimal occupational engagement (see fulfilment in Figure 30.1).

If the environment is challenging, people may raise their own capability to meet those demands, but this is not always possible and impairments may result in a reduction of 'fit' between the self and the environment, as illustrated in Figure 30.2.

Reduced ability in the biological self can be met by a more supportive environment. In relation to the physical environment, this can be through the use of assistive devices where the approach is to '… replace or support an impaired function of the user

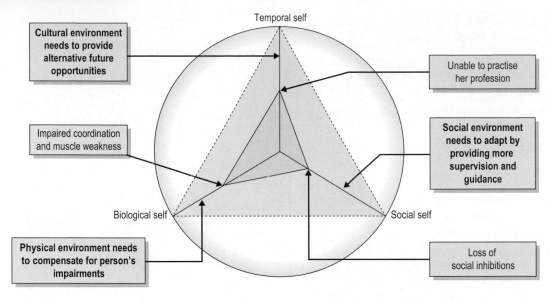

Figure 30.2 • The three-dimensional model of self with adjustments to maintain occupational performance following head injury, created by Helen Pain and Sue Pengelly

Policy context

There are many drivers for the increased use of assistive technology, including assistive devices, which include:

- the aging population and resultant pressure on systems of care

- increased aspirations of disabled and older people for full participation and social inclusion

- government policies – anti-discrimination, promoting choice and independence

- future opportunities from developments in design and technology together with increased public familiarity with technology, which facilitates the uptake of innovation.

Within the United Kingdom, the Audit Commission (2004) argued that assistive technology has huge potential to help people to remain independent and that public services should make use of it when delivering policies and the National Service Frameworks' (NSF) priorities. Assistive devices can increase choice, make remaining at home possible, ease the challenges of daily living, and increase security and confidence, while also relieving pressures on informal carers. Assistive devices may increase cost effectiveness of health and social care by easing the pressure on existing services through reducing risk at home, the need for home care, hospital admis-

sions, and places required in care homes, while also promoting earlier supported discharges and healthier living (Audit Commission 2004, Kings Fund 2006).

There are also potential disadvantages and barriers to the effective use of assistive devices. Their function should be to complement rather than replace human care, to avoid further social isolation amongst older people (Kings Fund 2006). Financing assistive devices for people with relatively low care needs is likely to produce the greatest cost benefits over the long term, which challenges the current tendency to prioritise resources for people with highest levels of need (Kings Fund 2006). Limited resources for rehabilitation or social care may increase pressure to use assistive devices when it is not actually the best option because it can be seen as a 'quick fix'. It should be remembered that while assistive devices are ideal for some people, for others they may cause additional fatigue, or they may prefer human assistance.

History of assistive device provision in occupational therapy

The history of assistive device provision within occupational therapy reveals a shift from the expert occupational therapist, prescribing specialist equipment to compensate for dysfunction, towards increased partnership working with disabled and older people to enable them to make informed decisions about assistive devices to promote their independence in occupations. This shift reflects broader changes in both the profession and society including a greater adoption of the social model of disability and person-centred practice.

The drive towards more inclusive design has resulted in assistive devices becoming more readily available. The simple long-handled shoe horn has moved from being categorised as specialist disability equipment issued by a professional, to becoming available to buy from suppliers of disabled equipment in the high street, to finally being stocked in mainstream shops.

A second significant change is that occupational therapy has moved from the former reductionist, medical approach to refocusing on enabling occupations. The purpose of any assistive device supplied is to enable people to undertake their chosen activities or occupations.

The third major change reflects the move away from maintaining control over the problem-solving process, which may serve as a barrier to the self determination of disabled people (Priestley 1999), towards an increased emphasis on partnership working and joint decision making. 'This type of person-centred decision making is based on an understanding of the occupational therapists' role as being a resource to enable people to make informed decisions, rather than themselves being expert decision makers' (Pengelly 2006, p. 59).

The key elements of person-centred practice, identified by Parker (2006), are essential when choosing assistive devices:

- Understanding and respect for uniqueness and diversity – active listening.

- Autonomy and choice – occupational therapists need to research options available and communicate clearly to provide full, timely and accessible information to enable people to make informed choices.

- Partnership and responsibility – focus on goals identified by the individual and work together to achieve them.

Problem solving and reasoning

The problem-solving process will be used to structure the next sections of the chapter to guide the

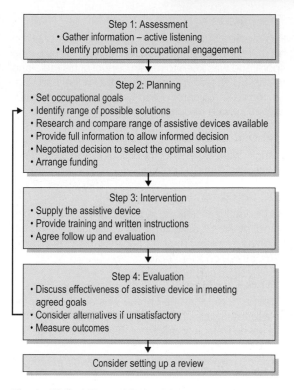

Figure 30.3 • The problem-solving process

reader through the application of these skills and professional reasoning in practice. Practice Scenario 30.1 provides an illustration of the full problem-solving process in the selection of assistive devices, which is outlined in Figure 30.3.

Practice Scenario 30.1
An illustration of the complete problem-solving process used to select assistive devices

Patrick was diagnosed with motor neurone disease (MND) 18 months ago and lives with his wife, Sarah. The MND nurse recently referred him to an occupational therapist specialising in environmental control systems.

Step 1: Assessment

Gemma, the occupational therapist, undertook an initial assessment based on the Canadian Model of Occupational Performance and Engagement, paying particular attention to his home environment and his control of movement.

The person

Patrick was frustrated by his decreased strength in his hands and arms. He also enjoyed music and sport, and was keen to regain control of his radio and television. The couple said the MND nurse had suggested having a carer but they described themselves as very private people.

The occupations

Patrick was experiencing difficulty using the telephone and remote controls.

The caregiver

Sarah was increasingly anxious about leaving him alone, making it difficult for her to shop or attend her local yoga class. They recognised this was placing extra stress on them both.

The environment

Gemma noted that their home was already adapted to accommodate the use of a powered wheelchair, but asked Patrick and Sarah if they were experiencing any difficulties.

Step 2: Planning

The occupational goals they prioritised were for Patrick to be able to operate the phone, television and radio, and for Sarah to be able to leave him for up to 1½ hours to attend her yoga and go shopping. The couple was satisfied with the accessibility of their home.

Potential solutions

Carers were not acceptable to the couple to solve the current issues. They were interested in the potential of environmental control systems. Gemma explained the range of facilities which could be controlled. They agreed Patrick needed to control the telephone and a pager which would operate within a mile of their house, along with the television and the radio. They looked at the literature from a number of firms that supplied environmental control systems. One important criterion was the versatility of the system to enable the addition of other facilities and to alter the type of control switch as needed in the future; and as Patrick was familiar with electronic technology and was keen to use a controller with a computerised screen and iconic display, these criteria enabled the selection of one company. A representative from this firm came, and after trying out the range of switches Patrick decided that a buddy button, using the side of his right hand, was the one which fitted best with his present control over movement. Further discussion with the representative led the

couple to request that an intercom and door-opening device for the front door should also be incorporated. The occupational therapist was in full agreement. The engineer later attended to provide a quotation for the necessary work to install the system.

Gemma completed the paperwork, and in due course, funding for the system was approved.

Step 3: Intervention

The engineer installed the system a fortnight later and taught both Patrick and Sarah how to use it. He left operating instructions for the system and a contact number to report any technical problems. Three weeks post installation Gemma telephoned to ask how it was going and Patrick reported that it was easier to operate the buddy button some days than others. She visited and discussed the optimum position for the buddy button so that he could always activate it effectively.

Step 4: Evaluation

After 8 weeks Gemma completed an evaluation by telephone and they reported that the environmental controls had met their present occupational goals and reduced stress. Ongoing review was agreed to monitor both the effectiveness of the input switch and the range of devices controlled by the system. Gemma arranged to review them in 4 months' time and ensured they had her contact number to get in touch with her beforehand if required.

This Practice Scenario was developed on the advice of Lyn Simpson. At the time of writing Lyn was working as a Clinical Specialist Therapist in Environmental Control Systems at the National Centre for Electronic Assistive Technology in Cardiff, UK.

For situations where an assistive device could meet part or all of an occupational challenge, the problem-solving process presented in the following sections is combined with insights drawn from occupational therapy, management and cognitive psychology literature (Carnevali 1995, Hagedorn 1996, Hardwick & Robbens 1998). This pays attention to all factors that affect the relevance, practicality and acceptance of an assistive device. This should help to maximise the use of the assistive device to promote effective occupational engagement and, therefore, prove cost-effective for the provider.

Throughout this process occupational therapists are encouraged to move beyond attempting to solve problems like rational technicians towards becoming reflective practitioners (Schön 1983) and to consciously utilise a range of different types of reasoning in practice. The integrated person-centred model offers a useful example of reasoning which combines cognition (use of discipline-specific knowledge); metacognition (reflection); and mutual decision-making between the therapist and the person, and, finally, acknowledges the importance of the environment (Paterson & Summerfield-Mann 2006). New practitioners are encouraged to utilise the following three different types of reasoning combined through reflective person-centred practice (Pengelly 2006):

- Theory-based reasoning (draws on theoretical knowledge to promote rational decision making, e.g. occupational therapy theory, ergonomics, bio-medical and social sciences).

- Meaning-based reasoning (understanding the subjective human world of the person, their home and family, work, occupations and values, understanding people's stories and possible futures).

- Pragmatic reasoning (understanding the practical reality of service delivery – what is possible within available resources and legislative/policy context).

Ranka and Chapparo (2000) identified five key dimensions for therapists in developing effective reasoning:

1. Development of stores of knowledge
2. Interpersonal skills
3. Ability to envisage the potential future for the people who require their services
4. Becoming aware of their own moral positions
5. Being able to reason the best course of action.

The last three were identified as the most important for understanding a person's perspective and were best enhanced through critical reflection. It is recommended that therapists adopt a structured approach to reasoning to help them develop these skills. It will also make their reasoning processes more overt and help them to justify decisions to fund holders.

Problem-solving process

Step 1: Assessment

Assessment is carried out in partnership with the person and carers and requires information gathering to identify problems in occupational engagement. The problem may have already been stated either in the broadest terms, for example a person following spinal injury needs a full assessment of their home situation, or in terms of a solution: 'I need a shower as I can't use the bath any longer'. This frames the information-gathering domain, but experience will suggest additional information gathering that may be very important; for example, a person may only talk about difficulty with dressing, but having seen her hand function, you would want to explore if preparing a meal, washing and other activities are also affected. The initial assessment could be structured around a model of occupational therapy, such as the Canadian Model of Occupational Performance and Engagement (Townsend & Polatajko 2007), and a standardised assessment such as the Canadian Occupational Performance Measure (Canadian Association of Occupational Therapists 2005) could be used to gain a meaning-based understanding of the person's occupational priorities. An overall assessment may require a walk-through with the person of their 24-hour day, but if the individual only identifies one activity as problematic, for example, using the toilet, it may be appropriate to limit assessment to that sphere.

Once the occupational challenges have been identified they need to be analysed in more detail, and pertinent information about the following must be collected:

- The occupation (especially the aspect(s) that the person finds difficult)

- The person's values, attitudes, motivation and physical impairment

- The environment (demands and resources) (Dutton 1995).

The *occupation* itself must be analysed, either to determine which particular aspects are the source of the difficulty, or to provide sub-goals in the journey towards restoration of occupational engagement. For example, if a person with tetraplegia wants to sail, then every component task of the sport must be examined to determine what adaptation or assistive device would be required.

The assessment of the *person* should include their skills and also their feelings and attitudes towards an assistive device. Reasoning solely based on overcoming dysfunction and pragmatic issues, such as available funding and structural feasibility, will fail to distinguish between one man who considers his stair lift to be the 'best thing since sliced bread' and another who refused to have one installed as it would have 'taken away his remaining shred of dignity' (Pengelly 2006, p. 58).

Thirdly, the *environment* needs to be investigated in detail. The *physical* environment can be described, sketched and measured where necessary. Photographs can also be useful, provided the individual gives their consent. Assessment of the *social* environment includes gathering information about the person's responsibilities, support received or available, including pertinent information about caregivers, especially if they will need to demonstrate, use or maintain any assistive device supplied. The social environment can make a major difference, for example people who live alone tend to use assistive devices more than those living with others (Hoffmann & McKenna 2004, Tomita & Mann 1997); the presence of a caregiver may affect motivation to remain occupationally active either positively through gentle encouragement and withdrawal of help, or negatively by being over-protective or impatient with slowness. The *cultural* environment also needs to be assessed as it may affect the solutions available, for instance it may be culturally unacceptable to clean oneself under continuous running water, so a shower would not be an appropriate solution.

Assessment tools specific to assistive devices are available. For example, assessment of the readiness to use an assistive device, the task and the person's needs can be guided by The Matching Person and Technology assessments (IMPT 2007). Another option could be the Individually Prioritised Problems Assessment (IPPA) (Efficiency of Assistive Technology and Services 1998), which, although designed as an outcome measure, can be used for assessment and reapplied after the delivery of the assistive device to evaluate its effectiveness. Some assessment issues are illustrated in Practice Scenario 30.2 by Mrs Johnson's need for an assistive device to bath her son Ryan.

Practice Scenario 30.2
Step 1: Assessment: Mrs Johnson and Ryan

Mrs Johnson is a single mother with a 3-year-old son who has severe learning difficulties and epilepsy. During an occupational therapist's visit one difficulty they identified was bathing, due to Ryan being unable to sit in the bath. The occupational therapist assessed

Ryan's sitting ability and discussed options with Mrs. Johnson, and they agreed on a bath seat to trial. Two days after delivering and demonstrating the seat, the occupational therapist got a telephone call saying the seat was fine for Ryan, but Mrs Johnson had always bathed him with his younger sister. The new seat was too big to have his sister in with him, and Mrs Johnson could not leave her on her own. The therapist realised this had not been taken into account during the initial assessment and that this was an extra factor which needed to be considered.

Using all the assessment information, problems in occupational engagement can then be identified in collaboration with the person. It is important that all interested parties are in agreement with the analysis of the problem, otherwise there will be misunderstanding and potential conflict in the selection and provision of a device.

Step 2: Planning

Planning involves setting occupational goals and identifying the range of potential solutions, of which an assistive device may be one. Whilst focusing on assistive devices in this chapter, bear in mind that these are often used in conjunction with personal assistance and rehabilitation. Alternatively a person may choose to avoid or delegate an activity, for instance deciding to live downstairs to avoid tackling the stairs, or asking their spouse to put on their shoes.

The first stage of planning is to have a clear shared image of potential future improvements. Anticipated occupational goals need to be agreed collaboratively and projected outcomes framed as objectives which are measurable, specific and relevant. This will help clarify the requirements for the assistive device. For example, a person whose goal is to go to the local shop may identify that he needs something that will enable him to travel the required distance, will have space for the shopping, and he will go twice a week.

It is important to make sure that all concerned are (Hardwick & Robbens 1998, Pain et al 2003):

- in agreement with the objectives

- involved in the review of possible solutions

- able to state their views and know they have been heard.

The next task is to generate possible solutions and evaluate them for their effectiveness in tackling the occupational dysfunction and likelihood of achieving the goals. A range of factors that may affect this process include (Crabtree & Lyons 1997, Kuipers et al 2006):

- the therapist's knowledge, experience and responsibilities
- the therapist's relationship with the person
- the ability to talk things over collaboratively
- responsibilities to guidelines and budgetary constraints of the therapist's employer.

When it has been agreed that an assistive device could be one of the possible solutions, then the range available needs to be researched. Catalogues, web-sites and centres dealing with specialist equipment are invaluable resources, but mainstream products should also be investigated. Creative thinking across boundaries can often yield positive results. This is illustrated in Practice Scenario 30.3 in the selection of an assistive device to enhance Mary's safety in the kitchen.

Practice Scenario 30.3
Step 2: Planning: Mary

Mary's balance was poor and her hip extensors were weak. She found standing while preparing food tiring and risky, and she was unable to carry things safely from one place to another. A wheeled walking frame with seat was too difficult to manoeuvre in the kitchen and a mobile commode with a padded over-seat did not move well when Mary tried to guide it when sitting on it. When the occupational therapist picked up an office catalogue for a new chair at work she realised that a wheeled adjustable-height office chair might be suitable for Mary, and it proved to be ideal.

Once the range of available devices has been identified, the optimal one has to be determined. The definitive way to compare and assess their suitability is to ask the potential user to actually try out each device in turn. This might be a straightforward task if there are only a few products and the person is able to trial them without difficulty. However, the range is often wide so options need to be narrowed to two or three possibilities before they can be tried out. Therapists will draw on their experience and knowledge to facilitate this process but care must

be taken to ensure that no factors which are important in the particular situation are missed (Hagedorn 1996).

Each potential assistive device must be judged on criteria that are the key to achieving a good match between a device and the person's requirements. The range of criteria includes:

- Usefulness (effectiveness) of the device
- The ease with which the person learns how to use and get the best from the device, including cognitive and physical components
- Usability which will include set up and use of all components in all likely situations, e.g. manoeuvring a wheelchair on various terrains
- Compatibility with the environment or other devices
- Acceptability to the person and other people involved
- Reliability
- Maintenance and servicing
- Whether the device meets local authority criteria for provision.

Prioritisation of these criteria is helpful to focus the search and to aid complex decisions. They should be applied flexibly to avoid discarding a possible solution because of a shortcoming in one area if that is not a high priority for the potential recipient. The importance of keeping options open is illustrated in Practice Scenario 30.4 in the selection of an appropriate chair for Fiona.

Practice Scenario 30.4
Step 2: Planning: Fiona

Fiona is a 5-year-old girl with cerebral palsy. The occupational therapist and her parents were seeking a supportive chair to enable her to engage in play and develop her hand-function skills. The parents grimaced at one particular chair in the catalogue, so the occupational therapist almost left it out of the picture. When all the advantages and disadvantages of the products were compared, both parents could see this 'ugly' chair was otherwise very suitable. They all agreed to see Fiona's reaction to it; she took to it immediately and the parents' satisfaction with its function and ease of use revised their attitude to its looks.

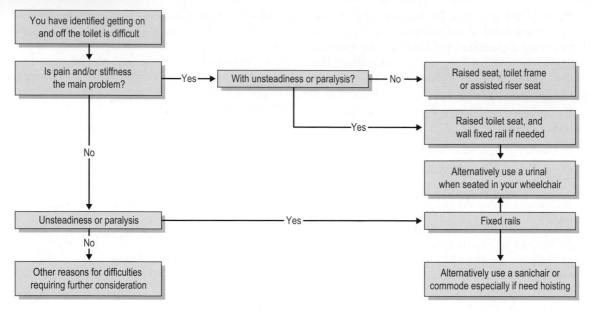

Figure 30.4 • Getting on and off the toilet (adapted from Pain, McLellan and Gore, *Choosing Assistive Devices: a guide for users and professionals*. Reproduced by permission of Jessica Kingsley Publishers)

There is some research evidence that guides the matching of person and assistive device for specific groups of products, but the coverage is patchy. The Centre for Evidence Purchasing (CEP) (2007) in the United Kingdom has a website that lists evaluations funded through the Department of Health since 2002. Earlier reports are available on request via email from CEP or held in health libraries in the United Kingdom. Evidence is sometimes used to compile flowcharts, also called decision trees or algorithms, which guide one's decisions as each successive question is answered. Pain et al (2003) reviewed literature and assessed evidence for devices related to the more commonly occurring aspects of daily living, and compiled flowcharts for straightforward decisions and matrices for more complex ones, to assist evidence-based decision-making. Figure 30.4 provides an example of a decision-making flowchart for the selection of an assistive device to enable a person to move onto and off a toilet, which could be used after the principle for such an item has been agreed with the person.

For other product areas, it is possible to compile a matrix oneself, with the essential user requirements down one axis and the potential products along the other. On the matrix is noted how well each product is expected to meet each user requirement, so building up a comprehensive picture. More detailed criteria can then be considered for those products that show good potential to meet the user's key needs. This exercise is time-consuming, so in practice it would mainly be used for novel or complex problems. The development of a decision-making matrix is illustrated in Practice Scenario 30.5, in the consideration of toilet needs of George.

Practice Scenario 30.5
Step 2: Planning: George

George is 62 and has multiple sclerosis. He and his wife were finalising the requirements for the major adaptations to their home with the occupational therapist. That day they were looking at automatic bidet toilets which would enable George to use the toilet and attend to subsequent hygiene needs without assistance. Five products had been researched by the therapist, and together they compiled a matrix (Table 30.3) to record the suitability of each against the criteria they had agreed as important. Products A and D had the greatest potential, so other criteria such as cost or delivery time, together with more information on reliability of Product D, would determine the final choice.

As has been stated above, trialling a product is the best way to decide the optimal product from a shortlist of two or three. However, this may be impractical, for example, when devices are not

Table 30.3 Matrix to compare automatic bidet systems for George (Practice Scenario 30.4)

User requirement	Product A	Product B	Product C	Product D	Product E
Elbow switch to operate wash/dry facility (ease of use)	Yes	No	Yes	Yes	Yes
Plumbed in so no connectors needed	Yes	Yes	No	Yes	Yes
Able to flush without wash/dry facility (for other users)	Yes	Yes	No	Yes	Yes
24-hour call out if system breaks down (post sales service)	Yes	Yes	No	Yes	No
Good track record for quality (reliability; low maintenance)	Yes	N/K	Yes	N/K	N/K
SCORES	5	3.5	2	4.5	3.5

Not known 'N/K' = 0.5, Yes = 1 and No = 0

available to test, or adaptation of the environment is needed as in George's case above. In such circumstances, alternative strategies are required, including an imaginary run-through of its use or simulation. Simulation can encompass:

- the use of scale plans, e.g. testing a new wheelchair's compatibility with the recipient's home with scale plan of the home and the proposed wheelchair (Abraham & Johnson (2006) highlight the impact of users' manoeuvring techniques on space required)

- testing a similar device so that unsatisfactory aspects can be identified (e.g. observing the user in a raiser recliner chair and discussing features that are suboptimal)

- visiting a centre where the device may be tested (e.g. taking the user to a show room that has a demonstration stair lift).

The ability to talk things through in detail is particularly important when the choice of solution is not clear-cut; in such cases, discussing and coming to agreement on why solutions are discarded and the relative merits of others, and applying the person's agreed priorities, will all increase confidence in the agreed solution. Everyone affected by the decision should be in agreement about the chosen solution. The person and any caregivers will have been involved from the outset, but it is necessary to bear in mind that the practitioner may still be regarded as the expert, and, therefore, will have to restore the balance by valuing people's contribution, and ensuring they understand any explanations and partake in the final decision. However much experience an occupational therapist has had, it is important to avoid the role of being the expert prescribing devices rather than a resource to enable people to make decisions. 'It is essential that, prior to making a final decision about equipment provision, the therapist ensures that the unique needs of the client have been fully considered' (Wielandt & Strong 2000, p. 72). This is illustrated in Practice Scenario 30.6 in the prescription of a wheelchair for Polly.

Practice Scenario 30.6
Step 2: Planning: Polly

John had been working in the wheelchair services for 8 years. When Polly, a 36-year-old mother with rheumatoid arthritis, came in for assessment, he quickly identified a chair he considered would be most appropriate, taking into account her strength, occupational needs and home situation. However, he was conscious that Polly was still pouring over wheelchair catalogues, so he asked her to tell him her goals for the new chair. Then he clearly explained the advantages and disadvantages of each model. When John asked which she thought was best, she indicated two, one of which was his original choice.

Funding for the agreed assistive device may be through a statutory authority, a charity, insurance firm or the person's own finances. If one potential device would necessitate using a different source of funding from another, the person must be fully aware of this during the decision-making process. Presentation of a reasoned decision and evidence of a full discussion of options with the potential recipient will help justify the recommendation to the funding body. Once a solution is identified and funding is agreed, a timescale should be specified for the provision of the assistive device.

Step 3: Intervention

Once the assistive device has been chosen and obtained, the intervention includes its delivery, provision of training, and all necessary information for its use and maintenance. It is also necessary to come to an agreement about the timing of follow-up, when the effectiveness of the assistive device will be evaluated.

The assimilation of an assistive device into the person's routine is an active process of adjustment with a number of components:

- Instruction in its use for all concerned, for instance a hoist for a person who has a succession of caregivers over the week would need a plan drawn up to ensure training for every caregiver
- Acquiring the new skill of using it
- Possible adaptation of the occupation with which it has been chosen to assist
- Acceptance by the person of it for the time, place and occupation for which it was selected.

Physical, psychological and cultural factors were considered in the choice of device because these are central to the acceptance and integrated use of the chosen product. It is also important that learning to use the device is not too difficult and that this process is adequately supported, because failure at this stage can frequently be the cause of rejection of an assistive device. This is illustrated in Practice Scenario 30.7 where Grace attempted to become independent in opening jars.

Practice Scenario 30.7
Step 3: Intervention: Grace

A year after having a stroke, Grace bought a jar opener through a mail-order catalogue. It was described as easy to use and looked ideal. When it arrived she was excited and tried it out straight away. She put the rubber strip around the lid, but as she was threading it into the handle, it slipped off. The instructions were in small print and had no pictures so Grace did not find them useful. She tried on several other occasions then gave up, and resumed asking her neighbour to open jars when he called in.

Acceptance of an assistive device can be thought of as a process similar to any other change, namely: trying it out; evaluating its usefulness and desirability; starting to use it regularly; and, finally, assimilation of the device into how one thinks of the occupation (see Kronlöff & Sonn 1999). Full involvement in the decision-making process can enhance the readiness for change and provide a positive attitude to cope with any teething problems the solution may pose (Pain et al 2003) and increase satisfaction with it (Nordenskiöld 1997). The need for adequate instruction is illustrated in Practice Scenario 30.8, when James learns to use an induction loop system for the television.

Practice Scenario 30.8
Step 3: Intervention: James

James was a mentally alert 90-year-old with severe hearing loss who lived alone in a terraced house. A member of the sensory impairment team had visited and supplied a device for listening to the television via a neck-worn induction loop. During the visit she explained it to him, he had successfully tried it out, and an instruction booklet was left. That evening, James tried it again, but for some reason it didn't work. He looked at the booklet but couldn't identify the problem. The following day he tried again and found that he had not had the neck loop on, and managed to use it successfully. However, the next day, there was another problem, so he rang the person who had delivered the device and explained he could not get it to work. She visited James again and went through the instructions, got James to try it out, and highlighted the step by step summary in the booklet. James and his neighbours were delighted that he could now use it confidently.

An appropriate level of support during the assimilation of an assistive device into the person's lifestyle can impact positively on a person's independence and quality of life, and also reduce the level of wastage of resources through infrequent or non-use of a product. This intervention does not have to be by the occupational therapist; peer modelling or tuition can be very effective as illustrated in Practice Scenario 30.9.

Practice Scenario 30.9
Step 3: Intervention: Daniel

Daniel was a 23-year-old who had sustained a spinal injury. He had been taught how to manage his wheelchair by therapists but did not feel confident. Seeing his therapists hop into a chair to demonstrate a manoeuvre just emphasised his disability. He was offered a wheelchair skills' class which he reluctantly agreed to attend. It was run by another person with paraplegia who was full of life and enthusiasm. Daniel found her to be a good instructor, because he knew she really used the skills she taught. For the first time he realised that his wheelchair could become an integral part of life rather than a hated necessity.

Step 4: Evaluation

Evaluation encompasses discussing the effectiveness of the assistive device in meeting goals; considering alternatives if it was unsatisfactory; measuring outcomes; and setting up a review system as appropriate.

The objectives agreed at the outset should be reviewed in discussion with all concerned, and the criteria used to assist selection of the device may be reapplied to evaluate its effectiveness. The time lag that is appropriate between supply and evaluation will depend on the product (the degree of learning it requires, the physical skill it requires and its effect on the way the occupation is undertaken), the frequency that the occupation is undertaken and the person's abilities. For example, a level-access shower may obviously meet the objective of independent ablutions, but questions about getting in and out, water containment, use of the shower controls and doors/curtains cannot be asked until the person has tried it out a few times. If the device involves caregivers, then their abilities and frequency of using the device must also be taken into account.

If the goal and objectives were not achieved, the reasons must be identified collaboratively, and the appropriate point on the problem-solving process returned to (Figure 30.3). For example, an unsatisfactory grip on a pick-up stick requires a look at alternative pick-up sticks, whereas failure to learn how to use a voice simulator may require more instruction, time for practice or a return to the decision-making cycle for an alternative solution. There is a body of research into the non-use of assistive devices which suggests that in the medium to long term, changing physical needs are the commonest reasons for cessation in use (Hocking 1999, Hoffmann & McKenna 2004, Pape et al 2002, Wessels et al 2003). However, there is still scope for more research to be done in this area to define more fully how attitudes and lifestyle affect usage, and how good design can address these needs as well as those of usability.

The method of evaluation will depend on the person concerned and the complexity of the intervention. In some cases a letter or telephone call is sufficient, while a visit is indicated for others. It has been acknowledged that developing outcome measures following provision of assistive devices can be difficult. This is because they are often provided for people with a progressive deteriorating condition to prevent or slow the loss of independence (Audit Commission 2004). Hence improvement with the device may not be discerned. However, there are measures specific to assistive devices that can be used to ensure systematic evaluation (Heaton & Bamford 2001). They include the:

- Quebec User Evaluation of Satisfaction with assistive Technology (QUEST), which evaluates the service which provided the product(s) and measures satisfaction with assistive devices (Demers et al 2000)

- Psychological Impact of Assistive Devices Scale (Day & Jutai 1996, PIADS 2007), a self-completion tool which has been designed to address the aspects of quality of life that devices affect. It has three subscales, namely competence, adaptability and self-esteem; these may not correlate directly with change in occupational performance (Buning et al 2001), but are factors that are important outcomes for the person concerned

- Efficiency of Assistive Technology and Services 6-D (EATS 1998). This is derived from EuroQol (2007) but amended to measure autonomy rather than physical ability. It provides a Quality of Life measure that its developers recommend as being more appropriate for assistive device users than other Quality of Life measures which are biased towards physical abilities

- KWAZO is a self-completion tool to evaluate the quality of service delivery to be applied after the provision of an assistive device. It is a seven-item questionnaire, and owes its name to a contraction of 'quality of care' in Dutch (Dijcks et al 2006).

The implementation of an evaluation is illustrated in Practice Scenario 30.10 with Graham.

Practice Scenario 30.10
Step 4: Evaluation: Graham

Graham was 52 and worked in the purchasing department of a large firm. He had been concerned that his Parkinson's disease was affecting his ability to use his computer. Following an assessment at work he had been provided with a tremor-resistant mouse and a voice-activated program which looked compatible with his personal computer and software. Since it had been supplied he had spent time using the online tutorials, training the voice recognition, and testing them out. Two weeks after delivery, the occupational therapist telephoned to ask how it was going and used the Psychological Impact of Assistive Devices Scale (PIADS) as an evaluation tool. Graham had mastered most aspects, but was having difficulty with spoken commands for one piece of software. The occupational therapist suggested some individualised tuition that could be arranged through Abilitynet (2007), which specialised in accessible computing. After this additional training, Graham became an expert user and had achieved his goal of continuing work. PIADS was reapplied and showed improved levels of competence and self-esteem using these devices.

Conclusion

The purpose of this chapter has been to present the theory, values and problem-solving process in relation to assistive technology. It has sought to provide a structure to assist new practitioners in the complex process of choosing optimal assistive devices to enable people to engage in occupations. The process of deciding which device is most effective demands theory-based, meaning-based and pragmatic reasoning, combined through reflective, person-centred practice. Active collaboration is required with the person at every stage. The problem has to be clearly defined regarding the person, occupation, and environment. Possible solutions need to be identified, clearly communicated and carefully compared using a structured approach to identify an optimal solution. The chosen device should be introduced with adequate instruction in its use, and support during the process of change during which it is incorporated into the person's life. Finally, the outcome must be evaluated against the objectives agreed at the outset, and outcome measures used to provide systematic evidence of the effectiveness of provision.

Engaging with the person to ensure psychological, social and cultural factors are all fully considered as well as the physical ones, minimises the risk of a device being inappropriate or unacceptable and, therefore, unused. This helps to ensure that resources are utilised effectively and that the person will experience assistive devices as desirable and satisfactory for enabling them to engage in their chosen occupations.

References

Abilitynet. Available online: http://www.abilitynet.org.uk. Accessed 7 Mar 2007.

Abraham, B. & Johnson, G. (2006). Constrained outlines: a method for creating access guidelines for individual wheelchair users. *British Journal of Occupational Therapy* 69(8), 379–385.

Anson, D. (2006). Assistive technology. In: H. McHugh Pendleton & W. Schultz-Krohn, (Eds). *Pedretti's occupational therapy practice skills for physical dysfunction.* (6th ed). Philadelphia, Elsevier, pp. 349–369.

Audit Commission. Assistive technology independence and well-being. (2004). Available online: www.audit-commission.gov.uk/reports/NATIONAL-REPORT. Accessed 24 Feb 2007.

Buning, M., Angelo, J. & Schmeler, M. (2001). Occupational performance and the transition to powered mobility: A pilot study. *American Journal of Occupational Therapy*, 55(3), 339–344.

Canadian Association of Occupational Therapists (2002). *Enabling occupation: an occupational perspective (revised edition)*. Ottawa, CAOT ACE Publications.

Canadian Association of Occupational Therapists (2005). Canadian occupational performance measure. (4th edn). Available online: http://www.caot.ca/copm/index.htm. Accessed 25 Nov 2007.

Carnevali, D. (1995). Self-monitoring of clinical reasoning behaviours: promoting professional growth. In: J. Higgs & M. Jones, (Eds). *Clinical reasoning in the health professions*. Oxford, Butterworth Heinemann, pp. 179–190.

Centre for Evidence based Purchasing. Available online: http://www.pasa.nhs.uk/PASAWeb/NHSprocurement/CentreforEvidencebasedPurchasing/CEPoutputs/Assistivetechnology/LandingPage.htm. Accessed 29 Jan 2007.

College of Occupational Therapists (2004). *Definitions and core skills for occupational therapy*. London, College of Occupational Therapists.

Crabtree, M. & Lyons, M. (1997). Focal points and relationships: a study of clinical reasoning. *British Journal of Occupational Therapy*, 60(2), 57–64.

Day, H. & Jutai, J. (1996). Measuring the psychosocial impact of assistive devices: the PIADS. *Canadian Journal of Rehabilitation*, 9(2), 159–168.

Demers, L., Weiss-Lambrou, R. & Ska B. (2000). *Quebec User Evaluation of Satisfaction with Assistive Technology (QUEST version 2.0) – An outcome measure for assistive technology devices*. Webster, NY, Institute for Matching Person and Technology.

Design for all. Available online: http://www.lboro.ac.uk/departments/cd/research/groups/erg/dfa/. Accessed 5 Jan 2007.

Dijcks, B., Wessels, R., de Vlieger, S., Post, M. (2006). KWAZO, a new instrument to assess the quality of service delivery in assistive technology provision. *Disabililty Rehabilitation*, 28(15), 909–914.

Dutton, R. (1995). *Clinical reasoning in physical disabilities*. Baltimore, Williams, Wilkins.

Efficiency of Assistive Technology and Services (EATS) (1998). Deliverable 3 includes the questionnaires for IPPA and EATS 6–D, and describes their use. Available online: www.siva.it/ftp/eats_deliverable3.pdf. Accessed 25 Nov 2007.

EuroQoL. Available online: www.euroqol.org. Accessed 22 Jan 2007.

Foundation for Assistive Technology (FAST) (2007). Definition of the term 'Assistive Technology'. Available online: http://www.fastuk.org/home.php. Accessed 21 Nov 2007.

Hagedorn, R. (1996). Clinical decision making in familiar cases: a model of the process and implications for practice. *British Journal of Occupational Therapy*, 59(5), 217–222.

Hardwick, R. & Robbens, G. (1998). *Creativity and decision making*. Oxford, Wolsey Hall.

Heaton, J. & Bamford, C. (2001). Assessing outcomes of equipment and adaptations: issues and approaches. *British Journal of Occupational Therapy*, 64(7), 346–356.

Helen Hamlyn Research Centre. Available online: http://www.rca.ac.uk/pages/research/helen_hamlyn_research_centre_748.html. Accessed 5 Jan 2007.

Hocking, C. (1999). Function or feelings: factors in abandonment of assistive devices. *Technology and Disability*, 11, 3–11.

Hoffmann, T. & McKenna, K. (2004). A survey of assistive equipment use by older people following hospital discharge. *British Journal of Occupational Therapy*, 67(2), 75–82.

IMPT (Institute for Matching Person & Technology). MPT Tools. Available online: http://members.aol.com/IMPT97/mptdesc.html. Accessed 18 Jan 2007.

Kielhofner, G. (1995). *A model of human occupation – theory and application*. (2nd ed). Baltimore, Williams and Wilkins.

Kings Fund (2006). Telecare and older people (background paper for securing good care for older people – Wanless Social Care Review). 2006. Available online: www.kingsfund.org.uk/publications. Accessed 24 Feb 2007.

Kronlöff, G. & Sonn, U. (1999). Elderly women's way of relating to assistive devices. *Technology in Disability*, 10, 161–168.

Kuipers, K., McKenna, K. & Carlson, G. (2006). Factors influencing Occupational Therapists' clinical decision making for clients with upper limb performance dysfunction. *British Journal of Occupational Therapy*, 69(3), 106–114.

Miyamae, T., Tsuru, S., Yoshikawa, H. & Johnson, N. (1998). *Application of three dimensional model of self for understanding activities and roles*. Montréal, 12th International Conference of the World Federation of Occupational Therapists.

Nordenskiöld, U. (1997). Daily activities in women with rheumatoid arthritis. Aspects of patient education, assistive devices and methods for disability and impairment assessment. *Scandinavian Journal of Rehabilitation Medicine*, 29, 37.

O'Brien P. (2006). Access standards: evolution of inclusive housing. In: S. Clutton, J. Grisbrooke & S. Pengelly (Eds). *Occupational therapy: building on firm foundations*. London, Whurr, pp. 109–138.

Pain, H., McLellan, D. L. & Gore, S. (2003). *Choosing assistive devices: a guide for users and professionals*. London, Jessica Kingsley.

Pape, T., Kim, J. & Weiner, B. (2002). The shaping of individual meanings assigned to assistive technology: a review of personal factors. *Disability Rehabilitation*, 24(1–3), 5–20.

Parker, D. (2006). The client-centred frame of reference. In: E. Duncan (Ed.). *Foundations for practice in occupational therapy*. (4th Ed). London, Elsevier Churchill Livingstone, 193–215.

Paterson, M. & Summerfield-Mann, L. (2006). Clinical reasoning. E. Duncan (Ed.). *Foundations for practice in occupational therapy*. (4th Ed). London, Elsevier Churchill Livingstone, 315–335.

Pengelly, S. (2006). The social model and clinical reasoning. In: S. Clutton, J. Grisbrooke, S. Pengelly (Eds). *Occupational therapy: building on firm foundations.* London, Whurr, 43–63.

Pheasant, S. (1996). *Bodyspace: anthropometry, ergonomics and the design of work.* (2nd edn). London, Taylor & Francis.

PIADS. Available online: http://www.piads.ca/index.asp. Accessed 24 Mar 2007.

Priestley, M. (1999). *Disability, politics and community care.* London, Jessica Kingsley.

Ranka, J. & Chapparo, C. (2000). Teaching clinical reasoning to occupational therapists. In: Higgs J & Jones M (Eds). *Clinical reasoning in the health professions.* (2nd edn). Oxford, Butterworth Heinemann, 191–197.

Schön, D. (1983). *The reflective practitioner: how professionals think in practice.* New York, Basic Books.

Tomita, M., Mann, W., Fraas, L. & Burns L. (1997). Racial differences of frail elders in assistive technology. *Assistive Technology*, 9(2), 140–151.

Townsend, E. & Polatajko, H. (2007). *Enabling occupation II: Advancing an occupational therapy vision for health, well-being and justice through occupation.* Ottawa, CAOT Publications ACE.

WAI (Web Accessibility Initiative). Available online: http://www.w3.org/WAI/guid-tech.html. Accessed 18 Jan 2007.

Wessels, R., Dijcks, B., Soede, M. et al. (2003). Non-use of provided assistive technology devices, a literature review. *Technology in Disability*, 15(4), 231–238.

Wielandt, T. & Strong, J. (2000). Compliance with prescribed adaptive equipment: a literature review. *British Journal of Occupational Therapy*, 63(2), 65–75.

Resources

Americans with Disabilities Act. (1990). Summary. Available online: www.jan.wvu.edu/links/adasummary.htm. Accessed 26 Jan 2007.

Gick, M. & Holyoak, K. (1980). Analogical problem solving. *Cognitive Psychology*, 12, 306–355.

Gray, D., Quatrano, L. & Lieberman, M. (Eds). (1998). *Designing and using assistive technology: the human perspective.* Baltimore, Paul Brooks.

National Service Frameworks. Available online: http://www.dh.gov.uk/en/Policyandguidance/index.htm. Accessed 24 Mar 2007.

Scherer, M. (2000). *Living in the state of stuck: how assistive technology impacts the lives of people with disabilities.* (3rd Ed). Cambridge, Mass, Brookline Books.

Sumison, T. (1997). Environmental challenges and opportunities of client-centred practice. *British Journal of Occupational Therapy*, 60(2), 53–56.

Sumison, T. (2000). A revised definition of client centred practice. *British Journal of Occupational Therapy*, 67(1), 304–310.

Internet resources

Abledata	www.abledata.com
Assist UK	www.assist-uk.org
AT for people with dementia	www.atdementia.org.uk
Disabled Living Foundation	www.dlf.org.uk
Foundation for Assistive Technology	www.fastuk.org
RADAR	www.radar.org.uk
Rehacare	www.rehacare.de
RICAbility	www.ricability.org.uk
Youre able	www.youreable.com

Wheelchairs: posture and mobility

Rachael L. McDonald

CHAPTER CONTENTS

Introduction 470

Occupation, person and environmental
factors 470

Health conditions of wheelchair users 471

Wheelchair prescription. 473

Enablement of mobility interventions 474

Self-propelling wheelchairs or independent
manual mobility systems 474

Attendant-propelled wheelchairs or
dependent mobility system. 474

Powered wheelchairs. 475

Children's wheelchairs and buggies 475

High-performance sports wheelchairs . . . 476

Bariatric wheelchairs 476

Stand-up wheelchairs 476

Elevating wheelchairs. 476

Assessment for wheeled mobility
systems 476

Seating interventions 476

Biomechanics and seating 478

Effect of force on seating. 478

Centre of mass. 478

Why is it important to know about forces
acting on the body of someone in a
wheelchair?. 479

Tissue integrity and pressure ulcers 479

Physical assessment and interventions
for postural management. 480

Cushioning within wheelchairs 482

Conclusion. 485

SUMMARY

People who have difficulty with, or are unable to, walk independently often require wheeled mobility devices or wheelchairs to assist with their mobility. People who have increasing impairments often need extra cushions or special cushions placed within their wheelchair. The prescription and evaluation of wheeled mobility devices and their accessories is a growing area of occupational therapy practice. The goal of providing wheelchairs and seating is to enable a person to engage in occupations, even though the provision itself is a technical intervention. Traditional approaches to wheelchair provision have tended towards a medical model; however, occupational therapists have been uncomfortable, only concentrating on the impairments of body functions and structures. It is the occupational therapist's role to address the cognitive, affective, and spiritual elements of the person, along with the self-care, leisure and productivity aspects of occupation and the cultural, institutional and social aspects of the environment. The occupational therapist is able to help the person by enabling mobility, and, therefore, a range of occupations, in a way which is person-centred. An integral part of the provision of wheeled mobility intervention is a detailed and thorough assessment, which takes into account the person's age, life stage and roles, funding considerations, environmental barriers and facilitators, and social and personal factors, as well as more technical considerations, such as body biomechanics and prevention of pressure ulcers. Collaboration between the occupational therapist and the person, education, and appropriate supports are essential in order for the wheelchair provision to be meaningful to the person and enable him to perform his desired activities.

KEY POINTS

- People with restricted mobility often require wheelchairs to enable them to perform occupations.
- Mobility is fundamental to occupational engagement and limitations to mobility can be enhanced or replaced by wheelchairs.
- Wheelchairs have a dual purpose, as a medicinal product and as a means of enabling participation in occupation.
- Seating assessment and intervention fall into three areas: seating for postural control, seating for tissue integrity and seating for comfort.
- When providing advice on mobility, occupational therapists should consider the person's age, life stage and stage of adjustment, funding, environmental barriers and facilitators, social and personal factors, collaboration, education and support.

Introduction

People with restricted mobility often require wheelchairs to enable them to perform the occupations they carry out in life (Best et al 2005). A growing area of occupational therapy practice involves the prescription and evaluation of wheeled mobility devices, as well as the seating that is placed within them. The provision of seating and wheeled mobility can be classified as a technical intervention, where the goal is to enable participation in occupations (Reid et al 2002). Traditional approaches to this technical intervention have tended towards a medical model of providing a piece of equipment that enables the person to be transported from one place to another (McDonald et al 2004). In the past, therapy practice and reasoning has focused on 'fixing' body functions and structures, and, in so doing, has not considered people's occupational needs.

Increasingly, the International Classification of Functioning, Disability and Health (ICF) (World Health Organisation 2001) is being taken up by therapists working in the field of seating and mobility (Cohen 2007, Sprigle 2007a, 2007b). The ICF fits well with the provision of wheelchairs and seating, because of the individualised contextual factors of personal preference, environmental limitations, and a person's activity and participation, which are given equal weight to the individual's health condition or impairments in body functions and structures (McDonald et al 2004).

The challenge of wheelchair provision is that wheeled mobility and seating devices have a dual purpose. The first is that of a medicinal product, prescribed and funded in the same manner as other aids and devices, with the role of compensating for or improving impairments of body functions and structure (Sprigle 2007b). The other role is that of performance, in which wheeled mobility and seating has the potential to enable a person without independent mobility to be independent. However, as wheeled mobility has the potential to cause harm, effective provision is essential. Effective provision of seating and wheeled mobility enables the user to have health, activity, occupational performance, and participation, and it reduces the burden on the health system by reducing further morbidity and increasing the person's ability to access and participate in occupational performance.

If the occupational therapist concentrates only on providing a piece of mobility equipment for physical aspects of the person, then, according to the Canadian Model of Occupational Performance and Engagement (Townsend & Polatajko 2007) the cognitive, affective, and spiritual elements of the person, along with the self-care, leisure and productivity aspects of occupation and the cultural, institutional and social aspects of the environment, are not considered. In other words, by concentrating on one aspect of occupational engagement, the person's capacity for success or change in their occupation engagement is not addressed. The effectiveness of wheelchair and seating provision is dependent upon person-centred practice, using the individual's seating and positioning devices as a way of enhancing his participation in occupational performance and engagement (Rudman et al 2006).

Occupation, person and environmental factors

The key to providing wheeled mobility is the setting of measurable and achievable goals which enable the individual to participate in occupations (Mortenson et al 2007), and this is mirrored in the philosophy of occupational therapy (Creek 2003, Law et al 1996, Townsend & Polatajko 2007). The impact of seating and positioning is complex, and an individual's underlying physical conditions have dominated the provision of seating and mobility devices. In the case of postural management, occupation, activity, and participation are enabled by equipment, which makes up for the difficulties in body functions and structures that the individual has. However, the dominance of body functions and structures has meant that occupational engagement, doing and participating in the occupations that people want and need to do, have been a secondary issue to treating the health of the individual.

Despite legislation to the contrary, commonplace physical environments, such as public transport, remain barriers to participation in everyday life for people who use wheelchairs (Hoenig et al 2003, Hunt 2005). There are wheelchairs available that have special facilities to overcome environmental barriers, such as those mentioned later in this chapter; however, these devices are usually expensive, and do not suit every individual. Furthermore, decreased access to the environment reduces an individual's ability to participate in all activities and occupations, which affects a person's self-esteem and world view.

Whether or not a wheelchair and seating system is useful is ultimately due to the personal factors and acceptance by the user. Research on compliance and agreement with all assistive technologies has shown that failure to consider the opinions and preferences, as well as degree of confidence in assistive technology devices results in abandonment and rejection of these devices (Cushman & Scherer 1996, Demers et al 1996, 2000, Hocking 1999). White (1999) showed that there is a need for greater collaboration between therapists and carers, and the users of special seating systems, partly for the very reason that collaboration and communication is likely to have an effect both on compliance in using the system, as well as overall satisfaction with the service the user receives (Pain et al 2000, White 1999). Collaboration where the wheelchair user is engaged in decision making every step of the way helps to optimise the provision of wheelchair and seating equipment to ensure the most optimal outcome.

Health conditions of wheelchair users

Health conditions that cause mobility impairment or seating difficulty range from a wheelchair user who needs a wheelchair occasionally to someone who is unable to sit upright independently and, therefore, needs not only wheeled mobility, but sophisticated positioning equipment within the wheelchair. Provision of wheelchairs and related equipment costs the National Health Service (NHS) of the United Kingdom (UK) approximately £40 to £80 million per year (AuditCommission 2000, 2002, Sanderson et al 2000). This does not account for private or charity funding of wheelchairs and seating equipment, nor the cost of many hours of therapist time required for assessment, evaluation, and re-evaluation (AuditCommission 2002).

Total population estimates of wheeled mobility users range from 0.61% of people living outside institutions in the United States of America (USA) (Kaye et al 2002) to 1.46% of the population in the UK (AuditCommission 2000, Sanderson et al 2000). Translating this into different populations, the number of wheelchair users in the USA may be anywhere between 1.8 to 4.4 million people, 900,000 users in the UK, and in Australia, between 125,000 and 300,000 users. The number of people using wheelchairs has doubled in the last 10 years, and is growing by approximately 7% per year (Audit-Commission 2000, 2002, Jelier & Turner-Smith 1997, Sanderson et al 2000). The proportion of people using wheelchairs increases with age. The highest rate of both manual and electric wheelchair use is amongst the elderly (65 years or above), with working-aged adults the next most prominent group, and children and young people having the least prevalence.

People who have neurological, musculoskeletal and/or cognitive impairments may have difficulty with their mobility. Often, the impact of these impairments will change throughout the lifespan or with progression of the disease, so the role of the occupational therapist may change as the individual's difficulties with his occupational performance and engagement change.

Conditions that are neurological or have neuro-muscular implications include: congenital or genetic disorders such as cerebral palsy, spina bifida or muscular dystrophy; acquired difficulties such as cerebral-vascular accident, traumatic brain injury or spinal cord injury; and other conditions such as multiple sclerosis, Parkinson's disease, Guillain–Barre syndrome or Huntington's chorea. The impact of the neurological impairment results in alterations of muscle tone, muscle weakness or paralysis, and sensory disorders. The group of users who have neurological problems will also have difficulties secondary to their original diagnosis. For example, a large proportion of children diagnosed with cerebral palsy will also have dislocating hips (Scrutton et al 2001) and in later life may develop scoliosis (Majd et al 1997), leading to extra positioning needs.

Musculoskeletal conditions may interfere with the mobility of the person. One of the most common symptoms of these conditions is acute or chronic pain (Bearne et al 2007, Estes et al 2000). Other symptoms of musculoskeletal disorders include painful, swollen and stiff joints with muscle wasting around the affected joints leading to contractures (Estes et al 2000).

Other health conditions that affect an individual's mobility are the cognitive disorders, such as pervasive developmental disorders, intellectual impairments, and Alzheimer's disease.

There are two other groups of people who use wheelchairs: frail elderly people and people with chronic health conditions. Frail elderly people are the most common users of wheelchairs due to their reduced capacity to safely cover short and/or long distances, in the absence of an underlying health condition or impairment.

A primary health condition is often the reason why the person may need a wheelchair. However, the individual's occupational performance and engagement is not dependent on the health condition alone. Personal and environmental factors, along with a person's activity and participation needs, contribute significantly to the successful provision of mobility equipment. The individual's health condition and impairments of body function and structure in the context of his desired activity, ability to participate, and various institutional and personal factors are illustrated in Practice Scenario 31.1. This scenario also illustrates how a change in one part of the process can have a major effect on a person's life.

Practice Scenario 31.1
Potential outcomes with wheeled mobility

This Practice Scenario illustrates the key role assistive technology plays in supporting body structure and function, as well as activities and participation. A criti-

cal path analysis allows comparison of likely outcomes for an individual with and without an optimal wheelchair and pressure cushion, and illustrates a complexity of other factors that must be considered alongside the wheelchair itself.

Critical path 1: optimal outcome

Orlando, 27, has a spinal cord injury resulting from a traffic accident, which means he is eligible for third-party funding. He undergoes rehabilitation and is discharged home with a combination of environmental adaptations, assistive technologies and personal care. These include stepless shower base and accessible toilet, both able to be accessed via padded, self-propelled over toilet/shower chair to minimise unnecessary transfers. His manual wheelchair is ultralight (8 kg), minimising the load he must propel, and light enough for him to pull into the passenger seat of a car and stow during car trips. The customised seat angle and rake support an active posture and wheel camber maximises self-propulsion. A lightweight, low-rise pressure cushion is fitted concurrently. Orlando is a 'beginner' now, but will develop high-level wheelchair skills over the next 12–18 months and the capacity to further adjust the wheelchair will ensure he does not 'grow out' of its capacity too soon. Orlando is actively involved in establishing his individualised package of personal care (hours and personnel) and in decreasing it over time as he becomes 'hardened' to daily activities. In the future, he is able to establish full independence, works full-time; plays sport; drives a car with hand controls; and can be said to engage in normal occupational opportunities for a man of his age.

Critical path 2: sub-optimal outcome

In this scenario, a fall from a ladder at home causes Orlando's spinal cord injury, thus he is not compensable. He undergoes the same rehabilitation process, but the environmental adaptations and assistive technologies provided are based upon public funding limits, which cap both type and cost of items regardless of individual client need. Orlando returns to a rental property where major modifications are not permitted, thus he needs to engage in multiple daily transfers onto the bath seat and toilet, and has a mid-cost, relatively heavy-pressure cushion and a 15 kg manual wheelchair, adjusted to fit, but not customised for him. His posture, therefore, tends to sacral sitting, with a resulting flexed position and slightly compressed chest cavity, which puts him at a slight biomechanical disadvantage when self-propelling and reaching. His personal care consists of twice-weekly visits from community nurses, which limit his capacity to make appointments or leave the house on those days, as they attend within a 4-hour window. Orlando performs multiple daily transfers onto hard surfaces, limits his hygiene to twice-weekly showers, and is propelling a mid-weight wheelchair. He has limited capacity to travel in vehicles as he requires assistance to lift and stow the wheelchair; therefore, his participation in community activities is minimal. Orlando's subsequent critical path thus includes frequent readmissions with pressure areas and compromised shoulder function. Bedrest to relieve pressure ulcers leads to a decrease in physical fitness, upper-limb strength, and independence. A powered wheelchair is required to enable independent mobility over distance, costing considerably more than an optimal manual wheelchair would have. Orlando's eventual outcome is a nursing home, where care costs plus his inability to work, decrease his disposable income to below pension level. He is no longer eligible for government funding for a replacement wheelchair as he is in residential care, further compounding his impoverished occupational opportunities and failure to accomplish life tasks.

Why the outcomes are different

The health condition is the same, but the outcomes are profoundly different. As we can see, an appropriate wheelchair is one essential component to ensure Orlando's critical path is on an upward trajectory. One critical difference is the resources available. Another is the professional reasoning of the prescribing occupational therapist. The occupational therapist who collaborates with the person to establish individualised occupational goals, and takes a whole-of-life approach can argue for best outcomes in view of the likely life trajectory of the person, enabling the achievement of occupational potential.

When providing advice on mobility, Orlando's occupational therapist must consider:
- age, life stage and stage of adjustment
- pragmatic constraints, such as funding
- environmental barriers and facilitators
- social and personal factors, which shape the individual's situation
- temporal aspects: the impact of the wheelchair and cushion through a day and into the future.
- collaboration, education, and support.

This Practice Scenario was provided by Natasha Layton. At the time of writing Natasha was working as an occupational therapist in Melbourne, Australia.

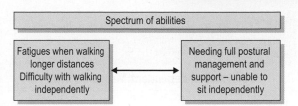

Figure 31.1 • Spectrum of abilities of people who use wheelchairs

It is useful to think of people who need to use wheeled mobility and seating equipment as on a continuum. Figure 31.1 illustrates the continuum of users of wheelchairs in terms of their physical abilities or body functions and structures. The role of the occupational therapist may be as simple as suggesting that the person looks into alternative mobility (towards the left of the diagram), or they may conduct an assessment and modify equipment for people who are unable to sit by themselves. Whatever the involvement of the occupational therapist, many individuals considering using a wheelchair will find this confronting and extremely challenging as it provides evidence of the severity of their impairment (Farley et al 2003).

Another way of framing this is to determine the amount of assistance the person using a wheelchair requires, by using the Wheelchair Independent Measure (WIM) (Kelly & Clements 2000) (Table 31.1). The WIM suggests that the abilities of people with mobility impairment can range from levels 1 and 2, indicating complete dependence on a carer, to 6 and 7, indicating independence with appropriate wheeled mobility or environmental adaptation.

Wheelchair prescription

For convenience, wheelchair prescription may be divided into two areas:

1. Interventions where the primary purpose is to enable mobility

2. Seating interventions where the primary purpose is to alleviate physical impairments in order to enhance the individual's seated occupational skills.

There is often overlap between the two, but generally on the continuum of physical difficulties, those with less care needs will need less intervention with their wheeled mobility.

Table 31.1 Range of abilities of people with mobility impairments (reproduced with kind permission by Gael Kelly and Jane Clements, 2000)

Wheelchair Independent Measure (WIM)			
Levels			
Independence			
7	Complete independence (timely, safely)	100%	NO
6	Modified independence (device)	100% −	HELPER
Modified Dependence			
5	Supervision	90% +	
4	Minimal assist	75% +	
3	Moderate assist	50% +	HELPER
Complete Dependence			
2	Maximal assist	25% +	
1	Total assist	0% +	

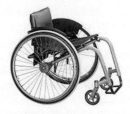

Figure 31.2 • Lightweight fixed-frame wheelchair. The increased seat to back angle and position of the seat decrease the stability of the chair but increase the mobility for a highly skilled user

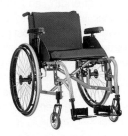

Figure 31.3 • Lightweight folding chair. Often used for people who need mobility help for short distances or are pushed by someone else.

Enablement of mobility interventions

Mobility is fundamental to the independent occupational engagement of individuals. Limitations to mobility can be enhanced or replaced by assistive technologies, in this case wheelchairs. Wheeled mobility may not need to have high specification cushions or seating devices, but when inappropriately prescribed can have a detrimental effect on the abilities and future body functions and structures of the user. There are three basic types of wheeled mobility base: self-propelling wheelchairs or independent manual mobility systems; attendant-propelled wheelchairs or dependent mobility systems; and powered wheelchairs.

Self-propelling wheelchairs or independent manual mobility systems

Many users fall into categories 6 or 7 on the WIM, or have been given wheelchairs to encourage the ability to self propel. These types of wheelchairs are for people who can propel the device by themselves. The chairs have either a 'fixed frame' (Figure 31.2) or 'folding frame' (Figure 31.3). The chairs have big wheels at the rear, and small wheels at the front to enable the user to push the chair in the most effective and efficient way. In general, fixed-frame chairs are easier to push and more sturdy, but unable to fold, and folding chairs have more apparatus and are heavier to push, but more convenient for storage. Recent studies have shown that it is imperative that the configuration of the wheelchair for the individual who self propels is correctly set up, as incorrect solutions can cause secondary problems with shoulder injuries (Boninger et al 2000, Curtis et al 1999, Robertson et al 1996). Thus, it is important to consider the occupational engagement needs of the user both in the short and the long term, to prevent this type of injury.

Attendant-propelled wheelchairs or dependent mobility system

These wheelchairs are used by people who are unable to push themselves independently, and include buggies or pushchairs for younger users, as well as wheelchairs that are purely for someone else to push. This type of chair tends to have small wheels at the back and the front, and is an essential

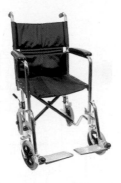

Figure 31.4 • Attendant-propelled manual wheelchair, which has increased stability, but no possibility for independent mobility

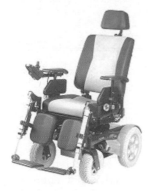

Figure 31.5 • Powered wheelchair, with joystick control on right hand side

back up if the person uses a powered wheelchair as their main form of independent mobility (Figure 31.4).

Powered wheelchairs

Powered wheelchairs are used by people who are capable of independent mobility, but are unable to achieve this through pushing themselves. They are usually driven using a joystick that controls the movement (Figure 31.5), but alternative controls are available for people who have limited upper-limb use.

Powered mobility, or electric indoor or outdoor wheelchairs and scooters enable the individual who either fatigues easily or does not have the physical skills to propel a wheelchair independently. They have, at times, been controversial: for example, parents of disabled children may not want their child to have powered mobility, as they may be

concerned about safety; professionals may be concerned that by giving a person powered mobility, that person will lose muscle power and skills, and may put on weight due to reduced exercise. However, recent studies have shown that people who begin to use powered wheelchairs do not increase their weight, but do increase their activities, and thus also their participation (Bottos et al 2001, Brandt et al 2004, Davies et al 2003, Kotsch 2003, Yang et al 2007). Additionally, the use of powered wheelchairs has been shown to improve wellness and quality of life.

It is important to recognise that powered mobility gives users the ability to have mobility, if they previously had none, and increase their opportunities to participate in daily activities. For example, the provision of a scooter to a person who cannot walk long distances may enable them to do grocery shopping.

There are different means of controlling powered mobility. The most common way is to 'drive' a chair using a joystick. For people who have weakness of the upper limb, the weight required to push a joystick may need to be modified, through the use of either a program in the computer system of the powered chair itself or a specially made joystick. If a person is unable to use their hands, then alternative controls for joysticks are available, such as single or multiple switches to operate a scanning interface (e.g. chin joysticks, light touch joysticks or integrated systems such as WiseDX or ClickToGo). Alternatives to standard joystick control of a powered wheelchair can be expensive and often complex. However, providing the means for independent mobility to disabled individuals makes an enormous difference to their quality of life and well-being.

Children's wheelchairs and buggies

Children who are unable to walk independently due to underlying difficulties still need to be transported. In this case, many parents want to transport their child as quickly and easily as possible; a range of buggies that have been made for a child of extra height and/or weight are available. These buggies look like standard buggies for younger children, but are usually larger and sturdier. Another special consideration for children is that their needs change as their bodies grow. Therefore, chairs and seating systems that grow with the child are an essential consideration.

High-performance sports wheelchairs

People who are very proficient at using their wheelchairs, such as people who have a low spinal cord injury, often use high-performance wheelchairs. These can significantly enhance the individual's ability to participate in their daily lives and occupations. These wheelchairs often have a rigid frame, so to transport the chair without the user in it often involves unclipping the wheels. In order to gain speed and manoeuvrability, the user may sacrifice some of the stability of the chair.

Bariatric wheelchairs

Bariatrics is the branch of medicine that deals with obesity. Regular wheelchairs can usually support a body weight up to 135 kg. Bariatric wheelchairs can accommodate people with body mass of up to 450 kg.

Stand-up wheelchairs

There are a number of environmental restrictions when using a wheelchair, due to the decreased height of the user. In order to promote independence and increase access to activities, some people like to use a stand-up wheelchair. They are a specialised device, and there are a number of pre-requisites for use, usually concerning safety. Biomechanical considerations of centre of gravity are extremely important here.

Elevating wheelchairs

The seated wheelchair position is a barrier to many activities that require standing height. An alternative to standing wheelchairs is those that elevate – instead of the individual assuming an assisted standing device, the whole seat is elevated.

Assessment for wheeled mobility systems

When assessing for even very basic wheeled mobility the occupational therapist still has to take into consideration the posture of the person. Figure 31.6 illustrates the most basic measurements that the therapist needs to take. This gives the therapist only a list of the basic size of the wheelchair and seating system. It does not give the individual information required about the person, their mobility goals or their underlying difficulties with body functions and structures, particularly in relation to an individual's

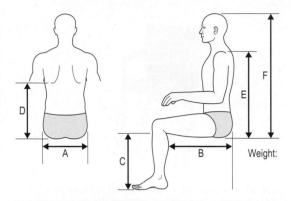

> Basic seating measurements
> A, Widest measure across the hips
> B, Rear of the buttocks to the inside of the bent knee
> C, Bottom of the heel to the inside of the bent knee
> D, Seat to scapula
> E, Seat to top of shoulder
> F, Seat to top of head

Figure 31.6 • Basic seating measurements

reduced sensitivity or movement and inability to correct their own position. The implications of this are that the person's independence and occupational engagement can be reduced if the mobility equipment provided is not appropriate. It is also important to assess the individual's occupational performance following provision of the wheelchair. Table 31.2 outlines some specific problems often found in wheelchairs and the potential implications of these problems.

Seating interventions

Seating intervention falls into three broad categories (Geyer et al 2003):

- Seating for postural control
- Seating for tissue integrity
- Seating for comfort.

Seating for postural control usually applies to people with neurological origins to their impairments of body functions and structures, whereas seating for tissue integrity and comfort apply to all wheeled mobility users. Helping wheelchair users sit as best they can is seen as a default position for the person to participate in their daily life. Thus, it fits into occupational therapy practice as an underlying skill that the person requires in order to achieve

Table 31.2 Examples of consequences of inappropriate seating provision

Inappropriate seating prescription	Leads to difficulties in body functions and structures and outcome	Leads to occupational performance difficulties in
Wheelchair seat too wide	Inability to reach wheels to self propel Encourages pelvic obliquity or unstable sitting base – hips and thighs move about	Poor stability in seating leads to decreased upper limb and head skills, leading to difficulties in eating, using hands and other IADL skills Decreases independence by hampering self propulsion or independent driving Environmental barriers increased
Wheelchair seat too narrow	Encourages pelvic obliquity, instability Discomfort Increased risk to tissue integrity	Discomfort decreases ability to perform independent functional activity Instability (as above) Pressure ulcer development decreased health and well-being of the user
Wheelchair seat too long	Pulls person forward in chair, increasing pressure on sacrum, encourages slumping and instability Compromises circulation of lower limb and creates pressure area behind knees Does not support the spine	Person unable to use their hands Pressure ulcer development – reduces person's health and well being
Wheelchair seat too short	Encourages instability by reducing base of support Increased pressure on thigh and supporting area	Pressure ulcer development reduces person's health and well-being Unstable sitting base leads to decreased ability to use hands and head to perform daily activities
Armrests too high	Elevates shoulders resulting in discomfort, encouragement of kyphosis and hyperextension of neck Reduces ability to use arms if relying on armrest for support	Reduces ability to self-propel or drive Reduces health and quality of life
Armrests too low	Encourages slumping either forward or to the side due to lack of support	Possible reduction of respiration, thus increasing fatigue Instability decreases physical ability to perform daily activities
Footplates too high	Discomfort in hips and knees Abduction of hips Adduction and internal rotation of hips, leading to increased risk of dislocation Increases pressure on buttocks and sacrum. Reduces base of support.	Instability decreases ability to perform daily activities Pressure ulcer reduces health and well-being of person
Footplates too low	May hit front castors, or hit pavements/curbs Pulls pelvis forward and encourages slumping and poor sitting stability	Potential environmental barriers increased

optimum occupational performance. However, it is a technical skill and requires some understanding of biomechanical principles.

Biomechanics and seating

When managing postural problems with the aim of enhancing an individual's ability to engage in various occupations, it is important to understand that the management of posture is governed by some basic biomechanical principles. The ability to sit and be stable comes from the underlying structural stability of the musculoskeletal system in conjunction with the body's biomechanical alignment, neurological, and vestibular systems. However, people with some spinal, neurological, orthopaedic, and other injuries do not have the underlying structural stability to support themselves in a regular seated position. Pre-requisites for stable sitting are a stable base of support through the pelvis and lower limbs, as well as stability throughout the trunk and upper body. In order to understand the concepts of managing posture, some understanding of how physical principles act on the human body is necessary.

Seating systems to manage posture have two aims:

- To prevent the development of deformity, secondary to the condition of the person

- To use the laws of biomechanics to give the person some stability so that they are able to participate in occupations.

Postural management devices work by applying forces to the body that counteract either the body's own internal forces or that of gravity.

Effect of force on seating

Forces can act either internally (e.g. a spastic muscle), or externally (e.g. a seating system). Stable or balanced seating is achieved if there is a balance of forces acting on a person. These forces include 'normal' or compression forces, 'shearing' force and gravitational force. Gravitational forces always act on a body. Most people are able to hold themselves up against gravity, but for people with low muscle tone, this is difficult and becomes an important consideration for seating and positioning.

The other two types of force which are essential to know about are 'normal or compression' forces and 'shearing' force (Figure 31.7). A normal force is

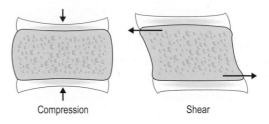

Figure 31.7 • Illustration of the effect of compressive and shear forces

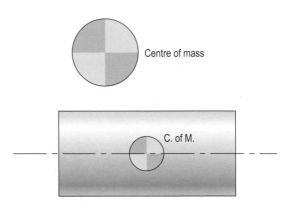

Figure 31.8 • Centre of mass of a cylinder

when the stress/force is ***perpendicular*** to the material/face (i.e. skin). In sitting, compression or normal force means that the blood vessels, muscles, and skin tissue are 'compressed'. This means oxygenation of the cells in the area being compressed is reduced. We will come back to the implications of this later in the chapter. Shear force is ***parallel or tangential*** to the face of the material (in this case skin). Shear force causes rubbing of the skin over the bone (think blisters from uncomfortable shoes). This leads to sores, which, combined with compression leads to pressure ulcers.

Centre of mass

The centre of mass, or composite mass, is the place where a person's weight is concentrated, in a downward way, together with gravity. A cylinder of constant diameter and density will have a centre of mass mid-way along the centre of the cylinder (Figure 31.8), but for a human being standing in the anatomical position, centre of mass is just in front of the spinal column at the level of S2 (Figure 31.9). When seated, the centre of mass changes – generally, it falls in front of the body, outside the trunk (Figure 31.10). However, we can manipulate the

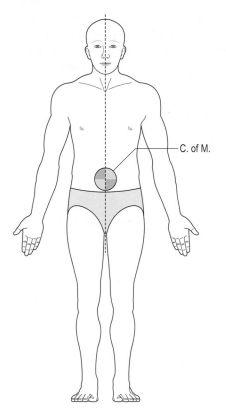

Figure 31.9 • Centre of mass of human body in anatomical position is in front of the spinal column at the level of S2

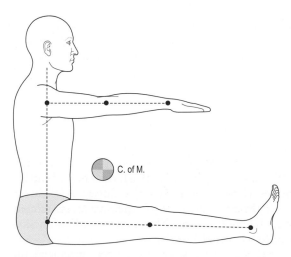

Figure 31.10 • Centre of mass changes as the body attains the seated position

centre of mass depending on the configuration of the wheelchair. For a person to be stable the centre of mass must fall within their base of support – in standing this is two feet, but in wheelchair seating, this is the base of the wheelchair. The centre of mass is very important in the provision of seating, as the effect of gravity together with where modifications are placed will determine how stable the person is in their seating system. If we make the wheels forward of the centre of mass, the person will tip backwards – such as when going up a curb. The position of the forward wheels is very important also; for example, if the width of the wheels is too narrow, the person is likely to tip sideways. If the front wheels are too far back, the person is at risk of tipping forward. Consideration of the centre of mass is essential for the safety and stability of a person, and thus their ability to perform activities.

Why is it important to know about forces acting on the body of someone in a wheelchair?

In assessment and provision of wheeled mobility and seating, the therapist must investigate, think and make a judgement about what effect mechanics have on the bodies of people who cannot move out of a sitting position. It is important to understand that the forces acting on the body are not always obvious, and that they may be internal as well as external. It is important to think about all the forces that are acting on the body not just the obvious ones. We use biomechanics and forces to:

- enable somebody to attain and maintain a stable position

- encourage comfort, so that the person is able to perform activities

- encourage occupation through comfort, stability and enabling the person to perform activities

- help prevent deformity by counteracting the forces that are acting on the body due to muscle tone, etc.

- help prevent the development of pressure ulcers.

Tissue integrity and pressure ulcers

Often, people who use wheelchairs and sit for long periods develop problems with their tissue integrity. Tissue integrity can be defined as the physiologic condition at which the skin and underlying tissues maintain function, structure, and viability (de Laat et al 2005). Impairments of the tissue or skin can lead to pressure ulcers (also known as decubitus ulcers and pressure sores). A pressure ulcer is an area of skin that breaks down, often when a person stays in one position for too long – as when sitting in a wheelchair all day. The constant pressure against the skin reduces blood supply, and the tissue that is supplied by that blood supply may die. A pressure ulcer starts by reddened skin (Stage 1), but then goes on to form a blister or an open sore (Stage 2), and then a sore that looks like a crater (Stage 3). Any further than this, the pressure ulcer becomes so deep that there is damage to the muscle and bone (Stage 4). The secondary effects of this include infection (Brillhart 2005, de Laat et al 2005). The consequences of developing pressure ulcers are poor health, but also restrictions in ability and opportunity to engage in occupations – through restrictions in mobility, enforced bed rest, and the need for surgery.

Pressure, which causes the blockage or occlusion of the vessels transporting blood to the tissues and removing the metabolic waste products away from the tissues, is the major factor causing pressure ulcers. As pressure increases, the length of time required to develop a blockage of the vessels decreases; so the aim of many interventions is to keep the amount of pressure to a minimum. Places where the individual bears weight through bony prominences, such as the ischial tuberosities and sacrum, are particularly at risk. So if the force is distributed over a small area (such as a bone) the pressure will be more than if it is distributed over a large area. Friction, where skin is pulled sideways over bone when moving, is a particular risk for developing pressure ulcers (Aissaoui et al 2001, Brillhart 2005). Tissue death can occur from shearing both inside and outside the body. The friction causes the surface of the skin to be rubbed away faster than it can be replaced (de Laat et al 2005).

Other factors that affect a person's susceptibility to or risk of developing pressure ulcers include heat and moisture of the skin. People who are incontinent, for example, have increased moisture in the same area that there are compressive and shearing forces. Age is another factor, as elasticity of skin decreases with age. Excess weight or malnourishment, inability to move parts of your body without assistance, and diseases that affect blood flow also increase the risk of pressure ulcer development (Apatsidis et al 2002, Stinson et al 2003). It is important that pressure ulcers are managed, as they can prevent a person participating in daily life activities.

Physical assessment and interventions for postural management

A thorough assessment for wheeled mobility, in addition to basic body measurements (Figure 31.6) should also involve activity, participation, and personal and environmental considerations as well. Consider Practice Scenario 31.1 and the fact that the difference between optimal and sub-optimal outcome has a great deal to do with considering all the contexts within which an individual operates, not just their body. Until recently, there were very few standardised assessments, but there has been recognition of the need for outcome measures in this field. A brief list of assessments can be found in Table 31.3. When considering only body functions and structure, or the physical aspects of the person, the physical assessment should be conducted in a seated position, outside of a chair, as well as in a supine position, to measure the person's underlying physical skills. The assessment should consider the individual's inherent postural control, as well as his underlying range of motion or orthopaedic factors.

Postural control

In relation to wheeled mobility, postural control refers to the way that a person sits, and is commonly evaluated by the person sitting on a plinth, a set of boxes or a chair without arms or back, in order to judge the level of competence in this position. There are some specific assessments which judge this postural control, mainly developed for children, and generally categorise an individual according to the ability of the person to sit by himself. Examples of these specific assessments include the Chailey Scales of Sitting (Mulcahy et al 1988), the Level of Sitting Scales (Fife et al 1991), the Sitting Assessment Scale (Myhr et al 1993) and the Sitting Assessment for Children with Neuromotor Dysfunction (SCAND) (Reid 1995).

Although these scales have been developed for children, what is common to all diagnoses and age ranges is the concept of progression from sitting without help, sitting with the hands free (i.e. the individual can use his hands to do activities without any external supports), sitting holding on (i.e. the

Table 31.3 Examples of assessment and outcome measurement tools to do with seating and wheelchairs

Name or type of assessment	What it does	Who is it for	Reference
Pressure Mapping Systems	Measure skin interface pressure between the seated surface and the skin of the user	All, but primarily adults	(Barbenel 1991, Pellow 1999, Brienza et al 2001, Crawford et al 2005)
Seating and Mobility Script Concordance Test of Spinal Cord Injury	Assesses competencies in professional reasoning of therapists providing seating equipment.	Seating Therapists	(Cohen 2003, Cohen et al 2005)
TAWC (Tool for Assessing Wheelchair disComfort)	Assessment to determine comfort within a wheelchair	Full-time wheelchair users with intact sensation (adult)	(Crane, Holm et al. 2007)
Seating assessment tool for community use	Guidelines for allocation of pressure cushions	Adult users at risk of compromised tissue integrity	(Shipperley & Collins 1999)
Wheelchair Outcome Measure (WhOM)	Client-specific tool which identifies individual goals for seating	Adult wheelchair users	(Mortenson et al 2007)
Functioning Everyday in a Wheelchair (FEW)	Questionnaire to assess everyday functioning from a wheelchair	Adult wheelchair users	(Mills et al 2002)
Functioning Everyday in a Wheelchair Performance (FEW-P)	Observational assessment of performance to accompany questionnaire	Adult wheelchair users	(Mills et al 2002)
Chailey level of ability Scales	7-point scale	Children with cerebral palsy	(Pountney et al 2000)
Seated Postural Control Measure	Observational assessment divided into two parts; physical assessment and seated function	Developed for children with neurological disorders but adapted recently for adults with neurological problems	(Fife et al 1991, Gagnon et al 2005)
The Sitting Assessment for Children with Neuromotor Dysfunction (SCAND)	Observational assessment using video camera to assess level of sitting	Children with neuromotor problems	(Reid 1995)
Wheelchair User's Shoulder Pain Index (WUSPI)	Index of shoulder pain and discomfort	Adult active wheelchair users	(Curtis et al 1995)
Obstacle Course Assessment of wheelchair user performance (OCAWUP)	10 items which represent environmental barriers to people using different types of wheelchairs	Any wheelchair user	(Routhier et al 2003, 2004, 2005)

individual needs extra help in sitting or will have to hold on, and thus not have hands free to do activities) to the person who is fully dependent and is unable to sit on a plinth or mat without falling over. Each of these levels requires different levels of seated support.

Orthopaedic factors

Measurement of orthopaedic factors involves measuring passive joint range of motion, often in supine and in sitting. It involves the identification of joints and body segments that are not symmetrical, and, therefore, at risk of developing deformity. There are three terms used to describe deformity: mobile deformity, fixed deformity, and structural deformity (Scrutton 1978, Williamson 2003). A mobile deformity is maintained by muscle power and/or gravity and can be corrected passively. This is the area in which correction by equipment is thought to be most useful. A fixed deformity (or contracture) is one that cannot be corrected passively as the soft tissue (muscle, ligament, etc.) does not allow a full range of movement at a joint. Structural deformity is one that is caused by abnormal bone shape or lack of joint integrity. Trying to correct a fixed or structural deformity by positioning may cause discomfort, and even stress and strain on the long bones of the individual, and increases their risk of pressure ulcer development (Brunner & Baumann 1994, Farley et al 2003).

The role of postural management is either to attempt to correct a deformity that is not fixed, or to accommodate a deformity that is fixed, thereby preventing the development of a secondary deformity. The examination should involve measurement of the joints of the hips, pelvis, knees, feet, upper limbs and head to decide which of these goals is most appropriate (Trefler & Taylor 1991, Trefler et al 1993). Table 31.4 identifies some possible secondary difficulties to individuals caused by inappropriate wheelchair provision, along with possible solutions to reduce/eliminate each identified difficulty.

Cushioning within wheelchairs

There are two main types of cushions for wheelchairs: adaptive seating and pressure cushion.

Adaptive seating systems

Adaptive seating systems are devices that seek, by using mechanical forces to correct or accommodate

to a person's postural difficulty. The purpose of providing adaptive seating is complex and varied. Research into adaptive seating systems remains largely descriptive and methodologically poor. Some authors assert that a seating system is an extended orthotic device, as it serves to support, align, prevent or correct deformities and improve the functions of body parts (Bergen et al 1990, Cook et al 2007, Healy et al 1997). Some authors claim that a 'good' adaptive seating system will reduce undesirable tone and reflexes, facilitate normal movement, maintain postural alignment, prevent tissue breakdown, decrease fatigue, enhance physiological function, and maximise stability (Cook & Hussey 2002, Healy et al 1997, Mulcahy et al 1988, Myhr & von Wendt 1990, Roxborough 1995). Others suggest that if the correct adaptive seating is not attained, then complications such as pressure sores, abrasions, shearing, and deformity, as well as reduced participation, will occur (Perr 1998). Postural management equipment needs to encourage the development of skills, and independence, and at the same time to respond to growth and changes in body shape, in environment and treatment plans (Cox 2003).

It is very difficult to summarise different types of adaptive seating systems, as the people who use them have complicated impairments of body functions and structures, and the configuration of adaptive seating must be on an individual basis.

It is important to remember that adaptive seating systems are used with people with complex physical problems, and the aim is to increase their ability to engage in occupations as well as prevent the development of secondary postural problems to ensure future occupational performance. An example of an adaptive seating system is shown in Figure 31.11. For an adaptive seating system, each body segment needs to be measured individually – it is an extension of the information in Table 31.2, but for individuals who have complex needs. Whatever the 'prescription', the adaptive seating system needs to be individually tailored to the individual's needs and goals.

Pressure cushions

A pressure ulcer refers to tissue necrosis caused by occlusion of blood supply usually caused when external pressure is put upon a bony prominence (Brienza et al 2001). In an attempt to reduce the pressure that may lead to an ulcer, pressure cushions are supplied (Brienza et al 2001). It has been found that pressure relieving/reducing seating surfaces are essential to the maintenance of skin integrity in a

Table 31.4 Examples of inappropriate wheelchair provision and the secondary difficulties caused to the individuals

Body part which presents difficulty with independent/ symmetrical seating	Description of movement	Secondary physical or occupational performance difficulties	Possible solutions
Posterior pelvic tilt	Pelvis is rotated or slumped backwards, due to spasticity in hip extensors, lack of muscle tone through the trunk	Pain where vertebrae are pushed together Protraction of shoulders reduce hand and upper limb activities Chin poking or hyperextension of neck occurs which may influence safety of swallowing	Check that length of seat is not too long Equipment such as pelvic belts, anti-thrust seats and pelvic bars can be employed
Anterior pelvic tilt	Pelvis is rotated forwards possibly due to weakness of trunk musculature, hip flexion contractures or hyper tonicity of lumbar extensors	Increased risk of hip dislocating anteriorly Instability of arms and head as both are pushed forwards Pain	Ensure seat is flat, not hammocked Hip belt positioned to counter the effect of the tilt
Pelvic obliquity	Pelvis is elevated on one side, judged by feeling the Anterior Sacro Iliac Spine (ASIS), and comparing line between them to the horizontal	Likelihood of secondary scoliosis increased Decreased stability of sitting position as balanced on one ischial tuberosity, often compensatory side flexion of trunk	Check the width of the seat
Pelvic rotation	Pelvis is rotated backwards on one side and forward on the other, due to asymmetry of muscle tone around the hip and trunk OR seat is too long on one side	Increases likelihood of developing secondary scoliosis Reduced stability in sitting Reduced ability to use hands – shoulder also rotated forward	Assess and accommodate for leg length discrepancy or hip ab/adduction contracture 45° bifurcate (Y-shaped) hip belt ASIS (Anterior Superior Iliac Spine) bar, rigid bar placed immediately below the ASIS
Scoliosis and kyphosis of spine	Neuromuscular or idiopathic curvature of the spine May be internally rotated around the vertebrae	Physical issues such as decreased respiration, increased gastro-oesophageal reflux Difficulty using one or both hands Difficulty holding head upright	Accommodation to fixed deformity, support of the body above and below the curve. Accommodation to spinal orthosis if worn May need to be reactive to spinal surgery
Side flexion (postural scoliosis) of trunk	Imbalance of tone throughout trunk, low tone of trunk and slumps to preferred side, or compensation for pelvic obliquity	Inability to use hands Increased susceptibility to develop fixed scoliosis Discomfort Poor head control	Firm seat base to reduce pelvic obliquity through hammocking Pads or moulded seat to counteract trunk position Spinal orthosis

(cont'd)

Table 31.4 Examples of inappropriate wheelchair provision and the secondary difficulties caused to the individuals—cont'd

Body part which presents difficulty with independent/symmetrical seating	Description of movement	Secondary physical or occupational performance difficulties	Possible solutions
Forward flexion (kyphosis) of trunk	Possible compensation for backwards pelvic tilt. Weight of arms pulls trunk forward with poor abdominal strength	Poor head and neck control, may influence safety in eating Discomfort or pain Difficulty using hands and arms for functional movement	Firm support of seat base and throughout the back Use of armrests and/or tray Accommodate if fixed kyphosis Tilt back in space
Hip extension	Spasticity of hip extensors, hamstring contractures	Unstable base of support means difficulty with all movements of upper limbs and head and neck	Firm seat and back Wedged or contoured seat Accommodate to fixed hamstring contractures in seat
Hip flexion	Spasticity of hip flexors, or hip flexion contractures	Unstable base of support means difficulty with all movements of upper limbs and head and neck	Ensure seat length and footplate height is correct Accommodate fixed contractures Firm seat, trial forward tilt
Adduction of hips	Due to spasticity of adductor muscles, contracture, subluxation or dislocation of hip Could be due to footplate height	Pain and discomfort as the hip begins to sublux Instability, poor use of arms, hands, head and neck Secondary issues at spine	Firm, contoured seat to support the thighs Use of pommel, or abduction straps Use of kneeblock and sacral pad Control pelvic rotation, but accommodate to fixed contracture
Abduction of hips	Due to spasticity of abductors, contracture or adduction of the opposite hip	Instability and discomfort May create environmental barriers	Accommodate to fixed contracture Use of hip guides or lateral supports along the thighs Control for pelvic rotation
Head and neck positioning	Flexion or extension of the neck, secondary to either poor positioning or lack of head control	May affect eating and drinking, communication, eye pointing May be unsafe	Good firm base of support/postural support throughout the whole body Possible head band or neck supports Tilt seating system in space

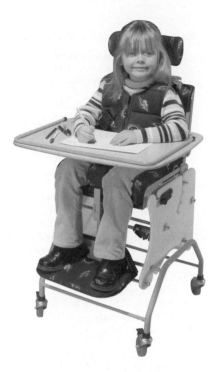

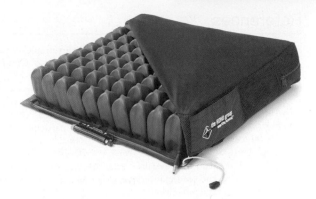

Figure 31.12 • Example of seat cushion designed to manage pressure in wheelchair seat. ROHO® QUADTRO SELECT® HIGH PROFILE® cushion, registered trademarks of ROHO, Inc (with kind permission of the RHO Group)

Figure 31.11 • Example of adaptive seating systems used to correct posture. MSS Tilt and Recline Chair (with kind permission of Wenzelite Re/hab Supplies)

person who is at risk (Dealey et al 1991). Cushions for pressure management are available, and use biomechanical principles of increasing the load-bearing area in order to reduce the pressure over a single surface.

When using a pressure cushion the aim is to:

*   distribute and decrease the pressure by increasing the area of support over a larger support surface (i.e. over the whole buttock rather than the ischial tuberosities)

*   take the weight, and compressive and shearing forces away from the bony prominences

*   control temperature and moisture.

The technologies for provision are rapidly developing, and involve air, pressure-relieving gel, and foam technologies (Brillhart 2005). Figure 31.12 shows a range of cushions, two of which use air and the other one uses a combination of memory foam and gel to increase the surface area and thus reduce pressure on the seated surface of the individual.

Conclusion

In terms of occupational engagement, the person is at the core, and the occupational therapist must ensure, above all, that the wheelchair and seating system meets the personal needs of the user. Age, life stage and stage of adjustment must all be considered. Collaboration with the person, so that their ability to participate in occupation is enhanced and developed is essential to the assessment and provision of a wheelchair and seating system. It is important to remember that 'the role of the occupational therapist in wheelchairs and seating is to enhance the user's participation in occupation through technical intervention' (Reid et al 2002, p. 261). All occupational therapists that participate in the assessment of wheelchair and seating systems have a responsibility to ensure that provision is cost-effective and safe for the person. Primarily though, the wheelchair must enhance the user's ability to access occupation.

Acknowledgements

Professor Robert Surtees, Gael Kelly, Jane Clements.

References

Aissaoui, R., Boucher, C., Bourbonnais, C., Lacoste, M. & Dansereau, J. (2001). Effect of seat cushion on dynamic stability in sitting during a reaching task in wheelchair users with paraplegia. *Archives of Physical Medicine and Rehabilitation*, 82(2), 274–281.

Apatsidis, D. P., Solomonidis, S. E., & Michael, S. M. (2002). Pressure distribution at the seating interface of custom-molded wheelchair seats: effect of various materials. *Archives of Physical Medicine and Rehabilitation*, 83(8), 1151–1156.

AuditCommission (2000). *Fully equipped – The provision of equipment services to older or disabled people by the NHS and social services in England and Wales*. (p. 106). London, Audit Commission.

AuditCommission (2002). *Fully equipped 2002 – Assisting independence*. (p. 63). London, Audit Commission.

Barbenel, J. C. (1991). Pressure management. *Prosthetics and Orthotics International*, 15(3), 225–231.

Bearnie, L. M., Coomer, A. F. & Hurley, M. V (2007). Upper limb sensorimotor function and functional performance in patients with rheumatoid arthritis. *Disability & Rehabilitation*, 29(13), 1035–1039.

Bergen, A. F., Presperin, J. & Tallman, T. (1990). *Positioning for function: wheelchairs and other assistive technologies*. New York, Valhalla.

Best, K. L., Kirby, R. L., Smith, C. & MacLeod, D. A. (2005). Wheelchair skills training for community-based manual wheelchair users: a randomized controlled trial. *Archives of Physical Medicine and Rehabilitation*, 86(12), 2316–2323.

Boninger, M. L., Baldwin, M., et al. (2000). Manual wheelchair pushrim biomechanics and axle position. *Archives of Physical Medicine and Rehabilitation*, 81(5), 608–613.

Bottos, M., Bolcati, C., Sciuto, L., Ruggori, C. & Feliciangel, A. (2001). Powered wheelchairs and independence in young children with tetraplegia. *Developmental Medicine & Child Neurology*, 43(11), 769–777.

Brandt, Å., Iwarsson, S. & Ståhle, A. (2004). Older people's use of powered wheelchairs for activity and participation. *Journal of Rehabilitation Medicine*, 36(2), 70–77.

Brienza, D. M., Karg, P. E., Geyer, M. J., Kelsey, S. & Trefler, E. (2001). The relationship between pressure ulcer incidence and buttock–seat cushion interface pressure in at-risk elderly wheelchair users. *Archives of Physical Medicine and Rehabilitation*, 82(4), 529–533.

Brillhart, B. (2005). Pressure sore and skin tear prevention and treatment during a 10-month program. *Rehabilitation Nursing*, 30(3), 85–91.

Brunner, R. & Baumann, J. U. (1994). Clinical benefit of reconstruction of dislocated or subluxated hip joints in patients with spastic cerebral palsy. *Journal of Paediatric Orthopaedics*, 14, 290–294.

Cohen, L. J. (2003). The development and validation of the seating and mobility script concordance test (SMSCT). *Unpublished doctoral thesis*. University of Pittsburgh.

Cohen, L. J., Fitzgerald, S. G., Lane, S. & Boninger, M. L. (2005). Development of the seating and mobility script concordance test for spinal cord injury: obtaining content validity evidence. *Assistive Technology*, 17(2), 122–132.

Cohen, L. (2007). Research priorities: Wheeled mobility. *Disability and Rehabilitation: Assistive Technology*, 2(3), 173–180.

Cook, A. M. & Hussey, S. M. (2002). *Assistive technologies principles and practice*. St Louis, Mosby.

Cook, A. M. & Polgar, J. M. (2007). *Cook & Hussey's assistive technologies: Principles and practice* (3rd ed.). St Louis, Mosby Elsevier.

Cox, D. L. (2003). Wheelchair needs for children and young people: a review. *British Journal of Occupational Therapy*, 66(5), 219–223.

Crane, B. A., Holm, M. B., Hobson, D., Cooper, R. A. & Reed, M. P.

(2007). A dynamic seating intervention for wheelchair seating discomfort. *American Journal of Physical Medicine and Rehabilitation*, 86(12), 988–993.

Crawford, S. A., Strain, B., Gregg, B., Walsh, D. M. & Porter-Armstrong, A. P. (2005). An investigation of the impact of the force sensing array pressure mapping system on the clinical judgement of occupational therapists. *Clinical Rehabilitation*, 19(2), 224–231.

Creek, J. (2003). *Occupational therapy defined as a complex intervention*. London, College of Occupational Therapists.

Curtis, K. A., Roach, K. E., Applegate, E. B., Amar, T., Benbow, C. S., Genecco, T. D. & Gualano, J. (1995). *Paraplegia*, 33(5), 290–293.

Curtis, K., Drysdale, G., Lanza, R., Kolber, M., Vitolo, R. & West, R. (1999). Shoulder pain in wheelchair users with tetraplegia and paraplegia. *Archives of Physical Medicine and Rehabilitation*, 80(4), 453–457.

Cushman, L. A. & Scherer, M. J. (1996). Measuring the relationship of assistive technology use, functional status over time, and consumer–therapist perceptions of ATs. *Assistive Technology*, 8(2), 103–109.

Davies, A., De Souza, L. H. & Frank, A. O. (2003). Changes in the quality of life in severely disabled people following provision of powered indoor/outdoor chairs. *Disability & Rehabilitation*, 25(6), 286–290.

de Laat, E. H., Scholte op Reimer, W. & van Achterberg, T. (2005). Pressure ulcers: diagnostics and interventions aimed at wound-related complaints: a review of the literature. *Journal of Clinical Nursing*, 14(4), 464–472.

Dealey, C., Earwaker, T. & Eden, L. (1991). Are your patients sitting comfortably? *Journal of Tissue Viability*, 1(2), 36–39.

Demers, L., Weiss-Lambrou, R. & Ska, L. (1996). Development of the Quebec User Evaluation of Satisfaction with Assistive Technology (QUEST). *Assistive Technology*, 8(1), 3–13.

Demers, L., Weiss-Lambrou, R. & Ska, L. (2000). Item analysis of the Quebec User Evaluation of Satisfaction with Assistive Technology (QUEST). *Assistive Technology*, 12(2), 96–105.

Estes, J. P., Bochenek, C. & Fassler, P. (2000). Osteoarthritis of the fingers. *Journal of Hand Therapy*, 13(2), 108–123.

Farley, R., Clark, J., Davidson, C., Evans, G., MacLennan, K., Michael, S., Morrow, M. & Thorpe, S. (1991). What is the evidence for the effectiveness of postural management?... including commentary by Roxborough L. *International Journal of Therapy and Rehabilitation*, 10(10), 449–455.

Fife, S. E., Roxborough, L. A., Armstrong, R. W., Harris, S. R., Gregson, S. C. & Field, D. (1991). Development of a clinical measure of postural control for assessment of adaptive seating in children with neuromotor disabilities. *Physical Therapy*, 71(12), 981–993.

Gagnon, B., Vincent, C. & Noreau, L. (2005). Adaptation of a seated postural control measure for adult wheelchair users. *Disability and Rehabilitation*, 27(16), 951–959.

Geyer, M. J., Brienza, D. M., Bertocci, G. E., Crane, B., Hobson, D., Karg, P., Schmeler, M. & Trefler, E. (2003). Wheelchair seating: a state of the science report. *Assistive Technology*, 15(2), 120–128.

Healy, A., Ramsey, C. & Sexsmith, E. (1997). Postural support systems: their fabrication and functional use. *Developmental Medicine & Child Neurology*, 39, 706–710.

Hocking, C. (1999). Function or feelings: factors in abandonment of assistive devices. *Technology and Disability*, 11, 3–11.

Hoenig, H., Landerman, L. R., Shipp, R. M. & George, L. (2003). Activity restriction among wheelchair users. *Journal of the American Geriatrics Society*, 51(9), 1244–1251.

Hunt, P. C. (2005). *Factors associated with wheelchair use and the impact on quality of life among individuals with spinal cord injury.* (p. 135). Pittsburgh, University of Pittsburgh, PhD.

Jelier, P. & Turner-Smith, A. (1997). Review of wheelchair services in England. *British Journal of Occupational Therapy*, 60(4), 150–155.

Kaye, H. S., Kang, T. & La Plante, M. P. (2002). Wheelchair use in the United States. *Disability Statistics Abstract*, 23, 1–4.

Kelly, G. & Clements, J. (2000). *Wheelchair independence measure.* (pp. 1–9). Caulfield General Medical Centre/Monash Medical Centre.

Kotsch, L. (2003). Wheelchair provision to the young disabled... Staincliffe's (vol 10(4), 2003, p. 151). *International Journal of Therapy and Rehabilitation*, 10(6), 285.

Law, M., Cooper, B. A., Strong, S., Stewart, D., Rigby, P. & Letts, L. (1996). The person-environment-occupational model: a transactive approach to occupational performance. *Canadian Journal of Occupational Therapy*, 63(1), 9–23.

Majd, M. E., Muldowny, D. S. & Holt, R. T. (1997). Natural history of scoliosis in the institutionalised adult cerebral palsy population. *Spine*, 22(13), 1461–1466.

McDonald, R., Surtees, R. & Wirz, S. (2004). The International Classification of Functioning, Disability and Health provides a model for adaptive seating interventions for children with cerebral palsy. *British Journal of Occupational Therapy*, 67(7), 293–302.

Mills, T., Holm, M. B., Trefler, E., Schmeler, M., Fitzgerald, S. & Boninger, M. (2002). Development and consumer validation of the functional evaluation in a wheelchair (FEW) instrument. *Disability and Rehabilitation*, 24(1), 38–46.

Mortenson, W. B., Miller, W. C. & Miller-Pogar, J. (2007). Measuring wheelchair intervention outcomes: Development of the Wheelchair Outcome Measure. *Disability and Rehabilitation: Assistive Technology*, 2(5), 275–285.

Mulcahy, C. M., Pountney, T. E., Nelham, R. L., Green, F. M. & Billington, G. D. (1988). Adaptive seating for motor handicap: problems, a solution, assessment

and prescription. *British Journal of Occupational Therapy*, 51, 347–352.

Myhr, U. & von Wendt, L. (1990). Reducing spasticity and enhancing postural control for the creation of a functional sitting position in children with cerebral palsy: A pilot study. *Physiotherapy Theory and Practice*, 6, 65–76.

Myhr, U., von-Wendt, L. & Sandberg, K. W. (1993). Assessment of sitting in children with cerebral palsy from videofilm: a reliability study. *Physical and Occupational Therapy in Pediatrics*, 12, 21–35.

Pain, H., Gore, S. & McLellan, D. L. (2000). Parents' and therapists' opinion on features that make a chair useful for a young disabled child. *International Journal of Rehabilitation Research*, 23(2), 75–80.

Pellow, T. R. (1999). A comparison of interface pressure readings to wheelchair cushions and positioning: a pilot study. *Canadian Journal of Occupational Therapy*, 66(3), 140–149.

Perr, A. (1998). Elements of seating and wheeled mobility intervention. *OT Practice*, 3, 16–24.

Pountney, T. E., Mulcahy, C. M., Clarke, S. & Green, E. (2000). *The Chailey Approach to Postural Management.* Birmingham: Active Design.

Reid, D. T. (1995). Development and preliminary validation of an instrument to assess quality of sitting of children with neuromotor dysfunction. *Physical & Occupational Therapy in Pediatrics*, 15(1), 53–82.

Reid, D., Laliberte-Rudman, D. & Herbert, D. (2002). Impact of wheeled seated mobility devices on adult users' and their caregivers' occupational performance: a critical literature review. *Canadian Journal of Occupational Therapy – Revue Canadienne d Ergotherapie*, 69(5), 261–280.

Robertson, R. N., Boninger, M. L., et al. (1996). Pushrim forces and joint kinetics during wheelchair propulsion. *Archives of Physical Medicine and Rehabilitation*, 77(9), 856–864.

Routhier, F., Vincent, C., Desrosiers, J. & Nadeau, S. (2003). Mobility of wheelchair users: a proposed performance assessment framework. *Disability and Rehabilitation*, 25(5–6), 19–34.

Routhier, F., Vincent, C., Desrosiers, J., Nadeau, S. & Cuerette, C. (2004). Development of an obstacle course assessment of wheelchair user performance. *Technology and Disability*, 16(1), 19–31.

Routhier, F., Vincent, C., Desrosiers, J. & Nadeau, S. (2005). Reliability and construct validity studies of an obstacle course assessment of wheelchair user performance. *International Journal of Rehabilitation Research*, 28(1), 49–56.

Roxborough, L. (1995). Review of the efficacy and effectiveness of adaptive seating for children with cerebral palsy. *Assistive Technology*, 7(1), 17–25.

Rudman, D. L., Hebert, D., et al. (2006). Living in a restricted occupational world: the occupational experiences of stroke survivors who are wheelchair users and their caregivers. *Canadian Journal of Occupational Therapy*, 73(3), 141–152.

Sanderson, D., Place, M. & Wright, D. (2000). *Evaluation of the powered wheelchair and voucher scheme initiatives*. (p. 72). York, York Health Economics Consortium, Department of Health.

Scrutton, D. R. (1978). Developmental deformity and the profoundly handicapped child. In: J. Apley (Ed.). *The care of the handicapped child*. London, Heinneman, pp. 83–89.

Scrutton, D., Baird, G. & Smeeton, N. (2001). Hip dysplasia in bilateral cerebral palsy: incidence and natural history in children aged 18 months to 5 years. *Developmental Medicine & Child Neurology*, 43, 601–608.

Shipperley, T. F. & Collins, F. (1999). A seating assessment tool for community use. *Wound Care*, 8(3), 119–120.

Sprigle, S. (2007a). Research priorities: Seating and positioning. *Disability and Rehabilitation: Assistive Technology*, 2(3), 181–187.

Sprigle, S. (2007b). State of the science on wheeled mobility and seating measuring the health, activity and participation of wheelchair users. *Disability and Rehabilitation: Assistive Technology*, 2(3), 133–135.

Stinson, M. D., Porter-Armstrong, A. & Eakin, P. (2003). Seat-interface pressure: a pilot study of the relationship to gender, body mass index, and seating position. *Archives of Physical Medicine and Rehabilitation*, 84(3), 405–409.

Townsend, E. & Polatajko, H. (2007). *Enabling occupation II: Advancing an occupational therapy vision for health, well-being & justice through occupation*. Ottawa, Canadian Association of Occupational Therapists.

Trefler, E. & Taylor, S. J. (1991). Prescription and positioning: evaluating the physically disabled individual for wheelchair seating. *Prosthetics & Orthotics International*, 15(3), 217–224.

Trefler, E., Hobson, D. A., Taylor, S. J., Monahan, L. C. & Shaw, C. G. (1993). *Seating and mobility for persons with physical disabilities*. Tucson, Therapy Skill Builders.

White, E. (1999). Wheelchair special seating: need and provision. *British Journal of Therapy & Rehabilitation*, 6(6), 285–286.

Williamson, J. B. (2003). Management of the spine in cerebral palsy. *Current Orthopaedics*, 17, 117–123.

World Health Organisation (2001). *International Classification of Functioning, Disability and Health*. Geneva, World Health Organisation.

Yang, W., Wilson, L., Oda, I. & Yan, J. (2007). The effect of providing power mobility on body weight change. *American Journal of Physical Medicine & Rehabilitation*, 86(9), 746–753.

Chapter
Thirty-Two

32

Driver assessment and rehabilitation within the context of community mobility

Marilyn Di Stefano and Wendy Macdonald

CHAPTER CONTENTS

Introduction 490

Driving, community mobility and health . . . 490

   Balancing road safety and an individual's
mobility needs 491

   Reporting of health and/or impairment-
related conditions that may impair
driving 492

   Driving as an information-processing
task 493

Role of non-driving-trained occupational
therapists in relation to driving 494

Occupational therapy driving specialist:
assessment and intervention 495

   The practice context 495

   Referral systems for specialist mobility
and driver-assessment services 495

   Characteristics of individuals referred for
driver assessment 496

   Driving-related assessments 496

   Off-road screening 497

   On-road assessment 498

   Possible driver evaluation outcomes 499

Emerging issues related to
occupational therapy driver assessment
and rehabilitation 503

Conclusion 503

SUMMARY

The ability to drive plays an important part in the
life roles of many people in industrially developed
countries, since it is often the preferred means of
maintaining good community mobility. Driving-
related issues can, therefore, be very important
for occupational therapists to address, since one
goal of occupational therapy is to improve the
occupational engagement of the people with
whom they work. Driving a motor vehicle is an
activity of daily living that requires a combination
of sensory, perceptual/cognitive, and motor
abilities, which together enable a driver to
develop the skills necessary to manoeuvre and
navigate their vehicle through complex, dynamic
environments. Occupational therapists working in
a number of areas of practice have responsibility
for identifying and educating individuals about
the potential impact of sensory, perceptual/
cognitive, and motor limitations on their driving
and community mobility; many also provide
training related to alternative community mobility.
Specialised individual assessments and
interventions that are more specific to driving are
usually the domain of occupational therapists
who have completed recognised post-graduate
training in driver assessment and rehabilitation.
Such professionals are referred to in this chapter
as 'occupational therapy driving specialists'. This
chapter describes some of the main theoretical
and empirically based foundations of
occupational therapy practice in these areas,
along with an outline of the limitations most likely
to impact upon driving and community mobility,
the content and general procedures involved in
driver assessments, and the associated
rehabilitation procedures.

KEY POINTS

- Driving is a common occupation in industrially
developed countries.

- The maintenance of independent driving and/or community mobility is important to support participation, socialisation and other forms of community engagement.
- A range of health, impairment, and ageing-related factors may impact upon safe driving and mobility.
- Occupational therapists play an important role in supporting individuals to maintain independence in these domains, and they assess and provide interventions related to community mobility.
- Occupational therapists educate and inform drivers about the impact of sensory, perceptual/cognitive, and motor impairment on driving.
- Occupational therapy driving specialists have a specific role in evaluating driver-related skills and devising customised rehabilitation programmes.
- There are many ways that drivers with limitations can be assisted to obtain, or maintain, their driving independence.

Introduction

In many industrialised societies, the rapid expansion of both suburban and rural populations based around regional shopping centres and industrial parks has contributed to increasing numbers of people being dependent on the car for transportation. In regions where there are very limited public or community transport options, or where long travel distances are involved, this reliance on personal vehicular modes of transport can create major problems for those unable to drive (Harris 1998, Rabbitt et al 2002). For these reasons driving an automobile is an important and valued occupation (Fricke & Unsworth 2001, Stacey & Kendig 1997).

Research on people's driving abilities in relation to their transport needs has focused largely on older drivers, most of whom have been driving regularly throughout their adult lives and expect to continue doing so indefinitely (Bailey 2004). There are various reasons why people's ability to drive safely may deteriorate significantly as they age – particularly beyond 75 or 80 years. However, people often do not plan for the time when they may need to reduce their driving, or perhaps cease driving altogether (Liddle & McKenna 2003). In addition, there are various health- and impairment-related causes of disruption to driving abilities, which may impact upon drivers across the lifespan (Dobbs 2005).

In this kind of context, occupational therapists can play several important roles. They may have an educational role in explaining the impact of impairment on driving abilities, and in explaining drivers' obligations within the relevant driver licensing jurisdiction. They may be required to develop remediation programmes to help people regain performance skills related to driving following injury or illness, and to facilitate and promote community mobility amongst those unable to drive. Occupational therapists with specialist training are responsible for assessing the driving-related abilities and driving performance of individual drivers as well as implementing interventions such as prescribing vehicle modifications and developing retraining programmes.

In pursuing these objectives, occupational therapists have multiple responsibilities – both to the individuals with whom they work and to the wider community. At an individual level, driving can be centrally important in maintaining a person's community mobility. At a societal level, drivers with some types of perceptual or cognitive impairments and certain health conditions can threaten both their own safety and that of others due to their increased risk of road accident involvement (Charlton et al 2004, Owsley et al 1998).

Driving, community mobility and health

'Community mobility' refers to the extent to which someone is able to travel within their community in accord with their needs and preferences. This can be accomplished by walking; or by using human-powered devices, such as bicycles, manual wheelchairs, or electric-powered versions of such devices; or by using public or community-based transportation systems (e.g. buses, taxis, trains); or by catching a ride with family or friends. But for many people, their preferred option is to drive independently (Macdonald et al 2006).

Coughlin (2001, p. v) highlighted the importance of transportation options to community mobility and the quality of people's lives:

> [Community] mobility, the ability to travel from point A to point B when and how one chooses, is the means by which individuals maintain their connection to society. Transportation has been described as the "glue" that holds together all the activities that we call life. Ready access to family, friends, social activities, health care, and goods and services are vital to full participation in daily life.

Many drivers see their ability to drive as centrally important to their well-being, and some evidence is available to support the reality of this view in cases where loss of a driver's licence has reduced the individual's community mobility. Such a loss has been associated with an increased incidence of illnesses, such as depression (Fonda et al 2001, Harris 2003, Marottoli et al 1997).

When people become unable to drive due to health problems, it might be thought that they should then start to walk rather than drive, or to use other options such as public or community-based transport to travel longer distances. However, for older individuals many of the most common ageing-related impairments have a greater effect on *personal* mobility (that is, their ability to walk around) than on driving performance (Whelan et al 2006). This means that for many older people, driving may be the most effective and sometimes the only means by which they can participate in activities outside their own homes, whether to perform essential tasks, such as shopping and visiting doctors, or to participate in social or recreational activities.

Figure 32.1 shows that, regardless of the particular transport mode, the primary determinant of community mobility is the quality of the match between an individual's personal characteristics and his transport options. As shown in the figure, both sides of this equation are influenced by the individual's own resources – both financial and social.[1] Among the personal characteristics shown here, sensory, perceptual/cognitive, and motor abilities are the most directly relevant, particularly if driving is the preferred transport option, because of the increased risk of road accidents if these abilities are inadequate. Some of the other personal characteristics, particularly driver age and a range of medical conditions, have been shown to influence a person's abilities (Charlton et al 2004, Dobbs 2005).

Figure 32.1 also highlights the potential effects of these factors on community mobility and more

general quality of life, which in turn have consequences for health, for road crash risk, and for the costs associated with both. This conceptualisation is consistent with the models of human occupation or activity engagement that have been developed to guide occupational therapy professional practice, a defining characteristic of which is the person-centred approach to service delivery. Such models are helpful in promoting understanding of the wide range of factors that influence driving and mobility engagement. The Model of Human Occupation (MOHO) (Kielhofner 2002), the Person-Environment-Occupation (PEO) model (Law et al 1996), the Occupational Adaptation model (Schultz & Schkade 2003) and the Canadian Model of Occupational Performance and Engagement (Townsend & Polatajko 2007) all identify relationships between human, task, social and environmental factors that change over the lifespan and impact upon successful performance in a particular situation. The Ecology of Human Performance (EHP) Framework (Dunn et al 1998), which is an inter-disciplinary model that shares some of the aforementioned characteristics, has also been applied to driver assessment and rehabilitation (Stav et al 2006b).

Balancing road safety and an individual's mobility needs

For occupational therapists working with drivers, a centrally important issue is the need to maintain a person's community mobility while at the same time maintaining road safety. This refers not only to the safety of the driver, but also the safety of passengers, along with other drivers and users of the road traffic system, including pedestrians and cyclists.

For many people, driving a vehicle in ordinary traffic is among the most hazardous activities routinely undertaken. The risk of death or serious injury due to road crashes is particularly high for drivers who are either very young or very old. The underlying reasons for these differences in crash risk are complex (e.g. see Braver & Trempel 2004, Hu et al 2000, Keall & Frith 2004). Older drivers are more likely than young ones to sustain the kind of illness-related impairments that commonly result in driving cessation. Apart from specific diagnosed illnesses, the more general 'ageing' process also leads eventually to impairments that are likely to increase crash risk substantially, as outlined below. This situation contrasts with that of *young* drivers, who are most

---

[1]This figure is based on the premise – drawn from the field of human factors psychology or ergonomics – that adequacy of system functioning is dependent on the 'goodness of fit' between individual characteristics (including physical, cognitive and psychomotor capacities, personal needs, and preferences) and the demands and other characteristics of the activities they wish to undertake (e.g. see Oborne 1982, Sanders & McCormick 1993). It is also consistent with Ecological Systems Theory as formulated by Bronfenbrenner (1979, 1989) and with European research on community mobility in relation to older people's quality of life (e.g. Mollenkopf 2003).

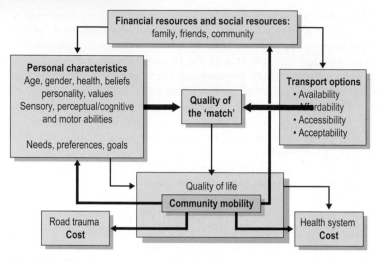

Figure 32.1 ● Determinants of community mobility

likely to require the services of specialist driver occupational therapists due to congenital impairments, or impairments resulting from accidents (including road crashes), such as acquired brain injuries or spinal injuries.

People presenting to occupational therapists for driver evaluations may have a variety of diagnoses and co-morbidities including stroke, closed head injuries, spinal injuries, dementia, and neurological conditions (Klavora et al 2000, Korner-Bitensky et al 2006, Lovell & Russell 2005). Across all age ranges, the following health conditions have been identified by researchers as associated with a substantial increase in crash risk: dementia, epilepsy, multiple sclerosis, psychiatric disorders (grouped into one category), sleep apnoea, alcohol abuse, and cataracts (Charlton et al 2004).

The driving performance of people with dementia has been a particular focus of research because the condition can develop quite rapidly and affected drivers may not be able to perceive and take account of decrements in their driving performance (Breen et al 2007). In light of the ageing populations in many countries, such issues have been widely discussed at both national and international levels (for example – Organisation for Economic Co-operative Development 2001, US Department of Transportation 2003, 2004).

Occupational therapists have considerable scope to help people develop and implement strategies to maintain reasonably good community mobility whilst reducing their exposure to mobility-related

accident risks. For example, better forward planning might lead to less frequent driving trips; or trips might be better planned to avoid high-risk situations such as driving at night, or in heavy or high-speed traffic, or when visibility is poor due to the weather. Apart from driving, potential means of maintaining community mobility for those without major cognitive-perceptual or musculo-skeletal difficulties may include use of public transport, motorised devices such as scooters, or use of a bicycle or tricycle. The remainder of this chapter focuses predominantly on driving as the preferred community mobility option.

Reporting of health and/or impairment-related conditions that may impair driving

In some jurisdictions, health professionals, such as occupational therapists, have legal obligations to report some types of health- and impairment-related conditions, including, for example, dementia, major visual field loss or cognitive/perceptual impairments.[2] It is, therefore, important for both generalist occupational therapists and those with specialist training in driver assessment to familiarise themselves with the licensing and medico-legal frameworks within which they practice (Green 2003).

---

[2]Apart from the reporting obligations of professionals, drivers may have self-reporting obligations.

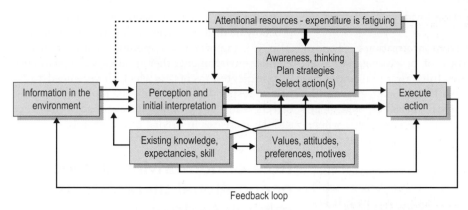

Figure 32.2 • How people 'process' information during activities. *Source:* Macdonald, W. 2004. Human Error: Causes and Countermeasures. Proceedings of the *Safety in Action Conference 2004.* Safety Institute of Australia, Victorian Division

Guidelines for medical and health professionals are readily available on the internet – see for example those produced by the American, Australian, British and Canadian transport or medical/health associations (American Medical Association & National Highway Traffic Safety Administration 2003, Austroads 2003, Canadian Medical Association 2006, Department of Transport UK 2007).

Whilst these documents provide some guidance, their usefulness is limited by wide variability in the type and severity of impairments that are associated with many medical diagnoses. Consequently, such guidelines are necessarily worded in quite general terms, and diagnosis of a specific medical condition, per se, is in reality likely to be a weak indicator of the quality of an individual's current driving performance (Di Stefano & Macdonald 2003a, Gallo et al 1999). To support the effective identification of those individuals whose driving is likely to present a substantial road-crash risk, it is, therefore, very important for occupational therapists to be able to assess the quality of the match between each individual's sensory, perceptual/cognitive, and motor abilities and the safe accessibility of driving as a transport option for that individual (see Figure 32.1).

Driving as an information-processing task

The safe accessibility of driving is determined by the demands that drivers have to cope with as they perform the task of driving a vehicle within the road traffic system. Although driving requires some phys-

ical abilities, such as adequate strength and range of motion of limbs required to move operational controls, it is visual, perceptual and cognitive functioning that are most important in enabling drivers to manage critical safety demands. To understand more about perceptual and cognitive abilities, it is helpful to view driving as an 'information-processing' task, as shown in Figure 32.2. The relationships between human information-processing capacities and limitations with interacting system characteristics have been well documented in the literature (e.g. Proctor & Van Zandt 1994, Wickens & Hollands 2000).

Figure 32.2 shows information from the environment (on the left) impinging on the driver's sensory organs, with some of this being registered in sensory stores, where it is very briefly retained. In the case of driving, *visual* information is clearly the most important type of sensory input, which means that effective visual sensory functioning is an important requirement for competent driving performance. It should be noted that *dynamic* visual acuity may be more important than the *static* acuity that is more routinely tested (Messinger-Rapport 2003).

Only a subset of the information registered in sensory stores progresses further into the system to be 'perceived'. Perception is the point where some initial interpretation occurs, based on the driver's pre-existing knowledge and skills, and influenced also by attitudes and motivational factors. This perceptual stage is critical for road safety since it sustains the driver's awareness of road and traffic conditions, and provides the basis for cognitive predictions of the immediate future road traffic situation to enable appropriate vehicle control actions and more general 'situation awareness' (Bolstad & Hess 2000).

Only a subset of *perceived* information goes on to the central, *cognitive* stage of processing, which is when the driver becomes fully aware or conscious of it. Processing of information at this stage requires the allocation of attentional resources, and since these resources are in limited supply, this is where humans' information-processing capacity is at its most limited. Associated with this, there is a maximum rate at which humans can process information. This limitation can result in drivers sometimes being at risk of information overload. It also makes it important that drivers allocate their available attentional resources optimally across different aspects of the task.

Some aspects of cognitive performance typically decline with old age: attentional limitations have been identified as being particularly important (Ball 1997, Ball et al 2002, Fisk & Rogers 1997). Also, sub-optimal *allocation* of available attentional resources becomes an increasingly common problem among the oldest drivers (Brayne et al 1999, 2000). As noted above, research has shown that it is perceptual and cognitive impairments rather than purely physical ones that are significantly linked to higher crash risk (Charlton et al 2004). Attentional issues may also be of concern with younger individuals who are cognitively compromised (e.g. those with congenital cognitive impairment, rapidly progressive neurological conditions or acquired brain injury).

Older people usually have the advantage of being highly experienced drivers. This means that when they are driving in familiar surroundings, a substantial part of the incoming information can be processed in an automatic, or partially automatic, fashion, indicated by the large arrow in Figure 32.2 connecting 'Perception and Initial Interpretation' directly to 'Execute Action'. Importantly, this arrow by-passes conscious awareness, which is the stage most demanding of attentional resources. Very experienced drivers are, therefore, able to cope with completely routine aspects of the driving task within highly familiar road environments without there being heavy demands on their attentional resources.

Regardless of age, the process of learning to drive (for young, cognitively compromised individuals), or re-learning to drive (for more experienced drivers following a major injury or illness) may place high demands on available attentional resources, since some of the required actions or performance strategies may not have been encountered or will probably be different from those previously learned. Also, it is important to remember that even in very familiar environments there is always the possibility of unexpected events to which drivers need to be able to respond quickly. Even the most experienced drivers can be temporarily overloaded by very sudden increases in driving task demands.

Role of non-driving-trained occupational therapists in relation to driving

All occupational therapists, whether they are generalists or specialist driver assessors, need to have a good understanding of the issues outlined above. For generalists, this is necessary because they routinely address a wide variety of issues with people and their families, including self-care, education, work, leisure, and social participation (Redepenning 2006). In many of these contexts, driving and/or community mobility issues may be important considerations.

The usual starting point for both generalist and specialist occupational therapists is to identify those people who may present an unacceptable crash risk as a driver, and independent of effects on crash risk, to identify whether they are likely to experience difficulties when driving. This is a complex process, and as yet there is no single battery of validated assessment tools or tests to support decision-making, although the use of diagnosis-related 'red flags' is emerging as a potentially useful approach. According to a recent review, current approaches are primarily opinion-based, such as consensus statements, or derived in other ways from experts' opinions (Molnar et al 2005). One simple tool that has acceptable face validity (its empirical validity is currently under investigation) is the 'SAFEDRIVE' checklist (Wiseman & Souder 1996). This tool is used by medical and allied health personnel to identify whether an individual's history and/or presenting signs and symptoms are indicative of the need to investigate driving-related abilities. The acronym is comprised of the following areas which should be reviewed:

S – safety record and history of crashes

A – attention deficits and skills

F – family report a history of driving-related problems

E – history of ethanol use

D – drug and/or medication use

R – reaction-time-related limitations associated with neurological or musculo-skeletal problems

I – intellectual impairment

V – vision-related problems

E – executive cognition limitations or concerns.

Factors impacting upon driving and/or community mobility may be identified in referral documentation and/or emerge from occupational therapy assessment procedures which are routinely conducted when working with a range of individuals. Concerns may also be raised by family or significant others. Various assessment checklists, including the SAFEDRIVE mentioned above, may trigger the need for further investigations. In such cases, the generalist occupational therapist's role may encompass:

- identification of individuals who may not meet the medical guidelines for drivers and who may require referral for medical assessment followed by specialist occupational therapy or mobility-centre driver evaluation

- occupational profile analysis, which will highlight the significance of independent driving and mobility in relation to the individual's roles and life goals

- occupational performance evaluation, which may identify specific gaps in performance abilities that also contribute to or impact upon driving performance

- remediation or compensation-related interventions aimed at improving abilities to enable driver or mobility assessment and rehabilitation

- education interventions for individuals, their families and significant others regarding driving and community mobility

- advocacy interventions that may be related to seeking approval or funding for driver or mobility assessment and rehabilitation as well as vehicle modifications or specialised mobility aides, if required.

In addition to considering issues that these tests address, there is a more general need to assess the level of driver insight. Individuals with any condition that demonstrate a lack of insight into major decrements may be a risk to public safety when driving, especially in re/licensing systems, which place the onus only on the individual to report their health/impairment status.

Occupational therapy driving specialist: assessment and intervention

The practice context

Occupational therapists specialising in driver assessment and rehabilitation rarely work *only* in this field. Typically, they also provide services for a range of other people, depending on the context of their practice. Such practice contexts include: private practice, rehabilitation units (e.g. for people who have had a stroke, spinal cord or acquired brain injury), geriatric assessment facilities, mental health units, and community health centres (French & Hanson 1999). They may also operate within 'mobility centres' that specialise in driver assessment and community mobility (Brooks & Hawley 2005).

In these various contexts, they are often part of formal or informal teams who are working together towards goals related to this aspect of human occupation (Stav et al 2006b). Team members usually include family members or caregivers, medical practitioners, driving instructors, other treating health practitioners (including generalist occupational therapists, physiotherapists, optometrists, orthotists), case managers, and mechanics who provide vehicle modifications (Pellerito & Blanc 2006). The degree to which different team members become involved will depend on the range and extent of health and impairment issues faced by individual drivers. In some driver licensing jurisdictions, these specialist occupational therapists may be required to register with the driver licensing authority, after having completed their specialist training, in order to offer their services (Di Stefano & Macdonald 2006b).

Referral systems for specialist mobility and driver assessment services

Individuals might be referred to occupational therapy driver specialists by personnel of medical, rehabilitation, educational, vocational training or other centres; by family members; and in some driver licensing jurisdictions, by the driver licensing authority. For individuals, the first part of the referral process might be undertaking a specific medical assessment, with the doctor completing an official report (e.g. see VicRoads 2000).

As part of this process, people might need to complete an 'Informed Consent' form, since privacy legislation in some jurisdictions limits the type of information about an individual that can be obtained or disseminated. Permission from the person might be required for the occupational therapist to contact the person's family members, medical practitioner, the referrer, or the driver licensing authority.

Characteristics of individuals referred for driver assessment

Occupational therapy driver assessments are commonly provided for individuals with a wide range of health impairment and ageing issues, which may impact upon their driving performance and activity participation (see Table 32.1). Referrals commonly fall into the following broad categories:

1. 'Learners': young adults with a congenital or acquired impairment who want to know if they have the capacity to drive (e.g. those with conditions such as spina bifida, cerebral palsy, intellectual impairment)

2. Individuals who are adapting to, or *recovering* from, physical, neurological or psycho-social conditions that often indicate a need to evaluate their driving performance (e.g. those with spinal cord injury, acquired brain impairment, long-term mental health problems)

3. Individuals with a *deteriorating* chronic illness (e.g. neurological conditions such as multiple sclerosis, muscular dystrophy, Parkinson's disease)

4. *Older* members of the community whose capacity has deteriorated due to the ageing process and/or a combination of other factors identified above.

Driving-related assessments

There are a number of published articles or booklets describing occupational therapy-related driver

assessment practices. These papers often present practice scenarios of specialist centres, or report on surveys of service characteristics (see for example Klavora et al 2000, Korner-Bitensky et al 2006, Redepenning 2006, Stav 2004, Wheatley 2001).

The evidence base for the application of specific assessments and interventions used in occupational therapy driver assessment is increasing. At times, the interpretation and general application of research findings is problematic because of the different methodologies, people and variable outcome measures used in the studies (Kua et al 2007). A wide range of screening and assessment procedures are currently used in the assessment of older drivers specifically (see for example: Dobbs 2005, Kua et al 2007, Molnar et al 2006, Redepenning 2006, Stav 2004). A general overview of the timing of referral and both components of the driver evaluation procedure is presented here.

The timing of driver assessments within the overall habilitation or rehabilitation process is determined by a number of factors including: requirements of medical or fitness-to-drive guidelines; the nature and extent of a person's injuries; the acute, chronic or progressive nature of a person's medical condition; concerns of the wider rehabilitation team; and individual factors including age, medication intake and compliance in taking prescribed medication, driving experience, financial status, and more general motivation and behavioural issues. For example, it would be inappropriate to assess someone who has experienced a major stroke within weeks of the event if they are likely to obtain the greatest extent of sensory, perceptual/cognitive, and motor return within 3 to 6 months. Undertaking the assessment *after* they have had sufficient time for recovery is more likely to reflect their longer-term abilities: an important consideration if the driver is considering expensive vehicle modifications.

In most cases, the specialist occupational therapy driver-assessment procedure consists of two components: off-road screening and on-road evaluation. Usually a core set of tests is used in the off-road screening to provide a consistent set of baseline measures across all individuals seen within the service (Lovell & Di Stefano 2007). For this purpose it is preferable to use tests that are standardised and are known to have good validity and reliability. Additional specific tests might be added to the battery, depending on an individual's presenting problems.

Table 32.1 Health or impairment issues and how they might influence driver-related performance. Based partly on Hatakka et al (1999) and the WHO International Classification of Functioning, Disability and Health (World Health Organisation 2001)

Health/impairment issue: abilities still compliant with requirements of relevant medical guidelines*	Planning of driving trip: timing and/or route	Driving performance		Participation/life roles, goals and skills for living
		Contextual factors/vehicle control, e.g. steering, use of accelerator or brake pedal	Interacting with traffic and other road users	
Reduced upper-limb movement, e.g. inco-ordination, pain or weakness	Performance may be influenced by diurnal fluctuations in pain/function Trip length may need to be extended to cope with need for more frequent rest breaks	Difficulties with ignition, use of steering wheel, indicators and secondary controls, slower movement time	May experience restricted ability to steer vehicle around objects quickly or respond to situations requiring skilful quick manoeuvring	Difficulties with driving independence may impact upon ability to retain previous or attempt new paid worker roles
Reduced or absent lower-limb movement, e.g. amputation, weakness		Difficulties with ingress/egress, use of foot operated pedals, seating balance	Sustained or quick acceleration or braking may be difficult	Reliance on aides for mobility may increase need to depend on vehicular-related mobility independence
Minor reduction in visual acuity, visuo-perceptual and/or cognitive abilities	May experience difficulties driving at night, in adverse weather, or peak hour conditions. Complex or new routes may create additional undesirable mental workload over and above reserves required to compensate for impairments	May not see, interpret or respond to important aspects of the road environment accurately, may not scan sufficiently to compensate, slower reaction time	May not be able to attend to environmental stimuli or recall appropriate strategies fast enough to cope with driving in complex conditions with many fast-moving, unpredictable road users. Reacting to unexpected movements/actions of vehicles or road users may be difficult or inconsistent	Difficulty with performance demands other than associated with routine day time driving may impact upon life roles as parent, carer or worker. May reduce occupational engagement with leisure, family, religious or community pursuits

*Note: Medical guidelines applicable to different countries/jurisdictions normally need to be met before drivers are eligible for licensure and assessed by occupational therapy driving specialists – see for example Austroads 2003, American Medical Association & National Highway Traffic Safety Administration 2003, Canadian Medical Association 2006, Department of Transport, UK, 2007.

Off-road screening

Off-road screening typically comprises the following elements:

- Review of the contents of medical or allied health reports

- Interview to obtain information regarding driving history, occupational profile, level of insight into the impact of impairments upon driving performance, types of vehicles driven and licences held

- Recording of medication taken and any side effects

- Assessment of:
  - vision (includes acuity, eye movement and co-ordination, visual fields, possibly contrast sensitivity)
  - hearing
  - other sensory abilities relevant to driving task demands (e.g. superficial sensation, proprioception, kinesthesia)
  - physical abilities relevant to driving task demands (e.g. muscle strength, range of motion, co-ordination, sitting balance, mobility and transfer abilities)
  - pain, physical and mental endurance
  - knowledge about road law and driving procedures (for example, via a written or computer-based test)
  - simple and choice reaction times (e.g. by use of a 'brake reaction' machine of some kind)
  - some perceptual/cognitive abilities by using tests such as the Mini-Mental State Examination (MMSE) (Folstein et al 1975), Trail making tests (Reitan 1985), the Useful Field of View (UFOV) (Owsley et al 1998), or other such tests as deemed appropriate
- Observations throughout the session, to assess more general perceptual/cognitive abilities or dysfunction (e.g. aspects of memory, attention, perception, visuo-perceptual, problem solving), which may be of concern in relation to driving task demands.

Off-road screening also offers the opportunity to observe and discuss as appropriate:

- a person's insight into their limitations
- a person's emotional status and contact with reality
- likely impact of the impairments on driving performance
- possible vehicle adaptations that may be needed
- nature of the on-road driving assessment
- driving requirements in relation to work, study, family, leisure, etc.
- impact of likely licence conditions on independence/life roles.

As a result of findings from this screening procedure, the occupational therapy driving specialist may sometimes require further information about a particular area of sensory, perceptual/cognitive or motor abilities. For example, more detailed visual assessment by an ophthalmologist or optometrist or an evaluation by a neuropsychologist. At times it may be appropriate for the individual being assessed to await further recovery or undertake intensive, targeted rehabilitation in order to maximise their potential. Of particular importance, is the need to ensure that the prospective driver meets minimum medical guidelines for fitness for driving, for example, the person meets minimum vision requirements (Austroads 2003). So that evaluation is efficient and interpretations of on-road behaviour are accurate, it is important that individuals perform whilst at their optimum (e.g. with vision corrected reflecting current status, having achieved maximum motor and sensory recovery after illness or trauma).

At the conclusion of the off-road screening, the occupational therapy driving specialist has a general idea of what to expect from the next stage of the driver assessment. The occupational therapist will also have clarified issues, such as:

- type of vehicle required, e.g. automatic transmission or manual
- adaptive devices that may be required, e.g. spinner knob, hand controls, modified seating
- type and duration of the on-road assessment route to be used
- special requirements of the driving instructor
- requirement for an interpreter
- the likely impact of presenting impairments on the person's ability to manage the various tasks associated with driving
- any specific cognitive-perceptual or other abilities to be tested during the drive.

Such information assists the occupational therapy driving specialist in the professional reasoning required to identify and interpret issues emerging during the on-road assessment, where an important focus is identifying possibilities for interventions. The off-road screen is thus a very important component of the overall occupational therapy driver evaluation.

On-road assessment

Many occupational therapy assessments include a component where the occupational therapist observes the individual whilst they attempt to

Table 32.2 Examples of behaviours/performance aspects assessed during on-road evaluation

Person: impact of impairment on driving skill components	Performance components	Road law application to the following	Road craft
Cognitive-perceptual function	Maintaining lane position	Speed limits	Vehicle position at intersections
Pain levels Endurance	Right and left turns at various intersections	Intersection give way laws	Application of indicators
Use of limbs to manage vehicle adaptations	Observations	Other road users (e.g. pedestrians)	Use of gears, accelerator and brake
Visual abilities	Slow-speed manoeuvres	Merging and lane changing	Manoeuvring in tight spaces

complete a task; the on-road driver evaluation involves just this in relation to driving. The assessment usually takes place in a vehicle with dual controls, with a driving instructor seated in the front passenger seat to provide navigational instructions and take responsibility for maintaining safety. The occupational therapist sits in the rear seat on the opposite side from the driver, and takes detailed notes using a checklist. Some examples of the areas of driver performance routinely evaluated are shown in Table 32.2.

In order to optimise safety, the driving course usually starts off in a low-demand situation, such as a quiet car park or segment of road in a suburban area with little or no traffic. It is graded in this way so that the driver can have some time to familiarise themselves with the vehicle by attempting basic operational tasks before venturing out into situations that are more complex and require interacting with greater numbers of road users under more demanding conditions. The road test can last up to 60 minutes, depending on the goals of the assessment and driver anxiety, fatigue and other characteristics.

On-road tests used in the evaluation of impaired drivers reported in the literature vary considerably. In some cases, licensing authority tests are used, with, or without, slight modification (e.g. Kantor et al 2004). In other cases, specific tests have been developed for particular populations (e.g. Dobbs et al 1998, Hunt et al 1997).

To ensure reliability and validity of any on-road assessment, adequate numbers and types of different test items should be included. These items include manoeuvres such as pulling to the curb, parking, completing turns at various intersections and merging or overtaking. In addition, the checklists used during on-road assessment should have route details and

pre-specification of particular points along the route at which observations are to be made, as well as documenting the specific behavioural items to be assessed (Di Stefano & Macdonald 2006b). To enable this degree of pre-specification, most occupational therapists have one or more 'standard' routes for their on-road assessments. Standard routes are usually those with sufficient item complexity and difficulty that would be consistent with the provision of an 'open area' license (allowing the driver to drive where they choose). This is to distinguish these routes from those used for a 'local area' test.

If a local area licence is being considered, a route around the person's home may be used, following the common and familiar travel paths to most frequent destinations, such as to shops, medical and recreational facilities. Commonly such local area tests and resultant licenses are used as either an interim measure for drivers who may be continuing to make improvements, but are still not able to deal with new or unpredictable driving situations, or as a step towards maintaining some degree of community mobility whilst gradually reducing driving privileges if the driver has a deteriorating condition. Depending on the occupational therapy service delivery model, personnel other than occupational therapy driver specialists may take responsibility for some aspects of the on-road assessment (Schold Davis 2003, Stav et al 2006a).

Possible driver evaluation outcomes

At the conclusion of the on-road driver assessment, the individual, driving instructor and occupational therapy driving specialist discuss the findings. A decision has to made about whether the person has passed, passed with provisions, needs further interventions prior to being re-assessed or has failed. Specific verbal feedback about driving behaviours is offered as well as relevant advice about vehicle choice, adaptations, planning and organising driving activities to accommodate functional limitations, transfer aids and seating considerations. The driver may be recommended to:

- await further recovery from illness or injury and/or undergo a period of remediation to optimise abilities prior to considering re-assessment and/or the continuation of driver rehabilitation

- undertake driving lessons, for the purpose of developing or improving general driving or other skills related to use of compensatory strategies and/or modified vehicle controls

- drive under restricted licence conditions, e.g. with a supervising driver, only within a local area limit, only in a vehicle of a certain type or fitted with specific devices such as a spinner knob, hand controls, automatic transmission, left external mirrors, or automatic transmission

- undertake occupational therapy, medical or other allied health re-assessments/reviews after specified amounts of time to track either improvement or deterioration in abilities.

Some examples of impairment issues and possible interventions and licensing considerations are presented in Table 32.3. All these strategies are targeted towards optimising driving independence by facilitating the execution of safe, consistent vehicle control and driver behaviours.

If the person fails the on-road assessment, the occupational therapist must decide what options, if any, are available to the driver. Professional reasoning, based on the referral and medical information, and results of both the off-road screening and on-road test, are used to evaluate available options. The occupational therapist must decide if there is any likelihood of further recovery, or if the driver might benefit from driver rehabilitation. If individuals have advanced forms of some conditions (e.g. dementia or other neurological conditions, such as Parkinson's disease or multiple sclerosis) and/or if there is a significant lack of insight into major limitations, the safety of the driver, passengers or the community at large may be at risk if the person continues to drive. In such cases, the occupational

therapist and driving instructor may recommend that a driver ceases driving altogether. Such recommendations are always based on sound, objective documented evidence and are usually forwarded to the licensing authority for further action. Decisions to recommend license suspension or cancellation are not undertaken lightly as this may impose significant practical transportation difficulties and lifestyle restrictions for the former driver. The research to date examining the effects of licence cancellation on older people has highlighted the detrimental effect this can have on psychosocial health and occupational roles (Marottoli et al 1997, 2000). The family, carers and other health personnel involved should always be advised of this outcome. A referral for counselling or other psychosocial support may be warranted. In addition, information about relevant funding schemes and advice related to alternative means of maintaining community mobility, including: walking, motorised devices (e.g. scooters), public and community-based transport services, and taxi services are provided.

Practice Scenario 32.1 involving Sue who sustained an acquired brain injury (ABI) highlights some of the driving-related issues that can be associated with multiple system impairments. Although Sue did not require vehicle modifications, she was tested, re-trained and eventually passed her second assessment, in a vehicle with automatic transmission. Driving an automatic car helps reduce the amount of both mental and physical workload associated with driving. Sue's progress through various types of health services also reinforces the importance of addressing driving-related issues very early in the rehabilitation process and depicts the collaborative and integrated efforts made by the three occupational therapists involved in her care.

Practice Scenario 32.1 Sue

Driver profile and relevant occupational history

Sue was a 21-year-old university student when she sustained an acquired brain injury (ABI) and multiple fractures (pelvis, left humerus and right clavicle) due to involvement in a motor vehicle accident. After spending 3 months in an acute-care setting, Sue was transferred to a rehabilitation facility. A further

Table 32.3 Examples of different impairments and possible occupational therapy interventions involving the person, vehicle, training and broader system (license) issues

Health or Impairment Issue: abilities still compliant with requirements of relevant medical guidelines*	Person	Vehicle options/ modifications	Training/task/road conditions	Licence conditions/ restrictions
Reduced upper limb movement, e.g. inco-ordination, pain or weakness	Remediation to improve movement related to range of motion Review pain management strategies	Use of automatic vehicle with power steering and steering aide Application of steering wheel cover to improve hand grip	Lessons for training related to use of vehicle modifications Grade exposure to driving tasks to evaluate stamina and improve endurance Initially avoid city or other driving environments requiring a lot of de/acceleration, turns or difficult parking manoeuvres	Driving only a certain type of car (e.g. automatic transmission) and/or with certain vehicle adaptations, requires a licence condition Check regulations re use of additional mirrors – may require a licence condition Licence restriction to drive only in familiar areas may be required to reduce likelihood of encountering unfamiliar and demanding driving situations Drivers with chronic and/or deteriorating conditions may be required to undertake periodic medical and/or license testing reviews
Reduced or absent lower limb movement, e.g. amputation, weakness	Remediation to optimise residual abilities If feasible, retraining of left foot to operate accelerator/brake	Use of automatic vehicle with either left foot accelerator or hand controls to replace foot-operated pedals		
Minor reduction in visual acuity, visuo-perceptual and/or cognitive abilities	Remediation to improve abilities Compensatory strategies to optimise performance Ensure optimal driver seating position and access/use of all controls	Automatic vehicle to simplify driving task Ensure optimal view out of all windows and size, number and placement of mirrors Additional mirrors may be installed to facilitate use of compensatory strategies	Lessons for training related to in-car compensatory strategies and use of mirrors or other aides Grade exposure to increasingly complex driving tasks to evaluate application of techniques and performance consistency over time Assess problem-solving skills when faced with common or unusual/more complex road scenarios	

*Note: Medical guidelines applicable to different countries/jurisdictions normally need to be met before drivers are eligible for licensure and assessed by occupational therapy driving specialists – see for example Austroads 2003, American Medical Association & National Highway Traffic Safety Administration 2003, Canadian Medical Association 2006, Department of Transport, UK, 2007.

3 months passed before Sue was fit enough to be discharged. She was making a good recovery having regained full sensory-motor function, although she still experienced mild upper-limb co-ordination difficulties and a neuropsychological assessment confirmed that she was still displaying some mild residual cognitive deficits, which impacted upon her executive skills (information-processing rate, divided attention, planning and problem solving). Sue was subsequently discharged to live at home with her family as she was independent with minimal support (e.g. adaptive devices, memory aides). After discharge she attended a community-based rehabilitation programme three mornings per week.

At the time of referral for occupational therapy driver assessment, some 9 months post accident, Sue expressed a desire to remain living at home whilst resuming her university studies, hopefully in the following year. She indicated that she wanted to return to driving in order to help her travel to university (she lived some 30 km from the campus) and assist her to lead a more independent lifestyle.

Prior to the accident, Sue had been living in a university hall of residence and had three years of driving experience in a manual car.

Generalist occupational therapy intervention: rehabilitation phases

Rehabilitation facility

During the rehabilitation phase of her recovery, the occupational therapist initially discussed driving and considered this in relation to Sue's self-care, study, and recreational pursuits. Driving was included in the rehabilitation plan goals and discussed at team and family meetings. The occupational therapist incorporated some computer-based driving-related games and education tools into Sue's programme, as well as relating some of the activities in the general rehabilitation programme to driving goals. For example, Sue was encouraged to play table soccer and use a sewing machine under supervision in order to test her memory, eye–hand co-ordination, visuo-spatial, and reaction-time abilities.

Community-based setting

Upon transfer to the service, the community-based occupational therapist reviewed the referral documentation and used the SAFEDRIVE checklist (Wiseman & Souder 1996) to confirm that attention deficits and skills, co-ordination, reaction time and executive cognitive limitations might impact upon Sue's driving abilities. Consequently, the occupational therapist also considered driving-related goals in the intervention plan, recommending that Sue:

- revise the content of the road rule handbook
- undertake a programme aimed at physical reconditioning (swimming and water aerobics)
- resume cycling in a graded programme (off-road initially, then low-demand open-road environment)
- play computer-based driving games.

These were implemented with the intention of improving co-ordination, hazard perception and road-awareness skills prior to considering driver assessment. In addition, a cognitive-perceptual programme (developed in conjunction with a neuropsychologist) was also commenced to improve skills relevant to this activity domain.

Occupational therapy driving specialist intervention

The community-based occupational therapist initially discussed referral with the occupational therapy driver specialist. Sue was reviewed by her rehabilitation medical specialist for the purpose of completing the specific 'medical assessment for drivers' prior to attempting the formal driver evaluation with the occupational therapy driver specialist.

Off-road screen

The off-road interview and assessment highlighted that Sue was very motivated to resume driving and her family were supportive. The screening tests revealed that Sue still experienced mild problems in relation to executive cognitive abilities and a slight reduction in her reaction time, although she had adequate upper-limb co-ordination, excellent insight, self-regulated her activities to avoid potential 'overload' situations, and was rigorously following her rehabilitation programme. No concerns were raised regarding road law knowledge and application.

On-road test and subsequent driver rehabilitation

The on-road test was undertaken in a car with automatic transmission to simplify the driving task. Sue did not require any other vehicle modifications. Only one half of the usual on-road assessment route was completed due to anxiety levels and errors. Sue agreed not to resume sole independent driving until a further assessment was completed and in the interim to undertake a programme of staged driver rehabilitation involving a series of graded lessons with a specialist driving instructor. In addition, with Sue as a passenger and her mother driving the car, Sue would practise some of the perceptual and cognitive skills involved in driving by providing a verbal commentary of the driving task, noting key elements and events, and identifying required driver responses. Over this period, the occupational therapy driving specialist liaised with Sue, her mother and the driving instructor to monitor progress.

Re-assessment post driver rehabilitation

After 3 months, and a total of 12 formal lessons, in addition to regular sessions with her mother, Sue was re-assessed by the occupational therapy driver specialist. This time the full on-road route was completed successfully and Sue was subsequently granted a licence to drive independently in an automatic car. A medical review to track her progress was recommended after 12 months, with further occupational therapy assessment dependent upon medical referral, if required.

Emerging issues related to occupational therapy driver assessment and rehabilitation

With increasing longevity and associated expectations that a high quality of life should be sustainable into old age, there will be an increasing demand for occupational therapy driver specialist services to assist individuals to maintain driving independence, despite impairment and advancing age (Schold Davis 2003). Concurrent with this, occupational therapy driver specialists will face the need to address a number of factors that are likely to impact upon mobility and driver independence. These factors include:

- In-vehicle technologies that may provide additional distractions/mental workload on individuals with compromised abilities, e.g. mobile phones, in-vehicle navigation systems (Di Stefano & Macdonald 2003b)

- In-vehicle technologies that support driving independence, e.g. cruise controls, crash avoidance systems, parking aides (Di Stefano & Macdonald 2006a)

- Technological developments associated with new types of individual mobility options that may become popular, e.g. motorised push bikes, the Segway Personal Tranporter (Segway 2008)

- New computer or simulator-based methods of evaluating mobility and driver pre-requisite skills.

Conclusion

Occupational therapists have a vital role to play in assisting people with sensory, perceptual/cognitive and/or motor limitations to maximise their independence by means of driving, or by whatever other means are most appropriate to achieve and sustain good community mobility. From a road safety viewpoint it is commonly a person's cognitive and perceptual limitations that are most important, but physical limitations also need to be addressed. In addition to directly supporting individuals to explore community mobility options, occupational therapists have an important role in educating and helping to optimise the abilities of the people they refer for specialist occupational therapy driver evaluations. Occupational therapists with specialist training in driver assessment and rehabilitation typically work in a team context in achieving driving-related objectives with individuals. Centrally important to the task of these occupational therapists is the careful evaluation of each driver's skills in relation to the requirements for consistently safe driving performance. To maximise the quality of the match between a person's characteristics and driving task demands, occupational therapists may utilise adaptive equipment, modified vehicle controls, remediation strategies, re-training and/or restricted licence conditions, with the aim of providing individuals with sensory, perceptual/cognitive and/or motor limitations opportunities to commence or resume safe driving.

References

American Medical Association, & National Highway Traffic Safety Administration (2003). *Physician's guide to assessing and counselling older drivers*. Available online: http://www.nhtsa.dot.gov/people/ injury/olddrive/OlderDriversBook/ pages/Contents.html. Accessed 2 Sept 2003.

Austroads (2003). *Assessing fitness to drive: for commercial and private vehicle drivers: Medical Standards for licensing and clinical management guidelines* (3rd ed.). Sydney, Austroads Incorporated.

Bailey, T. (2004). *Older motorists' perceptions of their information needs*. Available online:

http://www.transport.sa.gov.au/rss/content/safer_people/programs_resources/documents/Bailey_Older_Motorists_Perceptions_2004.pdf. Accessed 26 Aug 2007.

Ball, K. (1997). Attentional problems and older drivers. *Alzheimer Disease and Associated Disorders*, 11(Supplement1), 42–47.

Ball, K., Berch, D. B., Helmers, K. F. et al. (2002). Effects of cognitive training interventions with older adults: A randomized controlled trial. *JAMA: Journal of the American Medical Association*, 288(18), 2271–2281.

Bolstad, C. A., & Hess, T. M. (2000). Situation awareness and aging. In: M. R. Endsley & D. J. Garland (Eds.), *Situation awareness, analysis and measurement*, (pp. 277–301). New Jersey, Lawrence Erlbaum Associates.

Braver, E. R., & Trempel, R. E. (2004). Are older drivers actually at higher risk of involvement in collisions resulting in deaths or non-fatal injuries among their passengers and other road users? *Injury Prevention*, 10, 27–32.

Brayne, C., Spiegelhalter, D. J., Dufouil, C. et al. (1999). Estimating the true extent of cognitive decline in the old. *Journal of the American Geriatrics Society*, 47, 1283–1288.

Brayne, C., Dufouil, C., Ahmed, A. et al. (2000). Very old drivers: findings from a population cohort of people aged 84 and over. *International Journal of Epidemiology*, 29, 704–707.

Breen, D. A., Breen, D. P., Moore, J. W., Breen, P. A., & O'Neill, D. (2007). Driving and dementia. *British Medical Journal*, 334, 1365–1369.

Bronfenbrenner, U. (1979). *The ecology of human development*. Cambridge, MA, Harvard University Press.

Bronfenbrenner, U. (1989). Ecological systems theory. In: R. Vasta (Ed.). *Annals of child development*, 6 (pp. 187–251). Greenwich, CT, JAI.

Brooks, N., & Hawley, C. A. (2005). Return to driving after traumatic brain injury: a British perspective. *Brain Injury*, 19(3), 165–175.

Canadian Medical Association. (2006). Determining medical fitness to operate motor vehicles. Available online: http://www.cma.ca/multimedia/CMA/Content_Images/Inside_cma/WhatWePublish/Drivers_Guide/Contents_e.pdf. Accessed September 14 2007.

Charlton, J., Koppel, S., O'Hare, M., Andrea, D., Smith, G., Khodr, B., Langford, J., Oldell, M., & Fildes, B. (2004). *Influence of chronic illness on crash involvement of motor vehicle drivers* (Literature review No. 213), Melbourne, Monash University Accident Research Centre. Available online: http://www.monash.edu.au/muarc/reports/muarc213.pdf. Accessed March 3 2004.

Coughlin, J. F. (2001). Transportation and Older Persons: Perceptions and Preferences. A report on focus groups. Available online: http://www.aarp.org/research/searchResults.html?search_keyword=coughlin&x=20&y=8. Accessed March 13 2008.

Department of Transport, UK (2007). At a glance: guide to the current medical standards of fitness to drive. Available online: http://www.dvla.gov.uk/medical/ataglance.aspx. Accessed September 14 2007.

Di Stefano, M., & Macdonald, W. (2003a). Assessment of older drivers: Relationships among on-road errors, medical conditions and test outcome. *Journal of Safety Research*, 34(5), 415–429.

Di Stefano, M., & Macdonald, W. (2003b). Intelligent transport systems and occupational therapy practice. *Occupational Therapy International*, 10(1), 56–74.

Di Stefano, M., & Macdonald, W. (2006a). *In-Vehicle Intelligent Transport Systems*. St. Louis, Missouri, Elsevier Mosby.

Di Stefano, M., & Macdonald, W. (2006b). On-the-road evaluation of driving performance. In: J. Pellerito (Ed.), *Driver rehabilitation and community mobility: principles and practice*. (pp. 255–274). St. Louis, Missouri, Elsevier Mosby.

Dobbs, B. (2005). *Medical conditions and driving: a review of the literature 1960–2000*. (Technical Report No. DOT HS 809 690). DC: US Department of Transportation. Available online: http://www.nhtsa.dot.gov/people/injury/research/Medical_Condition_Driving/pages/Sec1-Intro.htm. Accessed 11 March 2008.

Dobbs, A., Heller, R., & Schopflocker, D. (1998). A comparative approach to identify unsafe older drivers. *Accident Analysis and Prevention*, 30(3), 363–370.

Dunn, W., McClain, L. H., Brown, C., & Youngstrom, M. J. (1998). The ecology of human performance. In: M. E. Neistadt & E. B. Crepeau (Eds.), *Willard and Spackman's occupational therapy*. (9th ed.) (pp. 525–535). Philadelphia, Lippincott, Williams & Wilkins.

Fisk, A. D., & Rogers, W. A. E. (1997). *Handbook of human factors and the older adult*. San Diego, Academic Press.

Folstein, M. F., Folstein, S. E., & McHugh, P. R. (1975). Mini mental state – a practical method for grading the cognitive state of patients for the clinician. *Journal of Psychiatric Research*, 12, 189–198.

Fonda, S. J., Wallace, R. B., & Herzog, A. R. (2001). Changes in driving patterns and worsening depressive symptoms among older adults. *The Journals of Gerontology Series B: Psychological Sciences and Social Sciences*, 56, S343–S351.

French, D., & Hanson, C. S. (1999). Survey of driver rehabilitation programs. *American Journal of Occupational Therapy*, 53(4), 394–397.

Fricke J., Unsworth, C.A. (2001). Time use and the importance of instrumental activities of daily living. *Australian Occupational Therapy Journal*, 48, 118–131.

Gallo, J. J., Rebok, G. W., & Lesikar, S. E. (1999). The driving habits of adults aged 60 years and older. *Journal of the American Geriatrics Society*, 47, 335–341.

Green, L. (2003). Keys to starting a driver rehabilitation program. *OT Practice* (October 5), 18–19.

Harris, A., (1998) Safety and mobility of older drivers living in rural Victoria. Available online: http://www.racv.com.au/images/pdf/safety_and_mobility_of_older_drivers_in_rural_victoria.pdf. Accessed May 17 2006.

Harris, A, (2003). *Transport research among non-driving older people.*

ARRB/REAAA Annual Conference May, 2003: Proceedings, Cairns, Australian Road Research Board: Melbourne, Victoria.

Hatakka, M., Keskinen, E., Gregersen, N. P., & Glad, A. (1999). Theories and aims of educational and training measures. In: S. E. Siegrist (Ed.), *Driver training, testing and licensing-towards theory-based management of young drivers' injury risk in road traffic.* (pp. 13–44). Berne, Switzerland: Human Research Department, Swiss Council for Accident Prevention bfu.

Hu, P Jones, D Reuscher, T Schmoyer, R & Truett, T (2000) *Projecting fatalities in crashes involving older drivers.* Report for the National Highway Traffic Safety Administration, Oak Ridge National Laboratory Tennessee, ONRL.

Hunt, L. A., Murphy, C., Carr, D. B., Duchek, J., Buckles, V., & Morris, J. (1997). Reliability of the Washington University Road Test: A performance-based assessment for drivers with dementia of the Alzheimer type. *Archives of Neurology*, 54(June, 1997), 707–712.

Kantor, B., Mauger, L., Richardson, V. E., & Tschantz-Unroe, K. (2004). An analysis of an Older Driver Evaluation Program. *Journal of the American Geriatrics Society*, 52(8), 1326–1330.

Keall, M. D., & Frith, W. J. (2004). Older driver crash rates in relation to type and quantity of travel. *Traffic Injury Prevention*, 5, 26–36.

Kielhofner, G. (2002). *A model of human occupation: Theory and application.* (3rd ed.). Baltimore, Williams and Wilkins.

Klavora, P., Young, M., & Heslegrave, R. J. (2000). A review of a major driver rehabilitation centre: A ten-year client profile. *Canadian Journal of Occupational Therapy*, April, 128–134.

Korner-Bitensky, N., Bitensky, J., Sofer, S., Man-Son-Hing, M., & Gelinas, I. (2006). Driving evaluation practices of clinicians working in the United States and Canada. *The American Journal of Occupational Therapy*, 60(4), 428–434.

Kua, A., Korner Bitensky, N., Desrosiers, J., Man-Son-Hing, M., & Marshall, S. (2007). Older driver retraining: A systematic review of evidence of effectiveness. *Journal of Safety Research*, 38, 81–90.

Law, M., Cooper, B. A., Strong, S., Stewart, C., Rigby, P., & Letts, L. (1996). The person-environment-occupation model: A transactive approach to occupational performance. *Canadian Journal of Occupational Therapy*, 63, 9–23.

Liddle, J., & McKenna, K. (2003). Older drivers and driving cessation. *British Journal of Occupational Therapy*, 66(3), 125–132.

Lococo, K. H., & Staplin, L. (2006). *Literature review of polypharmacy and older drivers: Identifying strategies to study drug usage and driving functioning among older drivers.* Available online: http://www.nhtsa.dot.gov/people/injury/olddrive/DrugUse_OlderDriver/pages/content.htm. Accessed 11 March 2008.

Lovell, R., & Di Stefano, M. (2007). *Driver education and rehabilitation course manual for occupational therapists.* Melbourne, School of Occupational Therapy, La Trobe University.

Lovell, R., & Russell, K. (2005). Developing referral and reassessment criteria for drivers with dementia. *Australian Occupational Therapy Journal*, 52, 26–33.

Macdonald, W. (2004). *Human error: Causes and countermeasures.* Paper presented at the Proceedings of the Safety in Action Conference 2004, Melbourne, Australia.

Macdonald, W., Pellerito, J., & Di Stefano, M. (2006). Introduction to driver rehabilitation and community mobility. In: J. Pellerito (Ed.), *Driver rehabilitation and community mobility: Principles and practice.* (pp. 5–35). Philadelphia, Elsevier.

Marottoli, R. A., Mendes de Leon, C., Glass, T. et al. (1997). Driving Cessation and Increased Depressive Symptoms: prospective Evidence from the New Haven EPESE. *Journal of the American Geriatric Society*, 45, 202–206.

Marottoli, R. A., Mendes de leon, C. F., Glass, T. A., Williams, C. S.,

Cooney, L. M., & Berkman, L. F. (2000). Consequences of driving cessation: decreased out-of-home activity levels. *Journal of Gerontology and Social Sciences*, 55B(6), S334–S340.

Messinger-Rapport, B. J. (2003). *Assessment and counseling of older drivers: a guide for primary care physicians – Primary care.* Available online: http://geriatrics.modernmedicine.com/geriatrics/data/articlestandard/geriatrics/502003/78791/article.pdf. Accessed May 2004.

Molnar, F. J., Byszewski, A. M., Marshall, S. C., & Man-Son-Hing, M. (2005). In-office evaluation of medical fitness to drive: practical approaches for assessing older people. *Canadian Family Physician*, 51(March), 372–379.

Molnar, F. J., Patel, A., Marshall, S., Man-Son-Hing, M., & Wilson, K. G. (2006). Clinical utility of office-based cognitive predictors of fitness to drive in persons with dementia: A systematic review. *Journal of the American Geriatric Society*, 54, 1809–1824.

Mollenkopf, H. (2003). *Mobility in later life – the European view.* Position paper presented at the Second Meeting of STELLA Focus Group 3: Society, Behavior, and Private/Public Transport, U.S. National Science Foundation, Arlington, Virginia, USA, January 13–14.

Oborne, D. J. (1982). *Ergonomics at work.* New York, John Wiley & Sons.

Organisation for Economic Co-operative Development. (2001). *Aging and transport: Mobility needs and transport issues; OECD Report.* Geneva, Switzerland: Organisation for Economic Co-operative Development.

Owsley, C., Ball, K., McGwin, G. et al. (1998). Visual processing impairment and risk of motor vehicle crash among older adults. *JAMA: Journal of the American Medical Association*, 279(14), 1083–1088.

Pellerito, J., & Blanc, C. A. (2006). The driver rehabilitation team. In: J. Pellerito (Ed.), *Driver rehabilitation and community mobility: principles and practice.*

(pp. 53–68). St. Louis, Missouri, Elsevier Mosby.

Proctor, R. W., & Van Zandt, T. (1994). *Human Factors in simple and complex systems*. Boston, Allyn and Bacon.

Rabbitt, P., Carmichael, A., Shilling, V., & Sutcliffe, P. (2002). *Age, health and driving: Longitudinally observed changes in reported general health, in mileage, self-rated competence and in attitudes of older drivers*. Manchester, Foundation for Road Safety Research: The University of Manchester Age and Cognitive Performance Research Centre.

Redepenning, S. (2006). *Driver Rehabilitation across age and disability: An occupational therapy guide*. Bethesda, MD, The American Occupational therapy Association, Inc.

Reitan, R. M. (1985). *The Halstead-Reitan neuropsychology battery: Theory and clinical practice*. Tucson, Neuropsychology Press.

Sanders, J. S., & McCormick, E. J. (1993). *Human factors in engineering and design*. (7th ed.). New York, McGraw Hill.

Schold Davis, E. (2003). Defining OT roles in driving. *OT Practice*, January 13, 15–18.

Schultz, S., & Schkade, J. K. (2003). Occupational adaptation. In: E. B. Crepeau, E. S. Cohn & B. A. Boyt Schell (Eds.), *Willard and Spackman's occupational therapy*. (pp. 220–227). Philadelphia, Lippincott Williams & Wilkins.

Segway (2008). About Segway: Dedicated to moving you. Available online: http://www.segway.com/. Accessed 13 March 2008.

Stacey, B. & Kendig, H. (1997) Driving, cessation of driving, and transport safety issues among older people. *Health Promotion Journal of Australia*, 7(3), 175–179.

Stav, W. B. (2004). *Driving rehabilitation: A guide for Assessment and Intervention*. San Antonio, PsychCorp.

Stav, W. B., Hunt, L. A., & Arbesman, M. (2006a). *Occupational therapy practice guidelines for driving and community mobility for older adults*. Tucson, Arizona, American Occupational Therapy Association Inc.

Stav, W. B., Justiss, M. D., Belchior, P., & Lanford, D. N. (2006b). Clinical practice in driving rehabilitation. *Topics in Geriatric Rehabilitation*, 22(2), 153–161.

Townsend, E. A., & Polatajko, H. J. (2007). *Enabling occupation II: Advancing an occupational therapy vision for health, well-being, & justice through occupation*. Ottawa, On, Canadian Association of Occupational Therapists.

US Department of Transportation. (2003). Safe mobility for a maturing society: challenges and opportunities. Available online: http://www.crag.uab.edu/safemobility/SafeMobility.pdf. Accessed 27 Aug 2007.

US Department of Transportation. (2004). Quantifying the relationships: Aging, driving cessation, health and costs. Available online: http://www.volpe.dot.gov/hf/docs/memo012804.doc. Accessed 27 Aug 2007.

VicRoads. (2000). *Resources and guidelines for OT driving assessors*. Melbourne, Roads Corporation.

Wheatley, C. J. (2001). Shifting into drive: Evaluating potential drivers with disabilities. *OT Practice*, July, 12–15.

Whelan, M., Langford, J., Oxley, J., Koppel, S., & Charlton, J. (2006). *The elderly and mobility: A review of the literature*. Available online: http://www.monash.edu.au/muarc/reports/muarc255.html. Accessed 11 March, 2008.

Wickens, C. D., & Hollands, J. G. (2000). *Engineering psychology and human performance* (3rd ed.). New Jersey, Prentice Hall.

Wiseman, E. J., & Souder, E. (1996). The older driver: a handy tool to assess competence behind the wheel. *Geriatrics*, 51(7), 36–38, 41–32, 45.

World Health Organisation (2001). *ICF International Classification of Functioning, Disability and Health*. Geneva, World Health Organisation.

Chapter Thirty-Three

33

Orthotics for occupational outcomes

Natasha Lannin and Iona Novak

CHAPTER CONTENTS

Introduction 508

What are orthoses? 508

Who needs orthoses? 509

The condition 510

The occupational goals of the person . . . 510

The structural properties of the upper
limb and hand 510

Types of orthoses 511

Static orthoses 511

Semi-dynamic orthoses 512

Dynamic orthoses 512

How to design orthoses 513

When to use orthoses 513

Immobilisation 513

Joint protection 513

Immobilisation for rest 513

Immobilisation for wound healing 513

Correcting deformities and preventing
contractures 515

Correcting deformities and preventing
scarring 516

Improving use of the hand 518

Reducing pain 521

Decreasing oedema 522

Conclusion 523

SUMMARY

Orthotics is the practice of designing, fabricating, fitting, and applying orthoses to restore or improve performance and structural characteristics. Orthoses are pieces of equipment applied externally to a body part to protect, immobilise or stabilise joints or to protect, correct and maintain skin integrity and/or movement. There are three types of orthoses: static, semi-dynamic, and dynamic. These orthoses are used to facilitate occupational engagement and the attainment of occupational goals for people with a variety of hand and upper-limb conditions. These can include neurological, inflammatory and degenerative conditions, burns and traumatic hand injuries among many others. Orthoses are used for a wide range of reasons. These include: immobilisation of the hand to promote joint protection, rest or wound healing; correction of deformity; prevention of scarring; improvement of hand use; reduction of pain; and reduction of oedema. This chapter introduces readers to the principles of orthoses prescription using these common reasons as examples. Indications, contraindications, assessment, design, materials, wearing, and review protocols are explored. In common with other specialised occupational therapy interventions, orthoses prescription is done within the context of person-centred reasoning. Orthoses are only used when they contribute to the attainment of relevant and meaningful occupational outcomes for the person and their family. Occupational therapists must, therefore, use sound reasoning when selecting orthotics as an intervention strategy. Every orthoses should thus: be customised to achieve the unique occupational goals of each person; use up-to-date information regarding efficacy, design, wearing protocol, materials, and monitoring regimes; and be relevant and practical in the person's life situation. Without careful attention to these three elements of orthoses prescription, even the most technically precise orthosis will not achieve occupational outcomes.

KEY POINTS

- Occupational therapists use orthoses to achieve occupational outcomes where equal attention is given to the scientific aspect of orthoses and to the person-centred aspect of practice.
- Orthoses are considered an adjunctive intervention as they are used to either 'establish or restore' a person's skills or prevent the occurrence or development of barriers to performance.
- Anyone who has a condition that affects the use of their hand/s may benefit from orthotic intervention.
- Occupational therapists conduct a comprehensive occupation-focused assessment which includes a review of relevant body structures and functions, and consideration of environmental factors to determine if an orthoses is appropriate.
- Orthoses may be prescribed to: immobilise and/or protect weak, painful or healing musculoskeletal structures; prevent or correct developing deformities, including contractures and scarring; assist in providing improved abilities and/or serve as an attachment for assistive devices; and reduce pain by limiting motion or weight-bearing.
- There are three classes of orthoses: static, semi-dynamic, and dynamic.
- The type of orthosis, the position of the hand or arm, and the wearing protocol will vary because each person is an individual, with unique occupational goals, unique injury or disease processes, and unique rehabilitation goals.
- Occupational therapists need to explicitly seek out and factor in scientifically gained knowledge into their daily decision-making, overcoming the inertia of practicing within the 'comfort zones', and constantly remain abreast of scientific evidence.

Introduction

Orthoses are used in the treatment of hand and upper-limb impairments by occupational therapists. Orthotics is the practice of designing, fabricating, fitting, and applying orthoses to restore or improve performance and structural characteristics. Occupational therapists use orthoses to achieve occupational outcomes. As a consequence, occupational therapists who use orthotic strategies must be able to synthesise the technical aspects of orthoses prescription, design, fabrication and application, with the inter-personal dimensions of understanding a person's performance and life role goals. The focus on occupational outcomes taken in this chapter, means that equal attention is given to the scientific aspect of orthoses and to the person-centred aspect of practice. Readers are encouraged to adopt an explicit attitude towards their reasoning when using orthoses in practice, so that the balance between the scientific and the personal occupation-focused dimension of therapy is maintained. Without this person-centred focus, the attainment of relevant, meaningful occupational outcomes through orthotics is unlikely.

This chapter does not aim to teach readers skills in splint or cast fabrication. There are specialist texts already available which meet this need and explain the biomechanical principles that underlie fabrication and the reader can refer to the list of further readings at the end of this chapter (e.g. Coppard & Lohman 1996, Goga-Eppenstien et al 1999, Hogan & Uditsky 1998, Wilton & Dival 1997). Rather, the chapter leads readers through foundation principles, provides examples, and points out important issues that should be explicitly considered in the reasoning process. In the Ecology of Human Performance Model there are five different approaches to intervention (Dunn et al 1994). Only two of these are pertinent to orthotic prescription, these are: 'establish or restore' interventions, which seek to improve the person's skills; and 'preventative' interventions, which aim to prevent the occurrence or development of barriers to performance (Dunn et al 1994). For this reason orthoses are thought of as an 'adjunctive' intervention (Copley & Kuipers 1999), that is they are always used in combination with other interventions designed to improve the person's occupational engagement.

What are orthoses?

Occupational therapists manufacture and prescribe orthoses as one specialised aspect of upper-limb intervention. Upper-limb orthoses are equipment applied externally to the body to restore or improve functional and structural characteristics of the musculoskeletal and nervous systems. They can be splints, casts, and garments. Splints and garments are external devices designed to immobilise the limb in a position or stabilise joints to encourage a movement (Copley & Kuipers 1999). Casts are made of plaster or fibreglass and are used to immobilise bones for fracture healing or to stretch muscles for reducing contractures (Lannin et al 2007b). The use of orthotics has developed largely from the experiences of therapists and is, therefore, predominantly expert opinion evidence (Kogler 2002). This means that the scientific evidence base for the design, application and evaluation of orthoses is both recent and rapidly growing in nature. It is vital, therefore, to maintain a working knowledge of developments and trends due to the dynamic nature of orthotic practice.

Orthoses can be made of a variety of materials and the development of new orthotic products is increasing all the time as specialist companies search for improved product range and performance. It is important, therefore, to seek out product information from local suppliers, benchmark this with recent evidence regarding performance of the material in clinical investigations and choose the material that will best suit a person's needs, therapeutic goals and resource constraints. Applying skills in appraisal of evidence helps therapists select not only what type of orthosis design could be used but also what type of material may be most appropriate. The types of materials mentioned in this chapter are only indicative of the range that may be available. Newer materials are constantly being developed which address factors such as ease of application, cosmesis, comfort, and durability.

Who needs orthoses?

Anyone who has a condition that affects the use of their hand/s may benefit from orthotic intervention. Occupational therapists use a range of information to determine if orthotic intervention is appropriate. They conduct a comprehensive occupation-focused assessment which includes a review of relevant body structures and functions, and consideration of environmental factors. Assessment may use a range of information sources including medical record review, standardised assessments, skilled observations, interview protocols, ecological measures, and activity analysis (Dunn 2000). People most likely to benefit from orthoses are those with musculoskeletal injury, neurological events such as stroke or spinal cord injury, burn injuries, as well as degenerative conditions such as arthritis. The goal in all of these circumstances is to enhance occupational

engagement through increased upper limb and hand use (Trombly & Ma 2002). Depending on the condition and the occupational goal, the person may require an orthosis that will support upper-limb structures such as joints, muscles or skin, or an orthosis that facilitates movement. The occupational goal always guides the selection of orthosis type and material – the same presenting condition may not require the same orthosis type as the occupational goals of the individual may vary. Unless the occupational goal is clear, the selection of orthosis type can not be well informed and may not be appropriate.

Occupational therapists need to have an excellent understanding of the condition, of the occupational goals of the person, and of the normal and abnormal structural properties of the upper limb and hand to inform the selection of orthoses as a suitable intervention strategy.

Practice Scenario 33.1 describes the professional practice of a certified hand therapist who maintains the person focus in orthotic practice.

Practice Scenario 33.1 Julia

Julia runs her own private hand therapy clinic in Sydney, Australia, where she carries a caseload in addition to supervising junior staff. In her daily practice, she sees a wide variety of people who have been referred for hand therapy – some with traumatic hand injuries, some who have a musculoskeletal condition, some who have had a stroke, and some who have had a brain injury. Being prepared to treat any upper-limb condition requires Julia to have a sound understanding of normal anatomy, normal healing processes, underlying pathology of a range of conditions, but most of all of problem solving. Julia maintains that the most important skill for a hand therapist to develop is that of reasoning. She states that therapists have,

> To be able to assess everything that is going on for each individual person, not only their injury and its usual healing processes, but also their work, domestic and leisure tasks, in order to know what intervention will provide the best possible outcome.

Excellent reasoning skills not only allow Julia to choose interventions to meet individualised goals, but also to be able to predict the timeframe for healing, to advise each individual of potential complications and when to address them, and to know that she will need to continually reassess her intervention plans. Unlike many junior therapists, Julia's experience in hand therapy has taught her that providing one splint is never the complete therapy programme. It is important to acknowledge that the natural tissue-healing process means that the splint will require adjustments, changes, or even prescription of a completely different splint in order to meet the ever-changing goals for the person. Experience has also taught Julia the benefits and limitations of different orthoses and flexibility to her approach to splinting, which allows her to know how to modify a design to suit each person's unique occupational requirements. Expert therapists such as Julia employ reasoning to ensure their interventions are not only evidence based, but that they are occupation focused and tailored to meet each person's unique and individual needs.

The condition

Any condition which adversely affects the use, comfort or cosmesis (aesthetic appearance) of the hand may indicate the need for an orthosis. Consideration of the disease process and pathology will allow the therapist to consider the extent to which the condition has affected normal structural features and processes, and the likely course or prognosis of the disease. For example, rheumatoid arthritis generally passes through one of three disease phases: acute, sub-acute, and chronic. The acute phase is characterised by inflamed, swollen, and painful joints, while during the sub-acute phase the disease is less active. In the sub-acute phase the person's condition remains stable for longer periods of time, but joint deformity is progressing. By the chronic phase the disease is no longer active, but the residual mechanical problems in and around the joint produce pain, instability, and stiffness, all resulting in a devastating loss of performance. Being aware of the disease process allows the therapist to educate the person about their condition and therapy goals, and to predict how therapy goals will need to change in the future to meet the occupational engagement goals of the person. The type of orthosis selected for different phases of the condition, the wearing regimen recommended and the likely structural outcomes will vary according to the disease process characteristics and phases.

The occupational goals of the person

The decision to use an orthoses will depend in part on the condition, but also to a great extent on personal goals. The starting point for any relationship between therapists and the people with who they work is in the establishing of goals, which should emerge from a collaborative rather than a prescriptive relationship. While some therapists find open-ended discussion a useful way to identify occupational goals and evaluation criteria, others use semi-structured interviewing focused around development of goal attainment scales (Hurn et al 2006, Ottenbacher & Cusick 1990), or structured approaches such as the Canadian Occupational Performance Measure (COPM) (Law et al 1990) to identify problems, priorities and impact measures. With or without structured instruments, the occupational therapist must identify how the altered hand performance is affecting the person's occupational engagement in self-care, productivity, and leisure and the person's desired occupational outcomes. Goals relating to orthotic prescription may include changes in: role performance, activity, particular desired movements, pain management, wound healing, and cosmetic appearance. The occupational goals of the person are paramount for occupational therapists. Body-structure problems, even when present, do not always translate to activities and participation impairments and, therefore, they may not need intervention (Bleck 1987, Copley & Kuipers 1999, Harris et al 1985).

The structural properties of the upper limb and hand

Occupational therapists need to have an excellent working knowledge of the anatomy and physiology of the upper limb and hand – it is the foundation to successful orthotic intervention. Therapists need to know how the 'normal' upper limb and hand is structured, how it works and the physiological processes that sustain it to be able to grasp the impact of disease or trauma and the likely mechanisms for recovery. As most orthoses use biomechanical principles in their design, a thorough understanding of biomechanical properties of the upper limb and hand is required. This is particularly important as biomechanical deficits are independent of specific disease processes that may be present in a condition.

Bone and joint injuries, infections, varying degrees of paralysis, joint diseases and trauma all have diverse causes and processes that may present similar biomechanical deficits. It is important to be mindful that biomechanical deficits do not necessarily translate into performance deficits and, therefore, comprehensive assessment that includes analysis of individual's goals is necessary.

Types of orthoses

All orthoses are prescribed for one or more of the following purposes, to:

- immobilise and/or protect weak, painful or healing musculoskeletal structures

- prevent or correct developing deformities, including contractures and scarring

- assist in providing improved abilities and/or serve as an attachment for assistive devices

- reduce pain by limiting motion or weight-bearing.

The individual assessment will indicate what particular objectives will be pursued through the orthosis design, application and wearing regimen in support of the desired overarching occupational outcome.

There are three classes of orthoses: static, semi-dynamic, and dynamic. This classification is based on the key purpose of the orthosis. Static orthoses aim to prevent any movement by immobilising a joint. Semi-dynamic orthoses limit an aspect of movement in a joint while facilitating another movement in other joints. Dynamic orthoses are designed to mobilise joints, muscles and/or skin to facilitate a desired movement.

Static orthoses

Static orthoses are also known as immobilisation splints (Figure 33.1). These have no moving parts and aim to immobilise to help prevent further deformity or soft-tissue contracture. Static orthoses immobilise a joint in a pre-determined position selected on the basis of the occupational goal, features of the presenting condition and structural

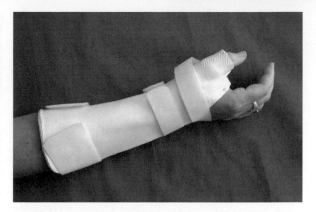

Figure 33.1 • Static splint

factors relating to the individual and the material used for fabrication. Static orthoses can rigidly support body structures as in the case of fractures, inflammatory conditions, and nerve injuries where the body part must be stabilised and protected. Static orthoses can also apply a prolonged stretch to muscles or skin when stretch is required to achieve structural change as in the case of neurological conditions or burns (Duncan 1989, Farmer & James 2001, Fess et al 2004, Hill 1988, Lowe 1995, Milazzo & Gillen 1998, Wilton & Dival 1997).

Examples of static orthoses include pressure splints (McKnight & Schomburg 1982), dorsal or volar wrist splints (Tenney & Lisak 1986, Wilton & Dival 1997), resting hand splints (Tenney & Lisak 1986, Wilton & Dival 1997), mallet splints (Handoll & Vaghela 2004) and buddy taping (Tenney & Lisak 1986).

The best known example is the resting splint (Figure 33.2). A resting splint does what the name suggests, it immobilises the wrist, fingers and thumb in a 'resting' position. The position of 'rest' is carefully determined for each individual. Resting splints are usually made of thermoplastic material, and are custom-moulded and secured onto the upper limb by adjustable strapping. They are commonly used with people with arthritis, but can be appropriate in other situations.

Orthoses that immobilise may allow a therapist to immobilise skin (e.g. immediately following skin graft surgery), to protect joints (e.g. in arthritic conditions), to promote tissue healing (e.g. following hand trauma), to stretch skin (e.g. as in the case of burns or hand trauma following wound healing), or

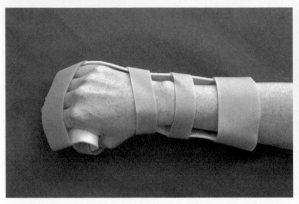

Figure 33.2 ● Resting splint

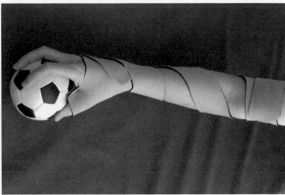

Figure 33.4 ● TAP splint

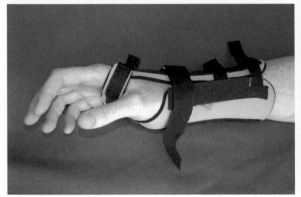

Figure 33.3 ● Semi-dynamic splint

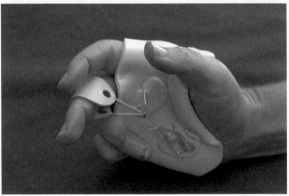

Figure 33.5 ● Dynamic splint

to stretch muscle (e.g. as in the case of neurological impairments).

Semi-dynamic orthoses

Semi-dynamic orthoses (Figure 33.3) restrict the force of a particular movement and facilitate another target movement using the intrinsic elastic property of the orthotic material. They can also substitute for loss of motor function by holding a joint in a position when the muscles do not have adequate strength or motor control. Materials such as Lycra®, neoprene, and rubber foam are used to manufacture semi-dynamic orthoses. Orthoses made from these materials are often named after the product, for example 'neoprene splint' or 'Lycra® garment'. Semi-dynamic orthoses are particularly useful for people with overuse injuries, burns, and neurological impairments. These orthoses tend to be circumferential in nature and either cover the target joint fully

or run parallel to the line of desired muscle pull. An example of this is the Tone and Positioning (TAP) splint shown in Figure 33.4.

Dynamic orthoses

Dynamic orthoses are also known as mobilisation splints (Figure 33.5). These have moving parts which promote, control or restore movement. They create an intermittent, gentle force on a segment of the upper limb resulting in motion of a joint or muscle. The force is created through the careful design of the orthoses so that the 'pull' of elastic bands, springs, or mechanical devices will create the desired therapeutic effect. Dynamic splints allow a therapist to control the direction and amount of movement in joints, tendons, and muscles. An example of a condition where dynamic splints are commonly used is in the rehabilitation phase after tendon repair. The therapist moulds a stable thermoplastic base splint from which they attach an 'outrigger', which pulls the target joint, tendons and muscles in a desired direction.

How to design orthoses

Many possibilities exist for static, semi-dynamic and dynamic orthosis design and fabrication. The choice of design is informed by a good working knowledge of upper-limb anatomy, a thorough assessment of the person that identifies problems which are limiting performance and, finally, by understanding the capabilities and limitations of each type of orthosis. Extensive reference material exists on orthoses designs and their indications for use. Some of this material can be found in the Further Reading section at the end of the chapter.

The biomechanical approach provides a logical method of analysing presenting structural problems and considering corrective options. In the biomechanical approach, the therapist aims to maintain or increase movement by controlling adverse movements and preventing or addressing the structural changes to joints, muscles, and soft issue caused by immobilisation and muscle imbalance (Copley & Kuipers 1999). Although a range of information sources may be used to determine if an orthotic intervention is potentially relevant, the actual design of the orthosis takes a particular approach. A biomechanical assessment is recommended, as this explores all factors relevant to orthosis fabrication: The biomechanical examination (Table 33.1) typically includes assessment of range of motion, muscle strength, sensation, pain, and analysis of the degree of voluntary movement possible (Bleck 1987, Gaubert & Mockett 2000). The factors of interest are only those which are causing movement loss, pain or concern to the person as they relate to the occupational goal of orthotic intervention.

When to use orthoses

Orthoses may be used with people in whom joint immobilisation and protection are required. This may arise from the need to rest, to heal wounds or facilitate performance. They may be required to correct deformities and prevent scarring or contractures. Orthoses may be used when there is a need to improve movement, reduce pain or decrease oedema. Each of these indications for orthotic intervention is now explored.

Immobilisation

Joint protection

Perhaps the most common use for an orthosis is to immobilise a body part, such as during fracture healing. Immobilising orthoses can also be used to protect joints, minimise joint damage or joint deformity, or help manage pain. Orthoses that are prescribed for joint protection may have wearing regimens governed by either presenting symptoms or featurens of the condition. For example, joint protection related to trauma may require an orthoses to be worn only when symptoms of pain may be present, while joint protection related to the pathology of an arthritic joint will require a wearing regimen independent of symptoms for the protective goals to be achieved.

Immobilisation for rest

Immobilisation may be undertaken to allow tissues to rest in a position which minimises any complications associated with inflammation, contracture or pain (Wilton & Dival 1997). Hand therapy literature maintains that at rest, the hand and wrist adopt a posture that allows a perfect balance of muscle and ligament tension (Wilton & Dival 1997). Therapists often use static splints to mimic this position, known as the 'resting' or 'functional' position. The resting position is 10–20° wrist extension, 20–45° flexion of MCP joints, and between 10 and 30° IP flexion (Wilton & Dival 1997).

The evidence for the use of splints to immobilise the hand for rest during the inflammatory phase of rheumatoid arthritis is controversial (Coppard & Lohman 1996). Rest is seen by therapists to be beneficial; however, this must be carefully balanced with movement to guard against loss of motion (Ouellette 1991).

Immobilisation for wound healing

Immobilisation may be undertaken to allow tissues to heal in a specific position, such as in skin healing following skin graft surgery. Immobilising orthoses may be used for healing skin, bone and ligamentous structures, and also surgically released nerves. The position of the hand will be determined primarily by the damaged structures and the surgeries (if any) performed. There needs to be a balance between the immobilisation of damaged structures and the maintenance of movement in structures which have not

Table 33.1 Biomechanical orthotic examination

Assessment	Rationale
Range of motion (ROM) assessment: ROM assessment is the numeric measurement of a joint's capability. Passive range of motion (PROM) is 'the amount of movement available at a joint when it is moved by an assistant' (Copley & Kuipers 1999, p. 298) and active range of motion (AROM) is, 'the amount of movement available at a joint when the limb is moved voluntarily by the person' (Copley & Kuipers 1999, p. 297). ROM is measured using a device called a 'goniometer'	ROM is routinely taken when hypertonicity, injury causing immobilisation, and joint conditions such as arthritis are present, because the risks of discomfort and joint contracture are elevated. ROM deficits can lead to a secondary loss of performance skills (Copley & Kuipers 1999)
Muscle strength assessment: A muscle group's strength can be graded in relation to its ability to provide resistance to fundamental forces such as gravity and then to an external force such as an assessor or weighted objects. Various scales exist to describe strength classifications, in addition to devices called 'dynamometers', which is the preferred methodology where possible (Bohannon 1997)	Muscle strength is an important element of AROM and endurance. Weakness affects movement and independence. Muscle weakness can be present as a primary impairment, for example, in muscle diseases and hypertonicity, but also occurs as a secondary impairment from immobilisation and lack of limb use
Pain assessment: Pain is assessed using a variety of tools. These include: Visual Analogue Scales (VAS); self-report survey measures (Farrar et al 2001); the McGill Pain Questionnaire (Melzack 1987); the Pain Behaviour Checklist (Kerns et al 1991); the West Haven-Yale Multidimensional Pain Inventory (WHYMPI) (Kerns et al 1985); and Pain-Free Function Questionnaire (Stratford et al 1989)	The presence of pain will affect the self-selected use of the limb and available ROM. Use may exacerbate pain and inflammation and discontinued use may result in secondary impairments of loss of ROM and strength
Voluntary movement assessment: Description: The quantity and quality of voluntary movement available to the person is measured using numerous standardised assessments. The selection of an appropriate tool depends on the person's diagnostic group and age, your purpose for measurement and the instrument's psychometric properties (Carey et al 1996, Fugl-Meyer et al 1975). Taxonomies exist to assist you to select appropriate instruments (Cole et al 1995, Law et al 1999, 2000)	The degree of voluntary movement possible affect the person's AROM, general limb use, quality of movement, compensatory movements adopted, and success with tasks
Person-Centred Self Assessment of Upper Limb Movement: There are a number of standardised tools that have been developed to help the therapist understand the upper limb impairment from the person's perspective, for example the Duruoz Hand Index (DHI) (Poole et al 2006) or the Disabilities of Arm Shoulder and Hand (DASH) (Hudak Amadio Bombardier 1996)	The person may conceptualise their occupational role loss in a different way to the therapist and this can bring new and insightful information to the assessment process

been damaged. Injuries may also warrant different immobilising positions for day and night. Therapists should remain aware of such potential complications which are all part of normal tissue-healing processes, and monitor the orthosis in order to make appropriate adjustments as required to ensure immobilisation (see Figure 33.6). For example, an orthosis applied in the first 72 hours after a traumatic injury may not fit the person shortly after application because of oedema. This is particularly the case in burn injuries which involve significant oedema.

The evidence for the effectiveness of immobilisation to facilitate wound healing is complex. Whilst immobilisation may facilitate wound closure it can cause secondary impairments. Such is the case in microsurgical repair of the hand following a digital nerve injury. In this condition immobilisation splinting is used to protect against possible damage to the

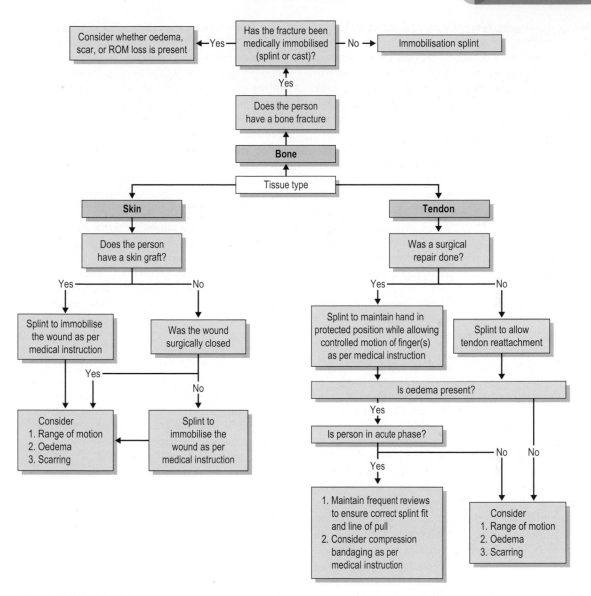

Figure 33.6 • Primary goal – tissue healing

repaired nerve sheath. Evidence, however, suggests that people who wear these splints have more adverse outcomes than those who are not splinted; they take longer to return to work and the unwanted symptoms of pain and loss of range of motion take longer to recover (Clare et al 2004). The choice of orthosis materials is also important to successful outcomes. Research now suggests that immobilisation of fractures using splints rather than casts is better tolerated and result in better hand recovery at the completion of the immobilisation period (O'Connor et al 2003, Plint et al 2006).

Correcting deformities and preventing contractures

If a body part is left immobile for a protracted period of time, joint capsule contraction and shortening of tendon and muscle groups that cross that joint occur. Such immobilisation occurs in many neurological conditions where the person loses the ability to activate their upper-limb muscles. However, recovery from acute injury may also dictate immobilisation (e.g. immediately following skin graft surgery, tendon repairs or fracture). Loss of extensibility in muscles and soft tissues acting across a joint is a common sequela of immobilisation. Such losses in extensibility will result in imbalance between structures and can result in quite dramatic impairments (e.g. a small loss of extensibility as a result of contracted structures will dramatically impair grasp).

Biomechanical theory maintains that anti-deformity positioning and stretching is able to minimise shortening of tendons, collateral ligaments, joint capsules, and muscle (Wilton & Dival 1997). In many conditions, several predictable contractures occur in the upper limb; these contractures are generally associated with the flexed position of comfort. A key aspect to the reasoning process when aiming to prevent deformity is an understanding of the disease or condition processes coupled with a sound understanding of the available interventions that have good supporting research evidence. While a strong history of practice supports the ability of an orthosis to correct deformity and prevent contracture, the evidence is less convincing.

Therapists may use static, semi-dynamic or dynamic orthoses to prevent the formation of, or to decrease, contracture (see Figure 33.7). The consistent aim, however, is to provide a stretch. Static orthoses, such as casts or resting splints, are used to position joints so that a stretch is maintained on soft tissues. For example, in people after severe burns, axillary contractures are usually prevented by positioning the shoulders widely abducted with axillary splints and elbow flexion contractures are minimised by statically splinting the elbow in extension. In adults after brain injury, therapists prevent contractures in the elbows using casts to maintain elbow extension, and use serial casts to increase range of motion in those people who have developed a contracture.

A semi-dynamic orthosis, such as a Lycra® garment or tone-and-positioning splint (see Figure 33.4), may also be used to provide a slow, low-force stretch, while allowing some movement. Gracies and colleagues (1997) found that individually made Lycra® garments can produce continuous stretch of muscles for several hours. Such garments are more commonly used with children, although they are used in burn and neurological rehabilitation as well.

A dynamic orthosis may also be applied for the purpose of preventing or treating contracture. A dynamic flexion splint following a flexor tendon repair provides controlled motion, protecting the healing tendon from excessive tension while allowing limited glide to prevent adherence of the tendon and the formation of a contracture.

The evidence of trials testing how effective splinting and casting is for the management of contracture is useful for therapists to review as an integral part of their reasoning process. There are research gaps which present challenges to evidence-based practice. Preliminary research has demonstrated that a daily total stretch time of more than 6 hours to address contracture in adults with hand fractures and tendon/soft-tissue contracture (Glasgow et al 2003). At the time of writing, however, there are no double-blind prospective randomised studies investigating the effectiveness of orthoses for contracture management in orthopaedic injuries. Harvey and Herbert (2002) completed a systematic review of stretch interventions for adults with spinal cord injury. This review also showed that there is insufficient evidence for the use of stretch for contracture management in this population. Perhaps the most research on contracture management to date, whilst still limited, has been with people with neurological conditions (Autti-Ramo et al 2006). Mixed results have been found in studies within this population. Trials have found that hand splints are unable to prevent or treat contracture in adults with stroke, brain injury or spinal cord injuries (Harvey et al 2006, Lannin et al 2003, 2007a). Studies investigating casting in the upper limb have shown improvement in range of movement (Hill 1993, Law et al 1997, Moseley et al 2006); however, in one study, the effects from cast-wear had disappeared 42 days after cast removal (Moseley et al 2006).

Such uncertainty clearly demonstrates the importance of remaining abreast of current literature. As more studies are conducted it is hoped that occupational therapists will have greater knowledge regarding when to use orthoses, for how long, and in what position the hand or arm should be positioned in order to address contracture.

Correcting deformities and preventing scarring

Wound healing from burns or open injuries is a multifaceted process, involving highly regulated cellular and chemical events intended to restore tissue integrity. Wound healing occurs through scar formation. Scar tissue integrity is challenged if the new

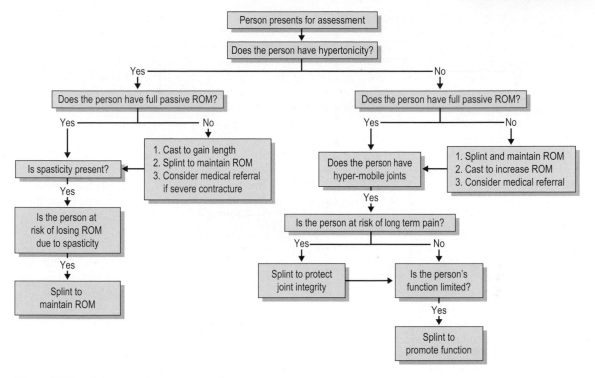

Figure 33.7 • Primary goal – range of motion

tissue structures are too weak, too strong or too abundant. This can result in hypertrophic scarring. Wounds are predisposed to hypertrophic scar formation when: the healing process is prolonged; inflammation is present; the wound is scratched; or if wound tension is excessive. Scar tissue is less elastic than normal soft tissue and thus can interfere with range of movement by preventing skin from moving adequately. Scar formation inside a wound can also cause adhesions that interfere with tendon gliding. Movement restrictions from lost skin elasticity or tendon glide both can lead to further performance loss in the hand, affecting occupational role performance. Scar formation can also significantly affect the cosmesis of the hand and, consequently, the person's feeling about their limb's appearance and likely use (Kasch 1998).

Intervention seeks to minimise scar formation; minimise scar adhesions, and promote scar remodelling. Whilst an effective rehabilitation programme will also emphasise activity, stretch and exercise to prevent contracture development, therapy may additionally include the use of splints and compression to prevent scarring (see Figure 33.8). Mechanical pressure has long been advocated as a way to influence scarring; ever since research found that

compression is able to rearrange the collagen in scars (Kischer et al 1975, Parks et al 1978). The reasoning behind using compression garments and splints on maturing scars is to apply perpendicular pressure that approximates capillary pressure (Carr-Collins 1992). This theory, has not, however, been empirically tested. Despite this, a range of specialised scar-management techniques are used, including: scar compression garments, which reduce the thickness of the resultant scar; massage, to promote scar softening and extensibility; ultrasound; casts; and splints with silicone-gel sheet linings, to promote scar elasticity and 'flattening'.

Scar management has been widely adopted in practice for reducing the performance and psychological effects of abnormal scar tissue. The evidence supporting the therapeutic approaches are inconclusive due to methodological weaknesses in the studies conducted (Mustoe et al 2002, O'Brien & Pandit 2006). Evidence-based guidelines recommend the use of silicone-gel sheeting and intralesional corticosteroids for abnormal scar management (Mustoe et al 2002), but a meta-analysis found no significant differences in efficacy between the varying approaches (Leventhal et al 2006). New evidence is constantly being developed in this field.

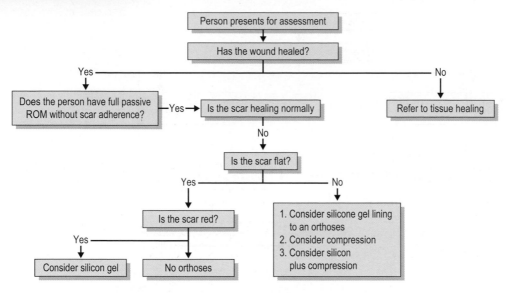

Figure 33.8 • Primary goal – scar management

Weak evidence suggests that silicone-gel sheeting reduces the incidence of scarring and improves scar elasticity (O'Brien & Pandit 2006). Research also suggests that the wearing of burns compression garments reduces scar thickness (Van den Kerckhove et al 2005). Research data show, however, that despite precise fitting techniques, pressure garments do not provide a consistent amount of pressure at the scar/garment interface (Mann et al 1997). Reasoning must be applied in the treatment of scars; scientific evidence is inconclusive and the therapist must work with the person to determine the most appropriate intervention plan.

Improving use of the hand

Occupational therapists prescribe orthoses to facilitate attainment of occupational outcomes. Dynamic, semi-dynamic, and static splints may be used to substitute for loss of movement (Fess et al 2004). Consequently, an orthoses that aims to improve use of the hand will be one that takes into account not only the structural characteristics of the upper limb and hand, but also the goals and preferences of the person who has the condition. As hand use is context- and task-specific, the selection, design and wearing protocol of a movement-enhancing orthoses must be based not only on the careful biomechanical assessment of upper limb and hand capacity, and individual goals, but also on the very best practice and research evidence available on the likely impact

on recovery. Currently, much orthotic practice for the upper limb and hand is based on practice tradition, theoretical assumptions and a still emerging body of empirical evidence. Orthoses have, for example, been used for decades in practice to help 'position' a joint in a 'functional position' with the belief that use of the hand can then be more easily facilitated. Theoretical assumptions have also been made that use of the hand will be improved with virtually all orthoses by diminishing pain, relieving movements and preventing deformity. These traditions and theoretical assumptions are being tested, and there is a condition-specific evidence base under rapid development. Occupational therapists must keep up to date to ensure their selection, design and wearing protocol prescriptions for appropriate orthoses are evidence based and relevant to varying conditions.

The types of hand movements that the therapist seeks to enhance through prescription of an orthoses include: reach, grasp, release, carry, bimanual hand movements, and in-hand manipulation (Exner 1996). The application of an orthosis to improve hand use is likely to be a long-term therapy decision. Providing such orthoses, therefore, requires great care in assessment to ensure that the orthosis will correct biomechanical deficits and improve performance without causing secondary problems that can range from skin breakdown to social stigma. Central to long-term orthotic success is the wearer's willingness and ability to maintain appropriate wearing protocols. Consequently, comfort, an observable

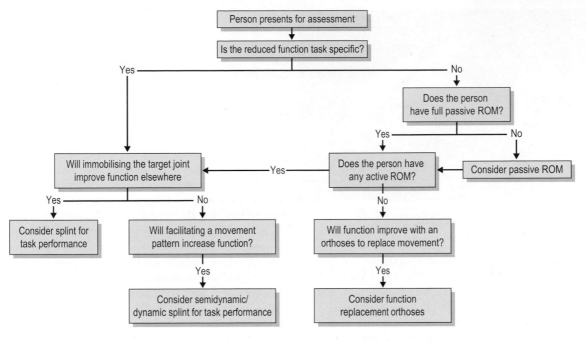

Figure 33.9 • Primary goal – improving hand movement

change in either the presenting symptoms or the level of hand use, ease of application, and cosmetic appearance will be important user factors that could affect occupational outcomes.

Orthoses that improve hand use may be static, semi-dynamic, or dynamic. The most common orthoses are static splints which aim to immobilise either part of or the whole of an upper limb or hand. Immobilisation can stabilise one component of the hand or arm in order to facilitate greater use of another aspect of the hand (Figure 33.9).

The 'wrist cock-up splint' (Figure 33.10) is such a splint and is seen commonly in practice, used with a wide variety of conditions. The rationale for the splint design is that if significant weakness exists in finger extensors, the hand can compensate for the weakness by using an alternative movement pattern called 'tenodesis'. Tenodesis is where the person uses wrist flexion and extension, instead of finger extension, to open and close the fingers for grasp. If the occupational outcome of therapy requires finger extensor rather than tenodesis movement patterns, then an orthosis is required to prevent the unwanted pattern and facilitate the desired pattern. The 'wrist cock-up splint' literally cocks the wrist to a desired angle, immobilises it to prevent wrist flexion and, in doing so, provides forced opportunities for active finger extension either as part of daily activity or as

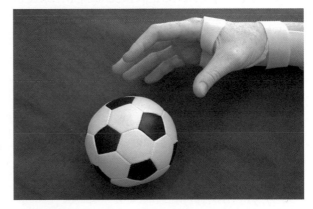

Figure 33.10 • Wrist cock-up splint

part of motor training intervention. The 'wrist cock-up splint' is, thus, commonly used when occupations requiring precise grasp and accurate hand aperture during prehension are therapy goals.

Another orthosis that operates on the basis of immobilising one joint in order to permit movement in another to achieve performance is the 'thumb post' splint (Figure 33.11). Here the central biomechanical challenge being met by the splint is that of supporting an unstable metacarpal phalangeal (MCP) joint or blocking undesired thumb adduction and flexion movements. The orthotic material is

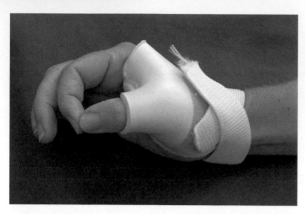

Figure 33.11 • Thumb post splint

figuratively moulded around the thumb forming a type of 'post' to immobilise the MCP joint of the thumb into mid-range flexion and abduction, and at times aiming to block MCP hyperextension. The orthoses modifies or restores the position of the hand and thumb to externally facilitate desired thumb opposition movement for the pincer grasp.

Hand use can also be improved using dynamic or semi-dynamic orthoses. These are particularly useful when the occupational outcome requires weak movements to be assisted. The selection of material for fabrication is critical in these splints as it is the degree of active or passive force being applied that must match the biomechanical goal to support the occupational outcome. Common fabrication materials are Lycra® or neoprene garments, or springs or elastic band components attached to thermoplastic base splints. An example of a common semi-dynamic orthosis used to promote a desired movement is the 'tone and positioning' (TAP) splint (see Figure 33.4). The TAP splint is made of neoprene. It helps the wearer to use supination and increase supination strength, as the splint 'wraps around' the upper limb and is anchored at key joints in such a way as to facilitate supination. It is the elastic properties of the neoprene that dynamically assist the movement.

Orthoses that improve hand use can also be developed to actually replace a movement that has been lost and is either unlikely to recover or is immediately needed by the person to achieve occupational goals. In these instances, the orthosis replaces the upper limb or hand movement in the task. Common examples are splints designed to hold a pen, pencil or eating instrument, orthoses to allow wheel control while driving a car, or orthoses to type on a computer. In addition, neural stimulation devices can be inserted into orthoses to facilitate muscle contractions for hand use. These developing sophisticated devices usually require multidisciplinary expertise including biomedical engineers or specialist prosthetic and orthotic professionals to devise safe and appropriate inclusions.

The literature researching the effectiveness of splinting in improving hand use is laden with methodological flaws. This is because the theoretical assumptions for orthotic intervention have changed so significantly over time, particularly in the field of hypertonicity management. Based on newer basic science evidence, no longer do occupational therapists believe that they reduce muscle spasticity associated with hypertonicity using orthoses. Yet the evidence base for orthoses for improving hand use lags behind, as research studies have included orthoses designed to simultaneously reduce spasticity and improve hand use. In addition to major problems with orthosis design, most of the studies lack methodological rigor and appropriate outcome measures. There is a pressing need for more research in this area of practice, where newer studies employ appropriate methodologies and are underpinned by sound theory. To date, the systematic review evidence about the efficacy of splinting people with hypertonicity to improve hand use is inconclusive. This is because of the low methodological design quality of research in this area, as discussed earlier (Autti-Ramo et al 2006, Teplicky et al 2002), and because orthoses need to be task-specific, making them difficult to compare in research studies. One study that has changed the field's understanding found that splinting the hand in the 'functional' position following brain injury, to reduce spasticity and pain, improve hand use and prevent contracture is not effective (Lannin et al 2003).

The evidence base for splinting to improve hand use in orthopaedic and trauma conditions is more favourable. Positive evidence supports the use of dynamic extensor bracing for lateral epicondylitis to reduce pain while improving upper-limb use and grip strength (Faes et al 2006). In addition, splinting the thumb joint of people with osteoarthritis leads to performance gain. These improvements are achieved no matter what thumb splint design is used (Wajon & Ada 2005), which accommodates for the personal preferences of the prescriber and wearer. Splinting is also useful for people with acute hand injuries. In this population, dynamic splinting initially produces the greatest rate of recovery, but by 6 months the performance outcomes of dynamic and static splints are equivalent (Mowlavi et al 2005).

There is moderate-quality evidence to support splints improving hand use for people with inflammatory disorders, such as arthritis. Evidence suggests that immobilisation of the wrist joint, in any variety of splint design, improves hand use and grip strength (Haskett et al 2004). The gains, however, are short-lived, and are equivalent to no splinting at all, after 6 months (Kjeken et al 1995).

Reducing pain

Orthoses may be appropriate when pain affects the attainment of occupational goals and the provision of external structural support can help alleviate it. Occupational therapists should have a good understanding of pain mechanisms and the person's condition to determine whether or not the use of an orthosis will assist or whether there could be adverse consequences from continued use (in a dynamic, semi-dynamic splint or static orthosis) or disuse (with a static splint). The occupational therapist also needs to have a good understanding of the underlying pathology of different conditions to inform this decision.

Musculoskeletal pain may be as a result of stretch of a muscle, ligament, tendon, irritation of the synovial membrane, or abnormal movement in a joint, muscle, or ligament. Joint pain may be caused by inflammation with resulting swelling and distension. Pain may be brought on by only the smallest amount of movement, or only at the extremes of range or upon actual stretching. When biomechanical factors and features of the condition are considered in the context of occupational goals, an orthosis will be only one of a range of pain-management options. If an orthosis is required, the design will focus on positions, structures and support that prevent movements that must be avoided, but permit stress or weight-bearing where it is allowed and contraction of those muscles that is safe and required in specified uses (Figure 33.12). In acute musculoskeletal conditions, or where pain is produced by overuse, fatigue, or stretch, the choice of orthosis may be restricted to static immobilisation splints to enforce rest.

The evidence about the effectiveness of orthoses achieving pain reduction is mostly favourable, but varies from one condition and joint to another. At the shoulder, the most effective treatments for reducing pain from subacromial impingement syndrome (SAIS) are not orthotics, but rather other techniques such as: exercise, joint mobilisation, and laser therapy (Michner et al 2004, Sauers 2005). If, however, the shoulder pain is secondary to cerebral vascular accident, the evidence to support pain reduction via orthoses such as shoulder slings is inconclusive because of poor methodological quality (Page & Lockwood 2003).

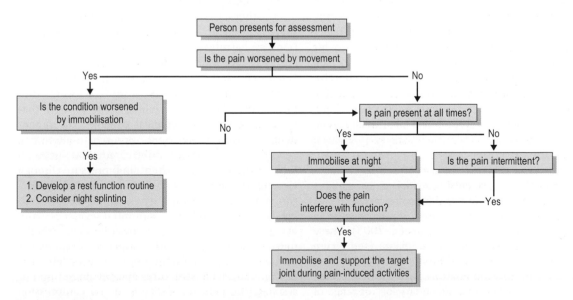

Figure 33.12 • Primary goal – pain management

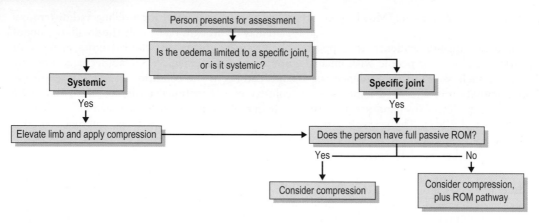

Figure 33.13 • Primary goal – oedema management

For the forearm, where pain is often associated with lateral epicondylosis (tennis elbow) orthoses are commonly prescribed to induce 'rest' by limiting movement, but the supporting scientific evidence is inconclusive (Borkholder et al 2004, Nimgade et al 2005). Steroid injections during the first 3 months provide the most relief of all available interventions. Active therapies such as acupuncture, exercise, and ultrasound are more effective than resting for reducing pain (Trudel et al 2004).

To reduce wrist pain associated with carpal tunnel syndrome (CTS) the following treatments are effective: splinting where wrist motion is immobilised without compressing the carpal tunnel, ultrasound, nerve-gliding exercises, magnetic therapy, and manual therapy (Muller et al 2004). Full-time splint wear is the most effective regimen (Walker et al 2000). Since immobilisation splints used for CTS reduce hand use, it is important for the person to know that wearing a night splint is more effective than not wearing a splint at all (Werner et al 2005). Splinting is proven to be equally as effective as oral steroid injections for reducing pain (Mishra et al 2006) but is less effective than surgery (Gerritsen et al 2002).

If, however, the wrist pain is caused by rheumatoid arthritis the scientific evidence to support orthoses reducing pain and increasing performance is inconclusive, despite people preferring to wear an orthosis than not wear one (Egan et al 2003). These splints are usually resting hand splints (see Figure 33.2), which immobilise the wrist and fingers. It is significant in this population that immobilisation does not appear to cause secondary loss of range of motion (Egan et al 2003). Also of importance, there

does not appear to be any added benefit of prescribing rest in an orthoses following intra-articular steroid injections to reduce pain (Wallen & Gilles 2006).

Decreasing oedema

When a person experiences burns, grafts, traumatic injury, or conditions that result in immobilised and dependent limbs, such as peripheral or central nerve damage, there is a risk of oedema. Oedema can contribute to joint stiffness and contracture and reducing oedema is an important preventative and rehabilitative strategy (see Figure 33.13).

Although there is little scientific evidence to help inform therapists in this area of the best approach, there is no evidence that commonly used interventions are harmful if compression garments are worn correctly and safely – instead a systematic review (Geurts et al 2000) reported that no specific treatment has yet proven its advantage over other physical methods for reducing hand oedema that occurs following neurological damage (i.e. dependent oedema). The current approach to alleviating oedema is the provision of retrograde massage, with limb elevation and consistent limb pressure through circumferential orthoses (e.g. custom-fitted Lycra® garments, tubular elastic dressings, or elastic wrap bandaging). As there is a limited evidence-base, occupational therapists who prescribe such orthoses must be alert to the safety aspects of splint and garment use, including the impact that oedema has had on underlying structures and the line-of-pull of a splint; the person's ability to don a compression garment correctly and safely when supervised, unsupervised, or with assistance; and the overall benefit balanced against purchasing and monitoring costs.

Conclusion

There is considerable variation in splinting practice. These variations include the design of the orthosis, critical period of orthotic use, wearing regimen, duration of use and the theoretical rationale behind the orthosis. In practice, no simple design or type of orthosis exists that applies to all people who present with the same diagnosis. Selecting the orthosis, the position of the hand or arm, and the wearing protocol will vary because each person is an individual, with unique occupational goals, unique injury or disease processes, and unique rehabilitation goals.

The ability to reason is based on the therapist's knowledge about the person's diagnosis, awareness of the person's occupational goals, motivation, and compliance, an understanding of orthotic protocols and techniques, and practice experience. The reasoning of a therapist is informed by an ever-increasing evidence base. Key to improving outcomes is encouraging individual therapists to explicitly seek out and factor in scientifically gained knowledge into their daily decision-making. Of course, this entails overcoming the inertia of practicing within the 'comfort zones' that we have developed based on our training, and constantly remaining abreast of scientific evidence.

Orthoses have historically been an integral part of the occupational therapy process when regaining performance or movement in the hand and upper limb. Each orthosis has a unique goal, and as the therapeutic goal changes, the design and use of the orthosis needs to be reconsidered in light of the person's occupational performance. As our body of research evidence also evolves, so too must our reasoning. In the future, it may be that therapists have more effective and efficient methods to produce better outcomes than those interventions we currently use.

References

Autti-Ramo, I. S. J., Anttila, H., Malmivaara, A. & Makela, M. (2006). Effectiveness of upper and lower limb casting and orthoses in children with cerebral palsy: an overview of review articles. *American Journal of Physical Medicine and Rehabilitation*, 85, 89–103.

Bleck, E. E. (1987). *Orthopaedic management in cerebral palsy*. London, MacKeith.

Bohannon, R. W. (1997). Internal consistency of manual muscle testing scores. *Perceptual and Motor Skills*, 85(2), 736–738.

Borkholder, C. D., Hill, V. A., Fess, E. E. (2004). The efficacy of splinting for lateral epicondylitis: a systematic review. *Journal of Hand Therapy*, 17(2),181–199.

Carey, L. M., Oke, L. E. & Matyas, T. A. (1996). Impaired limb position sense after stroke: a quantitative test for clinical use. *Archives of Physical Medicine and Rehabilitation*, 77(12), 1271–1278.

Carr-Collins, J. A. (1992). Pressure techniques for the prevention of hypertrophic scar. *Clinics in Plastic Surgery*, 19(3), 733–743.

Chong, P. S. T. & Cros, D. P. (2007). *Quantitative sensory testing equipment and reproducibility studies review*. American Association of Electrodiagnostic Medicine. Available online: http://www. aanem.org. Accessed 12 Feb 2007.

Clare, T. D., de Haviland Mee, S. & Belcher, H. J. C. R. (2004). Rehabilitation of digital nerve repair: is splinting necessary? *Journal of Hand Surgery*, 29B(6), 552–556.

Cole, B., Finch, E., Gowland, C. & Mayo, N. (1995). *Physical rehabilitation outcome measures*. Baltimore, Williams and Wilkins.

Copley, J. & Kuipers, K. (1999). *Management of upper limb hypertonicity*. San Antonio, Therapy Skill Builders.

Coppard, B. M. & Lohman, H. (1996). *Introduction to splinting: A critical-thinking and problem-solving approach*. St. Louis, Mosby-Year Book.

Duncan, R. M. (1989). Basic principles of splinting the hand.

Physical Therapy, 69, 1104–1116.

Dunn, W. (2000). *Best practice occupational therapy*. Thorofare, NJ, Slack Inc.

Dunn, W., Brown, C. & McGuigan, A. (1994). The ecology of human performance: A framework for thought and action. *American Journal of Occupational Therapy*, 48(7), 595–607.

Egan, M., Brosseau, L., Ouimet, M. A., Rees, S., Wells, G. & Tugwell, P. (2003). Splints/orthoses in the treatment of rheumatoid arthritis. *Cochrane Database of Systematic Reviews*, 1, CD004018.

Exner, C. (1996). Development of hand skills. In: J. Case-Smith, A. S. Allen & P. N. Pratt (Eds). *Occupational therapy for children*, (3rd ed.) (pp. 268–306). St Louis, Mosby-Year Book.

Faes, M., van den Akker, B., de Lint, J. A., Kooloos, J. G. & Hopman, M. T. (2006). Dynamic extensor brace for lateral epicondylitis. *Clinical Orthopaedics and Related Research*, 443, 149–157.

Farmer, S. E. & James, M. (2001). Contractures in orthopaedic and neurological conditions: a review of causes and treatment. *Disability and Rehabilitation*, 23, 549–558.

Farrar, J. T., Young, J. P., LaMoreaux, L., Werth, J. L. & Michael, P. R. (2001). Clinical importance of changes in chronic pain intensity measured on an 11-point numerical pain rating scale. *Pain*, 94, 149–158.

Fess, E. E., Gettle, K., Philips, C. A. & Janson, R. (2004). *Hand and upper extremity splinting principles and methods*, (3rd ed.) St Louis, Mosby.

Fugl-Meyer, A. R., Jaasko, L., Leyman, I., Olsson, S. & Steglind, S. (1975). The post-stroke hemiplegic patient. *Scandinavian Journal of Rehabilitation Medicine*, 7, 13–31.

Gaubert, C. S. & Mockett, S. P. (2000). Inter-rater reliability of the Nottingham method of stereognosis assessment. *Clinical Rehabilitation*, 14(2), 213–227.

Gerritsen, A. A. M., de Vet, H. C. W., Scholten, R. J. P. M., Bertelsmann, F. W., de Krom M. C. T. F. M., & Bouter, L. M. (2002). Splinting vs surgery in the treatment of carpal tunnel syndrome. *Journal of the American Medical Association*, 288(10), 1245–1251.

Geurts, A. C., Visschers, B. A., van Limbeek, J. & Ribbers, G. M. (2000). Systematic review of aetiology and treatment of post-stroke hand oedema and shoulder-hand syndrome. *Scandinavian Journal of Rehabilitation Medicine*, 32(1), 4–10.

Glasgow, C., Wilton, J. & Tooth, L. (2003). Optimal daily total end range time for contracture: resolution in hand splinting. *Journal of Hand Therapy*, 16, 207–218.

Goga-Eppenstien, P., Hill, J. P., Philip, P. A., Philip, M., Seifert, T. M. & Yasukawa, A. M. (1999). *Casting protocols for the upper and lower extremities*. Gaithersburg, Aspen.

Gracies, J. M., Fitzpatrick, R., Wilson, L., Burke, D. & Gandevia, S. C. (1997). Lycra garments designed for patients with upper limb spasticity: Mechanical effects in normal subjects. *Archives of Physical Medicine and Rehabilitation*, 78(10), 1066–1071.

Handoll, H. H. G. & Vaghela, M. V. (2004). Interventions for treating mallet finger injuries. *Cochrane Database of Systematic Reviews*, 3, CD004574.

Harris, S. R., Smith, L. H. & Krukowski, L. (1985). Goniometric reliability for a child with spastic quadriplegia. *Journal of Pediatric Orthopaedics*, 5, 348–351.

Harvey, L. A. & Herbert, R. D. (2002). Muscle stretching for treatment and prevention of contracture in people with spinal cord injury. *Spinal Cord*, 40(1), 1–9.

Harvey, L., de Jong, I., Goehl, G. & Mardwedel, S. (2006). Twelve weeks of nightly stretch does not reduce thumb web-space contractures in people with a neurological condition: a randomised controlled trial. *Australian Journal of Physiotherapy*, 52(4), 251–258.

Haskett, S., Backman, C., Porter, B., Goyert, J. & Palejko, G. (2004). A crossover trial of custom-made and commercially available wrist splints in adults with inflammatory arthritis. *Arthritis Rheumatology*, 15(5), 792–799.

Hill, J. (1988). Management of abnormal tone through casting and orthotics. In: Kovich, K. M. & Bermann, D. E. (eds) *Head injury: a guide to functional outcomes in occupational therapy* (pp. 107–124). Rockville, Aspen.

Hill, J. (1993). The effects of casting on upper extremity motor disorders after brain injury. *American Journal of Occupational Therapy*, 48, 219–224.

Hogan, L. & Uditsky, T. (1998). *Pediatric splinting-selection, fabrication, and clinical application of upper extremity splints*. San Antonio, Therapy Skill Builders.

Hudak, P. L., Amadio, P. C. & Bombardier, C. (1996). Development of an upper extremity outcome measure: the DASH (disabilities of the arm, shoulder and hand) [corrected]. The Upper Extremity Collaborative Group (UECG). *American Journal of Industrial Medicine*, 29(6), 602–608.

Hurn, J., Kneebone, I. & Cropley, M. (2006). Goal setting as an outcome measure: A systematic review. *Clinical Rehabilitation*, 20(9), 756–772.

Kasch, M. A. (1998). Clinical management of scar tissue. In: F. S. Cromwell & J. Bear-Lehman (Eds). *Hand rehabilitation in occupational therapy*. (pp. 37–52). Philadelphia, PA, Haworth Press.

Kerns, R. D., Turk, D. C. & Rudy, T. E. (1985). The West Haven-Yale Mulidimensional Pain Inventory (WHYMPI). *Pain*, 23, 345–356.

Kerns, R. D., Haythorthwarte, J., Roseberg, R., Southwick, S., Geller, E. L, Jacob, M. C. (1991). *The Pain Behaviour Checklist (PBCL)*. West Haven, Psychology Service.

Kischer, C. W., Shetlar, M. R. & Shetlar, C. L. (1975). Alteration of hypertrophic scars induced by mechanical pressure. *Archives of Dermatology*, 111, 60–64.

Kjeken, I., Moller, G. & Kvien, T. K. (1995). Use of commercially produced elastic wrist orthoses in chronic arthritis: a controlled study. *Arthritis Care and Research*, 8(2), 108–113.

Kogler, G. F. (2002). Orthotic management. In: D. A. Gelber & D. R. Jeffery (Eds). *Clinical evaluation and management of spasticity*. (pp. 67–91). Totowa, NJ, Humana.

Lannin, N., Horsley, S., Herbert, R., McCluskey, A. & Cusick, A. (2003). Splinting the hand in the functional position after brain impairment: a randomized controlled trial. *Archives of Physical Medicine and Rehabilitation*, 84, 297–302.

Lannin, N. A., Cusick, A., McCluskey, A. & Herbert, R. D. (2007a). Effects of splinting on wrist contracture after stroke: a randomized controlled trial. *Stroke*, 38(1), 111–116.

Lannin, N. A., Novak, I. & Cusick, A. (2007b). A systematic review of upper extremity casting for children and adults with central nervous system motor disorders. *Clinical Rehabilitation*, 21, 963–976.

Law, M., Baptiste, S., McColl, M., Opzoomer, A., Polatajko, H. & Polloock, N. (1990). The Canadian Occupational Performance Measure: An outcome measure for occupational therapy. *Canadian Journal of Occupational Therapy*, 57(2), 82–87.

Law, M., Russell, D., Pollock, N., Rosenbaum, P., Walter, S. & King, G. (1997). A comparison of intensive neurodevelopmental therapy plus casting and a regular occupational therapy program for children with cerebral palsy. *Developmental Medicine and Child Neurology*, 39, 664–670.

Law, M., King, G., Russell, D., Stewart, D., Hurley, P. & Bosch, E. (1999). *All about outcomes: an educational program to help you understand, evaluate, and choose pediatric outcome measures*. Thorofare, NJ, Slack Inc.

Law, M., King, G., Russell, D., Stewart, D., Hurley, P. & Bosch, E. (2000). *All about outcomes: an educational program to help you understand, evaluate, and choose adult outcome measures*. Thorofare, NJ, Slack.

Leventhal, D., Furr, M. & Reiter, D. (2006). Treatment of keloids and hypertrophic scars: a meta-analysis and review of the literature. *Archives of Facial and Plastic Surgery*, 8(6), 362–368.

Lowe, C. T. (1995). Construction of hand splints. In: C. A. Trombly (Ed.). *Occupational therapy for physical dysfunction*, (4th ed). (pp. 583–597). Baltimore, Williams & Wilkins.

McKnight, P. T. & Schomburg, F. L. (1982). Air pressure splint effects on hand symptoms of patients with rheumatoid arthritis. *Archives of Physical Medicine and Rehabilitation*, 63(11), 560–564.

Mann, R., Yeong, E. K., Moore. M., Colescott. D. & Engrav, L. H. (1997). Do custom-fitted pressure garments provide adequate pressure? *Journal of Burn Care Rehabilitation*, 18(3), 247–249.

Melzack, R. (1987). The short-form McGill pain questionnaire. *Pain*, 30, 193.

Michner, L. A., Walsworth, M. K. & Burnet, E. N. (2004). Effectiveness of rehabilitation for patients with subacromial impingement syndrome: a systematic review. *Journal of Hand Therapy*, 17, 152–164.

Milazzo, S. & Gillen, G. (1998). Splinting applications. In: G. Gillen & A. Burkhardt (Eds). *Stroke rehabilitation: a function-based approach*. (pp. 161–184). St Louis, Mosby.

Mishra, S., Prabhakar, S., Lal, V. & Modi, M. (2006). Efficacy of splinting and oral steroids in the treatment of carpal tunnel syndrome: a prospective randomized clinical and electrophysiological study. *Neurology India*, 54(3), 286–290.

Moseley, A., Herbert, R., Harvey, L., Hassett, L., Clare, J. & Leung, J. (2006). *Clinical trial of stretching after traumatic brain injury: Final report*. Sydney, Motor Accidents Authority.

Mowlavi, A., Burns, M. & Brown, R. E. (2005). Dynamic versus static splinting of simple zone V and zone IV extensor tendon repairs: a prospective, randomized, controlled study. *Plastic Reconstructive Surgery*, 115(2), 482–487.

Muller, M., Tsui, D., Schnurr, R., Biddulph-Deisroth, L., Hard, J. & MacDermid, J. C. (2004). Effectiveness of hand therapy interventions in primary management of carpal tunnel syndrome: a systematic review. *Journal of Hand Therapy*, 17, 210–228.

Mustoe, T. A., Cooter, R. D., Gold, M. H., Hobbs, F. D., Ramlet, A. A., Shakesphere, P. G., Stella, M., Wood, F. M., Ziegler, U. E. & International Advisory Panel on Scar Management (2002). International clinical recommendations on scar management. *Plastic Reconstructive Surgery*, 110(2), 560–571.

Nimgade, A., Sullivan, M. & Goldman, R. (2005). Physiotherapy, steroid injections, or rest for lateral epicondylosis? What the evidence suggests. *World Institute of Pain*, 5(3), 203–215.

O'Brien, L. & Pandit, A. (2006). Silicone gel sheeting for preventing and treating hypertrophic and keloid scars. *Cochrane Database of Systematic Reviews*, 25(1), CD003826.

O'Connor, D., Mullett, H., Doyle, M., Mofidi, A., Kutty, S. & O'Sullivan, M. (2003). Minimally displaced

Colles' fractures: a prospective randomized trial of treatment with a wrist splint or a plaster cast. *Journal of Hand Surgery*, 28(1), 50–53.

Ottenbacher, K. J. & Cusick, A. (1990). Goal attainment scaling as a method of clinical service evaluation. *American Journal of Occupational Therapy*, 44(6), 519–525.

Ouellette, E. A. (1991). The rheumatoid hand: orthotics as preventative. *Seminars in Arthritis and Rheumatism*, 21, 65–71.

Page, T. & Lockwood, C. (2003). Systematic review: prevention and management of shoulder pain in the hemiplegic patient. *Joanna Briggs Institute Reports*, 1, 149–165.

Parks, D. H., Evans, E. B. & Larson, D. L. (1978). Prevention and correction of deformity after severe burns. *The Surgery Clinics of North America*, 58(6), 1279–1289.

Plint, A. C., Perry, J. J., Correll, R., Gaboury, I. & Lawton, L. (2006). A randomized, controlled trial of removable splinting versus casting for wrist buckle fractures in children. *Pediatrics*, 117(3), 691–697.

Poole, J. L., Cordova, K. J. & Brower, L. M. (2006). Reliability and validity of a self-report of hand function in persons with rheumatoid arthritis. *Journal of Hand Therapy*, 19(1), 12–16.

Sauers, E. L. (2005). Effectiveness of rehabilitation for patients with subacromial impingement syndrome. *Journal of Athletic Training*, 40(3), 221–223.

Stratford, P. W., Norman, G. R. & McIntosh, J. M. (1989). Generalizability of grip strength measurements in patients with tennis elbow. *Physical Therapy*, 69, 276–281.

Tenney, C. G. & Lisak, J. M. (1986). *Atlas of hand splinting*. Boston, Little, Brown and Company.

Teplicky, R., Law, M. & Russell, D. (2002). The effectiveness of casts, orthoses, and splints for children with neurological disorders. *Infants and Young Children*, 15, 42–50.

Trombly, C. A. & Ma, H. (2002). A synthesis of the effects of occupational therapy for persons with stroke, part 1: Restoration of roles, tasks and activities. *American Journal of Occupational Therapy*, 56, 250–259.

Trudel, D., Duley, J., Zastrow, I., Kerr, E. W., Davidson, R. & MacDermid, J. C. (2004). Rehabilitation for patients with lateral epicondylitis: a systematic review. *Journal of Hand Therapy*, 17(2), 243–266.

Van den Kerckhove, E., Stappaerts, K., Fieuws, S., Laperre, J., Massage, P., Flour, M. & Boeckx, W. (2005). The assessment of erytherma and thickness on burn related scars during pressure garment therapy as a preventative measure for hypertrophic scarring. *Burns*, 31(6), 696–702.

Wajon, A. & Ada, L. (2005). No difference between two splint and exercise regimens for people with osteoarthritis of the thumb: a randomized controlled trial. *Australian Journal of Physiotherapy*, 52(1), 60.

Walker, W. C., Metzler, M., Cifu, D. X. & Swartz, Z. (2000). Neutral wrist splinting in carpal tunnel syndrome: a comparison of night-only versus full-time wear instructions. *Archives of Physical Medicine and Rehabilitation*, 81, 424–429.

Wallen, M. & Gilles, D. (2006). Intra-articular steroids and splints/rests for children with juvenile idiopathic arthritis and adults with rheumatoid arthritis. *Cochrane Database of Systematic Reviews*, 1, CD002824.

Werner, R. A., Franzblau, A. & Gell, N. (2005). Randomized controlled trail of nocturnal splinting for active workers with symptoms of carpal tunnel syndrome. *Archives of Physical Medicine and Rehabilitation*, 86(1), 1–7.

Wilton, J.C. & Dival, T. A. (1997). *Hand splinting: Principles of design and fabrication*. London, WB Saunders Company.

Further reading

American Society of Hand Therapists (ASHT) (1992). *Splint Classification System*. Chicago, ASHT.

Coppard, B. M. & Lohman, H. (1996). *Introduction to splinting: A critical-thinking and problem-solving approach*. St. Louis, Mosby-Year Book.

Fess, E. E., Gettle, K., Philips, C. A. & Janson, R. (2004). *Hand and upper extremity splinting principles and methods*. (3rd edn). St Louis, Mosby.

Goga-Eppenstien, P., Hill, J. P., Philip, P. A., Philip, M., Seifert, T. M. & Yasukawa, A. M. (1999). *Casting protocols for the upper and lower extremities*. Gaithersburg, Aspen.

Hogan, L. & Uditsky, T. (1998). *Pediatric splinting-selection, fabrication, and clinical application of upper extremity splints*. San Antonio, Therapy Skill Builders.

Tenney, C. G. & Lisak, J. M. (1986). *Atlas of hand splinting*. Boston, Little, Brown and Company.

Wilton, J. C. & Dival, T. A. (1997). *Hand splinting: Principles of design and fabrication*. WB London, Saunders Company.

Biomechanical strategies

Janet Golledge

CHAPTER CONTENTS

Introduction 527
    Defining terms 528
    Kinesiology 528
    Biomechanics 528
    Kinematics and kinetics 528
Rationale for biomechanical strategies . . . 529
Professional reasoning 535
Assessment 535
    Assessment of meaning 535
    Assessment of function 535
    Assessment of form 536
Implementing strategies 536
    Overall aims 538
    Strength 538
    Endurance 539
    Enhancing voluntary movements 539
Conclusion. 540

SUMMARY

When therapists use biomechanical strategies,
they use the principles of biomechanics to
understand human function. This chapter
presents an explanation of biomechanical
strategies and how they may be used
therapeutically. The strategies focus on
overcoming impaired voluntary movement,
inadequate muscle strength or reduced
endurance. These impairments adversely impact
on ability and may arise from varied pathologies,
some acute and others that have longer-term
consequences. Occupations are the vehicle for
applying biomechanical strategies when an
individual experiences occupation and role
disruption. Therapists use the principles from
biomechanics to select or modify equipment/
tools used in occupations, evaluate
environmental safety, construct splints (orthoses),
and ensure benefit from therapy. One detailed
Practice Scenario is presented to illustrate the
application of biomechanical strategies and
demonstrate the integration of these principles
within ergonomics. A further two brief and
contrasting examples alert the reader to the
scope of strategy application.

KEY POINTS

- Biomechanical strategies focus on the central
  concerns of voluntary movement, strength, and
  endurance.
- Understanding biomechanics informs the
  application of strategies.
- Strategies are implemented within an
  occupational framework.
- Assessments for skills and limitations reflect
  meaning, ability and form.
- Ergonomics capitalises on biomechanical
  strategies.
- Joint protection and energy conservation
  strategies utilise the principles of biomechanics.

Introduction

Biomechanics uses mechanical principles to understand human movement. When therapists use

biomechanical strategies, they use the principles of biomechanics for solving problems related to the structure and function of humans (Hall 2007). The three central concerns of biomechanical strategies are strength, endurance, and voluntary movement. Therapists focus on how these adversely affect occupational performance and an individual's satisfaction with that performance.

Knowledge of biomechanics enables therapists to analyse movement, weakness, and diminished endurance, and facilitates problem solving when observing an individual attempting to complete occupations. Carefully structured, adapted and graded occupations are used to overcome these problems.

Understanding theory is essential for effective application of biomechanical strategies. Theory from the physiological, psychological, and educational frames of reference (Hagedorn 2001) informs the strategies, with interventions applied within the context of occupational performance and engagement, using a top-down approach. The underpinning theory for biomechanical strategies was not constructed by occupational therapists and translation of the principles is necessary in order to use them within an occupational framework (Greene & Roberts 1999, McMillan 2006). Therapists use knowledge from biomechanics to analyse, formulate, and implement therapy and evaluate the outcomes for individuals in relation to their roles and occupations. Although therapists are interested in all influences on occupational performance and engagement, biomechanics attends solely to the capacity for movement. Different theoretical frameworks should be investigated to understand other influences on a person's ability (e.g. cognitive, emotional).

Defining terms

Kinesiology

Kinesiology refers to the study of movement (Rybski 2004). It uses scientific knowledge of musculoskeletal anatomy, neuromuscular physiology, and biomechanics. Kinesiology informs our understanding of biomechanics by explaining the forces impacting on movement and how the physiological state of active and passive structures (joints, muscles, tendons) influences the quality of movements. Various types of muscle action (concentric, eccentric, isometric) enable joints to move smoothly and accurately or remain in stable positions to support

occupational performance. By understanding forces and their impact on the body, therapy can be structured to facilitate recovery, prevent deterioration and/or promote compensation for lost skills.

Biomechanics

Biomechanics refers to both internal and external forces acting on the body (Freivalds 2004, Greene & Roberts 1999) and informs therapists about how these forces affect movement. These forces include gravity, friction, torque, resistance, leverage, stability, and equilibrium. Biomechanics has two divisions, *statics* and *dynamics*, both identifying stresses on anatomical structures (Rybski 2004, Spaulding 2008). Statics is concerned with equilibrium and forces impacting on the body at rest, whilst dynamics focuses on movement and acceleration. Dynamics, which is of most interest for this chapter, includes kinematics and kinetics.

Kinematics and kinetics

Kinematics describes motion and examines the results of movements in space and over time. It includes the noting of body position, joint angles, velocity, and acceleration. Kinetics studies the interacting forces that cause or affect movement (Chaffin et al 2006, Hamill & Knutzen 2003, Rybski 2004, Winter 2005).

Practice Scenario 34.1 illustrates the application of kinematics and kinetics within the context of an occupation.

Practice Scenario 34.1 Illustrating kinematics and kinetics whilst supermarket shopping

A woman enters a supermarket, selecting a trolley to collect her shopping.

Kinematics

She walks at a slow velocity as she negotiates the space and obstacles. She is able to decelerate her pace as she scans the shelves and avoid collisions with aisles, or accelerate as she rushes back to her car. Angular movements occur around the axis of joints – she reaches out to select foods from shelves using shoulder flexion, abduction, and elbow extension. Angular velocity slows as her hand nears the foods to enable her thumb to oppose to her fingers for grip on each item without knocking it over. Swing and stance phases in walking are executed effectively, with different lower-limb segments demonstrating co-ordinated movement to maintain an upright posture and move safely through the environment.

Kinetics

She generates push and pull forces on the trolley as she negotiates the aisles and other people. If she pushes too quickly, she may bump into obstacles but if she does not exert enough force, she will be unable to move the trolley. Isotonic contraction is developed in prime mover muscles with increasing recruitment of muscle fibres when items are heavy. Isometric action in antigravity muscles enables her to maintain standing whilst reading ingredients in products. Friction from the wheels on the floor generates resistance which she needs to overcome with increasing strength as the weight of food in the trolley mounts over time. She becomes thirsty so uses torque to twist the bottle top off a drink, creating tension in muscle fibres to generate enough strength to release the top. She calibrates the force to avoid spillage. Kinetics enables her to apply forces effectively to complete the occupation.

Rationale for biomechanical strategies

An occupational therapist needs to be aware of how different impairments can have an impact on the efficiency of the musculoskeletal and cardiopulmonary systems. The impairment that a person has will invariably have some influence on therapeutic decisions (Rogers 2004). Impaired voluntary movement may result from damaged bone or soft tissues, amputation, pain, congenital conditions, inflammation, or oedema. Inadequate muscle strength is often due to atrophy, disease processes, pain, and/or peripheral nerve damage. Reduced endurance is a consequence of cardiopulmonary disorders, pain, decreased strength and/or limited range of movement at joints (James 2003, McMillan 2006, Rybski 2004). Often, reduced voluntary movements, and limited strength and endurance are all apparent in individuals to varying degrees, and are further compromised by environments that do not facilitate occupational performance.

The occupational therapist implements strategies that aim to resolve these occupational performance limitations and enable participation in roles. This is achieved by enhancing or maintaining endurance and strength. Therapy often aims to increase voluntary movements but, equally, may guide individuals to limit movements that exceed task demands and are creating health problems. This is outlined in Practice Scenario 34.2.

Practice Scenario 34.2 Kasia

Kasia is 25 years old and moved to England from Poland 18 months ago for employment opportunities. She has been working in the offices of an insurance company for one year, completing computer-based work. For six months, Kasia has experienced pain in her shoulders, neck and wrists. Her general practitioner diagnosed extensor tenosynovitis at her wrists and rotator cuff tendinitis in her shoulders. Kasia has been referred to an outpatient occupational therapist by her occupational health department for a workstation assessment, to ascertain the influence of the environment on her problems. Her discomfort is worse in the afternoon and evening. Kasia lives alone, has a close group of friends, enjoys socialising and going to the cinema. She joined a rural conservation group and amateur dramatic group to develop her language skills. Maintaining her employment is important, to support her lifestyle and assist her family in Poland. Kasia hopes to start a business degree in England and perceives that consolidating her work skills is essential to achieving this long-term aim.

Assessment

The therapist conducted an initial interview, to explore Kasia's lifestyle, roles and occupations, using interactive reasoning to appreciate Kasia's perspective. Using procedural reasoning, the Canadian Occupational Performance Measure (COPM) (Law et al 2008) was selected as an outcome measure to record Kasia's concerns and priorities. The COPM identifies participation restrictions in self-care, productivity and leisure, and records change after interventions. Kasia was asked to think about a typical day and reflect upon what she wanted and needed to do to support her lifestyle. Her responses were recorded. She was then asked to rate how important each occupation she selected was to her, as well as how well she felt she performed, and how satisfied she was with her

Table 34.1 Initial Canadian Occupational Performance Measure results for Kasia

Occupational performance problems	Performance score*	Satisfaction score*
Four priorities (most important areas selected by Kasia)		
1. Use of computer and keyboard at work	3	3
2. Reading for leisure and work	5	4
3. Writing for work and conservation group	6	4
4. Preparing food for cooking	6	4
Average score	20/4 = 5	15/4 = 3.7

*1 = not important/unable to do/not satisfied at all; 10 = extremely important/do extremely well/extremely satisfied

performance of each occupation on a scale of 1 to 10 to establish priorities. Four priorities were noted (Table 34.1).

Scores were calculated by adding all the performance scores and dividing by four (four priorities) and the same was done for her satisfaction scores (Table 34.1).

The therapist conducted further investigation by completing a workplace ergonomic risk assessment (Open Ergonomics Ltd. 2000) and an analysis of Kasia preparing food in her own home using the Occupational Therapy Practice Framework (American Occupational Therapy Association 2002). In addition an assessment recording Kasia's experience of pain was also conducted (Strong et al 2002).

Workplace ergonomic risk assessment

The therapist liaised with the workplace manager to complete an ergonomic risk assessment (Health and Safety Executive 2002).

Ergonomics analyses individuals interacting with their environments, the tools/equipment they use, room layout, work methods, safety, and productivity (Berg Rice 2008). Ergonomics is the 'science concerned with the fit between people and their work' and aims to ensure that 'tasks, equipment, information and the environment suit each user' (Health and Safety Executive 2003, p. 3). Ergonomics draws significantly on the application of biomechanics (Kumar 1999) aiming to improve performance, reduce accidents, and ill health. Ergonomic principles apply to all occupations and design of tools/equipment, not just employment (Haims & Carayon 1998, Health and Safety Executive 1999, 2003).

Kasia's anthropometric measurements (dimensions of relevant body segments) were completed

and compared to measurements of her work station (Baker 2008, Pheasant 1990). Using procedural reasoning, the therapist observed Kasia working for 45 minutes, recording information about working style to ascertain the influence of workplace ergonomics on her symptoms. Interactive reasoning enabled the therapist to elicit Kasia's perspective before analysing her posture, use of equipment, space, ambient factors and opportunities for breaks. Kasia was asked about training and information she had received about working with computer equipment (Health and Safety Executive 1999, 2002, 2006). Results showed that ambient factors (lighting, temperature, humidity) and work load were acceptable. However, Kasia's posture and interaction with equipment were incompatible with effective occupational performance (Figure 34.1). The most significant issues contributing to Kasia's pain, impaired voluntary movement, and endurance were:

Posture:

1. She looked down at the screen; she had excessive neck flexion as her screen was too low.
2. Her shoulder joints were maintained in flexion; her upper arms were not in line with her trunk; she sat too far from her desk, compromising her keyboard work and writing tasks.
3. Her elbows were not at right angles as she sat too high for the keyboard and desk. Her trunk was flexed and she leant forward to do desk tasks.
4. Her wrists were extended over the keyboard, whereas they should be in a neutral position.

Desk and chair:

1. Her seat was too high, placing her elbows above keyboard height.

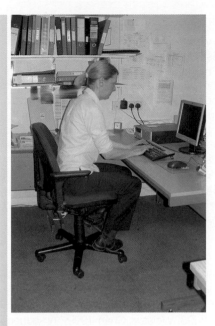

Figure 34.1 • Kasia's posture at her desk

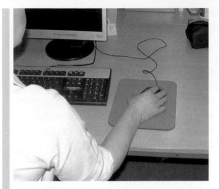

Figure 34.2 • Excessive wrist adduction required to move mouse

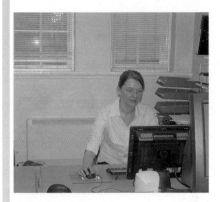

Figure 34.3 • Kasia uses excessive shoulder abduction for mouse work

2. There was insufficient clearance under her desk, placing her knees too close to the underside of her desk.
3. Her arm rests did not support her forearms indicating that they were incorrectly adjusted.
4. She had pressure at the back of her thighs as her seat was too high and her feet did not rest comfortably on floor.
5. She did not use her backrest for lumbar support; instead she leant forward, increasing her hip flexion.
6. Her chair was too far from the desk edge, requiring her to flex her shoulders to use the keyboard.

Monitor, keyboard and mouse:

1. Her monitor was too low; however, the distance from her eyes to the monitor was acceptable (56 cm).
2. Her keyboard was too far forward and raised at the back edge, creating stressful wrist extension.
3. Her wrists demonstrated excessive adduction, particularly on the right side when using a mouse (Figure 34.2).
4. The mouse was placed too far to her right, resulting in shoulder abduction for prolonged mouse work (Figure 34.3).

The assessment results informed the planning of the therapy sessions aiming to maximise the fit between Kasia, her work environment and occupations, linking the principles of biomechanics and ergonomics.

Analysis of food preparation

The therapist also observed Kasia preparing vegetables and chicken at home using the Occupational Therapy Performance Framework (American Occupational Therapy Association 2002). Her skills and deficits were identified.

Motor skills

Posture She positioned herself too far from the work surfaces resulting in excessive shoulder flexion.
Mobility There was a tendency to excessively reach during retrieval of food and utensils. She was able to walk and bend to retrieve items out of cupboards without any problem.

Co-ordination She demonstrated dexterity and good co-ordination of her upper limbs. However, the pain and her slowness had an impact on the flow of movements.

Strength and effort She was able to transport objects, but felt pain and weakness when carrying heavy bags and cooking equipment, causing pain in her wrists. She avoided preparing large vegetables and was unable to calibrate enough pressure for chopping. Maintaining her power grip was painful. She held items in her fingertips instead of her whole hand, which required more effort and force. She rinsed vegetables in a pan which caused her to use excessive wrist adduction.

Energy She worked at a slow pace, but had sufficient endurance. Her pain increased as she fatigued.

Process skills

Energy She was able to pace her work appropriately and was attentive throughout the whole task.

Knowledge She demonstrated no problem in knowing what to do. She chose and used appropriate objects and was able to heed task demands. She sometimes struggled to handle objects effectively and safely.

Temporal organisation She initiated, terminated, and sequenced stages appropriately.

Organising space, objects She was not able to organise tools and food items to make best use of working space and to limit painful movements. She searched effectively for items and gathered the required items appropriately. She navigated safely around obstacles and was able to tidy the kitchen afterwards.

Adaptation She struggled to accommodate her difficulties and made minimal adjustments to her occupational style. She did anticipate some problems showing that she utilised past experience.

Noticed and responded She responded appropriately to various environmental cues.

As a result of both assessments, the therapist was able to describe the functional problems and identified relevant cues. This enabled the formulation of logical hypotheses to explain Kasia's occupational dysfunction within the context of her pathology.

Plan

Assessment results were analysed to formulate person-centred goals. Priorities that were noted from the COPM and Kasia's identified hopes for the future (reflecting interactive and conditional reasoning) focused interventions on enhancing performance, modifying environments and occupational style, and preventing further activity limitations.

Therapy implementation

Kasia's pain was exacerbated by poor posture, intensive episodes of typing and repetitive reaching at work and home. She was advised to attend to her alignment in occupations, limit static positions in upper limb joints and use energy conservation strategies to avoid overuse of muscles and limit fatigue. For example, Kasia did not use her chair armrests and maintained shoulder flexion during work tasks resulting in her shoulder muscles working excessively to support her arms and counteract the force of gravity (Jensen et al 1999). It was suggested that Kasia could limit her shoulder flexion and abduction to reduce pain and promote efficient occupational engagement.

Work place interventions

Kasia's attention was drawn to ergonomic principles that she could use to ensure the best position for her when sitting at her desk (Eklund 1999, Engstrom 2002, Smith 2008, Weiss & Chan 1999). An education package, including directions to helpful internet sites was provided, alerting Kasia to her position at the desk, correct adjustment of her chair and using a foot rest. Anthropometric measurements, clearance (knees under desk, elbows over desk) and reach (to whole desk surface, feet to floor/foot rest) criteria, guided the correct adjustment of equipment (Claiborne et al 1999, Kroemer & Grandjean 1997, Smith 2008) (Figure 34.4).

Some key points that were shared with Kasia were:

1. Sit closer to her desk with her hips, knees and ankles at approximately 90°

2. Adjust her backrest to the correct height and angle the backrest to seat pan to an optimum of 105°

3. Lean against the backrest to ease fatigue on her trunk musculature and facilitate her endurance to complete her working day

4. Ensure the seat pan tilts to approximately 5° forwards/back

5. Ensure that her elbows were level with the keyboard

6. Ensure her armrests are correctly adjusted to support her elbows

7. Keep her upper arms in alignment with her trunk to ensure her shoulders are not abducted or flexed

8. Ensure the keyboard slopes down towards back edge and use a wrist rest to promote a neutral (not extended) wrist position

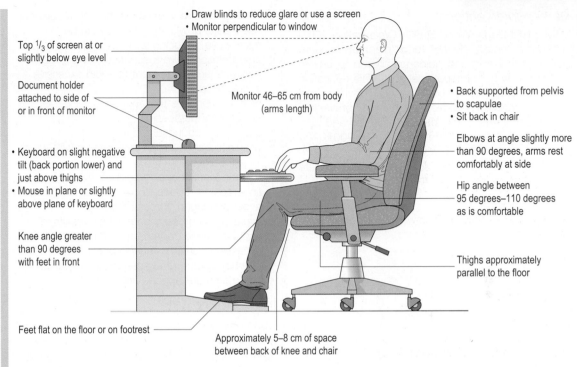

• Draw blinds to reduce glare or use a screen
• Monitor perpendicular to window

Top ¹/₃ of screen at or slightly below eye level

Document holder attached to side of or in front of monitor

Monitor 46–65 cm from body (arms length)

• Back supported from pelvis to scapulae
• Sit back in chair

Elbows at angle slightly more than 90 degrees, arms rest comfortably at side

• Keyboard on slight negative tilt (back portion lower) and just above thighs
• Mouse in plane or slightly above plane of keyboard

Hip angle between 95 degrees–110 degrees as is comfortable

Knee angle greater than 90 degrees with feet in front

Thighs approximately parallel to the floor

Feet flat on the floor or on footrest

Approximately 5–8 cm of space between back of knee and chair

Figure 34.4 • Ergonomics for the computer workstation

9. Monitor her wrists to prevent adduction and use a neutral position for keyboard and mouse tasks

10. Place the mouse more centrally on her desk when using the mouse for an extended period of time; she could also minimise the use of the mouse by using quick keys and templates to limit shoulder flexion and abduction

11. Have regular rest breaks – a few minutes every 30 minutes.

Biomechanical strategies reflecting ergonomic principles were promoted for Kasia's other priorities, to generalise her learning. For example, Kasia was encouraged to use a sloping surface for writing and reading (Figures 34.5 and 34.6). The optimum writing angle is between 10° and 20° above horizontal and the optimum reading angle is approximately 60° (Back Designs Inc 2002). This eased the pain in her shoulders, reduced her neck flexion and ensured she did not use unnecessary isometric muscle action to hold books or rehearsal notes for plays.

Biomechanical strategies were reflected in the principles of workspace layout at her office and kitchen (Stein et al 2006). Kasia was guided to place the most important and frequently used items in the most accessible locations, preventing unnecessary shoulder flexion and promoting comfortable voluntary

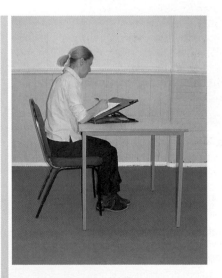

Figure 34.5 • Good ergonomic position for writing

movement. Kasia was advised to place items with closely related functions/actions together (e.g. kettle and sink, toiletries on a shelf, telephone and note pad). These principles were stressed during all occupations to facilitate energy conservation, a fundamental biomechanical strategy (McMillan 2006).

Kitchen interventions

Activity limitations (World Health Organisation 2001) that were noted during food preparation were explained to Kasia and guidance offered to enable her to modify her occupational style. This education prevented exacerbation of endurance difficulties and impaired voluntary movement, whilst preventing potential long-term musculoskeletal damage and further pain (Rochman & Kennedy-Spaien 2007). The therapist promoted a more efficient and comfortable occupational performance so Kasia could complete her roles effectively (Green & Roberts 1999).

When working in the kitchen Kasia was advised to:

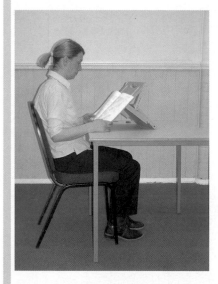

Figure 34.6 • Better ergonomic position for reading

- wash and drain vegetables through a colander
- use plastic bowls for vegetables in her microwave, reducing weight
- stand closer to work surfaces and organise materials and equipment to avoid excessive shoulder flexion
- work on surfaces that limit shoulder girdle elevation or depression
- avoid wrist adduction
- use both hands to lift heavier items with wrists in slight extension
- use the whole hand to hold items (not fingertips) to reduce force
- avoid prolonged, forceful gripping
- avoid carrying heavy bags which results in shoulder girdle depression and consequent excessive isometric muscle action
- purchase some ready-prepared vegetables
- use a smaller-capacity, lighter kettle.

In summary

Using interactive reasoning, interventions reflected Kasia's preferred option of altering her occupational style to limit difficulties rather than using adaptive equipment to compensate for loss of performance (McMillan 2006). New behaviours and habits were promoted whilst modifying performance skills and patterns (Rybski 2004, Stein et al 2006). Kasia hoped her symptoms would resolve as the problems were not longstanding. Conditional reasoning enabled the therapist to discuss potential use of splints to support Kasia's wrists, should her problems continue. Evaluation after two months included completion of the COPM again, to compare scores to those established at first contact. Results at two months indicated that there were positive outcomes (Table 34.2).

Table 34.2 Canadian Occupational Performance Measure Results for Kasia after two months

Occupational performance problems	Performance score*	Satisfaction score*
Four priorities		
1. Use of computer and keyboard at work	7	8
2. Reading for leisure and work	8	8
3. Writing for work and conservation group	8	8
4. Preparing food for cooking	7	8
Average score	30/4 = 7.5	32/4 = 8

*1 = not important/unable to do/not satisfied at all; 10 = extremely important/do extremely well/extremely satisfied

Professional reasoning

Employing professional reasoning to foster reflection on the therapist's performance and the uniqueness of each person limits exclusive dependence on past experiences to guide future interventions (Chapparo & Ranka 2000, Paterson & Summerfield-Mann 2006). Professional reasoning enables imaginative, person-centred therapy, rather than routine, formulaic interventions. Rogers (2004) describes occupational diagnosis as part of the reasoning process. She outlines the application of an 'occupational therapy diagnostic statement' (p. 19), which includes a description of the problems, an explanation of possible causes of the problem (hypotheses), identification of significant cues and any relevant pathological components. This aids analysis and synthesis of assessment data to plan effectively and implement intervention. Reference will be made to these elements of the occupational therapy diagnostic statement throughout the remainder of this chapter. Additionally, three track reasoning (procedural, interactive and conditional reasoning) (Mattingly & Fleming 1994) will be used to illustrate the professional reasoning process.

Assessment

In order to reflect the central concerns of biomechanics, assessments are used to investigate the consequences of impaired voluntary movement, inadequate strength or reduced endurance. Therapists have professional and ethical responsibilities to conduct assessments that provide valid results to form the basis for planning and therapy. Assessments need to gather information about skillfulness, effectiveness and difficulties with performance. As therapists understand individuals as occupational beings, influenced by contexts, assessments investigate the meaning, function and form inherent within occupations for each individual (Hocking 2001). Adopting this focus helps to guide the therapist's procedural, interactive and conditional reasoning, selecting assessments to explore each individual's life situation. Standardised assessments that have undergone rigorous evaluation are valuable for justifying interventions and providing objective evidence in the current climate of evidence-based practice (Lorch & Herge 2007). This should not devalue the use of structured non-standardised assessments,

using skilled observation and analysis. Sometimes, standardised tools are not available but the therapist must be alert to potential subjectivity and arriving at conclusions without a sound theoretical foundation. The latter will impact on effective occupational diagnosis as incorrect hypotheses will be generated (Rogers 2004).

Assessment of meaning

The meaning that people experience from participation in their repertoire of daily occupations is a reflection of their sense of identity. The varied impairments with which individuals present have considerable impact on occupational behaviour and the sense of who they are and what they hope to become. Christiansen (2004, p. 122) noted that 'who we are, is best understood by knowing what we do'. As such, the therapist must explore this concept in the initial interview using interactive reasoning, asking questions that clarify occupations to support necessary and valued life roles. Alternatively, the therapist may utilise a standardised assessment to obtain information about meaning and volition (e.g. Occupational Circumstances Assessment Interview Rating Scale [OCAIRS] (Haglund et al 2001), or the Occupational Performance History Interview II [OPHI-II] (Kielhofner et al 1997)).

Assessment of function

Assessments focusing on function ascertain why individuals wish to complete particular occupations: the purpose, importance, and contribution of the occupations to that person's lifestyle. Since individuals do not act in isolation, assessments investigate the needs of dependants (family members, pets, co-workers) and occupations that are completed to support or care for others. Informal questioning may provide many answers and may include such questions as: Which occupations are problematic?; Does pain impact on ability?; Do particular environments impede or support occupational behaviour?; Are relationships (and roles) disrupted as a result of difficulties completing occupations?

A more formalised assessment such as the Canadian Occupational Performance Measure (COPM) (Law et al 2008) may be used. This reflects categories of occupations (self-care, productivity and leisure) and includes outcome measurement to aid evaluation of interventions. There are numerous questionnaire-based standardised assessments, often self-administered, that collect relevant occupation-focused details, including the Arthritis Impact Measurement Scales (Meenan & Mason 1994), and the Short Form-36 Health Survey Questionnaire (Ware et al 1997). Problems amenable to occupational therapy intervention are identified and described through these informal and formal assessments (Rogers 2004).

Assessment of form

Form-focused assessments analyse 'the nature and extent of any observable disruption to performance' (Hocking 2001, p. 465). As a foundation for this type of assessment, the therapist needs an understanding of the capacities required to complete different occupations. Therapists need to understand what capacities a person needs to do various occupations. The occupational therapist needs to understand what the expected outcomes might be for each of these occupations.

Occupational performance is the product of the person, the occupation and the environment (Kielhofner 2002). As a result the therapist observes individuals completing occupations in the appropriate environment to identify and analyse any disruptions to the person's performance. Cues are recognised and hypotheses are generated about the most likely cause of the disruption (Rogers 2004). The therapist might be trying to answer questions such as: Are environmental conditions imposing restrictions on accomplishment?; Does the quality of performance match what is needed or desired?

Any adaptations an individual makes to accommodate for difficulties they are experiencing should be noted, as these helpfully indicate a person's capacity for change during future therapy. This is required for implementing many biomechanical strategies which may aim to adapt the occupational style or environment to support successful completion of occupations. Appropriate assessments that gather data on occupational skillfulness and effectiveness include the standardised Assessment of Motor and Process Skills (Fisher 2003) and non-

standardised observation using structured analysis methods. In employing these assessments procedural reasoning is actively employed.

Whilst analysing an individual's performance (Rogers 2004), deficits in components of function are noted (e.g. limited range of shoulder flexion impacting on reach within occupations, reduced strength in forearm muscles necessitates use of both hands for lifting heavy objects). The analysis of specific components may sometimes be necessary, and may include measuring range of joint movement, recording sensory loss in digits, or noting weakness of power grips (Wilby 2007). In contrast, Tyler et al (2005) note that measuring static and dynamic grip strength cannot be reliably used as an indicator of occupational hand function. Re-assessment of these components over time may contribute to evaluation of interventions, but these should always be done alongside occupation-focused evaluation. The reader is advised to be alert to the many standardised assessments that focus on components of function rather than having occupations as their core construct. Hocking (2001) stresses that if the intention of occupational therapy intervention is to alter occupational performance/engagement, then the focus should be on measuring and describing occupations, not specific components. The World Health Organisation (2001) also promotes focus at the activity and participation levels, not the impairment level which concentrates on components of function.

Implementing strategies

Using occupations, therapy is structured, graded and adapted to overcome difficulties caused by inadequate strength, restricted voluntary movement, and reduced endurance. These may all impact on a person's ability to complete occupations efficiently, in comfort and with satisfaction. Within therapy, a top-down approach is adopted (Boyt Schell et al 2003), exploring limitations at an occupational level, not at an impairment level. Movement, strength and endurance are components of function and are investigated within the context of occupational performance and engagement, not in isolation. This is encouraged by the World Health Organisation (2003, p. 4) who stress that assessment and therapy should focus on 'participation in life situations' and 'execution of activity' whilst noting the impact of personal and environmental factors. Practice Scenarios 34.3 and 34.4 illustrate how biomechanical strategies may be integrated into everyday life situations.

rhythmical movements, utilised large muscle groups and promoted postures against gravity. Dressing, showering, preparing food, cooking, vacuuming, washing dishes, playing bingo all presented opportunities for re-establishing voluntary movements. They offered resistance to varying degrees, building strength, endurance and promoting re-engagement with her lifestyle.

Practice Scenario 34.3 Eleanor

Eleanor, aged 70 years, has had a stroke which has left her with a movement deficit on her right side. She is married and has a supportive group of friends. She took pride in looking after her house and herself. Reading, playing bingo and line dancing were valued leisure pursuits.

The Functional Independence Measure (Guide for Uniform Dataset for Medical Rehabilitation 1997) and the Assessment of Motor and Process Skills (Fisher 2003) were administered. Both these assessments focus on assessing form. The results confirmed that Eleanor's movements were effortful, slow and lacked dexterity, with incorrect timing of prime movers and antagonists. Co-ordinating movements at numerous joints simultaneously in her right arm was challenging and fatiguing, limiting her endurance. Biomechanical changes in muscles (as a result of altered use after the stroke) and reduced joint movements had an impact on her motor control.

Other intervention strategies specific to working with a person who has had a stroke were employed. However, it was important to incorporate biomechanical strategies to enhance Eleanor's control of voluntary movement and increase her strength and endurance. The weakness in her muscles is a result of the reduced descending motor drive from the damaged motor cortex to lower motor neurones, with subsequent inadequate muscle activation (Golledge 2006). Strategies to increase her strength and voluntary movement are advocated by the Intercollegiate Stroke Working Party (2008) and other research (Canning et al 2000, Carr & Shepherd 2003, McCrea et al 2002, Ng & Shepherd 2000, O'Dwyer et al 1996, Patten et al 2004). Professional reasoning was also used to inform decisions.

Eleanor's posture and alignment to occupations, and the location of objects while doing occupations, was structured to increase shoulder flexion and abduction, elbow extension, mid-prone forearm and wrist extension, and to promote reach and grasp. Bringing items towards herself improved her control of elbow flexion. Increasing the duration and intensity of the tasks restored her strength and endurance. Other activities such as line dancing, using slow

Practice Scenario 34.4 Jacob

Jacob, a hair stylist, is 40 years old and has had rheumatoid arthritis for seven years. He enjoys cycling, eating out, and computer games. He has experienced increasing problems with wrist and hand pain.

Assessments confirm that pain and joint pathology have reduced his voluntary movement, grip strength and endurance, all affecting his work. His work tools required static grips and excessive pressure from his digits. Using procedural reasoning, the therapist selected the Occupational Performance History Interview–II (OPHI–II) (Kielhofner et al 1997) to explore meaning and the Disabilities of the Arm, Shoulder and Hand (DASH) assessment (Hadek et al 1996), investigating form and function. The DASH is a specific assessment tool designed for individuals who have rheumatological conditions (Adams et al 2005) with questions exploring physical abilities, symptoms and social roles. A work-place ergonomic assessment was also completed.

Jacob received guidance for modifying his grip on tools and bicycle handlebars, as a way to reduce pain and limit any potential musculoskeletal damage (Chaffin et al 2006, Greene & Roberts 1999, MacLeod et al 1990). He was advised, where possible, to grip with his forearm in supination or neutral (mid-prone) as these are the strongest and more efficient positions (Richards 1996). Joint protection strategies advocated by systematic reviews (Egan et al 2001, Steultjens et al 2004), national surveys (Cross et al 2006) and clinical trials (Hammond et al 2004, Stamm et al 2002) were recommended. Energy conservation principles were applied at work, home, whilst cycling, and when using the computer. Jacob purchased a cordless iron to reduce weight, thereby averting weakness and increasing endurance. Whilst eating, Jacob was advised to regularly put down his cutlery to avoid static grips. At home, he used adapted cutlery with large handles to reduce excessive flexion in his hand joints. Jacob was advised to wear wrist splints to rest and support his joints, reduce pain, maintain structural integrity and improve grip strength (MacDonald & Sorby 2006). Appropriate splints can enable optimal occupational performance (McKee & Rivard 2007) but Niederman et al (2004) have questioned the use of such splints long term, so this intervention has to be carefully evaluated, utilising conditional reasoning.

Overall aims

The aims for intervention will reflect the person's life situation but may include:

- preventing further deterioration in strength or endurance by maintaining these in the presence of a deteriorating pathology, such as osteoarthritis

- preventing further pain to enable individuals to maintain roles and successfully accomplish occupational demands

- reducing or eliminating unnecessary forces on musculoskeletal tissues to enable a person to do specific occupations

- restoring abilities that are temporarily compromised due to a more acute diagnosis or trauma. For example, the emphasis may be to improve range of movement at the shoulder joint once a fractured humerus has healed

- increasing strength which may be required in antigravity muscles after hip arthroplasty to maintain upright posture during domestic occupations or to enable safe transfers on/off seats

- enhancing endurance may be essential for return to work after a myocardial infarction. For these individuals, the recovery is more likely and therapy aims to assist the journey to the previous level of competence where possible

- implementing compensatory strategies to enable some people to adjust their occupational style or to accommodate the use of adaptive equipment to enable them to do occupations

- establishing skills to meet novel occupations for some individuals who may never have had opportunities to complete some occupations because of developmental difficulties. This situation may be evident with children or

adolescents with a range of pathologies, but their unfolding life situation requires acquisition of occupations to meet the demands of new roles within the family, school or perhaps a sheltered work environment.

Individuals may have a varied range of pathologies. Traditionally, these diagnoses only included damage to the musculoskeletal or cardiopulmonary systems (Hagedorn 2001, McMillan 2006), but people with damage to the central nervous system also acquire problems with voluntary movement, strength and endurance. Avoidance of biomechanical strategies for individuals after stroke was customary but the historical reasoning behind this decision is acknowledged as being flawed. Therapists are directed to attend to biomechanical consequences in clinical guidelines (Intercollegiate Stroke Working Party 2008) and national strategies (Department of Health 2001, 2007) in contrast to erroneous guidance in the past that did not include evidence-based or reflective practice (Blair & Robertson 2005). A prevalent idea was that providing resistance during therapy to improve strength and endurance would increase spasticity, even though evidence to support this notion was, and remains, lacking. Understanding theory enables therapists to utilise literature effectively rather than relying on outdated or misguided instruction. For all individuals, the application of strategies within the context of occupations is paramount.

Strength

Strength is required for isotonic and isometric activity and denotes the amount of force that can be produced in muscles. Strategies to improve strength capitalise on theory from kinetics which is concerned with forces and their interactions. Strength is increased by adding stress (demand) to muscles to the point of fatigue, to promote recruitment of maximal motor units (McMillan 2006, Rybski 2004). Some points to note when the aim is to increase strength are:

- The intensity, frequency and duration of the stress acting on a muscle can lead to adaptation in muscle tissue (e.g. hypertrophy of muscle fibres) with a subsequent improvement in strength.

- Increasing the time a person participates in occupations causes fatigue within the muscle, and can result in recruitment of more motor units. This needs to be carefully graded.

- Slow velocity (speed) in occupations increases strength more quickly than high-velocity activity.

- Strengthening relevant muscles requires occupational analysis to promote training specificity (Rybski 2004) so that biomechanical strategies reflect individual need.

- Slow concentric contractions produce more torque in muscles, so additional force can be generated.

It is not always possible to increase strength. When strength (and/or endurance) cannot be increased because of pathology, joint protection strategies may be implemented to prevent further dysfunction. MacDonald and Sorby (2006) and McMillan (2006) summarise the key features. They advise people to:

- respect pain and avoid placing joints in deforming positions. This is particularly relevant for people with pathologies resulting in rheumatoid arthritis and osteoarthritis

- keep joints, such as the elbow and hand joints, in their most stable position, and as much as possible avoid the extremes of joint range

- distribute the strain over multiple joints. For example, use all the hand joints to curve the digits around an item and place it securely in the palm rather than only gripping with fingertips

- avoid gripping objects too tightly to prevent damage to musculoskeletal tissues in the wrist and hand. Torque can be reduced by using lever taps instead of twist-turn taps or using specialised equipment for opening lids to limit the effects of torque on joints

- wear splints to support joints in non-damaging positions and to facilitate available strength

- avoid maintaining one position for too long as this generates isometric muscle action which is fatiguing, impacting on strength and endurance

- seek easier methods to do tasks by adapting occupational style

- work on the principle of doing valued occupations for short periods but frequently (little and often), as this will help to maintain available muscle strength and voluntary ranges of movement

- ensure a balance between rest and activity as this will inhibit a sense of weakness and promote endurance for a day's repertoire of occupations.

Endurance

Cardiopulmonary and muscular endurance is enhanced using occupations that impose low load on muscles, but are done over a longer duration, particularly using rhythmic, dynamic contractions in large muscle groups (Rybski 2004). Therapy to enhance endurance uses an understanding of kinetics. Inadequate muscle strength must be remedied before endurance can be developed, to capitalise on the necessary increasing time and repetitions required. Unlike strategies to increase strength, less than maximal stress is applied to sustain exertion over time. Engagement in occupations over progressively longer periods of time is greatly enhanced when occupations are meaningful and purposeful.

When problems with endurance have long-term implications, implementing energy-conservation strategies is advised to limit fatigue, reduce pain and enhance occupation tolerance, for greater productivity and quality of life (National Association of Rheumatological Occupational Therapists/College of Occupational Therapists 2003). Some suggested energy conservation principles include:

- planning and organising occupations

- establishing priorities

- eliminating unnecessary tasks

- using good postures

- avoiding unnecessary energy expenditure

- applying ergonomic principles

- using assistive devices

- resting regularly.

Enhancing voluntary movements

Enhancing voluntary movement incorporates theory from kinematics to identify impaired movements. Often, the problem is to do with limited range of movement at specific joints, depending on pathology. Improving the range of movement to meet occupational requirements may be achieved by

individuals with acquired brain injury. *Disability and Rehabilitation*, 24(10), 534–541.

MacDonald, R. & Sorby, K. (2006). Protection and preservation: maintaining occupational independence in clients with rheumatoid arthritis. In L. Addy (Ed.) *Occupational therapy evidence in practice for physical rehabilitation*. (pp. 101–127). Oxford, Blackwell.

MacLeod, D., Jacobs, P. & Larson, N. (1990). *The Ergonomics Manual*. Chaska MN, The Saunders Group. Available online: www.thesaundersgroup.com. Accessed 10 Nov 2006.

McKee, P. & Rivard, A. (2007). Orthoses as enablers of occupation: client centred splinting for better outcomes. *Canadian Journal of Occupational Therapy*, 71(5), 306–314.

McMillan, I. R. (2006). Assumptions underpinning a biomechanical frame of reference in occupational therapy. In E. A. S. Duncan (Ed.) *Foundations for practice in occupational therapy*. (pp. 255–275). Edinburgh, Elsevier Churchill Livingstone.

Mattingly, C. & Fleming, M. H. (1994). *Clinical reasoning. Forms of enquiry in therapeutic practice*. Philadelphia, FA Davis.

Meenan, R. F. & Mason, J. H. (1994). *AIMS2 Users Guide (revised)*. Boston University School of Medicine, Boston University Arthritis Center and Public Health Department.

National Association of Rheumatological Occupational Therapists/College of Occupational Therapists (2003). *Clinical guidelines 1. Occupational therapy in the management of rheumatic diseases*. London, NAROT/COT.

Niedermann, K., Fransen, J., Knols, R. & Uebelhart, D. (2004). Gap between short and long term effects of patient education in rheumatoid arthritis patients: a systematic review. *Arthritis and Rheumatism*, 51(3), 388–398.

Ng, S. S. & Shepherd, R. B. (2000). Weakness in patients post stroke: implications for strength training in neuro-rehabilitation. *Physical Therapy Reviews*, 5, 227–238.

O'Dwyer, N. J., Ada, L. & Neilson, P. D. (1996). Spasticity and muscle contracture following stroke. *Brain*, 119, 1737–1749.

Open Ergonomics Ltd (2000). *Workstation assessment*. Available online: www.openerg.com. Accessed 19 Oct 2006.

Paterson, M. & Summerfield-Mann, L. (2006). Clinical reasoning. In E. A. S. Duncan (Ed.) *Foundations for practice in occupational therapy*. (pp. 315–335). Edinburgh, Elsevier Churchill Livingstone.

Patten, C., Lexell, J. & Brown, H. E. (2004). Weakness and strength training in persons with post stroke hemiplegia: rationale, method and efficacy. *Journal of Rehabilitation Research and Development*, 41(3a), 293–312.

Pheasant, S. (1990). *Anthropometrics. An introduction*. Milton Keynes, British Standards Institution.

Richards, L. G., Olson, B. & Palmiter-Thomas, P. (1996). How forearm position affects grip strength. *American Journal of Occupational Therapy*, 50(2), 133–138.

Rochman, D. L. & Kennedy-Spaien, E. (2007). Chronic pain management. Approaches and tools for occupational therapy. *OT Practice*, 12(13), 9–15.

Rogers, J. C. (2004). Occupational diagnosis. In: M. Molineux (Ed.) *Occupation for occupational therapists*. (pp. 17–31). Oxford, Blackwell Publishing.

Rybski, M. (2004). *Kinesiology for occupational therapists*. Thorofare NJ, Slack Inc.

Smith, E. R. (2008). Seating. In K. Jacobs (Ed.). *Ergonomics for therapists*. (3rd ed.) (pp. 191–220). St. Louis, MS, Mosby Elsevier.

Spaulding, S. J. (2008). Basic biomechanics. In K. Jacobs (Ed.). *Ergonomics for therapists*, (3rd Ed.). (pp. 94–101). St. Louis, Mosby Elsevier.

Stamm, T. A., Machold, K. P., Smolen, J. S., Fischer, S., Redlich, K., Graninger, W., Ebner, W. & Erlacher, L. (2002). Joint protection and home hand exercises improve hand function in patients with hand osteoarthritis: a randomised controlled trial. *Arthritis and Rheumatism*, 47(1), 44–49.

Stein, F., Soderbach, I., Cutler, S. & Larson, B. (2006). *Occupational therapy and ergonomics*. London, Whurr.

Steultjens, E. E. M. J., Bouter, L. L. M., Deckkler, J. J., Kujk, M. M. A. H., Schaardenburg, D. D. & Van den Ende, E. C. H. M. (2004). Occupational therapy for rheumatoid arthritis. *The Cochrane Database of Systematic Reviews*, 1, CD 0033114.PUB2.DOI: 10. 1002/14651858.CD003114.pub2.

Strong, J., Sturgess, J., Unruh, A. & Vincenzio, B. (2002). Pain assessment and measurement. In Strong, J., Unruh, A., Wright, A. & Baxter, G. (Eds) *Pain: a textbook for therapists*. (pp. 123–147). London, Churchill Livingstone.

Tyler, H., Adams, J. & Ellis, B. (2005). What can hand grip strength tell the therapist about function? *British Journal of Hand Therapy*, 10(1), 4–9.

Ware, J. E., Snow, K. K., Kosinski, M. & Gandek, B. (1997). *SF–36 health survey: manual and interpretation guide*. Revised ed. Boston, Health Institute, New England Medical Centre.

Weiss, T. P. L. & Chan, C. C. H. (1999). Computers and assistive technology. In K. Jacobs (Ed.) *Ergonomics for therapists*. (pp. 240–268). Boston, Butterworth Heinemann.

Wilby, H. J. (2007). The importance of maintaining a focus on performance components in occupational therapy practice. *British Journal of Occupational Therapy*, 70(3), 129–132.

Winter, D. A. (2005). *Biomechanics and motor control of human movement*, (3rd edn). Hoboken NJ, John Wiley.

World Health Organisation (2001). *International classification of functioning, disability and health*. Geneva, World Health Organisation.

World Health Organisation (2003). *ICF Checklist Version 2.1a, Clinician form*. Geneva, World Health Organisation.

Chapter Thirty-Five

35

Skills for addressing sensory impairments

Farieda Adams and Michelle Morcom

CHAPTER CONTENTS

Introduction 543

Sensory system impairments 544

Sensory system impairments 544
Neuropraxia 544
Axonotmesis 544
Neurotmesis 544

Assessment 545

Assessment of specific modalities 545
Light touch 545
Temperature 545
Pain 546
Proprioception 546
Vibration sense 547
Two point discrimination 547
Moving two point discrimination 547
Touch localisation 547
Stereognosis 548
Standardised assessments 548

Addressing sensory impairments 548

Peripheral nerve injuries 548

Spinal cord injuries 549

Brainstem, thalamus and sensory cortex . . 550

Conclusion 550

SUMMARY

Although at first glance addressing sensory impairments may seem far removed from the occupational needs of people, it can be an important component of occupational therapy. The ability to receive and process sensory information is vital if an individual is to be able to understand the environment and orchestrate appropriate occupational responses. Occupational therapists, therefore, need to have an understanding of the anatomy and physiology that underpins sensation, as well as the ability to assess sensory abilities and plan appropriate intervention programmes. This chapter will provide a brief review of anatomy and physiology, but focus primarily on the essential skills and knowledge to enable sensory impairments to be addressed, within an occupation-focused programme.

KEY POINTS

- The ability to perceive and process sensory information is vital for occupational engagement.
- Assessment of sensation and sensibility can be conducted at different levels depending on the situation.
- Intervention to address sensory problems can include compensatory, rehabilitative, or educative approaches, or a combination.
- Intervention needs to be planned taking into account the person's condition, occupational difficulties, and prognosis.

Introduction

The human ability to interpret sensory stimuli forms the basis of our connection with the outside world, and, therefore, is an important aspect of occupational engagement. In order to devise and implement appropriate intervention for people with impaired sensory abilities it is important for the occupational therapist to have a thorough understanding of the anatomy and physiology of the nervous system, the common pathologies affecting the sensory system and the resulting impact of sensory impairment on occupational engagement. The aim of this chapter is to provide an introduction to the sensory system, outline evidence-based approaches for the assessment of sensation and sensibility, and consider some of the strategies used to address sensory impairment. It is important that readers appreciate that, although this chapter focuses on the details of sensation and sensibility, assessment and intervention are ultimately aimed at improving occupational engagement.

Sensory system impairments

Before proceeding, it is necessary to define two terms which have consistently been used in the literature, as they form the basis of this chapter. Omer (1980, p. 3) describes *sensation* as 'the acceptance and activation of impulses in the afferents of the nervous system'. Four modalities of sensation are recognised, namely touch-pressure, pain, warmth and cold. *Sensibility* has been described as 'the conscious appreciation and precise interpretation of sensation' (Omer 1980, p. 3). In order to make sense of sensory information an individual must draw on these two distinct, yet related, processes/abilities. While it is beyond the scope of this chapter to provide a detailed review of the sensory system, it is important to recognise that sensation and sensibility are complex processes that are made possible by the central nervous system and peripheral nervous system. The central nervous system (CNS) comprises the brain and spinal cord, and the peripheral nervous system (PNS) is made up of cranial nerves, ganglia, nerve plexuses, and peripheral nerves.

Sensory receptors in the skin, joints, muscles, and organs are activated by sensory stimuli. There are different sensory receptors that respond to different sensory stimuli, for example light touch, proprioception, and temperature. Some receptors, called exteroceptors, are located close to the surface of the body and detect information about how the body is interacting with the environment. In contrast interoceptors detect information about the internal state of the body, such as oxygen saturation levels. Proprioceptors are located in muscles, tendons, and joints (Patestas & Gartner 2006), and provide

information which is used to appreciate 'the precise position of body parts, the shape and size of an object being held in the hand, the mass of objects and the range and direction of movement' (Reid 1996, p. 52). This information is transmitted via the PNS to the CNS where it is interpreted and an appropriate response is generated. In some situations, the sensory information may only be transmitted as far as the motor neurons in the spinal cord, where an involuntary reflex movement is generated in response to the sensory stimulus. Sensory pathways are the routes taken by sensory information as it passes between the receptors, PNS, and CNS. These pathways are classified according to the sensory modalities they carry and their anatomical location. The dorsal column pathway is responsible for transmitting discriminatory light touch, vibration, and joint position sense. Pain, temperature, and some information about light touch are carried via the spinothalamic tract.

Sensory system impairments

Injuries to the peripheral nerves vary in nature. Prognosis normally varies according to the severity of the injury. Severity of nerve injuries is determined by the level at which injury has occurred as well as the type of injury (Callahan 2002). Seddon's classification is a recognised way of describing peripheral nerve injuries (Smith 2002).

Neuropraxia

The nerve has been damaged, but the axons remain in continuity and so nerve conduction is preserved proximal and distal to the level of injury. Injuries of this sort are usually caused by traction, friction or compression.

Axonotmesis

Damage to the nerve disrupts continuity of axons and results in degeneration of the axon and its myelin sheath distal to the site of the injury (Wallerian degeneration). Common causes of axonotmesis are stretching, compression, direct trauma, friction, and ischaemia.

Neurotmesis

Neurotmesis is the most severe form of peripheral nerve injury, as there is complete division of all elements of the nerve, hence, there can be no recovery without surgical repair.

Following injury or repair, nerves regenerate proximally to distally at a rate of approximately 1 mm per day (Callahan 2002). Damage to peripheral nerves can result in motor, sensory, and sympathetic changes. Sensory changes following injury can include alteration in pain, touch, temperature, stereognosis, and two-point discrimination (Van Velze 1994, Wynn Parry 1981). The precise pattern of sensory change will vary according to the level at which interruption of the sensory pathway has occurred, therefore, presentation will vary amongst individuals.

Impairments of the CNS may disrupt the sensory pathways at the level of the spinal cord or brain and, therefore, will result in altered sensation in accordance with the areas of damage and may present in a specific pattern of altered sensation based on the location of the disruption to the sensory pathway. Impairments to the nervous system are complex and may result in problems with the reception of sensory information via receptors in the skin, disruption of the sensory pathways, and/or problems with the cortical interpretation of sensory information. Considering the functional impact of sensory impairment, it is clear to see, for example, that it can result in reduced 'exploration of the environment and have detrimental effects on spontaneous use of hands, object manipulation, and precision grip. Moreover, sensory loss has a negative effect on personal safety, functional outcome and quality of life…' (Carey & Matyas 2005, p. 429). Specifically, upper-limb sensory impairment may result in difficulties such as:

- reduced ability to achieve and maintain grip, which may make holding delicate objects difficult or may cause objects to be dropped

- inability to recognise objects based on touch, such as objects in one's pocket or handbag

- reduced ability to manipulate small objects such as tools, buttons.

Assessment

Occupational therapists must assess sensation and sensibility as significant components of occupational engagement. Professional reasoning must be used to first determine the type of sensory assessment required. For example, assessment may be used as a gross screening of sensory function or may need to be more specific, such as in the assessment of sensation and sensibility in complex hand injuries. Assessments may be standardised or non-standardised. Evaluation of sensory function can be carried out to aid in diagnosis, to monitor recovery, and to determine readiness for sensory re-education (Callahan 2002).

Evaluation of sensation and sensibility remains mainly subjective and occupational therapists need to consider all influencing variables prior to testing. Several general principles of assessment should be considered when planning/conducting an assessment of sensation or sensory ability and these are presented in Table 35.1.

Assessment of specific modalities

Light touch

Light touch sensibility is a necessary component of fine discrimination and it is tested in order to determine whether the skin is anaesthetic, hyperanaesthetic or hypoanaesthetic (Callahan 2002, Leveridge 1996). Before testing, with the person's eyes open, touch an area of unaffected skin with cotton wool using a dabbing motion. Ask them to respond 'yes' each time they sense being touched with the cotton wool. Repeat this procedure with the person's eyes closed (or with the hand hidden by a screen such as in Figure 35.1), randomly applying the stimulus. Ensure consistency in the intensity of the stimulus provided. The test may be carried out to assess areas within specific dermatomes or within a specific nerve distribution (Fuller 2004). Use a diagram to record where light touch is intact, impaired/diminished or absent. It is also advisable to make a note of irregular responses whilst testing, e.g. the person saying 'yes' when no stimulus has been applied.

Temperature

To assess temperature, the person is required to tell the therapist if they detect hot or cold when they are touched with a test tube of warm or cold water. Ask the person to close their eyes and randomly apply the warm and cold test tubes by working from distal to proximal. Assess the areas within each dermatome or within a specific nerve distribution and record areas of intact, impaired/diminished or absent temperature sensation on a diagram (Fuller 2004). Bentzel (2007) describes Waylett-Rendall's

Table 35.1 General principles of sensory assessment (Callahan 2002, Fuller 2004, Leveridge 1996, Van Velze 1994, Wynn Parry 1981)

- Ask the person about the nature of their sensory change
- Explain the purpose and procedure of assessment
- Select assessments according to diagnosis/affected area, if known, but it can be better to approach assessment with a battery of tests
- Testing should be carried out in a quiet room
- Monitor the person's concentration and anxiety
- Provide standard instructions before each test
- Check that the person understands the instructions and how they are required to respond
- Prior to formal testing, perform the test with the person's eyes open to ensure understanding, demonstrating on an area of the person's skin that has intact sensation
- Start assessment with low-threshold stimuli
- Assess and record differences/similarities in sensation between the left and right
- When assessing the hand, where possible, use the unaffected hand as the control
- Use a standard method of supporting the hand when assessing sensibility in the hand
- Eliminate the person's vision during testing through the use of a screen or by asking the person to close their eyes. Blindfolds should be avoided as these can increase anxiety
- In people with cognitive/perceptual or communication impairments, it may not be possible to carry out a formal sensory assessment. The assessment technique should be adapted to suit the needs of the person
- Use a standard method to document findings
- Record sensation as intact, impaired/diminished or absent
- Assess the impact of sensory change on occupational engagement
- Review sensation regularly

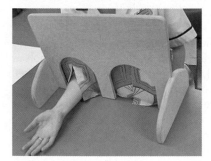

Figure 35.1 • Example of a screen that can be used to occlude vision during testing

recommendations for temperature sense assessment. It is recommended that the test tube filled with warm water measures 115–120°F (46–49°C) and the test tube filled with cold water measures 40°F (4°C). However, in the clinical environment, achieving these specific temperatures is not always possible.

Pain

Commercially available kits or safety pins may be used to assess pinprick sensation (Callahan 2002).

To begin, with the person's eyes open, touch an area of unaffected skin with the sharp end and blunt end of the tool, and ask the person to indicate 'sharp' or 'blunt'. Fuller (2004) recommends consistency in the intensity of the stimulus provided during testing. Use the amount of pressure required to elicit a correct response on the unaffected side as a guide for pressure to be applied when testing the affected side (Callahan 2002). For the assessment, vision should be eliminated, and sharp and blunt stimuli randomly applied from distal to proximal (Fuller 2004). A diagram may be used to record the findings. In the hand it is useful for the therapist to map the area of impairment. It should be remembered, that if the person is experiencing hyperanalgesia following nerve repair, they may be hypersensitive to the pin prick (Callahan 2002).

Proprioception

To assess proprioception the therapist should, with the person's eyes open, hold the lateral aspect of the person's distal phalanx of any digit between two fingers. Move the digit indicating what is 'up' and what is 'down'. Ask the person to report the position of the digit as 'up' or 'down' (Fuller 2004). Repeat

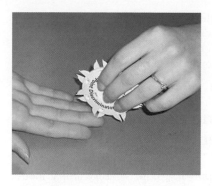

Figure 35.2 • Two point discriminator

this for the testing procedure with vision occluded, working from distal joints to proximal joints. Compare joint position sense on the left and right. Start with large movements then move to smaller movements, being careful to avoid the impact of pressure sensation during assessment (Fuller 2004). The test should be repeated several times for each joint to ensure consistency of responses. Results are recorded according to the most distal joint where joint position sense is intact and/or the differences between right and left.

Vibration sense

Before carrying out the test, strike a 128-Hz tuning fork, and with the person's eyes open, touch an intact bony area such as the chin or sternum, and ask the person to indicate if they feel the vibration. For the testing procedure, vision should be eliminated and the tuning fork placed on key bony prominences working from distal to proximal. If vibration sense is intact distally there is no need to continue assessing proximally (Fuller 2004). Record the most distal point where vibration sense is intact or record differences between left and right as appropriate.

Two point discrimination

Two point discrimination is the ability to recognise whether the skin is being touched by one or two points simultaneously (Fuller 2004). Callahan (2002) describes the test for two point discrimination as the classic test of functional sensibility, as it relates to the ability to use the hand for fine motor tasks. Assessment is carried out with a blunted compass or two point discriminator (Figure 35.2), which is recommended for hand assessment. Before

testing, with the person's eyes open, touch an area of unaffected skin with either one or two points. Ask the person to indicate whether you have touched them with one or two points. For the test, with the person's vision occluded, gradually decrease the distance between the two points of the tool and ask the person to indicate if they are being touched by one or two points (Fuller 2004). As this is light touch discrimination, do not apply too much pressure with the testing tool. For hand assessment, Callahan (2002) recommends only the fingertips need to be assessed as they are involved in tactile scanning of objects. Begin the test with a 5 mm distance between the two points, applying the two point discriminator longitudinally on the finger to avoid overlap of digital nerves. If responses are inaccurate, increase the distance between the points by 1, 2 or 5 mm until a correct response is achieved (Callahan 2002). Record the last distance between the two points where the person is able to sense being touched by two points and according to the area being assessed. Norms are available for interpreting the results of assessment (American Society of Surgery of the Hand 1990).

Moving two point discrimination

According to Callahan (2002, p. 234), Dellon's rationale for assessment of moving two point discrimination is that 'fingertip sensibility is dependent on motion and the stimulus for discrimination testing should be moving'. Begin by setting a distance of 8 mm between the two points of the discriminator and move from proximal to distal on the fingertip, longitudinally. The distance can only be narrowed if 7 out of 10 accurate responses are achieved. Testing is stopped at 2 mm, which represents normal moving two point discrimination.

Touch localisation

Touch localisation, or locognosia, is the 'the ability to identify correctly an area which has been marked out on an exact point on the skin where a person has been touched'. (Jerosch-Herold et al 2006, p. 1048). With the person's eyes open, use cotton wool to touch an area of unaffected skin with a dabbing motion and ask 'where am I touching you?' For testing, randomly apply the stimulus while the person's vision is occluded, asking 'where am I touching you?' Assess areas within each dermatome and/or compare left and right depending on the

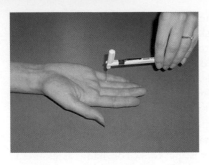

Figure 35.3 • Testing touch localisation using Semmes–Weinstein monofilament

person's impairment. Use a diagram to indicate areas of intact, impaired/diminished or absent touch localisation.

Stereognosis

A collection of common household items, such as a key, coin and pen are used for this assessment. With the person's eyes open, place an object in their unaffected hand, asking them to explore and name the object. During testing, with the person's vision occluded, place an object in their affected hand, asking them to explore the object and name it. Record the object presented and the person's ability to identify it through touch. The inability to recognise objects by touch is recorded as astereognosis.

Standardised assessments

There are a number of standardised assessments that can be used for indepth sensory assessment. These include:

- *The Rivermead Assessment of Somatosensory Performance (RASP)* is a standardised battery of tests that aims to provide a quantifiable measure of somatosensory function in neurological disorders (Winward et al 2002).

- *The Semmes–Weinstein monofilaments* are an objective measurement tool and according to Bell-Krotoski (2002, p. 194), they provide an 'absolute numerical and pictorial record for serial measurements of the same patients...'. The monofilaments indicate areas of normal and impaired sensibility within a spectrum of normal touch, and the loss of protective sensation (see Figure 35.3).

- *The Moberg pick up test* is a timed, practical test of functional sensibility. An assortment of

everyday objects is placed in front of the person, who is then asked to pick up the objects with their affected hand and place them in a box as quickly as possible (Callahan 2002).

Addressing sensory impairments

Intervention approaches for sensory impairments may include compensatory, rehabilitative, educative approaches, or a combination. When making a decision regarding the approach to be taken, careful thought must be given to the cause of the impairment and the likely prognosis. Rehabilitation programmes for sensory loss or change are based on the premise that the brain is plastic, that the non-affected areas of the brain can be trained to take over functions of affected areas, and that this neuroplasticity is dependent on stimulation of neuronal pathways (Elbert & Rockstroh 2004, Yekutiel 2000).

Yekutiel (2000, p. 65) defines sensory rehabilitation as 'a process in which the patient learns with the therapist's help to discover and use whatever somatic sensations are available to him and whatever reduced or distorted form they may "filter through"'. Furthermore, she suggests that the aim of sensory re-education is 'to challenge the brain with interesting sensory problems and provide it with information that it can use' (Yekutiel 2000, p. 13). Approaches to the treatment of sensory change in peripheral nerve injuries, injuries to the spinal cord and injuries to the brain vary due to the nature or site of injury, surgical/medical management, and prognosis.

Peripheral nerve injuries

The role of the therapist when the person lacks protective sensation is to teach them how to compensate with intact vision sense. The person should be educated on potential dangers of heat, cold, sharp objects, or risks associated with using tools or leisure equipment, in order to prevent burns and other injuries (Leveridge 1996). Regular visual inspection for any signs of injury to the skin should also be encouraged. In addition, the therapist should discuss with the person the possibility that they may experience muscle wasting, paraesthesia, and hyperaesthesia during recovery (Leveridge 1996). In the recovery phase, there is progressive reinnervation and the ongoing monitoring and assessment of motor, sensory and sympathetic function is vital. According to Ewing Fess (2002, p. 635) 'functional sensibility in the hand improves over time, with use and with training'. Sensory retraining should commence when light touch has returned over the palm and proximal phalanges in the hand (Van Velze 1994).

According to Ewing Fess (2002, p. 635) the process of sensory reeducation in peripheral nerve injuries is defined as 'a method of teaching a patient to reinterpret the altered profile of neural impulses reaching his conscious level after his injured hand has been stimulated'. Dellon and Curtis (1980) recommend that a programme of sensory rehabilitation is introduced as soon as possible. The programme is divided into early and late phases, but essential to both is the person observing the stimulus, thinking about it and focusing on how it feels whilst watching it.

During the early phase, slowly and quickly adapting sensory fibres are stimulated by the person touching his/her hand with the rubber end of a pencil, applying varying pressures. The person watches what is going on and considers how it feels with both eyes open and eyes closed. In order to stimulate quickly adapting fibres, the person moves the rubber end of the pencil over the skin, proximally to distally, again, with both eyes open and then closed, and considers how it feels. Early phase activities should be repeated for 5–10 minutes, three to five times each day.

During the late phase, the person is able to perceive touch at the distal phalanx. During this phase, nuts of different sizes and shapes are used in two ways. First, the person is asked to discriminate between large and small nuts. This task is graded to discriminating between nuts more similar in size. The person then discriminates between the four sharp sides of a square nut and the six blunt sides of a hexagonal nut, rolling them across the finger with the unaffected hand. Finally, the person is required to discriminate between the round and flat cap of a nut. This is graded to smaller cap nuts, until the person is able to identify the groove in a button. During the late stage of the programme, the person follows the same principles as in the early stage, watching first and then repeating the task with closed eyes, and also considering how it feels. These activities are carried out for 10–15 minutes, repeated three to five times each day. This programme has the benefits of being simple,

repetitive and can be carried out independently by the person.

Wynn Parry (1973, 1981) has also described a method of sensory rehabilitation following peripheral nerve injury. In this approach, the person is exposed to moving touch, constant touch and pressure with vision occluded, and is asked to discuss what they feel. The same process is then repeated with vision. These two steps are repeated until the person is able to correctly interpret the sensations, without the use of vision. Also, objects are placed in the hand, and the person is asked to describe the properties of each object without vision, and then again with vision. Once again, these steps are repeated until the person is able to correctly interpret the sensations without relying on vision. Once the person is able to successfully describe the properties of the object, new objects can be used which are more difficult to identify by touch. Grading of objects can progress from wooden blocks to cubes of different sizes and materials, three-dimensional shapes, objects with different textures, familiar everyday objects, objects with complex shapes and finally, objects buried in a bowl of sand. Wynn Parry described the grading of object use from large to small objects, heavy to light, coarse to fine and simple to complex. The final stage is for the person to participate in occupations such as dressing (perhaps focusing on fastening buttons, and tying shoe laces) and writing. Wynn Parry recommends that evaluation is performed throughout rehabilitation. The programme may last from just one week up to six weeks, depending on the motivation and concentration of the person. Throughout intervention following peripheral nerve injury, the therapist educates the person on the reasons for participating in a sensory rehabilitation programme, the risks associated with reduced sensation in the limb and may also teach compensation through the use of assistive devices and the use of intact sensations such as vision.

Spinal cord injuries

The two main approaches used in the treatment of sensory change following spinal cord injury are education and compensation, but the exact nature of intervention will vary depending on the location and extent of the injury. The role of the occupational therapist in managing sensory change after spinal cord injury is to provide continuous education regarding the risks associated with absent or altered sensation, including development of pressure areas, burns and injury to skin (Umphred 2001). The therapist teaches compensatory techniques, utilising intact sensation to compensate for altered/absent sensation. This can be done for example by using vision to check for redness or areas of skin break-down. Similarly, a limb with intact sensation can be used to test water temperature before bathing. For people with incomplete spinal cord lesions or spinal cord compression, areas of sensory change may be patchy, but still impact on occupational engagement. In these circumstances, using vision to observe the movement of the affected limb may increase occupational engagement. If appropriate, the occupational therapist may also teach assertiveness skills, empowering the person to ask for assistance in the monitoring of pressure areas and requesting assistance for pressure relief.

Brainstem, thalamus and sensory cortex

When damage to the brainstem, thalamus or sensory cortex has resulted in sensory impairment, rehabilitative (sensory re-education), compensatory, educational or a combination of approaches may be used. The approach chosen is determined by the particular condition. For example, a rehabilitation approach should be considered where there is the potential for improvement, as may be the case in a person who has had a stroke. In people with high-grade brain tumours affecting the sensory cortex, for example, a compensatory and educative approach may be most appropriate. General principles in the management of sensory changes following brainstem, thalamic or sensory cortex lesions include encouraging the use of the affected upper limb during bilateral and unilateral occupations. The occupational therapist should allow opportunities to increase tactile awareness, stereognosis and sensory discrimination using a variety of sensory inputs. In the compensatory approach, the occupational therapist facilitates the use of intact sensory systems such as vision and hearing to compensate for reduced sensation, hence facilitating occupational engagement. Assistive devices and environmental modification can be used to facilitate occupations and prevent injury. The occupational therapist should also educate continuously regarding risks associated with absent sensation including development of pressure areas, burns and injury to skin (Umphred 2001).

Yekutiel (2000) has highlighted additional principles to be used in sensory re-education programmes for the hand, following stroke. In setting up a sensory re-education programme, the focus should be on success and achievement. Activities should be chosen according to the person's abilities, with the person acting as the leader and the therapist as the facilitator. The person should choose tasks which he feels will be successful, and which he will be able to do alone. Tasks should be graded slowly, ensuring success and preventing failure. Yekutiel (2000) has provided detailed outlines of intervention sessions with lessons in touch, lessons in proprioception and lessons in the recognition of objects and their qualities. She has reinforced that sensory re-education requires motivation and achievement to be successful. It should be a conscious process, something that the person does, rather than something that is done to the person. In order for sensory rehabilitation to be successful, the person must have intact cognitive, perceptual and communication skills. Johansson (2004, p. 238) concurs that 'rehabilitation strategies that are meaningful for the individual patient are likely to be the most effective'.

In her sensory re-education programme of the hand after stroke, Yekutiel (2000) has stated that for each chosen activity, the therapist should start by discussing with the person the qualities of an object, to focus attention on the task. The person should then feel the object with the unaffected hand, with eyes closed. The person and therapist spend time working with the unaffected hand to assist in preparing for use of the affected hand. The object is then felt with the affected hand with the eyes open and then with the eyes closed. Verbalising, using vision and feeling during the tasks, utilises different pathways to the brain and maximises potential for change.

Conclusion

Intervention for people with sensory impairment following peripheral or central nervous system lesions requires a thorough understanding of anatomy and physiology relating to the sensory system, the assessment and treatment techniques to be employed, and functional implications of altered sensation. It is also imperative that the occupational therapist be able to appreciate the impact of impairments to the sensory system and the resultant disruption to occupations that make up the person's life. Impairments of the sensory system do not usually occur in isolation, but rather occur in combination with other physical impairments. The therapist needs to always assess the person as a whole and remember that sensory assessments are only a small part of the overall assessment. Similarly, interventions for sensory impairments are only a small part of restoring a person's function. It can be easy to lose sight of the occupations the person needs or wants to do, and so working in this area can be challenging to ensure an occupational focus.

References

American Society of Surgery of the Hand (1990). *The hand: examination and diagnosis*. (3rd ed.). New York, Churchill Livingstone.

Bell-Krotoski, J.A. (2002). Sensibility testing with the Semmes–Weinstein monofilaments. In E. J. Mackin, A. D. Callahan, T. M. Skirven et al (Eds.), *Hunter–Mackin–Callahan Rehabilitation of the hand and upper extremity* (5th ed.). (pp. 194–213). Missouri, Mosby.

Bentzel, K. (2007). Assessing abilities and capabilities: Sensation. In M. Radomski & C. Trombly (Eds.). *Occupational therapy for physical dysfunction* (pp. 212–233). Philadelphia, Lippincott, Williams and Wilkins.

Callahan, A. D. (2002). Sensibility assessment for nerve lesions-in-continuity and nerve lacerations. In E. J. Mackin, A. D. Callahan, T. M. Skirven et al (Eds.), *Hunter–Mackin–Callahan rehabilitation of the hand and upper extremity* (5th ed.). (pp. 214–239). Missouri, Mosby.

Carey, L. M. & Matyas, T. A. (2005). Training of somatosensory discrimination after stroke: Facilitation of stimulus generalisation. *American Journal of Physical Medicine and Rehabilitation*, 84, 428–442.

Dellon, A. L. & Curtis, R. M. (1980). Sensory reeducation after peripheral nerve injury. In G. Omer & M. Spinner (Eds.), *Management of peripheral nerve problems*.

(pp. 769–778). Philadelphia, WB Saunders.

Elbert, T. & Rockstroh, B. (2004). Reorganisation of the human cerebral cortex: The range of changes following use and injury. *Neuroscientist*, 10(2), 129–141.

Ewing Fess, E. (2002). Sensory reeducation. In E. J. Mackin, A. D. Callahan, T. M. Skirven et al (Eds.), *Hunter–Mackin–Callahan rehabilitation of the hand and upper extremity*. (5th ed.). (pp. 635–639). Missouri, Mosby.

Fuller, G. (2004). *Neurological examination made easy*. (3rd ed.). Edinburgh, Churchill Livingstone.

Jerosch-Herold, C., Rosén, B. & Shepstone, L. (2006). The reliability of the locognosia test after injuries to peripheral nerves in the hand. *Journal of Bone and Joint Surgery (Br)*, 88–B, 1048–1052.

Johansson, B. B. (2004). Brain plasticity in health and disease. *The Keio Journal of Medicine*, 53(4), 231–246.

Leveridge, A. C. (1996). Peripheral nerve injuries. In A. Turner, M. Foster & S. E. Johnson (Eds.), *Occupational therapy and physical dysfuntion – principles, skills and practice*. (4th ed.). (pp. 571–598). United Kingdom, Harcourt Publishers Limited.

Omer, G. (1980). Sensibility testing. In G. Omer & M. Spinner (Eds.), *Management of peripheral nerve problems*. (pp. 3–15). Philadelphia, WB Saunders.

Patestas, M. A., & Gartner, L. P. (2006). *A textbook of neuroanatomy*. (1st ed.). Oxford, Blackwell Publishing.

Reid, C. (1996). *A primer of human neuroanatomy*. Pretoria, JL van Schaik.

Smith, K. L. (2002). Nerve response to injury and repair. In E. J. Mackin, A. D. Callahan, T. M. Skirven et al (Eds.), *Hunter–Mackin–Callahan rehabilitation of the hand and upper extremity*. (5th ed.). (pp. 583–598). Missouri, Mosby.

Umphred, D. A. (2001). *Neurological rehabilitation*. (4th ed.). Missouri, Mosby.

Van Velze, C. A. (1994). Rehabilitation of the injured hand. In U. Mennen (Ed.), *The handbook – A practical approach to common hand problems*. (1st ed.). (pp. 201–239). South Africa, Southern Book Publishers.

Winward, C. E., Halligan, P. W. & Wade, D. T. (2002). The Rivermead Assessment of Somatosensory Performance (RASP): standardization and reliability data. *Clinical Rehabilitation*, 16, 523–533.

Wynn Parry, C. B. (1973). *Rehabilitation of the hand*. (3rd ed.). London, Butterworths.

Wynn Parry, C. B. (1981). *Rehabilitation of the hand*. (4th ed.). London, Butterworths.

Yekutiel, M. (2000). *Sensory re-education of the hand after stroke*. London, Whurr.

Moving and handling strategies

Maggie Bracher and April Brooks

CHAPTER CONTENTS

Introduction 554

Impact of moving and handling on the
body – risks to the occupational therapist . . 555

Principles of movement. 556

   Biomechanical principles 558
   Stability. 558
   Base of support 558
   Centre of gravity and line of gravity. 558
   Friction 560
   Levers and forces 561

Risk assessment 562

   Focusing the risk assessment. 565
   MHQ1: What is normal movement for
   this task?. 566
   MHQ2: Can I teach the person to do this
   unaided? 566
   MHQ3: If not completely unaided, is there
   equipment available that would mean the
   person *could* do this for themselves? 566
   MHQ4: If unable to perform the task
   themselves, even with equipment, what is
   the minimum assistance one and then two
   people can give: a) without equipment and
   b) with equipment?. 567
   MHQ5: Are there unsafe ways of doing this
   I must avoid? If so, what are they?. 567
   MHQ6 and MHQ7 567
   MHQs in practice. 567

Equipment provision and use 568

   Standing equipment. 569
   Hoists 569
   Competency to use equipment 570

Principles of safer handling. 570

Legislation 571

Conclusion. 574

SUMMARY

Manual handling remains one of the major
causes of occupational injuries in many
countries. In the United Kingdom, in 2001 to
2002, manual handling was associated with more
'over-three-day' injuries reported to the Health
and Safety Executive (HSE) (38%) than any other
occupational task (Health and Safety Executive
2007a). The handling of people is a particular
risk factor (Health and Safety Executive 2007b)
due to the unpredictable nature of the task.
People vary in size, shape, and physical/
cognitive abilities and the adult human form is
difficult to hold due to an uneven distribution of
weight. The potential for uncooperative/
aggressive behaviour increases risk of injury for
therapists and carers (Anonymous 1965, Nelson
2006). Additionally, the psychosocial impact of
organisational and other work issues, such as
high levels of demand, low levels of support or
lack of control over workload have been shown
to increase stress in employees, exacerbating
symptoms of existing musculoskeletal disorder,
or heightening awareness of musculoskeletal
pain (Devereux 2003, Devereux & Buckle 2000,
Erez & Lindgren 1999). While there is a dearth of
research regarding work-related musculoskeletal
disorders in occupational therapists, much exists
for both nursing and physiotherapy. Considering
the nature of occupational therapy, it is likely that
injuries in this profession are comparable to
those for nursing and physiotherapy (Cromie et al
2000, Royal College of Nursing 1996).

KEY POINTS

- Understanding of biomechanics and normal human movement is essential in the analysis and safe facilitation of moving and handling people.
- Moving and handling practice and policy must be underpinned by legislation and risk assessment.
- Therapists and all those who assist people to move need to have an awareness of personal joint and back care, and mechanisms of injury.
- Independence in movement should be encouraged when possible, using rehabilitation or compensatory approaches or a combination of both.
- Care handling and therapeutic handling can be used together.
- Active participation of individuals can be encouraged by the appropriate use of equipment – this also reduces the risk of injury to all involved.
- Balanced decision-making in risk assessment must take account of the needs and protection of everyone involved in the moving and handling task.

Introduction

Independent normal movement is taken for granted by most of us. People do not think about how they are going to turn in bed or stand up, as all these movement patterns are learned at the pre-verbal stage of development in infancy. When mobility is restricted by injury or disease, the occupational therapist plays a key role in the analysis of the demands of daily occupations, assessing the abilities of the individual affected and identifying social and environmental factors which may enable or disable that person in their daily routines (World Health Organisation 2001). Manual handling is an intrinsic part of this process and includes direct handling of the individual and guidance/instruction to other carers (Cromie et al 2000, Royal College of Nursing 1996). The understanding of normal movement and biomechanics is crucial when developing the most appropriate and safe interventions. When considering manual-handling interventions with an individual, a balance must be maintained between the needs and human rights of that individual and the safety of those assisting them to move (Mandelstam 2005).

Manual handling involves transporting or supporting a load by applying force with any part of the human body, either directly or indirectly. These actions include lifting, putting down, steadying, positioning, pushing or pulling (Health and Safety Executive 2004b). It encompasses all aspects of assisting a person to move any part of their body; therefore, activities ranging from supporting a limb, while splinting, through to hoisting a person from the floor, all require knowledge and skill to maintain safety for the therapist and individual concerned. Application of safe moving and handling principles is essential if therapists are to protect themselves and those with whom they are working. This application of safe moving and handling principles will be illustrated throughout the practice scenarios presented in this chapter, starting with Practice Scenario 36.1.

Practice Scenario 36.1
Introducing Caroline

Caroline is 54 years old. She is in hospital following a fall. She has multiple sclerosis, is intermittently ambulant, no longer able to work and lives in a two-bedroom house with her husband who works long hours from Mondays to Fridays. The occupational therapist involved with Caroline is responsible for ensuring her safe discharge and continuing care in the community. Safe mobility and assistance with moving are key areas of concern for Caroline, as she is on her own for periods during the day and her husband is often physically and mentally exhausted when he finishes work at the end of each day. Her interests are gardening and painting, and she wishes to continue engaging in these occupations for as long as possible.

Caroline's diagnosis and prognosis are important considerations when shaping any interventions. Using the medical model to consider the future effects of the disease process signposts her potential medical needs; however, occupational therapists are also concerned with any psychosocial and environmental effects on Caroline's occupational performance and engagement. Using the Social Model of Function and Disability (World Health Organisation 2001), social and environmental aspects of her lifestyle and surroundings need to be assessed to establish which may enable or disable her in the immediate and longer term. With this in mind the potential need for equipment/adaptation needs to be considered, taking into account environmental and social issues, in order to facilitate safe mobility for as long as possible for the sake of Caroline, her husband and any other carers.

Occupational analysis will be central to the interventions used with Caroline and her family. Issues of mobility and assistance with moving will have a significant impact on the way she manages her daily life and carries out her chosen occupations. In order to facilitate optimum conditions for Caroline's mobility and handling needs, and to protect those who assist her, the occupational therapist needs to have knowledge of the following:

- Normal movement for each task/activity she wishes to carry out
- Changes in her abilities which may affect the way in which she carries out these tasks
- Compensatory approaches used to enable her to carry out chosen tasks
- Her priorities for task completion
- Structure, components and order of the tasks she carries out
- The ability of Caroline's husband, and other carers, to assist her
- Equipment and resources available for her mobility/activity needs
- Skill levels required to enable movement or use of equipment.

This chapter will provide an overview of moving and handling principles. It is not within the remit of this chapter to discuss the wide variety of methods and equipment available for safer moving and handling. This is dealt with comprehensively in other texts (see Aitchison 1999, Smith 2005).

Impact of moving and handling on the body – risks to the occupational therapist

Musculoskeletal disorders (MSD) are the most common of all reported work-related health problems in the European Union: one in four workers reported suffering from back pain in 2005 (European Agency for Safety and Health at Work 2007). Occupational therapists are at risk of musculoskeletal injury because of the nature of their work: back pain, neck pain and work-related upper-limb disorders (WRULD) are all conditions that characteristically result from overuse of muscles and other soft tissues. The major contributory factors for work-related injury are known, and it is possible to put measures in place to try to prevent these factors or injuries (Pheasant 1996).

Students and newly qualified therapists can be particularly at risk of an MSD. Smith et al (2006) investigated a cross-section of Australian occupational therapy students, and found that three-quarters of all students (75.5%) reported an MSD occurring in at least one body region during the previous 12 months. Almost 40% (39.5%) reported an MSD that had affected their daily life. Studies involving chartered physiotherapists also identify that newly qualified graduates and younger therapists (under 30 years of age) are at particular risk (Cromie et al 2000, Glover 2005, Mierzejewski & Kumar 1997, Molumphy et al 1985, Scholey & Hair 1989).

Glover (2005) refers to a 'can do' attitude and the 'good therapist' who 'just gets on with it', and there is evidence of 'client first' pressure. It is suggested that cultural values within the health service make it difficult for therapists to do their jobs in a way that minimises risk (Cromie et al 2000). A great deal of research has now been done, and therapists are much better informed regarding best practice and coping strategies within the field of moving and handling, and strategies for reduction of risk of musculoskeletal injury (Bork et al 1996, Glover et al 2005, Holder et al 1999, Molumphy et al 1985, Scholey & Hair 1989). Possible sources of back pain that can affect therapists can be found in Box 36.1.

Moving a person has to take into consideration a multitude of factors, such as weight distribution, asymmetric body mass, unpredictable behaviour, medical issues such as muscle spasms or loss of spatial awareness, and so on. The amount of assistance the individual can offer at any point in time may vary, so every time the task is performed the risks may be different. Added to this are the problems of clutter, confined spaces, and, not least, how the therapist is feeling in themselves, and about the task and the person. Lifting, turning, and positioning of people can then lead to fatigue, muscle strain, and, ultimately, injury (Nelson 2003).

Not all stressful tasks involve straightforward direct lifts of people. Owen and Garg (1990) identified 16 stressful person-handling tasks which may apply to occupational therapists, especially when teaching family members or carers (Practice Scenario 36.2). The most stressful tasks that were identified are shown in rank order in Box 36.2.

Box 36.1

Possible sources of back pain in the workplace

Examples of known sources of back pain (for therapists) in the workplace:

- Heavy manual labour (e.g. lifting equipment into the back of a car, lifting or transferring heavy clients)
- Manual handling in awkward places (e.g. bathrooms or toilets)
- Repetitive tasks (e.g. carrying out exercises with a person)
- Working in the same position for long periods (e.g. sitting at a workstation for a long period of time if the workstation is not correctly arranged or adjusted to fit the person)
- Driving long distances, particularly if the seat is not properly adjusted
- Inadequate training in injury prevention
- Treating a large number of people in one day
- Difficulty in performing safe handling techniques due to a person's condition, size and/or shape.

Examples of physical activities that can aggravate back pain:

- Continuing to work when injured or hurt
- Stooping, bending over or crouching, including poor posture when working at computers
- Lifting objects which are heavy or bulky, carrying objects awkwardly
- Pushing, pulling or dragging excessive loads
- Working beyond or at normal abilities and limits, when physically overtired
- Using poor lifting techniques (or when posture is compromised due to other risk factors)
- Stretching, twisting and reaching
- Spending prolonged periods in one position, leading to postural strain
- Understaffing which leads to psychosocial risk stressors.

Adapted from Health and Safety Executive 2007, Glover, Sullivan & Hague 2005

Practice Scenario 36.2
Beginning to identify risks

For the safety of Caroline and her carers, the occupational therapist needs to be aware of mechanisms of injury and how the daily activities for this couple may potentially increase the risk of injury to either Caroline or any of her carers. By listing Caroline's essential and chosen daily activities, when these occur and how they are prioritised, the therapist can begin to identify where risks may be higher; for example, Caroline needing physical assistance to get into bed at night. Manual-handling activities such as this may place her husband at increased risk of musculo-skeletal disorders, as he is often exhausted from work at the end of the day. Her husband, therefore, risks injury through trying to work beyond his physical capability at that time.

The therapist needs to help the couple prioritise where formal care or careful use of equipment (such as transfer board or later, a ceiling track hoist) is needed in order to protect both Caroline and her husband from injury and to facilitate maximum participation and independence for Caroline. Once activities have been identified and prioritised, the therapist needs to look at Caroline's performance and the fluctuations in her ability. Application of normal movement and biomechanical principles will help identify areas of risk for her and her carers during mobility tasks. From this, more detailed risk assessment can be carried out in order to develop a personal handling profile.

The combination of a high injury prevalence associated with handling people, and the large estimates of biomechanical stress associated with manual handling techniques in these situations have led to the use of risk assessment tools such as Rapid Entire Body Assessment (REBA) (Hignett & McAtamney 2000), in order to analyse the biomechanics of handling techniques. At the same time safer handling techniques have been developed and equipment designed to facilitate independence and minimise risk to the handler.

Principles of movement

It is not the remit of this chapter to discuss the neuro-physiological principles of movement, but in order to make decisions related to moving or handling people, it is necessary to understand how a person would move themselves if they were able to. In the context of moving and handling a person, this is called 'normal movement'. Put simply, it is the way that a person would normally move: the voluntary and automatic movements produced by the nerve pathways and action of muscles on bones and joints, which then achieve a movement task in an energy-efficient, co-ordinated way. Patterns of movement are sequences of movement for the

Box 36.2

People handling tasks identified as increasing musculoskeletal stress

Stressful handling tasks (Owen & Garg 1990)

1. Transferring person from chair-to-toilet-to-chair
2. Transferring person from chair-to-bed-to-chair
3. Transferring a person into/out of a bath
4. Weighing a person
5. Repositioning a person in bed
6. Repositioning a person in a chair
7. Undressing a person
8. Feeding a bed-ridden person.

High-risk tasks (Nelson et al 2006)

1. Bathing person in bed
2. Making an occupied bed
3. Dressing a person in bed
4. Transferring a person from bed to stretcher
5. Transferring from bed to wheelchair
6. Transferring from bed to dependency chair
7. Repositioning a person in a chair
8. Repositioning a person in bed
9. Applying anti-embolism stockings.

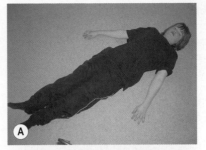

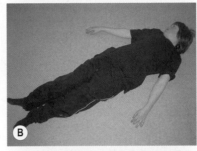

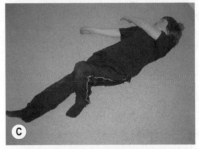

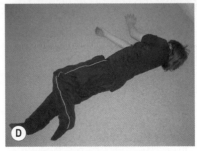

Figure 36.1 • Normal movement sequence for turning onto the side in supine lying. (a) Supine lying. (b) Turning the head in the direction of the move. (c) Bending the knee and placing foot flat on the floor while reaching across the chest with the arm. (d) Reaching with the arm and pushing with the foot to turn onto the side

achievement of a motor goal. Normal movement requires combinations of movement patterns.

If a whole-year group of occupational therapy students were lying supine on a floor, arms by their sides, legs straight, and on a given cue they turned onto their right sides, there would be many common components to their methods of completing the task. Movement generally starts with the head – looking to the right in this instance. The left shoulder girdle will follow the rotation of the cervical spine and the left arm reach across the chest. In order for the body mass to move, it is likely that the left knee will bend, the foot will be placed on the floor, and the 'reach' with the arm, and the 'push' with the foot, will cause the body to roll onto its side. Figure 36.1 illustrates the above sequence of 'normal' movement for turning to the side from supine lying.

Variations will of course occur – due to previous injury, body shape, age, medical condition and so on – but since the human form is generally made up of the same component parts, movement patterns are somewhat predictable. If therapists are going to ask a person to move, and perhaps give them instructions to do so, unless therapists first understand how a person would normally achieve the task (i.e. the most effective, efficient way for them), they can actually *dis*-able them and negatively impact on their abilities.

The objective of the therapist is usually to enable the person to do as much for themselves as possible. Placing the person in an optimum starting position, making use of biomechanical advantage, and giving opportunity for recruitment of muscles and joints, may be sufficient to enable the person to complete a moving task; or help the therapist to identify the missing components or which compensatory movements the person is using. In order to meet this objective, therapists need to have a sound knowledge of anatomy and basic principles of biomechanics.

Biomechanical principles

Stability

The stability of an object is its ability to withstand external and internal forces and remain in its current position or shape. Stability in the human body is dependent upon a number of factors, such as the size of the base of support, location of the body's (or body segment's) centre of gravity, and, as a consequence, where the line of gravity falls within the base of support (Tyldesley & Grieve 2002). Stability is also affected to a degree by friction and internal/external forces acting on the body.

Base of support

The base of support is denoted by the contact points of an object or person with the ground and all the area inside those contact points, as in Figure 36.2. A large base of support gives greater stability (Figure 36.3). A small base of support means that the person is less stable (Figure 36.4).

Stability is also linked to the position of the centre of gravity and line of gravity relative to the base of support.

Centre of gravity and line of gravity

The point at which gravity is thought to act on an object is described as its centre of gravity. In the adult human body, while standing or lying in the anatomical position, the centre of gravity of the whole body is estimated to be anterior to the second sacral vertebra (Norkin & Levangie 2005). Each segment in the human body has its own centre of gravity; however, within the remit of moving and

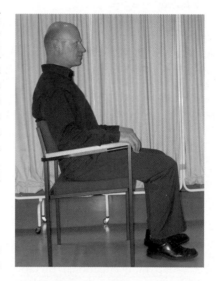

Figure 36.3 • Large base of support (BOS) from back legs of chair to front of person's feet

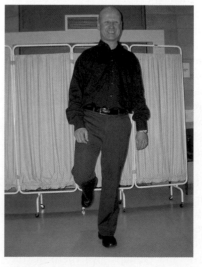

Figure 36.4 • Small base of support (BOS) denoted by one foot in contact with the ground

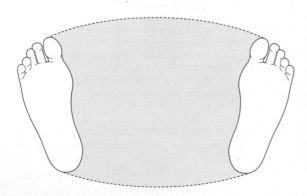

Figure 36.2 • Base of support

handling, the centre of gravity of the whole body is generally referred to. The line of gravity is an imaginary line drawn vertically from the centre of gravity to the ground and helps us estimate, at any time, where the centre of gravity is relative to the base of support. Knowing this helps us estimate the stability of a person. The more central the centre of gravity and line of gravity are within the base of support, the greater a person's stability (Figure 36.5). A low centre of gravity increases a person's stability, therefore when people are lying in prone or supine they are at their most stable (Figure 36.6).

Conversely, raising the centre of gravity (Figure 36.7) will decrease stability. In addition, as people rearrange the segments of their bodies, the centre of gravity of the whole body moves. It can move in any direction and can be outside the physical body (Norkin & Levangie 2005). If this movement results in the line of gravity moving toward the edge of or outside the base of support, the person becomes unstable as in Figure 36.8.

In summary, if a person has a small base of support (Figure 36.4) it will take very little movement of the body in order for the line of gravity to fall towards or outside the edge of the base of support, thus destabilising them. Equally changing

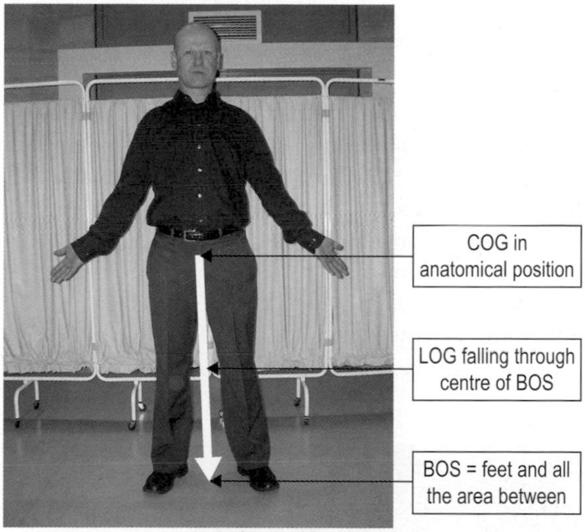

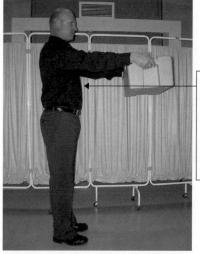

Due to rearrangement of body segments and addition of weight on the arms, the COG moves up and forward decreasing the person's stability

Figure 36.7 • Position of decreased stability due to a higher centre of gravity

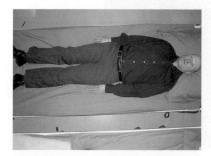

COG in anatomical position

LOG falling through centre of BOS

BOS = feet and all the area between

Figure 36.5 • Centre of gravity (COG) in anatomical position and line of gravity (LOG) falling within centre of the BOS

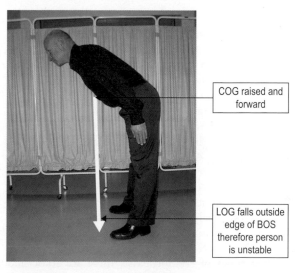

COG raised and forward

LOG falls outside edge of BOS therefore person is unstable

Figure 36.6 • Position of maximum stability with large BOS and low COG (level with S2); low COG falls centrally within BOS

Figure 36.8 • Position of LOG outside BOS creates instability

the weight distribution of the body may raise the centre of gravity, which will also reduce stability. While a high degree of stability is necessary for safety when, for example, a person is supporting a load, reduced stability is necessary in order for movement to occur. If a person was to keep his centre of gravity and line of gravity centrally within a wide base of support all the time (Figure 36.3) he would find it very difficult to change position.

In rehabilitation, interventions generally begin with the person in a position of maximum stability. Having a low centre of gravity, and large base of support, requires the least amount of energy consumption and muscle tone (e.g. in supine lying Figure 36.6). The objective may be to progress to movement in a position of less stability, in order to re-train muscle tone, balance, reactions, etc. An example of this would be the person ultimately being able to stand on tip-toe with arms raised to lift an object into a high cupboard. This position is one of reduced stability as the centre of gravity is raised (due to re-organisation of body segments and added weight through the arms) and the base of support is small. Any shift in position of the centre of gravity now, will more easily result in the line of gravity falling outside the base of support, thus destabilising the person. In order to maintain balance in this position of reduced stability, the person is dependent on recruitment of appropriate muscle groups, vestibular and visual function, and intact proprioception.

Friction

Another factor potentially affecting a person's ability to move, the effort required and the quality of movement is friction. Where two objects are in contact with each other, friction will occur to a greater or lesser extent, depending on the type of surfaces in contact and the pressure between them. It is important to understand the effects of friction coefficients in different materials and their effects on movement. A surface with a high friction coefficient will resist movement across it, for example a deep-pile wool carpet. Alternatively a surface with a low friction coefficient will enable movement to occur more easily and reduce the degree of shearing forces on the moving object, for example a slide sheet (Norkin & Levangie 2005).

Two types of friction exist: these are static and dynamic friction. Static friction resists movement.

Therefore, when a person sits still in a chair (Figure 36.3), static friction between the thighs/buttocks and the chair seat prevents slipping out of the chair. In order to overcome this static friction a person must create movement through internal or external forces. Once movement begins, dynamic friction occurs between the surfaces in contact with each other. For the therapist and person, this can be either beneficial or a hindrance. If the person in Figure 36.3 wishes to get out of the chair, the high friction coefficient and his body weight will necessitate greater internal/external forces to enable him to move. Therefore, a high friction coefficient will be beneficial in enabling him to stay in the chair, but will make moving out of the chair more difficult. This is often the case when people are in bed (Figure 36.6). Static friction between the person's body and the bed means that the person is very stable; however, when he needs to move the dynamic friction between the two surfaces increases the risk of shearing forces on the person's skin. The therapist also has to exert much larger external forces to help initiate movement, increasing her risk of musculoskeletal injury. Using slide sheets, which have a very low friction coefficient, reduces the impact of shearing forces and requires less external force to create movement (Figure 36.9). This principle applies equally where people are able to sit up and move themselves on a bed. Using small slide sheets between themselves and the bed reduces

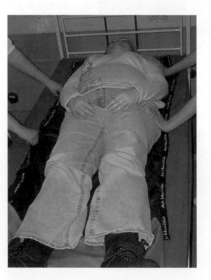

Figure 36.9 • Reducing dynamic friction using slide sheets to make movement easier

shearing forces and minimises the amount of effort required to move.

Levers and forces

In order to understand how people move, it is important to understand levers. A lever system comprises an axis, an effort force and a resistance force. In the human body, the axis is commonly a joint. The effort force is directed so as to produce movement of the body or body part and the resistance force opposes the movement. The process of standing from sitting illustrates all these aspects and enables us to start analysing why this activity can sometimes be difficult and how to make it easier. In order for this movement to be easy, the distance of the effort force from the axis should be as large as possible, as the larger the distance of a force from an axis, the greater its mechanical advantage. The effort force in this case is provided by the quadriceps muscles which extend the knee. The axis is the knee joint and the resistance force is the body weight, the central point of which is the centre of gravity. Figures 36.10A and 36.10B show that the distance of the resistance force from the axis is greater than the distance of the effort force, which is common, as muscle attachments cannot move and, therefore, are generally close to a joint.

When a person sits upright in a chair, he has a large base of support with his line of gravity falling near the centre of this support. The person is, therefore, very stable. In order to stand up, he needs to *de*-stabilise his body. Figures 36.10A and 36.10B illustrate the biomechanical differences between static upright sitting and preparation for standing and explain how changing the position of the body's centre of gravity facilitates standing.

To make standing even easier for a person, therapists can ask or assist him to move his hips forward in the chair to bring the line of gravity closer to the edge of the base of support, thus destabilising him further. Additionally, by using chair raisers to increase the height of the chair, the angles at the hips and knees when sitting are increased and the body's centre of gravity (line of resistance force) is automatically closer to the knees (axis). Its mechanical advantage is therefore decreased even further in relation to that of the quadriceps muscles (effort force).

Having an understanding of biomechanics and normal patterns of movement in an able-bodied

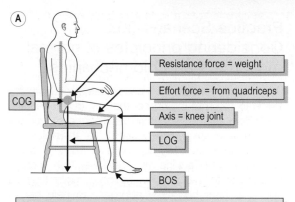

In the upright sitting position, the resistance force (weight) is much further from the axis (knee) than the effort force (from quadriceps). The resistance force therefore has greater mechanical advantage and more effort is required to overcome gravity in order to stand.
The line of gravity also falls from the COG near to the centre of the BOS therefore stability is high.

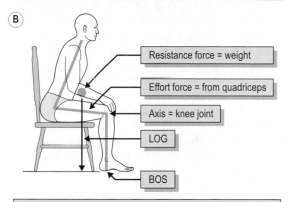

By leaning forward the resistance force (weight) is brought closer to the axis (knee), reducing its mechanical advantage relative to the effort force (from quadriceps)
The LOG now falls closer to the edge of the BOS, therefore stability is decreased.
This results in reduced effort for standing.

Figure 36.10 • Biomechanical principles related to upright sitting and preparation for standing (A) Upright sitting (B) Leaning forward in preparation to stand

adult of average body mass, provides a working base line from which it is possible to understand the effect of changes in tone (increased or decreased), body mass (increased or decreased, as in pregnancy or amputation) or joint function (pain, etc.) on movement. Application of this understanding of biomechanics and normal patterns of movement is illustrated in Practice Scenario 36.3.

Practice Scenario 36.3
Considering principles of normal movement and biomechanics

Caroline's condition may necessitate greater assistance to move at the end of the day, due to fatigue. By understanding the principles of normal movement and biomechanics, the occupational therapist can reduce potential injury for both Caroline and her carers. Should Caroline wish to transfer from a chair/wheelchair to the bed, her husband might typically adopt a 'bear hug'-type approach to help her to stand. As is common in these situations he may not encourage her to move to the edge of the chair. By standing in front of her and grasping her round the waist he reduces Caroline's ability to use normal movement by blocking her potential to lean forward. He becomes the effort force. However, Caroline's centre of gravity (resistance force) is a significant distance from her knees (axis). As a result, he will need to use extra effort to bring her centre of gravity toward the edge of her base of support, thus destabilising her enough to move. Through careful task analysis, the occupational therapist should be able to offer training in alternatives, such as those described below:

- Use chair raisers to raise the height of the chair. Caroline to utilise normal movement as described above to position herself ready to stand. Her husband can then position himself at her side and provide minimal assistance to enable her to lean forward and stand to transfer.
- Reduce the risk of falls through fatigue, by training the couple in the safe use of a transfer board. This enables Caroline to continue using normal movement to transfer from chair/wheelchair into bed in the evenings.
- In terms of assisting a person to move, a distinction is made between 'therapeutic handling' and 'care handling'. The differences are listed in Table 36.1. By Health and Safety Executive (2004b) definition, handling of a person involves the application of human effort using the hands or any other part of the body, either directly or indirectly, to transport, support, move, steady, or position a load. For therapists this includes guiding, facilitating, manipulating or providing resistance (Chartered Society of Physiotherapy 2003). So in fact *all* physical contact with a person, wherever that takes place, will potentially involve manual handling – including work with rehabilitation equipment.

NOTE: When defining an intervention programme, which involves specific methods of moving and handling with the person, the therapist is responsible for carrying out those handling techniques. A therapist must not expect other professionals or untrained staff to carry out treatment handling techniques with a person unless the therapist has specifically trained and assessed the competence of individuals in methods specific to that person (College of Occupational Therapists 2006a, The Chartered Society of Physiotherapy 2008). It is also important to remember that the code of professional conduct empowers the therapist to say 'no' to performing a task if they are not competent to complete it safely, and this also applies to moving and handling tasks (College of Occupational Therapists 2005).

For the most part there is no single 'correct' way of moving a person to achieve a task. Most importantly having a sound knowledge of biomechanics and human movement enables us to assess risk accurately, achieve completion of tasks while promoting maximum ability and facilitating occupational engagement.

Risk assessment

Approximately half the manual-handling injuries reported in healthcare services happen during tasks involving moving and handling people (Health and Safety Executive 2007a). Avoidance of injury through manual handling should be a primary concern for employers and staff alike. Under health and safety legislation, employers must take measures to eliminate manual-handling tasks which put staff at risk of injury. Where this is not possible risks must be assessed and reduced to the lowest level that is reasonably practicable. This must be regularly reviewed. A useful acronym for this is AARR: **A**void **A**ssess **R**educe and **R**eview (Health and Safety Executive 2004b).

People live in a world full of hazards; therefore, every time a person gets out of bed, he takes risks as he is exposed to the hazards around him. It is unreasonable to assume that a person can always eliminate risks and this is particularly true in the work environment. Therefore, risk assessments need to be carried out in order to reduce the potential for accidents and injury, particularly in the case of handling people. When carrying out risk assessments therapists need to strike a balance between

Table 36.1 Types of person handling

Therapeutic handling	Care handling
Takes place within a structured setting or therapy session, usually by a therapist in a department, hospital ward or within a person's home	Takes place in wards, residential settings, a person's home, school or other day facility
Is of short duration and may include active/passive moving, use of equipment, or positioning with a specific goal in mind	Is potentially carried out a number of times throughout a 24-hour period and may include active/passive moving, use of equipment, or positioning of the patient/person
Requires co-operation from the individual	While co-operation is encouraged, care handling of necessity may not involve active participation from the person due to limitations in physical or cognitive ability
Improves or maintains performance	Maintains performance, with or without the use of equipment and may help improve overall mobility and quality of life. Can involve compensatory approaches
Involves highly trained qualified staff	Involves formal/informal carers, family members, school assistants, etc., who have received training from a qualified moving and handling trainer
Involves calculated risks in order to improve performance. Requires professional reasoning and expertise and completion of risk assessment documentation to support this. Needs to take account of required performance in a variety of environments	Involves completion of detailed risk assessments and individual handling profiles for standard handling tasks to assist with essential activities of daily living. Usually occurs where limited change is anticipated in the person's functional ability. Carers and environment may be relatively constant

the potential benefits to the person being moved, against the risk of injury to the handler (The Chartered Society of Physiotherapy 2008, College of Occupational Therapists 2006a).

For the occupational therapist, personal risks will be high where active rehabilitation (therapeutic handling) is taking place. In this situation the therapist will be testing the boundaries of the person's abilities in order to optimise occupational performance. Professional reasoning and expertise will enable the therapist to decide what is reasonable in terms of risk and balance this with the potential benefit to each individual.

In care handling situations the therapist may be making detailed risk assessments of the everyday handling needs of each individual to ensure safest practice for carers. These differing approaches form the basis of the 'care–therapy handling continuum' which is illustrated in Table 36.1.

Risk assessment involves identifying hazards within a given situation and deciding whether these hazards pose a risk of injury to those carrying out associated tasks. Risk assessment should be undertaken where any manual-handling task is considered to present a health risk to those involved (Health and Safety Executive 2004a). Risk assessments may be *generic* or *individual*; however, the process is much the same for both.

Generic risk assessments cover all common tasks carried out within an area, including people and inanimate load handling, and can be divided into themes in order to manage the identified risks (Hignett 2001). For example, in a residential setting, profiling beds may be recommended to replace manually adjustable beds. Increasing a resident's independent movement on the bed reduces the need for manual assistance from staff, for activities such as sitting up in bed. This results in reduced risk of musculoskeletal injury to both staff and residents (Ferguson-Burt 2007) while encouraging residents to be more independent, improving self-esteem and encouraging occupational engagement. As can be seen from this example *generic risk assessments* are important tools for managers and their teams, as they can provide the basis for prioritising funds for additional resources. Box 36.3 summarises the stages of generic risk assessment.

Individual risk assessments are carried out where individuals have specific or complex needs (either therapists or the people who require their services) which fall outside generic protocols. From these, personal handling profiles are developed, providing more specific detail about processes, equipment, numbers and skill base of handlers, and type of assistance required for each given handling task. Personal handling profiles should take into account the individual's wishes and needs (Human Rights Act 1998), their fluctuating ability, plus the physical and psychosocial influences on all those involved in the tasks (Devereux 2003, Pheasant 1991). Before embarking on handling tasks, the therapist should be conversant with guidance on weights, lifting positions, and other manual-handling activities such as pushing and pulling. An example of such guidance is the risk assessment filter described in the Manual Handling Operations Regulations (1992): Guidance on Regulations (Health and Safety Executive 2004b). This will help the therapist decide whether further detailed risk assessment of each identified task is necessary. Box 36.4 summarises the individual risk-assessment process.

A simple and easily applied risk-assessment tool is TILE (Health and Safety Executive 2004b). This ergonomic approach to risk assessment requires analysis of the Task, Individual, Load, and Environment (TILE). These components are described in Table 36.2. The reader is referred to Pearce and Cassar (1999) for a more detailed description of the individual elements of a TILE risk assessment.

In addition to the four factors listed in the TILE tool, other considerations are psychosocial, religious or cultural issues, pressure of work, time constraints, and the time of day that the task is being carried out by either the person or therapist. The human body's circadian rhythms have been shown to be slower in reaction and performance times, particularly between the hours of 2 a.m. and 4 a.m. (Colquhoun 1971, Rodahl et al 1976). Because of these physiological changes, therapists/carers may be at increased risk of injury when carrying out manual handling tasks at these times. The risk assessment process should account for this, and alternative methods or equipment may be required to assist people to move at night, as opposed to those used during the day.

In addition to the above, therapists need to consider potential *triggers* for adverse behaviour, particularly when handling people with complex needs or challenging behaviour. Fear of equipment or experiences of pain from poor handling procedures or use of equipment, may trigger physiological responses, such as muscle spasm or behavioural responses, such as aggression. These all increase the risk of injury to individuals and their handlers. Therefore, the acronym TILE may be changed to TITLE (Task, Individual, Triggers, Load and Environment) for these situations.

Having completed the risk assessment, clear documentation showing action plans and instructions for handling procedures are essential. These must be dated and signed, and must also indicate a timescale for review, or be reviewed whenever there is significant change in a person's or carer's circumstances (Health and Safety Executive 2004b, Pearce & Cassar 1999).

Table 36.2 TILE Assessment Tool (Health and Safety Executive 2004b)

Task	Does it need to be done?
	What does it entail?
	Are there inherent risks to the handler or others from carrying it out?
Individual	This refers to the handler(s)
	Do they have correct/sufficient skills and training?
	Are they in an at-risk group for injury?
	Are they wearing the correct clothing and footwear?
Load	Is this inanimate or a person?
	What is the weight of the load and the distribution of this weight?
	What is the ability/diagnosis of the person?
	Are there factors of unpredictability?
	What clothing is the person wearing?
	What are the effects of present condition; of the medication, etc.?
	Is the person co-operative?
Environment	What are the levels of lighting, ambient temperature and humidity and do these enable safe handling?
	Are there any slip or trip hazards; inanimate or otherwise?
	Is the floor or ground surface safe for moving on?
	This section also includes an assessment of the equipment to be used for moving and handling

It is not always appropriate to use only one risk-assessment tool where there are complex handling situations. A risk-assessment filter is initially required to establish the need for formal risk assessment. The choice of assessment tool will then depend on the activity and the circumstances in which it is being used. Qualitative tools such as Task Individual Load Environment (TILE) (Health and Safety Executive 2004b) and the ARJO Mobility Gallery (ARJO 2005) allow us to create a picture of potential risk related to individuals and activities. Where prioritisation of resources or funding is crucial, more detailed quantitative risk assessments, such as Rapid Entire Body Assessment (REBA) (Hignett & McAtamney 2000) or Manual handling Assessment Charts (MAC) (Health and Safety Executive 2003) may be required to identify the level of risk present for each activity. A range of possible assessments is listed in Box 36.5. When conducting risk assessments, it is important to remember the issue of sustained static postures, such as supporting a load, as referred to in the Health and Safety Executive (2004b) definition of manual handling. In these cases, assessment tools such as Rapid Upper Limb Assessment (RULA) (McAtamney & Corlett 1993) and Ergonomic Workplace Analysis (Ahonen et al 1989) are useful assessment tools.

Additional qualitative and quantitative assessment tools are described in the *Guide to the Handling of People* (Smith 2005).

Box 36.5

Examples of qualitative and quantitative risk assessments

Rapid Entire Body Assessment (REBA) (Hignet & McAtamney 2000)

ARJO Mobility Gallery (ARJO 2005)

Finnish Work Ability Index (Ilmarinen 1998)

Ergonomic Workplace Analysis (Ahonen et al 1989)

Benner Scale (Benner 1984)

Functional Independence Measure (FIM) (Granger et al 1993)

Manual Tasks Risk Assessment Tool (ManTRA) (Straker et al 2004)

Rapid Upper Limb Assessment (RULA) (McAtamney & Corlett 1993)

NIOSH equation for lifting tasks (NIOSH 1981)

Manual Handling Assessment Chart (MAC) (Health and Safety Executive 2003)

Ovako Working Posture System (OWAS 2007).

Practice Scenario 36.4 illustrates the risk assessment process with Caroline.

Focusing the risk assessment

Manual Handling Questions (MHQs) provide a logical, hierarchical, principle-based approach to

Table 36.3 Manual Handling Questions (MHQs) for people handling	
MHQ1	What is normal movement for this task?
MHQ2	Can I teach the person to do this unaided? (Yes [how?] or No [move to Q3])
MHQ3	If not completely unaided, is there equipment available that would mean the person could do this for themselves? (Yes [how] or No [move to Q4])
MHQ4	If unable to perform the task themselves, what is the minimum assistance one and then two people can give: a) without equipment and b) with equipment?
MHQ5	Are there unsafe ways of doing this I must avoid? (If so, what are they?)
MHQ6	Do the tasks need to be delegated to another medical professional or more junior staff? If so, what measures must be put in place?
MHQ7	Do the tasks need to be delegated to non-medical personnel? If so, what measures must be put in place?

assessment and decision-making prior to moving or handling a person. The questions that make up the tool are asked by the therapist (handler) and prompt a sequence of thinking that should result in any intervention regarding the moving or handling of the person being at the level which is most appropriate.

The MHQs were developed as a means of introducing people to moving and handling, and to the complexity of risk assessment and practical handling. No matter what the task or person's ability, the therapist can use the tool as an aide memoire in the process of decision-making, and the tool will always encourage optimum ability and independence where possible, for the individual. The hierarchy of MHQs is illustrated in Table 36.3.

MHQ1: What is normal movement for this task?

This is the primary question – all others are built from this one. Understanding how people move (that is, the way in which people move themselves physically, and the biomechanical principles that apply when they do so), makes it possible to promote optimal, efficient and effective activity. Chapter 6

in the *Guide to the Handling of People* (Smith 2005) is recommended reading here.

MHQ2: Can I teach the person to do this unaided?

Teaching someone to move in a way that will produce predicted movement relies on an understanding of MHQ1 and on good communication skills. The instructions should enable the person to use appropriate sequential movement patterns that result in achievement of the task. Vocal emphasis on dynamic words encourages the person to understand that this will require effort on their part. It is helpful if all the instructions are given first to prepare the person and begin the process of engaging relevant muscle groups and movement pattern recognition. In this way consent and understanding may also be gained. For example, using a movement pattern for a roll to the right in supine lying by an unimpaired adult, the therapist should ensure that the person is in an optimum starting position (in this case lying supine, left knee bent with left foot flat on the surface, left arm across their body, head turned towards the handler who is positioned on their right), and say: 'When I say 'Ready, Steady, Roll' I want you to *reach* with your arm and *push* with your foot and roll towards me. Is that OK?' (the person agrees), 'Ready, Steady, *Roll*'. While this basic system of commands requires cognitive, perceptual and sequencing ability, physical demonstration of the activity, pictures, minimal physical assistance, etc., may also enable the person with cognitive/perceptual deficit to understand what is required for the task.

MHQ3: If not completely unaided, is there equipment available that would mean the person *could* do this for themselves?

Any of the inhibitors affecting movement described in MHQ1 may result in the person being unable to achieve the required move even if the principles of MHQ2 are applied. If so, moving and handling equipment may make up for the deficit. The person is still encouraged to begin in the optimum biomechanical starting position, and instructions are still given as in MHQ2. Where the objective is to encourage improvement it is important to reinforce normal movement patterns even when equipment is used. In some cases, however, moving and handling equipment may enable the person to move independently in a way that is *not* using the same muscle groups in the same way as the person would to move *without* the equipment – for example, when issuing bed levers and some stand-aids. The balance of abilities, independence and normal movement is reached through mutual decision-making between therapist, person and any others involved in their therapy/care.

MHQ4: If unable to perform the task themselves, even with equipment, what is the minimum assistance one and then two people can give: a) without equipment and b) with equipment?

At this stage the therapist needs to assess the person to enable them to achieve the movement task, applying biomechanical principles in a way that minimises risk of injury, promotes safety for all involved and which compensates for any deficit. This may be done in combination with equipment such as stand aids, transfer boards, hoists, etc. The principles of safer handling are used, hazards identified are managed, and risks reduced to the minimum. Again, instructions are given to the person as for MHQ2 and movement patterns encouraged that meet the principles of MHQ1 to promote maximum activity, produce movement in a controlled and efficient way, and minimise effort for the therapist/carers.

MHQ5: Are there unsafe ways of doing this I must avoid? If so, what are they?

MHQ5 is used to prompt the risk-assessment process as it applies to the technique, the individual handler(s), the person and the environment. This will also remind therapists of the biomechanical safer-handling principles compromised in any controversial handling that they may have previously used and now need to avoid (Smith 2005).

MHQ 6 and MHQ7

MHQ6 and MHQ7 are two additional questions that can be used to prompt therapists to follow protocols or pathways for delegating therapy or care handling tasks – to medical and non-medical personnel, for example. These are included when the MHQs arc to be used as part of the therapists' risk-assessment process.

Further information regarding documentation, protocols and pathways can be found in The Chartered Society of Physiotherapy (2008) *Guidance on Manual Handling in Physiotherapy* and the College of Occupational Therapists (2006a) *Manual Handling Guidance 3*.

MHQs in practice

The value of MHQs is that whatever the task is or whoever the personnel involved, the therapist has a reasoned, progressive series of problem-solving questions that should enable them to decide on an appropriate course of action.

The tool should not be used in isolation. An understanding of normal movement patterns, the effect of incapacity on movement, and the use of basic biomechanical principles are required. This has become the foundation of a principle-based, ergonomic approach to moving and handling training.

Practice Scenario 36.4
Detailed risk assessment

Regular assessment of Caroline's performance and needs will be required as her ability will potentially fluctuate, as well as deteriorate. It is not appropriate to introduce equipment too early, as she will want to retain as much independence as possible, for both her and her husband's sake. Interprofessional collaboration will be the key to enabling her to retain her abilities and the occupational therapist will possibly be the co-ordinating professional, ensuring contact with statutory and voluntary bodies to provide support. Task analysis will enable us to identify elements of daily activities in which Caroline may be independent, partially dependent or totally dependent. Maintenance of mobility through analysis of normal movement and application of biomechanical principles to tasks will enable Caroline to focus her energy on activities which are most important to her.

Having established Caroline's priorities for activities and identified those that may present a risk of injury to her or her carers, application of the risk-assessment filter will help the therapist to decide which activities present risks significant enough to apply formal risk assessment. From here the therapist must select the most appropriate tools to use. Box 36.5 lists a number of risk assessments. Generally the TI(T)LE assessment is used initially to establish presence of significant risk; however, in Caroline's case, it may also be useful to use the ARJO Mobility Gallery to establish her general performance at different times and for different activities. Along with this, the Benner scale (Benner 1984) would indicate the skill level required for those assisting her and would direct the therapist to potential training and equipment needs.

At this point it is also important to consider the Manual Handling Questions protocol (Brooks 2008) to identify activities which can be carried out with minimal or no assistance; those which may require Caroline to use compensatory techniques or small equipment or those for which equipment may be necessary to assist with mobility. For example, when Caroline transfers from a chair to bed at night it is important to know how to stand to transfer (MHQ1) and then what instructions carers could give Caroline for her to safely achieve this with minimum effort (MHQ2). If standing becomes unsafe, there is a need to identify how normal movement could be utilised to enable Caroline to use a transfer board (MHQ3). In the longer term, she may be too fatigued to even use a transfer board and then consideration should be given to what equipment the carers may need to use (e.g. hoist) and what physical assistance Caroline may need in order to move her from her chair to the bed (MHQ4). Despite potentially needing to be hoisted, there may be some aspects of the task which Caroline can contribute to, such as leaning forward in the chair and helping to place the sling leg pieces under her legs. She may also be able to roll when on the bed, to assist with removal of the sling. The therapist and carers must utilise normal movement or person-initiated compensatory techniques wherever possible, even when large equipment is required to move the more dependent person.

Following manual handling risk assessments for all activities where assistance is required and where there may be risk of injury to Caroline, her carers or therapists working to maintain her mobility will be in a position to produce a personal handling profile. This should detail how and when Caroline needs assistance with mobility, methods to be used and equipment required. The personal handling profile should give clear indication of how and when equipment is to be used, what the criteria are for this and who is able to use it. It will be important to gain consent from Caroline for both manual assistance and introduction of equipment to aid mobility. Environmental issues such as access, circulation space for equipment, aesthetics, and potential hazards must all be assessed, particularly with regards to any mobility aids used by Caroline. The occupational therapist must consider alternative approaches to be used at different times of the day/night in order to facilitate safest practice for anyone assisting Caroline with mobility. There must also be a clear indication of any specific treatment handling which takes place, when this happens and with whom.

The therapist must be careful to provide or source appropriate training and assessment of competence for all carers, in both techniques and equipment use in order to reduce the risk of musculoskeletal injury. While the Manual Handling Operations Regulations (1992) (as amended, Health and Safety Executive 2004b) serve to protect the formal carers, the Human Rights Act (1998) must be considered, particularly when recommending formal care or equipment. Balanced decision-making (Mandelstam 2005) is important in order to enable Caroline to feel an active participant rather than a passive recipient. This will help to minimise the risk of triggers (Bracher 2007) such as anxiety-induced muscle spasm or emotional rejection of recommendations, which may impact on both Caroline's and her carer's safety. More detailed risk assessments such as REBA (Hignett & McAtamney 2000) may be required for specific tasks, particularly where a case for purchasing equipment or additional resources is presented. Most importantly, the personal handling profile and risk assessment must be regularly reviewed, adapted and signed, to account for changes in Caroline's or her carer's functional ability or needs.

Equipment provision and use

The provision of equipment for moving and handling is often considered to be one of the first options when people experience mobility problems. While equipment may be essential, the therapist should first address mobility problems using detailed task analysis, risk assessment, and manual handling questions. It is important to establish those elements of the task which are problematic and those which the individual can carry out with minimal or no assistance, always encouraging as much active participation as possible.

Having completed a baseline task analysis for an activity, identified normal movement requirements, any physical, cognitive, and sensory limitations for the person, and risks associated with task completion for the person and carers, there is a need to identify equipment which either the person can use for themselves or which can be used by carers to safely move them. Box 36.6 provides examples of equipment which may be used either by the person to assist movement or by carers, where the person is more dependent.

Box 36.6

Examples of equipment used to facilitate independent or assisted movement

- Rope ladders, bed levers, mattress variators and profiling beds facilitate turning or sitting up in bed.
- Bed hand blocks or slide sheets reduce friction between the body and bed, enabling easier movement on the bed while sitting or lying.
- Transfer boards enable safer less effortful movement from one surface to another (e.g. bed to chair; wheelchair to car). Where a person is unsteady in standing a turntable placed under the feet will reduce rotational forces on the knees and hips for those who have weakness or pain in the lower limbs.
- Leg lifters or handling slings enable the person or carers to lift legs into baths, onto beds or wheelchair footplates, reducing the risk of bruising through finger pressure on the legs and limiting the risk of back pain for carers through stooping to reach patients' feet.
- Chair raisers increase the height of chairs, thus reducing the mechanical advantage of gravity against which the person is moving (Chan et al 1999a, 1999b) and making standing easier.

The careful assessment of motor, sensory, and cognitive ability is essential prior to the provision of equipment. The therapist must be confident that the person and carers can follow instructions and understand safety principles when using equipment, and that the equipment and environment are compatible with the target activity. The therapist must also be clear about the rationale and potential risks related to the use of such equipment and that any equipment selected meets safety criteria as set out by the Medical and Health Care Products Regulations Agency (2008).

Standing equipment

For those people unable to achieve independent part or entire movement using small equipment, the therapist may consider a greater degree of manual intervention, including larger handling equipment. Even at this stage, hoists are not the immediate answer for those with limited mobility.

People are often able to stand for short periods, if provided with a biomechanical advantage for sitting to standing. However, maintenance of

standing or walking may be unreliable due to underlying pathology, environmental risks or anxiety as a result of previous falls. Numerous studies have identified risk factors for falling and strategies for dealing with this in older people (Brace et al 2003, College of Occupational Therapists 2006b, McIntyre 1999, Simpson et al 1998). However, many of the underlying principles could be applied to younger people.

Where standing and walking are unreliable, but minimal weight bearing is possible, standing aids may be considered for certain transfers. Thorough assessment of the person's physical and cognitive ability is essential to ensure safety for all, when using this equipment. The therapist must also understand the functions and purpose of the chosen equipment, within the individual's personal context, to prevent misuse and risk of injury, particularly when delegating tasks to carers or other professionals. Standing aids may be manual or electric. Manual stand aids require the individual to pull themselves into standing on a platform, to be transferred from one seated position to another. Electric stand aids pull the individual into a semi-stand or standing position by the use of specifically designed slings.

It is important to remember that stand aids generally do not encourage normal movement patterns during sit-to-stand; therefore, thorough needs analysis is required to direct the use of these, either as an alternative to normal movement or as part of a rehabilitation programme. Some electric stand aids can be used to encourage weight bearing and mobility, having provided the movement for standing. In these cases the footplate is removed and the person is encouraged to take weight through their lower limbs. Use of stand aids in this way requires skilled analysis of the task and person to be moved. Stand aids should never be used inappropriately in the absence of a hoist or as a means of saving time, as opposed to encouraging mobility.

Hoists

Where weight bearing and trunk stability are very limited or absent, it may be necessary to use a hoist for some or all transfers or, for example, to lift people from the floor following a fall. As with other equipment, it is essential to complete a full needs analysis and physical/cognitive assessment of the person to establish the most appropriate type of hoist/slings for the required transfers. Examples of issues to consider when making decisions about use of hoists include:

- Environmental issues, such as circulation and storage space, convenience of access, risk of injury from equipment

- Personal attitude. This may be expressed as fear through loss of control or resentment/anger, particularly where the use of the hoist may emphasise irreversible physical deterioration

- Ability of other carers/health care professionals who may be required to operate the hoist

- Infection control where hoists are being used for a number of different people.

Hignett (1998) suggests that the introduction of hoists for moving and handling does not automatically reduce risk of injury for the therapist/carer. Lack of understanding in the use of a hoist may result in musculoskeletal injuries at sites other than the back. In addition, Conneeley (1998) identifies a range of factors influencing acceptance or rejection of hoists by individuals who have been prescribed them. The introduction of hoists to people and their families, whether in the hospital or home environment, requires a skilled and sensitive approach by the therapist.

While hoists are traditionally perceived as the equipment of choice for transferring more dependent people, there has recently been an increase in their use with specialist walking harnesses to facilitate therapeutic intervention. Skilled use of a hoist with a walking harness enables the therapist to test and improve trunk stability and mobility in standing. In addition, it reduces the risk of musculoskeletal injury for the therapist, who would otherwise be manually supporting the person during standing activities (LIKO UK 2008). Appropriate use of standing harnesses with hoists reinforces the positive philosophy of encouraging as much independence as possible and facilitating occupational engagement, while reducing risk of injury to both the person and therapist.

Competency to use equipment

It is important for therapists to have access to standard moving and handling equipment to be able to deal with mobility issues in both departments and the community. Hignett (2003) identifies examples of equipment considered essential for

hospital environments where people moving and handling takes place. These include hoists (for people unable to weight bear), stand aids, sliding sheets, lateral transfer boards, handling belts, and adjustable-height beds and baths.

Occupational therapists should only provide services and use techniques/equipment for which they are qualified by education, training and/or experience and which are within their professional competence (College of Occupational Therapists 2005). This is particularly true of moving and handling equipment, as professional qualification alone does not automatically imply expertise in this area.

Principles of safer handling

The application of safer handling principles is dependent upon sound departmental or service moving and handling policies. In the United Kingdom these are a legal requirement under Sections 2 and 3 of the Health and Safety at Work Act and Regulation 5 of the Management of Health and Safety at Work Regulations (Health and Safety Executive 1999). Manual handling of people is complex and, therefore, clear guidance appropriate to each service is important. The following are principles of risk assessment identified by the Health and Safety Executive (2004b):

- Manual handling should be *avoided* where there is a risk of injury to those involved.

- If manual handling cannot be avoided, tasks should be *assessed*.

- Action should be taken to *reduce* identified risks.

- All risks should be regularly *reviewed*.

Where there are exceptional or emergency circumstances, safest practice for the therapist is not always possible. An example of an *exceptional situation* may be if an individual exhibits excessive anxiety or aggressive behaviour whenever therapists/carers attempt to use handling equipment. Following risk assessment of the situation, manual handling techniques may need to be used in the immediate term, to reduce anxiety or adverse behaviour, and thus reduce risk of injury to therapists/carers. An *emergency situation* is one that is life threatening to the individual (e.g. cardiac arrest, building collapse, fire/flood, danger from traffic in immediate proximity, etc.). While there should be provision for these situations within the service moving and handling policy, handling procedures may not always reflect the lowest risk to handlers. In these cases, clear documentation of events and actions is required to facilitate improved planning for similar future events. The Reporting of Injuries, Diseases and Dangerous Occurrences Regulations (RIDDOR) (Health and Safety Executive 2008) is particularly appropriate in this situation. This is because it enables, in addition to accidents, the identification of incidents which may have presented a risk of injury, but which may not have resulted in specific injury at that time.

As previously identified, there is no single correct way to move a person/load (Health and Safety Executive 2004b). Each situation will demand a different approach. Therefore, basic principles are important to ensure optimum safety for handlers and the people being moved. Before engaging in a moving and handling task, the therapist should consider the following:

- Understanding biomechanical and normal movement principles will enable the therapist to establish normal movement for the given tasks and analyse internal and external factors that inhibit normal movement for the individual, or, indeed, the therapist.

- Use of the Manual Handling Questions check list (Table 36.3) (Brooks 2008) will help the therapist establish appropriate levels of intervention for either themselves or carers, whilst maintaining as much independence for the individual as possible.

A balanced approach to handling tasks ensuring the rights of the person as well as the safety of handlers encourages co-operation, thus reducing the risk of adverse reactions and the subsequent risk of injury (College of Occupational Therapists 2006a). These issues are illustrated in Practice Scenario 36.5.

Practice Scenario 36.5

Consent, cultural awareness and clear communication are paramount if changes to Caroline's environment/routine are implemented or equipment/ alternative practices are introduced to ensure safer handling. The environment must be safe for carers to work in and they must be sufficiently trained to enable them to apply safe handling principles when working

with Caroline. There needs to be a clear distinction between when therapy handling and care handling approaches are to be used. In addition, given her deteriorating condition, a falls management strategy may need to be considered. Careful introduction and use of equipment will reduce the risk of negative physiological or psychological responses during handling tasks (College of Occupational Therapists 2006c, Lofthouse & Charlesworth 2006). The Manual Handling Questions protocol (Brooks 2008) and risk assessment process should continue to be used throughout.

If after careful consideration of the situation, it is necessary to assist Caroline to move, either manually or with the use of equipment, the principles outlined in Figure 36.11 should be applied to ensure best practice and safety during and after the manoeuvre.

Legislation

The law regarding the moving and handling of people has two main objectives: prevention of injury and compensation for those injured through manual handling activities (Richmond 2005). The Manual Handling Operations Regulations (Health and Safety Executive 1992) within the United Kingdom sits under the umbrella of the Health and Safety at Work Act (1974) which is part of criminal law (College of Occupational Therapists 2006a). The Manual Handling Operations Regulations (Health and Safety Executive 1992) were developed as a result of a European Union (EU) directive in Health and Safety for member states, established in 1990. Interpretations of these regulations have ranged from minimal application to blanket 'no-lift' policies. Extremes of application such as the latter have been subject to scrutiny in the United Kingdom due to their perceived inflexible nature and lack of consideration for the human rights of the individual concerned.

In tackling these issues, particularly in the community, legislation such as The Human Rights Act (1998), The National Health Service and Community Care Act (1990), The Disabled Persons (Services, Consultation and Representation) Act (1986) and the Chronically Sick and Disabled Person's Act (1970) need to be considered in order to make suitable assessment of people's manual handling needs in the home, at work, in education and leisure pursuits. Application of these Acts alongside those

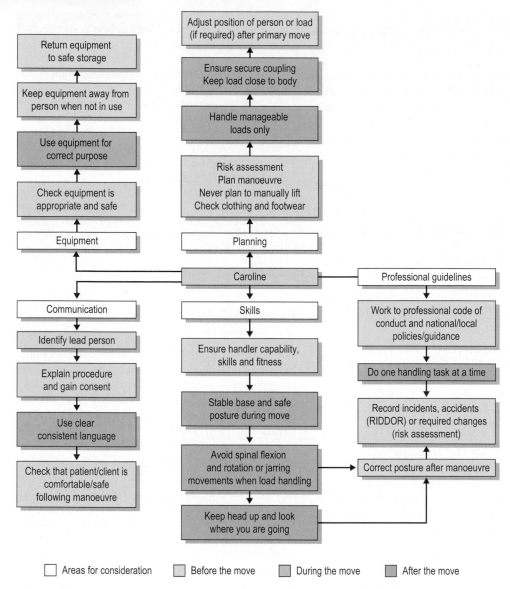

□ Areas for consideration	▨ Before the move	▨ During the move ▨ After the move

Figure 36.11 • Safer handling principles (modified from Health and Safety Executive 2004a)

outlined in Box 36.7 allows for balanced decision-making, when considering the needs of both the people being moved and those carrying out moving and handling tasks with them (Mandelstam 2003). Dimond (1997) suggests it would be very difficult for occupational therapists to eliminate risk of injury from manual handling, without an unacceptable reduction in personal choice. Within civil law therapists have a duty of care to anyone who may be affected by our actions or omissions. Therefore, therapists should aim to reduce risk of injury through

manual handling to the lowest level reasonably practicable (Richmond 2005) while also taking into account the needs and rights of the person.

It is not within the remit of this chapter to provide detailed description/application of all legislation pertaining to manual handling. It is important for the occupational therapist to investigate and understand the context of national, regional and local legislation to protect themselves, carers and individuals under their care, when assessing manual-handling risks and recommending intervention.

Box 36.7

Summary of United Kingdom legislation relevant to moving and handling

Health and Safety at Work Act (HSWA) 1974 (Health and Safety Executive 1974)	The employer is to ensure so far as is reasonably practicable, the health, safety and welfare of all his employees. Employees must also take reasonable care for the health and safety of themselves and others while at work
Manual Handling Operations Regulations (MHOR) 1992 (Health and Safety Executive 2004b)	Employers must ensure that employees: • Avoid hazardous manual handling • Assess that which cannot be avoided • Take action to reduce the risk to the lowest level reasonably practicable • Review risks regularly
Provision and Use of Work Equipment Regulations (PUWER) 1992 (Health and Safety Executive 1998a)	Employers must ensure that all work equipment is suitable for its intended use and is regularly serviced
Workplace Health, Safety and Welfare Regulations (W(HSW)R) 1992	Employers must ensure a suitable environment for employees to work in, including appropriate light, temperature, ventilation, flooring and suitable workstations (which may include treatment plinths etc.)
Lifting Operations and Lifting Equipment Regulations (LOLER) 1998 (Health and Safety Executive 1998b)	Requires employers to ensure that lifting equipment: • Is adequate for the tasks required; • Is positioned/installed safely; • Displays safe working load; • Is in good working order when installed; and • Is examined by a competent person every 6 months
Human Rights Act (HRA) 1998	Most relevant to health and personal injury are: • Article 2 – right to life • Article 3 – prohibition of torture, inhumane or degrading treatment or punishment • Article 8 – right to respect for private and family life
Management of Health and Safety at Work Regulations (MHSWR) 1999 (Health and Safety Executive 1999)	Requires employers to make suitable and sufficient assessment of all risks to the health and safety of employees while at work and provide training where appropriate

Box 36.7 provides an outline and brief explanation of key legislation relevant to manual handling in the United Kingdom. The reader is directed to Chapters 1 and 2 of the *Guide to the Handling of People* (Smith 2005), and to *The College of Occupational Therapists Manual Handling Guidance 3* (College of Occupational Therapists 2006a) for more detailed application of this legislation within the context of general treatment and rehabilitation settings.

The occupational therapist should also understand the importance of reporting injuries sustained at work, in order for safety and risk management to be improved. In the United Kingdom, the *Reporting of Injuries, Diseases and Dangerous Occurrences Regulations* (RIDDOR) (Health and Safety Executive 1995 Reg. 3) requires employers to notify an enforcing authority of any over-three-day injuries/illnesses to employees, caused at or by work.

Therapists need to be aware of their professional boundaries when providing services to people and training or supporting others in moving and handling. This is particularly important in the community, where therapists may be working with staff/carers from a wide range of other services, including agencies, volunteers, and informal carers.

Occupational therapists may often be perceived as the experts in the provision and use of equipment. However, professional status does not necessarily imply expertise in this area, and training and delegation of tasks to others must be carefully considered within the realms of personal skills and knowledge. Where there is doubt about personal levels of experience/expertise in this area, the occupational therapist should not engage in training others or delegation of tasks related to moving and handling/use of equipment. Principles of training, equipment provision and of delegation and guidance to others in moving and handling are discussed in *Manual Handling Guidance 3* (College of Occupational Therapists 2006a) and in the *Code of Ethics and Professional Conduct* (College of Occupational Therapists 2005).

To ensure best practice when dealing with the manual handling needs of people, the occupational therapist should have access to regular training in safe manual handling as required in Regulation 13 of the *Management of Health and Safety at Work Regulations* (Health and Safety Executive 1999). Interprofessional collaboration is essential when dealing with manual handling issues and the occupational therapist should be working closely with other professionals, such as physiotherapists, back care/manual handling advisers, and tissue viability nurses to assess risks to people and staff, and develop realistic and safe handling protocols. Practice Scenario 36.6 illustrates the consideration of legislation in relation to the moving and handling of Caroline.

Practice Scenario 36.6 Consideration of relevant legislation

The therapist will need to balance the wishes and needs of Caroline with the safety of the therapist, Caroline's husband and others involved in her care, taking account of relevant legislation. Central to this is adherence to the Code of Ethics and Professional Conduct (College of Occupational Therapists 2005) in order to ensure the safety and dignity of Caroline and the safety of her carers. In addition, local policies and procedures related to moving and handling and equipment provision must be available and applied in all moving and handling situations. This applies to both general care handling and, more specifically, to treatment handling protocols. Underpinning the

occupational therapists safe practice will be up-to-date training in person handling, either through local service provision or attendance at a nationally recognised course. It is imperative that the therapist has experience and expertise in assessing for and recommending appropriate equipment and handling techniques, if this is to be part of the intervention plan for Caroline. Along with this is the therapist's responsibility to ensure adequate training, assessment of competence and documentation in the safe use of any equipment and specific handling techniques recommended for carers.

Conclusion

This chapter has addressed the issues of moving and handling people ranging from facilitating independent movement in order to maximise occupational engagement, through assisted movement in order to enable completion of essential activities of daily living, to the use of specialist techniques/equipment in order to move the more dependent person. Introduction of the *Manual Handling Operations Regulations* and other guidance from 1992 onward focused assessment on reducing risks to professionals and carers who manually assist people to move. Since then, the introduction of the Human Rights Act (1998) has encouraged more balanced decision-making (Mandelstam 2005) in terms of the rights of both the professional/carer and the people who require their services, and has encouraged a more collaborative approach between professionals and those receiving therapy or care. We have combined the principles of risk assessment, legislation and safe handling with those of normal movement, biomechanics and a Manual Handling Questions Protocol. This provides the therapist with a 'toolbox' of principles with which to analyse moving and handling tasks, and to establish appropriate levels of intervention across the continuum from care handling to treatment/therapeutic handling. We emphasise that there is no one correct way to move or handle a person and that the therapist should be guided by sound principles, to establish safe approaches within the boundaries of professional practice and expertise. Task analysis forms the basis of occupational therapy practice and this should always be applied in the field of people handling to guide decision-making and enable the best outcome for both individuals and therapists/carers.

References

Ahonen, M., Launis, M. & Kuorinka, T. (1989). *Ergonomic workplace analysis*. (p. 33).Transl. by Georgianna Oja. Helsinki, Finland, Ergonomics Section Finnish Institute of Occupational Health.

Aitchison, L. (Ed.). (1999). *Safer handling of people in the community*. Middlesex, BackCare

Anonymous (1965) The nurse's load (editorial). *The Lancet*, ii, 422–423.

ARJO Mobility Gallery. (2005). Available online: http://www.arjo.co.uk/uk/Page.asp?PageNumber= 804. Accessed 16 July 2007.

Benner, P. (1984). *From novice to expert: Excellence and power in clinical nursing practice*. Menlo-Park, Addison-Wesley.

Brace, C.L., Haslam, R.A., Brook–Wavell, K. & Howarth, P.A. (2003). *Being led up the garden path: Why older people are still falling at home. Contemporary ergonomics*. London, Taylor & Francis.

Bork, B., Cook, T., Rosencrance, J., et al. (1996). Work-related musculoskeletal disorders among physical pherapists. *Physical Therapy*, 76(8), 827–835.

Brooks, A. (2008). Manual handling questions: A tool for training, assessment and decision-making in person handling. *The Column* 20.1, 11–13.

Chan, D., Laporte, M. & Sveistrup, H. (1999a) Rising from sitting in elderly people, Part 1: Implications of biomechanics and physiology. *British Journal of Occupational Therapy*, 62(1), 36–42.

Chan, D., Laporte, M. & Sveistrup, H. (1999b) Rising from sitting in elderly people, Part 2: Strategies to facilitate rising. *British Journal of Occupational Therapy*, 62(2), 64–68.

Chartered Society of Physiotherapy (2002). *Guidance in manual handling for chartered physiotherapists*. London, Chartered Society of Physiotherapy.

Chartered Society of Physiotherapy (2008). Guidance in manual handling for physiotherapists. London, Chartered Society of Physiotherapy.

Chronically Sick and Disabled Persons Act (1970). Available online: http://www.opsi.gov.uk/RevisedStatutes/Acts/ukpga/1970/cukpga_19700044_en_1. Accessed 27 March 2008.

College of Occupational Therapists (2005). *Code of Ethics and Professional Conduct for Occupational Therapists*. London, College of Occupational Therapists.

College of Occupational Therapists (2006a). *Manual handling (Guidance 3)*. London, College of Occupational Therapists.

College of Occupational Therapists (2006b) *Falls management (Guidance)*. London, College of Occupational Therapists. Available oline: http://www.cot.org.uk/members/profpractice/guidelines/pdf/FALLS_MANAGEMENT.pdf. Accessed 18 July 2007.

College of Occupational Therapists (2006c). *Risk management college of occupational therapists (Guidance 1)*. London, College of Occupational Therapists. Available online: http://www.cot.org.uk/members/publications/list/patients/standards/pdf/136-Risk_Management.pdf. Accessed 18 July 2007.

Colquhoun, E.H. (1971). Circadian variations in mental efficiency. *Biological rhythms and human performance*. (pp. 39–108). London, Academic Press Inc.

Conneeley, A.L. (1998). The impact of the Manual Handling Operations Regulations 1992 on the use of hoists in the home: The patient's perspective. *The British Journal of Occupational Therapy*, 61(1), 17–21.

Cromie, J.E., Robertson, V.J. & Best, M.O. (2000). Work related musculoskeletal disorders in physical therapists: Prevalence, severity, risks and responses. *Physical Therapy*, 80(4), 336–351.

Devereux, J. (2003) *Work related stress as a risk factor for WRMSDs: Implications for ergonomics interventions. Contemporary ergonomics*. (pp. 59–64). London, Taylor & Francis.

Devereux, J. J. & Buckle, P.W. (2000). Adverse work stress reactions – A review of the potential influence of work related musculoskeletal disorders (WRMDS). *Proceedings of the IEA 2000/HFES 2000 Congress*, 5, 457–460.

Dimond, B.C. (1997). Legal aspects of occupational therapy. Oxford, Blackwell Science.

Disabled Person's Act (1986). *Statutory Instrument 1987 No. 564 (C.13)*. Available online: http://www.opsi.gov.uk/si/si1987/Uksi_19870564_en_1.htm. Accessed 27 March 2008.

Erez, A. B. & Lindgren, K. N. (1999). Psychosocial factors in work related musculoskeletal disorders. In: K. Jacobs (1999). *Ergonomics for therapists*. (2nd ed.). Boston, Butterworth-Heinemann.

European Agency for Safety and Health at Work (2007). *Factsheet 73 – Hazards and risks associated with manual handling of loads in the workplace*. Available online: http://osha.europa.eu/publications/factsheets/73?language=en. Accessed July 20 2007.

Ferguson-Burt, L. (2007). The potential benefits of the introduction of electric profiling beds in preference to manually height-adjustable Kings Fund beds within the NHS: A literature review. *Column*, 19(2), 12–15.

Glover, W., Sullivan, C. & Hague, J. (2005). *Work-related musculoskeletal disorders affecting members of the Chartered Society of Physiotherapy*. London: Chartered Society of Physiotherapy.

Granger, C. V., Hamilton, B. B., Linacre, J. M., Heinemann, A. W. & Wright, B. D. (1993). Performance profiles of the functional independence measure. *American Journal of Physiotherapy Medicine Rehabilitation*, 72, 84–89.

Health and Safety Executive (1974). *Health and Safety at Work Act*. Available online: http://www.healthandsafety.co.uk/haswa.htm. Accessed 20 July 2007.

Health and Safety Executive (1992). *Workplace (Health Safety and Welfare) Regulations. A Short Guide for Managers*. Available online: http://www.hse.gov.uk/

pubns/indg244.pdf. Accessed 20
July 2007.

Health and Safety Executive (1995).
*Statutory Instrument No. 3163.
Reporting of Injuries, Diseases and
Dangerous Occurrences Regulations
(RIDDOR)*. Available online:
http://www.opsi.gov.uk/SI/si1995/
Uksi_19953163_en_1.htm#end.
Accessed 27 July 2007.

Health and Safety Executive (1998a).
*Simple Guide to the Provision and
Use of work Equipment Regulations*.
Available online: http://www.hse.
gov.uk/pubns/indg291.pdf.
Accessed 20 July 2007.

Health and Safety Executive (1998b).
*Simple Guide to the Lifting
Operations and Lifting Equipment
Regulations*. Available online: http://
www.hse.gov.uk/pubns/indg290.
pdf. Accessed 20 July 2007.

Health and Safety Executive (1999).
*Management of health and safety at
work. The Management of Health
and Safety at Work Regulations.
Approved Code of Practice and
Guidance L21* (2nd ed.). London,
Health and Safety Executive.

Health and Safety Executive (2004a).
*Getting to Grips with Manual
Handling: A short guide*. Available
online: http://www.hse.gov.uk/
pubns/indg143.pdf. Accessed 16
July 2007.

Health and Safety Executive (2004b).
*Manual Handling Operations
Regulations 1992 (as amended)
Guidance on Regulations. L23*.
Norwich, HMSO.

Health and Safety Executive (2006).
Five steps to risk assessment.
Available at: http://www.hse.gov.
uk/pubns/ing163.pdf, accessed 24
June 2007.

Health and Safety Executive (2007a).
*Musculoskeletal disorders – Advice
for employers*. Available online:
http://www.hse.gov.uk/
healthservices/msd/employers.htm.
Accessed 20 July 2007.

Health and Safety Executive (2007b).
*What can lead to back pain in the
workplace*. Available online: http://
www.hse.gov.uk/msd/backpain/
wkp.htm. Accessed 14 Aug 2007.

Health and Safety Executive (2008). *A
guide to the reporting of injuries,
diseases and dangerous occurrences
regulations 1995* (3rd ed.).
Norwich, HMSO.

Hignett, S. (1998). Ergonomic
evaluation of electric mobile hoists.
*British Journal of Occupational
Therapy*, 61(11), 509–516.

Hignett, S. (2001). Manual handling
risk assessments in occupational
therapy. *British Journal of
Occupational Therapy*, 64(2),
81–86.

Hignett S. (2003). Systematic review
of patient handling activities
starting in lying, sitting and standing
positions. *Journal of Advanced
Nursing*, 41(6), 545–552.

Hignett, S. & McAtamney, L. (2000).
Rapid entire body assessment.
Applied Ergonomics, 31,
201–205.

Hignett, S., Fray, M., Rossi, M. A.,
Tamminen-Peter, L., Hermann, S.,
Lomi, C., Dockrell, S., Cotrim, T.,
Cantineau J. B. & Johnsson, C.
(2007). Implementation of the
Manual Handling Directive in the
Healthcare Industry in the
European Union for Patient
Handling Tasks. *International
Journal of Industrial Ergonomics*,
37(5), 415–423.

Holder, N., Clark, H., DiBlasio, J.
et al. (1999). Cause, prevalence,
and response to occupational
musculoskeletal injuries reported by
physical therapists and physical
therapist assistants. *Physical
Therapy*, 79(7), 642–652.

Human Rights Act (1998). Available
online: http://www.opsi.gov.uk/
ACTS/acts1998/19980042.htm.
Accessed 221 July 2007.

Ilmarinen, J. (1998). *Work Ability
Index*. Finland, Finnish Institute of
Occupational Health.

LIKO UK (2008). Raising with an
overhead lift. Available online:
www.liko.com/uk. Accessed 30
March 2008.

Lofthouse, A. & Charlesworth, S.
(2006). *Moving and handling in
challenging situations* (unpublished
document).

Mandelstam, M. (2003). Disabled
people, manual handling and human
rights. *British Journal of
Occupational Therapy*, 66(11),
528–530.

Mandelstam, M. (2005). Manual
handling in social care: law, practice
and balanced decision making. In
J. Smith (Ed.). *The Guide to the
Handling of People*. (5th ed.).

Middlesex, BackCare and Royal
College of Nursing.

McAtamney, L. & Corlett, E. N.
(1993). RULA: a survey method
for the investigation of work-related
upper limb disorders. *Applied
Ergonomics*, 24, 91–99.

McIntyre, A. (1999). Elderly fallers: A
baseline audit of admissions to a
day hospital for elderly people.
*British Journal of Occupational
Therapy*, 62(6), 244–248.

Medical and Health Care Products
Regulations Agency (2008).
*Medicine and Medical Devices
Regulations: What you need to
know*. Available online: www.mhra.
gov.uk/Aboutus/index.htm.
Accessed 28 March 2008.

Mierzejewski, M. & Kumar, S.
(1997). Prevalence of low back
pain among physical therapists in
Edmonton. *Canada Disability
and Rehabilitation*, 19(8),
309–317.

Molumphy, M., Unger, B., Jensen, G.
& Lopopolo, R. (1985). Incidence
of work-related low-back pain in
physical therapists. *Physical
Therapy*, 65(4), 482–486.

National Health Service and
Community Care Act (1990).
http://www.opsi.gov.uk/acts/
acts1990/ukpga_19900019_en_1.

Nelson, A. (ed.) (2003). *Patient care
ergonomics resource guide: safe
patient handling and movement*.
Tampa, Ergonomics Technical
Advisory Group, Veterans Health
Administration.

Nelson, A. (2006). Evidence-based
practices for safe patient handling
and movement. *Orthopaedic
Nursing*, 25(6), 366–379.

NIOSH (1981) *Work Practices Guide
for Manual Lifting*. Cincinnati,
National Institute for Occupational
Safety and Health.

Norkin, C. C. & Levangie, P. K.
(2005). *Joint structure and
function: a comprehensive analysis*.
(4th ed.). Philadelphia, PA., FA
Davis Co.

OWAS (WinOWAS) (2007). *A
computerized system for the analysis
of work postures*. Available online:
http://turva1.me.tut.fi/owas/index.
html. Accessed 1 Aug 2007.

Owen, B. & Garg, A. (1990). Assistive
devices for use with patient
handling tasks. In: B. Das (Ed).

Advances in industrial ergonomics and safety. Philadelphia, PA, Taylor & Francis.

Pearce, J. & Cassar, S. (1999). In: L Aitchison (Ed.). *Safer handling of people in the community*. Middlesex, BackCare.

Pheasant, S. (1991). Ergonomics, work and health. London, MacMillan Press.

Pheasant, S. (1996). *Bodyspace: anthropometry, ergonomics and the design of work*. London, Taylor and Francis.

Ramadan, P. A. & Ferreira, M. (2006). Risk factors associated with the reporting of musculoskeletal symptoms in workers at a laboratory of clinical pathology. *Annals of Occupational Hygiene*, 50(3), 297–303.

Rodahl, A., O'Brien, M. & Firth, R. G. R. (1976). Diurnal variation in performance of competitive swimmers. *Journal of Sports Medicine and Physical Fitness*, 16(72), 72–76.

Richmond, H. (2005). Legal and professional responsibilities. In: J. Smith (Ed.). *The guide to the handling of people*. (5th ed.). Middlesex, BackCare and Royal College of Nursing.

Royal College of Nursing (1996). *Working well initiative – introducing a safer handling policy*. London, RCN (revised 2000).

Scholey, M. & Hair, M. (1989). Back pain in physiotherapists involved in back care education. *Ergonomics*, 32(2), 179–190.

Simpson, J. M., Marsh, N. & Harrington, R. (1998). *Guidelines for managing falls among elderly people*. British Journal of Occupational Therapy, 61(4), 165–168.

Smith, D., Leggat, P. A. & Clark, M. (2006). Upper body musculoskeletal disorders among Australian Occupational Therapy students. *British Journal of Occupational Therapy*, 69(8), 365–372.

Smith, J. (Ed.). (2005). *The guide to the handling of people* (5th ed). Middlesex, BackCare and Royal College of Nursing.

Spencer, J., Denton, D. & Smith, J. (2001). A Lateral Transfer Investigation with the person in supine. *The Column*, 13(2), 19–21.

Straker, L., Burgess-Limerick, R., Pollock, C. & Egeskov, R. (2004). A randomized and controlled trial of a participative ergonomics intervention to reduce injuries associated with manual tasks: physical risk and legislative compliance. *Ergonomics*, 47(2), 166–188.

Tyldesley, B., Grieve, J. I. (2002). *Muscles, nerves & movement in human occupation*. (3rd ed.). Oxford, Blackwell Science Ltd.

World Health Organisation (2001). *International Classification of Functioning, Disability and Health (ICF)*. Available online: http://www.who.int/classifications/icf/en/. Accessed 20 May 2007.

Further reading

Bell, F. (1998). *Principles of mechanics and biomechanics*. Cheltenham, Stanley Thornes.

College of Occupational Therapists (2006c). *Risk management college of occupational therapists (Guidance 1)*. London, College of Occupational Therapists. Available online: http://www.cot.org.uk/members/publications/list/patients/standards/pdf/136-Risk_Management.pdf. Accessed 18 July 2007.

Disabled Living Foundation (2006). *Choosing an overhead hoist. DLF Factsheet*. Available online: www.dlf.org.uk.

Essex Back Exchange (2002) *Unsafe handling techniques (Video)*. Essex, Back Exchange.

Green, L. & Williams, K. (1992). Differences in developmental movement patterns used by active versus sedentary middle-aged adults coming from a supine position to erect stance. *Physical Therapy*, 72(8/August), 660–568.

Health and Safety Executive (2003). *Manual Handling Assessment Charts (MAC)*. London, Health and Safety Executive.

Health and Safety Executive (2006). *Public Sector Programme 2006/7; Musculoskeletal Disorders in the Health Services*. Available online: http://www.hse.gov.uk/foi/internalops/sectors/public/7_06_05.pdf. Accessed 21 July 2007.

Hignett, S. (1999). East Midlands ergonomic product evaluation; sliding sheets. *The Column*, 11.1, 20–24.

Hignett, S., Chipchase, S., Tetley, A. & Griffiths, P. (2007). *Risk assessment and process planning for bariatric patient handling pathways*. Available online: http://www.hse.gov.uk/research/rrpdf/rr573.pdf. Accessed 18 July 2007.

Hignett, S., Fray, M., Rossi, M.A., Tamminen-Peter, L., Hermann, S., Lomi, C., Dockrell, S., Cotrim, T., Cantineau, J. B. & Johnsson, C. (2007). Implementation of the manual handling directive in the healthcare industry in the European Union for patient handling tasks. *International Journal of Industrial Ergonomics*, 37(5), 415–423.

Nelson, A. L., Matz, M., Chen, F., Siddharthan, K., Lloyd, J. & Fragala, G. (2006). Development and evaluation of a multifaceted ergonomics program to prevent injuries associated with patient handling tasks. *International Journal of Nursing Studies*, 43(6), 717–733.

Norkin, C. C. & Levangie, P. K. (2005). *Joint structure and function: A comprehensive analysis*. (4th ed.). Philadelphia, PA, FA Davis Co.

Statutory Instrument (1992). *No. 2051 The Management of Health and Safety at Work Regulations*. London, The Stationary Office Ltd. Available online: http://www.opsi.gov.uk/si/si1992/Uksi_19922051_en_1.htm. Accessed 20 July 2007.

Chapter
Thirty-Seven

37

Optimising motor performance following brain impairment

Annie McCluskey, Natasha Lannin and Karl Schurr

CHAPTER CONTENTS

Introduction 580

Essential skills, knowledge and attitudes
for improving motor performance 580

Analysing movement 580

Normal reaching to grasp 580

Postural adjustments in sitting 583

Focus on 'positive' versus 'negative'
impairments 585

Recognising contractures 585

Recognising compensatory strategies . . . 587

Hypothesising about compensatory
strategies 588

Teaching motor skills 589

The stages of motor learning 589

Making training task-specific 590

Maximising practise 590

Giving feedback 591

Evaluating change in motor
performance 591

Evidence-based intervention to improve
upper-limb motor performance 593

Strength training for weak or paralysed
muscles 594

Electrical stimulation 594

Constraint-induced movement therapy . . . 594

Mental practice 595

Reducing muscle force during grasp 595

Dexterity training 598

Preventing and managing contractures . . . 599

Improving reaching and postural control
in sitting 601

Future directions 602

Conclusion 603

SUMMARY

This chapter provides a framework for optimising the motor performance of children and adults with brain impairment. Conditions such as stroke, traumatic brain injury, and cerebral palsy are mainly focused upon; however, the content can be applied to people with other progressive neurological conditions, such as multiple sclerosis. The occupations of eating and drinking are used as examples throughout the chapter. Skills and knowledge required by graduates are identified, including knowledge of motor behaviour, the features of reaching to grasp and postural adjustments required when reaching in sitting. Common movement compensations are explained, followed by secondary musculoskeletal complications such as contracture, which need to be anticipated and managed. Factors which enhance motor learning, skill acquisition and engagement are discussed, with implications for therapists' teaching skills. Finally, a summary is provided of interventions to improve motor performance after brain impairment. The best currently available evidence is provided, from systematic reviews and randomised trials.

KEY POINTS

- Essential knowledge in neurological
  rehabilitation includes an understanding of

normal motor behaviour, muscle biology, and
skill acquisition.
- Abnormal motor performance can be observed
during a task such as reaching for a cup, and
compared with expected performance.
Hypotheses about the cause(s) of observed
movement differences can be made and
tested.
- Paralysis, weakness, and loss of dexterity
negatively affect upper-limb motor
performance and occupational engagement.
These impairments should be the focus of
the therapists' attention rather than spasticity,
which is not correlated with reduced
performance.
- Many people with brain impairment have
difficulty understanding instructions and
feedback, and do not practise well. To help
people learn, each therapist needs to become
an effective coach.
- Motor performance should be remediated
using evidence-based strategies including
task-specific training (as opposed to
generalised, non-specific training).

Introduction

Some people are born with cerebral palsy; others
may sustain a stroke or brain injury later in life.
These types of brain impairment can lead to paralysis and muscle weakness, and disrupt occupational engagement. Motor control is a term
commonly used in rehabilitation (Dickson 2002)
and refers to the complex neural mechanisms
responsible for movements such as reaching-
to-grasp, and sitting-to-standing. Occupational
therapists and physiotherapists retrain motor
impairments which interfere with tasks such as
sitting safely on the toilet or picking up a cup. The
aim in this chapter is to encourage therapists to
systematically observe, analyse and measure motor
impairments and use targeted evidence-based
interventions.

Participation in rehabilitation, and later in community occupations such as eating in a restaurant,
may be restricted by paralysis or contractures. These
impairments need to be actively managed. It is not
enough to teach a person how to compensate using
one-handed techniques, or wait for recovery.
Instead, therapists need to proactively seek muscle
activity and anticipate secondary problems such as
contractures.

Essential skills, knowledge and attitudes for improving motor performance

To improve motor performance, therapists should
think of themselves as 'movement scientists' (Carr
et al 1987, Refshauge et al 2005). Just as occupational science refers to the science of occupation,
movement science refers to the science of
movement.

A movement scientist uses specialist knowledge
from basic science (e.g. neuroplasticity, muscle
biology), applied science (e.g. normal movement or
motor control), education and adult learning (e.g.
coaching strategies, feedback, and practise). This
knowledge is combined with critical appraisal of
systematic reviews and randomised controlled trials
to inform intervention decisions. Valid and reliable
instruments are used to measure motor performance, and determine the effectiveness of those
intervention decisions. Systematic reviews and randomised controlled trials are critically appraised and
implications of those reviews and trials are used to
inform treatment decisions. Movement scientists
use this background knowledge to observe and
analyse movement, plan intervention, and evaluate
the success (or failure) of intervention. The first step
in this process involves analysing movement.

Analysing movement

Movement analysis involves watching a person as
they attempt a task, then comparing the details of
that attempt with 'normal' movement. Therefore,
therapists need to understand the biomechanics of
normal movement, including kinematics and kinetics. The biomechanics of reaching to grasp a cup in
sitting will be described, to illustrate the process of
movement analysis. Reaching to grasp for a cup has
been chosen because drinking is an everyday
occupation.

Normal reaching to grasp

The kinematics and kinetics of reaching to grasp
have been described elsewhere (e.g. Jeannerod
1984, 1986, Martenuik et al 1987, 1990, Wing et al
1986). *Kinematics* refers to the observable features
of a movement (i.e. the angular displacements, the
trajectory that body parts take during movement,

velocity and acceleration). Kinematics are what we see. For example, we see increasing shoulder flexion and thumb abduction when a person reaches for a cup (Figures 37.1A–C). While kinematics can be seen, the *kinetics* (or forces) that cause these displacements cannot be directly observed.

When reaching for a cup, our brain automatically selects the most appropriate hand trajectory (the 'path' our arm will take as it moves through space), decides when to begin forming the appropriate shape and how much grip force to use, based on experience and visual input. In addition, adaptations are made to disturbances and inertial forces on the

cup when it is grasped. Also, selection is made of the appropriate arm trajectory to transport the cup to an end point, and control the release of the cup.

This process of reaching occurs with little or no conscious thought. Final grasp is based on the *intrinsic properties* of the cup, such as the shape, size and perceived fragility (e.g. a plastic cup versus a wine glass) as well as *extrinsic factors*, such as distance from the object, and whether the person is sitting or standing. Hand shape and grasp position are selected early in reach. Normally, we produce a smooth trajectory, control forces at all joints involved, and resist disturbances to our grasp.

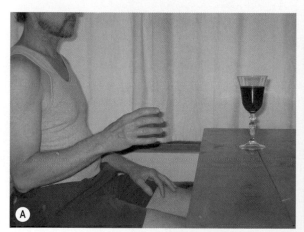
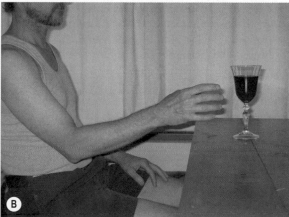

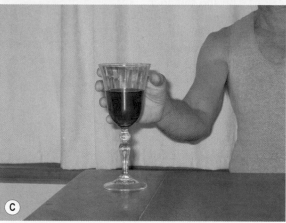

Figure 37.1 • Transport and pre-shaping of the hand during reaching to grasp a glass
These illustrations present the kinematics of reaching (i.e. what we see).
Figures 37.1A and 37.1B show the trajectory of the arm (the transport phase), and pre-shaping of the fingers and thumb. As the hand is transported forwards, the shoulder moves into forward flexion, external rotation (enabling the hand and thumb to reach the glass), elbow flexion then elbow extension.
Figure 37.1C shows wrist extension, and the forearm held midway between pronation and supination. As pre-shaping occurs, the fingers are slightly flexed and rotated (at the metacarpal joints), producing pad-to-pad opposition in preparation for contact with the glass. The thumb is abducted to make a space for the glass, but also rotated at the base of the thumb, allowing pad-to-pad opposition.

The timing and synchronisation of reaching requires careful observation, particularly the timing of the hand's pre-shaping and transport, acceleration and deceleration, and the size of hand aperture, if abnormalities are to be identified. For example, we know that in healthy adults, hand pre-shaping and transport of the arm *do not* begin at exactly the same time (van Vliet 1998). Rather, *our arm* begins to move (particularly shoulder forward flexion and external rotation) slightly *before the thumb, fingers and hand open* to form the grasp shape.

Reaching to grasp in children has also been investigated (e.g. Zoia et al 2006). Even when object size and distance reached vary, 5-year-old children and adults show more similarities than differences in their reach (e.g. grasp formation and timing). The major differences include longer movement duration and deceleration times in 5-year-olds compared to adults, and a larger hand aperture (opening) in children, particularly when visual feedback is missing. Zoia and colleagues propose that younger children may naturally compensate by reaching with a larger 'safety margin' than necessary (hand aperture) while developing reaching skills.

Finally, when adults reach for a cup which is close (i.e. within 60% of arm's length), there is minimal hip flexion and trunk movement (Dean et al 1999a). When reaching for a cup or object further away (i.e. 100% or 140% of arm's length), movement occurs first at the trunk (via hip flexion). Hip and shoulder flexion, and elbow extension all contribute to transport the hand forwards. Trunk displacement via hip flexion, and upper-arm movements are observed earlier when people reach for objects further away. The elbow does not fully extend at the end of reach, except when this is the only way the object can be reached (Figures 37.2A–C).

Therefore, it is normal, and biomechanically more efficient, for people to move their trunk forwards to assist with arm placement during many reaching tasks. Similarly, it is abnormal, and biomechanically inefficient, for people to fully extend their elbow when reaching for a cup which is close to them, unless that is the only way to accomplish the task.

In summary, in people without brain impairment, the hand begins to make an appropriate hand shape and aperture shortly after the upper arm begins to move. During near reaching, the elbow remains flexed, with minimal hip and trunk movement. When reaching for distant objects, the trunk moves first, via hip flexion. These features are characteristic of

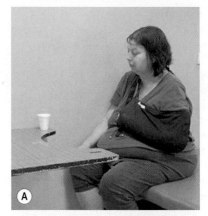

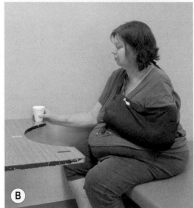

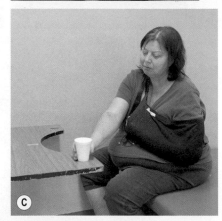

Figure 37.2 • Transporting the hand forward during seated reaching (cup within arms length then at 100% of arms length)

In Figures 37.2A and 37.2B, there is minimal hip flexion and trunk displacement when this lady reaches for a cup which is close and within arms length. Note also that her elbow remains flexed even when grasping the cup.

In Figure 37.2C, the cup has been placed at arms length, and on her affected side. Hip and shoulder flexion, and elbow extension all help this lady to successfully transport her hand forward.

many observed reaching tasks, not just reaching for a cup, and are consequently often called *essential components*.

Postural adjustments in sitting

In the next section, we discuss adjustments required to maintain upright sitting when reaching for a cup, and what to look for when analysing this task. We have intentionally chosen the term 'postural adjustments' to encourage a shift in thinking (and therapy) away from muscles of the trunk, to muscles of the lower limb. It is the leg, not the trunk, muscles that prevent falling when a person reaches forward or to the side. In this section, we also discuss environmental factors such as *base of support, reaching distance* and *direction*. Each of these factors can be manipulated during analysis, to make seated reaching easier or more challenging.

When reaching for a cup in sitting, we anticipate the effect that gravity will have on our body prior to moving. We intuitively know, and can anticipate, what will happen when we reach forwards, sideways or towards the floor because of the effect of gravity. Consequently, we adjust our bodies to maintain balance and avoid falling. These adjustments are required during dressing and toileting. Our base of support, the direction and speed of reaching all influence reaching in sitting (Dean et al 1999a, 1999b).

Our *base of support* comes from our feet and thighs when we sit with both feet on the floor. When reaching forwards beyond this base of support, the leg muscles are critical for maintaining upright sitting (Chari & Kirby 1986, Dean et al 1999a, 1999b). For example, when reaching for a cup at 140% of arm's length, tibialis anterior contracts prior to anterior deltoid in the arm. Soleus and biceps femoris muscles contract soon after, to control the forward movement of our body mass (Dean et al 1999a, Crosbie et al 1995) (Figures 37.3A–F).

If thigh support is reduced when reaching forwards, the contribution of the leg muscles increases to compensate (Dean et al 1999b). If both feet are off the floor (e.g. when sitting on a high bed or plinth), our base of support is reduced considerably. We can no longer push with our feet. We cannot make postural adjustments using the large muscles which cross our knees and reach our feet. Instead, we have to rely on muscles around the hip to keep

us from falling. Reaching distance is significantly reduced when both feet are off the ground, and becomes difficult even for healthy adults.

Reaching direction also influences leg muscle activity. Reaching for a cup on the right side of the body results in increased right leg extensor activity (Chari & Kirby 1986, Dean et al 1999b). Reaching in front, or to the opposite side, results in increasing leg extensor activity on the side opposite to the reaching arm (Dean et al 1999b). Absence of one leg (e.g. following amputation) also reduces the distance that can be reached to that side (Chari & Kirby 1986).

This research on normal reaching in sitting can be applied when training people who have difficulty staying upright while reaching. For example, if a person is unable to generate sufficient leg extensor force to prevent him/herself from falling forward while reaching, they will need to learn to activate their leg extensor muscles in order to be successful at this task. Reaching forward will be easiest when there is maximal thigh support, both feet are on the floor and the chair/bed height is low. A person's practise will be more successful if they are asked to reach to a target within arm's reach, so they can control their trunk movement before reaching further forward (i.e. beyond arms reach).

Less muscle activity is required from the affected leg extensors if a person reaches to the unaffected side. Therefore, it is likely to be easier for a person to practise reaching for a cup on their unaffected side first. Task difficulty can be progressed by reaching further forward, reaching first to the unaffected side, then to the front, then to the affected side. As the person becomes more successful, the amount of thigh support can be reduced and the seat height increased to increase the force required from the legs.

Feedback during training also helps to increase learning. If a person is unable to push effectively on their affected leg, they may need specific feedback about whether their leg muscles are working. Bathroom scales can be used to give feedback about the force being generated through the affected leg (e.g. weight in kilograms). Bathroom scales can also provide information about timing. For example, are the leg muscles pushing at the appropriate time (i.e. anticipating the transfer of weight forward) to prevent the person falling? Systematic and persistent practise of reaching in this way has been shown to improve reaching ability and the ability to

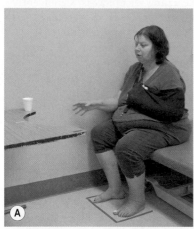

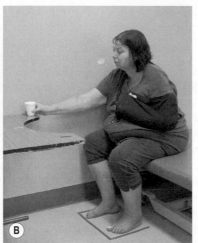

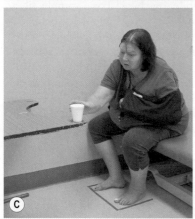

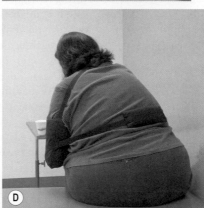

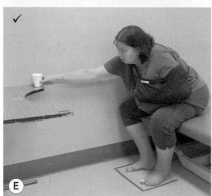

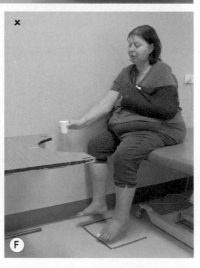

Figure 37.3 • Postural adjustments required to stay upright in sitting, when reaching for a cup at distances greater than arms length

This lady has been asked to reach for, and pick up a cup on her unaffected side, beyond arms length. Her thighs and feet form her base of support. She looks at the object, begins to pre-shape her hand, anticipates the effect that gravity will have on her base of support as she lifts her arm, then transports her arm forwards. To avoid falling forwards when lifting her arm, she pushes with her feet (Figures 37.3A and 37.3B).

In Figure 37.3C, this lady is reaching for a cup placed beyond arms length, and on her affected side. This task is difficult for her, requiring greater leg extensor activity from her left leg. If she does not push through her left leg and foot, she will fall forwards and to her left.

Figure 37.3D illustrates her weight shift forwards and to her left side. Figure 37.3E shows a training session which involves practice of seated reaching. This lady is practicing reaching for a cup placed beyond arms length and to her unaffected side. When her skill and motor control improve, she will practice placing the cup across to the left side of the table. Her feet are on the floor and her thighs well supported. Electrical tape marks correct foot position.

In Figure 37.3F, the seat height has been raised, and this lady's feet are now off the floor. She cannot push with her feet. Consequently, she is unable to reach as far forward as when her feet are one the floor. To optimise successful reaching, the base of support available to a person needs to be considered and planned.

stand-up in people who have had a stroke in both acute (Dean et al 2007) and chronic settings (Dean & Shepherd 1997).

Before concluding this section, we want to argue strongly against the practice of 'facilitating' movement. Training postural adjustments and sitting balance by pushing a person in one direction (external perturbations by the therapist) will result in very different muscle activation patterns compared to self-generated movement (Forssberg & Hirschfield 1994). The person cannot anticipate what direction or force of perturbation will be used by the therapist, nor when these disturbances will occur. Training postural adjustments by pushing a person from side to side in sitting is unlikely to help them activate appropriate muscles necessary for self-generated movement (for example, when cleaning themself on the toilet). Such 'training' strategies may cause the person to become rigid and fearful of moving during therapy, and should be avoided. The anticipatory muscle activity that occurs during reaching while seating, and the possible intervention implications and strategies, are presented in Table 37.1.

Training strategies should aim to mimic the normal sequence of muscle activity specific to the task for which the person is being trained (see Table 37.1 for some examples). If a person is unable to sit, the therapist will need to accurately analyse the reasons why they cannot sit, then develop training strategies which are specific to those difficulties.

In summary, seated reach can be progressed by gradually increasing the distance, and changing the direction of reach (i.e. to the affected side, then forwards, then to the contralateral or unaffected side), decreasing the amount of thigh support and increasing seat height. However, 'tapping' or pushing a person off balance as part of training is unhelpful and may interfere with their recovery. By systematically increasing the demands of a reaching task as suggested previously, people with neurological conditions can learn to engage more successfully in occupations such as dressing and bathing.

Focus on 'positive' versus 'negative' impairments

Neurological conditions, such as stroke and cerebral palsy, lead to impairments which can be classified as either 'positive' or 'negative' (Ada et al 2000, Burke 1988, O'Dwyer et al 1996). 'Positive'

impairments include abnormal postures, exaggerated proprioceptive reflexes producing spasticity, and exaggerated cutaneous reflexes of the limbs producing flexion withdrawal spasms. 'Negative' impairments include paralysis, weakness, loss of coordination and loss of dexterity. In practice, it is the 'negative' impairments or characteristics, such as paralysis, that most concern people with stroke and other conditions, not spasticity and abnormal reflexes.

Therapy textbooks (and many experienced practitioners), focus on the management of spasticity (a 'negative' impairment), but provide less guidance to students and new graduates on strength or dexterity training. However, research indicates that reducing spasticity does not automatically improve performance (McLellan 1977, Neilson & McCaughey 1982). There appears to be little correlation between spasticity and function (Ada et al 2006b, O'Dwyer et al 1996, Sommerfield et al 2003). Thus, while acknowledging the presence of spasticity, we question its emphasis. In this chapter, we provide examples of strategies which focus on strength and dexterity ('positive' impairments), which therapists are more likely to be able to influence.

Here is a final note about analysing and labelling motor impairments. Therapists often use the term 'spasticity' or 'high tone' to refer to stiff or tight muscles in the hand or arm, or to stiff joints. The cause of such stiffness or tightness needs to be determined so that intervention can be planned (Boyd & Ada 2001). Often what therapists describe as spasticity or high tone is a shortening of muscles or contracture. Therapists need to be able to recognise and diagnose a contracture, because muscle contractures, unlike spasticity, may be amenable to therapy.

Recognising contractures

A contracture can be recognised by loss of joint range and increased resistance to passive movement at a joint (Ada & Canning 2005). Resistance to movement is typically due to peripheral changes in muscle fibres and connective tissue (O'Dwyer et al 1996, Pandyan et al 2003), not to central nervous system changes or spasticity. Animal studies show that muscles shorten and lengthen in response to immobilisation. Animal muscles increase in length when immobilised in a lengthened position, and decrease in length when immobilised in a shortened

Table 37.1 Summary of seated reaching without back support, feet on or off the floor

Reaching forward in sitting without back support, feet on the floor	Anticipatory muscle activity		Implications for intervention	Possible training strategies
	Leg/trunk	Arm		
Within arm's length	Back extensors Hip extensors	**Transport** Shoulder forward flexion and external rotation **Pre-shaping** Wrist and finger extension, radial deviation, thumb abduction and opposition	• Begin to train reaching within arm's length if person is unable to activate hip extensors • Sit with back supported to minimise initial task difficulty • Provide trunk support if unable to sit without assistance	Practice set-up • Sitting with back support: practise moving forward from (hip flexors) and back to (hip extensors) the back support • Sit next to wall on the non-affected side for a vertical cue
Greater than arm's length	Hip extensors Knee extensors Plantarflexors		• Practise sitting on a stable surface • Specific training of hip and knee extensor strength and endurance on affected side • Maximise thigh support • Practise with feet supported before training with feet unsupported	Feedback: • Provide vertical cue for sitting alignment (i.e. if the person is falling towards their left, position them with a wall at their right side to provide a close vertical cue and feedback when they begin to fall) • Provide visual cue (e.g. line on wall for appropriate shoulder position) • Place bathroom scales under affected foot for feedback about weight bearing • Sitting on lower surface to decrease extensor force required
Ipsilaterally (i.e. to the unaffected or intact side)	Ipsilateral (unaffected) hip, knee and ankle extensors		• Train reaching to ipsilateral side if person is unable to reach to contralateral side • Gradually increase distance the person is attempting to reach ipsilaterally • Gradually introduce reaching across the midline towards contralateral side	
Contralaterally (i.e. to affected side)	Contralateral hip, knee and ankle extensors		• Ensure appropriate alignment of weight-bearing leg (i.e. knee over foot, leg not abducted) • Ensure person begins to use leg extensors in anticipation of weight transference to affected side	Progress difficulty by: ○ increasing time ○ increasing distance from wall ○ decreasing thigh support ○ increasing height of surface ○ increasing distance reached ○ increasing contralateral distance

Table 37.1 Summary of seated reaching without back support, feet on or off the floor—cont'd

Reaching forward in sitting, without back support, feet off the floor	Anticipatory muscle activity	Implications for intervention	Possible training strategies
Within arm's length	Back extensors Hip extensors	• Provide back support if the primary purpose is to train reaching.	Feedback: • Provide vertical cue for sitting alignment (i.e. if the person is falling towards their left side position them with a wall at their right side to give them feedback when they begin to fall)
Greater than arm's length	Hip extensors Back extensors	• Specific training of hip extensors if unable to elicit hip extensor activity • Maximise thigh support • Gradually and systematically increase the distance reached • Practise with feet supported before training with feet unsupported	• Bathroom scales under the affected thigh for weight-bearing feedback Progress difficulty by: ○ increasing distance from wall ○ decreasing thigh support
Ipsilaterally	Ipsilateral hip extensors	• As above concentrate on ipsilateral hip extensors	○ increasing distance reached ○ increasing contralateral distance
Contralaterally	Contralateral hip extensors	• Concentrate training on contralateral hip extensors	

position, for example, in a plaster cast, by adding or losing sarcomeres, respectively (Tabary et al 1972, Williams & Goldspink 1978). A sarcomere is the contractile part of a myofibril, within skeletal muscle (Gossman et al 1982). When immobilised in a short-ened position, muscles generate tension at a new, shorter resting length (Herbert & Balnave 1993).

These structural changes lead to disorganisation of connective tissue within a muscle (Goldspink & Williams 1990), disrupting the synovial fluid, joint membrane and articular cartilage (Trudel et al 2003). Changes in the mechanical-elastic properties of muscles and connective tissue limit joint range of movement after stroke (Vattanaslip et al 2000), and probably also after other neurological conditions. This joint stiffness leads to resistance. Therapists often (inappropriately) call this resistance to move-ment 'high tone' or 'spasticity'.

While it remains unknown how long contractures take to develop after brain impairment, there is no doubt that they do develop. Contractures are unde-sirable for many reasons, including their effect on occupational performance. For example, a person with contractures of the wrist and finger flexor muscles will be unable to extend their wrist to achieve normal grasp and release. Nor will they be

able to open their hand wide enough to pick up a cup. Such contractures will need to be reversed using strategies such as positioning, passive stretch-ing and plaster casting. There is, however, still uncertainty about the effectiveness of these inter-ventions, and how long stretches or positioning need to be maintained per day to adequately reverse contracture. Nonetheless, it is unlikely that short-duration stretch methods such as passive ranging of joints, will change tissue structure. Therefore, methods for applying long-duration stretch are required, and are discussed later in this chapter.

Recognising compensatory strategies

When analysing motor and occupational perfor-mance, therapists need to be able to recognise com-pensations. Compensatory strategies are movement solutions that allow a person to compensate for loss of normal muscle activity (Carr & Shepherd 1989). Compensations may be caused by a muscle contrac-ture, muscle weakness or both. For example, a person who cannot successfully reach forward to grasp a cup may use hip flexion and/or shoulder abduction to compensate for poor shoulder flexion. In previous years, these patterns of muscle contraction were called 'abnormal synergies', and believed to be a normal stage of recovery after stroke or brain injury. However, there is no neurophysiological explanation for these synergies. Rather, this combination of muscle activity appears to be more biomechanically advantageous to the person who cannot activate weak or paralysed muscles (Carr & Shepherd 1989).

The problem with compensations is that they become learned. The more a person practises using these inappropriate movement solutions, the more difficult it becomes to change behaviour. In the long term, compensatory strategies are inefficient and inflexible. Therefore, therapists need to help people to contract their muscles more appropriately when reaching. When observing a person reach to grasp a cup, we also need to compare what we see (kinematics) with our knowledge of normal movement.

For example, when pre-shaping to reach for a cup within arm's reach, we need to determine if a person is opening their hand and abducting their thumb at the beginning of reaching. Thumb abduction and metacarpo-phalangeal extension of the fingers are essential, and result in a web space large enough to accommodate the cup. Typically, people who have difficulty abducting their thumb, and/or extending their fingers and wrist will compensate by *extending* their thumb, *pronating* their forearm and/or *abducting* their shoulder (Carr & Shepherd 1987, 2003) (Figures 37.4A–B). These strategies may lead to successful contact with a cup, but are inefficient and compensatory.

When a person transports their arm towards a cup which is nearby (i.e. within arm's reach), we watch to see if they are using their shoulder flexors and external rotators, without using excessive shoulder elevation, internal rotation or abduction. The latter three compensatory movements may suggest weakness or paralysis of the person's shoulder flexors and/or external rotators. Alternatively, these shoulder movements may be helping to compensate for poor control of forearm, wrist, thumb or finger muscles. For a full discussion and analysis, see Carr and Shepherd (1987).

When reaching in sitting, it is normal to flex at the hips to reach distances at arm's length or greater (Dean et al 1999a). However, it is not normal to use hip flexion when reaching for an object such as a cup which is very close to the body. In that case, hip

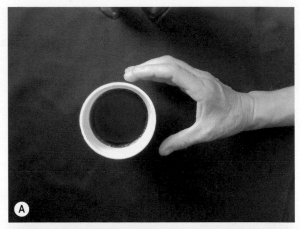

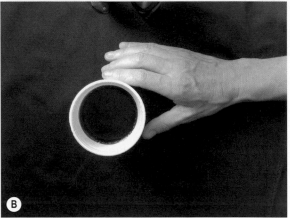

Figure 37.4 • Normal pre-shaping while reaching for a cup and commonly observed compensations
Figure 37.4A illustrates normal pre-shaping during reaching, with the thumb abducted and opposed, and the person's wrist extended ready to grasp the cup.
However, in Figure 37.4B the person is compensating during reaching for poor control of thumb abduction (a missing essential component). Instead, they are extending their thumb and pronating their forearm (both are compensations) to try to grasp the cup.

flexion and trunk movement may be compensations for weak shoulder flexors.

Hypothesising about compensatory strategies

The final step in the process of analysing movement is developing then testing the movement hypotheses. Developing a hypothesis (or hypotheses) about a person's movement compensations will help us to plan treatment. One hypothesis might be that a person's shoulder muscles are paralysed or too weak to lift the limb up against gravity, to reach for a cup. This hypothesis can be tested by assessing muscle strength (i.e. palpating the muscle belly during a movement attempt). If a person cannot easily reach forwards, two key muscles to check are anterior deltoid (a shoulder flexor) and infraspinatus (an external rotator). If these muscles are weak, strengthening exercises will be required. In the absence of a muscle contraction, we might use electrical stimulation (Ada & Foongchomcheay 2002, Pomeroy et al 2006) and/or mental practise to elicit muscle contractions (see Bell & Murray 2005, Braun et al 2006).

A second hypothesis might be that muscles such as the internal rotators, elbow, wrist and finger flexors are short and/or stiff due to contractures. The opposing muscles may be incapable of generating the necessary force to lift the arm, extend the wrist or open the hand. This hypothesis can be tested by manually checking the available range of external rotation; forward flexion; elbow, wrist and finger extension; and thumb abduction. Loss of range at any one of these joints will change the person's ability to reach for an object such as a cup.

A third possible hypothesis might be that the person is using excessive muscle force to achieve the task (i.e. to pick up the cup). They may be using too many muscles, too much force, or both. A group of muscles such as the finger and wrist flexors may be overactive and contract with excessive force when movement is attempted. Overactivity may occur (e.g. all the muscles of the arm switch on with effort) to help compensate for weakness in other muscle groups, such as the shoulder flexors. We can test our hypothesis by setting up the practice task to minimise effort. For example, the person could practise reaching with their arm supported on a table, and a sheet of paper or cloth under their hand to reduce friction.

A fourth hypothesis might be that the task and/or environmental set-up are too challenging. The cup may be positioned too far in front or to the side for the person to grasp without compensating. Or the table may be too high. We can test these hypotheses by placing the cup closer or lowering the table. Another example is changing the person's position, allowing muscles to contract more easily (e.g. moving the person from a sitting to lying position). This change will lessen the effect of gravity on their weak shoulder flexors, and decrease the amount of

muscle force required. Taping a light polystyrene cup into their hand will also decrease task demands and eliminate the need to pre-shape the hand. The person can then concentrate on transporting the cup rather than worrying about pre-shaping. Each movement hypothesis can be tested in turn.

Assuming we have correctly analysed the person's movement problems, identified the missing essential components and compensations, and tested our hypotheses, the next step is to design a programme to improve motor performance.

Teaching motor skills

People with brain impairment often have difficulty understanding instructions, using feedback, remembering their practice and learning motor skills. Therefore, therapists need to develop critical teaching skills and become effective coaches. We need to understand how motor learning progresses, provide training that is task-specific, ensure learners practise well and often, and provide useful, timely feedback. Each of these factors will influence learning.

The stages of motor learning

There is considerable literature on motor learning. The Fitts and Posner model of motor learning (1967) is most often used to inform rehabilitation practice. The three stages described by Fitts and Posner are: (1) the verbal-cognitive stage; (2) the motor stage; and (3) the autonomous stage. In the first stage, learners rely on verbal feedback and external environmental information to achieve goals and understand the demands of a task (Haggard 2001, Prinz 1997). In the second stage, the focus is on the quality of movement, mass practice (Mastos et al 2007) and decreasing mistakes (McNevin et al 2000). Finally, in the third stage the learner is able to perform the task with less cognitive effort, cope more effectively with distractions and draw on their problem-solving skills when performing the task in novel situations (Mastos et al 2007, McNevin et al 2000). At each stage, learners need timely feedback about performance and goal achievement, and increasing amounts of practise (Lee & White 1990, McNevin et al 2000, Shea et al 2000).

Using our previous training example of reaching for a cup in sitting, a goal might be for the person to sit upright for 30 seconds without falling to the affected side. In the first stage of learning, they may require continual feedback about pushing with their affected leg, to avoid falling to their affected side. In the second stage, they may recognise when they are beginning to fall, make an attempt to prevent this but require occasional assistance or prompting. In the third stage, they can sit without assistance, conduct a concurrent conversation and reach forward to pick up a cup of water with their non-affected hand without falling to the affected side. If practise tasks are too demanding in the early stages of learning, the person may be unable to achieve the goal. For example, asking the person to reach to their contralateral (affected) side before they can sit upright for 5 seconds would be unrealistic.

Making training task-specific

The terms 'task-specific training', 'task-related practise' and 'specificity of training' are used in the literature (e.g. Blennerhassett & Dite 2004, Dean & Shepherd 1997, Michaelsen et al 2006, van der Lee et al 2001). These terms refer to therapy involving intentional practise of a specific movement, action or task, versus repetition of non-specific tasks (Bayona et al 2005) such as lifting your arm up high for no reason, touching your head or nose (in response to an instruction by a professional) or stacking cones instead of practising reaching for a cup. Examples of task-specific training include practise of pen or cutlery manipulation to improve writing and eating respectively, or picking up and transporting a cup to improve the occupation of drinking. In the early stages of motor recovery, when a person cannot hold objects, implements can be taped into the affected hand (e.g. a fork or cup), or placed in front to encourage reaching.

Research shows that we learn (or relearn) motor skills through engagement in tasks and activities. For example, when people practised reaching to pick up a pen and write their name, compared to *pretending* or imagining themselves picking up a pen to write, the quality of reach and grasp improved significantly (Wu et al 1994). Although that writing study involved healthy adults, the implication is that people need to practise real-life tasks, not simulate them. Studies involving adults with brain injury also demonstrate the importance of using real-life tasks for motor training (Neistadt 1994, Sietsema et al 1993). For instance, people with a brain injury produced a greater range of movement when reaching

out to control a computer game (Sietsema et al 1993), and demonstrated improved dexterity when engaging in kitchen activities versus table-top therapy activities (Neistadt 1994).

The bottom line is that people learn what they practise. If a person wants to learn to drink from a cup, they should practise reaching for and transporting a cup, not a plastic shape or cone that vaguely resembles a cup. Early training might involve sliding or placing a lightweight plastic cup forwards on a low table, with the cup taped into the person's hand if they have no active hand movement. Advanced dexterity training might involve moving and manipulating objects of interest, such as garments, eyeglasses, cutlery and writing implements, not beans or plastic counters. Training should replicate the skill or task that a person wants to learn. Valuable time should not be wasted on non-specific practise.

Maximising practise

More time spent practising leads to improved performance across many skill areas including chess (Charness 1981), typing (Ericsson 2004), sports performance (Helsen-Starkes & Hodges 1998) and playing musical instruments (Ericsson 2004, Lehmann & Ericsson 1996). In a study involving 20-year-old violinists (Ericsson 2004), the best performers, as judged by conservatory teachers averaged 10,000 hours of practise during their lives. The second-best performers averaged 7,500 hours, the next-best, 5,000 hours and so forth.

A similar commitment to practise is required by learners with acquired brain impairment and their therapists, if motor performance is to improve. In a randomised controlled trial evaluating the effect of seated reaching (Dean & Shepherd 1997), people with stroke each performed 2,970 reaches beyond arm's length during a 2-week training period. Participants in the intervention group could reach further and faster than the control group after task-specific training, and improved their ability to stand-up.

Repetition of practise tasks is also integral to learning. Multiple repetitions of a movement can significantly improve upper limb strength in people following stroke. In one study, people with stroke practised repetitive finger flexion and extension against resistance, twice daily for 15-minute periods (Butefisch et al 1995). This task-specific practise led to greater grip strength, improved contraction velocities and peak acceleration in the extensor muscles, compared to a control group receiving standard Bobath therapy. Another study by Feys and colleagues (1998, 2004) included adults with minimal arm function after stroke, who were required to protract and retract their affected shoulder while seated in a rocking chair, for 30 minutes daily over 6 weeks. This practise was intended to help improve forward reaching. The treatment had greatest effect in people with more severe motor deficits. Improvements in upper-limb motor function were retained at 5 years' follow-up.

Mass practise and multiple repetitions are also features of constraint-induced movement therapy (CIMT; see Morris et al 1997 for a summary). CIMT involves restraining the unimpaired arm and hand to encourage intensive practise of tasks using the affected arm. Although CIMT studies require participants to practise for up to 6 hours a day, the amount of practise required to improve function remains unknown. However, we do know that a minimum dose of 16 hours additional practise is needed to improve motor outcome following stroke, according to a recent systematic review (Kwakkel 2006).

Finally, practice which involves lots of repetitions but no transfer of learning may limit skill development. For example, using a fork with a built-up handle to repeatedly pick up pieces of soft bread will not enable a person to eat a meal successfully in a restaurant with a normal fork. Motor learning theory suggests that people improve their performance by practising in a variety of situations, and experiencing errors during learning. In order to move beyond the first two stages of motor learning, people need to practise in different settings, with different movement parameters (for example, forks with different handles, and different foods). Increasing demands in this way helps learners to problem solve and fathom the rules underlying task performance (Schmidt & Lee 1999).

Giving feedback

Accurate feedback is critical to the teaching and learning of motor skills. Feedback can be provided by the task itself (intrinsic feedback), or by an outside source such as the therapist, biofeedback device or timer (extrinsic feedback). Extrinsic feedback has been further classified into two types:

knowledge of performance and knowledge of results (Kilduski & Rice 2003).

Knowledge of performance refers to information about the movement process or attempt, for example 'Your wrist was flexed' or 'You kept your elbow close to your body'. *Knowledge of results* refers to information about the movement outcome, for example 'You picked up the cup'. Knowledge of results is usually obvious to the person performing the task; they either achieved the desired outcome or they did not. The bigger problem is how to change the next attempt. This is where the therapist as coach can provide knowledge about performance, and suggest ways to make the next attempt more successful.

Extrinsic feedback can be very helpful to learners, particularly corrections that need to be made, and features to focus on during subsequent attempts (Kernodle & Carlton 1992). The timing of feedback is important, relative to performance. Concurrent knowledge of results – that is, feedback provided during performance – appears to impede motor learning (Annett 1959). Talking during performance may be distracting (although motivational comments such as 'Keep going' or 'That's right' can be helpful). However, feedback given after task completion has a positive influence on motor learning (Adams 1971, Bilodeau 1966, Newell 1976). The amount and frequency of extrinsic feedback also affects performance. Intermittent feedback is more effective than constant feedback (Ho & Shea 1978, Winstein & Schmidt 1990), whereas too much feedback may negatively influence learning (van Vliet & Wulf 2006). People appear to benefit from watching others demonstrate a task, and then receive feedback about their movement outcome (Reo & Mercer 2004). This form of modelling seems to be most effective when presented at intervals during skill acquisition, before practise commences, and at various intervals thereafter.

Evaluating change in motor performance

Therapists need to re-evaluate motor (and occupational) performance at regular intervals. Objective measures need to be taken before and during training. Ideally, a review of performance and goals will occur at every session. Performance can be measured using complex or simple equipment. For example, to determine if a person with sitting balance problems is weight-bearing equally through both legs, a therapist may use bathroom scales. Other simple measures of performance include the number of movement repetitions per session, the number of correctly performed movements versus those performed with compensations, and distance reached.

If performance is not changing, the problem may lie with the therapist rather than the person with brain impairment. Common reasons for lack of improvement include unclear instructions, feedback and goals. If instructions are unclear, off-target, or too detailed, the person with stroke or brain injury may not understand the expected goal. Similarly, if verbal feedback is unclear (or even absent), the person may not understand how to alter their next movement attempt to achieve success.

In addition to carefully considering the words we use to explain and correct movement attempts, the task chosen to elicit a movement attempt is also important. If the task is too difficult (or too easy) progress may not be seen. If our initial movement hypothesis was wrong, we miss the main cause of a movement problem, and change in performance may not be seen. When re-measurement of performance shows little or no progress, we need to reassess the person's abilities before hypothesising again about the possible causes of their movement problems. If the movement hypotheses are correct, therapists can then reflect critically on their teaching skills. Alternatively, if a different movement hypothesis is made new training strategies and an intervention plan will be needed. Therapists should not underestimate the importance of re-measuring performance, reflecting on their teaching skills, and, above all, persisting and expecting to see improved motor performance at every session.

Practice Scenario 37.1 shows how Leo, an occupational therapist, developed his teaching and analysis skills, and applied evidence-based practice in adult rehabilitation.

Practice Scenario 37.1 Leo and Mary

Leo is an experienced occupational therapist working in a large district hospital in rural Australia. He has over 10 years experience in adult neurological rehabilitation. Leo is dedicated to developing his skills. He has attended upper-limb motor training workshops,

videotaped clients, and discussed his training programmes with peers. He has organised fortnightly peer review sessions where staff observe each other conducting a therapy session, and provide feedback about analysis and teaching skills. Leo regularly attends rehabilitation conferences as he feels they 'are a great pick-me-up'. More recently, Leo increased his knowledge and skills by commencing a major research project, a randomised controlled trial of task-specific training, as part of a Masters degree.

Here, Leo gives an example of a lady, Mary, he saw recently following her stroke. He describes her motor control problems and compensations, and the upper-limb training programme provided over several months to improve occupational performance. Mary could not use her affected arm much when engaging in daily occupations. She could not hold or transport objects such as a cup or a knife during meals.

Mary

"I saw Mary recently. She had recovery of some muscles in her arm, but a lot of overactivity, many compensations and little control in her hand. For example, when attempting to reach forwards to grasp a cup, she elevated her shoulder and abducted her arm, clenched her fingers, flexed her elbow, and moved her whole body forwards instead of just her arm and hand. She compensated for poor shoulder flexion, loss of external rotation and thumb adduction by using every muscle possible in her arm. It was hard work.

Training sessions targeted Mary's shoulder flexors in a lying position, which reduced the effect of gravity. We focused on the anterior deltoid muscle. Mary was asked to rest her hand on her forehead with the elbow flexed, and control her anterior deltoid in that position. When she could hold her arm there, she started sliding her hand back from her forehead to the pillow and the crown of her head, to control anterior deltoid in lying, then reaching higher to the wall to touch a marker. It was too hard in sitting. She couldn't lift her arm up against gravity without compensating. Other practice tasks focused on her shoulder external rotation, elbow, wrist and finger extension and thumb abduction. We pieced each component together, then eventually began working on functional reaching in a seated position (see Figure 37.5).

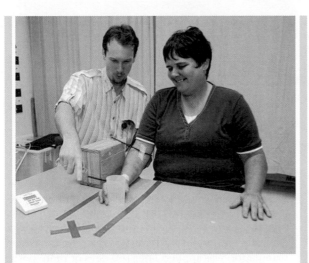

Figure 37.5 • Practice of essential components required for reaching (forward flexion and external rotation) and drinking from a cup

Since her stroke, this woman has had limited opportunities to engage in occupations such as drinking from a cup with her dominant right hand. She has weak shoulder flexors and external rotators, and cannot open her thumb or fingers to pre-shape correctly. The occupational therapist is helping her to practise shoulder flexion and external rotation – essential components of reaching – while also maintaining wrist extension and forearm supination.

In this photograph, she is sliding the cup forwards while staying inside the black lines (electrical tape stuck to the table). The practice environment encourages external rotation, wrist extension and supination, and discourages compensations such as internal rotation and abduction. Two drinking straws have been applied to her arm, one to the inner elbow and another on to the back of her wrist. These straws act as visual cues, reminding her to maintain shoulder external rotation (the straw stays in contact with the wooden block) and wrist extension (her knuckles stay in contact with the flexible straw). She is also learning to monitor her own performance, so that she can practise alone outside of therapy sessions. Notice the timer near the therapist's right hand, to record practice time and repetitions

Mary practised for about two hours a day for three months (unsupervised for some of the time); then one hour daily for another three months; then about three hours a week for the last three months. It took 36 weeks or six months before she had a functional grasp and release. In the first six weeks she completed 12,810 repetitions, with an average of 427 reps per session or 85 per exercise. After 36 weeks, she achieved a score of 16/57 on the Action Research Arm Test, compared to 2/57 at the

beginning, a 14 point change. With a combination of task–specific training, persistence on both our parts, objective measurement, intensive practice and feedback, Mary achieved improved hand function. Without this persistence and practice, I don't think she would have achieved this outcome."

Ensuring enough practice by people with a stroke or brain injury is always a challenge: to help ensure individuals spend plenty of time each day practising, Leo uses typed practice records with imported digital photographs. The rehabilitation team runs a cross-disciplinary upper-limb group several times a week, where people with stroke or brain injury follow their own practice programme with co-learners, and supervision from therapists. Therapy assistants and relatives also help supervise individual practice after this has been documented with instructions, goals and illustrations by the therapist. Family members are involved in helping with practice as early as possible, because of the limited time available for one-to-one therapy.

Evidence-based intervention to improve upper-limb motor performance

There are several reasons why a person may be unable to reach for, grasp and drink from a cup. Different causes will require different intervention/s. A person with a paralysed arm, who is unable to elicit any muscle contractions, will require intervention targeting muscle strength. A person with a contracture will require intervention to lengthen, and then strengthen, their weak overstretched muscles.

In this chapter, we have emphasised the importance of identifying the correct motor control problem, in order to select appropriate, targeted intervention. A number of interventions have now been tested in randomised trials, and the collective findings synthesised in systematic reviews. It is the effective interventions we highlight here. Where interventions and training strategies have not been tested using more rigorous research, we will indicate if we are relying on lower level evidence or personal experience.

In adult rehabilitation, interventions that improve performance of upper-limb motor control appear to involve greater intensity of practise and repetitions (Kwakkel 2006, van der Lee et al 2001), and use task-specific training strategies to improve strength (Ada et al 2006b). However, the evidence is still scattered and limited. By definition, more intense practise and repetitions requires active involvement of the learner. One of the biggest challenges in rehabilitation (and this is not limited to motor rehabilitation) is how to increase the amount of practise a person completes in the hospital and community. For a thoughtful discussion of the feasibility of providing intensive practise, see Kwakkel (2006). It is important that people spend as much time as possible practising. One hour of therapy doing 100 repetitions is better than 1 hour of therapy doing 10 or 20 repetitions. Keeping a record of repetitions completed during each therapy session is one way of ensuring practise intensity. Such records provide an insight into just how much practise is needed before people acquire particular skills.

Strength training for weak or paralysed muscles

Some individuals may be unable to elicit a muscle contraction due to paralysis or weakness. They need practise which helps them elicit a single muscle contraction then gradually increase the duration and strength of contractions. There is a growing body of evidence demonstrating that muscle strengthening and repetitions improve strength and function without any increase in spasticity (e.g. Ada et al 2006a, Butefisch et al 1995).

One of the few randomised trials targeting very weak muscles has already been highlighted (Feys et al 1998). These researchers recruited 100 people early after stroke, and provided a novel training strategy to improve shoulder control. Participants were seated in a rocking chair with their affected arm in an airsplint, and practised protraction and retraction for 30 minutes daily for 6 weeks. The median score on the Action Research Arm Test (ARAT) was 0 at baseline for control and experimental groups (total maximum score = 57). At the 5-year follow-up, the mean difference in improvements between groups was 17 points on the ARAT (Feys et al 2004). As previously noted, greater gains were seen in people with severe motor deficits at baseline. While there was a wide range and variability in responses, the mean effect in this very weak population was large.

Examples of practice tasks aimed at increasing muscle strength are shown in Figures 37.6–37.9.

Electrical stimulation

Electrical stimulation should be provided to people with no palpable muscle activity after a stroke. Ada and Foongchomcheay (2002) conducted a meta-analysis involving four trials of electrical stimulation to prevent subluxation early after stroke (average 17 days post-stroke), involving a total of 145 subjects. Electrical stimulation reduced subluxation by an average of 6.5 mm, but had no worthwhile effect on reducing pain or improving functional recovery. No clinically important differences were found when stimulation was applied later (60 days or more post-stroke), based on meta-analysis of data from three randomised trials.

More recently, Pomeroy and colleagues (2006) examined the effect of electrical stimulation on upper- and lower-limb motor recovery. A total of 24 randomised trials were included, involving 888 participants from 9 days to 4 years post stroke. When compared to no treatment, function was improved (statistically significant difference between groups) on the Box and Block tests, motor reaction time and isometric muscle torque. Another exploratory study involving nine people with chronic stroke who had moderate-to-severe motor weakness and intact sensation reported improved motor function after only 2 hours of electrical stimulation to the sensory nerves of the hand (Wu et al 2006). In summary, electrical stimulation is being used increasingly in adult neurological rehabilitation, although further research is still needed, including research involving children.

Constraint-induced movement therapy

Constraint-induced movement therapy (CIMT) is a relatively new and popular treatment aimed at increasing use of the affected hand after stroke, brain injury, and cerebral palsy in children and adults. Typically, a splint or mitt and a sling are used to restrain the unaffected hand for up to 6 hours a day, for 2 weeks, during which time the person intensively practises using their hand. The aim is to discourage use of the 'good' hand and greater use of the affected hand. For a detailed description of a CIMT protocol, see Morris and colleagues (1997).

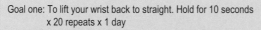

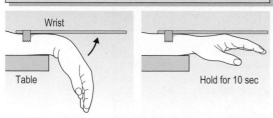

Goal one: To lift your wrist back to straight. Hold for 10 seconds
x 20 repeats x 1 day

Wrist

Table

Hold for 10 sec

Instructions
1. Tape straw on forearm
2. Hand on table; elbow straight
3. Let wrist drop down so fingers hang over edge of table
4. Keep fingers **straight**
5. Bring your hand back to straight by moving your wrist

Critical features
• Wrist back **evenly**
• Fingers straight throughout
• Thumb does not move outwards away from hand

* Record number correct/number of attempts

Date	No. correct
17/7	14/20
17/7	15/20
26/7	21/25
30/7	9–10
	7–10
02/8	20/25
03/8	22/25

Figure 37.6 • Wrist extension
Wrist extension is essential for most activities involving reaching, such as picking up a cup to drink. The page shown above is taken from a practice book and illustrates the wrist extension exercise, where the goal is to lift the wrist back to the 'straight' position and hold for 10 seconds, and to repeat this exercise 20 times in one session.

The collective research in stroke rehabilitation (14 randomised trials and four systematic reviews) shows a moderate effect of CIMT on upper-limb motor performance, as measured by the Action Research Arm Test (Hakkennes & Keating 2005). However, all participants have had active wrist and finger extension at study commencement. We do not yet know if this intervention can drive recovery in people with a paralysed arm, as occurred in early studies involving monkeys. Currently in adult stroke rehabilitation, CIMT is used with small cohorts of individuals but may have the potential to drive recovery if used more widely.

CIMT for paediatric populations has been studied less. A small number of randomised controlled trials with low methodological quality and small sample sizes have been reported (e.g. Taub et al 2004, Willis et al 2002). Consequently, the effect remains uncertain (Hoare et al 2007, see Wallen 2007 for an overview and key references). Readers should follow the work of Eliasson and colleagues in Sweden. They describe a programme of CIMT, which involves shorter periods of restraint using a mitt, for 2 hours over 8 weeks with adolescents who had cerebral palsy (Eliasson et al 2003). More recently, they evaluated the effect with young children with cerebral palsy using a non-randomised study design (Eliasson et al 2005).

Mental practice

Mental practice and imagery have been used to promote motor recovery. This type of practice is used routinely in sports training to improve skill acquisition. In rehabilitation, a person with stroke or brain injury might mentally rehearse the task of picking up a cup and imagine the transport and pre-shaping actions, without physically attempting the actions (Bell & Murray 2005). A recent systematic review (Braun et al 2006) summarised the effects of several studies in stroke rehabilitation but again found underpowered studies with small sample sizes. No definite conclusions could be reached, but this intervention is promising for people with no active movement. Interested therapists will need to devise their own script and tape to give to interested people. For an example see Dijkerman and colleagues (2004).

Reducing muscle force during grasp

Some individuals turn on too many muscles, or the wrong muscles, when reaching for and grasping objects. This is a normal response to skill acquisition (not spasticity) in most cases. Until we have mastered or refined a new skill, we will try a range of strategies, and use too many muscles. Therefore, one aim in therapy is to reduce effort, and help the person focus on the muscle actions required for task performance.

Changing the demands of a task and the environment can reduce effort. For example, asking a

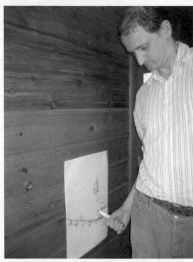

Goal one: Keep texter pentip touching the X mark for 5 seconds
 x 3 times in a row
Goal two: Draw a line with the texter 5 cm up the wall
 x 3 times in a row

Instructions
1. Stick the paper onto the wall with tape (X mark at hip height).
2. Stand beside the poster with pen in hand.
3. Rotate the pen out so the pentip touches the X mark.
 keep shoulder rotated out.
4. Hold for 5 seconds, rest and repeat.
5. Try drawing a line up the wall – no further than 5 cm initially

Check
• Look ahead – don't turn inwards, towards the wall or
 bend your trunk.
• Remember to breathe while practicing.
• Keep your elbow straight/lengthened.

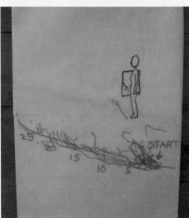

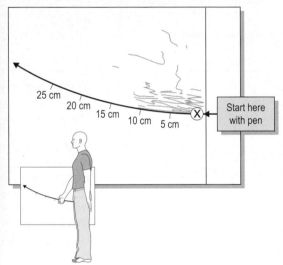

25 cm 20 cm 15 cm 10 cm 5 cm Ⓧ Start here with pen

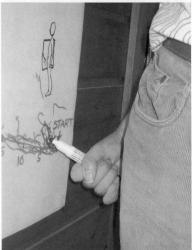

Figure 37.7 • Practice for shoulder external rotation and forward flexion in standing

Both external rotation and shoulder forward flexion are essential for transporting the arm and hand forwards to reach for a cup or telephone. While this man is using extra muscle force to hold the pen (increased finger flexion), his response is typical of new skill acquisition, and is not a concern to the therapist.

The first goal (Goal 1: Keep the texta pentip touching the X mark on the paper for 5 seconds) demands a sustained contraction of his external rotators combined with full supination. Without some external rotation, the goal cannot be achieved (except by trunk rotation). The second goal (Goal 2: Draw a line 5 cm up the wall) demands sustained external rotation and shoulder flexion

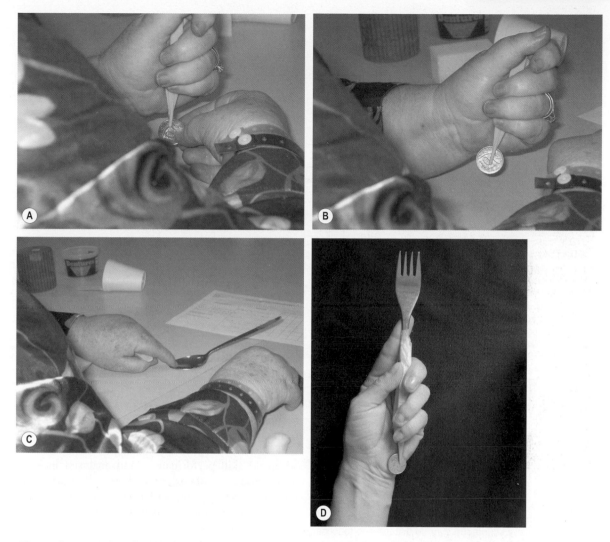

Figure 37.8 • Practice to improve fork control

This lady cannot sustain flexion of her fourth and fifth digits around a fork handle when trying to pick up food. When she tries to use her fork, the handle rotates and she loses her grasp. Part-practice has been devised to help improve flexion of her ring and little fingers around a fork handle. Figures 37.8A and 37.8B show her setting up the practice. She has been asked to hold a coin between plastic tweezers for 5 seconds. This task sustains her attention. She gets feedback instantly if her grasp weakens, because the coin drops onto the table.

Figure 37.8C shows her still holding the tweezers and coin (coin no longer visible), flexing her wrist and fingers, and pressing the index finger down on the end of a spoon. She finds it much more challenging to keep her fourth and fifth digits flexed in this position while her index finger is extended, as it needs to be while using a fork. Again, she receives instant feedback if her grasp weakens because the coin drops out of the tweezers – feedback which would not be provided by a standard fork.

Figure 37.8D illustrates how the tweezers and fork handle can be taped together, to enable fork practice to progress. This lady can continue her practice with the coin held between plastic tweezers, and learn to transport small pieces of soft vegetable or bread squares from plate to plate, without dropping the coin

Goal: After 10 minutes stretch, to move your forearm over so that the cup touches the blue 'blob', hold for 10 seconds x 30 repeats

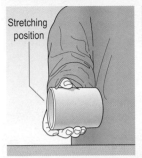

Stretching position

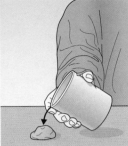

Instructions
1. Sitting with your right arm supported on a table, elbow straight
2. Tape a cup into your hand so that your thumb web space is stretched
3. Use your left hand to take your arm over and hold it in a stretch
4. Take your left hand off, hold the cup on the 'blob' for 10 seconds
5. Come back so that the cup is upright
6. Move the cup back so that the lip touches the 'blob'

Date	No. correct
10/7	0/30
21/7	0/30
27/7	0/20
30/7	3/30
03/8	5/30

Figure 37.9 ● Supination practice
Practice book showing the exercise (Forearm Supination) and goal, in the learners own words: 'After 10 minutes stretch, to move your forearm over so that the cup touches the blue 'blob', hold for 10 seconds'. Additional instructions have also been added, and a section for recording practice attempts

person to lift a light plastic cup off the table instead of a glass, or slide rather than lift a cup along the table will help to reduce effort. If a person is unable to grasp while reaching, taping a cup into their hand will reduce the task demands and help the person to concentrate on specific features of reaching. If too much force is used, use a disposable polystyrene cup which deforms easily when grasped, to give the person feedback about their force production (Figures 37.10 and 37.11).

Different instructions may also help the person to become more self-aware, and learn to use some muscles more and others with less force. For example:

'When you next reach forwards for the cup, slide rather than lift your hand. Watch your hand and keep it the same shape as the cup. Notice if your fingers and thumb are closing as you reach. If they are, see if you can keep your fingers and thumb 'soft' as you reach.'

or:

'This time, when you close your fingers around the polystyrene cup, don't press so hard. Try not to squash or deform the cup. If you press too hard, the water will come up above the marked line. Just use light pressure on the sides of the cup'.

Dexterity training

Some individuals can grasp and pick up objects, such as a cup, knife or fork, but cannot manipulate them. Training of advanced hand function involves more than cutting up slices of bread or repeatedly copying lines of writing. Careful analysis enables therapists to determine which components of skilled performance are missing or altered, in comparison to normal manipulation. This stage of analysis and training is most interesting but demands careful observation and problem solving. Tasks requiring advanced skill performance (and analysis) include handwriting, use of cutlery or chopsticks, putting on jewellery, applying contact lenses, tying shoes, doing up buttons, using a screwdriver or mobile phone.

With small objects, training of grip force during lift-off and manipulation will be required, with repetitions and feedback. Healthy adults typically apply a force slightly higher than the minimum required in order to prevent object slippage (Nowak & Hermsdorfer 2003). However, people with chronic stroke and intact sensation ($n = 10$) have been shown to apply significantly greater mean grip forces ($\geq$ 39%) at lift-off compared to healthy adults (Quaney et al 2005). The participants with stroke used a greater safety margin. Blennerhassett and colleagues (2006) reported different findings for 45 people with stroke and 45 healthy adults, who were able to pick up a pen lid concealed from view, using a pinch grip. These authors reported prolonged time and excessive grip force prior to commencing the lift in half the people with stroke, as well as fluctuating forces and extreme slowness, but excessive safety margins were not present in all cases.

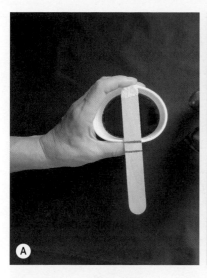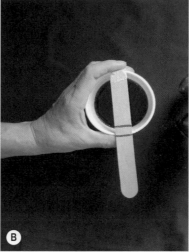

Figure 37.10 • Practice to decrease finger and wrist flexion force while transporting a cup to drink or while carrying liquid

The person has been asked to gently press the side of the polystyrene cup, and move the cup edge between the two lines on the wooden stick (Figure 37.10A).

When the short-term goal has been achieved, the person can progress to transporting the cup of liquid up onto a box, stand up while holding the cup, and, finally, walk while carrying the cup.

Short-term goal: Press the cup inwards 1 cm to the second pen mark, release and repeat 3 times.

Medium-term goal: In sitting, maintain the round shape of the cup (see Figure 37.10B) and lift onto a 5 cm box.

Medium-term goal: Maintain the round shape of the cup (Figure 37.10B) while standing up and sitting down 5 times from a 45 cm chair.

Long-term goal: Carry a full cup of water 3 times, from the kitchen to the dining room table, without spilling any liquid

The combined message for therapists from these studies is that people with stroke typically have difficulty preparing a suitable grip force and using the normal feed-forward mechanisms. Impaired sensation is likely to compound these problems. However, training strategies are likely to be similar for people with and without sensory impairment. Training needs to involve task-specific practice, with many repetitions and feedback. If a person has difficulty using a knife, fork or pen, they need to engage in part-practise with these utensils. For example, picking up an object precisely without spinning or rotating the handle, cutting food and writing all require appropriate force production and accurate opposition of the forces of the thumb and fingers to be successful. See Figure 37.12 as one example.

Preventing and managing contractures

During the therapy planning process, therapists need to not only consider the contractures that are present, but also anticipate contractures that may develop in the future. Loss of shoulder external rotation range of movement is common after stroke. In one study ($n = 25$), people with stroke experienced an average of 30% loss of external rotation (Andrews & Bohannon 1989), with some experiencing a loss of up to 60% of their range. This loss of range correlates with shoulder pain (Bohannon 1988) and impacts on occupational performance, particularly self-care tasks. Therefore, it is important for therapists to anticipate and prevent contractures.

Muscle stretching has become the main intervention for managing muscle-length changes and contracture. Animal studies suggest that muscle stretches need to be sustained for more than a few minutes to reverse length-related changes from immobilisation (Goldspink & Williams 1990, Williams 1990). However, it is not possible or economical for stretches to be provided manually by therapists for extended periods. Instead, stretches need to be integrated into routine positioning programmes. For example, shoulder extensors and

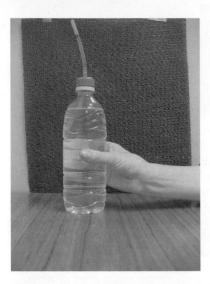

Figure 37.11 • Practice to modulate finger and thumb flexion force while holding a plastic bottle which deforms easily

The person has been asked to gently press the sides of the plastic bottle, and control the water levels between the two black lines on the tube. Too much pressure causes a jet of water to shoot out the top, which gives immediate feedback to the learner about the amount of force being generated. The practice demands attention for successful performance.

To construct the training device, first drill a hole in the top of a plastic bottle cap. The hole should be just large enough to accommodate the suction tubing. Insert tubing down through the hole, fill the bottle with water and seal the unit tightly with the screw top. If necessary, seal the unit with tape to prevent air escaping.

Short-term goal: In sitting, push water up and down between the two black lines 5 times, without water escaping from the tube.

Medium-term goal: In sitting, keep the water level with the upper black line and lift the bottle up onto a 5 cm box, 5 times, without water escaping from the tube

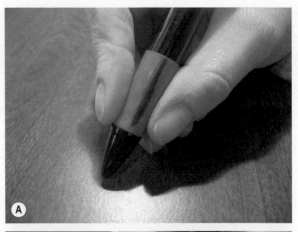

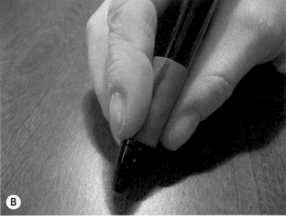

Figure 37.12 • Practice of pen rotation

This practice aims to improve pen control and handwriting. The *short-term* goal is to rotate the pen/pencil 10 times in 30 seconds by the end of one week. The *medium-term goal is to* rotate the pen/pencil 10 times in 20 seconds by the end of 2 weeks.

Instructions remind the person to:

• roll the pen/pencil a 1/2 turn in each direction
• aim to cover then uncover a pen mark along the barrel of the pen (see Figures 37.12A and 37.12B)
• allow the pen/pencil to rest against the webspace while practicing
• use the middle finger to re-adjust pen position when necessary
• avoid using the other hand to help
• aim to practise for 5 minutes x 3 times daily (15 minutes daily)
• try not to hold the pen tightly
• practise with different pens/pencils to help generalise this skill

internal rotator muscles can easily be stretched by positioning the arm on a table, out to the side in supine in bed or on the floor (Figure 37.13). Range of movement can be monitored with simple measures as illustrated.

More sustained stretches can be applied with serial casts to immobilise joints in their stretched position. Serial casts should only be considered for more severe contractures of the elbow, wrist or fingers because they impede motor training and may reinforce learned non-use. Studies investigating the effect of hand splinting to prevent contracture after stroke and brain injury have shown no difference in

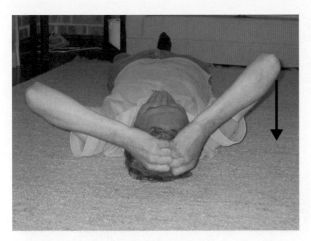

Figure 37.13 • Shoulder stretch to increase external rotation for reaching
This is a gravity-assisted stretch aimed at lengthening the right internal rotator muscles and increasing the range of available external rotation. Limited external rotation is very common after stroke and reduces reaching performance during daily occupations such as eating and drinking. This stretch can be done independently for up to 30 minutes daily, lying on the bed or floor. Some people find this stretch more comfortable if a pillow or rolled-up towel is placed under the humerus, as they can relax into the stretch more easily.

In this figure, this man's goal was to relax both shoulders during the stretch so that his right elbow was 20 cm above the floor (comparable with his unaffected left shoulder). At the beginning of his outpatient therapy sessions, his right elbow was 38 cm above the floor due to shortening of his internal rotators.

wrist extensibility compared to controls (no splint), even when splints were worn for many hours over 4 weeks (Lannin et al 2003, 2007) and 3 months (Harvey et al 2006). A recent Cochrane review also concluded that hand splinting had no effect on function, finger or wirst flexibility or pain, although this conclusion was based on a small number of trials (Tyson & Kent 2009).

Although anecdotal evidence suggests that contractures are a common secondary complication after brain impairment, evidence that long-duration stretch lengthens shortened muscles or maintains their length is limited (Harvey et al 2002). Two trials involving adults with stroke (Ada et al 2005a, de Jong et al 2006) reported that shoulder and arm positioning to promote stretch slowed down, but did not prevent, contracture development. Other studies involving stroke populations were either underpowered (e.g. Dean et al 2000, Turton &

Britton 2005) or found no difference following stretch/positioning.

There is, therefore, still uncertainty about whether stretch interventions are effective in the long term and, if they are, how long stretches should be held for and how often they should be administered. Animal research suggests that if stretches are being used, they should be sustained for as long as practically feasible (Harvey 2008). It may be that stretches in humans need to be administered for many hours a day, rather than minutes, and continued indefinitely in people with minimal motor recovery.

Shoulder strapping appears to reduce shoulder pain but not function. A Cochrane systematic review (Ada et al 2005b) found that shoulder strapping with adhesive tape delayed the onset of shoulder pain but did not reduce pain, improve function or contracture development. A more recent randomised controlled trial post stroke ($n = 33$) confirmed the effect of strapping (Griffin & Bernhardt 2006). These authors reported a mean of 26 pain-free days for the intervention group compared to 19 pain-free days in a placebo controlled group, and 16 in the control group.

Shoulder slings and supports have not been well researched despite their frequent use in practise (Ada et al 2005b,c). Current expert opinion is that external supports such as wheelchair and chair attachments are needed to support the weight of the arm (Foongchomcheay et al 2005). Triangular bandages and collar and cuff slings may help to protect the arm during transfers but do not physically reduce a joint subluxation. Electrical stimulation shows more promise as an intervention than slings and supports; however, ultimately individuals need active motor training, in supine and side lying to help them learn to switch on paralysed muscles around the shoulder and upper arm.

Improving reaching and postural control in sitting

Limited research has been conducted on sitting balance training. A Cochrane review (Pollock et al 2003) highlighted the need for task-specific training strategies instead of generalised 'approaches' which have been used in the past. Task-specific training strategies have been shown to be effective in randomised trials involving people with stroke (Dean & Shepherd 1997, Dean et al 2007). These studies, which have already been discussed, involved reaching in sitting to the affected side at distances greater than arm's length. The 'sham' training or control group received an equivalent amount of reaching practise but within arm's reach. After 2 weeks' training participants in the intervention group all improved in the distance and speed with which they could reach in comparison to the control group. In addition, the increased weight-bearing practise improved the participants' ability to stand up.

General principles for training reaching in sitting include the following: minimise the effort required to sit; check that both feet are on the ground; provide good thigh support to maximise the base of support; limit the distance reached initially; introduce forward reaching, and reaching to the unaffected side before reaching across to the affected side which requires maximum leg extensor muscle control; if unable to activate the leg extensor muscles on the affected side, the person will be unable to control movement onto the affected side; help people learn to activate their leg extensor muscles, and anticipate the need to turn those muscles on prior to beginning to moving towards that side; as the person improves their ability to turn their leg extensor muscles on, task difficulty can be increased. This can be done by reaching across to the affected side, increasing the distance reached, decreasing the amount of thigh support and increasing the chair height (which increases the force required from the

leg extensors). Table 37.2 presents a detailed analysis and training suggestions.

Future directions

These are exciting times. New technologies and more rigorous methodologies provide increasing support for theories of movement rehabilitation. We know that the earlier rehabilitation begins, the better the recovery from conditions such as stroke and brain injury. Greater intensity of treatment translates into better outcomes. Gains in motor control and recovery continue for many years. Therapists are moving away from one-on-one, hands-on therapy and making better use of circuit and group training programmes. And as rehabilitation research continues to grow, so too will the evidence on which therapists base their practice.

The need for increased intensity of practice has led to the testing of two more novel rehabilitation techniques, CIMT and robotics. Reinkensmeyer and colleagues (2004) report that robotic therapy allows for some of the labour-intensive training tasks performed currently by therapists to be performed by automated devices, thereby providing people with greater access to therapy. As the evidence grows in support of more intensive therapy, constraint and robotics will be used more often because they can increase practise and may lead

Table 37.2 Summary of motor control problems affecting the upper limb and seated reaching, and possible interventions for people with neurological conditions

Motor control problem	Possible interventions and evidence from key studies
Eliciting movement in paralysed muscles	• Repetitive contractions and practice of shoulder protraction in sitting (Feys et al 1998, 2004) • Electrical stimulation of the wrist extensor and forearm (Powell et al 1999), and shoulder muscles (Ada & Foongchomcheay 2002) • Mental practice (Braun et al 2006, Dijkerman et al 2004) • Mirror box therapy (Altschuler et al 1999, Yavuzer et al 2008)
Increasing force generation or strength in weak muscles	• Electrical stimulation of the wrist extensor and forearm (Powell et al 1999), and shoulder muscles (Ada & Foongchomcheay 2002, Pomeroy et al 2006)
Decreasing force in overactive muscles	• Repetitive contractions and practice, wrist and forearm muscles (Butefisch et al 1995)
Increasing dexterity, speed and control	• Constraint-induced movement therapy (Eliasson et al 2005, Hakkennes et al 2005) • Task-related training in groups (Blennerhassett et al 2004)
Preventing or reversing muscle contractures	• Stretching internal rotators in supine for 30 minutes daily may help to decrease loss of external rotation range of movement (Ada et al 2005)

to greater motor recovery. Mirror box therapy is another intervention which is supported by two randomised trials (Altschuler et al, 1999; Yavuzer et al, 2008). Like CIMT, this intervention allows independent practice by people with stroke. With technologies improving all the time, it is not possible to predict what advances will become routine practice in the future. The important message is, therefore, to remain abreast of current scientific evidence.

Conclusion

This chapter has focused on the process of analysing and retraining motor performance in children and adults with brain impairment. The content is necessarily impairment-focused because much of upper-limb rehabilitation, particularly in hospital settings, focuses on eliciting muscle activity and strength training prior to return of functional grasp. At this stage, therapists need to remind themselves and the people they work with of the occupational goals of training, for example, eating a meal with family members using cutlery in both hands. Once a person has an effective grasp, can hold and manipulate objects, tasks and goals are more obvious. While the overall goal of occupational therapy is to increase engagement in occupations, we cannot and should not ignore impairment-focused intervention.

References

Ada, L. & Canning, C. (2005). Changing the way we view the contribution of motor impairments to physical disability after stroke. In: K. Refshauge, L. Ada & E. Ellis (Eds). *Science-based rehabilitation: theories into practice.* (pp. 87–106). Edinburgh, Elsevier, Butterworth-Heinemann.

Ada, L., Canning, C. & Dwyer, T. (2000). Effect of muscle length on strength and dexterity after stroke. *Clinical Rehabilitation*, 14, 55–61.

Ada, L. & Foongchomcheay, A. (2002). Efficacy of electrical stimulation in preventing or reducing subluxation of the shoulder after stroke: a meta-analysis. *Australian Journal of Physiotherapy*, 48, 257–267.

Ada, L., Foongchomcheay, A. & Canning, C. (2005a). Supportive devices for preventing and treating subluxation of the shoulder after stroke. *The Cochrane Database of Systematic Reviews Issue 1.*

Ada, L., Foongchomcheay, A. & Canning, C. (2005b). Use of devices to prevent subluxation of the shoulder after stroke. *Physiotherapy Research International*, 10, 134–145.

Ada, L., Goddard, E., McCully, J., Stavrinos, T. & Bampton, J. (2005c). Thirty minutes of positioning reduces the development of external rotation but not flexion contracture in the shoulder after stroke: a randomised controlled trial. *Archives of Physical Medicine and Rehabilitation*, 86, 230–234.

Ada, L., Dorsch, S. & Canning, C. (2006a). Strengthening interventions to increase strength and improve activity after stroke: a systematic review. *Australian Journal of Physiotherapy*, 52, 241–248.

Ada, L., O'Dwyer, N. & O'Neill, E. (2006b). Relation between spasticity, weakness and contracture of the elbow flexors and upper limb activity after stroke: an observational study. *Disability and Rehabilitation*, 28, 891–897.

Adams, J. A. (1971). A closed-loop theory of motor learning. *Journal of Motor Behavior*, 3, 111–150.

Altschuler, E. L., Wisdom, S. B. & Stone, L. (1999). Rehabilitation of hemiparesis after stroke with a mirror. *Lancet*, 353, 2035–2036.

Andrews, A. W. & Bohannon, R. W. (1989). Decreased range of motion on paretic side after stroke. *Physical Therapy*, 69, 768–722.

Annett, J. (1959). Learning a pressure under conditions of immediate and delayed knowledge of results. *Quarterly Journal of Experimental Psychology*, 11, 3–15.

Bayona, N. A., Bitensky, J., Salter, K. & Teasell, R. (2005). The role of task-specific training in rehabilitation therapies. *Topics in Stroke Rehabilitation*, 12, 58–65.

Bell, A. R. & Murray, B. J. (2005). Improvement in upper limb motor performance following stroke: The use of mental practice. *British Journal of Occupational Therapy*, 67, 501–507.

Bilodeau, I. M. (1966). Information feedback. In E. A. Bilodeau (Ed.). *Acquisition of skill.* (pp. 225–296). New York, Academic Press.

Blennerhassett, J. & Dite, W. (2004). Additional task-related practice improves mobility and upper limb function early after stroke: a randomised controlled trial. *Australian Journal of Physiotherapy*, 50, 219–224.

Blennerhassett, J. M., Carey, L. M. & Matyas, T. A. (2006). Grip force regulation during pinch grip lifts under somatosensory guidance: comparison between people with stroke and healthy controls. *Archives of Physical Medicine and Rehabilitation*, 87, 418–429.

Bohannon, R. W. (1988). Relationship between shoulder pain and selected variables in patients with hemiplegia. *Clinical Rehabilitation*, 2, 111–117.

Boyd, R. N. & Ada, L. (2001). Physiotherapy management of spasticity. In M. P. Barnes & G. R. Johnson (Eds). *Upper motor neurone syndrome and spasticity.* (pp. 96–103). Cambridge, Cambridge University Press.

Braun, S. M., Beurskens, A. J., Borm, P. J. et al (2006). The effects of mental practice in stroke rehabilitation: a systematic review. *Archives of Physical Medicine and Rehabilitation*, 87, 842–852.

Burke, D. (1988). Spasticity as an adaptation to pyramidal tract injury. *Advances in Neurology*, 47, 401–423.

Butefisch, C., Hummelsheim, H., Denzler, P. et al. (1995). Repetitive training of isolated movements improves the outcome of motor rehabilitation of the centrally paretic hand. *Journal of the Neurological Sciences*, 130, 59–68.

Carr, J. H. & Shepherd, R. B. (1987). *A motor relearning programme for stroke*. (2nd ed). Oxford, Heinemann Medical.

Carr, J. H. & Shepherd, R. B. (1989). A motor learning model for stroke rehabilitation. *Physiotherapy*, 75(7), 372–380.

Carr, J. H., Shepherd, R. B., Gordon, J. et al (1987). *Movement science: foundations for physical therapy in rehabilitation*. Rockville, MD, Aspen.

Carr, J. H. & Shepherd, R. B. (2003). Reaching and manipulation. In: *Stroke rehabilitation: guidelines for exercise and training to optimize motor performance*. (pp. 159–206). London, Butterworth-Heinemann.

Chari, V. R. & Kirby, R. L. (1986). Lower-limb influence on sitting balance while reaching forward. *Archives of Physical Medicine and Rehabilitation*, 67, 73–733.

Charness, N. (1981). Search in chess: age and skill differences. *Journal of Experimental Psychology: Human Perception and Performance*, 7, 467–476.

Crosbie, J., Shepherd, R. & Squire, T. (1995). Postural and voluntary movement during reaching in sitting: the role of the lower limbs. *Journal of Human Movement Studies*, 28, 103–126.

de Jong, L. D., Nieuwboer, A. & Aufdemkampe, G. (2006). Contracture preventive positioning of the hemiplegic arm in subacute stroke patients: a pilot randomized controlled trial. *Clinical Rehabilitation*, 20, 656–667.

Dean, C. & Shepherd, R. (1997). Task related training improves performance of seated reaching tasks after stroke: a randomised

controlled trial. *Stroke*, 28, 722–728.

Dean, C., Shepherd, R. & Adam, R. (1999a) Sitting balance I: trunk and arm coordination and the contribution of the lower limbs during self-paced reaching in sitting. *Gait and Posture*, 10, 135–146.

Dean, C., Shepherd, R. & Adam, R. (1999b). Sitting balance II: reach direction and thigh support affect the contribution of the lower limbs when reaching beyond arm's length in sitting. *Gait and Posture*, 10, 147–153.

Dean, C., Katrak, P. & Mackey, F. (2000). Examination of shoulder positioning after stroke: a randomized controlled pilot trial. *Australian Journal of Physiotherapy*, 46, 35–40.

Dean, C., Channon, E. & Hall, J. (2007). Sitting training early after stroke improves sitting ability and quality and carries over to standing up but not to walking: a randomised controlled trial. *Australian Journal of Physiotherapy*, 53, 97–102.

Dickson, M. (2002). Rehabilitation of motor control following stroke: searching the evidence. *British Journal of Occupational Therapy*, 65, 269–274.

Djikerman, H. C., Letswaart, M., Johnston, M. et al. (2004). Does motor imagery training improve hand function in chronic stroke patients? A pilot study. *Clinical Rehabilitation*, 18, 538–549.

Eliasson, A. C., Bonnier, B. & Krumlinde-Sundholm, L. (2003). Clinical experience of constraint induced movement therapy in adolescents with hemiplegic cerebral palsy – A day camp model. *Developmental Medicine and Child Neurology*, 45, 357–359.

Eliasson, A. C., Krumlinde-Sundholm, L., Shaw, K. et al (2005). Effects of constraint-induced movement therapy in young children with hemiplegic cerebral palsy: An adapted model. *Developmental Medicine and Child Neurology*, 47, 266–275.

Ericsson, K. A. (2004). Deliberate practice and the acquisition and maintenance of expert performance in medicine and related domains. *Academic Medicine*, 79, S70–S81.

Feys, H. M., de Weerdt, W. J., Selz, B. E. et al (1998). Effect of a therapeutic intervention for the hemiplegic upper limb in the acute phase after stroke: a single-blind randomized multicentre trial. *Stroke*, 29, 785–792.

Feys, H. M., de Weerdt, W. J., Verbeke, G. et al (2004). Early and repetitive stimulation of the arm can substantially improve the long-term outcome after stroke: a 5-year follow-up study of a randomized trial. *Stroke*, 35, 924–929.

Fitts, P. M. & Posner, M. I. (1967). *Human performance*. Belmont, CA, Brooks/Cole.

Foongchomcheay, A., Ada, L. & Canning, C. (2005). Use of devices to prevent subluxation of the shoulder after stroke. *Physiotherapy Research International*, 10(3), 134–145.

Forssberg, H. & Hirschfeld, H. (1994). Postural adjustments in sitting humans following external perturbations: muscle activity and kinematics. *Experimental Brain Research*, 97, 515–527.

Goldspink, G. & Williams, P. (1990). Muscle fibre and connective tissue changes associated with use and disuse. In L. Ada & C. Canning (Eds.) *Key issues in neurological physiotherapy*. (pp. 197–218). Oxford, Butterworth-Heinemann.

Gossman, M. R., Sahrmann, S. A. & Rose, S. J. (1982). Review of length associated changes in muscle. *Physical Therapy*, 62, 1799–1808.

Griffin, A. & Bernhardt, J. (2006). Strapping the hemiplegic shoulder prevents development of pain during rehabilitation: a randomized controlled trial. *Clinical Rehabilitation*, 20, 287–295.

Haggard, P. (2001). The psychology of action. *British Journal of Psychology*, 92, 113–128.

Hakkennes, S. & Keating, J. L. (2005). Constraint-induced movement therapy following stroke: A systematic review of randomised controlled trials. *Australian Journal of Physiotherapy*, 51, 221–231.

Harvey, L. (2008). *Management of spinal cord injuries: a guide for physiotherapists*. United States, Butterworth Heinemann.

Harvey, L., Herbert, R. & Crosbie, J. (2002). Does stretching induce lasting increases in joint ROM? A systematic review. *Physiotherapy Research International*, 7, 1–13.

Harvey, L., de Jong, I., Goehl, G. & Mardwedel, S. (2006). Twelve weeks of nightly stretch does not reduce thumb web-space contractures in people with a neurological condition: a randomised controlled trial. *The Australian Journal of Physiotherapy*. 52, 251–258.

Helsen-Starkes, J. L. & Hodges, N. J. (1998). Team sports and the theory of deliberate practice. *Journal of Sport and Exercise Psychology*, 20, 12–34.

Herbert, R. B. & Balnave, R. J. (1993). The effect of position of immobilisation on the resting length, resting stiffness and weight of rabbit soleus muscle. *Journal of Orthopaedic Research*, 11, 358–366.

Ho, L. & Shea, J. B. (1978). Effects of relative frequency of knowledge of results on retention of a motor skill. *Perceptual and Motor Skills*, 46, 859–866.

Hoare, B., Imms, C., Carey, L. & Wasiak, J. (2007). Constraint-induced movement therapy in the treatment of the upper limb in children with hemiplegic cerebral palsy: a Cochrane systematic review. *Clinical Rehabilitation*, 21, 675–685.

Jeannerod, M. (1984). The timing of natural prehension movements. *Journal of Motor Behaviour*, 26, 235–254.

Jeannerod, M. (1986). The formation of finger grip during prehension: a cortically mediated visuomotor pattern. *Behaviour and Brain Research*, 19, 99–116.

Kernodle, M. W. & Carlton, L. G. (1992). Information feedback and the learning of multiple-degree-of-freedom activities. *Journal of Motor Behaviour*, 24, 187–196.

Kilduski, N. C. & Rice, M. S. (2003). Qualitative and quantitative knowledge of results: Effects on motor learning. *American Journal of Occupational Therapy*, 57, 329–336.

Kwakkel, G. (2006). Impact of intensity of practice after stroke: Issues for consideration. *Disability and Rehabilitation*, 28, 823–830.

Lannin, N. A., Horsley, S. A., Herbert, R. et al (2003). Hand splinting in the functional position after brain impairment: A randomised controlled trial. *Archives of Physical Medicine and Rehabilitation*, 84, 297–302.

Lannin, N. A., Cusick, A., McCluskey, A. & Herbert, R. (2007). Effects of splinting on wrist contracture following stroke: a randomised controlled trial. *Stroke*, 38, 111–116.

Lee, T. D. & White, M. A. (1990). Influence of an unskilled model's practice schedule on observational motor learning. *Human Movement Science*, 9, 349–367.

Lehmann, A. C. & Ericsson, K.A. (1996). Music performance without preparation: Structure acquisition of expert sight reading. *Psychomusicology*, 15, 1–29.

Martenuik, R. G., Mackenzie, C. L., Jeannerod, M. et al (1987). Constraints on human arm movement trajectories. *Canadian Journal of Physiotherapy*, 4, 365–378.

Martenuik, R. G., Leavitt, J. L., Mackenzie, C. L. et al (1990). Functional relationships between grasp and transport components in a prehension task. *Human Movement Science*, 9, 149–176.

Mastos, M., Miller, K., Eliasson, A. C. et al (2007). Goal-directed training: linking theories of treatment to clinical practice for improved functional activities in daily life. *Clinical Rehabilitation*, 21, 47–55.

McLellan, D. L. (1977). Co-contraction and stretch reflexes in spasticity during treatment with Baclofen. *Journal of Neurology, Neurosurgery, and Psychiatry*, 40, 30–38.

McNevin, N. H., Wulf, G. & Carlson, C. (2000). Effects of attentional focus, self-control, and dyad training on motor learning: implications for physical rehabilitation. *Physical Therapy*, 80, 373–385.

Michaelsen, S. M., Dannenbaum, R. & Levin, M. F. (2006). Task-specific training with trunk restraint on arm recovery in stroke. *Stroke*, 27, 186–192.

Morris, D. M., Crago, J. E., Deluca, S. et al (1997). Constraint induced movement therapy for motor recovery after stroke. *Neurorehabilitation*, 9, 29–43.

Neilson, P. & McCaughey, J. (1982). Self-regulation of spasm in cerebral palsy. *Journal of Neurology, Neurosurgery and Psychiatry*, 45, 320–330.

Neistadt, M. (1994). The effect of different treatment activities on functional fine motor coordination in adults with brain injury. *American Journal of Occupational Therapy*, 48(10), 877–882.

Newell, K. M. (1976). Knowledge of results and motor learning. *Exercise and Sport Sciences Reviews*, 4, 195–228.

Nowak, D. A. & Hermsdorfer, J. (2003). Selective deficits of grip force during object manipulation in patients with reduced sensibility of the grasping digits. *Neuroscience Research*, 47, 65–72.

O'Dwyer, N. J., Ada, L. & Neilson, P. D. (1996). Spasticity and muscle contracture following stroke. *Brain*, 119, 1737–1749.

Pandyan, A. D., Cameron, M., Powell, J. et al (2003). Contractures in the post-stroke wrist: a pilot study of its time course of development and its association with upper limb recovery. *Clinical Rehabilitation*, 17(1), 88–95.

Pollock, A., Baer, G., Pomeroy, V. et al (2003). Physiotherapy treatment approaches for postural control and lower limb function following stroke. *The Cochrane Database of Systematic Reviews*, Issue 2.

Pomeroy, V. M., King, L., Pollock, A. et al (2006). Electrostimulation for promoting recovery of movement or functional ability after stroke. *The Cochrane Database of Systematic Reviews*, Issue 2.

Powell, J., Pandyan, D., Granat, M. et al (1999). Electrical stimulation of wrist extensors on poststroke hemiplegia. *Stroke*, 30, 1384–1389.

Prinz, W. (1997). Perception and action planning. *European Journal of Cognitive Psychology*, 9, 129–154.

Quaney, B. M., Perera, S., Maletsky, R., Luchies, C. W. & Nudo, R. J. (2005). Impaired grip force modulation in the ipsilesional hand after unilateral middle cerebral artery stroke. *Neurorehabilitation and Neural Repair*, 19, 338–349.

Refshauge, K. M., Ada, L. & Ellis, E. (Eds) (2005). *Science-based rehabilitation: theories into practice.* Edinburgh, Elsevier, Butterworth-Heinemann.

Reinkensmeyer, D. J., Emken, J. L. & Cramer, S. C. (2004). Robotics, motor learning, and neurologic recovery. *Annual Review of Biomedical Engineering*, 6, 497–525.

Reo, J. A. & Mercer, V. S. (2004). Effects of live, videotaped, or written instruction on learning an upper-extremity exercise program. *Physical Therapy*, 84, 622–633.

Schmidt, R. A. & Lee, T. D. (1999). *Motor control and learning. A behavioral emphasis.* Human Kinetics Champaign, IL.

Shea, C. H., Wright, D. L., Wulf, G. et al (2000). Physical and observational practice afford unique learning opportunities. *Journal of Motor Behavior*, 32, 27–36.

Sietsema, J. M., Nelson, D. L., Mulder, R. M. et al (1993). The use of a frame to promote arm reach in persons with traumatic brain injury. *American Journal of Occupational Therapy*, 47(1), 19–24.

Sommerfield, D. K., Eek, E. U. B., Svensson, A. K. et al (2003). Spasticity after stroke: its occurrence and association with motor impairments and activity limitations. *Stroke*, 35, 134–140.

Tabary, J. C., Tabary, J. C., Tardieu, C. et al (1972) Physiological and structural changes in the cat's soleus muscle due to immobilization at different lengths by plaster case. *Journal of Physiology (London)*, 224, 231–244.

Taub, E., Landesman Ramey, S., DeLuca, S. et al (2004). Efficacy of constraint-induced movement therapy for children with cerebral palsy with symmetric motor

impairment. *Pediatrics*, 113, 305–312.

Trudel, G., Himori, K., Goudreau, L. et al (2003). Measurement of articular cartilage surface irregularity in rat knee contracture. *Journal of Rheumatology*, 30, 2218–2225.

Turton, A. & Britton, E. (2005). A pilot randomized controlled trial of a daily muscle stretch regime to prevent contractures in the arm after stroke. *Clinical Rehabilitation*, 19, 600–612.

Tyson, S. & Kent, R. (2009). Orthotic devices after stroke and other non-progressive brain lesions. *The Cochrane Database of Systematic Reviews*, Issue 1, Art. No.: CD003694. DOI: 003610.001002/14651858. CD14003694.pub14651852.

van der Lee, J., Snels, I. A. K., Beckerman, H. et al (2001). Exercise therapy for arm function in stroke patients: A systematic review of randomised controlled trials. *Clinical Rehabilitation*, 15, 20–31.

van Vliet, P. M. (1998). *An investigation of reaching movements following stroke.* PhD thesis, University of Nottingham, Nottingham.

van Vliet, P. M. & Wulf, G. (2006). Extrinsic feedback for motor learning after stroke: what is the evidence? *Disability and Rehabilitation*, 28, 831–840.

Vattanasilp, W., Ada, L. & Crosbie, J. (2000). Contribution of thixotropy, spasticity and contracture to ankle stiffness after stroke. *Journal of Neurology, Neurosurgery and Psychiatry*, 69, 34–39.

Wallen, M., Ziviani, J., Herbert, R., Evans, R. & Novak, I. (2007). Modified constraint-induced therapy for children with hemiplegic cerebral palsy: A feasibility study. *Developmental Neurorehabilitation*, Oct 15, 1–10.

Williams, P. (1990). Use of intermittent stretch in the prevention of serial sarcomere loss in immobilised muscle. *Annals of Rheumatological Disease*, 49, 316–317.

Williams, P. E. & Goldspink, G. (1978) Changes in sarcomere length and physiological properties in immobilized muscle. *Journal of Anatomy*, 127, 459–468.

Willis, J. K., Morello, A., Davie, A. et al (2002). Forced use treatment of childhood hemiparesis. *Pediatrics*, 110, 94–96.

Wing, A. M., Turton, A., Fraser, C. (1986). Grasp size and accuracy of approach in reaching. *Journal of Motor Behaviour*, 18, 81–260.

Winstein, C. J. & Schmidt, R. A. (1990). Reduced frequency of knowledge of result enhances motor skill learning. *Journal of Experimental Psychology*, 16, 677–691.

Wu, C. Y., Trombly, C. A. & Lin, K. C. (1994). The relationship between occupational form and occupational performance: A kinematic perspective. *American Journal of Occupational Therapy*, 48, 679–688.

Wu, C. W., Seo, H. J. & Cohen, L. G. (2006). Influence of electric somatosensory stimulation on paretic-hand function in chronic stroke. *Archives of Physical Medicine and Rehabilitation Medicine*, 87, 351–357.

Yavuzer, G., Selles, R., Sezer, N. et al (2008). Mirror therapy improves hand function in subacute stroke: A randomized controlled trial. *Archives of Physical Medicine and Rehabilitation*, 89(3), 393–398.

Zoia, S., Pezzetta, E., Blason, L. et al (2006). A comparison of the reach-to-grasp movement between children and adults: a kinematic study. *Developmental Neuropsychology*, 30(2), 719–738.

Cognitive and perceptual strategies

Carolyn A. Unsworth

CHAPTER CONTENTS

Introduction 608

Why do people have problems with
cognition and perception? 608

How we make sense of the world:
Normal and abnormal cognition and
perception 609

   Attention and concentration. 609

   Memory and learning 609

   Metacognition and executive functions . . . 610

   Perception of a whole world – unilateral
   neglect 610

   Simple and complex perception 610

   Praxis 611

Frameworks for occupational therapy
when people have cognitive and
perceptual problems 611

Assessment strategies 613

   Pre-assessment considerations 614

   Standardised assessments 614

   Observation of performance (hypothesis
   testing) 620

Intervention strategies 621

Intervention strategies for specific
problems 628

   Problems with attention and
   concentration 628

   Remedial approach 628

   Compensatory approach 628

   Problems with memory and learning 628

Remedial approach 628

Compensatory approach 629

Problems with metacognition and
executive functions 629

Remedial approach 629

Compensatory approach 629

Problems with unilateral neglect 629

Remedial approach 629

Compensatory approach 630

Problems with simple and complex
   perception 630

Visual object agnosia 630

Anosognosia 630

Somatoagnosia 630

Right and left discrimination 630

Figure ground disorder 630

Form discrimination 630

Problems with praxis 631

Remedial approach 631

Compensatory approach 631

Community integration: the ultimate
goal of cognitive and perceptual
rehabilitation 631

Conclusion 631

SUMMARY

At some point during their career, nearly all
occupational therapists will work with a person
who has a cognitive or perceptual impairment
that produces difficulties in occupational
engagement. This person may be a child,
teenager, adult or older person, and the
occupational therapist may be working in a

hospital, community centre, school or residential care facility. The purpose of this chapter is to provide the reader with an overview of different types of cognitive and perceptual problems, a range of evaluation strategies that an occupational therapist may use, and ideas for implementing and evaluating therapy. The chapter is illustrated with the story of Jill and Vivian to provide detailed information on how an occupational therapist works with one individual who is experiencing occupational performance problems as a result of cognitive and perceptual problems. An occupational perspective is taken, so the chapter focuses on practical ideas for occupation-based assessment and intervention. However, the chapter also draws on the work of neuropsychologists, speech and language therapists, and occupational therapists (Árnadóttir 1990, Bradshaw & Mattingley 1995, Katz 1998, Lezak 1995, Ponsford 2004, Unsworth 1999).

KEY POINTS

- Following acquired brain damage, problems with thinking (cognition) and making sense of the world (perception) are relatively common.
- A variety of cognitive and perceptual problems can impact on peoples' ability to perform the occupations they want or need to do.
- People may have problems with attention and concentration, memory, executive functions, apraxia, unilateral neglect, agnosias, and complex perceptual problems.
- Occupational therapists who work with people who have cognitive and perceptual problems use a variety of theoretical approaches, such as theories of occupation and models of cognitive and perceptual rehabilitation, to guide therapy.
- There is a growing body of evidence to support a variety of interventions for people with cognitive and perceptual problems.

Introduction

Cognition and perception are capacities we take for granted. Being able to think, remember, learn and make sense of the world are fundamental to carrying out all our daily occupations. However, when disease, trauma, tumours, toxins or infection affect these abilities, the consequences can be devastating. While some degree of habilitation or rehabilitation is often possible, many people with cognitive and perceptual problems are not able to live alone, hold down paid employment or sustain a family life and relationships. These problems can produce great

personal difficulties, hardships and burden for family, and considerable financial cost to the individual, his or her family and the community (Unsworth 1999). Cognitive and perceptual problems are also very puzzling, and individuals and their family may be very confused about why, for example, the individual:

- can 'see' the breakfast tray on some occasions but not others
- can not put clothes on the correct body parts
- can not brush teeth despite intact motor skills and a perfect description of what to do
- can not seem to be able to learn to use a walking aid.

Occupational therapists are well placed to assist individuals who experience cognitive and perceptual problems to minimise or overcome the occupational impact of these problems and continue to lead meaningful lives as part of the community.

Cognition is usually defined as the capacities that enable us to 'think', which includes concentrating or paying attention, reasoning, remembering, and learning. Executive functions are sometimes discussed under this heading as well. Executive functions include the capacity to plan, manipulate information, initiate and terminate activities, recognise errors, problem solve, and think abstractly. Perception is the dynamic process of receiving the environment through sensory impulses (e.g. visual, auditory, tactile) and translating those impulses into meaning based on previous environmental experience/learning (Árnadóttir 1990, Grieve 1993). The resulting awareness of objects and experiences within the environment enables the individual to make sense out of a complex and constantly changing internal and external sensory environment (Sharpless 1982).

Why do people have problems with cognition and perception?

Occupational therapists work with individuals across the lifespan. Children may have problems with cognition and perception due to a variety of factors such as exposure to toxins while in utero or birth trauma. People with mental health disorders such as schizophrenia or chronic depression, neurological conditions such as Parkinson's disease or multiple sclerosis, and other degenerative diseases such as Alzheimer's disease, may also experience cognitive and perceptual problems. While the information contained in this chapter may be relevant to working with individuals who have these problems, the focus of this chapter is on working with adults who have acquired brain damage through the following mechanisms:

- tumours that are benign or malignant

- trauma resulting from motor vehicle accidents, falls, or violent incidents (e.g. sport, or gunshot)

- infections such as encephalitis

- anoxia as may occur following near-drowning, cardiopulmonary arrest or carbon monoxide poisoning

- toxins such as alcohol or substance abuse

- vascular disease, which may produce an infarct or haemorrhagic stroke.

The largest two groups of people who acquire cognitive and perceptual problems are persons who experience stroke and traumatic brain injury. Figures from the United States of America, United Kingdom and Australia are all similar, with Australian data provided here. Using self-reports from the 2001 National Health Survey, approximately 1.2% of those surveyed have had a stroke sometime in their lives, or 217,500 Australians. It is estimated that approximately 40,000–48,000 individuals have a stroke event annually. The majority (around 70%) of these are first-ever strokes. In addition, about 12,000 people who have previously experienced a stroke suffer another stroke every year (AIHW, 10 Mar 2007). It is estimated that in Australia, there are approximately 27,991 incidents of traumatic brain injury (TBI) each year (O'Connor & Cripps 1999) and from these, 4,368 people experience long-term disability as a result of TBI (Fortune & Wen 1999).

How we make sense of the world: Normal and abnormal cognition and perception

We make sense of the world by taking in information through our senses and combining it with what we already know and think. When these capacities are interrupted, the individual needs to learn new ways to understand the world, or adapt to it. Therapists must have a good understanding of the capacities normal individuals possess in order to work with individuals who are having problems. This section of the chapter provides an overview of some of the main kinds of cognitive and perceptual capacities and problems.

Attention and concentration

Following brain damage, problems with attention/concentration are the most frequently reported deficits (Cicerone 1996, van Zomeren & Brouwer 1994). Even individuals with mild brain damage often complain of slowed thinking, being more easily distracted, and having trouble doing more than one thing at a time (Cicerone 1996). Attention/concentration is generally referred to as existing in three forms: sustained, focused (selective), and divided/alternating.

Sometimes referred to as a concentration span, sustained concentration is the capacity to attend to relevant information during occupations. A person who has problems with this kind of concentration may report that they start to read the newspaper and then 'just drift off'.

Problems with focused attention/concentration are often referred to as distractibility. The capacity to selectively attend/concentrate requires the individual to disregard irrelevant environmental visual or auditory stimuli.

Alternating attention/concentration is the capacity to move flexibly between tasks and respond appropriately to the demands of each task. Divided attention is the capacity to respond simultaneously to two or more tasks. Divided attention is required when more than one response is required or more than one stimulus needs to be monitored (Mateer 1996). Individuals who have difficulty with alternating and divided forms of attention/concentration may also have great difficulties with more complex daily living activities such as cooking a meal or driving.

Memory and learning

Memory may be broadly defined as the capacity to store experiences and perceptions for recall and recognition. Memory comprises acquisition or learning, storage or retention, and retrieval or recall (Abreu 1999).

Learning has been described as a relatively permanent change in the capacity for responding which, resulting from practice and experience, persists with time, resists environmental changes, and can be generalised in response to new tasks and situations (Schmidt 1988). Learning is crucial in rehabilitation.

Using a temporal taxonomy, three levels of memory are often described: immediate recall, short-term memory, and long-term memory (Abreu 1999). Immediate recall involves retention of information that has been stored for a few seconds. Short-term memory mediates retention of events or learning that has taken place within a few minutes, hours or days (Lezak 1995). Long-term memory consists of early experiences and information acquired over a period of years. Individuals who do not have long-term memory are often described as having amnesia.

Metacognition and executive functions

Metacognition is generally the term used to describe an individual's knowledge about their ability to think. Executive functions are often referred to as an individual's ability to start and stop behaviour, persist at a task or switch as needed, plan, be flexible, self monitor and think abstractly (Winegardner 1993, Zinn et al 2007).

Lezak (1995) proposed that executive functions consist of four overlapping components: volition (the capacity to determine what one needs and wants to do and conceptualise a future realisation of one's needs and wants); planning (identifying and organising the steps and elements such as skills, material or other people needed to do something or achieve a goal); purposive action (capacities for productivity and self-regulation, including the ability to structure an effective and fluent course of action by initiating, maintaining, switching, and stopping complex action sequences in an orderly manner to realise a goal); and effective performance (capacity for quality control, including the ability to self-monitor and self-correct one's behaviour).

Perception of a whole world – unilateral neglect

Intact perception enables us to perceive the whole world and attend to all the information in it. Following acquired brain damage, difficulties with attending to the body or space in one hemisphere is termed unilateral neglect. Unilateral neglect (some-times referred to as hemi inattention, unilateral visual inattention or visual neglect) is most often seen following damage to the right cerebral hemisphere (Vallar 1993).

Persons with neglect may appear not to perceive or to ignore auditory, visual or tactile stimuli coming from the opposite (contralesional) side of space, despite intact sensory abilities. Paradoxically, such persons may be over-attentive to and distracted by stimuli coming from the ipsilesional side.

Perhaps the most perplexing aspect of the phenomenon of neglect is that individuals can be unaware of this deficit. It seems as though half of the world has ceased to exist. In some cases, this may extend to the point where a person may deny any dysfunction or the presence of paresis. This particular problem is referred to as anosognosia (Gialanella et al 2005, Halligan & Marshall 1993).

Simple and complex perception

Disorders of perception are often classified as either simple or complex. Individuals with simple perceptual problems are often described as having an agnosia or an inability to recognise or make sense of incoming information despite intact sensory capacities (Bauer & Rubens 1993).

Agnosias are often classified according to the sensory modality that is affected. The main types of agnosias are alexia or 'word blindness' (an acquired inability to comprehend written language) (Friedman et al 1993); auditory agnosia (the inability to distinguish between sounds, or to recognise familiar sounds); colour agnosia (the inability to associate objects with particular colours); prosopagnosia (the inability to recognise familiar faces despite intact sensory abilities (Bauer & Rubens 1993)); simultanagnosia (difficulty in recognising the elements of a visual array (Ellis & Young 1988)); tactile agnosia or astereognosis (inability to recognise objects by touch alone with vision occluded); and visual object agnosia (the inability to recognise objects by looking at them, despite intact vision).

Complex perceptual functions include body scheme abilities and visuospatial functioning. Body scheme abilities are defined as perception of body position, including and involving relation of body parts to each other. Unilateral neglect, as described above, is frequently described as a difficulty with complex perception. Visuospatial abilities are defined as the ability to relate objects to each other, or to the self. This includes spatial perceptions, object relationships (sometimes combined and referred to as spatial relations), constructional abilities, figure ground discrimination, form discrimination, perception of depth, unilateral spatial attention, as well as topographical orientation.

Praxis

Praxis is the capacity to carry out learned skilled movements. Apraxia then, is an inability to perform purposeful movements and these difficulties cannot be accounted for by inadequate strength, loss of coordination, impaired sensation, attentional difficulties, abnormal tone, movement disorders, intellectual deterioration, poor comprehension, or uncooperativeness (Croce 1993, Kirshner 1991, Tate & McDonald 1995). Apraxia is more common following left hemisphere damage, and so many individuals with this problem also present with aphasia (Lezak 1995). Two main forms of apraxia discussed in the literature are ideomotor and ideational apraxia. A third form, buccofacial or oral apraxia, is actually a type of ideomotor apraxia and is characterised by difficulties with performing the purposeful movements that involve facial muscles related to the mouth (Bradshaw & Mattingley 1995).

Ideomotor apraxia refers to a breakdown between the concept of what to do and the actual performance. An individual with ideomotor apraxia may be able to carry out habitual tasks automatically and describe how they are done but is unable to imitate gestures or perform on command (Mozaz et al 1990, Raade et al 1991).

On the other hand, ideational apraxia is a failure to conceptualise what is to be done. The individual is unable to perform a purposeful movement either automatically or on command. In many cases, the individual can perform isolated components of a task, but can not combine them into a complete act. Finally, the person can not verbally describe the process of performing an activity (Mayer et al 1990).

Frameworks for occupational therapy when people have cognitive and perceptual problems

In 2001, the World Health Organisation (WHO) revised its classification of health states and proposed the International Classification of Function (ICF). This system is adopted widely by health care professionals and provides an ideal foundation for occupational therapists to organise practice and describe it to others (see for example, College of Occupational Therapists 2004 and Australian Institute of Health and Welfare 2003). For example, using ICF terminology for individuals who have cognitive and perceptual problems, impairment (or problems with body structure and function) is the term used to describe memory problems, apraxia or perceptual problems. These impairments produce activity limitations which are the resulting problems an individual may experience when performing daily occupations such as dressing, driving, or typing on the computer. Depending on how the individual is able to interact with society, activity limitations may lead to participation restrictions, or handicap. Once impairments have been identified, the emphasis for occupational therapists is on assessing and treating the individual's activity limitations/occupational performance and assisting the individual to minimise the participation restrictions that may result. These levels of function are also mitigated by barriers and facilitators and the environment.

In addition to using an ICF framework, an occupational therapist will select an overarching occupational therapy theory to guide practice such as the Canadian Model of Occupational Performance and Engagement (Townsend & Polatajko 2007), or the Model of Human Occupation (Kielhofner 2002) and a practice model specific to working with people who have cognitive and perceptual problems. The selection of a practice model is particularly crucial as this will guide the kinds of evaluations and interventions that the therapist will undertake (Unsworth 1999). One of the main differences between practice models is whether they adopt a remedial and adaptive approach to therapy.

The main practice models that a therapist could use when working with individuals who have cognitive and perceptual problems have been comprehensively reviewed (Katz 1998, Unsworth 1999) and include; the Dynamic Interaction Approach (Toglia 1992), the Retraining Approach (Averbuch & Katz 1992), which are primarily remedial; the Neurofunctional Approach (Giles & Wilson 1992), and Compensatory/Rehabilitation Approach (Fisher 1997a, Trombly 1995) which are primarily adaptive; and the Quadraphonic Approach (Abreu 1990) which combines aspects that are both remedial and adaptive.

The Practice Scenario of Vivian and her occupational therapist, Jill, is used to illustrate this chapter (see Practice Scenario 38.1). Following an introduction to Vivian and Jill, the theoretical frameworks adopted by Jill are described. Since Jill uses the Occupational Performance process Model (Townsend et al 1997) the case study follows the seven stages of practice outlined in the model (Table 38.1). These stages are clearly identified throughout the Practice Scenario. This model is currently in revision (Townsend & Polatajko 2007).

Practice Scenario 38.1
Introducing Vivian and her occupational therapist, Jill

Stage 1 – Issues

Vivian was assigned to Jill's caseload. Jill is a senior therapist and has worked on the neurological rehabilitation team at the facility for 17 years. Jill consulted Vivian's medical record where some notes had been made by the admission team. Vivian is a 65-year-old

Table 38.1 The seven stages of the Occupational Performance Process Model (Fearing et al 1997, Townsend et al 1997)

Stage number	Topic	Description
1	Identify occupational performance issues known	Through reading case notes and meeting with the individual, identify occupational performance issues related to self care, productivity and leisure Simply put: Identify why the person has come to see you
2	Select theoretical approaches to guide practice	Choose an overarching model and specific practice models that can guide your practice. For example you might use the Model of Human Occupation (MOHO) or the Canadian Model of Occupational Performance and Engagement (CMOP-E) as an overarching model and then the Occupational Performance Process Model and Retraining Model or Rehabilitation Model as practice models Simply put: Select theories to provide a framework for practice
3	Identify occupational performance components and environmental conditions	Through a variety of evaluation processes, the therapist and person identify the occupational performance components and environmental conditions that contribute to the occupational issues identified in Stage 1 Simply put: Choose assessments to be used, administer them and summarise the findings
4	Nominate strengths and weaknesses	This is the problem list, and also information on strengths and resources of the individual and the therapist Simply put: Develop a list of the individual's strengths and weaknesses, and identify therapist strengths as well
5	Negotiate targeted outcomes and develop a plan of action	The therapist and individual develop an action plan for therapy Simply put: Develop long-term goals and short-term objectives to guide therapy
6	Implement plans through occupation	Intervention plans are implemented, reviewed and modified on an ongoing basis Simply put: Implement intervention programme
7	Evaluate occupational performance outcomes	Outcomes are identified. If targeted outcomes have been achieved, the service ends. If outcomes have not been achieved targets are reviewed and a new plan may be made, repeating the above process Simply put: Evaluate the success of intervention: did you meet goals and objectives? Is the person satisfied with the outcomes? Are significant others satisfied with the outcomes?

Resolved: the individual is discharged
Unresolved: return to Stage 1

divorced woman who was admitted to an acute care facility following a right parietal infarct (stroke). After 4 days, she was discharged to the current specialist rehabilitation facility. On admission to the facility, she showed signs of mild, resolving hemiparesis of the left upper and lower limbs and some reduced co-ordination. Jill read that Vivian had been previously in good health, although she had been involved in a minor car accident 5 years ago in which her right leg was broken. It appears that as a result of this injury she experiences ongoing stiffness and minor pain, which seems to be aggravated by cold weather.

Jill conducted an interview with Vivian. Jill gathered information about Vivian's family and family commitments, daily life routines, habits, work, home life and interests, and began to form a picture of who Vivian is as a person and what she wants to achieve. Jill learned that Vivian retired 1 year ago from her job as a secondary school teacher of Spanish and history, and lives with one of her three sons in a single-level home that she rents. She also has a 36-year-old son who lives interstate, and a 40-year-old son with schizophrenia and an intellectual disability who recently moved from living with Jill to residential care. Vivian disclosed that her financial situation was adequate and that she did not have any worries about this hospital stay. Vivian stated that she enjoys lawn bowls, reading the daily papers, painting and drawing, and often goes to the local community centre where there is a Spanish club and discussion group.

Through administering the Canadian Occupational Performance Measure (Law et al 1998) with Vivian, Jill finds that Vivian does not think her problems are very severe, and that she should be able to return home in a few days. Vivian identifies that what she most looks forward to doing on her return home is being able to attend her Spanish group where she has many friends, visit her son in the residential care facility and return to her usual home jobs such as caring for the house and cooking evening meals for her son. Vivian previously drove to Spanish group and to visit her son, and thinks there will be no problems with this.

During the interview Jill became concerned that Vivian seemed to focus just on the right side, and that her clothing was falling off on the left. When Jill moved to a chair on the left of Vivian, Vivian seemed to think Jill had left the room. This information indicated to Jill that Vivian might be experiencing a unilateral neglect. Jill considered that this was consistent with the site of Vivian's stroke in the right parietal lobe.

Stage 2 – Select theoretical approaches

Jill uses the Occupational Performance Process Model from the Canadian Model of Occupational Performance and Engagement (Townsend & Polatajko 2007) to guide her therapy and adopts the retraining approach (Averbuch & Katz 1992) as a practice model. When an individual's performance in daily occupations has plateaued and she is working towards a home discharge, Jill often turns to a rehabilitation frame of reference (Trombly 1995) to finalise her therapeutic interventions. Hence, Jill believes in neural plasticity of the brain, and that skills taught in one environment can generalise to others. However, when an individual's performance has plateaued and discharge is imminent, Jill becomes more pragmatic in her approach and begins to modify the environment and arrange for home services to do the tasks the person cannot complete.

Consistent with these theoretical approaches, Jill usually administers standardised cognitive and perceptual assessments such as those identified in Table 38.2 during Stage 3, and a Canadian Occupational Performance Measure (COPM) (Law et al 1998) during Stage 1. However, since many people with cognitive and perceptual problems can have limited insight into the nature and extent of their problems, Jill has found articles such as the one by Hobson (1996), which discusses enhancing person-centred practice when the person has cognitive and perceptual problems, useful in guiding practice.

Assessment strategies

Once the therapist has selected an appropriate theoretical orientation, the assessments and interventions that follow are logically linked to that approach. Hence, a therapist using a remedial retraining approach will probably select assessments such as the Lowenstein Occupational Therapy Cognitive Assessment (LOTCA) (Averbuch & Katz 1992), or the Rivermead Behavioural Memory Test (RBMT) (Wilson et al 1991). Conversely, a therapist using a compensatory rehabilitative approach may consider the Assessment of Motor and Process Skills (AMPS) (Fisher 1997b) as the assessment of choice.

The purpose of administering an assessment may include one or more of the following; identify the individual's problem areas, establish a baseline for intervention, provide information for intervention planning, or to predict performance in activities of daily living. The assessments described in this chapter will assist the therapist to determine which cognitive and perceptual abilities are intact and which are limited. The importance of accurate and thorough assessment cannot be over-emphasised. Hence, this section of the chapter describes the importance of screening the person for motor and sensory problems prior to assessment of cognitive and perceptual problems, and discusses some of the non-cognitive/perceptual related issues that may influence assessment results and therefore must be factored into the evaluation process. Finally, a selection of standardised assessments is presented, and a hypothesis-testing approach to identifying an individual's cognitive and perceptual problems is outlined.

Pre-assessment considerations

Before assessing an individual for the presence of cognitive or perceptual problems, the therapist must have initially determined if the person has any sensory or physical deficits such as a sensory loss, language impairment, hearing loss, motor loss (weakness, spasticity, incoordination), visual disturbance (poor eyesight, homonymous hemianopia), disorientation, or lack of comprehension. The therapist needs to be able to distinguish between these kinds of physical and sensory problems and problems which are of a cognitive or perceptual nature. For example, if the therapist has not completed a sensory assessment, she will be unable to determine if a person with stroke wearing a blindfold cannot recognise the item before them due to a tactile sensory loss or an agnosia.

Assessment should also not commence until the individual is medically stable, not in a state of post-traumatic amnesia (a period of confusion and disorientation which follows traumatic brain injury, but not stroke, during which a person does not have the capacity to form new memories), and is psychologically and emotionally ready for assessment. The therapist needs to be aware of behaviours that reflect a person's psychological response to illness rather than particular cognitive or perceptual abilities. Anxiety over capabilities may inhibit a person's optimal performance during assessment and therapy, and therapists should spend time reassuring individuals of a positive outcome, regardless of assessment results. Finally, depression, fatigue and medication can also reduce an individual's performance during assessment and the therapist should try to take these factors into account when interpreting assessment results. For example, following stroke, 30 to 50% (Pak & Dombrovy 1994) of people are said to experience depression, and these symptoms can easily be mistaken for cognitive or perceptual problems.

Finally, it should be noted that not all areas of performance loss are typically detected within the hospital setting. It is not uncommon for the person to perform adequately in self-care skills after therapy in the hospital but to fail on the same tasks in other environmental contexts, such as the home. Higher-level tasks, such as driving, banking, or planning a meal may only emerge as areas of difficulty once the person is discharged home. When appropriate, the person's competence in these areas should be considered within the context of instrumental activities of daily living (IADL) assessment.

Standardised assessments

A standardised assessment has a uniform procedure to administer and score the assessment so that the tester can be confident that every time the assessment is administered, it is done so in the same way. Standardised assessments also have a method for referencing an individual's scores, or determining how well or badly they have done (Anastasi 1988, de Clive-Lowe 1996) using normative data (a norm-referenced assessment) (de Clive-Lowe 1996) or pre-determined criteria (criterion-referenced assessment).

When selecting a standardised assessment the therapist must consider many factors such as what the therapist wants to learn about the person, and what the assessment can potentially reveal (Unsworth 1999). In many cases a single assessment will not provide all the information required by a therapist to plan intervention, so several assessments may be administered. Table 38.2 outlines several screening or battery assessments that are commonly used by occupational therapists to assess an individual's cognitive and perceptual status.

Several other global outcome measures could also be used to measure the outcome of the person's rehabilitation such as the Medical Outcomes Study (MOS), Short Form Health Survey (SF-36) (Ware & Sherbourne 1992), Australian Therapy Outcome Measures AusTOMs (Unsworth & Duncombe 2007, Unsworth, 2005), The Canadian Occupational Performance Measure (COPM) (Law et al 1998), Rivermead Rehabilitation Centre Life Goals

Table 38.2 Summary of key features of standardised assessments used with people who have cognitive and perceptual problems

Assessment	Purpose/content	Developed by an OT	Used with remedial, adaptive or both approaches	Training required	Uses ADL	Is partial administration recommended	Evidence of test–retest reliability, inter-rater reliability	Evidence of content validity, criterion validity, construct validity	Time to administer (minutes)
1. A-ONE (Árnadóttir 1990)	Developed to measure a person's neurobehaviour through daily living tasks (dressing, grooming, hygiene, transfer and mobility, feeding, and communication). A wide variety of cognitive and perceptual impairments can be detected with this assessment	Yes	Remedial (both)	Yes	Yes	Yes	Preliminary data / Yes	Yes / No / Yes	30–40
2. SOTOF (Laver Powell 1995)	Designed to assess older persons' level of occupational performance and neuropsychological functioning following neurological damage of cortical origin. Consists of a screening assessment, neuropsychological checklist, and four ADL scales (eating from a bowl, pouring a drink and drinking, putting on an upper body garment, and washing and drying hands)	Yes	Remedial (both)	No	Yes	No	Yes / Yes	Yes / Yes / Preliminary	45

(cont'd)

Table 38.2 Summary of key features of standardised assessments used with people who have cognitive and perceptual problems—cont'd

Assessment	Purpose/content	Developed by an OT	Used with remedial, adaptive or both approaches	Training required	Uses ADL	Is partial administration recommended	Evidence of test-retest reliability, inter-rater reliability	Evidence of content validity, criterion validity, construct validity	Time to administer (minutes)
3. AMPS (Fisher 1997a)	A structured, observational evaluation of a person's performance in daily living activities. The therapist observes the person's performance on two or three familiar personal or instrumental activities of daily living of their choice and then rates the quality of this performance in terms of how effortless, efficient, safe, or independent the person's ADL motor and ADL process skills are in the context of the task performance (the dynamic interaction of the person with the environment)	Yes	Adaptive (both)	Yes	Yes	No	Yes Yes	Yes Yes Yes	30–60
4. ACL (Allen 1990)	Following an interview to gain information concerning the person's educational and work background, the person is observed performing the visuomotor task of leather lacing. Used as a screening tool to estimate a person's cognitive level. Although originally developed for use with people who have psychiatric problems, this assessment is also used with people who have acquired brain damage, or experience a dementing illness such as Alzheimer's disease	Yes	Adaptive	No	Yes	No	Yes Yes	Preliminary Yes Preliminary	20

5. COTNAB (Tyerman et al 1986)	Designed to assess cognitive and perceptual deficits in individuals aged 16 years and over following stroke or head injury. Consists of 12 tests divided into four sections assessing visual perception, constructional ability, sensory-motor ability, and ability to follow instructions	Yes	Remedial (both)	No	No	No	Yes Preliminary data	No No Preliminary	60–80
6. RPAB (Whiting et al 1985)	Assesses visual perceptual deficits in people following head injury or stroke. Consists of 16 performance tests that assess form discrimination, colour constancy, sequencing, object completion, figure-ground discrimination, body image, inattention, and spatial awareness	Yes	Remedial (both)	No	No	No	Yes Yes	Yes Yes Yes	60
7. BIT (Wilson et al 1987)	Assesses individuals for the presence of unilateral visual neglect and provides the therapist with information concerning how the neglect impacts the person's ability to perform everyday occupations. The BIT consists of nine activity-based subtests and six pen-and-paper subtests	No	Remedial (both)	No	No	Yes	Yes Yes	Preliminary Yes No	60

(cont'd)

Table 38.2 Summary of key features of standardised assessments used with people who have cognitive and perceptual problems—cont'd

Assessment	Purpose/content	Developed by an OT	Used with remedial, adaptive or both approaches	Training required	Uses ADL	Is partial administration recommended	Evidence of test–retest reliability, inter-rater reliability	Evidence of content validity, criterion validity, construct validity	Time to administer (minutes)
8. LOTCA (Itzkovich et al 1990)	Battery-style assessment composed of 20 subtests that assess four areas: orientation, visual and spatial perception, visuomotor organisation, and thinking operations	Yes	Remedial (both)	No	No	No	No Yes	Yes Yes Yes	30–45
9. RBMT (Wilson et al 1991)	Assesses a person's everyday memory abilities. It offers the therapist an initial assessment of the individual's memory function, an indication of appropriate areas for treatment, and enables the therapist to monitor memory skills throughout the treatment programme	No	Remedial (both)	No	No	No	Yes Yes	Yes Yes Yes	30
10. BADS (Wilson et al 1996)	Measures everyday executive function and higher-level cognitive functions. Includes six subtests and a 20-item questionnaire	No	Remedial	No	Some	No	Yes Yes	Yes Yes Yes	30–45

	Description											Time
11. TEA (Robertson et al 1994)	Measures selective attention, sustained attention, and attentional switching. Includes eight ADL-based subtests such as elevator counting, map and telephone book searching, and lottery tickets	No	Remedial	No	Some	No	Yes	Preliminary	Yes	Yes	Yes	45–60
12. COGNISTAT (Kiernan et al 1987)	Cognitive screening assessment. Items include measures of attention, level of consciousness and orientation, language, memory, calculations, and reasoning	No	Remedial	No	No	No	Yes	Yes	Yes	Yes	Yes	10–30
13. OT-APST (Cook 2005)	Visual perception screening assessment of 25 items in the areas of agnosia, visuospatial skill (including awareness of body scheme and unilateral neglect, constructional skill, apraxia and acalculia	Yes	Remedial (both)	No	No	No	Yes	Yes	Yes	Yes	Yes	20–25

A-ONE (Árnadóttir – Occupational Therapy Neurobehavioural Evaluation); SOTOF (Structured Observational Test of Function); ACL (Allen Cognitive Level Test); COTNAB (Chessington Occupational Therapy Neurological Assessment Battery); LOTCA (Loewenstein Occupational Therapy Cognitive Assessment); BIT tthe Behavioural Inattention Test); RPAB (Rivermead Perceptual Assessment Battery); RBMT (Rivermead Behavioural Memory Test); TEA (Test of Everyday Attention); COGNISTAT (Neurobehavioral Cognitive Status Screening Examination); OT-APST (Occupational Therapy Adult Perceptual Screening Test).

Questionnaire (Davis et al 1992), Reintegration to Normal Living Index (RNL) (Wood-Dauphinee 1988) or the Functional Independence Measure (Adult FIM SM) (Guide for the Uniform Data Set for Medical Rehabilitation 1999). Some of these assessments also incorporate items that measure cognition and perception. For example, the FIM includes three cognition-related items: memory, problem solving, and social interaction.

Observation of performance (hypothesis testing)

Gathering information about an individual's cognitive and perceptual problems while they are engaged in everyday occupations can be another useful way to assess a person. Referred to as hypothesis testing, this is a systematic approach to observing an individual's performance and considering the kinds of cognitive and perceptual impairments that may be present. A detailed description of this process is documented in Unsworth (1999) and an overview is presented here.

This approach has many similarities to the dynamic interaction approach to assessment developed by Toglia (1992). In both of these assessment procedures, the therapist selects an activity to undertake with the person, and proposes a hypothesis which is then tested. While the hypothesis-testing approach cannot replace standardised assessments, the approach remains useful for therapists who are not trained to use assessments such as the A-ONE or AMPS, or for students and less experienced therapists to use in conjunction with other standardised assessments. The steps in the hypothesis-testing approach include:

1. Observe the person performing an occupation (such as dressing or grooming or making a snack) and identify problem areas.

2. Consider the individual's strengths and weaknesses known at this stage.

3. Generate a single or multiple hypotheses that explain the individual's problems.

4. Select an occupation of daily living to test the hypothesis/es.

5. The therapist structures the occupation in order to control some of the variables present and manipulate or alter the relative presence or absence of others. In this way, changes can be

introduced which allow the therapist to exclude alternative or competing explanations or hypotheses for the person's difficulties. This will lead to confirmation or rejection of the hypotheses.

6. The therapist examines the data and accepts or rejects each hypothesis, or may return to the first step to re-define the problem and generate new hypotheses. The information gained during hypothesis testing supplements information gained during standardised assessment.

Practice Scenario 38.2 illustrates several approaches to assessment, including standardised assessments and hypothesis testing.

Practice Scenario 38.2 Assessing Vivian

Stage 3 – Identify occupational components and environmental conditions

Given the issues noted by Jill during the initial interview, she decided to conduct a Visual Confrontation Test (Gainotti et al 1991, Pedretti 1985) and Extinction Test (as developed by Lynn Robertson and cited in Rafal 1994) a Behavioural Inattention Test (BIT) (Wilson et al 1987) (Figure 38.1) and hypothesis testing assessment during making a cup of tea (Figures 38.2 and Table 38.3). Table 38.3 outlines the first three steps in the hypothesis identification process.

In Table 38.3, the hypotheses that Jill thinks are the best at this stage are underlined in the third column. Following this, Jill will select a new activity and test out her hypotheses. For example, Jill could test out these hypotheses during grooming. Jill needs to manipulate task demands in order to test her hypotheses. Since Jill has hypothesised that Vivian may have some short-term memory problems, she could test this out by asking Vivian the steps she needs to follow for grooming and then provide a written or pictorial list of these steps. If Vivian's performance improves when following the chart, this supports the hypothesis of a short-term memory problem.

Jill could also quickly test out her competing hypotheses of whether Vivian has a unilateral neglect or visual object agnosia by laying out three objects on Vivian's right side (toothpaste, lipstick and deodorant) and three on her left (brush, comb, soap). Jill could then ask Vivian to name all the items in front of her. If Vivian can name the three items on her right, this disconfirms the hypothesis of visual object either side as presented during the confrontation test. However, when presented with simultaneous stimuli (that is stimuli from both sides) the individual may respond only to the stimulus on the non-neglected side, thus 'extinguishing' stimuli on the neglected side. It has also been noted that extinction may be more subtle and resilient than a unilateral neglect (Robertson & Eglin 1993). In people with HH, simultaneous extinction is not present, since individuals will never see stimuli on the left side. Finally, during activities of daily living, a consistent loss is noted in individuals with HH. However, people with UN show an inconsistent performance as they are able to respond appropriately to some stimuli but not others.

Jill also conducted a brief physical and sensory evaluation with Vivian and found Vivian's right body side had normal sensation and motor control (although some stiffness resulting from the orthopaedic injuries sustained in the car accident). While Vivian has full passive and active range of motion in her left arm, her strength was reduced. She also demonstrated some reduced co-ordination and fine motor skills, and altered sensation on the left. Jill also worked on these issues with Vivian; however, it is beyond the scope of this chapter to include discussions on assessment and treatment of Vivian's physical and sensory problems.

Stage 4 – Identify strengths and resources

Following all assessments (initial interview, COPM, the BIT, Extinction Test, Visual Confrontation Test and hypothesis testing) Jill reasoned that while Vivian did have a neglect with extinction, there was no evidence of homonymous hemianopia. The assessments also revealed some difficulties with divided attention/concentration, mild short-term memory problems and difficulties with insight to her problems. Jill felt confident in identifying these problems and decided to pursue goal setting rather than conduct further standardised tests such as the Rivermead Behavioural Memory Test (RBMT) (Wilson et al 1991).

Jill drew up Table 38.4 as a summary of Vivian's strengths and problems to work on in therapy based on the ICF framework (please note that this table omits sensory and physical problems).

Intervention strategies

Once a particular theoretical orientation has been decided upon, therapists can confidently direct therapy towards remedial or compensatory interventions. However, many therapists who commence intervention using a remedial approach may

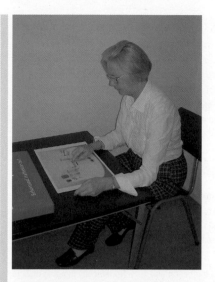

Figure 38.1 • Vivian undertaking the Behavioural Inattention Test (Wilson et al 1987)

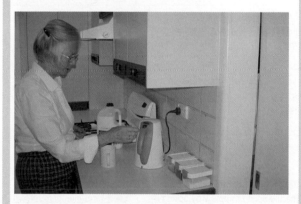

Figure 38.2 • Vivian making a cup of tea during the hypothesis testing procedure

agnosia and supports the hypothesis of unilateral neglect.

When administering the visual confrontation test, Jill looks to see if the person may have a left homonymous hemianopia (HH) as well as a left unilateral neglect (UN). When a person has an HH, the person has a sensory-based, visual problem meaning that she/he can not see. However, in a unilateral neglect, the person can 'see' but cannot attend to this information. Other differences between an HH and a UN are that individuals with HH often have insight to their visual loss and people with UN, like Vivian, do not.

Another way to distinguish between individuals with HH and UN is whether the phenomenon of extinction is present. Extinction is evident when the person can attend to isolated stimuli coming from

Table 38.3 Findings from hypothesis testing activity of making a cup of tea

Problem occupation	Observations	Hypotheses
Vivian (V) chose to make a cup of tea with milk and sugar in the occupational therapy kitchen	Jill shows V where the tea-making things are located in the OT kitchen. V talks about liking tea and how she takes it (white with half a teaspoon of sugar). She says she needs to get a tea bag, sugar and spoon and milk, and comments that the tea bags and sugar are on the bench	Good planning skills
	V then turns on the kettle, Jill reminds her to check if it's full first	Unfamiliar kitchen – Vivian probably has her jug full at home Problem-solving difficulties
	V turns kettle off, opens the lid and states that it is sufficiently full	Shows some problem-solving skills
	V finds the tea bags and sugar containers on the right side of the bench and opens these. States 'I'm just waiting for the kettle to boil'	No difficulty locating objects on the right side
	Jill asks if she needs anything else. Vivian states 'Oh yes, I need milk'	Short-term memory problem
	V turns around and seems to look around the kitchen. She asks Jill where the fridge is (the fridge is on V's left side). Jill prompts V to look at each object around the kitchen and she then locates the fridge	Unilateral neglect Visual object agnosia
	V opens the fridge with her right hand. The fridge handle is at waist height on the right side of the fridge, and the door opens to the left. The milk is on the door on V's left. V spends several minutes looking in the fridge and moves several objects on her right side to look behind them	Unilateral neglect Visual object agnosia
	On hearing the kettle boil, splutter and turn off, Vivian shuts the fridge, and walks back to the kettle saying 'The water's ready now'	Concentration problem (selective) Short-term memory problem
	V then asks the therapist for a cup. The therapist tells her the location and V finds one easily in the cupboard above. The therapist prompts V by asking if they have everything they need. With prompting, V eventually replies they need milk	Unilateral neglect Short-term memory problem
	V finds the fridge again, and with prompting, and positioning of V's hand on the top of the fridge door, V takes several minutes to locate the milk. V and Jill walk back to the bench. V places the large milk container in the middle of the bench and Jill moves it to the left	
	V then takes out a tea bag and places it in the cup, pours in water, and then asks where the milk has gone. Jill stands on V's left and taps the bench next to the milk and asks V to draw her attention to that side of the bench. V states again that she cannot find the milk, and Jill guides V's right hand over to it. V 'states 'Oh! there it is'	Unilateral neglect
	V then asks Jill for a spoon for the sugar, and Jill directs V to find the drawers on V's right. The spoon is located on the left side of the drawer. V states this must be the wrong drawer, she turns to Jill and then when she turns back to the drawer sees the spoon which is now on her right side. V places the sugar in the cup, stirs and drinks the tea. She uses her right hand throughout the task	Unilateral neglect

Table 38.4 Vivian's strength and problem list drawn from hypothesis testing and standardised assessments – using ICF framework

IMPAIRMENTS	CAPACITIES
• Unilateral neglect (with extinction) • Concentration/attention (some distractibility) • Memory – short term	• Communication (expressive and receptive) • Walks independently • Intact vision
ACTIVITY LIMITATIONS (DISABILITIES)	ACTIVITY STRENGTHS (ABILITIES)
• Personal Activities of Daily Living (ADL) (e.g. showering, grooming, dressing, eating) • Instrumental ADL (e.g. domestic activities such as cooking, telephone use and cleaning the house, and community activities such as driving, shopping, banking)	• Aspects of personal ADL, such as toileting
PARTICIPATION/PARTICIPATION RESTRICTIONS	ENVIRONMENTAL RESOURCES (family, community and organisational supports):
• These are unknown at this stage and require examination closer to the time of discharge	• Spanish group members (have visited) • Son (with whom Vivian lives) • Vivian's son is being cared for in a residential care facility (Vivian is very happy with the care provided)

introduce compensatory ideas and strategies with the individual once progress has plateaued, or when discharge is imminent. The following section of the chapter introduces a variety of remedial and compensatory intervention ideas and strategies when working with individuals who have cognitive and perceptual dysfunction. While there is research evidence to support some of these techniques, a great deal more research is required to support occupational therapy practice in this area. Possible interventions that may be used with Vivian are presented in Practice Scenario 38.3.

Practice Scenario 38.3
Intervention and evaluation of therapy outcomes with Vivian

Stage 5 – Negotiate targeted outcomes and developing action plans

Based on her problem list and the findings from administering a Canadian Occupational Performance Measure (COPM) (Law et al 1998), Jill and Vivian began to set goals and map out intervention activities. Jill and Vivian set long-term goals in relation to performing activities of daily living (both personal and instrumental).

Initially, Jill found she needed to set quite simple goals such as getting dressed, since Vivian was not able to understand how the unilateral neglect impacted on her activities of daily living. Once Vivian became more involved and Jill was able to provide video feedback of her performance, Vivian became more insightful to the nature of her difficulties. As Vivian gained insight and understood that she would need to stay in rehabilitation for several weeks, Jill was able to work with Vivian to develop goals that were more closely related to her abilities.

Intervention occupations

Vivian and Jill began to work on a variety of personal and domestic activities of daily living in therapy. Jill and Vivian also talked of her wish to visit her son and to be able to attend her weekly Spanish Group. In this Practice Scenario, one intervention session has been written in detail to give the reader an idea of the kinds of techniques and strategies Jill used with Vivian.

Rationale: Selection of a treatment occupation

Jill and the medical rehabilitation consultant have explained to Jill that she cannot drive when she returns home, and that she will need a specialised driving assessment with an occupational therapist before resuming driving, if this is possible. This specialist assessment has been scheduled for 6 months after her stroke so that Jill is aware of this process and begins to think about alternative transport. The rehabilitation consultant has told Jill that he expects Vivian's unilateral neglect will not resolve. Therefore, while Vivian wants to be able to use public transport in the short term, Jill is making sure that Vivian is as independent as possible so that she will be able to manage in the short term or long term as a public transport user. Jill also spoke to the son who lives with Vivian. Vivian's son explained that while he could help with shopping, he couldn't drive Vivian to her Spanish group as he was at work at this time, and that it was better for Vivian to visit the residential care facility during the day rather than in the evenings (when he was able to drive her), since her son in residential care was better able to cope with visitors during the day. Vivian and Jill planned to purchase a 6-month local ticket just prior to her discharge so that Vivian would only need to validate rather than purchase a ticket for each journey.

In addition to the fact that Vivian wants to be a competent public transport user to access the community (visit her son and attend her Spanish Group), Jill reasoned that Vivian would also need to be able to use public transport to shop. Jill thought that this was an ideal activity as it gives plenty of opportunity to determine how Vivian's unilateral neglect affects her performance and develop strategies to overcome these problems. In addition to demanding Vivian attend to both hemispaces, peripersonal spaces and both her body sides, this activity requires many other cognitive and perceptual skills such as concentration (Vivian needs to sustain concentration on the whole activity and when she is using public transport and she needs to be able to follow the directions so she knows when to alight the bus), executive function (planning, problem solving and judgement to determine the route and what to do when a bus does not arrive), memory (names of suburbs and addresses of where she needs to go), and complex perceptual skills (route finding and map use).

Therefore, one long-term goal and one short-term objective documented by Jill in consultation with Vivian were:

Long-term goal: For Vivian to be able to use the local public bus (to attend Spanish Group, to shop and to visit her son in residential care).

Short-term objective:
Who: Vivian
Given what: Precursor activity of bean bag toss game using left upper limb (this limb activation will promote attention to the left hemispace during this, and subsequent activities (Robertson et al 1994)), use of a perceptual anchor and red ribbon and all necessary equipment (street directory, bus maps and timetable, pen and pencil)
Does what: Plans the buses to take, and the timetables for taking public transport to visit her son

How well: Vivian will have prepared a written daily schedule of suitable buses and times to visit her son, and be able to follow the route on a map (prior to discharge, Jill and Vivian will try out these plans on a day outing)
By when: The end of a 60-minute therapy session.

Stage 6 – Implement plans through occupation

Table 38.5 provides information on the kinds of therapy activities that Jill and Vivian will undertake during her 4 week stay. Included in Table 38.5 are details about a home visit, and a family meeting so that Vivian's sons have a chance to talk with Vivian and the whole team about her progress, discharge plans, and the ongoing difficulties Vivian may experience and supports that may assist her.

In addition, details have been provided for one therapy session in Table 38.6, to demonstrate the kinds of strategies and grading processes that might be used with Vivian. In Table 38.6, the steps for the activity are detailed in the first column. The second column describes the problems that Vivian might have with this activity. The third column provides details of the treatment strategies used to address Vivian's cognitive and perceptual difficulties at each step.

Stage 7 – Evaluate outcomes

The final stage of the intervention process is to evaluate outcomes with the individual, and determine if the individual would like, and benefit from, follow-up services such as outpatient therapy or community links. Jill evaluated the outcome of each session as she progressed with Jill. For example, after the first bus route finding session, Jill and Vivian concluded that, although Vivian had successfully completed the task (thus meeting the objective), they would repeat this session in a few days to refine Vivian's skills and continue to work on attending to the left hemispace. While insight was initially a problem, as Vivian progressed her insight to her problems increased. However, as Vivian became more aware of her problems she also became more depressed.

Jill also evaluated the programme at the time of Vivian's discharge by talking with Vivian, her sons and other therapy colleagues to determine if they thought Vivian had improved, and documenting that the generalisation of skills learned in occupational therapy had transferred to other aspects of Vivian's life. In addition, Jill re-administered the standardised assessments used on Vivian's admission (the BIT and COPM) and un-standardised assessments (interview, Extinction Test and Visual Confrontation Test) to

Table 38.5 Example of a 4-week occupational therapy programme for Vivian. Jill also spent time with Vivian each morning working on dressing and grooming

Day	Week 1	Week 2	Week 3	Week 4
MON Session 1	Initial interview assessment	IADL session Simple meal preparation (sandwich and cold drink)	Drawing session (see Figure 38.3)	Feedback with Vivian from home visit. Practise skills related to any problems from home visit
MON Session 2	Visual Confrontation test BIT assessment	Cooking activity with scanning (Vivian to choose a type of biscuit or scones with opportunity for spacing on the baking tray)	Money management session (role play shopping, and check money handling). Preparation for outing to use public transport	Indoor lawn bowls and reassessment using visual confrontation test
TUE Session 1	Breakfast time – Hypothesis testing making tea and toast	Newspaper reading. Video taping of session with play-back to gain insight to neglect	Indoor lawn bowls Video taping of session with play-back to gain insight to neglect	Morning outing to test out use of public transport to visit her son (as developed in Table 38.6)
TUE Session 2	COPM and Goal setting	Indoor lawn bowls. Video-record this and play back to increase Vivian's insight to her neglect	Variety of simple games such as balloon tennis, bean bag throwing, floor maze challenge	As above
WED Session 1	Scanning board game of Vivian's choice (e.g. Scrabble, Monopoly)	Bean bag toss activity (limb activation on left side as precursor activity for Session 2)	IADL session Telephone use	Newspaper reading
WED Session 2	Drawing session (layout of equipment/attending to the whole drawing, such as a vase of flowers) (Figure 38.3)	Planning to use public transport to visit her son (see detailed notes in Practice Scenario and Table 38.6)	Newspaper reading, and planning to use public transport to shop and go to Spanish group	Reassessment using COPM
THU Session 1	Indoor lawn bowls (also serves as a precursor activity for newspaper reading)	Drawing session (this is one of Vivian's hobbies and provides opportunity to attend to both halves of the page)	IADL session Main meal preparation	Family meeting with Vivian, and her sons to plan discharge
THU Session 2	Newspaper reading. Video-record this and play back to increase Vivian's insight to her neglect	Variety of simple games such as balloon tennis, bean bag throwing, floor maze challenge to encourage left turn taking. Video taping of session with play-back to gain insight to neglect	Scanning board game of Vivian's choice (e.g. Scrabble, Monopoly)	Discharge planning session, including linking with follow-up outpatient services
FRI Session 1	Extension of goal-setting activity using video feedback to increase Vivian's insight	Drawing session	Home visit	Re-assessment using BIT
FRI Session 2	Review of progress. Video taping of a game of memory cards and play-back to gain insight to neglect	IADL session Main meal preparation, and eat this for evening meal	Home visit	Cake baking activity to take a cake home on discharge

Table 38.6 Outline of a session to enable Vivian to use a bus to visit her son: Activity steps, difficulties Vivian may have, strategies and grading used to facilitate performance (focus on unilateral neglect), using remedial and some compensatory strategies

Activity steps (what is to be done/achieved)	Possible problems the person will have with this step	Strategies or grading to overcome the problem, or facilitate performance
1. Precursor activity to stimulate left limb activation (Robertson et al 1994). Bean bag toss: Vivian throws the beanbags with her left arm onto a score board on the floor (there are circles with points written inside, and the highest points are on the left of the board)	Vivian tries to throw with her right hand. Vivian misses throwing to the left of the board	Verbal prompting to use left hand, and to throw to the higher scores on the left of the board. Place a wide red strip of card or ribbon on the left of the score board on the floor and prompt Vivian to scan for this prior to throwing a bean bag. The use of this precursor activity (which stimulates motor circuits on the left should also lead to improved performance in the main activity for the session which is planning to use public transport. Up- and downgrade the activity during the whole session by manipulating variables related to the environment, the therapist and the task. Some examples have been provided below, although these are not exhaustive
2. Plan the activity with Vivian, and gather all the necessary equipment. Start by discussing the objective for the session: Vivian, given a precursor activity of bean bag toss game, use of a perceptual anchor and red ribbon and all necessary equipment, will plan the buses to take, and the timetables for taking public transport to visit her son, so that Vivian will have prepared a written daily schedule of suitable buses and times to visit her son, and be able to follow the route on a map, by the end of the 60-minute therapy session	Jill and Vivian have agreed on the objective for the session, so this should be a straightforward discussion on what the session will involve. Vivian may forget the objective is to plan transport to visit her son (for example, another session will also need to plan transport to get to Spanish group). Vivian needs to gather relevant materials for the activity (street directory, bus maps and timetable, pen and pencil), and some of these are placed in the left side of the cupboard, or in a cupboard on the left side of the room, which she may not attend to. Additionally, she may forget to gather some of these items	Provide verbal prompts to gather items and where they are located. Verbal prompts can be downgraded to provide Vivian with a written checklist of things she needs to gather for the activity, or the goal and steps of the activity. Since Vivian may have difficulty locating cupboards on the left, or items in the left side of the cupboard, Jill can assist by guiding Vivian to the relevant cupboards, and then prompting Vivian to scan for all edges of the cupboard prior to locating the equipment. The activity can be downgraded by Jill gathering all the items for Vivian, or by placing the items in cupboards on the right side of the room, and the middle or right side of the cupboard
3. Use the street directory and find Vivian's street and house and the street and the residential care facility where her son lives. Make a colour photocopy of this page of the map. Vivian's home is on the right side of the double map page, and the residential facility is on the far left	Difficulty locating the index pages on the left side to find her street and the residential care facility. Forget the grid reference for her street and the residential care facility	Perceptual 'anchoring' can be used, and Vivian can place her left arm at the edge of the page and be prompted to scan across to her arm at each step. This can be used when finding the street names in the index and also when finding the streets on the actual map. Verbally prompt Vivian to write the grid reference for the maps she needs. Use a highlighter pen to mark her house (street) and the residential care facility (and street) If Vivian is managing well, walk down to the administration office of the facility and make a colour copy of the map. Downgrade: Jill to have a copy that she made earlier ready for use

Table 38.6 Outline of a session to enable Vivian to use a bus to visit her son: Activity steps, difficulties Vivian may have, strategies and grading used to facilitate performance (focus on unilateral neglect), using remedial and some compensatory strategies —cont'd

Activity steps (what is to be done/achieved)	Possible problems the person will have with this step	Strategies or grading to overcome the problem, or facilitate performance
4. Use the notes on the street directory to determine which bus line and number operates in the area. Trace the bus route onto a photocopy of the street directory. The bus leaves from the end of Vivian's street, and there is a bus stop at the entrance to the residential care facility. Do activity seated at table with all equipment (map, ruler, highlighter pen, bus timetable, pen, paper)	Difficulty locating the residential care facility on the left of the map, and the bus numbers. Difficulty with tracing from her home (on the right) towards the residential care facility (on the left of the map)	Jill to sit at the table on Vivian's left side. Verbal prompts to locate the bus symbols and bus numbers in blue on the map. As above, use perceptual anchor to the left of the street directory map. Prompt Vivian to place her left index finger on the care facility, and she can trace towards this when highlighting the route with a pen. Downgrade by adding red ribbon to the left margin of the page if needed
5. Look up the bus number in the bus timetable booklet and decide on the bus times that best suit Vivian's routine, and suitable visiting times at the residential care facility	The bus timetable book is quite small, and therefore is quite central in Vivian's spatial field. However, Vivian may have some difficulty in scanning the columns and locating the right bus and reading the times	Verbally prompt Vivian to locate the left side of the schedule and use her left hand as a perceptual anchor to hold the book open, then place a clear ruler over the page and hold with left hand, and use right finger to point to relevant bus times. Vivian to identify suitable times, and Jill to write these down (days, departure times and arrival times). Upgrade by asking Vivian to look up the schedule and record the details on paper. Downgrade by having another pre-prepared bus timetable with the relevant bus and times highlighted
6. Vivian can practice tracing out the bus route on the map using her finger. Identify landmarks that will be on the right (library, park and large house with two palm trees at the entrance) and left (police station, three shops together, post box and house with the high green fence) of the bus on the journey. Plan a strategy to prompt looking to the left	Vivian may have difficulty tracing her finger over the map all the way to the residential care facility. It may be difficult for Vivian to identify landmarks on the left of the bus and then recognise when she arrives at the residential facility which will also be on the left of the bus. When she returns home, her home will be on the right of the bus, so she should not have difficulty with this	Place left arm as a perceptual anchor and verbally prompt Vivian to scan to her arm as she traces with her right index finger along the bus route. Verbally prompt Vivian to look to the residential care facility as marked on the map as she commences the task. Downgrade by placing the map on a cork board and sticking coloured pins at the site of her home and the residential care facility. If Vivian is able to monitor the progress of the bus as they drive, then she will be able to practice 'Look Left' and search specifically for the landmarks she has identified with Jill. Downgrade: If Vivian is unable to locate the residential care facility on the left side, she will need to ask the bus driver to tell her they are at the residential care facility bus stop.
7. Evaluate the session by reviewing if the objective has been met. Plan for the outing in the final week to test out using the bus		Downgrade. If Vivian is unable to catch the bus independently, arrange for half-price taxi voucher so that Vivian has an alternative means of transport

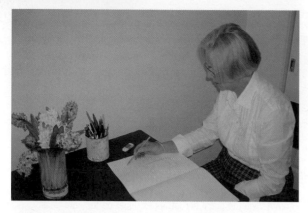

Figure 38.3 • Vivian draws during a therapy session. The therapist will ask Vivian to place her left arm on the left edge of the page to serve as a perceptual anchor

document improvements made. Finally, Jill examined the long-term goals she had set with Vivian and determined which had been met.

Vivian wanted to continue some outpatient therapy at the centre and Jill supported an outpatient programme of two visits per week for a month with a review and possible extension of this. With Vivian's approval, Jill also arranged for Vivian to receive home help to assist with cleaning from the local council, and a half-price taxi voucher so that Vivian would have access to affordable taxi transport in the evenings, or if she chose not to use the bus.

Intervention strategies for specific problems

Problems with attention and concentration

While attention/concentration as defined earlier in the chapter was divided into the categories of sustained, focused (selective) and divided/alternating, there is limited empirical evidence to support interventions with these specific forms. Hence, the interventions described below may be tried with different presentations of the problem.

Remedial approach

The purpose of therapy is to increase the individual's attention to appropriate stimuli, and disregard inappropriate stimuli. Individuals can be trained to scan the visual environment in a slow and systematic manner. It may also be useful to set time or speed limits, amplify critical stimuli, and make the crucial stimuli salient (noticeable) to the individual (Diller & Weinberg 1972). A Cochrane review (Lincoln et al 2000) revealed only two controlled trials of attention training in stroke. The review found that training improved alertness and sustained attention on measures of these capacities, but there was no evidence to support or refute the use of cognitive rehabilitation for attention deficits to improve independence.

Compensatory approach

The inability to attend to significant stimuli is compounded for many individuals by distraction due to extraneous stimuli in the environment such as noise. Therefore, the environment can be controlled to maximise the individual's ability to concentrate (Ponsford et al 1995). Fasotti et al (2000) have reported successfully teaching people with head injury to compensate for slowed information processing by using time pressure management (TPM), while Sohlberg et al (2000) documented the effectiveness of attention process training (APT).

Problems with memory and learning

Remedial approach

The aim of memory retraining is to enable the individual to effectively encode and recall information so that learning can occur. One of the foundation skills for this is to be able to attend and concentrate. Therefore, when working on memory skill, therapists should also be working with individuals to improve attention (Abreu 1999). When working with the individual to effectively code information it is important to teach the person strategies to organise material to be remembered, and making logical associations. A determination should be made of how the individual used to remember information and build on these past strategies. While there is little evidence to support the use of computer games in the rehabilitation of memory skills, the therapist may be able to help the individual identify skills gained and reinforce these during everyday occupations. A recent Cochrane review (Majid et al 2000) found only one controlled trial exploring memory interventions. This trial by Doornheim and

De Haan (1998) showed that memory training had no significant effect on memory impairment or subjective memory complaints. The Cochrane reviewers concluded that there was insufficient evidence at that time to support or refute the effectiveness of cognitive rehabilitation for memory problems after stroke.

Compensatory approach

The use of a diary or notebook system (memory log) can help many individuals to manage their daily living activities (Ownsworth & McFarland 1999). Environmental prompts such as a beeper or a wall calendar can be useful to assist individuals to remember their routine, or to look at their diary. Mnemonics training may be successful with some individuals (Kaschel et al 2002).

Problems with metacognition and executive functions

Remedial approach

The provision of a structured environment, feedback, and routine, can enable a person to reduce the impact of their problems with executive functions (e.g. providing the individual with steps to follow, assisting the task to become routine by repeated practice, or providing immediate feedback about the individual's behaviour and the effect it has on others). The therapist initially acts as the individual's frontal lobes, and gradually transfers these responsibilities to the person. However, unless the person has some awareness of the problems (insight), a remedial approach will not be particularly successful (Ponsford et al 1995). Honda (1999) recently reported a study with three individuals who were provided with self-instructional training, a problem-solving procedure and physical-set changing exercises over a 6-month period. While two of the subjects showed improvements on the neuropsychological test used as an outcome measure, all subjects improved in personal and instrumental activities of daily living. Limitations of this study include the small sample size and lack of control subjects, since it could be expected that these individuals would make spontaneous recovery over the 6-month study period.

Compensatory approach

When using this approach, intervention focuses on working with the client to use other intact cognitive functions and/or modify the environment in order to complete the occupation. For example, the therapist might ask the person to perform a task in a room with minimal distractions, or change the demands of the person's work, home, or community to diminish the need to employ executive functions. A beeper or alarm clock may be used to assist a person overcome poor initiation, and there are a range of other compensatory techniques (Duran & Fisher 1999, Ponsford et al 1995). Zinn et al (2007) report they are currently developing compensatory rehabilitation techniques for use with people who have problems with executive functions following stroke.

Problems with unilateral neglect

Remedial approach

Unlike some of the other cognitive and perceptual impairments, a great deal of research has been conducted to identify interventions for unilateral neglect. In particular, the reader is referred to two excellent reviews by Bowen et al (2005) and Pierce and Buxbaum (2002) which describe and evaluate the effectiveness of several of the interventions outlined below. Asking the individual with unilateral neglect to move their left body side (hemispheric activation approaches), such as simply clenching and unclenching the fist, can improve attention to the left body side and hemispace (Eskes et al 2003). In one of the first studies using this technique, Robertson et al (1994) carried out a study with six individuals who were asked to walk through a doorway. Each of the individual's walking trajectories (pathways) was measured, and it was found that all trajectories were significantly deviated to the right of centre. Participants were then asked to clench and unclench their left hands prior to, and during, walking through the doorway. The researchers found that this procedure significantly assisted participants to centre their walking trajectories.

Other techniques that have been used successfully with individuals with unilateral neglect include eye-patching (Ari et al 1997), prism glasses (Keane et al 2006), neck vibration therapy (Karnath et al 1993), phasic alerting (Robertson et al 1998), constraint-induced therapy (Taub 1999) and caloric stimulation (where cold water is irrigated contralesionally and warm water ipsilesionally into the external ear canal) (Rode et al 1998). However, these techniques are not yet common in occupational therapy and further research to support their effectiveness is required. It is also suggested that the use of verbal instructions should be minimised with individuals who experience neglect, and simple verbal instructions should be used to encourage the person to turn the head to the left to anchor his or her attention to that side of space (Herman 1992).

Compensatory approach

Initially, the therapist educates the individual and carers about the condition, and then strategies to manage everyday activities are devised. For example, when reading a book or newspaper, a red ribbon may be placed on the left margin and the person is taught to scan back to this point after completing each line (Van Deusen 1993). The environment may also be adapted to facilitate left turn-taking. Hospital staff can place the person's call button, telephone, and other essential items on the unaffected side. A mirror may be placed in front of the person while he or she is dressing or ambulating to draw attention to the neglected side.

Problems with simple and complex perception

Some of the intervention ideas used to address simple perceptual problems (the agnosias) are presented prior to techniques used with individuals who have complex perceptual problems (spatial-relations disorder). These ideas are not exhaustive and a mixture of both remedial and compensatory techniques is suggested.

Visual object agnosia

Individuals are usually able to compensate for visual object agnosia by using information from other senses such as touch, audition and smell to recognise the object.

Anosognosia

Anosognosia is not a particularly common condition and often resolves spontaneously in the first 3 months following stroke (Maeshima et al 1997). However, until the condition resolves, it seriously hampers rehabilitation (Maeshima et al 1997). It is extremely difficult to compensate for if the condition persists long term. Safety is of paramount importance in intervention and discharge planning, because individuals typically do not acknowledge

that they have a disability and will therefore refuse to take care during potentially dangerous daily occupations such as cooking, or even adjusting water temperature when showering (Sharpless 1982).

Somatoagnosia

Using a remedial approach the therapist aims for the individual with somatoagnosia to associate sensory input with an adaptive motor response. Facilitation of body awareness is accomplished through sensory stimulation to the body part affected. For example, the individual can rub the affected body side with a rough cloth as the therapist names it or points to it (Fisher 1991).

Right and left discrimination

If using a compensatory approach for people with right/left discrimination problems, the words 'right' and 'left' should be avoided. Instead, pointing or providing cues using distinguishing features of the limb are more effective (e.g. 'the arm with the watch'). These guidelines are particularly salient for the therapist teaching locomotion or transfers, where confusing instructions may have dangerous consequences. The right side of all common objects such as shoes and clothing can be marked with red tape or seam binding.

Figure ground disorder

If using a remedial approach to address figure ground disorder, the therapist can arrange for practise in visually locating objects in a simple array (such as three very different objects), and progress to more complex arrays (four or five dissimilar objects and three similar ones). If using a compensatory approach, the person can be taught to use other, intact senses (e.g. touch) when searching for items such as clothing or grooming items. When learning to lock a wheelchair, the person can be advised to locate the brake levers by touch rather than by searching for them visually. Brightly coloured tape can be used to mark the edges on stairs.

Form discrimination

In a remedial approach, the person with form discrimination difficulties can practice describing, identifying, and demonstrating the use of similarly shaped and sized objects. The individual can sort like objects and should be assisted to focus on differentiating cues. When using a compensatory approach with individuals who can read, frequently used and confused objects can be labelled. The individual can be encouraged to use vision, touch, and self-verbalisation in combination when objects are confused.

Problems with praxis

Although therapists tend to use similar interventions whether the person has an ideomotor or ideational apraxia, a Cochrane review is currently underway to investigate if therapy is effective to reduce ideomotor aparaxia after stroke (West et al 2008).

Remedial approach

The therapist needs to speak slowly, and provide one-step commands only. When teaching a new task, it should be broken down into its component parts. In one approach, the person is taught one component at a time, with the therapist physically guiding the person through the task if necessary. It should be completed in precisely the same manner each time. When all the individual units are mastered, an attempt to combine them should be made. A great deal of repetition may be necessary (Wall 1982). Family members can be advised to use the same approach. An example of a young woman re-learning how to drink from a cup using this technique is provided by Butler (1999). Using the sensorimotor approach, multiple sensory inputs are used on the affected body parts to enhance the production of appropriate motor responses.

Compensatory approach

A randomised controlled reported by Donkervoort et al (2001) reported that occupational therapy 'strategy training' was an effective intervention with people who have apraxia. In strategy training, the individual is taught compensatory techniques to overcome the apraxia in ADLs such as the use of pictures in the correct sequence to support everyday occupations.

Community integration: the ultimate goal of cognitive and perceptual rehabilitation

Occupational therapists work with individuals to improve cognitive and perceptual function so that the person can return to their community and lead a fulfilling life through occupational engagement. Therefore, therapists are increasingly focused on community integration as the ultimate outcome of rehabilitation in this field (Doig et al 2001, Fleming et al 1999, McColl et al 1998, Willer et al 1993). Community integration may be defined as:

- assimilation, or being able to fit in with other people, knowing your way around and being accepted (McColl et al 1998, 2001)

- occupation which includes meaningful and productive activity to be involved in as well as having things to do for fun (McColl et al 1998, 2001, Willer et al 1993)

- independent living including making everyday decisions and life choices (McColl et al 1998, 2001), and

- having social support, or being part of a network of family, friends and acquaintances (McColl et al 1998, 2001, Willer et al 1993).

Increasingly, community integration is seen as the best outcome measure of rehabilitation for people, particularly following head injury. However, a great deal more research is required to examine whether people with cognitive and perceptual problems manage their home and community living activities, and whether they are satisfied with their lives and their ability to engage in these activities (Willer et al 1993). Specifically, research is required to identify and measure the types of community integration difficulties people face, and factors that predict community integration. The findings of such studies will assist occupational therapists to develop interventions that will promote long-term community integration.

Conclusion

Occupational therapists work with individuals to improve cognitive and perceptual capacities so they can engage in the occupations they want or need to do and thus lead fulfilling lives as part of the community. This chapter provided an overview of a range of cognitive and perceptual problems, the kinds of diseases or accidents that can lead to such problems, theories that guide an occupational therapist when working with individuals who experience problems in this area, ways therapists can evaluate these problems and finally, the kinds of evidence-based interventions that can be used to assist individuals overcome these problems. The chapter has been illustrated with the detailed case study of Vivian. This case study outlines aspects of therapy undertaken by the occupational therapist, and provides the reader with clear

guidelines for the use of the Occupational Performance Process Model (Townsend et al 1997) to structure therapy. The chapter also provides extensive references and resources so the reader can pursue excellence in practice when working with people who have cognitive and perceptual problems.

References

Abreu, B. C. (1990). *The quadraphonic approach: Management of cognitive and postural dysfunction*. New York, NY: Therapeutic Service Systems.

Abreu, B.C. (1999) Evaluation and intervention with memory and learning impairment. In C.A. Unsworth (Ed.). *Cognitive and perceptual dysfunction: a clinical reasoning approach to evaluation and intervention.* (pp. 163–208). Philadelphia, FA Davis.

AIHW (2007). Incidence and prevalence of chronic disease. Available online: http://www.aihw. gov.au/cdarf/data_pages/incidence_ prevalence/index.cfm#Stroke. Accessed 10 Mar 2007.

Allen, C. K. (1990). *Allen Cognitive Level Test Manual*. Colchester, CT, S & S Worldwide.

Anastasi, A. (1988). *Psychological testing* (6th ed.). New York, Macmillan Publishing Co.

Ari, T., Ohi, H., Sasaki, H., Nobuto, H., & Tanaka, K. (1997). Hemispatial sunglasses: Effect on unilateral spatial neglect. *Archives of Physical Medicine and Rehabilitation*, 78, 230–232.

Árnadóttir, G. (1990). *The brain and behavior: Assessing cortical dysfunction through activities of daily living*. St. Louis, MO, CV Mosby.

Australian Institute of Health and Welfare (2003). *ICF Australian user guide. Version 1*. Canberra, Australian Institute of Health and Welfare.

Averbuch, S. & Katz, N. (1992). Cognitive rehabilitation: A retraining approach for brain-injured adults. In N. Katz (Ed.), *Cognitive rehabilitation: Models for intervention in occupational therapy*. (pp. 219 –239). Boston, Andover Medical.

Bauer, R.M. & Rubens, A.B. (1993). Agnosia. In K.M. Heilman & E. Valenstein (Eds.), *Clinical neuropsychology* (3rd ed.) (pp. 215– 278). Oxford, Oxford University Press.

Bowen, A., Lincoln, N.B. & Dewey, M. (2005). *Cognitive rehabilitation for spatial neglect following stroke – Cochrane Review*. The Cochrane Library, Update Software.

Bradshaw, J.L. & Mattingley, J.B. (1995). *Clinical neuropsychology: behavioral and brain science*. San Diego, Academic Press, 1995.

Butler, J. (1999). Evaluation and intervention with apraxia. In C.A. Unsworth (ed). *Cognitive and perceptual dysfunction: a clinical reasoning approach to evaluation and intervention*. (pp. 257–297). Philadelphia, FA Davis.

Cicerone, K.D. (1996). Attention deficits and dual task demands after mild traumatic brain injury. *Brain injury*, 10, 79–89.

College of Occupational Therapists (2004). *Guidance on the use of The International Classification of Functioning, Disability and Health (ICF) and the Ottawa Charter for Health Promotion in occupational therapy services*. London, College of Occupational Therapists.

Cook, D.M. (2005). *Occupational Therapy – Adult Perceptual Screening Test (OT – APST)*. Brisbane, Function for Life.

Croce, R. (1993). A review of the neural basis of apractic disorders with implications for remediation. *Adapted Physical Activity Quarterly*, 10, 173.

Davis, A., Davis, S., Moss, N., Marks, J., McGrath, J., Hovard, L., Axon, J. & Wade, D. (1992). First steps towards an interdisciplinary approach to rehabilitation.

Clinical Rehabilitation, 6, 237–244.

de Clive-Lowe, S. (1996). Outcome measurement, cost-effectiveness and clinical audit: The importance of standardised assessment to occupational therapists in meeting these new demands. *British Journal of Occupational Therapy*, 59, 357–362.

Diller, L. & Weinberg, J (1972). Differential aspects of attention in brain-damaged persons. *Perceptual and Motor Skills*, 35, 71–80.

Doig, E., Fleming, J. & Tooth, L. (2001). Patterns of community integration 2–5 years post-discharge from brain injury rehabilitation. *Brain Injury*, 15, 747–762.

Donkervoort, M., Dekker, J., Stehmann-Saris, F.C. & Deelman, B.G. (2001). Efficacy of strategy training in left hemisphere stroke patients with apraxia: A randomized clinical trial. *Neuropsychological Rehabilitation*, 11, 549–566.

Doornheim, K. & De Haan, E.H.F. (1998). Cognitive training for memory deficits in stroke patients. *Neuropsychological Rehabilitation*, 8, 393.

Duran, L. & Fisher, A.G. (1999). Evaluation and intervention with executive functions impairment. In C.A. Unsworth (ed). *Cognitive and perceptual dysfunction: A clinical reasoning approach to evaluation and intervention*. (pp. 209–254). Philadelphia, FA Davis.

Ellis, A.W. & Young, A.W. (1988). *Human cognitive neuropsychology*. Hillsdale, NJ, Lawrence Erlbaum Associates.

Eskes, G.A., Butler, B., McDonald, A., Harrison, E.R. & Phillips, S.J. (2003). Limb activation effects in hemispatial neglect. *Archives of*

Physical Medicine and Rehabilitation, 84, 323–328.

Fasotti, L., Kovacs, F., Eling, P.A. & Brouwer, W.H. (2000). Time pressure management as a compensatory strategy training after closed head injury. *Neuropsychological Rehabilitation,* 10, 47–65.

Fearing, V. G., Law M. & Clark J. (1997). An occupational performance process model: Fostering client and therapist alliances. *Canadian Journal of Occupational Therapy,* 64(1), 7–15.

Fisher, A. G. (1997a). An expanded rehabilitative model of practice. In A. G. Fisher (Ed.), *Assessment of motor and process skills.* (2nd ed.) (pp. 73–85). Fort Collins, CO, Three Star Press.

Fisher, A. G. (1997b). *Assessment of motor and process skills.* (2nd ed.). Fort Collins, CO, Three Star Press.

Fisher, A. G., Murray, E. A. & Bundy, A. C. (1991). *Sensory integration: Theory and practice.* Philadelphia, FA Davis.

Fleming, J., Tooth L., Hassell, M. & Chan., W. (1999). Prediction of community integration and vocational outcome 2–5 years after traumatic brain injury rehabilitation in Australia. *Brain Injury,* 13(6), 417–431.

Fortune, N. & Wen, X. (1999). *The definition, incidence and prevalence of acquired brain injury in Australia.* Canberra, Australian Institute of Health and Welfare.

Friedman, R.B., Ween, J.E. & Albert, M.L. (1993). Alexia. In K. M. Heilman & E. Valenstein (Eds.), *Clinical neuropsychology.* (3rd ed.) (pp. 37–62). Oxford, Oxford University Press.

Gainotti, G., D'Erme, P. & Bartolomeo, P. (1991). Early orientation of attention toward the half space ipsilateral to the lesion in patients with unilateral brain damage. *Journal of Neurology, Neurosurgery and Psychiatry,* 54, 1082–1089.

Gialanella, B., Monguzzi, V., Santoro, R. & Rocchi, S. (2005). Functional recovery after hemiplegia in patients with neglect: the rehabilitative role of anosognosia. *Stroke,* 36, 2687–2690.

Giles, G. M. & Wilson, J. C (1992). *Occupational therapy for the brain injured adult: A neurofunctional approach.* London, Chapman and Hall.

Grieve, J. (1993). *Neuropsychology for occupational therapists: Assessment of perception and cognition.* Oxford, Blackwell Scientific Publications.

Guide for the Uniform Data Set for Medical Rehabilitation (Adult FIM SM). (1999). Version 5.0. State Univ of New York at Buffalo, Buffalo.

Halligan, P. W. & Marshall, J. C. (1993). The history and clinical presentation of neglect. In I. H. Robertson & J. C. Marshall (Eds.), *Unilateral neglect: Clinical and experimental studies* (pp. 3–25). Hove, Lawrence Erlbaum Associates Ltd.

Herman, E. W. M. (1992). Spatial neglect: New issues and their implications for occupational therapy practice. *American Journal of Occupational Therapy,* 46, 207–212.

Hobson, S. (1996). Reflections on being client-centred when the client is cognitively impaired. *Canadian Journal of Occupational Therapy,* 63(2), 133–137.

Honda, T. (1999). Rehabilitation of executive function impairment after stroke. *Topics in Stroke Rehabilitation,* 6, 15–22.

Itzkovich, M., Elazar, B., Averbuch, S. & Katz, N. (1990). *The Loewenstein Occupational Therapy Assessment (LOTCA).* NJ, Pequanock.

Karnath, H.O., Christ, K. & Hartje, W. (1993). Decrease of contralesional neglect by neck muscle vibration and spatial orientation of trunk midline. *Brain,* 116, 383–396.

Kaschel, R., Della Sala, S., Cantagallo, A., Fahlbock, A., Laaksonen, R. & Kazen, M. (2002). Imagery mnemonics for the rehabilitation of memory: A randomised group controlled trial. *Neuropsychological Rehabilitation,* 12, 127–153.

Katz, N. (Ed.). (1998). *Cognition and occupation in rehabilitation: Cognitive models for intervention in rehabilitation.* Bethesda, American Association of Occupational Therapy.

Keane, S., Turner, C., Sherrington, C. & Beard, J.R. (2006). Use of Fresnel Prism glasses to treat stroke patients with hemispatial neglect. *Archives of Physical Medicine and Rehabilitation,* 87, 1668–1672.

Kielhofner, G. (2002). *A model of human occupation: Theory and application* (3rd ed.). Baltimore, MD, William and Wilkins.

Kiernan, R.J., Mueller, J., Langston, J.W. & Van Dyke, C. (1987). The Neurobehavioral Cognitive Status Examination: A brief but differentiated approach to cognitive assessment. *Annals of Internal Medicine,* 107, 481–485.

Kirshner, H. (1991). The apraxias. In W. Bradley, R. Daroff, G. Fenichel & C. Marsden (Eds.), *Neurology in clinical practice: Principles of diagnosis and management* (Vol. 1) (pp. 117–122). London, Butterworth-Heinmann.

Laver, A. J. & Powell, G. E (1995). *The Structured Observational Test of Function (SOTOF).* Windsor, England, NFER–NELSON.

Law, M., Baptiste, S., Carswell, A., McColl, M., Polatajko, H. & Pollock, N. (1998). *The Canadian Occupational Performance Measure* (3rd ed.). Toronto, Canadian Association of Occupational Therapy.

Lezak, M. D. (1995). *Neuropsychological assessment* (3rd ed.). New York, Oxford University Press.

Lincoln, N. B., Majid, M. J. & Weyman, N. (2000). *Cognitive rehabilitation for attention deficits following stroke (Cochrane review).* In *The Cochrane Library,* Issue 3, Update Software, Oxford, 2000.

Maeshima, S, Dohi, N., Funahashi, K., Nakai, K., Itakura, T. & Komai, N. (1997). Rehabilitation of patients with anosognosia for hemiplegia due to intracerebral haemorrhage. *Brain Injury,* 11, 691–706.

Majid, M. J. Lincoln, N. B. & Weyman, N. (2000). *Cognitive rehabilitation for memory deficits following stroke* (Cochrane Review). In *The Cochrane Library,* Issue 4. Oxford: Update Software.

Mateer, C. A., Kerns, K. A. & Eso, K. L. (1996). Management of attention and memory disorders following traumatic brain injury.

Journal of Learning Disabilities, 29, 618–632.

Mayer, N. H., Reed, E., Schwartz, M. F., Montgomery, C. & Palmer, C. (1990). Buttering a hot cup of coffee: An approach to the study of errors of action in patients with brain damage. In: D. E. Tupper & K. D. Cicerone (Eds). *The neuropsychology of everyday life: Assessment and basic competencies*. (pp. 94–295). London, Kluwer.

McColl, M. A., Carlson, P., Johnston, J. et al. (1998). The definition of community integration: perspectives of people with brain injuries. *Brain Injury*, 12, 15–30.

McColl, M. A., Davies, D., Carlson, P., Johnston, J. & Minnes, P. (2001). The community integration measure: development and preliminary validation. *Archives of Physical Medicine and Rehabilitation*, 82, 429–434.

Mozaz, M., Marti, J., Carrera, E. & de la Puente, E. (1990). Apraxia in a patient with lesion located in right sub-cortical area: Analysis of errors. *Cortex*, 26, 651–655.

O'Connor, P. & Cripps, R. (1999). *Needs and opportunities for improved surveillance of brain injury – a progress report*. Adelaide, Australian Institute of Health and Welfare.

Ownsworth, T. L. & McFarland, K. (1999). Memory remediation in long-term acquired brain injury: two approaches in diary training. *Brain Injury*, 13, 605–626.

Pak, R. & Dombrovy, M. L. (1994). Stroke. In: D. C. Good & J. R. Couch (Eds). *Handbook of neurorehabilitation*. (pp. 461–480). New York, Marcel Dekker.

Pedretti, L. R. (Ed.), (1985). *Occupational therapy: Practice skills for physical dysfunction* (3rd ed.). St. Louis, C.V. Mosby Company.

Pierce, S. R. & Buxbaum, L. J. (2002). Treatments of unilateral neglect: A review. *Archives of Physical Medicine and Rehabilitation*, 83, 256–268.

Ponsford, J. (2004). *Cognitive and behavioral rehabilitation*. New York, The Guilford Press.

Ponsford, J., Sloan, S. & Snow, P. (1995). *Traumatic brain injury: Rehabilitation for everyday adaptive living*. Hove, Lawrence Erlbaum.

Raade, A. S., Gonzalez Rothi, L. J. & Heilman, K. M. (1991). The relationship between buccofacial and limb apraxia. *Brain and Cognition*, 16, 130–146.

Rafal, R. (1994). Neglect. *Current Opinion in Neurobiology*, 4, 321–326.

Robertson, I. H., Tegnér, R., Goodrich, S. J. & Wilson, C. (1994). Walking trajectory and hand movements in unilateral left neglect: A vestibular hypothesis. *Neuropsychologia*, 32, 1495–1502.

Robertson, I., Ward, T., Ridgeway, Y. & Nimmo-Smith, I. (1994). *The test of everyday attention*. Bury St. Edwards, Thames Valley Test Co.

Roberton, I. H., Mattingley, J. B., Rorden, C. & Driver, J. (1998). Phasic alerting of neglect patients overcomes their spatial deficits in visual awareness. *Nature*, 395, 169–172.

Robertson, L. C. & Eglin, M. (1993). Attentional search in unilateral visual neglect. In I. H. Robertson & J. C. Marshall (Eds.), *Unilateral neglect: Clinical and experimental studies* (pp. 169–192). Hove, Lawrence Erlbaum Associates.

Rode, G., Perenin, M. T., Honore, J. & Boisson, D. (1998). Improvements of the motor defect of neglect patients through verstibular stimulation: Evidence for a motor neglect component. *Cortex*, 34, 253–261.

Schmidt, R. A. (1988). *Motor control and learning: A behavioral emphasis* (2nd ed.). Champaign, IL, Human Kinetics.

Sharpless, J. W. (1982). *Mossman's a problem oriented approach to stroke rehabilitation* (2nd ed.). Springfield, IL, Charles C Thomas, Springfield.

Sohlberg, M. M., McLaughlin, K. A., Pavese, A., Heidrich, A. & Posner, M. I. (2000). Evaluation of attention process training and brain injury education in persons with acquired brain injury. *Journal of Clinical Experimental Neuropsychology*, 22, 656–676.

Tate, R. & McDonald, S. (1995). What is apraxia? The clinician's dilemma. *Neuropsychological Rehabilitation*, 5, 273–297.

Taub, E. (1999). New discovery equals change in clinical practice. *Journal of Rehabilitation Research Development*, 36, vii–viii.

Toglia, J. P. (1992). A dynamic interactional approach to cognitive retraining. In N. Katz (Ed.), *Cognitive rehabilitation: Models for intervention in occupational therapy*. (pp. 104–143). Boston, Andover Medical Publishers.

Townsend, E. A. & Polatajko, H. J. (2007). *Enabling occupation II: Advancing an occupational therapy vision for health, well-being, and justice through occupation*. Ottawa, Canadian Association of Occupational Therapists.

Townsend, E., Stanton, S., Law, M. et al (1997). *Enabling occupation: An occupational therapy perspective*. Ottawa, Canadian Association of Occupational Therapists.

Trombly, C. A. (1995). Theoretical foundations for practice. In C. A. Trombly (Ed.), *Occupational therapy for physical dysfunction* (4th ed.) (pp. 15–27). Baltimore, MD, Williams and Wilkins.

Tyerman, R., Tyerman, A., Howard, P. & Hadfield, C. (1986). *COTNAB – Chessington Occupational Therapy Neurological Assessment Battery introductory manual*. Nottingham, Nottingham Rehab Limited.

Unsworth, C. A. (1999). *Cognitive and perceptual dysfunction: A clinical reasoning approach to evaluation and intervention*. Philadelphia, FA Davis.

Unsworth, C. A. (2005). Measuring outcomes using the Australian Therapy Outcome Measures for Occupational Therapy (AusTOMs – OT): Data description and tool sensitivity. *British Journal of Occupational Therapy*, 68(8), 354–366

Unsworth, C. A., & Duncombe, D. (2007). *AusTOMs for Occupational Therapy* (2nd ed.). Melbourne, La Trobe University.

Vallar, G. (1993). The anatomical basis of spatial hemineglect in humans. In: I. H. Robertson & J. C. Marshall (Eds.), *Unilateral neglect: Clinical and experimental studies* (pp. 27–59). Hove, Lawrence Erlbaum Associates Ltd.

Van Deusen, J. (1993). *Body image and perceptual dysfunction in adults*. Philadelphia, Saunders.

van Zomeren, A. H. & Brouwer, W. H. (1994). *The clinical neuropsychology of attention*. New York, Oxford University Press.

Wall, N. (1982). Stroke rehabilitation. In Logigian, M. K. (Ed.). *Adult rehabilitation: A team approach for therapists* (pp. 225–240). Boston, Little.

Ware, J. E. & Sherbourne, C. D. (1992). The MOS 36 item short-form health survey (SF36): Conceptual framework and item selection. *Medical Care*, 30, 473–483.

West, C., Bowen, A., Hesketh, A. & Vail, A. (2008). *Interventions for motor apraxia following stroke (Protocol)*. Cochrane Database of Systematic Reviews, Issue 2.

Whiting, S., Lincoln, N., Bhavnani, G. & Cockburn, J. (1985). *RPAB-Rivermead Perceptual Assessment Battery*. Windsor, NFER–NELSON.

Willer, B., Rosenthal, M., Kreutzer, J., Gordon, W. & Rempel, R. (1993). Assessment of community integration following rehabilitation for TBI. *Journal of Head Trauma Rehabilitation*, 8, 11–23.

Wilson, B., Cockburn, J. & Halligan, P. W. (1987). *Behavioural Inattention Test*. Bury St. Edmunds, Thames Valley Test Company.

Wilson, B., Cockburn, J. & Baddely, A. (1991). *RBMT – The Rivermead Behavioural Memory Test*. Bury St Edmunds, Thames Valley Test Company.

Wilson, B., Alderman, N., Burgess, P., Emslie, H. & Evans, S. S. (1996). *Behavioural assessment of the dysexecutive*. Bury St Edmonds, Thames Valley Test Company.

Wilson, B., Greenfield, E., Clare, L., Baddeley, A., Cockburn, J., Watson, P., Tate, R., Sopena, S., Nannery, R. & Crawford, J. (2008). *The Rivermead Behavioural Memory Test (RBMT-3)* (3rd Ed.). London, Pearson.

Winegardner, J. (1993). Executive functions. In: H. Cohen (Ed.), *Neuroscience for rehabilitation* (pp. 346–353). Philadelphia, Lippencott.

Wood-Dauphinee, S. L., Opzoomer, M. A., Williams, J. L., Marchand, B. & Spitzer, W. O. (1988). Assessment of global function: The Reintegration to Normal Living Index. *Archives of Physical Medicine and Rehabilitation*, 69, 583–590.

World Health Organisation (2001). *International Classification of Function*. Geneva.

Zinn, S., Bosworth, H. B., Hoenig, H. M. & Swartzwelder, S. (2007). Executive function deficits after stroke. *Archives of Physical Medicine and Rehabilitation*, 88, 173–180.

39

Strategies for sensory processing disorders

Deborah Windley

CHAPTER CONTENTS

Introduction 638

An introduction to sensory integration
theory 638

Sensory registration 639

Sensory modulation 639

Arousal levels 639

Sensory systems 639

Inhibitory and facilitatory stimuli 640

Sensory processing disorders 640

Sensory discrimination disorders 640

Sensory modulation disorder 643

Sensory-based motor disorder 644

Sensory processing disorders and
occupation 645

Occupational therapy sensory
integration intervention 647

The person. 647

The occupation 648

The environment. 648

Conclusion. 648

SUMMARY

The ability to process sensory information is the
basis for all our interactions with the external
environment. Sensory processing skills shape our
occupational choices and roles. Sensory
processing disorders affect our ability to attend
and respond appropriately as they can impact
upon arousal level, motor co-ordination and
spatial awareness. This has a significant
consequence for occupational performance and
engagement. The relationship between sensory
integration theory and how it informs
occupational therapy intervention with people
with sensory processing disorders is discussed.
By using Practice Scenarios with a child and with
an adult with a learning disability, developmental
and compensatory strategies are explored as a
way of meeting occupational and sensory
processing needs.

KEY POINTS

- Occupational choices and roles are influenced
  by sensory processing skills.
- The term 'sensory processing disorder' is used
  rather than 'sensory integration dysfunction' in
  order to clearly distinguish the *disorders* from
  the *theory* and the *intervention*.
- Sensory integration theory describes how the
  central nervous system processes sensory
  information and facilitates motor learning,
  behaviour, emotions and attention.
- Sensory registration and sensory modulation are
  two of the core processes involved in the ability
  to process sensory information.
- The tactile, visual, vestibular and proprioceptive
  systems are relevant to sensory integration
  theory as they have a significant impact upon
  normal development and occupational
  engagement.
- There are three categories of sensory processing
  disorders: sensory discrimination disorders;
  sensory modulation disorder; and sensory-based
  motor disorder.

- Sensory processing disorders have an impact upon a person's ability to interpret and interact with stimuli, and have a global impact on occupational performance components involving physical, cognitive, psychological and emotional factors.
- There are three ways of addressing sensory processing disorders: developing the sensory processing abilities of the individual; adapting the environment to assist in optimal arousal; and designing and grading occupations to allow maximum participation.

Introduction

The ability to be aware of sensation and to respond to it appropriately could be said to be the foundation of all occupations (Dunn 2001). This ability to process sensory input is what enables humans to register what is happening in the environment, and to learn how to interact with that information in a meaningful way. Without this ability to process sensory information humans are unable to make sense of the world; preventing learning and mastery. Hence the relationship between sensory preferences and sensory processing skills may underpin occupational choices. For some a rock concert may be an exciting stimulation of their tactile, auditory, vestibular, proprioceptive and visual senses; for others it is just unpleasant and over-stimulating.

The roots of sensory integration theory (SIT) and its use within occupational therapy lie in the work of Jean Ayres. Ayres, an occupational therapist and neuroscientist, formulated SIT from her observations of children with learning, developmental and emotional difficulties (Ayres 1972). She theorised that various problems may be due to impaired sensory processing, which she termed 'sensory integration dysfunction' (Ayres 1979). Subsequent research has suggested new models and diagnostic categories for sensory integration dysfunction (Dunn 2001, McIntosh et al 1999, Miller et al 1999, 2001, 2007). Furthermore, the diversity in the group of people benefiting from sensory integration interventions has led to the need for clarification and consistency in terminology. As a result a new classification of the diagnosis of sensory processing disorders has been proposed and will be used within this chapter (Miller et al 2007). This uses the term 'sensory processing disorder' rather than 'sensory integration dysfunction' in order to clearly distinguish the *disorders* (SPD) from the *theory* (SIT) and the

intervention (occupational therapy – sensory integration (OT-SI)) (Miller et al 2007).

This chapter will explore the concepts underpinning sensory integration theory (SIT) and how these manifest in sensory processing disorders (SPD). Two practice scenarios will be used to illustrate how SPD can affect the occupational performance and engagement of a child and an adult with learning disabilities, and how occupational therapists can use SIT to enable occupational performance and engagement.

An introduction to sensory integration theory

The development of sensory processing skills is part of normal development and continues to be refined throughout life. This process is unconscious, and enables individuals to register and respond to information from the sensory systems in order to interact with the environment and make sense of the world (Bogdashina 2003).

SIT describes how the central nervous system (CNS) processes this sensory information and facilitates motor learning, behaviour, emotions and attention. Figure 39.1 illustrates the circular process which SIT describes. Firstly the CNS receives internal (vestibular and proprioceptive) and external (taste, smell, touch, vision and hearing) sensory input; secondly sensory integration takes place whereby the amount of sensory input registered is selected and enhanced or inhibited in response to the activity and the context. As Ayres (1989, p. 11) stated, 'the brain must select, enhance, inhibit, compare, and associate sensory information in a flexible, constantly changing pattern; in other words the brain must integrate it'. The CNS can then plan and organise an adaptive response appropriate to the

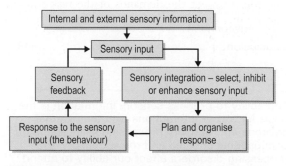

Figure 39.1 ● Circular process of sensory integration

sensory input. Adaptive behaviour can be physical or affective. Physically this is observed in the changes in muscle tone affecting movement and posture; affectively it can be seen in the emotional or stress response (Spitzer & Smith Roley 2001). This response or behaviour in itself provides feedback to the sensory system and continues the process.

Sensory registration and sensory modulation are two of the core processes involved in the ability to process sensory information. The relationship between registration, modulation and arousal levels affects the ability to respond to the environment adaptively.

Sensory registration

Although we may all have sensory preferences, our responses to sensation tend to fall within certain parameters (Williams & Shellenberger 1996). For instance walking barefoot on the sand for some is a pleasure and for others something to endure on the way to the sun bed. For an individual who is sensitive to tactile stimulation and has maladaptive registration, walking on sand may be experienced as if walking on broken glass; clearly this experience is likely to lead to a non-adaptive response to being on the beach (e.g. fearful of the sand or being very slow and cautious when walking across it). Levels of sensory awareness, or registration, are central to how we interact with stimuli from the environment.

Sensory modulation

At any one time we are bombarded by a myriad of sensations such as the touch of our clothing, the deep pressure through our seat or background noise. Sensory modulation enables the CNS to regulate and organise responses to sensory input adaptively in order to meet the demands of the task and the environment (Miller et al 2001). This is hypothesised as involving inhibition and facilitation of sensory input at a neural level, slowing and limiting the sensation that does not require attention and enhancing that which does (Dahl Reeves 2001). For instance when absorbed in a good book we may not hear someone talking to us. Yet if we were caring for a young child we can hear their cry from quite a distance away. Someone who is unable to modulate sensory input effectively may become overloaded with sensations, causing them to carry out behaviours which block out as much sensation as possible.

This ability to modulate sensory input varies dependent upon the amount of sensory demands and also on state of mind or health (Williams & Shellenberger 1996). One's tolerance to noise and distraction can be considerably affected after a late night, making it harder to shut out sensation in order to focus on studies.

Arousal levels

The CNS has been described as functioning at four different levels of arousal: asleep, awake, attending and alert (Moore 1985 cited in Williams & Shellenberger 1996). Arousal levels are regulated in order to enable attention to focus selectively on the most important stimuli for that particular context (Dahl Reeves 2001). Being in a profoundly low arousal state will mean that our reactions are slow, whereas being in an alert state means that our reactions are more heightened. Consider the body language of a tennis player awaiting a serve, they are primed to respond to the first movement of the opposing player and adapt their body in response to the speed and direction of the ball. They are in an alert state of arousal optimal to that environment and occupation.

The relationship between sensory processing and arousal levels involves the hypothalamus and the autonomic nervous system (ANS) which controls the fight-or-flight mechanism (Lane 2002). Therefore, problems associated with sensory modulation are likely to result in a stress reaction.

Sensory systems

In order to understand the relationship between sensory processing, behaviour, learning and emotions one needs to be aware of the functions of the different sensory systems. The tactile, visual, vestibular and proprioceptive systems are of particular relevance to SIT as they impact upon normal development and occupational performance most significantly.

The *tactile system* has five different types of receptors in the skin (light touch, pressure, pain, heat and cold). The tactile system contributes to the development of body schema and awareness of the body in relation to the external environment, and it also has a defensive function (Bogdashina 2003).

Through its connection with the ANS it helps to regulate arousal levels.

The *visual system* provides constant, detailed information about the social and physical environment. Its functions are closely aligned with the vestibular and proprioceptive systems and include spatiotemporal orientation, anticipation, adaptation and to support memory and learning (Smith Roley & Schneck 2001). The visual system provides extensive information on which motor planning relies such as the distance, speed, size, weight, height and nature of an object with which one needs to interact.

The *vestibular system* provides unconscious awareness of the position of the head in space via the semicircular canals located in the inner ear (Bogdashina 2003). This is stimulated by movement of the head and gravitational pull. This sensation enables the individual to maintain balance and perform co-ordinated movements. The vestibular system has a central function in arousal levels through its direct relationship with the ANS and 'primes' the entire CNS (Ayres 1979). Consequently arousal levels can be significantly affected by vestibular stimulation (e.g. being spun around (raising arousal levels) or being gently rocked (lowering arousal levels)).

The *proprioceptive system* is located in muscle fibres and receptors in the joint capsule. It is stimulated by: movement of, weight through, and pressure to, joints and muscles. This enables the individual to be aware of their body position in order to carry out co-ordinated movement and maintain posture by monitoring and adapting muscle tone (Blanche & Schaaf 2001, Bogdashina 2003).

Together these sensory systems enable the individual to adapt their level of arousal and respond to the demands of their environment and engage in occupations. The systems are all interrelated as the sensory and motor nerve fibres pass through the brain stem, a conduction pathway between the brain and the spinal cord. Within the brain stem, the reticular formation influences and is influenced by all areas of the CNS (Dahl Reeves 2001). Here positioning and postural reflexes are integrated to co-ordinate muscle tone. The reticular formation maintains equilibrium and arousal levels in response to internal and external sensory input by filtering the amount of sensory input that passes to the higher brain, interacting with the limbic structures (resulting in emotional responses to sensation), and the hypothalamus which regulates the ANS (Dahl Reeves 2001, Moore 1985).

Inhibitory and facilitatory stimuli

Different types of sensory input produce inhibitory or facilitatory effects upon the reticular formation and either raise or lower arousal levels (Dahl Reeves 2001). Table 39.1 outlines the inhibitory or facilitatory function of different forms of sensory stimulation. Inhibitory stimulation is calming and relaxing; facilitatory is alerting and arousing. The examples used in Table 39.1 are not universal as there may be individual differences but it does provide a guide to the type of stimuli in each category.

Sensory processing disorders

Individual sensory processing skills are on a continuum, with professional footballers and ballet dancers having very highly tuned sensory processing skills whilst others may 'have two left feet' (Williams & Shellenberger 1996). Our sensory preferences and tolerance to sensory input are also individually determined based on our sensory processing skills and experience. This *difference* only becomes a *disorder* when it has a severe impact upon global occupational performance and engagement, and the ability to learn new behaviour. Miller et al (2007) propose three categories of SPD: sensory discrimination disorders (SDD); sensory modulation disorder (SMD); and sensory-based motor disorder (SBMD) (Table 39.2).

Sensory discrimination disorders

Normal sensory discrimination enables the individual to effectively plan movement and postural responses in relation to any sensory information. For example, running to catch a ball requires the simultaneous registration of the visual stimuli of the ball, as well as proprioceptive and vestibular stimuli in order to move towards the ball and prepare to catch it. People with SDD have difficulty in registering sensation and being able to interpret it (Miller et al 2007). They may, therefore, need extra time to process sensation, resulting in slower and perhaps dysfunctional performance. This lack of motor skill can have psychosocial consequences as repeated failures can result in a loss of self-confidence (Miller et al 2007).

Table 39.1 Inhibitory and facilitatory sensory stimuli

Sensory modality	Tactile	Vestibular	Proprioception	Visual	Auditory	Smell and taste
Inhibitory	Deep pressure Warm air/ water	Slow linear movement (e.g. rocking)	Static weight bearing (e.g. heavy blanket) Pressure through joints and muscles (e.g. hand biting)	Low light Neutral colours Uncluttered	Soft, low voice Calming repetitive music	Bland food
Facilitatory	Light, brisk touch Varied textures	Fast movement Spinning or jumping	Movement against gravity (e.g. pushing a shopping trolley) Jumping	Bright, coloured lights Moving lights	Loud, high-pitched voice Music with strong base	Strong tastes (e.g. spicy or sour)

Table 39.2 Proposed classification for SPD (based on Miller et al 2007)

Sensory processing disorders					
Sensory modulation disorder			Sensory-based motor disorder		Sensory discrimination disorder
Sensory over-responsive	Sensory under-responsive	Sensory seeking	Dyspraxia	Postural disorders	Affects any of the six senses

Sarah, in Practice Scenario 39.1, presents with SDD affecting her ability to process vestibular and proprioceptive stimuli and, as a consequence, her occupational performance and engagement are affected (i.e. productivity (educational performance), self care (getting dressed) and leisure (being excluded from games with her friends and learning new dance routines)).

Practice Scenario 39.1 Sarah

Background to referral

Sarah was five years old when she was referred to occupational therapy, following concerns by her teacher about her poor co-ordination during physical education and the number of minor accidents she has in the playground. Sarah was also highly distractible and frequently in trouble for wandering around the classroom when she should be sitting and working.

Assessment

Sarah was assessed by:
- interviewing her parents and teacher about her occupational performance and engagement
- observation in the school environment
- carrying out a standardised developmental assessment
- the Sensory Profile (Dunn 1999).

The assessment indicated that Sarah's gross and fine motor skills were lower than her age would suggest, and that she had predominantly low muscle tone. She was struggling with reading and handwriting, and Sarah indicated that she did not like school and became tearful when talking about being in class. Despite her difficulties in physical education Sarah enjoyed singing and dancing, and went to a dance class at the weekend. Her parents reported that they often helped her get dressed in the morning in order to be out of the house in time.

Diagnosis

Sarah was diagnosed with a sensory discrimination disorder due to poor vestibular and proprioceptive processing. She was identified as being under-responsive to sensory input affecting her postural stability, spatial awareness, and motor planning skills. This resulted in poor gross motor skills and difficulties in maintaining postures, such as sitting still. She was also found to have a sensory modulation disorder resulting in being easily distracted and a poor attention span, as she would seek out sensory stimulation in her environment in order to raise her arousal levels, by wandering around the room.

Intervention

Sarah wanted to be included in more games in the playground as her friends often ran off and left her. She also wanted to be able to take part in the next stage show being held by the dance class, but found it hard to remember the three-minute routine. Sarah's parents wanted her to be more confident and independent, and her teacher wanted Sarah to be able to focus for longer on her work to develop her writing skills.

Sarah needed the opportunity to experience vestibular and proprioceptive stimulation to enable her to develop her sensory processing skills. This would allow her to organise the sensory input and facilitate the development of mastery and self-confidence in her occupations.

Sarah, her parents, and her teacher all required education in order to understand what the underlying causes of her difficulties were. They required advice to facilitate Sarah's sensory processing skills and promote her occupational performance and engagement. Sarah needed to be able to identify her own regulation needs and access the correct type of sensory input as required.

Individual occupational therapy sessions

Individual sessions focused on providing vestibular stimulation (e.g. spinning and swinging in a net hammock), swing in conjunction with inhibitory stimulation (the deep pressure from the net hammock itself). The spinning was controlled by Sarah by pushing herself around. Over time the intervention developed at Sarah's pace and facilitated postural control by increasing demands on sitting balance (e.g. reaching and throwing whilst on a platform swing with no proprioceptive input). These activities were graded to include more demands in motor planning (e.g. negotiating an obstacle course).

Sensory diet

Discussions took place with Sarah and her parents about what would help her to reach optimal arousal to enable her to engage in her occupations. She was given an individualised sensory diet to maximise her access to the sensory input she required (vestibular and proprioceptive) and advised how to use inhibitory and facilitatory sensory input to maximise her occupational performance. The 'diets' for home, school and dance class can be seen in Table 39.3.

The arousing sensory input shown in the table can be used to prepare Sarah for carrying out activities and facilitate her ability to attend to the task. Before getting dressed each morning her CNS can be 'woken up' with a cool shower and being briskly towel dried. This will aid her organisational skills in order to dress herself in conjunction with the inhibitory strategies of reducing distraction. Encouraging the use of the mini trampoline and space hopper at home were means of Sarah receiving more vestibular and proprioceptive feedback.

Table 39.3 Sensory diet for Sarah (adapted from Wilbarger 1995)

Tactile	Vestibular	Proprioception	Visual	Auditory
Calming				
		Tight lycra leotard for dance class – provides deep pressure	Minimise visual distractions Black out curtains Low-light hiding place in classroom for Sarah to retreat when over-stimulated	Minimal verbal communication Soft voice Repeated phrases
Arousing				
Cool shower Body scrubs or briskly towel dried	Mini trampoline Space hopper Dancing Bouncy cushion for school chair	Mini trampoline Space hopper Dancing Bouncy cushion for school chair		

Sarah was encouraged to be aware of her own arousal levels and to recognise what type of activities would help her to 'wake up' or 'calm down'.

Compensatory methods

Sarah required the minimum of distraction when carrying out focused activity. Therefore, noise, movement and light should be reduced as much as possible. For instance, when getting dressed in the morning her parents were advised that Sarah should be with one of them on her own with the door closed. Using a minimum of discussion Sarah should be prompted to get dressed and by placing the clothes in sequence the demands of motor planning are reduced. Strategies to overcome current priorities such as videoing the dance routine for Sarah to practice at home, or facilitating structured imaginative play with her friends as opposed to more demanding physical activities were discussed with the parents and teacher.

Sensory modulation disorder

Sensory modulation enables individuals to be flexible, responsive and able to adapt to changing conditions (Miller et al 2001). For instance on picking up a box which we assume to be heavy only to find it is empty, the response is modulated quickly, re-arranging posture and muscle tone to avoid falling over or throwing the box in the air. SMD exists when there is a problem in the regulation and organisation of the response to sensory input affecting occupational performance (Miller et al 2001). Miller et al (2007) identify three disorders related to sensory modulation: under responsivity, over responsivity and sensory seeking.

People with SMD demonstrate sensory avoiding or sensory seeking behaviours usually dependent upon their ability to register sensory input (Dunn 2001). Those with a low sensory awareness usually crave sensory input and seek it out in order to raise their arousal levels and interact with the environment successfully. Those with over responsivity may avoid sensory input or seek out inhibitory stimulation in order to reduce arousal levels (Dunn 2001). Peter in Practice Scenario 39.2 avoids engaging in any activity, quickly becomes over aroused and distressed resulting in biting his hand to provide deep pressure and reduce arousal levels. This is indicative of being over-responsive.

Practice Scenario 39.2 Peter

Background to referral

Peter is 28 years old, has a severe learning disability and lives in 24-hour supported accommodation. He was referred to occupational therapy because the support staff found him difficult to engage in occupations due to extreme fluctuations in his arousal levels and challenging behaviours, such as biting his hand and hitting his head. Peter spent the majority of his time alone in bed and his support staff were concerned about his lack of engagement. These were long-standing difficulties and there was no indication that Peter had any physical or mental health problems.

Assessment

Assessment of Peter's occupational performance and sensory processing was carried out through discussion with support staff and observation of Peter carrying out his activities of daily living, using the Sensory Integration Inventory-Revised for Individuals with Developmental Disabilities (Reisman & Hanschu 1992), and the Adult/Adolescent Sensory Profile (Brown & Dunn 2002). Peter's limited communication and cognitive skills made it difficult to obtain information directly from him. His occupational performance also needed to be assessed in relation to his learning disability.

Peter enjoyed walking and running in the park, going for coffee in the local café, watching staff make dinner and doing certain puzzles. However, he was inconsistent in his willingness to do these occupations, had a very short attention span and would frequently become distressed and self-injure by biting his hand.

Assessment by the psychologist had not indicated any specific environmental triggers for these behaviours, the speech and language therapist introduced a visual reference communication system to facilitate Peter's ability to make choices.

Diagnosis

Peter had a sensory modulation disorder indicated by fluctuating arousal levels, resulting in Peter seeking inhibitory stimulation by retiring to his room where it was quiet, wrapping himself up in his duvet and avoiding any form of interaction.

Intervention

The aim of occupational therapy intervention was to enable Peter to participate in more occupations, reduce the time spent alone in his room and reduce the incidence of self-injury.

Sensory diet

Peter required assistance to modulate his sensory input by access to stimulation which raised his arousal levels to facilitate awareness and then reduce arousal to prevent over-stimulation and anxiety. The support staff had to be trained to know how to meet these needs.

Grading and adapting

Activities and the environment needed to be designed to provide optimal proprioceptive, vestibular, visual and tactile sensory input. These ensured that there was inhibitory stimulation included in each activity. Ideas for activities can be seen in Table 39.4. By Peter wearing a weighted rucksack when walking or a heavy cushion on his lap when doing a table-top activity it was possible to provide inhibitory stimulation for Peter to enable him to continue to engage with an activity and not become over-stimulated.

The pattern of his day needed to take into account high and low arousal type activities, so that he could gradually raise his arousal levels followed by a period of withdrawal to his room to reduce them again. Support staff were given general guidelines about carrying out activities, such as to give time to Peter to process information and assist this by establishing: a daily routine, a set of visual cues for each activity, a consistent location, and a routine for each activity. This assisted Peter in being aware of what was expected of him and preparing himself to respond appropriately.

Table 39.4 Activities that meet Peter's sensory processing needs

Occupations	Ideas
Cooking	• Using electric whisk/hand blender to make smoothies or soups (P, Vest, T) • Kneading dough (P, T) • Rolling out scones (P, T)
Domestic	• Take laundry basket to washing machine/load machine (P, T, Vest) • Empty rubbish bins (P, T, Vest) • Putting tins away in cupboard. (P, T, Vest)
Garden	• Digging (P) • Pushing wheelbarrow (P)
Gym	• Trampolining (P, Vest) • Weight training (P) • Running (P, Vest)
Outdoor leisure	• Hill walking (P) • Parachute-type games (V, Vest, P, T)
Indoor leisure	• Collage making (T, V) • Table top games (V) • Wind instruments (P)
Relaxation	• Chanting music (Vest) • Rocking chair (Vest)

P – proprioceptive; Vest – vestibular; V – visual; T – tactile

Table 39.5 illustrates examples of responses to high or low registration of tactile and vestibular sensory input. The type of stimulation which is sought out will reflect whether it has an inhibitory or facilitatory function (Table 39.1). Someone with SMD is likely to swing between low and high arousal states affecting their levels of anxiety when presented with particular stimuli (Porter 2002, Stagnitti et al 1999). People with SMD exhibit emotional problems (e.g. anxiety, depression, lability); attentional problems (e.g. hyperactivity); difficulties in carrying out activities of daily living and poor social interaction skills (Miller et al 2001). Peter, in Practice Scenario 39.2, is exhibiting some of these factors as he isolates himself and becomes anxious and stressed, very quickly leading to self-injury.

Sensory-based motor disorder

Skilled movement requires the ability to register and modulate sensory input adaptively. People with SBMD have occupational performance difficulties related to poor motor co-ordination and motor planning. This is often related to either a SMD or SDD and is manifest as either a postural disorder, difficulty in stabilising posture in order to carry out a task or, dyspraxia, being unable to effectively plan the movements required (Miller et al 2007). These children are often labelled clumsy or lazy as their finished work often seem messy and incomplete, and they find physical activities such as sport extremely challenging.

Table 39.5 Behaviours resulting from sensory processing disorders

Sensory modality	Misperception	Examples of behaviour
Tactile	Misperception of touch and/or pain	**Over-responsive** Withdrawing when touched, refusing to eat certain 'textured' foods and/or to wear certain types of clothing, complaining about having hair or face washed, avoiding getting hands dirty, using finger tips rather than whole hands to manipulate objects, self-imposed isolation, general irritability, distractibility, and hyperactivity
		Under-responsive Mouthing, touching objects constantly, unexplained cuts, scratches and burns
Vestibular	Misperception of movement and changes in position of the head	**Over-responsive** Fearful reactions to ordinary movement activities (e.g. swings, slides, ramps, inclines), trouble learning to climb or descend stairs or hills, apprehensive walking or crawling on uneven or unstable surfaces, fearful in open space, clumsy
		Under-responsive Actively seek very intense sensory experiences such as excessive body whirling, jumping, and/or spinning
Proprioception	Misperception of muscle tone, joint, and tendon components affecting subconscious awareness of body position and posture	Clumsiness, tendency to fall, lack of awareness of body position in space, odd body posturing, difficulty manipulating small objects, eating in a sloppy manner, resistance to new motor movement activities, poor motor planning

Sensory processing disorders and occupation

Occupational performance is determined by the interrelationship between the person the environment and the occupation (Law et al 1996). SPD impacts upon the *person's* ability to interpret and interact with stimuli, and has a global impact on occupational performance components including physical, cognitive, psychological and emotional factors. Consequently children with SPD often have additional diagnoses/labels such as minimal brain dysfunction, clumsy child syndrome, specific language disability, pervasive developmental disorder, dyslexia, dyspraxia, developmental co-ordination disorder and attention deficit hyperactivity disorder (Ayres 1972, Chu 1996, Kientz & Dunn 1997, Mulligan 1996). These children experience delay in mastery of skills in relation to their peers.

Occupational roles are dynamic and change throughout life, and childhood is characterised by extreme occupational role changes (Baum & Christiansen 2005). This ability to acquire new roles relies upon learning new skills which arise from past and new experiences (Moyers 2005). Establishing appropriate occupational roles at different life stages is essential for successful socialisation and is the result of learning adaptive role behaviour (Baum & Christiansen 2005). The ability to carry expected roles has an impact upon self-esteem and is particularly relevant in childhood, where self concept is still developing.

The primary school child who is able to sit still and pay attention during class may adapt more easily to secondary and higher education than the highly distractible child, regardless of intellectual abilities, and so will benefit from the positive regard of their teachers and family. However, children who lack the sensory processing skills to be involved in games and sports may be last to be picked for a team or even excluded from playground games. A child with SPD can easily be thought of as rough due to their poor co-ordination and modulation skills leading to over hitting, over throwing or running into people. Exclusion and possible social isolation may influence other aspects of their personality. For those without other compensatory resources such as intellectual skills or an understanding and supportive family, the long-term consequences can be poor self-esteem and confidence which may in turn impact in the long term on mental health.

However, the relationship between SPD and occupational performance is a complex one. Whilst literature indicates a relationship between SPD and decreased social skills, immature play, impaired self concept, decreased motor skills, poor school performance and deficits in activities of daily living (Bundy 2002, Parham & Mailloux 2005), studies are not conclusive. White et al (2007) found a statistically significant relationship between sensory processing and occupational performance, particularly in relation to those tasks requiring motor co-ordination in children between 5 and 13 years. However, the study by Bundy et al (2007) did not find a correlation between SPD and playfulness, indicating a more complex relationship between SPD and the type of play children may choose to engage in rather than overall playfulness.

People with SMD may experience great fluctuations in their arousal levels and this has been linked to attention deficit disorder or problems of impulse control (Chu 1996). Many individuals will present with significant behavioural problems as their ability to concentrate and modulate their behaviour is challenged. Childhood occupational dysfunction can have severe consequences not only for the individual and their family but for society itself. Studies indicate that low educational attainment often associated with impulsivity and hyperactivity are risk factors for juvenile delinquency (Farrington 1999). Small studies of young offenders have found an association with factors indicative of SPD (Meltzer et al 1984, Snyder & Fanchiang 1990).

Behaviours that the individual with SPD discovers assist in optimising arousal levels may be seen as maladaptive by others. For a child with SPD the demands within the classroom to sit still and be quiet may be incompatible with their sensory processing needs; so that the child who needs to move about is apparently disruptive and is excluded from school. Such socially unacceptable behaviours come to prevent integration and participation in occupations. This is particularly the case for adults and children with SPD and learning disabilities whose cognitive impairment may prevent them from understanding the consequences of their behaviours. In some instances this can result in a predominance of self-stimulatory or self-injurious behaviours in order to access the inhibitory or facilitatory stimuli they require (Brocklehurst-Woods 1990, Reisman 1993). Triggers for challenging behaviour are very closely related to arousal levels (Emerson 2001). Head banging, teeth grinding, and hand biting can all reduce arousal levels and cause self-injury. Furthermore, a preoccupation with self-stimulation can exclude the person from engaging with opportunities for learning and participation, placing the individual at risk of occupational deprivation (Whiteford 2000), if they are not enabled to access occupations which meet sensory processing needs.

There is growing evidence that a high proportion of adults and children with learning disabilities have SPD (Bogdashina 2003, Green et al 2003, Reisman & Hanschu 1992). Investigations into the psychophysiological responses to sensory input indicate that atypical sensory responses are a common feature of autism, fragile X syndrome and Down's syndrome (McIntosh et al 1999, Miller et al 1999). For people on the autistic spectrum, estimates for abnormal responses to sensory stimuli range between 30 and 100% (Dawson & Watling 2000). A survey of 30 people on the autistic spectrum revealed that 70% reported a sensitivity to touch, 87% sensitivity to auditory experiences, and 81% reported differences in their visual perception having an impact on their spatial awareness (Walker & Cantello 1994). The consequences of this can be severe self injury, seclusion from society, harm to others and a very limited quality of life.

The multiple pathologies which a person with a severe learning disability may present with make any one diagnosis very difficult. Some behaviour may be a manifestation of an underlying physical or mental health problem. Furthermore, the person may have developed behaviours which meet sensory, communication or physical needs and have become embedded in their routines. It is essential that any assessment of such behaviour is multi-disciplinary, encompassing health, communication, environmental, and occupational needs.

Occupational therapy sensory integration intervention

Miller et al (2007) use the term occupational therapy-sensory integration (OT-SI) to indicate occupational therapy intervention which is informed by SIT. As with other frames of reference, the occupational therapist should use SIT in order to maximise the individual's ability to participate in occupations. Returning to the person-environment-occupation (Law et al 1996) model shows us that there are three ways of addressing these needs:

1. Developing the sensory processing abilities of the individual

2. Adapting the environment to assist in optimal arousal

3. Designing and grading occupations to allow maximum participation.

OT-SI-based interventions have been traditionally guided by the following principles:

- Sensory processing skills are developmental and emerge with the maturation of the CNS and sensory experience. OT-SI intervention promotes the normal development of neural processes, and organisation of the brain (Bundy & Murray 2002).

- These interventions are based on neural plasticity, or the ability of the brain structures to change and develop following adaptive responses to stimuli. OT-SI intervention addresses the underlying dysfunction rather than training in specific skills or behaviour (Bundy & Murray 2002).

- Adaptive behaviour facilitates sensory processing skills as the CNS receives sensory feedback from adaptive behaviour. OT-SI intervention uses planned and controlled sensory input to elicit an adaptive response and facilitate brain organisation (Bundy & Murray 2002).

- People have an inner drive to achieve mastery over their environment (Bundy & Murray 2002); the service user initiates, directs and engages in therapeutic activities at their own level of ability.

The first three principles adopt a purely developmental perspective. However, SIT can be applied in a compensatory manner with adaptations made to the environment or the occupation itself to enable the individual to maximise his occupational engagement. In Practice Scenario 39.1, when working with Sarah a 5-year-old child, more emphasis is placed upon the developmental aspect of the intervention seeking to promote the development of her sensory processing skills. In Practice Scenario 39.2, when working with Peter a 28-year-old adult with a learning disability, emphasis is placed on a compensatory approach in order to promote interaction and minimise self-injury and withdrawal.

The person

Practice Scenario 39.1 demonstrates how OT-SI encourages Sarah to experience an adaptive response to previously challenging sensory input by providing a secure and safe environment, and maintaining optimum arousal levels (Bundy & Koomar 2002). For example, a child who is over-responsive to vestibular stimulation will have a maladaptive response to movement, resulting in them avoiding physical play. By wrapping them up tightly in a blanket and providing inhibitory deep pressure whilst on a swing the child's arousal levels will be reduced. This will allow the child to experience the vestibular sensation of swinging and begin to process the sensation in an adaptive way. Although Sarah is under-responsive to sensory input, her immature modulation skills mean that she could easily change from being under-stimulated to being over-stimulated once she starts to use the swing and register the vestibular stimulation.

By providing deep pressure through the net hammock the occupational therapist controls the sensory input encouraging child-led exploration and tapping into the child's 'inner drive'. The occupational therapist will provide more challenging opportunities for the child to test and develop vestibular processing within a fun-filled child-centred play environment. OT-SI is child-directed, in this instance facilitating vestibular stimulation, which provides the enjoyment and exhilaration that a child without SPD can experience every day in the playground. The OT-SI goal will be to enable the child to pursue these experiences in a more adaptive manner independently once neural development has taken place.

The occupation

Although it is a developmental framework, SIT can underpin a compensatory approach and facilitate greater participation and engagement in occupations. 'Sensory diets' are personalised sensory-based activity schedules (Wilbarger 1995), which aim to provide the sensory input an individual's CNS requires to stay focused and organised in order to carry out occupations. A person whose CNS is over-responsive will need more calming input, while someone who is under-responsive will need more arousing input. Therefore, a diet is designed to enable the individual to access appropriate sensory stimuli and facilitate optimum arousal in preparation for carrying out an occupation (Dunn 1999). For example, someone who is under-responsive may need highly stimulatory tactile input to raise arousal levels in order to prepare the CNS to carry out the motor co-ordination demands of getting dressed. This could be integrated into their daily routine (e.g. by briskly rubbing moisturiser onto their arms and legs before getting dressed, or using a body scrub in the shower each morning). This may lead to more developed sensory processing skills or become a long-term management strategy. Williams and Shellenberger (1996) adopt this approach as a way of empowering children and their carers in understanding their sensory processing needs and developing their own strategies for optimising arousal in order to achieve success and independence.

The principles of inhibitory and facilitatory stimulation in Table 39.1 can be applied to the individual based on daily activities carried out in order to ensure appropriate sensory input to facilitate occupational engagement. Table 39.6 shows some examples of the types of items which can be included in such a diet. Some may become an occupation in themselves (e.g. trampolining), others may be necessary before, during or after an activity as appropriate (e.g. someone with a SMD where they are predominantly over-responsive may require a lot of calming activities before, during and after a task requiring concentration). The sensory diet could recommend head massage (tactile deep pressure) beforehand, a stress ball to squeeze during the activity (proprioception) and a quiet dark space to retreat to after the activity. Using similar principles, OT-SI can identify activities to promote engagement and encourage participation, as they will be meeting and not challenging sensory processing needs. Practice Scenario 39.2 illustrates how activities

can be individually designed to meet the needs of someone with SMD, and incorporate appropriate sensory input throughout the day.

The environment

Sensory 'adaptation' requires examination of the environment and the occupation from a sensory perspective and identifying where the barriers to participation may be for someone with SPD. OT-SI can provide guidance on the optimum sensory environment for particular tasks or the way in which they are carried out (Bundy & Koomar 2002, Williams & Shellenberger 1996). For example, an individual on the autistic spectrum who has a SMD may become over-aroused in visually and aurally stimulating environments. In order for them to be able to focus on an individual task requiring concentration the amount of stimulation may need to be minimised. They would benefit from having either a quiet room or a screened off area in order to successfully carry out certain tasks, such as art work or completing a jigsaw. Peter in Practice Scenario 39.2 is required to have on-going access to a room with minimal sensory input in order to enable him to reduce his arousal levels at periods throughout the day.

Conclusion

Understanding a diagnosis of SPD has evolved considerably since Ayres' first formulation of sensory integration dysfunction (Ayres 1972). Models of practice emphasise the importance of self-regulation (Dahl Reeves 2001, Dunn 2001, Williams & Shellenberger 1996) and how this can be applied with diverse populations. OT-SI intervention can work directly with the individual to develop sensory processing skills. However, it can also empower individuals and their carers by them learning how to regulate modulation of the CNS through compensatory methods, grading and adapting to maximise participation in occupation.

The development of a classification of SPD (Miller et al 2007) is an important step in creating a unified approach to diagnosis. It could be argued that some of the difficulty occupational therapists have had in developing a sound research base for SIT has been because the group of people who have SPD has been poorly defined, leading to SIT being used

Table 39.6 Sensory diet (adapted from Wilbarger 1995)

Tactile	Vestibular	Proprioception	Visual	Auditory	Taste/smell
Calming					
Brushing hair Foot spa Massage with warm oils Warm bath	Rocking chair	Deep massage/pressure Heavy blanket Squashy objects to hold Supportive/squashy seating	Minimise objects in environment	Minimal verbal communication Soft voice Repeated phrases	Bland food
Arousing					
Sherbert and fizzy drinks Feathers Vibrating products Electric fan Nail care Body scrubs	Trampolining Walking and opportunity for movement Vibrating products Dancing	Tug of war games Parachute games Laughing Musical instruments to bang or blow Balloons to hit Dancing	Lava lamps Projected images Bubble tube Sun catchers/ mobiles Mirrors Bright lights Hide and seek games	Lively upbeat voice Music with strong beat	Strong contrasting tastes and smells (e.g. pickles, spicy, garlic, citrus)

for diverse applications. More defined diagnostic categories and procedures for intervention may assist this research (Parnham et al 2007). This chapter has argued for an inclusive approach to addressing SPD which may or may not address the underlying sensory processing skills. This highlights the role of a compensatory approach in order to facilitate occupation.

References

Ayres, J. (1972). *Sensory integration and learning disorders*. Los Angeles, Western Psychological Services.

Ayres, J. (1979). *Sensory integration and the child*. Los Angeles, Western Psychological Services.

Ayres, J. (1989). *Sensory integration and praxis tests*. Los Angeles, Western Psychological Services.

Baum, C. M. & Christiansen, C. H. (2005). Person-environment-occupation-performance: An occupation-based framework for practice. In C. M. Baum, C. H. Christiansen & J. Bass-Haugen (Eds.) *Occupational therapy: performance, participation and well being* (3rd ed) (pp. 243–266). Thorofare, NJ, Slack Inc.

Blanche, E. I. & Schaaf, R. C. (2001) Proprioception: A cornerstone of sensory integration intervention. In S. Smith Roley, E. Blanche & R. Schaaf (Eds.). *Sensory integration*

with diverse populations (pp. 109–124). San Antonio, USA, Therapy Skill Builders.

Bogdashina, O. (2003). *Sensory perceptual issues in autism and Aspergers syndrome* London and Philadelphia, Jessica Kingsley Publishers.

Brocklehurst-Woods, J. (1990) The use of tactile and vestibular stimulation to reduce stereotypic behaviours in two adults with mental retardation. *American Journal of Occupational Therapy*, 44(6), 536–541.

Brown, C. E. & Dunn, W. (2002). *Adolescent/adult sensory profile*. San Antonio, USA, Psychological Corporation: Therapy Skill Builders.

Bundy, A. (2002). Using sensory integration theory in schools: sensory integration and consultation. In A. Bundy, S. J. Lane & E. A. Murray (Eds.) *Sensory*

integration theory and practice (2nd Ed.). (pp. 310–331). Philadelphia, F.A. Davis.

Bundy, A. & Koomar, J. (2002). *Orchestrating intervention: The art of practice*. In A. Bundy, S. J. Lane & E. A. Murray (Eds.). *Sensory integration theory and practice* (2nd Ed.). (pp. 242–259). Philadelphia, F.A. Davis.

Bundy, A. & Murray, S. L. (2002). *Sensory Integration: A. Jean Ayres revisited*. In A. Bundy, S. J. Lane & E. A. Murray (Eds.) *Sensory integration theory and practice* (2nd Ed) (pp. 3–33). Philadelphia, F.A. Davis.

Bundy, A., Shia, S., Qi, L. & Miller, L. J. (2007). How does sensory processing dysfunction affect play? *American Journal of Occupational Therapy*, 61, 201–208.

Chu, S. (1996) Evaluating the sensory integrative functions of mainstream schoolchildren with specific developmental disorders. *British Journal of Occupational Therapy*, 59(10), 465–474.

Dahl Reeves, G. (2001). From neuron to behaviour. In: S. Smith Roley, E. Blanche & R. Schaaf (Eds.). *Sensory integration with diverse populations* (pp. 89–108). San Antonio, USA, Therapy Skill Builders.

Dawson, G. & Watling, R. (2000). Interventions to facilitate auditory, visual and motor integration in autism: A review of the evidence. *Journal of Autism and Developmental Disorders*, 30(5), 415–422.

Dunn, W. (1999). *The sensory profile*. San Antonio, TX, Psychological Corporation.

Dunn, W. (2001) 2001 Eleanor Clarke Slagle Lecture – The sensations of everyday life: Empirical, theoretical & pragmatic considerations. *American Journal of Occupational Therapy*, 55, 608–620.

Emerson, E. (2001). *Challenging behaviour: Analysis and intervention in people with severe intellectual disabilities*. Cambridge, Cambridge University Press.

Farrington, D. (1996). *Social Policy Research Findings* No. 3. York, Joseph Rowntree Foundation.

Green, D., Beaton, L., Moore, D., Warren, L., Wick, V., Sanford, J. & Santosh, P. (2003). Clinical incidents of sensory integration difficulties in adults with intellectual disabilities and illustration of management. *British Journal of Occupational Therapy*, 66(10), 454–463.

Hare, D. J., Chapman, M., Fraser, J., Gore, S. & Burton, M. (2003). The prevalence of autistic spectrum disorders in people using a community intellectual disabilities service. *Journal of Intellectual Disabilities*, 7(3), 267–281.

Kientz, M. A. & Dunn, W. (1997). A comparison of the performance of children with and without autism on the sensory profile. *American Journal of Occupational Therapy*, 51, 494–503.

Koomar, J. & Bundy, A. (1991). The art and science of creating direct intervention from theory. In: A. G. Fisher, E. A. Murray & A. C. Bundy (Eds.) *Sensory integration:*

Theory and practice (pp. 251–317). Philadelphia, FA Davis Company.

Lane, S. (2002). Structure and function of the sensory systems. In A. Bundy, S. J. Lane & E. A. Murray (Eds.) *Sensory integration theory and practice* (2nd Ed). (pp. 35–70). Philadelphia, F.A, Davis.

Law, M., Cooper, B., Strong, S., Stewart, D., Rigby, P. & Letts, L. (1996). The person-environment-occupation model: A transactive approach to occupational performance. *Canadian Journal of Occupational Therapy*, 63, 9–23.

McIntosh, D. N., Miller, L. J., Shyu, V. & Hagerman, R. J. (1999) Sensory-modulation disruption, electrodermal responses, and functional behaviours. *Developmental Medicine and Child Neurology*, 41, 608–615.

Meltzer, H., Levine, M. D., Karniski, W., Palfrey, A. & Clarke, S. (1984). An analysis of learning styles of adolescent delinquents. *Journal of Learning Disabilities*, 17, 600–608.

Miller, L. J., McIntosh, D. N., McGrath, J., Shyu, V., Lampe, M., Taylor, A. K., Tassone, F., Neitzel, K., Stackhouse, T. & Hagerman, R. J. (1999) Electrodermal responses to sensory stimuli in individuals with fragile X syndrome: a preliminary report. *American Journal of Medical Genetics*, 83, 268–279.

Miller, L. J., Reisman, J. E., McIntosh, D. N. & Simon, J. (2001). An ecological model of sensory modulation: Performance of children with fragile X syndrome, autism, attention deficit/hyperactivity disorder and sensory modulation disorder. In A. Smith Roley, E. Blanche & R. Schaaf (Eds.). *Sensory integration with diverse populations* (pp. 57–88). San Antonio, USA, Therapy Skill Builders.

Miller, L. J., Anzalone, M. E., Lane, S., Cermak, S. A & Osten, E. T. (2007). Concept evolution in SI: A proposed nosology for diagnosis. *American Journal of Occupational Therapy*, 61(2), 135–140.

Moyers, P. (2005). Introduction to occupation based practice. In

Baum, C. M., Christiansen, C. H. & Bass-Haugen J. (Eds.) *Occupational therapy: performance, participation and well being* (3rd ed). (pp. 221–234). Thorofare, NJ, Slack Inc.

Mulligan, S. (1996). An analysis of score patterns of children with attention disorders on the Sensory Integration and Praxis Tests. *American Journal of Occupational Therapy*, 50, 647–654.

Parham, L. D. & Mailloux, Z. (2005). *Sensory integration*. In J. Case-Smith (Ed.). *Occupational therapy for children* (5th Ed.). (pp. 356–409). St Louis, MO, Mosby.

Parnham, L. D, Cohn, E. S., Spitzer, S., Koomar, J., Miller, L. J., Burke, J. P., Brett-Green, B., Mailloux, Z., May-Benson, T. A., Smith Roley, S., Schaaf, R. C, Schoen, S. A. & Summers, C.A. (2007). Fidelity in sensory integration intervention research. *American Journal of Occupational Therapy*, 61(2), 216–227.

Porter, J. L. (2002) *Sensory modulation disorder – A case study*. Sensor Net Newsletter, 16, 4–8.

Reisman, J. (1993) Using a sensory integrative approach to treat self injurious behaviour in an adult with profound mental retardation. *American Journal of Occupational Therapy*, 47(5), 403–411.

Reisman, J. E. & Hanschu, B. (1992) *Sensory integration inventory – revised for individuals with developmental disabilities*. Hugo, MN, POP Press.

Smith Roley, S. & Schneck, C. (2001). Sensory integration and visual deficits including blindness. In S. Smith Roley, E. Blanche & R. Schaaf (Eds.). *Sensory integration with diverse populations* (pp. 313–344). San Antonio, TX, Therapy Skill Builders.

Spitzer, S. & Smith Roley, S. (2001). Sensory Integration revisited: A philosophy of practice. In S. Smith Roley, E. Blanche & R. Schaaf (Eds) *Sensory integration with diverse populations* (pp. 3–23). Therapy Skill Builders: San Antonio, TX.

Stagnitti, K., Raison, P. & Ryan, P. (1999). Sensory defensiveness syndrome: A paediatric perspective and case study. *Australian*

Occupational Therapy Journal, 46, 175–187.

Snyder, C. & Fanchiang, S. P. (1990). Sensory integration and delinquency. *Sensory Integration Special Interest Section Newsletter*, 13(3), 4–6.

Walker, N. & Cantello, J. (1994). *You don't have the words to describe what I experience. The sensory experience of individuals with autism, based on first hand accounts*. The

Geneva Centre for Autism. Available: http://www.autism.net/html/nowords.html. Accessed 18/6/02.

White, B. P., Mulligan, S., Merrill, K. & Wright, J. (2007). An examination of the relationships between motor process skills and scores on the sensory profile. *American Journal of Occupational Therapy*, 61(2), 154–162.

Whiteford, G. (2000). Occupational deprivation: Global Challenge in

the New Millennium. *British Journal of Occupational Therapy*, 63(5), 200–204.

Wilbarger, P. (1995). The sensory diet: Activity programs based upon sensory processing theory. *Sensory Integration Special Interest Section Newsletter*, 18(2), 1–3.

Williams, S. W. & Shellenberger, S. (1996) *How does your engine run? A leaders guide to the alert program for self regulation*. Albuquerque, TherapyWorks, Inc.

Index

A-ONE, **615**
AARR (Avoid Assess Reduce Review),
manual-handling injuries
prevention, 562, 570
Ableism, 45
Access
housing design, 411
building regulations/standards,
413–414
universal design, 411, 413
Accomplishment of natural growth,
137, 138
Accountability of therapists, 42
ACL, **616**
Action Research Arm Test (ARAT),
594, 595
Active engagement, nature of
occupation, 19
Active listening, 154, 207, 457
Active participation model, 226
Activism, 215
Activities of daily living, 342
Activity analysis, home modification
assessment, **424**
Activity Card Sort, 365
Hong Kong version, 84
Activity demands
influence on performance, 178, **179**
work rehabilitation assessment
process, 401, 402
Activity Index, 365, 366
Adaptation
as enabling skill, **117**
joint protection strategies, 539
process skills, **170**
strength improvement strategies, 538
see also Adjustment to physical
impairment
Adaptations, environmental
enabling leisure activities, 367
as enabling skill, **118**
Adaptive equipment
enabling leisure activities, 367
work rehabilitation, 405
Adaptive role behaviour, 645
Adaptive seating systems, 482, **485**
Adjustable height beds/baths, 570

Adjustment disorders, 191
Adjustment to physical impairment,
194, 200
enabling strategies, 200
perceived personal control, 201
psychosocial intervention strategies,
201–202
Adult learning, 223–224
Advocacy, 211–219, 272, 282, 284,
287, 328
community-based rehabilitation, 316
concept, 214–215
definitions, 215
driving/community mobility, 495
as enabling skill, **117**
occupational justice, **289**
in occupational therapy practice,
214–215, **217**
barriers to incorporation, 287–288
managing associated conflicts, 218
promoting disabled peoples'
participation, 288, **289**
therapist as agent of change,
215–216
social model of disability, 213
types, **216**
Affirmative model of disability, 31–32,
35
Age-associated cognitive decline,
occupational group work, 258
Age-friendly environments, 431
Agnosias, 610
intervention strategies, 630
Alcohol abuse, driving safety
considerations, 492
Alexia (word blindness), 610
Alzheimer's disease, 472, 608–609
Americans with Disabilities Act, 413
Anger management, 202
Anosognosia, 610
intervention strategies, 630
Anthropometrics, 415, 417, 420
assistive device design, 455
home modification interventions,
421, 422
performance measurements, 420
structural measurements, 420

Anxiety
cognitive/perceptual problems
assessment, 614
management, 202
Anxiety disorder, 190, 191
Aphasia, 611
Appliance height, 448, **448**
Appropriate paper technology (APT),
334
Apraxia, 611
intervention strategies, 631
Architectural drawings, 426
Argumentative reasoning, 64
ARJO Mobility Gallery, 565
Arousal levels, 639, 640
inhibitory/facilitatory effects of
sensory stimulation, 640, **641**
sensory processing disorders, 646,
648
sensory diets, **642**, **644**, 648, **649**
Arthritis Impact Measurement Scales
(AIMS2), 536
Arthritis, use of orthoses, 509, 511
Articulate practice, 7, 330
Arts-based activities, community
development, 274
Assertiveness training, 202
Assessment, 81–91, 96, 97
assistive device selection, 28,
459–460
biomechanical strategies, 535–536
cognitive/perceptual problems,
613–620, **615–619**
consent, 83
data gathering, 82
as continuous process, 85
methods, 59–60, 88–91
procedure, 87
tools, 86
driving safety, 494
specialist occupational therapist's
role *see* Driving
ethical issues, 87, 89
evidence-based practice, 83
home modification, 414, 416–417
activity analysis, **424**
occupational basis, 415

impairments, 84
informal/formal, 348
informational needs, 227
leisure occupations, 364–366
meaningfulness of occupation, 82
non-standardised, 90–91, 348
   limitations, 91
occupation analysis, 165, 182
occupation-based, 84–85
   goals/strategies, 87
   top-down approach, 83–84, 165,
      166
occupational therapy process, 59–60
orthoses prescription, 509, 511
   biomechanical examination, **514**
person-centred, 83
person–environment–occupation fit,
   98–99, **100**
play as means in children, 379, 382
reporting, 87
screening, 85–87
self-care, 346–350
   practice scenario, **349**
sensory impairments, 545–548, **546**
   indepth standardised instruments,
      548
standardised, 88–89, 99, 348
   professional responsibility, 89–90
   psychometric properties, 89
   review, 90
   validity/reliability, 88, 99
steps, 85, **86**
wheelchair users' spectrum of
   abilities, 473, **473**
wheeled mobility systems
      prescription, 476
   basic measurements, **476**
   orthopaedic factors, 482
   postural control evaluation, 480,
      482
   postural management, 480
   tools, **481**
work rehabilitation process, 401–403
Assessment of Communication and
   Interaction Skills (ACIS), 162,
   167, 182
Assessment of Computer-Related
   Skills, 84
Assessment of Ludic Behaviours, 383
Assessment of Motor and Process
   Skills (AMPS), 84, 89, 162,
   167, 182, 536, 613, **616**
Assistive devices, 421, 453–466, **454**,
   455

assessment, 459–460, **460**
   tools, 460
assimilation into person's routine,
   464, 465
enabling occupation, 454, 457
evaluation of effectiveness, 465–466,
   466
   formal measures, 465
funding, 464
goals selection, 460
historical development, 456–457
intervention, 464, **464**
joint protection strategies, 539
matching person's requirements and
   device, 461, 462–463, **462**, **463**
   evidence-based decision-making,
      462
   use of simulations, 463
mobility-related, 89
non-use, 465, 471
occupational reasoning, 457,
   458–459
person-centred practice, 457
planning, 460–463, **461**
policy context, 456
practice scenarios, **457–458**, **460**,
   461, **462**, **463**, **464**, 466
problem-solving process, 457, **457**
   occupation analysis, 459
product selection criteria, 461
training in use, 464, **464**, **465**
universal design, 455, 457
Assistive technology, 59, 84, 453
   cost–benefit considerations, 456
   definition, 454
   policy context, 456
   self-care enabling strategies, **351**
Assumptions, influence on
   communication, 155
Astereognosis (tactile agnosia), 548,
   610
Asylum seekers, 268, 299
Attachment to home, 412
Attendant-propelled wheelchairs/
   dependent mobility systems,
   474–475, **475**
Attention
   arousal level relationship, 639
   divided/alternating, 609
   focused (selective), 609
   sustained (concentration span), 609
Attention deficit hyperactivity
   disorder, 645, 646
Attention process training (APT), 628

Attention training, 628
Attention/concentration problems, 609
   intervention strategies, 628–629
Audio recordings, information
   provision, 228, 230
Auditory agnosia, 610
Australian Classification of
   Occupations, 403
Australian Therapy Outcome Measures
   (AusTOMS), 614
Autism-spectrum disorders
   associated sensory processing
      disorders, 646, 648
   play as therapy, 385, 386
Autonomic nervous system, 639, 640
Autonomy of individuals, 129, 152,
   153, 226, 457
Axonotmesis, 544

Back pain, workplace related
   generic risk assessment, **556**
   risk to occupational therapists, 555
BADS, **618**
Bariatric wheelchairs, 476
Base of support
   effects on reaching to grasp when
      seated, 583
   movement biomechanics, 558, **558**,
      559, 560
Bathrooms
   common barriers, **445**
   universal design, 444–447, **446**
      bathing fixtures, 445, **447**
      lavatories, 444
      offset controls, 445–446
      reinforcing for grab bars, 446–447
      toilets, 444, **447**
      water controls, 447
Bathtubs, 445
Beattie model of health promotion,
   244–245, **245**
Bed levers, **569**
Behaviour change, 248–249
   educational interventions, 248
   Health Belief Model, 224
   health promotion, 240, 244
   self-efficacy theory, 224–225
   social cognition models, 248–249
   transtheoretical (stages of change)
      model, 225, **226**, 249, **249**
Behavioural demands, job analysis,
   403
Beneficence, 42
Biomechanical model, 77

Biomechanical strategies, 527–540
  assessment, 535–536
    form-focused, 536
    function, 535–536
    meaning, 535
  implementation, 536–537
    aims, 538
    endurance enhancement strategies,
      539
    energy-conservation strategies, 539
    joint protection strategies, 539
    occupational performance focus,
      536
    strength improvement strategies,
      538–539
    voluntary movements
      enhancement, 539–540
  occupational reasoning, 535
  practice scenarios, **529–534**,
    537–538
    ergonomic analysis, 530–531, 533,
      534
  rationale, 529
  terminology, 528
Biomechanics, 528
  dynamic, 528
  static, 528
  voluntary movement, 558–561
    base of support, 558, **558**, 559,
      560
    centre of gravity, 558–559, **559**,
      560, 561, **561**
    friction, 560–561, **560**
    lever systems, 561–562, **561**
    line of gravity, 558–559, **559**
    stability, 558
BIT, **617**
Body function/structure, 178–179
  performance skills relationship, 173
  work rehabilitation assessment
    process, 401, 402
Body positions, relevance to motor
  skills, **168**
Body scheme abilities, 610
Brain injury, acquired/traumatic, 471
  cognitive/perceptual problems, 609
    see also Cognitive problems;
      Perceptual problems
  motor performance optimisation *see*
    Motor performance
    rehabilitation
  occupational-therapy driving
    specialist referral, 496
  post-traumatic amnesia, 614

screening assessment, 86
sensory impairments, 545
stretch interventions for contractures
  prevention, 516
Brainstem
  injury, sensory change management,
    550
  reticular formation, 640
Buccofacial (oral) apraxia, 611
Buddy taping, 511
Buggies, 475
Building contracts, 425
Building regulations, 413
  reinforcing for grab bars, 446
Built environment, 140–141
Bureaucracy-led services, 42
Burns injury, 59
  contractures prevention, 516
  immobilisation for wound healing, 514
  orthoses, 509, 514, 516–517
    semi-dynamic, 512
  prolonged stretch application, 511,
    516
  scar compression garments, 518
  scar formation prevention, 516–517

Cabinets, universal design, 441, 443,
  443, **444**
Calgary Cambridge Model of History
  Taking, 155–157, **156**
Canadian Model of Occupational
  Performance and Engagement,
  74, 129, 459, 470, 491, 611
Canadian Occupational Performance
  Measure (COPM), 59, 89, 90,
  101, 129, 157–158, 366, 459,
  510, **530**, 535, 614
Capabilities, 306–307, **307**
Capacities
  cognitive, 609–611
  performance skills relationship, 173
Capacity building
  community development, 306–308
  core capabilities, 306–307, **307**
  practice scenario, **307–308**
Cardiopulmonary disorders,
  biomechanical strategies, 538
Cardiopulmonary endurance
  enhancement, 539
Care pathways, 345
Caritas Europe, 298
Carpal tunnel syndrome, 522
Case method, 58
Casts, 508, 509

continuous stretch maintenance for
  contractures prevention, 516,
  600
scar management, 517
Cataract, driving safety considerations,
  492
Centre of gravity, movement
  biomechanics, 558–559, **559**,
  560, 561, **561**
Centre of mass, seating biomechanics,
  478–479, **478**, **479**
Cerebral palsy, 84, 471, 472, 496
  constraint-induced movement
    therapy, 594, 595
  positive versus negative impairments,
    585
Cerebrovascular accident *see* Stroke
Chailey Scales of Sitting, 480
Chair raisers, **569**
Challenge, relation to health, 240
Child Occupational Self Assessment
  (COSA), 89
Child-centred therapy, 386
Child-Initiated Pretend Play
  Assessment, 383
Children
  cognitive/perceptual problems, 608
  collaborative goal setting, 101
  constraint-induced movement
    therapy, 594, 595
  play *see* Play
  reaching to grasp, 582
  sensory processing disorders,
    645–646, 647, 648
    challenging behaviour, 646
    educational impact, 645–646
Children's wheelchairs, 475
Choice of occupation, 115
  influence on self-care, 342, 345–346
  see also Decision-making
Chronic care model, 226
Chronically Sick and Disabled Persons
  Act (1970), 571
Clarifying, advanced communication
  skills, **197–199**
Client-centred therapy, 32–34, 41, 42
  assessment, 90, 91
  critical appraisal, 42–43
    discrimination, 42–43
    needs-led versus bureaucracy-led,
      42
    needs-led versus economic-led, 42
    outcome assessment, 42
  see also Person-centred practice

Closet storage, universal design, 448, **449**
Clumsy child syndrome, 645
Coaching as enabling skill, **117**
Code of Ethics and Professional Conduct, 190, 193, 195
Cognition, definition, 608
Cognitive ability
  driving performance, 494
    off-road screening, 498
  job analysis for work rehabilitation, 403
  normal capacities, 609–611
Cognitive behavioural approaches, 77, 201, 202
Cognitive client libraries, 62–63
Cognitive dissonance, 248
Cognitive problems, 472, 608–609
  apraxia, 611
  assessment, 87, 613–619, **615–619**
    observation of performance (hypothesis testing), 620, **622–623**
    pre-assessment identification of physical/sensory deficits, 614
    standardised, 614, 620
  attention/concentration deficits, 609
  children with sensory processing disorders, 646
  community integration following rehabilitation, 631
  driving abilities
    attentional resources, 494
    reporting of conditions causing problems, 492
  educational interventions, 230
  home modification, 410, 412
  intervention strategies, 621, 623, **625–627**
    attention/concentration problems, 628
    executive function problems, 629
    memory/learning problems, 628–629
    metacognition problems, 629
    praxis problems, 631
    unilateral neglect problems, 629
  kitchen controls, universal design, 443
  occupational impact, 608
  occupational therapy frameworks, 611–612

outcome measures, 614
practice scenarios, **612–613**, **620–621**, **623–624**, **627**
wheelchair use, 471, 472
COGNSTAT, **619**
Collaboration, 115, 152, 154, 192–193, 226, 227
  communication processes, 192, 193
    therapeutic use of self, 199–200
  as enabling skill, **118**
  health promotion considerations, 246
  orthoses prescription, occupational goals, 510
  person-centred approach, 193
    decisions concerning risk-taking, 345
    goal-setting, 350
  promoting disabled people's participation, **289**
  seating systems use, 471
  therapist flexibility, 120
  wheelchair users, 471
Collectivism (versus individualism), 144
Colour agnosia, 610
Commitment, relation to health, 240
Communication, 151–159, 191–192, 227
  barriers, 155
  contextual considerations, **158**
  elements of interpersonal interaction, 192
  enabling strategies, 153–154
  home modification, 423–426
  non-verbal, 154, **158**, 196
  occupational therapy process, 192–193
  therapeutic relationships, 192, 193
  verbal, **159**, 196
  work rehabilitation, 395
  see also Information gathering
Communication skills, 162, 167, 170–171, **172**, 192, 194–195, 196
  advanced, 196, **197–199**
  application, 193–194
  development, 154
  person-centred practice, 193
  silence, **159**
  training/development, 193
  see also Interpersonal interaction skills

Communities
  as care setting, 269
  as context of occupation, 136, 139–145
    built spaces, 140–141
    cultural differences, 143–144
    geographic features, 139–140
    sociocultural aspects, 141–142
  disabled people's rights to participation, 282
  inclusiveness, 297–311
  key features, 268–269
  occupational therapist consultancy, 329
Community development, 120, 267–277
  arts/cultural action, 274
  co-operative enterprises, 276
  community-based rehabilitation strategies, 315
  educational opportunities, 275
    inclusive education facilitation, 308–309
  environmental action, 274–275
  evaluation, 310
  forms, 273–274
  key features, 269
  occupational therapist roles, 273–274, 302–303
  participation
    programme planning, 269
    Third Way policies, 273
  practical aspects, 304
    capacity building, 306–308, **307–308**
    establishing partnerships, 303–306, **303**, **304–306**
    Managing for Impact approach, 310–311, **310**
  practice scenarios, **269–271**, **304–306**, **307–308**, **309–310**
  rationale, 271–272, 302
Community mobility, 490–491, **492**
  alternatives to driving, 492, 500
  road safety/mobility needs balance, 491–492
Community-based interventions, 246
  social change, 294
  tele-consultations, 335–336, **336**
  see also Community-based rehabilitation
Community-based rehabilitation, 311–321

collaborative implementation, 312, 317–319
    practice scenario, **317–318**
core strategy, 312
    evolution, 313, **315**
early medically framed approaches, 313
matrix (strategy components), 318, **319**
occupational therapists' role, 320–321
    facilitating collaboration, 321
    programme development/ implementation, 321
    provision of direct therapy, 320
    referral services, 320–321
    transfer of rehabilitation knowledge/skills, 320
occupational therapy synergy, 319–320
programme development guidelines, 318, **318**
re-conceptualisation, community development strategy, 315
    practice scenario, **314–315**
role of disabled people's organisations, 316
    practice scenario, **316–317**
Comparative reasoning, 62–63
Compensatory strategies, 587–589, 611
    enabling strategies, **121**
    self-care, **352**, **353**
    hypothesis development/testing, 589
    reaching to grasp, 588, **588**
Compression forces
    pressure ulcers, 478
    seating biomechanics, 478, **478**
Computer programs, information provision, 229
Conceptual frameworks, 58–59
    acquisitional/developmental, 59
    biomechanical, 59
    rehabilitation, 59
Concerted cultivation, 137, 138
Conditional reasoning, 63
Conditions management teams, 272
Consent, 83, 496
Constraint-induced movement therapy (CIMT), 59, 591, 602
    children, 594, 595
    upper limb motor performance remediation, 594–595
Consultation as enabling skill, **118**

Contextual factors, 21–22
    assessment process, 85
        work rehabilitation, 401, 402
    communities, 136, 139–145
    group work, 256, 257
Contractures, 585, 587
    hypothesis development/testing, 589
    management approach, 580, 587
        long duration stretch application, 587, 599–600, **601**
    prevention, 599–600
        evidence-based practice, 516
        immobilisation orthoses, 515–516, **517**
        oedema reduction, 522
Control, relation to health, 240
    empowerment, 247
    self-care, collaborative goal-setting, 350
Controls, kitchen universal design, 443
Co-operative enterprises, 276
Coordination as enabling skill, **118**
Corticosteroid injections
    lateral epicondylitis, 522
    scar management, 517
Cost–benefit considerations, assistive technology, 456
COTNAB, **617**
Council of Europe Disability Action Plan, **301**
Council of Europe social cohesion policy, 302
Counselling, 222
Counters/work surfaces, kitchen universal design, 437, 441, 443, **443**, **444**
Creativity, pretend play associations, 379
Cultural activities, community development, 274
Cultural factors
    assessment processes, 87, 89–90, 348, 349
    assistive device selection, 460
    categories of occupation, 47
    community context of occupation, 143–144
        colonization, 144
        universality, 144
    doing/being relationship, 144
    environmental interactions, 48
    goal-directed/socially sanctioned occupation, 46

independence versus dependence, 45, 344
interpersonal interactions, 195
language influences, 139
leisure activities, 47, 365
performance context, 177
professional assumptions impact, 41
self-care, 344, 346, 348, 349
therapist understanding enhancement, 82
see also Sociocultural context of occupation
Curbless shower design, 445
Cushioning for wheelchairs, 482
    adaptive seating systems, 482, **485**
    pressure cushions, 482–483, **485**

Decision-making
    clients' information needs, 227
    partnership/participation, 131, 227
    person-centred practice, 130, 131
    see also Choice of occupation
Decubitus ulcers *see* Pressure ulcers
Definitions, 4–13, 28
    advocacy, 215
    assistive technology, 454
    enablement, 115
    leisure, 358
    occupation, 17–19, **18**, 47
    occupation analysis, 163, 164
    person-centred approach, 128
    play, 372
    poverty, 298
    well-being, 49
Deformity, 482
    evaluation for wheeled mobility/ seating interventions, 482
    orthoses prescription, 511, 515–516
Dementia, 88
    driving performance, 492, 500
    home modification, 410
    performance in home environment, 178
Denver II, 90
Depression, 190, 191
    cognitive/perceptual problems assessment, 614
Descriptors of occupational therapy practice, 7, 8, 9, 10–11
Developmental coordination disorder, 84, 89, 645
Developmental delay, 86
Developmental programmes, 382
Dexterity training, 598–599, **600**

Diagnosis, occupational therapy process, 60–61, **60**
Dignity, 129, 130, 302
Disability, 27–36, 145, 146
  affirmative model, 31–32, 35
  building regulations/accessibility standards, 413
  goals of therapy
    normality, 28, 29, 31, 32, 35, 43–44, 45
    physical independence, 28, 32, 35, 44–45
  individual model, 30, 34, 213
  models, 212–213
  occupational therapy services
    citizen-centred, 34–35
    client-centred, 32–34, 42
    disabled people's perspective, 28–29
    traditional services, 28
  poverty association, 298, 299, **300**, 312, 316
  social model, 30–31, 33, 34, 35, 213
  therapist as agent of change, 215–216
    strategies, 216
  therapist–client power relationships, 29–30, 33, 34, 42
  tragedy model, 30, 31, 213
  see also Disabled people
Disability Discrimination Act (1995), 30
Disability Equality Training, 34
Disabled people, **300**
  access to resources, 276
  barriers to participation, 282, 283–284
    built environment, 140–141
  community-based activities, 274–275
  decision-making, 194
  educational opportunities, 275
  home modification, 410, 411, 412
  mainstreaming, 302
  partnerships development, 281–295
  social activism, 275–276
  social marginalisation/vulnerability, 213–214, **214**, 272, 298, 302
  see also Disability
Disabled people's organisations, role in community-based rehabilitation, 316
  practice scenario, **316–317**

Disabled Persons (Services, Consultation and Representation) Act (1986), 571
Disaster preparedness and response, 336, **336–337**
Discrimination in services provision, 42–43
Displaced persons strategy, 306
Distractibility, 609
Domains of Occupational Therapy, 162, **163**
Doors, universal design, 434
Doorways, universal design, 448, **448**
Dorsal column pathway, 544
Down's syndrome, 646
Driving, 489–503
  generalist occupational therapist's role, 494–495
    crash risk assessment, 494–495
  in-vehicle technologies, 503
  individual's insight into limitations, 495, 498, 500
  as information processing task, 493–494, **493**
  licensing
    local area licences, 499
    medical-legal aspects, 492
    suspension recommendation, 500
  rehabilitation, 500, 503
    practice scenario, **500**, **502–503**
  reporting of conditions causing impairment, 492–493
  road safety/mobility needs balance, 491–492
  specialist occupational therapist's role, 495–496, 503
    driving evaluation outcomes, 499–500, **501**
    driving-related assessments, 496
    informed consent for information-sharing, 496
    off-road screening, 497–498
    on-road assessment, 498–499, **499**
    practice context, 495
    referral systems, 495–496
    referred individuals/health and impairment issues, 496, **497**
DVDs, information provision, 228
Dynamic Interaction Approach, 611
Dynamic orthoses (mobilisation splints), 512–513, **512**
  contractures prevention, 516

hand use improvement, 518, 519, 520
  pain relief, 521
  range of movement improvement, 540
Dynamic performance analysis, 90
Dynamic play family therapy, 386
Dyslexia, 645
Dyspraxia, 644, 645

Early Years Study, 377–378
Ecology of Human Performance Model, 491, 508
Economic environment, context of occupation, 136, 145–147
Economic self-sufficiency, professional assumptions, 47
Economic-led services, 42
Education/training
  assistive device use, 464
    practice scenario, **464**
  barriers to participation by disabled people (educational deprivation), 272, 283, 284
  community development activities, 275
  driving/community mobility activities, 495
  as enabling skill, **119**
  health promotion, 244
  home modification services, 412
  inclusive, 302
    facilitation, 308–309
    practice scenario, **309–310**
  occupation analysis applications, 166
  rights-based approach, 309
  self-care enabling strategies, **351**, **353**
  sensory change management, 548, 549
    brainstem/thalamus/sensory cortex injury, 550
    spinal cord injury, 549
  work rehabilitation interventions, 405
Educational interventions, 221–234, 247–248
  aims, 222–223
  educational needs/objectives determination, 227–228
    content needs, 227
    topic checklist, 227
  formats, 223, 227, 228–229, 230

for clients with impairments impacting receiving/processing information, 230
group programmes, 223, 229
health literacy considerations, 230
outcome evaluation, 227, 231, 233
   formal, 231, 233
   informal, 231
partnership working, 225–227
planning, 227–231
practice scenarios, **234–235**
setting objectives, 227
theories/models, 223–225
timing, 229–230
Effectiveness of occupational therapy, 4, 9
evaluation *see* Evaluation of effectiveness
evidence base, 22–24
Efficiency of Assistive Technology and Services 6-D, 465
Elastic dressings, oedema reduction, 522
Elderly people
cognitive performance decline, 494
driving, 490, 491, 496
   attentional resources, 494
   license suspension effects, 500
   road safety/mobility needs balance, 491–492
falls, 417
health/mobility maintenance, 364
home modification, 410, 411
leisure occupations, 364
occupational therapy programmes, 335, **335**
personal mobility, 491
relevance of universal design concept, 411, 431
value of occupational group work, 257–258
wheelchair use, 471, 472
Electric stand aids, 569
Electrical stimulation, upper limb motor performance remediation, 593–594
Elevating wheelchairs, 476
Emotional intelligence, 200–201
facilitating occupational therapy activities, 202
self-management abilities, 202
Emotional issues, 190
adjustment to physical impairment, 191, 194

cultural differences, 195
enabling strategies, 200
cognitive/perceptual problems assessment, 614
difficulties, intervention strategies, 201
relationship building skills, 196
Emotional skills, 201
Empathy, 154–155, 195, 196, 207
therapeutic use of self, 199
Employment *see* Productive occupation; Work (paid work)
Empowerment, 120, 194
active participation in care, 226, 227
adult learning theory, 223
barriers, 131
clients' information needs, 227
control over health, 247
disabled persons organisations, 302
facilitating strategies, 131
health promotion, 244
participation relationship, 247, **247**
person-centred practice, 130–131
social policy aspects, 301
Enablement of occupational engagement/performance, 6, 9, 10, 12, 13, 115–116
assistive devices, 454, 457
person-centred practice, 129
Enabling choice, 130
Enabling skills, 116, **117–119**
Enabling strategies, 114, 116, **121**, 190, 194
adjustment to physical impairment, 200
collaborative practice, 115
empowerment, 131
practice scenarios, **116, 202–207**
psychosocial support, 200–207, **202–207**
top-down versus bottom-up, 116, 120
wise practice concept, 114
Endurance
biomechanical strategies, 528, 529, 536
   energy-conservation, 539
   implementation, 539
impairment, 529, 538
   assessment, 535
Energy, motor skills, **168**
Energy-conservation strategies, 539
enabling leisure activities, 367

Engagement as enabling skill, **119**
Entrances
common barriers, **435**
modification, 435, **436**, **437**
   integrated site solutions, 436–437, **440, 441**
   platform lifts, 435–435, **439**
   ramps, 435, **437, 438**
repositioning, 435, **436**
universal design, 434–435
   additional features, 434
Entrepreneurial practice, 329–332
with elderly people, 335, **335**
forward planning, 332
marketing, 331, 332–333
occupational therapist consultancy services, 334, **334–335**
strategic intent, 332
tele-consultations, 335–336, **336**
use of technology, 333, 334
   appropriate paper technology (APT), **334**
   Information and Communication Technology (ICT), 333, **333–334**
Entrepreneurs
key features, 331–332
types, **332**
Environmental action, community development, 274–275
Environmental aesthetics, 141
Environmental factors, 112
adaptations
   enabling leisure activities, 367
   as enabling skill, **118**
assessment, 99, 348
   biomechanical strategies, 536
   work rehabilitation, 401, 403
assistive device selection, 459, 460
barriers to participation by disabled people, 282, 284, 316, 471
as context of occupation
   built spaces, 140–141
   geographic features, 139–140
   group work, 256, 257
influence on performance, 177–178
   intrinsic/extrinsic factors, 178
interpersonal interaction facilitation, 194–195
job analysis for work rehabilitation, 403
occupational therapy-sensory integration intervention (OT-SI), 648

play, 376–377
professional assumptions, critical appraisal, 48
reaching to grasp when seated, 583
selection of occupation-focused strategies, 105–106
self-care influence, 342, 346, 348
goal-setting, 350
see also Person–environment fit
Environmental mastery, 48
Environmental press, 139–140
Epilepsy, 492
Equality, 42
Equitable service delivery, 115
Ergonomic analysis
practice scenarios, **530–531, 533, 534**
see also Biomechanical strategies
Ergonomic Workplace Analysis, 565
Ergonomics, assistive device design, 455
Ethical practice, 83
assessment processes, 87, 89
Ethnocentrism, 41, 46, 144
European Social Agenda, 301
Council of Europe Disability Action Plan, **301**
Evaluation of effectiveness, 87–88, 97, 99, 245–246
assistive devices, 465–466, **466**
educational interventions, 227, 231, 233
group work, 257–258, 261
motor performance remediation, 591–592
person–environment–occupation fit, 106–107, **107**
reporting outcomes, 88, 107
screening assessments, 86
SMART goals, 103
progress reviews, 103
Evidence-based practice, 22–23, 40–41, 43, 68–69, 114
assessment, 83
screening, 87
assessment tools evaluation, 89
health promotion, 245–246
orthoses, 518, 520–521
selection of occupation-focused strategies, 106
spinting/casting, 516
upper limb motor performance remediation, 593–594
Evidence-based reasoning, 64

Evolutionary aspects, 23
Executive functions, 610
components, 610
definition, 608
problems, intervention strategies, 629
Expectancy-value models, 248
Exploring, advanced communication skills, 192, 196, **196, 197–199**
Extrinsic purpose, 164
Eye contact, 154

Facial expression, 154
Fair Housing laws, 413
Families
access to occupational pursuits, 137
routines/rituals, influence on performance patterns, 175–176
time-use patterns, 138–139
Family history, 136
influence on occupational development, 136–139
Figure ground disorder, 630
Filial therapy, 386
Financial aspects
assistive devices funding, 464
home modification, 411–412, 424
wheelchair costs, 471
Finger flexion force modulation exercises, **599, 600**
FirstSTEP Screening Test for Evaluating Preschoolers, 86
Flesch Reading Ease formula, 231
Flow concept, experience of leisure, 361
Forearm supination exercise, **598**
Fork control practice, **597**
Form discrimination, intervention strategies, 630–631
Forward planning, 332
Fragile X syndrome, 646
Freedom, 49, 360
Friction
movement biomechanics, 560–561, **560**
static/dynamic, 560
'Function' as descriptor of practice, 10
case study, **10–11**
Functional capacity, work rehabilitation assessment, 401–402
Functional Group Model, 258
Functional Independence Measure (FIM), 59, 620

Gardening activities, community development, 274–275
Garments, orthotic, 508
scar management, 517
Gender issues, 7
Gender-related norms, 142
Genuineness, 195, 196, 199
Geographical differences, performance context, 177
Geriatric Depression Scale, 60
Global entrepreneurial opportunities, 327–337
Globalization, 44
Goal Attainment Scale (GAS), 101, 106
Goal-setting
assistive device requirements, 460
collaborative approach, 100, 101
with children, 101
documentation, 101
occupation-focused, 100–101
orthoses prescription, 510
prioritisation, 101
self-care, 350–351
SMART method see SMART goals
work rehabilitation, 395, 403–404
written documentation, 101
Goals of occupational therapy, critical appraisal, 43–44
Grab bars, reinforcing for bathrooms, 446–447
Grasp
movement analysis, 581–582, **581, 582**
see also Reaching to grasp
Group work, 253–262
aims, 258
content/context, 258
cost-effectiveness, 258
creating the group, 258
educational programmes, 223, 229
effectiveness evaluation, 257–258, 261
engaging, 259
format, 258
group leader's role, 260
health promotion, 254, 255
managing the group, 259–261
membership establishment, 259
occupational, 254, 255–256, **256**
creative/productive opportunities, 256, 257
social interaction facilitation, 256
planning, 258, **262–264**

practical aspects, 259
practice scenarios, **255**, **256**, **262–264**
psycho-educational, 254, 255–256, **255**
psychosocial support, 201
session preparations, 259, **260**
types, 254–255
value, 256–257
  community connectedness, 256, 257
  in physical rehabilitation, 254
Guillain–Barre syndrome, 471

Habits
  influence on performance patterns, 175–176
  leisure occupations incorporation, 367
Hand
  contractures prevention, 599–600
  dexterity training, 598–599, **600**
  holding objects, motor skills, **168**
  movement analysis, 598
    reaching to grasp, 581, **581**, 582, **582**
  orthoses
    resting splints, 511
    for use improvement, 518–521, **519**
    see also Orthoses
  sensation assessment, 546, **546**, 547, **547**
  sensory re-education, 548–549
  strength, 62, 63
Handling belts, 570
Health
  determinants, 242, **242**, 243
  impact of occupation, 11–12, 13, 49, 112, 113, 114
    paid work, 45–46
    professional assumptions, critical appraisal, 47–48
  inequalities, 240–241, 271
  Labonte model, 240, **241**
  play relationship, 377–378
  recreation relationship, 361–362
  WHO definition, 241
Health Assessment Questionnaire, 59
Health Belief Model, 224, 249
Health education, 242, 243, 247–248
Health literacy, 230
Health promotion, 239–249
  Beattie model, 244–245, **245**
  core philosophy, 243

education, 247–248
evaluation of effectiveness, 245–246
evidence-based approach, 245–246
group work, 254, 255
key concepts, 240–243
Naidoo and Wills' five approaches, 243–244
Ottawa Charter, 242–243, 245
preventive focus, 240, 241
relation to occupational therapy, 246–247
settings approach, 245
Health Promotion Forum of New Zealand, 243
Health and Safety at Work Act (1974), 570, 571
Hearing
  driving performance off-road screening, 498
  impairment, educational interventions, 230
High-performance sports wheelchairs, 476
Hoists, 569–570
  with walking harness, 570
Holding objects, motor skills, **168**
Holism/holistic practice, 9, 71, 190, **208**
Holistic framework, 33, 34
Home Enabler, 417, **418–419**
Home modification, 409–427
  activity analysis, **424**
  architectural drawings, 426
  bathrooms, 444, **446**
  building contracts, 425
  by homeowners, 410–411
  communication, 423–426
    construction/design documentation, 425, 426–427
  effectiveness, 410
  emotional dimension, 412
  entrances, 435
  financial aspects, 411–412, 424
  home assessment, 414, 416–417
    hazard identification, 417
    home visiting, 417
    occupational basis, 415
    purpose, 417, **420**
    tools, 417, **418–419**
  interventions, 414, 420–423
    anthropometric considerations, 422
    practice scenarios, **421**, **422–423**
    use of reflective framework, **423**, **425**

key features, 410
kitchens, 437
legislation, 413–414, **413**
modification reasoning, 414–415, **416**
modification recommendations, 426–427
  documentation of professional reasoning, 426, **426**
psychological barriers, 412
tenants' responsibilities, 411
Home Visitability legislation, 411
HOMEFAST, 417, **418–419**
Housing design, 411
  accessibility standards, 413
  building regulations, 413
Human rights, 49, 50, 145, 213, 214, 282, 287, 298, 302, 345
  community-based rehabilitation strategies, 312, 313, 316
  manual handling issues, 571, 572
Human Rights Act (1998), 571
Humerus fracture, 538
Huntington's chorea, 471
Hypertonicity, orthoses in management, 520
Hypothalamus, 639, 640
Hypothesis development/testing
  cognitive/perceptual problems assessment, 620, **622–623**
  motor performance rehabilitation, 589
  occupational reasoning, 63

Ideational apraxia, 611
Identity
  attachment to home, 412
  employment/worker role, 392, 393
  impact of occupation, 114
  influence on self-care, 342, 343
  play in children, 376
  relation to leisure activities, 361, 362
  self-concept, 343
Ideomotor apraxia, 611
  intervention strategies, 631
Immobilisation splints, 511, **511**
  contractures prevention, 515–516
  deformity correction, 515–516
  joint protection, 513
  pain relief, 522
  use for rest, 513
  wound healing, 513–515, **515**
  see also Static orthoses

Impairment
  assessment, 99
  associated negative affectivity, 191
  emotional adjustment, 194
    enabling strategies, 200
  psychological sequelae, 191
  psychosocial adjustment, 190, 191
In-home services, 431
Inclusive design see Universal design
Inclusive education, 302
  facilitation, 308–309
    practice scenario, **309–310**
Independence
  cultural aspects, 45, 344
  as goal of therapy, 28, 32, 35, 44–45
  quality of life enhancement, 45
  self-care, 342, 343–344
    assessment processes, 348
    goal-setting, 350
Individual model of disability, 30, 34,
    213
Individual Prioritised Problems
    Assessment (IPPA), 460
Individualism (versus collectivism),
    144
Induction loop system, 464, **464**
Inferential reasoning, 63
Information and Communication
    Technology (ICT), 333
  practice scenario, **333–334**
Information gathering
  for assessment, 59–60
  communication skills, 153, 154
  occupation analysis, 182–183
    indirect/direct assessment, 182
  practice scenario, **158**
  tools, 155–158
Information processing, driving
    performance, 493–494
Informational needs
  assessment, 227
  work rehabilitation, 395
Institutional environment, goal-setting
    for self-care, 350
Intellectual impairment see Cognitive
    problems
Interdependence, 44–45, 47, 49–50
Interest Checklist, 365
Interest checklists, 365
International Classification of
    Functioning, Disability and
    Health (ICF), 43, 58, 59, 84,
    96, **97**, 105, 284–285, 315,
    328–329, 470

activity and participation, 179, **180**
application to occupation analysis,
    179
  practice scenario, **185**
body functions/structures, 179,
    180–181, **185**
cognitive/perceptual problems, 611
work rehabilitation framework, 395,
    401
Internet information, 229
Interpersonal interaction skills, 192,
    207
  advanced communication skills, 196,
    197–199
  application, 193–194, **194**
  environment-creating skills, 194–195
  relationship building skills, 195–196
  therapeutic use of self, 199
  training/development, 193
Intervention planning, 96–97
  assistive device selection, 460–461
  enabling strategies see Enabling
    strategies
  goals documentation, 101
  occupation analysis, 183
  review and administration of
    oucome measures, 103
  selection of occupation-focused
    strategies, 105–106
  steps in process, **97**
Intervention strategies
  assistive devices, 464
  occupational therapy process, 61
  play activities in children, 382,
    385
  psychosocial support, 201
  sensory rehabilitation, 548–550
  work rehabilitation, 394, 404–405
Interviews, **159**
  assessment of occupational
    performance and engagement,
    59
  communication skills training, 193
  occupation analysis, 182
  screening assessment, 86
  work rehabilitation assessment
    process
    manager/supervisor, 402–403
    worker, 401
Intrinsic purpose, 164

Job classification systems, 403
Job dissatisfaction, therapist, 4–5
Joint pain, orthotic management, 521

Joint position sense assessment,
    546–547
Joint protection, 539
  immobilisation orthoses, 513
Justice, 42, 50
  redistributive, 120
  see also Occupational justice; Social
    justice

Kawa model of occupation, 41, 74
Keitel Function Test, 59
Kinematics, 528, 580–581
  compensatory strategies recognition,
    588
  movement improvement strategies,
    539–540
  practice scenario, **528–529**
Kinesiology, 528
Kinetics, 528, 580, 581
  endurance improvement strategies,
    539
  practice scenario, **528–529**
  strength improvement strategies,
    538
Kitchens
  universal design, 437, 441–443,
    442
    cabinets, 441, 443, **443**
    controls, 443–444
    counters/work surfaces, 437, 441,
      443
    refrigerated storage, 441
    self-storage doors, **444**
    sinks, 443
    water controls, 447
Knowledge base supporting
    occupational practice, 22,
    40–41
  critical appraisal, 41, 50
Knox Preschool Play Scale, 383
KWAZO, 466

Lalonde report, 242
Language
  development, pretend play
    associations, 378
  impairment, educational
    interventions, 230
Lateral epicondylitis (tennis elbow),
    orthoses in management, 520,
    522
Lavatories, universal design, 444
Learn to Play programme, 385–386,
    386

Learning, 67, 68, 70, 609
  assistive device use, 464
  childhood occupational role change,
    645
  community development
    approaches, 275, 310–311
  environmental context, 309
  problems, intervention strategies,
    628–629
  see also Motor learning
Learning disability, associated sensory
    processing disorders, 646
Leg lifters, **569**
Leg muscles, activity during reaching
    to grasp when seated, 583
Legislation, 146, **146**, 216
  home modification, 413–414, **413**
  moving and handling, 571–574, **573**
    practice scenario, **574**
Leisure, 20, 162, 357–368
  as activity, 359
  application to practice, 362–364
    practice scenarios, **362–363**
  assessment tools, 364
    interest checklists, 365
    limitations, 365–366
    measurement of time, 364–365
    qualitative interview approaches,
      366
    satisfaction measures, 366
  cultural considerations, 47, 365
  enabling participation, 366–368
    environment/occupation
      adaptation, 367
    temporal aspects, 367
  experience of engagement, 359,
    360–361, 366
    awareness of time/concept of
      flow, 360–361
    enjoyment, 360
    intrinsic reward, 360
    perceived freedom, 360
    qualitative data collection, 366
    relaxation, 360
  families' access to opportunities, 137
  health relationship, 361–362
  key features, 358–359
  occupation analysis, 166
  performance components as means
    of therapy, 367–368
  professional assumptions, critical
    appraisal, 46, 47, 48
  recreation relationship, 361
  as residual/free time, 358–359

Leisure bordom, 359
Leisure Interest Profile for
    Adolescents, 365
Leisure Interest Profile for Seniors,
    365
Leisure Satisfaction Scale, 366
Level of Sitting Scales, 480
Lever systems, movement
    biomechanics, 561–562, **561**
Lever taps, 539
Lid opening equipment, 539
Light touch sensation, 545, 639
Line of gravity, movement
    biomechanics, 558–559, **559**
Listening, 153, 154, 155, 192, 196,
    196, **197**, 199
  active, 154, 207, 457
Literacy, 272, 275
  educational interventions, 230
  pretend play associations, 378
Lobbying, 211–219
  in occupational therapy, 215, **217**
    managing associated conflicts,
      218
    therapist as agent of change,
      215–216
  promoting disabled people's
    participation, **289**
  social model of disability, 213
Local area driving licences, 499
Locognosia (touch localisation)
    assessment, 547–548, **548**
Locus of control, 247
Lowenstein Occupational Therapy
    Cognitive Assessment
    (LOTCA), 613, **618**
Lycra garments, 512
  continuous stretch application, 516
  hand use improvement, 520
  oedema reduction, 522

Mallet splints, 511
Management of Health and Safety at
    Work Regulations, 570, 574
Manual handling see Moving and
    handling
Manual handling Assessment Charts
    (MAC), 565
Manual Handling Operations
    regulations, 564, 571, 574
Manual Handling Questions (MHQ),
    565–567, **566**, 571, 574
Manual stand aids, 569
Marketing, 331, 332–333

Massage
  oedema reduction, 522
  scar management, 517
Matching Person and Technology
    assessment, 460
Meaningfulness of Activity Scale, 366
Meaningfulness of occupation, 20–21,
    112, 113, 114, 115, 152, 165
  assessment, 82, 84–85, 86, 535
  context of performance, 177, 178
  influence of roles, 175
  play in children, 376
  selecting occupation-focused
    strategies, 105
  self-care occupations, 342, 345–346
  sociocultural aspects, 141
  work (paid work), 392–393
    professional assumptions, 46–47
Medical Achievement Reading Test
    (MART), 230
Medical model, 6, 7, 9, 241, 470
  of disability, 213
Memory, 609
  immediate recall, 610
  long-term, 610
  problems, intervention strategies,
    628–629
  short-term, 610
Memory log, 629
Memory retraining, 628–629
Mental activity, nature of occupation,
    19–20
Mental health disorders
  cognitive/perceptual problems, 608
  sequelae of physical impairment,
    191, 200, 208
Mental practice, upper limb motor
    performance remediation, 595
Metacognition, 610
  problems, intervention strategies,
    629
Migrants, 269, 271, 299
Millenium Development Goals, 328,
    328
Miller Function and Participation
    Scales, 382
Mini-Mental State Examination
    (MMSE), 60, 498
Minimal brain dysfunction, 645
Mnemonics training, 629
Moberg pick up test, 548
Mobilisation splints see Dynamic
    orthoses
Mobility aids, 410

Mobility cues, 414
Mobility skills, 44
Model of Human Occupation, 74, 491, 611
Modelling
  motor learning, 591–592
  self-efficacy enhancement, 225
Models of disability, 212–213
Models of practice, 67–78, 105
  cognitive/perceptual problem approaches, 611
  educational interventions, 223
  generic, 71, 73–74, **74**, 77
  intervention, 71, 73, 74, **75–76**, 77
  overview, 71–73, **72**
  terminology, 69–70, 71
  therapist education, 68–69, 70
Moral model of disability, 213
Motivation, 164
  adult learning theory, 224
  influence on self-care, 342, 344–345
    collaborative goal-setting, 350, 351
Motor learning
  autonomous stage, 589, 590
  dexterity training, 598–599
  feedback, 589, 590, 591–592, 599
    knowledge of performance, 591
    knowledge of results, 591
  modelling, 591–592
  motor stage, 589–590
  practice, 589, 590, 594, 599
    maximisation, 590–591
    record-keeping, 594
  repetition, 590–591, 594, 599
  stages, 589
  task-specific training, 590, 594, 599, 601
  verbal-cognitive stage, 589
Motor performance rehabilitation, 579–603
  contractures prevention/management, 599–600
  evaluation of change, 591–592
  motor skills teaching, 589–590
    maximising practice, 590–591
    stages of motor learning, 589–590
    task-specific training, 590
  movement analysis, 580–581, **581**, **582**
    compensatory strategies recognition, 587–589
    contractures recognition, 585, 587

hypothesis development/testing, 589
  movement science approach, 580
  positive versus negative impairments, 585
  practice scenarios, **591–592**
  reaching to grasp, 580–583, **581**, **582**
  seated reaching
    anticipatory muscle activity, **586–587**
    postural adjustments, 583–585, **584**
    sitting balance training, 601–602
    training strategies, **586–587**
  upper limb, 593–594
    constraint-induced movement therapy, 594–595
    dexterity training, 598–599, **600**
    electrical stimulation, 594
    mental practice, 595
    reducing muscle force during grasp, 595, 598, **599**, **600**
    strength training, 594, **595**
Motor skills, 162, 167, **168**
Motor skills teaching, 589
  stages of motor learning, 589
  task-specific training, 590
Movement analysis, 580–581
  compensatory strategies recognition, 587–589
  contractures recognition, 585, 587
  hypothesis development/testing, 589
  reaching to grasp, 580–583, **581**, **582**
  postural adjustments in sitting, 583–585, **584**
Movement (voluntary movement)
  biomechanical principles, 558–561
  base of support, 558, **558**, 559
  centre of gravity, 558–559, **559**, 560, 561, **561**
  friction, 560–561, **560**
  lever systems, 561, **561**
  line of gravity, 558–559, **559**
  stability, 558
  biomechanical strategies, 528, 529, 536, 539–540
  impairment, 529, 538
    assessment, 535
  normal patterns, 556–557, **557**
Moving and handling, 553–574
  care handling, 563, **563**
  care–therapy handling continuum, 563

equipment, **569**
  competency in use, 570, 574
  hoists, 569–570
  needs analysis, 566–567, 569
  physical/cognitive limitation assessment, 271, 272
  provision/use, 568–569
  standing, 569
  legislation, 571–574, **573**
  Manual Handling Questions (MHQ), 565–567, **566**, 571
  movement principles/biomechanics, 571
  practice scenarios, **554–555**, **556**, **562**, **567–568**, **571**, 574
  risk assessment, 563–568, **567–568**, 570
    AARR (Avoid Assess Reduce Review) approach, 562
    documentation, 564
    generic, 563
    individual/personal handling profiles, 564, **564**
    stages, **564**
    stressful/high-risk tasks, **557**
    time of day considerations, 564
    tools, 556, 564–565, **565**
    triggers for adverse behaviour, 564
  risks to occupational therapist, 555, 556
  safer handling principles, 570–571, **572**
  therapeutic handling, 563, **563**
  training needs, 574
Moving self/objects, motor skills, **168**
Moving two point discrimination assessment, 547
Multiple sclerosis, 471, 608
  driving safety considerations, 492, 496, 500
Muscle endurance enhancement, 539
Muscular dystrophy, 471, 496
Musculoskeletal disorders
  biomechanical strategies, 538
  orthoses, 509
  wheelchair use, 471, 472
  work-related risk to occupational therapists, 555
Musculoskeletal pain, orthotic management, 521
Muslim clients, 63
Myocardial infarction, 538

Naidoo and Wills' model of health promotion, 243–244
Narrative competence, pretend play associations, 378–379
Narrative play therapy, 386
National Health Service and Community Care Act (1990), 571
Neck pain, work-related risk to therapists, 555
Needs-led therapy, 41, 42
  critical appraisal, 42–43
  see also Client-centred therapy
Neglect phenomenon, 610
Neoprene splints, 512
  hand use improvement, 520
Neurodevelopmental model, 77
Neurofunctional Approach, 611
Neurological disorders
  biomechanical strategies, 538
  cognitive/perceptual problems, 608
  contractures, 515
    prolonged stretch application, 511, 516
  driving performance considerations, 496, 500
  orthoses, 509, 511
    semi-dynamic, 512
  wheelchair use, 471–472
    seating interventions, 476
Neuropraxia, 544
Neurotmesis, 544–545
Non-verbal communication, 154, **158**, 196
Normality as goal of therapy, 28, 29, 31, 32, 35, 43–44, 45, 275
Normative re-education strategy, 217
Norms, 21, 43, 45, 142, 248
  gender divisions, 142
  influence on forms of occupational performance, 142
  performance context, 177
Nottingham Leisure Questionnaire, 365

O*NET, 403
Observation
  assessment measures, 59–60
  form-focused assessment (analysis of performance), 536
  home modification assessment, 415, 417
  occupation analysis, 182
    for work rehabilitation, 403

play, 375
screening assessment, 86
self-care assessment, 347–348
Observation skills, **197**
Occupation, 17–24
  categories, 47
  core concept, 5, 6, 11, 13, 71
  definitions, 17–19, **18**, 47
  impact on health, 22–24, 47–48, 49, 112, 113
    occupational problems, 112, **113**
  impact on social change, 112–113
  Kawa model, 41
  key characteristics, 19
    active engagement, 19–20
    contextual nature, 21–22
    purposefulness, 20
    specifically human nature, 22
  meaningfulness, 20–21, 46–47, 82
  professional assumptions, critical appraisal, 45–49
    ableism, 45
    economic self-sufficiency, 47
    environmental interaction, 48
    environmental mastery, 48
    goal-directed/socially sanctioned activity, 46–47
    occupational balance, 47–48
    paid work, 45–46
  therapist as experts, 10, 11
Occupation analysis, 161–184, **164**
  application, 182, 183
  assistive device selection, 459
  definitions, 163, 165
  'doing' emphasis, 162, 163, 166
  information gathering, 182–183
  key features, 162–165
  performance areas, 166, **166**
  performance contexts, 177–178
  performance patterns, 162, 174–177
  performance skills, 166–172
  person factors, body function impairments, 179
  person-centred approach, 173
  practice scenario, **183–184**, **186**
  role in assessment, 165
  strength improvement strategies, 539
  work rehabilitation process, 403
Occupation transitions
  leisure occupations, 364
  time use evaluation, 367
Occupation-focused plans, 96–97
  overview, 97, **97**

Occupation-focused practice, 6, 8, 12, 71, 95–96, 112–113, 152–153
  assessment process, 87
  constraints of medical model, 9–10
Occupational Adaptation model, 491
Occupational apartheid, 299, 300–301
Occupational balance, 112, 113
Occupational Circumstances Assessment-Interview Rating Scale (OCAIRS), 535
Occupational deprivation, 299, 300–301
  children with sensory processing disorders, 646
  community-based rehabilitation approaches, 313–314
Occupational diagnostic statement, 60–61, **60**, 535
Occupational history, 21–22, 182
Occupational justice, 50, 282, 285, 287, 299–300, 302
  partnership approach, 288
    actions, **289**, 294
    practice scenarios, **288–294**
Occupational Performance History Interview, 366, 535
Occupational Performance Model, 612, **612**
Occupational persona, 136
Occupational reasoning, 57–65, 96, 105
  argumentative reasoning, 64
  assessment data interpretation, 349–350
  assistive device selection, 457, 458–459
  biomechanical strategies, 535
  comparative analysis, 62–63
  conditional reasoning, 63
  decision-making, **62**
  deductive, 96–97
  driving performance, 500
    off-road screening, 498
  evidence-based reasoning, 64
  home modification, 414–415, **416**
  hypothesizing, 63
  inductive reasoning, 97
  inferential reasoning, 63
  orthotics prescription, 508
  reframing, 64
  self-care assessment, 347
  sensory impairments assessment, 545

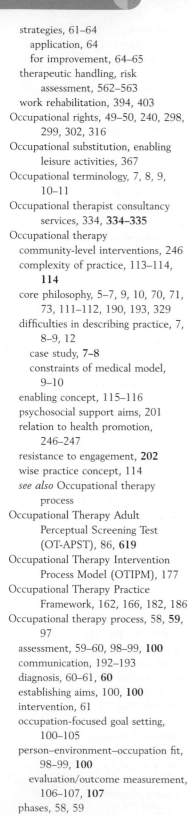

strategies, 61–64
  application, 64
  for improvement, 64–65
  therapeutic handling, risk
    assessment, 562–563
  work rehabilitation, 394, 403
Occupational rights, 49–50, 240, 298,
  299, 302, 316
Occupational substitution, enabling
  leisure activities, 367
Occupational terminology, 7, 8, 9,
  10–11
Occupational therapist consultancy
  services, 334, **334–335**
Occupational therapy
  community-level interventions, 246
  complexity of practice, 113–114,
    114
  core philosophy, 5–7, 9, 10, 70, 71,
    73, 111–112, 190, 193, 329
  difficulties in describing practice, 7,
    8–9, 12
    case study, **7–8**
    constraints of medical model,
      9–10
  enabling concept, 115–116
  psychosocial support aims, 201
  relation to health promotion,
    246–247
  resistance to engagement, **202**
  wise practice concept, 114
  see also Occupational therapy
    process
Occupational Therapy Adult
  Perceptual Screening Test
  (OT-APST), 86, **619**
Occupational Therapy Intervention
  Process Model (OTIPM), 177
Occupational Therapy Practice
  Framework, 162, 166, 182, 186
Occupational therapy process, 58, **59**,
  97
  assessment, 59–60, 98–99, **100**
  communication, 192–193
  diagnosis, 60–61, **60**
  establishing aims, 100, **100**
  intervention, 61
  occupation-focused goal setting,
    100–105
  person–environment–occupation fit,
    98–99, **100**
    evaluation/outcome measurement,
      106–107, **107**
  phases, 58, 59

practice scenarios, **98**, **99–100**
  re-assessment, 61
  referral, 97–98
  selecting occupation-focused
    strategies, 105–106, **106**
  steps, 97, **97**
Occupational therapy–sensory
  integration (OT-SI), 638, 647
  environment, 648
  occupation, 648
  person, 647
  principles, 647
  sensory diets, **642**, **644**, 648
Occupational-therapy driving
  specialists *see* Driving
Oedema reduction, orthoses, 522–523,
  522
Oral (buccofacial) apraxia, 611
Organisational factors
  barriers to empowerment, 131
  job analysis for work rehabilitation,
    403
  return-to-work programme, 405
Orthopaedic factors, evaluation for
  wheeled mobility/seating
  interventions, 482
Orthoses, 507–523
  assessment for prescription, 509,
    511, **514**
  contractures prevention, 515–516,
    517
  deformity correction, 515–516
  design, 513
    biomechanical approach, 513, **514**
  dynamic, 511, 512–513, **512**
  evidence-based practice, 518,
    520–521
  hand use improvement, 518–521, **519**
  hypertonicity management, 520
  immobilisation for rest, 513
  indications, 509, 513
    conditions, 510
  joint protection, 513
  key features, 508–509
  materials, 509
  occupational goals, 509, 510
  oedema reduction, 522–523, **522**
  pain relief, 521, **521**
  practice scenario, **509–510**
  purposes, 511
  scar formation prevention, 516–518,
    518
  semi-dynamic, 511, 512, **512**
  static, 511, **511**, **512**

types, 511
  upper limb/hand biomechanics,
    510–511
  wound healing promotion, 513–515,
    515
Osteoarthritis, 520, 538
  joint protection strategies, 539
Ottawa Charter on Health Promotion,
  242–243, 245
Outcome measures, 85, 96
  cognitive/perceptual problems, 614
  educational interventions, 231, 233
  evaluation of person–environment–
    occupation fit, 106–107, **107**
  group work, 257–258
  SMART goals, 102, 103
  wheelchair prescription/seating
    interventions, **481**
  work rehabilitation, 395, 403–404
Outcome statements (occupational
  goals), 61
Overuse injury, semi-dynamic orthoses,
  512

Pain receptors, 639
Pain relief, orthoses, 521, **521**
Pain Self Efficacy Questionnaire, 344
Pain sensation, 544
  changes following peripheral nerve
    damage, 545
  pinprick testing, 546
Paralysis
  management approach, 580
  strength training, 594, **595**
Parenthood, 364
Parkinson's disease, 471, 608
  driving abilities, 496, 500
Partnership approach, 152
  assistive device selection, 457, 463
  barriers, 131
  community development, 303–306
    phases, 303, **303**
    practice scenario, **304–306**
  community-based rehabilitation
    strategies, 316
  educational interventions, 225–227
  health promotion relationship,
    246–247
  person-centred practice, 128, 130,
    131
  promoting disabled peoples'
    participation, 131, 281–295
    actions, **289**, 294
    practice scenarios, **288–294**

trust establishment, 130
United Nations Convention on the
    Rights of Persons with
    Disabilities, 287
Paternalism, 226
Pathways to Work policy, 272
Patient-centred care model, 226
Pediatric Evaluation of Disability
    Inventory (PEDI), 90
Perceived Efficacy and Goal Setting
    System (PEGS), 101
Perceived personal control, 201
Perception
    definition, 608
    driving performance off-road
        screening, 498
    normal capacities, 609–611
    simple/complex functions, 610–611
Perceptual problems, 84, 608–609
    assessment, 613–620, **615–619**
        observation of performance, 620,
            622–623
        pre-assessment identification of
            physical/sensory deficits, 614
        standardised, 614, 620
    community integration following
        rehabilitation, 631
    intervention strategies, 621, 623,
        625–627, 630–631
    occupational impact, 608
    occupational therapy frameworks,
        611–612
    outcome measures, 614
    practice scenarios, **612–613**,
        620–621, 623–624, 627
    reporting of conditions causing
        driving impairment, 492
    simple/complex disorders, 610,
        630–631
Perceptual processing, driving
    performance, 493–494
Performance accomplishment
    assessment process, 85, 182
    occupation analysis, 182
    self-efficacy enhancement, 225
Performance areas, 162, 179
    occupation analysis, 166, **166**
Performance Assessment of Self-Care
    Skills, 59
Performance context, 162, 177–178
    activity demands, 178, **179**
    environment, 177–178
    person factors, 177, 178–179
Performance patterns, 162, 174–177

habits/routines, 175–176
    observation, 183
    roles, 175, **175**
Performance skills, 162, 163–164, 165,
    166
    body structure impairment
        influence, 165
    capacities (body functions)
        relationship, 173
    communication/interaction, 170,
        172–173, **172**
    identification, **174**
    motor, 167, **168**
    observation, 183
    occupation analysis, 166–172
    process, 167, **168–170**
Peripheral nerve injuries, 544–545
    sensory re-education, 548–549
Person-centred goals, 97
Person-centred practice, 71, 83, 115,
    127–132, **129**, 152, 153, 190,
    226
    assistive device selection, 457
        assessment, 459–460
    collaborative approach, 193
        decisions concerning risk-taking,
            345, 348
        goal-setting, 350
    communication skills, 154, 155, 193
    definition, 128
    empathy, 154
    habits/routines, influence on
        performance patterns, 176, **176**
    health promotion relationship, 246
    implementation, 129–130
    leisure activities, 367–368
    occupation analysis, 173
    occupational reasoning, 535
    orthotics, 508
    practical aspects, 131–132
        practice scenario, **132**
    psychosocial support, 201
    relationship building skills, 195, 196
    self-care assessment processes, 348
    therapeutic use of self, 199
    wheelchair and seating provision,
        470
Person–environment fit, **415**, 455,
    455, 456
    home modification assessment, 415
Person-Environment-Occupation
    Model, 96, 105, 177, 491
Person-Environment-Occupation-
    Performance Model, 177, 376

Personal handling profiles, 564
Personalisation of space, 412
Pervasive developmental disorders,
    472, 645
Physical activity, nature of occupation,
    19–20
Physical capacity
    driving performance off-road
        screening, 498
    work rehabilitation
        assessment, 401–402
        job analysis, 403
Physical impairments
    identification prior to cognitive/
        perceptual impairment
        assessment, 614
    leisure occupations, 364
    self-care assessment, 348
Pie diagrams, leisure assessment,
    365
Pinch strength, 63
Pinprick sensation testing, 546
Platform lifts, 435, **439**
Play, 371–387, 646
    analysis of engagement, 377
    assessment, 383, **384–385**, 385
    with conventional toys, 372
    development, 373, **374**
    environmental factors, 376–377
    health/well-being relationship,
        377–378
    key features, 372
    occupation analysis, 166
    occupational perspective, 373,
        375–376
        'becoming', 376
        'belonging', 376
        'doing' versus 'being', 373,
            375–376
    practical applications, 379–382
        as ends in therapy, **380–381**,
            383–384, **386–387**
        as means in therapy, 379,
            380–381, 382, **382–383**
        practice scenarios, **382–383**,
            386–387
    pretend, 372, 383
        conventional-imaginative, 372
        creativity associations, 379
        interventions, 385
        language development associations,
            378
        literacy associations, 378
        mental representation ability, 378

narrative competence association, 378–379
problem solving associations, 379
social competence associations, 379
symbolic, 372
theories, 372–373
time requirement, 373
types, 373, **375**
with unstructured objects, 372
value, 377–378
Play Assessment for Group Settings (PAGS), 84, 383
Play History, 383, 385
Policy issues, 268, 282, 287
assistive technology, 456
facilitation of disabled people's participation, **289**, 301–302
mainstreaming strategy, 302
influence of occupational participation, 147
therapist as agent of change, 216
strategies, 217–218
Political activity, 120
Political issues, 268
context of occupation, 136, 145–147
lobbying see Lobbying
Post traumatic stress disorder, 191
Postural management, 471
Posture, 154
Posture control, seating interventions, 476, 478
aims, 478
importance, 479
physical assessment/interventions, 480
tools/outcome measures, **481**
Poverty, 46, 47, 241, 271–272, 276, 301
assessment methods, 298
community-based rehabilitation strategies, 316
definitions, 298
disability association, 298, 299, **300**, 312, 316
United Nations Millenium Development Goals, 328, **328**
Power relationships, therapist–client, 29–30, 33, 34, 196
client-centred therapy evaluation, 42
Power-coercive strategy to effect change, 217–218

Power-sharing partnership, 115
Powered wheelchairs, 475, **475**
joystick control, 475
Praxis, 611
problems, intervention strategies, 631
Pre-discharge home-assessment visits, 90
Preschool Activity Card Sort, 84
Pressure areas, educational interventions with sensory impairment, 549, 550
Pressure cushions, 482–483, **485**
Pressure sensation, 544, 639
see also Touch sensation
Pressure splints, 511
Pressure ulcers, 478, 480, 482
risk factors, 480
risk in wheelchair users, 480
stages in development, 480
Preventive care, 240
health promotion, 240, 241
Primates, non-human, 23
Private occupational therapy practice, 42
Problem solving, pretend play relationship, 379
Process skills, 162, 163, 167, **168–170**, 170
Productive occupation, 20, 162
meaningfulness, 46–47, 392–393
occupation analysis, 166
professional assumptions, critical appraisal, 46–47
as therapy, 392
see also Work (paid work); Work rehabilitation
Professional assumptions, critical appraisal, 40, 41–50
client-centred practice, 42–43
global perspective, 41
goals of occupational therapy, 43–45
normality, 43–44
paid employment, 46
physical independence, 44–45
quality of life enhancement, 45
well-being promotion, 49
nature of occupation, 45–49
nature of occupational therapy profession, 41–42
Professional experience, 62
Professional image, 4, 5, 42
see also Professional assumptions

Professional self-talk, 64
Professional status, 7, 10
Profiling beds, **569**
Proprioception, 640
assessment, 546–547
Proprioceptors, 544
Prosopagnosia, 610
Proto-occupations, 22, 23
Psychiatric disorders, driving safety considerations, 492
Psycho-educational group work, 254, 255–256
occupational potential of activities, 255
practice scenarios, **255**
Psychodynamic model, 77
Psychodynamic play therapy, 386
Psychological Impact of Assistive Devices Scale, 465
Psychological issues, 190
sequelae of physical illness/impairment, 191, 200
Psychosocial impairment, 191
Psychosocial issues
adjustment to impairment, 190, 191
job analysis for work rehabilitation, 403
Psychosocial support, 189–208
communication skills, 192, 194–195
enabling strategies, 200–207
practice scenarios, **202–207**
group interventions, 201
intervention strategies, 201
rehabilitation, 200
role of emotional intelligence, 200–201
therapeutic use of self, 196, 199
value of group work, 257
Psychosocial well-being monitoring, 191
Purposefulness of occupation, 20, 112, 115, 163, 165
intrinsic/extrinsic purpose, 164

Quadraphonic approach, 611
Quality of life, 114
enhancement as goal of therapy, 45
role of interdependence, 47
Quebec User Evaluation of Satisfaction with Assistive Technology (QUEST), 465

Questioning, 192
  assessment of occupational
    performance and engagement,
    59
  leisure activities, 366
  skills, 196, **197**
Questionnaires, 59

Rails, 410, 421, 422
  location for fitting, 415, **416**
Ramps, 410, 435, **437**, **438**
Randomised controlled trials, 88
  health promotion effectiveness
    evaluation, 246
Range of motion, 63
  measurement, 106
Rapid Entire Body Assessment
    (REBA), 556, 565
Rapid Estimate of Adult Literacy in
    Medicine (REALM), 230
Rapid Upper Limb Assessment
    (RULA), 565
Rapport, 154
Rational-empirical strategy to effect
    change, 217
Reaching to grasp
  anticipatory muscle activity, **586**
  compensatory strategies, 588, **588**
  movement analysis, 580–583, **581**,
    582
    associated trunk movement/hip
      flexion, 582
    base of support effects, 583
    children, 582
    essential components, 582–583
    hypothesis development/testing,
      589
    postural adjustments in sitting,
      583–585, **584**
    reaching distance/direction
      effects, 583
    sitting balance training, 601–602,
      602
    training postural adjustments, 583,
      585
    upper limb motor performance
      remediation, 593–594
Readability of written material, 231
Reasoning *see* Occupational reasoning
Re-assessment, occupational therapy
    process, 61
Records, 97
  assessment, 87
  evaluation findings, 87–88

home modifications documentation,
    425, 426–427
occupation analysis for work
    rehabilitation, 403
Recreational activities, 361
Redistributive justice, 120
Referral, 97–98
  to mental health services, 191
Reflection, 114, 115, 128, 154
Reframing, occupational reasoning, 64
Refrigerated storage, kitchen universal
    design, 441
Rehabilitative/compensatory model,
    77
Reintegration to Normal Living Index
    (RNL), 620
Relationship building skills, 195–196
Remediation as enabling strategy, **121**
Reporting of Injuries Diseases and
    Dangerous Occurrences
    Regulations (RIDDOR), 571,
    573
Resistance to engagement in
    occupational therapy, **202**
Resource limitation, 42
Respect, 129, 130, 152, 153, 195,
    268
Resting position, immobilisation
    orthoses, 513
Resting splints, 511, **512**, 513
  contractures prevention, 516
Reticular formation, 640
Retirement, 364
Retraining Approach, 611
Return-to-work programmes, 404–405
  'time-waster' programmes, 405
    practice scenarios, **405–406**
Rheumatoid arthritis, 61, 77
  joint protection strategies, 539
  orthoses, 510
    pain relief, 522
    resting splints, 513
Right/left discrimination problems,
    630
Rights to occupation, 115
  see also Human rights
Risk assessment
  job analysis for work rehabilitation,
    403
  moving and handling *see* Moving and
    handling
Risk-taking, 115
  collaborative decision-making, 345,
    348

Rituals, influence on performance
    patterns, 175–177
Rivermead Assessment of
    Somatosensory Performance
    (RASP), 548
Rivermead Behavioural Memory Tesst
    (RBMT), 613, **618**
Rivermead Rehabilitation Centre Life
    Goals Questionnaire, 614–620
Robotic therapy, motor performance
    rehabilitation, 602
Role stress, 5, 11
Roles, influence on performance
    patterns, 175, **175**
Routines
  assimilation of assistive devices,
    464
  influence on performance patterns,
    175–176
  internalisaed, 176
  leisure occupations incorporation,
    367
RPAB, **617**

SAFEDRIVE checklist, 494–495
SAFER, 417, **418–419**
Safer handling principles, 570–571,
    572
Safety aids, 410
Scar compression garments, 517, 518
Scars
  formation prevention, immobilisation
    orthoses, 516–518, **518**
  hypertrophic, 517
Screening assessment, 85–87
Seating biomechanics, 478
  centre of mass, 478–479, **479**
  gravitational forces, 478
  importance for wheelchair
    prescription, 479
  normal (compression) forces, 478,
    478
  shear forces, 478, **478**
Seating interventions, wheelchair
    prescription *see* Wheelchair
    prescription
Self-awareness, 199, **200**, 201
Self-care, 20, 44, 162, 341–353
  assessment, 346–348
    data interpretation, 349–350
    decision-making, 347
    occupational profile development,
      348–349
    practical approaches, 347–348

practice scenario, **349**
purpose, 346–347
choice, 342, 345–346
definition, 342
environmental factors, 342, 346
establishing goals, 350–351
identity impact, 342, 343
independence, 342, 343–344
meaning, 342, 345–346
motivation, 342, 344–345
multiple elements, 342
practice scenarios, **342–343**
occupation analysis, 166
professional assumptions, critical
appraisal, 46, 47
self-efficacy, 342, 344
strategies for enabling engagement,
351–352
assistive technology, **351**
compensation, **352, 353**
education, **351, 353**
Self-concept, 343
Self-efficacy, 224–225, 247
enhancement strategies, 225
self-care, 342, 344
Self-Efficacy Gauge, 344
Self-esteem, 343
Self-maintenance, 20, 342
see also Self-care
Self-propelling wheelchairs/
independent manual mobility
systems, 474
fixed frame, 474, **474**
folding frame, 474, **474**
shoulder injury avoidance, 474
Self-report, self-care assessment, 348
Semi-dynamic orthoses, 511, 512,
512
contractures prevention, 516
hand use improvement, 518, 519,
520
materials, 512
pain relief, 521
Semmes–Weinstein monofilaments,
548
Sensation
assessment, 545
definition, 544
modalities, 544
Sensibility
assessment, 545
driving performance off-road
screening, 498
definition, 544

Sensory based motor disorder, 644
Sensory cortex injury, sensory change
management, 550
Sensory diets, **642, 644,** 648, **649**
Sensory discrimination disorders, 640
practice scenario, **640–641**
Sensory impairments, 543–551
assessment, 545–548, **546**
indepth standardised instruments,
548
functional impact, 545
home modification, 410
identification prior to cognitive/
perceptual impairment
assessment, 614
intervention strategies, 548–549
brainstem/thalamus/sensory
cortex, 550
ongoing monitoring, 549
peripheral nerve injuries, 548–549
spinal cord injuries, 549–550
protective sensation loss, 548, 549
terminology, 544
Sensory integration dysfunction, 638
Sensory integration theory (SIT), 382,
638, **638**
Sensory modulation, 639
Sensory modulation disorder, 643–644,
644
arousal level relationship, 646
over responsivity, 643
practice scenario, **643–644**
sensory seeking, 643
under responsivity, 643
Sensory pathways, 544
Sensory processing
arousal level relationship, 639
inhibitory/facilitatory effects of
sensory stimulation, 640, **641**
sensory integration theory (SIT),
638, **638**
sensory modulation, 639
sensory registration, 639
Sensory processing disorders, 637–649
arousal level relationship, 646
inhibitory/facility stimulation,
648
sensory diets, **642, 644,** 648, **649**
classification, 640, **641**
occupational performance impact,
645–646
sensory based motor disorder, 644
sensory discrimination disorders, 640
practice scenario, **640–641**

sensory modulation disorders, 639,
643–644, **644**
practice scenario, **643–644**
sensory registration disorders, 639
Sensory receptors, 544
Sensory registration, 639
Sensory rehabilitation, 548–549
cerebrovascular accident, 550
peripheral nerve injuries, 548–549
spinal cord injuries, 549–550
Sensory system, 544, 639–640
Shared decision-making model, 226
Shear forces
movement biomechanics, 560
pressure ulcers, 478
seating biomechanics, 478, **478**
Short Form Health Survey (SF-36),
536, 614
Shoulder external rotation/forward
flexion exercise in standing,
596
Shoulder slings/supports, 601
Shoulder strapping, 601
Showers, 445
Signals/signage, universal design
entrances, 434
kitchens, 443
Signs/symptoms interpretation,
self-efficacy enhancement, 225
Silence, communication skills, **159**
Silicone-gel sheeting, scar management,
518
Simultanagnosia, 610
Sinks, kitchen universal design, 443
Sitting Assessment for Children with
Neuromotor Dysfunction
(SCAND), 480
Sitting Assessment Scale, 480
Sitting balance, reaching to grasp
training, 601–602, **602**
Skill mastery, self-efficacy
enhancement, 225
Skin graft healing, immobilisation
orthoses, 513
Sleep apnoea, 492
Slide sheets, 560, **560, 569,** 570
SMART goals, 101–105
domains, 101
Activity-based strategies,
102–103
Measurable, 102
Review, 103–104
Specific, 101–102
Timeframe, 104

key steps, **105**
work rehabilitation, 404
SMOG, 231
Social action, 283
Social activism, 268, 269
Social capital, 272–274
Social change, 112–113, 268, 282, 283
  community-based interventions, 294
  global trends, 329
  health promotion, 244
  occupational therapists' role,
    302–303
Social cognition models, 248–249
Social cohesion, 302
Social communication/interaction
    skills, 170, 172–173, **172**
  pretend play associations, 379
Social exclusion, 283, 299, 302
  occupational deprivation association,
    301
Social justice, 213, 215, 218, 268,
    299–300, 302
Social model of disability, 30–31, 33,
    34, 35, 213
Social networks, 256, 257
Social opportunities, 272–274
  inequalities, 271–272
Social participation, occupation
    analysis, 165, 166
Social policy see Policy issues
Sociocultural context of occupation,
    141–142, 177
  influence on norms/forms of
    occupational performance, 142
  place/space associations, 143
  time constructs, 143
Somatoagnosia, 630
SOTOF, **615**
Space and objects, process skills, **169**
Spasticity (high tone), 585, 587
Spatial relations perception, 610
Specialised techniques as enabling
    skills, **119**
Specific language disability, 645
Speech impairment, educational
    interventions, 230
Spina bifida, 471, 496
Spinal cord injury, 471, 496, 509
  contractures prevention, 516
  sensory impairments, 545
    management, 549–550
Spinothalamic tract, 544
Spiritual factors, performance context,
    177

Splints, 508
  continuous muscle stretching for
    contractures prevention, 600
  immobilisation see Immobilisation
    splints; Static orthoses
  joint protection strategies, 539
  mobilisation see Dynamic orthoses
  range of movement improvement,
    540
  scar management, 517
  semi-dynamic see Semi-dynamic
    orthoses
Sports high-performance wheelchairs,
    476
Stand-up wheelchairs, 476
Standing aids, 569
  hoist with standing/walking harness,
    570
Static orthoses, 511, **511**, **512**
  contractures prevention, 516
  hand use improvement, 518, 519
  pain relief, 521
  range of movement improvement,
    540
  see also Immobilisation splints
Stereognosis
  assessment, 548
  changes following peripheral nerve
    damage, 545
Strength impairment, 529, 538
  assessment, 535
  biomechanical strategies, 528, 529
    implementation, 536, 538–539
Strength training
  motor performance remediation,
    589
  upper limb paralysis/weakness, 594,
    595, **596**, **597**
Stress reduction, 362
Stretch interventions
  contractures prevention, 511, 516,
    587, 599–600
  range of movement improvement
    strategies, 540
Stroke, 59, 62, 63, 86, 471
  associated depression, 614
  attention training, 628
  biomechanical strategies, 538
  cognitive/perceptual problems,
    609
  grip force, 598
  motor performance remediation
    constraint-induced movement
    therapy, 595

electrical stimulation, 594
  strength training, 594
  orthoses, 509, 516
  positive versus negative impairments,
    585
  reporting outcomes, 88
  sensory re-education programmes for
    the hand, 550
  stretch interventions for contractures
    prevention, 516, 599–601
Subacromial Impingement Syndrome,
    521
Suitability of Assessment Materials
    (SAM), 231
Supervision, 199
Support groups, 201
Sustaining performance, process skills,
    168–170
Swing-way hinges, 448, **448**
Symbolic and Imaginative Play
    Development Checklist, 383
Sympathy, 154

Tactile agnosia (astereognosis), 548,
    610
Tactile receptors, 639
Tactile system, 639–640
  sensory processing disorders,
    associated behaviours, **645**
Task analysis, 163, 404
Task knowledge, 164
  application, process skills, **169**
TEA, **619**
Teaching skills, 68
Teamworking (team-based practice), 5,
    152, 153
  communication skills, 153
  psycho-educational groups, 255
Tele-consultations, 335–336, **336**
Tele-health, 335–336
Temperature receptors, 639
Temperature sensation, 544
  assessment, 545–546
  changes following peripheral nerve
    damage, 545
Tendon repair rehabilitation, dynamic
    orthoses, 512, 516
Terminology
  definitions of occupation, 18,
    18
  models of practice, 69–70, 71
Test of Functional Health Literacy in
    Adults (TOFHLA), 230
Test of Playfulness, 383

Thalamus injury, sensory change management, 550
Theoretical models *see* Models of practice
Theory of mind, pretend play associations, 379
Theory of reasoned action/planned behaviour, 248
Theory–practice gap, 69
Therapeutic alliance, 85, 154
 power relationships, 196
 see also Interpersonal interaction skills
Therapeutic use of self, 196, 199
Thumb flexion force modulation exercise, **600**
Thumb joint osteoarthritis, 520
Thumb post splint, 519–520, **520**
TILE (Task Individual Load Environment) Assessment Tool, 564, **565**
Time
 constraints, selection of occupation-focused strategies, 105
 context of performance, 177
 organisation, process skills, **169**
 sociocultural construction, 143, 144–145
 use evaluation, 367
 use patterns, 138–139
Time diaries, leisure assessment, 364–365
Time measurement, leisure assessment tools, 364–365
Time pressure management (TPM), 628
Timeframe for goal achievement, work rehabilitation, 395, 404
Timing of tasks, occupation analysis, 403
Tissue integrity, wheelchair users, 479–480
Toilets
 assistive device selection, 462, **462**, **463**
 practice scenario, **462**
 universal design, 444, **447**
Tone of voice, 154
Tone-and-positioning splints, 512, **512**
 continuous stretch application, 516
 hand use improvement, 520
Touch Inventory for Elementary School-Aged Children (TIE), 90

Touch sensation, 544
 assessment
  light touch, 545, 639
  localisation (locognosia), 547–548, **548**
  moving two point discrimination, 547
  two point discrimination, 547, **547**
 changes following peripheral nerve damage, 545
Tragedy model of disability, 30, 31, 213
Training *see* Education/training
Transfer boards, **569**, 570
Transportation, 140
Transtheoretical (stages of change) model, 225, 249, **249**
 stages of behaviour change, **226**
Trust, 195, 196
 person-centred practice, 130
Two point discrimination
 assessment, 547, **547**
  moving two points, 547
 changes following peripheral nerve damage, 545

Ultrasound, scar management, 517
Umbrella Framework for Understanding Models (UFUM), 71, **72**, 74, 77
Unconditional positive regard, 195–196
Unemployment
 disabled people, 283
 as occupational deprivation, 301
 professional assumptions, 46
Unilateral neglect, 610
 intervention strategies, 629–630
Uniqueness of individuals, 129
United Nations Convention on the Rights of Persons with Disabilities, 282, **285–287**, 316, 394
 as advocacy tool, 284, 287–288, 294
United Nations Human Development Index (HDI), 298
United Nations Millenium Development Goals, 328, **328**
Universal design, 141, 411, 413, 431–451
 assistive devices, 455, 457
 bathrooms, 444–447, **446**

closet storage, 448, **449**
doors with swing-way hinges, 448, **448**
entrances, 434–435, **435**, **436**, **437**, **438**, **439**, **440**, **441**
goals, 431
kitchens, 437, 441–443, **442**
practical applications, 448, **450**
practice scenarios, **449–450**
principles, 433, **433–434**
raised appliances, 448, **448**
washing-machine height, 448
water controls, 447
Upper limb
 contractures prevention, muscle stretching, 599, **601**
 functional impact of sensory impairments, 545
 motor performance remediation, 593–594
  constraint-induced movement therapy, 594–595
  dexterity training, 598–599, **600**
  electrical stimulation, 594
  mental practice, 595
  reducing muscle force during grasp, 595, 598, **599**, **600**
  strength training, 594, **595**
 movement analysis of reaching to grasp, 580–583, **581**, **582**
 compensatory strategies, 588
 orthoses *see* Orthoses
 work-related damage risk to occupational therapists, 555
Useful Field of View (UFOV), 498

Value of occupational therapy, 4, 9, 40, 330
 marketing, 332–333
Value of play, 377–378
Values of clients, 137
Values of occupational therapists, 212
 congruence with actions, 218, **218**
Verbal education, 228
Verbal persuasion, self-efficacy enhancement, 225
Vestibular system, 640
 sensory processing disorders, 647
 associated behaviours, **645**
Vibration sense assessment, 547
Video recordings, information provision, 228
Virtual driving assessment, 88

Virtual environment, context of performance, 177–178
Visitable Homes Act (1998), 413
Visual field loss, 492
Visual function for driving performance, 493
Visual impairment
  driving performance off-road screening, 498
  educational interventions, 228, 230
  mobility cues, 414
Visual object agnosia, 610
  intervention strategies, 630
Visual system, 640
Visuospatial functioning, 610–611
Vulnerable groups, 268, 269, 298–299
  mainstreaming strategy, 302

Walking harness, with hoists, 570
Washing-machine height, 448
Water controls, universal design, 447
Weakness see Strength impairment
The Well Elderly Study, 257–258
Well-being, 73
  definition, 49
  driving ability/community mobility relationship, 491
  impact of occupation, 112, 113, 114
  monitoring psychosocial aspects, 191
  play relationship, 377–378
  promotion as goal of occupational therapy, 49
  relation to leisure activities, 362
Westmead Home Safety Inventory, 417, **418–419**
Wheelchair Independent Measure (WIM), 473, **474**
Wheelchair prescription, 473–485
  assessment, 476
    basic measurements, **476**
  collaborative decision-making, 471
  cushioning, 482
    adaptive seating systems, 482, **485**
    pressure cushions, 482–483, **485**
  inappropriate, secondary difficulties caused to individuals, **483–484**
  mobility enablement, 474–476
  seating biomechanics, 478
    centre of mass, 478–479, **479**
    gravitational forces, 478
    importance, 479
    normal (compression) forces, 478, **478**
    shearing forces, 478, **478**

seating inadequacies
  consequences, **477**
  pressure ulcer risk, 480
seating interventions, 473, 476, 478
  for comfort, 476, 479
  orthopaedic factors evaluation, 482
  outcome measures, **481**
  physical assessment, 480, **481**
  for postural control, 476, 478, 479
  postural control evaluation, 480, 482
  for tissue integrity, 476, 479–480
Wheelchair users
  bathtub/shower use, 445
  environmental barriers to participation, 471
  health conditions, 471–472
  kitchen design, knee space under counters/work surfaces, 437, 441, 443
  matching person's requirements and device, 463
    practice scenario, **463**
  practice scenarios, **472–473**
  spectrum of abilities, 473, **473**
    assessment, 473, **473**
Wheelchairs, 42, 469–485
  acceptance by user, 471
  attendant-propelled/dependent mobility systems, 474–475, **475**
  bariatric, 476
  building accessibility standards, 413
  children's, 475
  costs, 471
  effective provision, 470
  elevating, 476
  footprints, 413
  frame flexibility, 413
  high-performance sports, 476
  matching person's requirements and device, 463
    practice scenario, **463**
  person-centred practice, 470
  powered, 475, **475**
  prevalence of use, 471
  self-propelling/independent manual mobility systems, 474
  stand-up, 476
  types, 474

Wise practice concept, 114
Work (paid work), 301, 392
  impact on health, 45–46
  meaningfulness, 46–47, 392–393
  professional assumptions, 45, 46–47
  economic self-sufficiency, 47
Work rehabilitation, 391–407
  aims, 394
  assessment, 401–403
    job analysis, 403
    setting, 401, 402
    worker, 401–402
    worker's capacity, 401–402
    workplace, 402–403
  communication, 395
  early referral, 394
  ergonomic principles, 394
  goal-setting, 395, 403–404
  key features, 394–395
  monitoring/review, 395, 407
  occupational reasoning, 394, 403
  outcome measurement, 395, 403–404
  process, 395
    key phases, 395, **396**
    practice scenarios, **396–401**
  return to work facilitation, 393–394
    hierarchy, 394, **394**
    matching worker and work tasks, 403
    work modification, 395
  role of occupational therapist, 393–394
  terminology, 392, **393**
  therapeutic interventions, 404–405
    education/training, 405
    environmental/task modification, 405
    implementation, 407
    return-to-work programme, 404–405
    'time-waster' programmes, 405, **405–406**
  workplace setting, 394–395
Working hours, 138
Working through, advanced communication skills, 192, 196, **196**, **197–199**
Workplace injury
  economic/human costs, 393
  prevention programmes, 394
  rehabilitation see Work rehabilitation

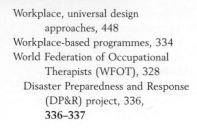

Workplace, universal design
approaches, 448
Workplace-based programmes, 334
World Federation of Occupational
Therapists (WFOT), 328
Disaster Preparedness and Response
(DP&R) project, 336,
336–337

World Programme of Action concerning
Disabled Persons, 282
Wound healing, immobilisation
orthoses, 513–515, **515**
scar formation prevention, 516–518,
518
Wrist cock-up splint, 519, **519**
Wrist extension exercise, **595**

Wrist flexion force modulation
exercise, **598**
Wrist splints, 511
see also Wrist cock-up splint
Written health education materials,
228, 230
content/design, 230–231, **232**
reading level (readability), 231